DIETARY REFERENCE INTAKES (DRIs): RECOMMENDED INTAKES FOR INDIVIDUALS, MINERALS FOOD AND NUTRITION BOARD, INSTITUTE OF MEDICINE, NATIONAL ACADEMIES

LIFE-STAGE GROUP	CALCIUM (mg/day)	CHROMIUM (mcg/day)	COPPER (mcg/day)	FLUORIDE (mg/day)	IODINE (mcg/day)	IRON (mg/day)	MAGNESIUM (mg/day)	MANGANESE (mg/day)	MOLYBDENUM (mcg/day)	PHOSPHORUS (mg/day)	SELENIUM (mcg/day)	ZINC (mg/day)	POTASSIUM (g/day)	SODIUM (g/day)	CHLORIDE (g/day)
Infants															
0-6 mo	210*	0.2*	200*	0.01*	110*	0.27*	30*	0.003*	2*	100*	15*	2*	0.4*	0.12*	0.18*
7-12 mo	270*	5.5*	220*	0.5*	130*	**11**	75*	0.6*	3*	275*	20*	**3**	0.7*	0.37*	0.57*
Children															
1-3 yr	500*	11*	**340**	0.7*	**90**	**7**	**80**	1.2*	**17**	**460**	**20**	**3**	3.0*	1.0*	1.5*
4-8 yr	800*	15*	**440**	1*	**90**	**10**	**130**	1.5*	**22**	**500**	**30**	**5**	3.8*	1.2*	1.9*
Males															
9-13 yr	1300*	25*	**700**	2*	**120**	**8**	**240**	1.9*	**34**	**1250**	**40**	**8**	4.5*	1.5*	2.3*
14-18 yr	1300*	35*	**890**	3*	**150**	**11**	**410**	2.2*	**43**	**1250**	**55**	**11**	4.7*	1.5*	2.3*
19-30 yr	1000*	35*	**900**	4*	**150**	**8**	**400**	2.3*	**45**	**700**	**55**	**11**	4.7*	1.5*	2.3*
31-50 yr	1000*	35*	**900**	4*	**150**	**8**	**420**	2.3*	**45**	**700**	**55**	**11**	4.7*	1.5*	2.3*
51-70 yr	1200*	30*	**900**	4*	**150**	**8**	**420**	2.3*	**45**	**700**	**55**	**11**	4.7*	1.3*	2.0*
>70 yr	1200*	30*	**900**	4*	**150**	**8**	**420**	2.3*	**45**	**700**	**55**	**11**	4.7*	1.2*	1.8*
Females															
9-13 yr	1300*	21*	**700**	2*	**120**	**8**	**240**	1.6*	**34**	**1250**	**40**	**8**	4.5*	1.5*	2.3*
14-18 yr	1300*	24*	**890**	3*	**150**	**15**	**360**	1.6*	**43**	**1250**	**55**	**9**	4.7*	1.5*	2.3*
19-30 yr	1000*	25*	**900**	3*	**150**	**18**	**310**	1.8*	**45**	**700**	**55**	**8**	4.7*	1.5*	2.3*
31-50 yr	1000*	25*	**900**	3*	**150**	**18**	**320**	1.8*	**45**	**700**	**55**	**8**	4.7*	1.5*	2.3*
51-70 yr	1200*	20*	**900**	3*	**150**	**8**	**320**	1.8*	**45**	**700**	**55**	**8**	4.7*	1.3*	2.0*
>70 yr	1200*	20*	**900**	3*	**150**	**8**	**320**	1.8*	**45**	**700**	**55**	**8**	4.7*	1.2*	1.8*
Pregnant															
≤18 yr	1300*	29*	**1000**	3*	**220**	**27**	**400**	2.0*	**50**	**1250**	**60**	**12**	4.7*	1.5*	2.3*
19-30 yr	1000*	30*	**1000**	3*	**220**	**27**	**350**	2.0*	**50**	**700**	**60**	**11**	4.7*	1.5*	2.3*
31-50 yr	1000*	30*	**1000**	3*	**220**	**27**	**360**	2.0*	**50**	**700**	**60**	**11**	4.7*	1.5*	2.3*
Lactating															
≤18 yr	1300*	44*	**1300**	3*	**290**	**10**	**360**	2.6*	**50**	**1250**	**70**	**13**	5.1*	1.5*	2.3*
19-30 yr	1000*	45*	**1300**	3*	**290**	**9**	**310**	2.6*	**50**	**700**	**70**	**12**	5.1*	1.5*	2.3*
31-50 yr	1000*	45*	**1300**	3*	**290**	**9**	**320**	2.6*	**50**	**700**	**70**	**12**	5.1*	1.5*	2.3*

Data from Food and Nutrition Board, Institute of Medicine: *Dietary Reference Intakes for calcium, phosphorus, magnesium, vitamin D, and fluoride* (1997); *Dietary Reference Intakes for thiamin, riboflavin, niacin, vitamin B_6, folate, vitamin B_{12}, pantothenic acid, biotin, and choline* (1998); *Dietary Reference Intakes for vitamin C, vitamin E, selenium, and carotenoids* (2000); *Dietary Reference Intakes for vitamin A, vitamin K, arsenic, boron, chromium, copper, iodine, iron, manganese, molybdenum, nickel, silicon, vanadium, and zinc* (2001), and *Dietary Reference Intakes for water, potassium, sodium, chloride, and sulfate* (2004), Washington, DC, National Academies Press (www.nap.edu).

Note: This table presents Recommended Dietary Allowances (RDAs) in **bold type** and Adequate Intakes (AIs) in ordinary type followed by an asterisk (*). RDAs and AIs may both be used as goals for individual intake. RDAs are set to meet the needs of almost all (97% to 98%) individuals in a group. For healthy breast-fed infants, the AI is the mean intake. The AI for other life-stage and gender groups is believed to cover needs of all individuals in the group, but lack of data or uncertainty in the data prevent being able to specify with confidence the percentage of individuals covered by this intake.

DIETARY REFERENCE INTAKES (DRIs): TOLERABLE UPPER INTAKE LEVELS (UL[a]), MINERALS FOOD AND NUTRITION BOARD, INSTITUTE OF MEDICINE, NATIONAL ACADEMIES

LIFE-STAGE GROUP	ARSENIC[b]	BORON (mg/day)	CALCIUM (g/day)	CHROMIUM	COPPER (mcg/day)	FLUORIDE (mg/day)	IODINE (mcg/day)	IRON (mg/day)	MAGNESIUM (mg/day)[c]	MANGANESE (mg/day)	MOLYBDENUM (mcg/day)	NICKEL (mg/day)	PHOSPHORUS (g/day)	SELENIUM (mcg/day)	SILICON[d]	VANADIUM (mg/day)[e]	ZINC (mg/day)	POTASSIUM	SULFATE	SODIUM (g/day)	CHLORIDE (g/day)
Infants																					
0-6 mo	ND[f]	ND	ND	ND	ND	0.7	ND	40	ND	ND	ND	ND	ND	45	ND	ND	4	ND	ND	ND	ND
7-12 mo	ND	ND	ND	ND	ND	0.9	ND	40	ND	ND	ND	ND	ND	60	ND	ND	5	ND	ND	ND	ND
Children																					
1-3 yr	ND	3	2.5	ND	1000	1.3	200	40	65	2	300	0.2	3	90	ND	ND	7	ND	ND	1.5	2.3
4-8 yr	ND	6	2.5	ND	3000	2.2	300	40	110	3	600	0.3	3	150	ND	ND	12	ND	ND	1.9	2.9
Males, Females																					
9-13 yr	ND	11	2.5	ND	5000	10	600	40	350	6	1100	0.6	4	280	ND	ND	23	ND	ND	2.2	3.4
14-18 yr	ND	17	2.5	ND	8000	10	900	45	350	9	1700	1.0	4	400	ND	ND	34	ND	ND	2.3	3.6
19-70 yr	ND	20	2.5	ND	10,000	10	1100	45	350	11	2000	1.0	4	400	ND	1.8	40	ND	ND	2.3	3.6
>70 yr	ND	20	2.5	ND	10,000	10	1100	45	350	11	2000	1.0	3	400	ND	1.8	40	ND	ND	2.3	3.6
Pregnant																					
≤18 yr	ND	17	2.5	ND	8000	10	900	45	350	9	1700	1.0	3.5	400	ND	ND	34	ND	ND	2.3	3.6
19-50 yr	ND	20	2.5	ND	10,000	10	1100	45	350	11	2000	1.0	3.5	400	ND	ND	40	ND	ND	2.3	3.6
Lactating																					
≤18 yr	ND	17	2.5	ND	8000	10	900	45	350	9	1700	1.0	4	400	ND	ND	34	ND	ND	2.3	3.6
19-50 yr	ND	20	2.5	ND	10,000	10	1100	45	350	11	2000	1.0	4	400	ND	ND	40	ND	ND	2.3	3.6

Data from Food and Nutrition Board, Institute of Medicine: *Dietary Reference Intakes for calcium, phosphorus, magnesium, vitamin D, and fluoride* (1997); *Dietary Reference Intakes for thiamin, riboflavin, niacin, vitamin B_6, folate, vitamin B_{12}, pantothenic acid, biotin, and choline* (1998); *Dietary Reference Intakes for vitamin C, vitamin E, selenium, and carotenoids* (2000); *Dietary Reference Intakes for vitamin A, vitamin K, arsenic, boron, chromium, copper, iodine, iron, manganese, molybdenum, nickel, silicon, vanadium, and zinc* (2001), and *Dietary Reference Intakes for water, potassium, sodium, chloride, and sulfate* (2004), Washington, DC, National Academies Press (www.nap.edu).

[a]UL = The maximum level of daily nutrient intake that is likely to pose no risk of adverse effects. Unless otherwise specified, the UL represents total intake from food, water, and supplements. Due to lack of suitable data, ULs could not be established for arsenic, chromium, and silicon. In the absence of ULs, extra caution may be warranted in consuming levels above recommended intakes.

[b]Although the UL was not determined for arsenic, there is no justification for adding arsenic to food or supplements.

[c]The ULs for magnesium represent intake from a pharmacologic agent only and do not include intake from food or water.

[d]Although silicon has not been shown to cause adverse effects in humans, there is no justification for adding silicon to supplements.

[e]Although vanadium in food has not been shown to cause adverse effects in humans, there is no justification for adding vanadium to food, and vanadium supplements should be used with caution. The UL is based on adverse effects in laboratory animals, and this data could be used to set a UL for adults but not children and adolescents.

[f]ND = Not determinable due to lack of data of adverse effects in this age-group and concern with regard to lack of ability to handle excess amounts. Source of intake should be from food only to prevent high levels of intake.

DIETARY REFERENCE INTAKES (DRIs): RECOMMENDED INTAKES FOR INDIVIDUALS, MACRONUTRIENTS[a] FOOD AND NUTRITION BOARD, INSTITUTE OF MEDICINE, NATIONAL ACADEMIES

	PROTEIN		CARBOHYDRATE		FIBER		FAT		n-6 POLYUNSATURATED FATTY ACIDS (LINOLEIC ACID)		n-3 POLYUNSATURATED FATTY ACIDS (α-LINOLENIC ACID)		TOTAL WATER[f]
LIFE-STAGE GROUP	RDA/AI (g/day)[b]	AMDR[c]	RDA/AI (g/day)	AMDR	RDA/AI (g/day)	AMDR	RDA/AI (g/day)	AMDR	RDA/AI (g/day)	AMDR	RDA/AI (g/day)	AMDR[d]	RDA/AI (L/day)
Infants													
0-6 mo	9.1*	ND[e]	60*	ND	ND		31*		4.4*	ND	0.5*	ND	0.7*
7-12 mo	**11**	ND	95*	ND	ND		30*		4.6*	ND	0.5*	ND	0.8*
Children													
1-3 yr	**13**	5-20	**130**	45-65	19*			30-40	7*	5-10	0.7*	0.6-1.2	1.3*
4-8 yr	**19**	10-30	**130**	45-65	25*			25-35	10*	5-10	0.9*	0.6-1.2	1.7*
Males													
9-13 yr	**34**	10-30	**130**	45-65	31*			25-35	12*	5-10	1.2*	0.6-1.2	2.4*
14-18 yr	**52**	10-30	**130**	45-65	38*			25-35	16*	5-10	1.6*	0.6-1.2	3.3*
19-30 yr	**56**	10-35	**130**	45-65	38*			20-35	17*	5-10	1.6*	0.6-1.2	3.7*
31-50 yr	**56**	10-35	**130**	45-65	38*			20-35	17*	5-10	1.6*	0.6-1.2	3.7*
51-70 yr	**56**	10-35	**130**	45-65	30*			20-35	14*	5-10	1.6*	0.6-1.2	3.7*
>70 yr	**56**	10-35	**130**	45-65	30*			20-35	14*	5-10	1.6*	0.6-1.2	3.7*
Females													
9-13 yr	**34**	10-30	**130**	45-65	26*			25-35	10*	5-10	1.0*	0.6-1.2	2.1*
14-18 yr	**46**	10-30	**130**	45-65	26*			25-35	11*	5-10	1.1*	0.6-1.2	2.3*
19-30 yr	**46**	10-35	**130**	45-65	25*			20-35	12*	5-10	1.1*	0.6-1.2	2.7*
31-50 yr	**46**	10-35	**130**	45-65	25*			20-35	12*	5-10	1.1*	0.6-1.2	2.7*
51-70 yr	**46**	10-35	**130**	45-65	21*			20-35	11*	5-10	1.1*	0.6-1.2	2.7*
>70 yr	**46**	10-35	**130**	45-65	21*			20-35	11*	5-10	1.1*	0.6-1.2	2.7*
Pregnant													
≤18 yr	**71**	10-35	**175**	45-65	28*			20-35	13*	5-10	1.4*	0.6-1.2	3.0*
19-30 yr	**71**	10-35	**175**	45-65	28*			20-35	13*	5-10	1.4*	0.6-1.2	3.0*
31-50 yr	**71**	10-35	**175**	45-65	28*			20-35	13*	5-10	1.4*	0.6-1.2	3.0*
Lactating													
≤18 yr	**71**	10-35	**210**	45-65	29*			20-35	13*	5-10	1.3*	0.6-1.2	3.8*
19-30 yr	**71**	10-35	**210**	45-65	29*			20-35	13*	5-10	1.3*	0.6-1.2	3.8*
31-50 yr	**71**	10-35	**210**	45-65	29*			20-35	13*	5-10	1.3*	0.6-1.2	3.8*

Data from *Dietary Reference Intakes for energy, carbohydrate, fiber, fat, fatty acids, cholesterol, protein, and amino acids (macronutrients)*, Washington, DC, 2002, The National Academies Press.

Note: This table presents Recommended Dietary Allowances (RDAs) in **bold type** and Adequate Intakes (AIs) in ordinary type followed by an asterisk(*). RDAs and AIs may both be used as goals for individual intake. RDAs are set to meet the needs of almost all (97% to 98%) individuals in a group. For healthy breast-fed infants, the AI is the mean intake. The AI for other life-stage and gender groups is believed to cover the needs of all individuals in the group, but lack of data prevents being able to specify with confidence the percentage of individuals covered by this intake.

[a]Intakes of dietary cholesterol, trans fatty acids, and saturated fatty acids should be as low as possible while consuming a nutritionally adequate diet; added sugars should be limited to no more than 25% of total energy.

[b]Based on 1.5 g/kg/day for infants, 1.1 g/kg/day for 1-3 yr, 0.95 g/kg/day for 4-13 yr, 0.85 g/kg/day for 14-18 yr, 0.8 g/kg/day for adults, and 1.1 g/kg/day for pregnant (using prepregnancy weight) and lactating women.

[c]Acceptable Macronutrient Distribution Range (AMDR) is the range of intake for a particular energy source that is associated with reduced risk of chronic disease while providing intakes of essential nutrients. If an individual has consumed in excess of the AMDR, there is a potential of increasing the risk of chronic diseases and insufficient intakes of essential nutrients.

[d]Approximately 10% of the total can come from longer-chain, n-3 fatty acids.

[e]ND = Not determinable due to lack of data of adverse effects in this age-group and concern with regard to lack of ability to handle excess amounts. Source of intake should be from food only to prevent high levels of intake.

[f]Includes all water contained in food, beverages, and drinking water.

Williams' Essentials of Nutrition and Diet Therapy

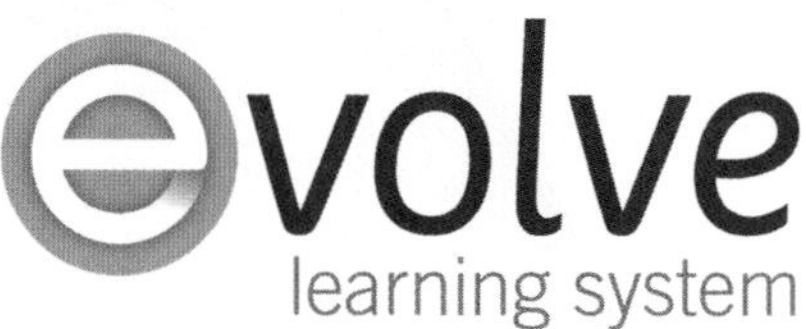

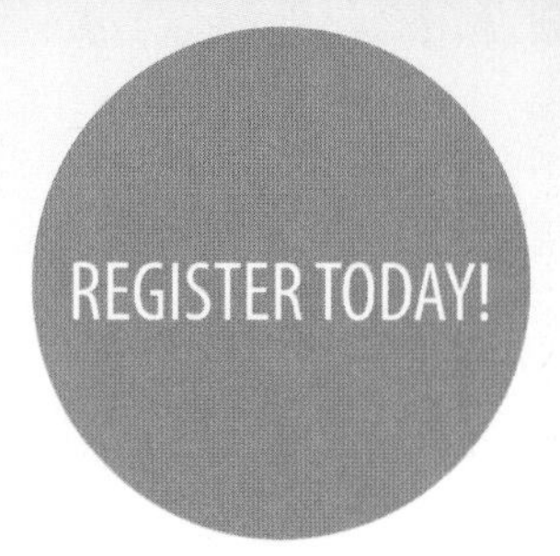

To access your Student Resources, visit:

http://evolve.elsevier.com/Williams/essentials/

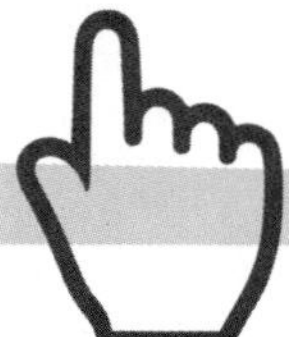

Evolve® Student Resources for Schlenker & Roth: *Williams' Essentials of Nutrition and Diet Therapy*, Tenth Edition, offer the following features:

- **Study Questions**
  Multiple-choice questions organized by chapter test your knowledge of pertient content and provide instant scoring and feedback for test preparation.
- **Case Studies**
  Real-life scenarios provide an opportunity to apply key information.
- **Flash Cards**
  Interactive study experience helps test your knowledge of key terms and concepts.
- **Nutritrac Nutrition Analysis 5.0**
  This food database contains over 5000 foods in 18 different categories and allows you to enter and edit their intake and output. It includes a weight management planner, a detailed energy expenditure section, and sample diets.
- **Food Composition Table**
  This detailed listing allows you to search the nutrient values of more than 5000 foods contained in the Nutritrac Nutrition Analysis Program, Version 5.0. This table is separated and alphabetized into 18 different food categories.
- **Appendixes**

ELSEVIER

tenth edition

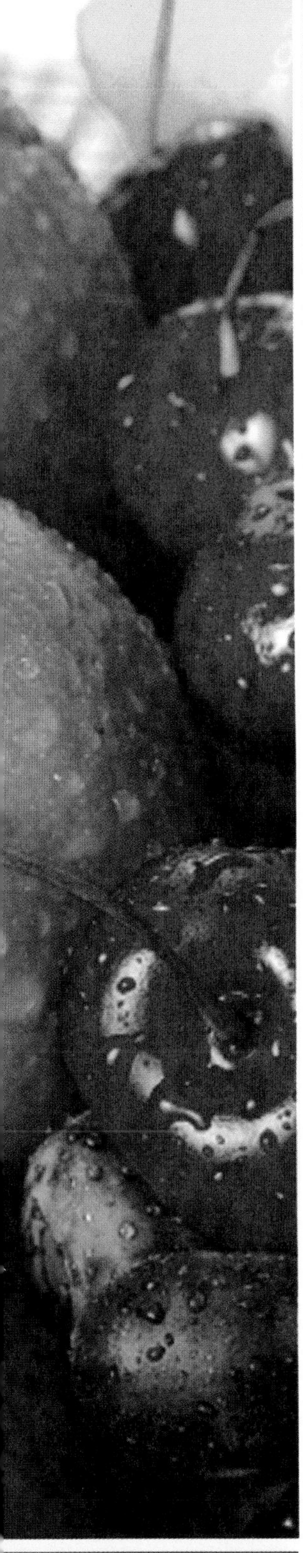

Williams' Essentials of Nutrition and Diet Therapy

Eleanor D. Schlenker, PhD, RD

Professor and Extension Specialist
Department of Human Nutrition, Foods, and Exercise
College of Agriculture and Life Sciences
Virginia Polytechnic Institute and State University
Blacksburg, Virginia

Sara Long Roth, PhD, RD

Professor
Director, Didactic Program in Dietetics
Department of Animal Science, Food, and Nutrition
Southern Illinois University Carbondale
Carbondale, Illinois

ELSEVIER
MOSBY

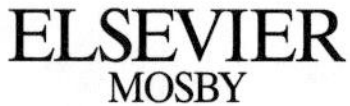

MOSBY

3251 Riverport Lane
St. Louis, Missouri 63043

WILLIAMS' ESSENTIALS OF NUTRITION & DIET THERAPY, TENTH EDITION ISBN: 978-0-323-06860-4

Notices

Knowledge and best practice in this field are constantly changing. As new research and experience broaden our understanding, changes in research methods, professional practices, or medical treatment may become necessary.

Practitioners and researchers must always rely on their own experience and knowledge in evaluating and using any information, methods, compounds, or experiments described herein. In using such information or methods they should be mindful of their own safety and the safety of others, including parties for whom they have a professional responsibility.

With respect to any drug or pharmaceutical products identified, readers are advised to check the most current information provided (i) on procedures featured or (ii) by the manufacturer of each product to be administered, to verify the recommended dose or formula, the method and duration of administration, and contraindications. It is the responsibility of practitioners, relying on their own experience and knowledge of their patients, to make diagnoses, to determine dosages and the best treatment for each individual patient, and to take all appropriate safety precautions.

To the fullest extent of the law, neither the Publisher nor the authors, contributors, or editors, assume any liability for any injury and/or damage to persons or property as a matter of products liability, negligence or otherwise, or from any use or operation of any methods, products, instructions, or ideas contained in the material herein.

Library of Congress Cataloging-in-Publication Data
Schlenker, Eleanor D.
Williams' essentials of nutrition and diet therapy. — 10th ed. / Eleanor D. Schlenker, Sara Long.
p. ; cm.
Essentials of nutrition and diet therapy
Rev. ed. of: Williams' essentials of nutrition & diet therapy. 9th ed. / Eleanor D. Schlenker, Sara Long. c2007.
Includes bibliographical references and index.
ISBN 978-0-323-06860-4 (pbk. : alk. paper) 1. Nutrition. 2. Diet therapy.
I. Roth, Sara Long. II. Williams, Sue Rodwell. Essentials of nutrition and diet therapy. III. Schlenker, Eleanor D. Williams' essentials of nutrition & diet therapy. IV. Title. V. Title: Essentials of nutrition and diet therapy.
[DNLM: 1. Nutritional Physiological Phenomena. 2. Diet Therapy. QU 145]
RM216.S358 2011
613.2—dc22

2010038867

Senior Editor: Yvonne Alexopoulos
Senior Developmental Editor: Danielle M. Frazier
Publishing Services Manager: Deborah L. Vogel
Senior Project Managers: Ann Rogers; Jodi M. Willard
Design Direction: Amy Buxton

Printed in United States of America

Last digit is the print number: 9 8 7 6 5 4 3 2 1

This edition is dedicated to Sue Rodwell Williams, who created the first eight editions and continues to be a source of inspiration.

The Authors

To my parents, Harold and Nora, who taught me to appreciate learning.

Eleanor D. Schlenker

To Harvey & Trish Welch for all you have done: "No one, but no one, could ask for better colleagues, mentors, and friends!"

Sara

Kenneth Byrne, BS
Graduate Student
Department of Animal Science, Food, and Nutrition
Southern Illinois University Carbondale
Carbondale, Illinois

Joyce Ann Gilbert, PhD, RD, LD
Director
Associate Professor
Marilyn Magaram Center for Food Science, Nutrition, and Health
California State University Northridge
Northridge, California

Allan Higginbotham, PhD, RD, LD
Director
Nutrition Matters
Hattiesburg, Mississippi

Sharon M. (Shelly) Nickols-Richardson, PhD, RD
Associate Professor
110 Chandlee Laboratory
Department of Nutritional Sciences
The Pennsylvania State University
University Park, Pennsylvania

Staci Nix, MS, RD, COI
Assistant Professor
Division of Nutrition
University of Utah
Salt Lake City, Utah

REVIEWERS

Melissa J. Benton, PhD, MSN, RN, CNS
Assistant Professor
College of Nursing
Valdosta State University
Valdosta, Georgia

Peter Beyer, MS, RD
Associate Professor
Department of Dietetics and Nutrition
University of Kansas Medical Center
Kansas City, Kansas

Bethany Derricott, MSN, RN
Assistant Professor of Nursing
Kent State University
Twinsburg, Ohio;
Adjunct Faculty
Chamberlain College of Nursing
Columbus, Ohio

Mary Flynn, PhD, RD, LDN
Assistant Professor of Medicine
Research Dietitian
Biomed Department
Brown University;
The Miriam Hospital
Providence, Rhode Island

Elizabeth K. Friedrich, MPH, RD, CSG, LDN
Nutrition and Health Promotion Consultant
Board Certified Specialist in Gerontological Nutrition
Salisbury, North Carolina

Delaine Curtis Furst, MS, EdS
Associate Professor
Foods and Nutrition
Indian River State College
Fort Pierce, Florida

Kathy Hammond, MS, RN, RD, LD
Consultant/Continuing Education and Nutrition
Chartwell Diversified Services, Inc.;
Adjunct Assistant Professor
Department of Foods and Nutrition
University of Georgia;
Georgia Nurses Association
Continuing Education Administrator and Nurse Planner
Atlanta, Georgia

Debra A. Indorato, RD, LDN, CLT
Associate Director
Food and Nutrition Services
Sentara Norfolk General Hospital
Norfolk, Virginia;
Owner
Approach Nutrition Food Allergy Management
Virginia Beach, Virginia

Katy Lenker, MS, RD, LD
Adjunct Instructor
Department of Nutrition, Dietetics and Food Management
University of Central Oklahoma
Edmond, Oklahoma

Edith Lerner, PhD, LD
Associate Professor and Vice Chair
Department of Nutrition
School of Medicine
Case Western Reserve University
Cleveland, Ohio

Patricia B. Lisk, BSN, RN
Retired
Nursing and Allied Health Departments
Augusta Technical College
Augusta, Georgia

Mary-Pat Maciolek, MBA, RD
Chairperson
Hotel, Restaurant and Institution Management Department
Director of Dietetic Technology Program
Middlesex County College
Edison, New Jersey

Marilyn K. Miller, RN, BSN, MSN
Associate Professor
St. Charles Community College
St. Charles, Missouri

Anita K. Reed, MSN, RN
Clinical Instructor
St. Elizabeth School of Nursing
Lafayette, Indiana

Tammy Stephenson, PhD
Faculty
Department of Nutrition and Food Science
University of Kentucky
Lexington, Kentucky

Eric Vlahov, PhD
Professor
Department of Exercise Science and Sport Studies
The University of Tampa
Tampa, Florida

Janelle Walter, BS, MEd, PhD
Professor
Baylor University
Waco, Texas

Through nine highly successful editions, this nutrition textbook has presented a sound approach to student learning and clinical practice in the health professions. It provides both a strong research base and a person-centered approach to the study and application of nutrition in human health. We have appreciated the suggestions and positive reception of this text by users in colleges, community colleges, and clinical settings throughout the United States and in other parts of the world.

Rapid changes are occurring in nutrition. New regulations and protocol are being proposed, with evidence-based practice becoming the standard for decision making. The science base in biology, biotechnology, and health is expanding. Terms such as nanotechnology, nutrigenomics, and functional foods have entered our sphere of practice. Social expectations and structures are changing, and patient populations are more culturally diverse. Health care systems and practices are very different from a generation or even a decade ago and will continue to change with new legislation in health care reform. Public interest and concern with nutrition and health are increasing. The Internet offers broad possibilities for health information that may or may not be appropriate. Nutrition has become prominent in the marketplace of competing ideas and expanding product lines. It is small wonder then that these changes are being reflected in nutrition education and professional practice because nutrition is fundamentally a very human applied science and art.

This new tenth edition reflects these far-reaching changes. As always, we are guided by a commitment to sound nutrition principles rooted in basic science and their application to human health and well-being. We have built on previous editions to produce this new book—updated and rewritten, with our new design and format—to meet the changing needs of students, faculty, and practitioners in the health professions.

NEW TO THIS EDITION

To accommodate the demands of a rapidly developing science and the needs of an increasingly diverse society, the entire text has been updated and rewritten. Changes and additions based on input from many teachers, students, and clinicians have been incorporated to increase its usefulness.

Chapter Changes

With the retirement of Dr. Sue Rodwell Williams, the founder and primary author of the first eight editions of this textbook, we continue to share the responsibility for the preparation of this tenth edition. Part 1, *Introduction to Human Nutrition,* provides the foundation for understanding the basic science of nutrition, which is applied to human nutritional needs in Part 2, *Community Nutrition and The Life Cycle.* Part 3, *Introduction to Clinical Nutrition,* addresses the nutritional care needs within specific illnesses and conditions and the appropriate application of medical nutrition therapy.

The problem of obesity has emerged as a growing health crisis among all age-groups and societies in all parts of the world. The chapter on obesity provides readers with a comprehensive review of this public health problem, its causes, and intervention strategies. We welcome contributing author Dr. Allan Higginbotham, who revised Chapter 15, "The Complexity of Obesity: Beyond Energy Balance." We also welcome Dr. Joyce Ann Gilbert, who revised Chapter 17: "Metabolic Stress" and Mr. Kenneth Byrne, who revised Chapter 19: "Nutrition Support: Enteral and Parenteral Nutrition" and Chapter 25: "Cancer." Dr. Sharon M. Nickols-Richardson has updated Chapters 11 and 12, which focus on nutrition in pregnancy and lactation and normal growth and development. Ms. Staci Nix, author of *Williams' Basic Nutrition & Diet Therapy,* contributed Chapter 14, which addresses nutrition and physical fitness.

New material has been incorporated throughout this edition, including not only recent scientific research findings and clinical treatment therapies, but also a continuing emphasis on preventive health and reducing the incidence of chronic disease. The importance of health promotion along with strategies for implementation is a recurring theme throughout the text, and students are encouraged to look for the *Health Promotion* heading in each chapter for special information to assist with the nutrition education of individuals and groups. A new feature in every chapter is an Evidence-Based Practice, which addresses this new paradigm in the practice of nutrition and dietetics. Each box builds on a practice issue pertinent to that chapter, posing the practice question and describing and evaluating current research findings. Feature boxes appearing in the previous edition addressing contemporary issues in nutrition and health have been updated for the new edition. *Complementary and Alternative Medicine (CAM)* boxes—found in all chapters in Part 3—review and evaluate new therapies relevant to chapter topics. *Focus on Culture* boxes introduce students to the concept of cultural competence and the special nutritional needs, health problems, and appropriate interventions applicable to different cultural, ethnic, racial, and age-groups. *Focus on Food Safety* boxes alert readers to food safety issues related to a particular nutrient, age-group, or medical condition. *Perspectives in Practice* boxes have been redesigned in a concise format to provide practical elements for nutrition education, and students will find these helpful in future professional roles in community or clinical settings. Tools that can be appropriately downloaded from government or other public sites have been included. "Websites of Interest" continue to connect students with Internet sources of accurate and appropriate information, which will be useful in finding answers to client or patient inquiries. "Further Readings and Resources" provide appropriate materials from the research and professional literature to enable further inquiry in a topic of interest.

Illustrations and Design

Numerous illustrations—anatomic figures, graphic line drawings, and photographs—most in full color, enhance the overall design and help students better understand the concepts and clinical practices presented.

Enhanced Readability and Student Interest

Continuing attention has been given to enhancing readability and enlivening the text stylistically with greater use of boxes, illustrations, and recurring themes to capture student interest and assist in comprehension. New material has been added, and remaining sections have been rewritten. Recent advances in basic and clinical science are explained and applied. Issues of public-professional controversy pertinent to students' future practice are discussed.

LEARNING AIDS WITHIN THE TEXT

This tenth edition continues to include many learning aids throughout the text.

Chapter Openers

To alert students to the content of each chapter and draw them into its study, each chapter opens with a preview of the chapter topics. In addition, an outline of the major chapter headings is included on this page.

Key Terms

Key terms important to the student's understanding and application of the chapter content are presented in two steps. First, they are identified in blue type in the body of the text. These terms are then grouped and defined in boxes in the lower corners of the pages close to their mention. This dual-level approach to vocabulary development greatly improves the overall study and usefulness of the text.

Pedagogy Boxes: *Perspectives in Practice, Focus on Culture, Complementary and Alternative Medicine (CAM), Focus on Food Safety, and NEW! Evidence-Based Practice*

These special features throughout the text introduce supplemental material—brief information on chapter-related issues or controversies, a deeper look at chapter topics, and illustrations of practical application of nutrition concepts. These interesting and motivating studies help the student comprehend the importance of scientific thinking and develop sound judgment and openness to varied points of view.

Case Studies

In Parts 2 and 3 realistic case studies lead the student to apply the text material to related nutrition care problems. Each chapter contains at least one case accompanied by questions for analysis and decision making. These case studies help students learn to apply community nutrition interventions and medical nutrition therapy to the individuals and groups they will encounter in their clinical assignments.

Chapter Summaries

To assist the student in drawing the chapter material together as a whole, each chapter concludes with a summary of the key concepts presented and their significance or application. The student can then return to any part of the chapter material for repeated study and clarification as needed.

Review Questions

To help students understand and learn to think critically about key parts of the chapter and apply it to community and patient needs or problems, review questions are provided at the end of each chapter.

Chapter References

A strength of this text is its range of current documentation of the topics presented, drawn from a wide selection of pertinent journals. To provide immediate access to all references cited in the chapter text, a full list of these key references is given at the end of each chapter rather than collected at the end of the book.

Further Readings and Resources

In addition to referenced material in the text, an annotated list of suggestions for further reading for added interest and study is provided at the end of each chapter. These selections extend or apply the text material according to student needs or areas of special interest. The annotations improve their usefulness to students by identifying the pertinent topics of the reference. An addition to each chapter is a list of reliable websites for further reference or study.

Appendixes

The revised appendixes include a number of materials for use as reference tools and guidelines in learning and practice. The most recent edition of the *Choose Your Foods: Exchange Lists for Diabetes* is included. A new addition is a recently developed summary of Cultural Dietary Patterns and Religious Dietary Practices, which includes both foods eaten and foods avoided within each food group. A summary of federal food assistance programs funded and supervised by the U.S. Department of Agriculture and the Administration on Aging, including the target audience, guidelines for participation, and food resources provided, has been added to the Appendix for easy reference.

SUPPLEMENTARY MATERIALS AVAILABLE ON EVOLVE

Our Evolve website is designed to provide supplemental online learning opportunities to complement the material in the book. The Evolve website contains sections for both instructor and student resources. The material was prepared by experienced nutrition writer, editor, and project coordinator Gill Robertson, MS, RD.

Instructor Resources

- Instructor's Manual with chapter overviews, objectives, chapter outlines with teaching notes, and individual/group activities
- Extensive Test Bank of about 1200 NCLEX-style multiple-choice examination questions
- Image Collection of approximately 100 images from the text
- PowerPoint presentations for each chapter, each containing approximately 20 to 30 text slides to guide classroom lecture
- **NEW!** Audience response questions, approximately 4 per chapter
- **NEW!** Answers and guidelines for the textbook case studies

Student Resources

- 250 Study questions with instant feedback
- **NEW!** Case Studies (1 to 3 per chapter)
- **NEW!** Flashcards (5 to 10 per chapter)
- Expanded Food Composition Table

Nutritrac Nutrition Analysis 5.0

- This food database contains over 5000 foods in 18 different categories: Baby Food, Baked Goods, Beverages, Breads/Grains and Pasta, Breakfast Foods/Cereals, Dairy and Eggs, Fats and Oils, Fruits and Vegetables, Meats and Beans, Nuts and Seeds, Frozen Entrees and Packaged Foods, Restaurant Chains–Fast Foods, Restaurant Chains–Other, Seafood and Fish, Snacks and Sweets, Soups, Supplements, and Toppings and Sauces.
- A complete listing of more than 150 activities—daily/common, sporting, recreational, and occupational—is included in the *Detailed Energy Expenditure* section.
- The profile feature allows users to enter and edit the intake and output of an unlimited number of individuals, and the weight management planner helps outline healthy lifestyles tailored to various personal profiles.
- In addition to foods and activities, features include an ideal body weight (IBW) calculator, a basal metabolic rate calculator to estimate total daily energy needs, and sample diets with nutrition recommendations for a variety of conditions.

PERSONAL APPROACH

The person-centered approach that has been a hallmark of previous editions continues to be emphasized in this new edition. The authors and contributors have continued to write in a personal style and to use materials and examples from personal research and clinical experience. Scientific knowledge is presented in human terms as a tool to develop practical solutions to individual problems.

ACKNOWLEDGMENTS

A textbook of this size is never the work of just authors and contributors. It develops into the planned product through the committed hands and hearts of a number of persons. It would be impossible to name all of the individuals involved, but several groups deserve special recognition.

First, the authors are grateful to the reviewers, who gave their valuable time and skills to strengthen the manuscript: Peter L. Beyer, Liz Friedrich, Delaine Curtis Furst, Kathy A. Hammond, Debra A. Indorato, Betty (Elizabeth) Kenyon, Bridget Klawitter, Kelly Kohls, Jane Kufus-Krump, Diane T. Kupensky, Edith Lerner, Jaimette A. McCulley, Jessie Pavlinac, Rena Quinton, and Jennifer M. Williams.

Second, we are indebted to Elsevier and the many persons there who had a part in this extensive project. We especially thank our senior editor of nutrition publications, Yvonne Alexopoulos, whose skills and support have always been invaluable; and our senior developmental editor, Danielle Frazier, whose creative and energetic talents helped shape the book's pages. We also thank our production project managers, Ann Rogers and Jodi Willard, for essential guidance; and our senior book designer, Amy Buxton, who helped to bring a new look to this tenth edition. To our marketing managers and the many fine Elsevier sales representatives throughout the country, we owe great appreciation for their help in ensuring the book's success with users.

Eleanor D. Schlenker
Blacksburg, Virginia
Sara Long Roth
Carbondale, Illinois

PART 1 INTRODUCTION TO HUMAN NUTRITION

APPENDIXES

Look for these appendixes on the Evolve website:
http://evolve.elsevier.com/Williams/essentials

Williams' Essentials of Nutrition and Diet Therapy

PART 1

Introduction to Human Nutrition

1

Nutrition and Health

Eleanor D. Schlenker

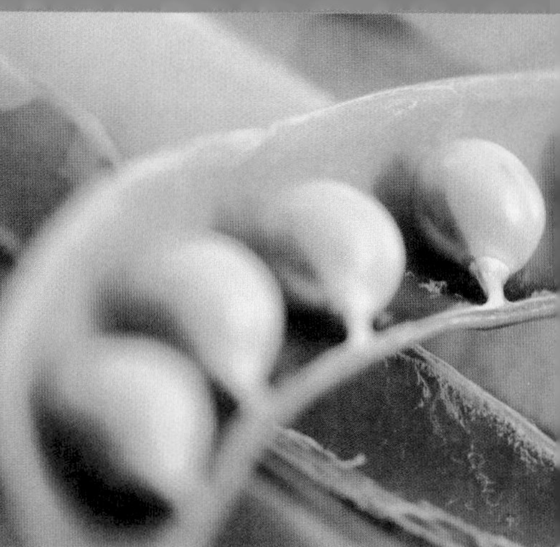

evolve WEBSITE
http://evolve.elsevier.com/Williams/essentials/

CHAPTER OUTLINE

With this chapter, we begin our study of nutrition and human health. Sound nutrition principles coupled with skills in food selection are the cornerstone of personal health. Current knowledge in nutrition rooted in basic science reflects our growing understanding of the relationship between food and health. What people are eating is receiving attention from government agencies charged with the enormous task of lowering chronic disease rates and containing health care costs. Ensuring access to a safe and wholesome food supply and the nutrition it provides must be our goal for all people. In our study we will emphasize a person-centered approach to education and intervention, keeping in mind individual needs, differences, and goals.

NEW CHALLENGES FOR NUTRITION PROFESSIONALS

The Obesity Epidemic

A major health problem in the United States and worldwide is the rising prevalence of obesity. Countries previously facing food shortages and undernutrition are now experiencing increasing overweight.[1] Changes in food and lifestyle patterns over the past 25 years have resulted in tremendous changes across the United States (Figure 1-1). Since 1980, body weights have increased by 20% even when corrected for age and increases in body height.[2] Seventy-one percent of men and 61% of women are overweight or obese,[3] and 32% of children are either overweight or at risk for overweight.[4] Persons ages 40 to 59 are more likely to be overweight or obese than adults younger or older, and children older than age 5 are at greater risk of overweight than preschoolers. The obesity among children and adolescents is increasing their risk of type 2 diabetes and metabolic syndrome, conditions seldom before seen in youth.[5] Apparently, however, body weight may be leveling off in women[3] and youth[4] while continuing to rise among men.[3]

This rise in obesity is related to environmental rather than genetic factors, although some individuals are more prone than others to gain weight.[5] In contrast to earlier times when humans survived as "hunter-gatherers," we now have a plentiful supply of good-tasting, energy-dense food, with little physical activity required to obtain it. The ever-present vending machine, special offers of two hamburgers for the price of one, and accessible food at most sporting and social events all contribute to food intake (Box 1-1). Portions served at fast-food restaurants are two to five times larger than those offered 20 years ago,[6] and food served at home often equals three to four times the serving size referred to in meal planning guides (Figure 1-2). People increase their portion size when more food is served,[6–8] adding to the potential for overeating at "all you can eat" food outlets.

As energy intake is rising, energy expenditure is falling. For many children, sedentary pastimes such as watching television or playing video games have replaced active games, and most children ride rather than walk to school. Many residential developments and most rural localities lack sidewalks, and other neighborhoods are unsafe for walking. Collaborative efforts among government agencies, schools, community planners, food service providers, and health professionals will be required to solve this problem.

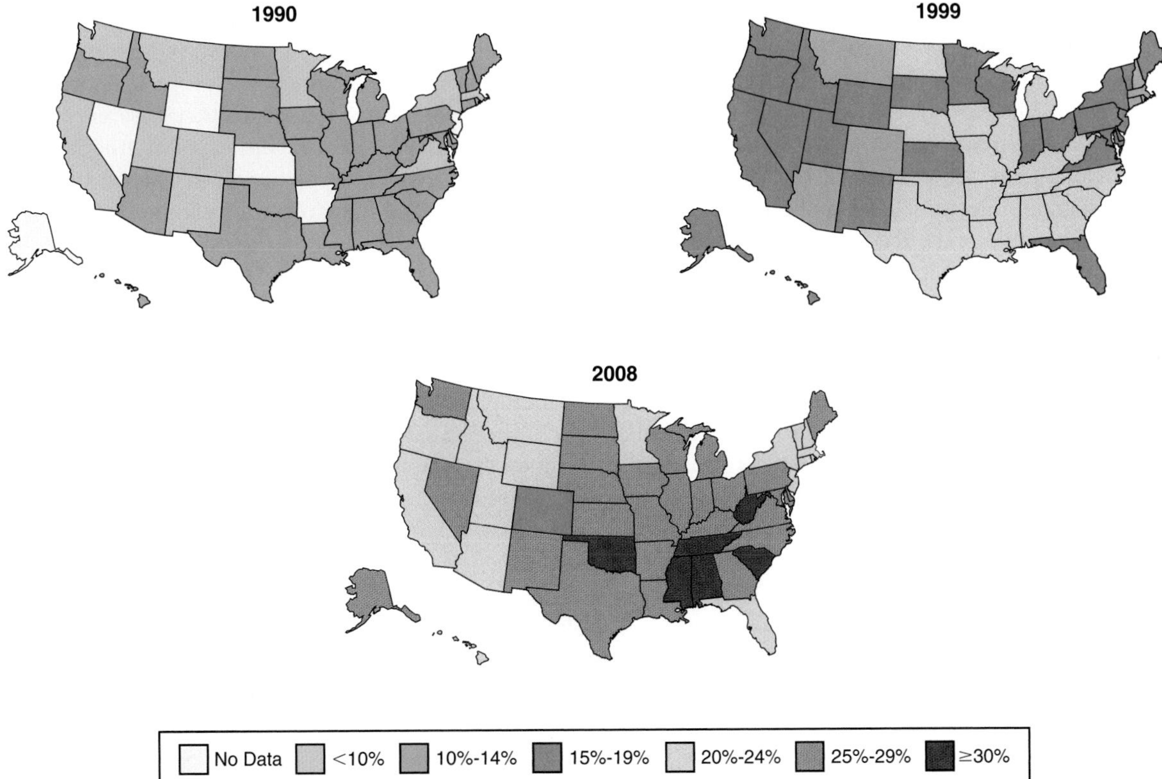

FIGURE 1-1 The obesity epidemic among U.S. adults. Notice the rise in the number of states in which at least one fourth (25%-29%) of the residents are obese. By 2008, only one state had an obesity prevalence below 20%, and 32 states had a prevalence of at least 25%. (Obesity is defined as a body mass index of 30 or greater, which is the equivalent of 30 lb overweight for a person 64 inches tall.) (Map data from the Behavioral Risk Factor Surveillance System, Centers for Disease Control and Prevention: *U.S. obesity trends: 1985-2008,* Atlanta, 2008, U.S. Department of Health and Human Services. Retrieved July 29, 2009, from www.cdc.gov/nccdphp/dnpa/obesity/trend/index.htm.)

BOX 1-1 FACTORS CONTRIBUTING TO INCREASED FOOD INTAKE

- Media advertising of high-sugar and high-calorie foods
- Greater access to vending machines selling high-sugar drinks and high-fat snacks
- More meals eaten away from home
- All-you-can-eat restaurant buffets
- Larger portion sizes—both at home and in restaurants
- Continuous snacking
- "Supersizing"—larger portions costing only a fraction more than the *normal* portion

Portion Distortion

CHEESEBURGER

20 Years Ago

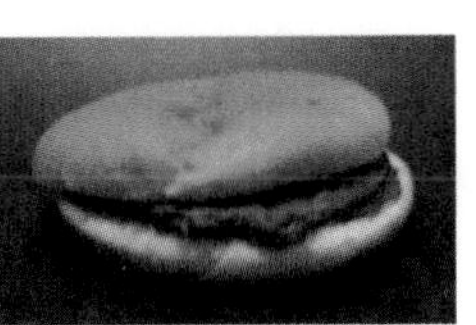

260 calories

Today

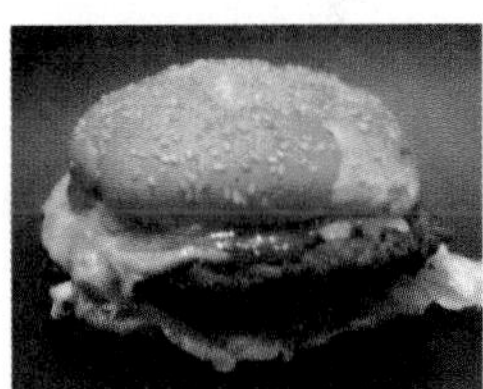

850 calories

FIGURE 1-2 Change in portion size of common foods. Over the last 20 years, portion sizes have almost tripled. A hamburger and roll that supplied 260 kcal may now contain 850 kcal. Visit the website of the National Heart, Lung and Blood Institute, National Institutes of Health *(http://hp2010.nhlbihin.net/portion/keep.htm)* to view photographs of many food items that have changed in size and kcalorie content. Take the quiz to learn how many minutes you would need to exercise to burn the extra kcalories. (Concept from U.S. Department of Health and Human Services, National Institutes of Health, National Heart, Lung and Blood Institute, Obesity Education Initiative: *Keep an eye on portion size,* Bethesda, Md, 2004, U.S. Government Printing Office. Retrieved from http://hp2010.nhlbihin.net/portion/keep.htm.)

Shifts in Population

Number of Older Adults

Over the past century, advances in sanitation and public health have raised life expectancy at birth from 45 years to nearly 80 years.[9] Infectious diseases such as influenza and pneumonia have been replaced by chronic diseases, heart disease, cancer, and stroke as leading causes of death. As life expectancy has risen, so has the number of people ages 65 and over. In fact, the number of older adults is increasing twice as rapidly as the general population (Figure 1-3),[9] and this tendency carries implications for health care. Although the 65-and-older group make up only 13% of the population, they incur nearly 30% of all health care costs.[9] As physical changes related to the aging process and chronic disease bring about losses in function, innovative food delivery systems to support homebound older adults in the community and medically compromised older adults in long-term care facilities will be urgently needed. Intervention programs directed toward young and middle-age adults emphasizing appropriate food and activity habits can slow the development of chronic disease and ensuing disability.

Ethnic and Racial Diversity

The United States is becoming increasingly diverse. Diverse racial and ethnic groups now make up one third of the general population, and this proportion is expected to rise.[10] Hispanic Americans, Asian Americans, and Pacific Islander Americans are increasing at the most rapid rates, and Hispanic Americans now surpass African Americans in number. These population shifts affect health care in several ways. First, certain racial and ethnic groups are at increased risk of developing particular chronic conditions, especially if they have moved away from their traditional diets toward the typical American diet higher in **kilocalories** (kcalories or kcal), fat, and protein. Asian Americans[11] and Hispanic Americans are at increased risk of diabetes, and African Americans are more likely than other groups to be *salt sensitive* and develop hypertension.[12] Second, health professionals must be knowledgeable about the eating patterns and favorite foods of different racial, ethnic, and cultural groups if they are to help these individuals develop a meal plan that will be accepted and implemented.[13]

The *Focus on Culture* box, "Diversity in Food Patterns," introduces the typical meal patterns and food group choices of various groups to begin your study of cultural and ethnic foods.

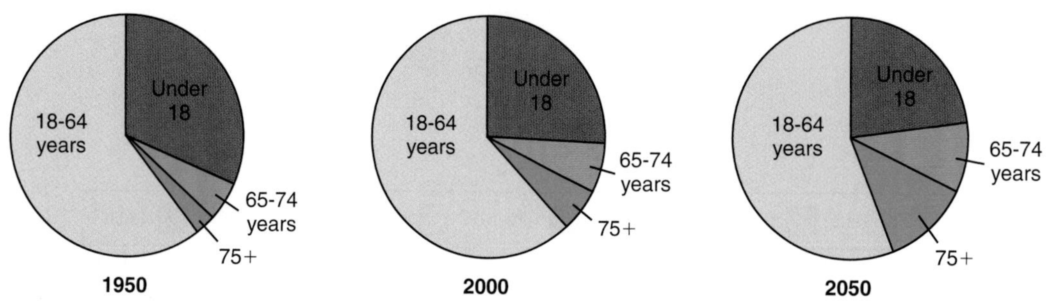

FIGURE 1-3 Projected increases in the number of persons age 65 and older. Between 1900 and 2000, the older age group grew from 3 million to 37 million and currently makes up 12% of the general population. By 2030, this group will number 70.5 million and represent almost 20% of the general population. By 2050, 21 million people will be at least age 85. (From Federal Interagency Forum on Aging-Related Statistics: *Older Americans 2008: Key indicators of well-being. Federal Interagency Forum on Aging-Related Statistics,* Washington, DC, 2008, U.S. Government Printing Office.)

FOCUS ON CULTURE

Diversity in Food Patterns

Regardless of their location and the foods available, people have survived the world over, receiving their nourishment from various protein foods, cereals and grains, and fruits and vegetables. The nutrients are important, not the individual foods; thus healthy diets can be obtained from a wide variety of foods. You will see these many different patterns as you work among various cultural and ethnic groups.

How Food Patterns Develop

Food provides the nutrients that sustain life, but for most of us, this is not the reason why we choose to eat what we do. Food habits—what we eat and when we eat it—have evolved over thousands of years. In all cultures and societies, several factors influence food patterns, as follows:

Agriculture: The available land for raising crops or animals led to the evolution of food patterns based on plant foods or animal foods. Raising cattle requires land for grazing. Lack of water resources or limited space led to increased emphasis on plant foods in some locations. Although parts of Europe were well adapted to raising cattle or pigs, other terrains were better suited to support goats and sheep for meat and milk. Feta cheese made from the milk of sheep or goats, a common food in Greece, Turkey, and other areas of southeastern Europe, has become a popular cheese in the United States as well.

A major influence on the food patterns of every culture is the cereal or grain traditionally grown in their region. Rice, the cereal indigenous to much of Southeast Asia, is served at every meal in traditional Chinese, Japanese, Hmong, and Cambodian households, much the same as bread is a staple in the American diet. Because of the limited supply of meat, the Asian food pattern usually combines a small amount of meat or fish with vegetables and rice for stew-like dishes. Chinese cooks believe that refrigeration diminishes natural flavors, thus they select the freshest foods available, hold them for the shortest time possible, and cook them quickly at a high temperature. Most foods are prepared in a wok with small amounts of fat and liquid, which preserves natural flavor, color, and texture.

Maize or field corn, along with rice, is the traditional cereal grown in the southern region of the United States and parts of Central and South America. Native-American foods made from corn—corn bread, corn cake, tortillas, cornmeal mush, and popcorn—were dietary staples. Sheep and goats thrived in the Native-American lands and offered meat and milk. The traditional southern or African-American food pattern also relied on corn as the early slaves adapted their African recipes to the food staples available in this country. Traditional hot breads made with corn included spoon bread, cornmeal muffins, and

FOCUS ON CULTURE

Diversity in Food Patterns—cont'd

skillet cornbread. Cooked cereals such as cornmeal mush and hominy grits along with rice were eaten regularly.

The Mexican food pattern also relied on corn as the basic grain, and bread took the form of tortillas, flat cakes baked on a hot griddle. Beans and peppers are also common foods in the traditional Mexican food pattern. Recognizing the differences between the Mexican food pattern and the Puerto Rican food pattern that relies on rice and tropical fruits and vegetables is important. When working with Latino clients, establishing their ethnic origin will be necessary, given that food habits will differ.

Climate: When people raised all of their own food, the length of the growing season, amount of rainfall, and general temperature defined what they ate. Root vegetables such as potatoes and cold-hardy cultivars such as cabbage and carrots made up a large part of the diet of persons in northern Europe where the growing season is relatively short. These vegetables, along with apples, could be stored in a root cellar to sustain families over the long winter. In contrast, grains and legumes, along with a bountiful supply of vegetables and fruits, provided the plant base of the healthful Mediterranean diet. Milder temperatures and longer growing seasons for fresh produce contributed to the frequent use of vegetable stews and salads in the typical Italian and Greek food patterns. Olives, olive oil, and dates remain important foods in Mediterranean cultures. Based on its promotion as a healthy fat, olive oil is now used in many parts of the world. The Caribbean region with its extended growing seasons is known for its tropical fruits and starchy vegetables. These foods are often imported for sale in street markets in U.S. cities with large populations from Puerto Rico and the Caribbean region.

Proximity to water: Populations living near water included fish or seafood in their daily diet. The typical Japanese meal in addition to steamed rice often included grilled, broiled, or pan-cooked fish or shellfish. Sushi, a traditional Japanese dish made with very fresh raw fish combined with rice and seaweed, is enjoying growing popularity in the United States. The French-American (Cajun) diet common to southeast Louisiana also made liberal use of the nearby seafood. The Cajuns descended from early French colonists who settled in Nova Scotia and eventually relocated to southern Louisiana. They blended their French culinary background with the Creole cookery found around New Orleans. Cajun foods are strongly flavored and spicy, with seafood as a base, and are usually cooked as a stew and served over rice. Tabasco sauce evolved from Cajun cookery. Seafood and chicken gumbo, jambalaya, blackened catfish, red snapper, oysters, and boiled crawfish appear frequently in the Cajun diet.

Religion: Religious beliefs define not only what the appropriate food is, but also when it may be eaten. Fasting can restrict certain foods or set periods when no foods shall be eaten. Judaism and Islam (Muslim) are two examples of religions with dietary laws. Within Judaism are three different groups whose food laws differ in degree of restriction: (1) the Orthodox follow a strict observance, (2) the Conservative are less strict, and (3) the Reformed have the fewest restrictions. The body of dietary laws is called the *Rules of Kashruth*. Foods selected and prepared according to these laws are called *kosher*, from the Hebrew word meaning *fit or proper*. Jewish law governs how animals are slaughtered, and supervision by a rabbi is required to certify that correct procedures have been followed. For Orthodox believers, meat and milk may not be combined, and Orthodox homes maintain two sets of dishes and cooking utensils—one for serving meat and the other for meals containing dairy foods. These dishes and cookware must be washed and stored separately. Many traditional Jewish foods such as matzo, a type of unleavened bread, relate to observances that commemorate significant events in Jewish history. Although bagels are a traditional Jewish food, they have become popular across the general population.

Muslim dietary laws were derived from Islamic teachings in the Koran. Food is considered to be a form of worship, and Muslims are urged to avoid self-indulgence. As with Judaism, pork is strictly forbidden, and other animals must be slaughtered under the supervision of a religious leader. In the United States, many Muslims use kosher meats. The Koran mentions certain foods as being of special value to physical and spiritual well-being, including figs, olives, dates, honey, milk, and buttermilk. Muslims celebrate Ramadan, a 30-day period of daylight fasting that occurs during the ninth month of the Islamic lunar calendar. During Ramadan, no food or beverages are eaten from dawn to sunset, but special meals are celebrated after sundown. Traditionally, these meals start with an appetizer such as dates or a fruit drink followed by the family's "evening breakfast," the *iftar*. At the end of Ramadan, a feast with special foods climaxes the observance.

Changes in Ethnic Patterns

Over time, people adapt to the food patterns around them and place less emphasis on their traditional foods. Unfortunately, popular American foods are often less healthy than were their native foods. Traditional meal patterns usually emphasize rice, legumes, and vegetables high in nutrients and fiber with small amounts of meat or fish. These foods are often replaced with soft drinks, fast foods, and snack foods high in sugar and fat, resulting in rapid weight gain and increased risk of chronic disease. A balance between the old and the new is the best way to preserve one's heritage and health.

For lists of specific foods from each food group common to various ethnic and religious groups, see Appendix E.

BIBLIOGRAPHY

Diabetes Care and Education Dietetic Practice Group, Goody CM, Drago L, editors: *Cultural food practices*, Chicago, 2010, American Dietetic Association.

Kittler PG, Sucher KP: *Cultural foods: traditions and trends*, Belmont, Calif, 2000, Wadsworth/Thomson Learning.

KEY TERMS

kilocalorie The general term *calorie* refers to a unit of heat and is used alone to designate the small calorie. The large calorie, 1000 calories or kilocalorie, is used in the study of metabolism to avoid the use of very large numbers in calculations.

New Products in the Marketplace

Growing concerns about increasing chronic disease and health care have attracted the attention of food scientists and food processors. New research has discovered that various foods contain naturally occurring substances other than nutrients that promote health, and these foods are known as *functional foods. Phytochemicals* (plant chemicals) found in fruits and vegetables appear to have cancer-fighting properties.[14] Dark chocolate, often considered a food to be avoided, is now known to contain phytochemicals that help prevent cardiovascular disease and can be included in a healthy diet.[15] Public interest in nutrients and other substances related to health has led to their addition to processed foods. Certain plant sterols that help lower blood cholesterol levels are being added to margarine, and orange juice has become an alternative source for calcium and vitamin D to help stem bone loss and associated disability. On the other hand, "energy drinks" with added herbs and stimulants, marketed to replace water or other healthful beverages, may be harmful and should be used with caution. As more and more products promising health benefits enter the marketplace, the task of assisting consumers in making appropriate choices will fall to the health professional.

Nutrition and Our Genes

The Human Genome Project, an international project to map all human genes and determine their deoxyribonucleic acid (DNA) sequence, is helping scientists learn how diet and environmental factors influence our genes (nutrigenomics) and, conversely, how slight variations in our genetic code affect our nutrient needs and susceptibility to particular diseases (nutrigenetics).[16] We hope to learn why some people cannot produce the enzyme needed to break down lactose or why others are allergic to certain proteins in wheat flour. Individuals with particular gene types are more likely than others to develop cardiovascular disease or osteoporosis and can lower their risk by adopting appropriate food patterns. The study of nutrigenomics will help us understand how particular substances in foods such as grapes or green tea influence diseases such as diabetes, arthritis, and cardiovascular disease.[17–18]

Genetic differences influence response to a health intervention. For example, a change in the amount or type of dietary fat that improves blood lipid levels in most people may actually worsen blood lipid levels in others.[19] In time, we may be able to individualize diets based on genetic predisposition to specific diseases and nutrient requirements, but we still have a lot to learn before this idea becomes a reality. Nevertheless, general recommendations relating to disease prevention are highly appropriate for individuals whose family history puts them at risk.

The Information Explosion

Consumer surveys indicate the majority of Americans believe that diet and health are related, and more than 80% of these individuals are choosing or would be interested in choosing foods or beverages benefiting health.[20] However, where are they getting their food and nutrition information? The Internet and other technology-based materials are expanding as sources of health and nutrition advice for the eager consumer; in fact, approximately one half of persons interviewed noted the Web as their major source.[20] Internet sites maintained by government agencies, universities, state extension services, and nonprofit health organizations contain science-based information and direct readers to other reliable resources. Reputable food companies provide helpful information on the nutrient content of their products; however, commercial sites devoted to sales often post misleading health claims, and Internet sales of herbs, drugs, and health devices are not monitored by government regulatory agencies. (See Chapter 9 for more information on government regulation.) Health professionals and responsible journalists using print and voice media must present balanced views of nutrition issues in ways that are easily understood. Based on the strongly negative view of dietary fat presented in the media, some consumers have decreased their intakes of "good" fats needed to supply important nutrients. At the close of each chapter you will find a list of websites recommended for clients or patients wishing additional information.

THE SCIENCE OF NUTRITION

Nutrition builds on two areas of science. The life sciences of biochemistry and physiology help us see how nutrition relates to our physical health and body function. The behavioral sciences help us understand how nutrition is interwoven with our psychosocial needs. Both aspects are at work in our lives.

Human organisms are highly complex groupings of chemical compounds constantly at work in an array of reactions that sustain life. Nutrients participate in and help control these chemical reactions. Various physiologic systems integrate the activities of the millions of individually functioning cells and organs, uniting them into a functioning whole. This highly sensitive internal control is called homeostasis.

We also have social and emotional qualities rooted in our earliest awareness of interpersonal interactions and life experiences. Eating patterns and attitudes toward food develop over our lifetime based on the acculturating influences of our primary family and friends, ethnic or cultural group, community, nation, and world. How we perceive food, what we choose to eat, why we eat what we do, and the ways in which we eat are all integral parts of human nutrition.

Working Definitions

Nutrition means *to nourish* and involves the food people eat and how it enriches their lives physically, socially, and personally. From the moment of conception until death, an appropriate supply of food supports optimal growth and maturation, mental and physical well-being, and resistance to disease. Good nutrition promotes health and reduces the risk of adverse conditions ranging from low birth weight to obesity to cardiovascular disease.[21] Food supplies energy to carry out body functions such as inhaling and exhaling, maintaining body temperature, and engaging in physical activity; food also nourishes the human spirit. We all have our particular "soul foods," certain comfort foods that connect us to our family and provide a sense of psychologic and emotional well-being.

To study nutrition, we need to define the terms that describe this body of knowledge and the health professionals who work within it. *Nutrition* refers to the food people eat and how it nourishes their bodies, whereas nutrition science defines the nutrient requirements for body maintenance, growth, activity, and reproduction. Dietetics is the health profession with the primary responsibility for the practical application of nutrition science in various conditions of health and disease. The registered dietitian (RD) is the nutrition expert on the health care team and, in collaboration with the physician and nurse, carries the major responsibility for patients' nutritional care. Public health nutritionists oversee programs that serve high-risk groups in the community, such as pregnant teens or homebound older adults, assessing needs and developing interventions. RDs may collaborate with school nurses to teach weight-management classes for children and parents, assist day care providers in planning menus and snacks, or help clients at fitness centers improve their body composition or athletic performance.

Functions of Food and Nutrients

Food serves as the vehicle for bringing nutrients into the body; however, the specific chemical compounds and elements found in food—the nutrients—are the substances the body requires. No one particular food or food combination is required to ensure health. The human race has survived for centuries on a wide variety of foods, depending on what was available and what the culture designated as appropriate. Approximately 50 nutrients have been found to be essential to human life and health, although countless other elements and molecules are being studied and may be essential. The identification of all essential nutrients is particularly important when developing formulas for enteral and parenteral feeding of critically ill patients.

Essential nutrients include the macronutrients—carbohydrates, fats, and proteins—and the micronutrients—vitamins and minerals. The macronutrients supply energy and build tissue, whereas the micronutrients are used in much smaller amounts to form specialized structures and regulate body processes. Water is the often-forgotten nutrient that sustains all of our life systems. The sum of all chemical reactions that use nutrients is known as metabolism. The first section of this text describes these important nutrients, and in later chapters, we learn how they participate in growth, maturation, aging, health, and nutrient-based interventions in acute and chronic illness.

Nutrients have three general functions in the body, as follows:

1. To provide energy
2. To build and repair body tissues and structures
3. To regulate the metabolic processes that maintain homeostasis and support life

Energy Sources

Carbohydrates. Dietary carbohydrates—starch and sugars—are the primary source of fuel for heat and energy. *Glycogen* is the body's storage form of carbohydrate used for quick energy. It is sometimes called *animal starch* because its structure is similar to that of plant starch. Each gram of carbohydrate when metabolized in the body yields 4 kcal, known as its *fuel factor.* In a well-balanced diet for a healthy person, 45% to 65% of total kcalories are supplied by carbohydrates.[22] The majority of these kcalories should come from complex carbohydrates (starch), with a smaller amount from simple carbohydrates (sugars). Another form of complex carbohydrate known as *fiber* does not yield energy but has other important body functions. Although the general public uses the word *calorie* to refer to the energy value of food, nutritionists use the technical term *kilocalorie* (kcalorie or kcal). Later in this chapter, you will notice that MyPyramid, the food guidance system developed for the general public,

KEY TERMS

nutrigenomics The study of the effects of nutrients and other bioactive substances found in food on genes, body proteins, and metabolites.

nutrigenetics The study of the effect of an individual's particular genetic variation on metabolic and physiologic function, including nutrient requirements, food digestion and absorption, or risk of certain diseases.

homeostasis State of dynamic equilibrium within the body's internal environment; a balance achieved through the control of various interrelated physiologic mechanisms.

nutrition The sum of the processes involved in taking in food, releasing the nutrients it contains, and assimilating and using these nutrients to provide energy and maintain body tissue.

nutrition science The body of scientific knowledge developed through controlled research that relates to all aspects of nutrition—national, international, community, and clinical.

dietetics The science concerned with the nutritional planning and preparation of foods and diets.

registered dietitian (RD) A health professional who has completed an accredited academic program and a minimum of 900 hours of postbaccalaureate supervised practice and has passed the National Registration Examination for Dietitians administered by the Commission on Dietetic Registration of the American Dietetic Association.

public health nutritionist A health professional who has completed an academic program in nutrition and a graduate degree (MPH or DrPH) in a school of public health accredited by the American Association of Public Health; he or she supervises the nutrition component of public health programs in county, state, national, or international community settings.

nutrients Substances in food that are essential for energy, growth, normal body function, and maintenance of life.

macronutrients The three energy-yielding nutrients: carbohydrate, fat, and protein.

micronutrients The two classes of non–energy-yielding elements and compounds—the minerals and vitamins. Minerals and vitamins are essential for regulation and control of cell metabolism and building body structures.

metabolism The sum of all the various biochemical and physiologic processes by which the body grows and maintains itself (anabolism), breaks down and reshapes tissue (catabolism), and transforms energy to do its work. Products of these various reactions are called metabolites.

and the *Dietary Guidelines for Americans* use the term *calorie* when indicating the energy value of foods or diets. We will learn more about these energy terms in Chapter 8.

Fats. Dietary fats from animal and plant sources provide an alternate or storage form of energy. Fat is a more concentrated fuel than carbohydrates, with a fuel factor of 9, yielding 9 kcal/g. Most nutrition experts recommend that fats supply no more than 20% to 35% of total kcalories.[22] Less than 10% of dietary fat should be saturated fat, with the remainder coming from unsaturated fats. Fats also contain the essential fatty acids required for life and health.

Proteins. The primary function of protein is tissue building, although it can be used for energy if needed. The body draws on dietary or tissue protein when the fuel supply from carbohydrates and fats is not sufficient to meet body needs. Protein yields 4 kcal/g, making its fuel factor 4. Protein can provide 10% to 35% of total kcalories in a well-balanced diet for healthy individuals.[22]

Tissue Building and Repair

Protein. Protein foods are broken down into amino acids, the building blocks for making and repairing body tissues. Body tissues are constantly being broken down and rebuilt to ensure growth and maintenance of body structure. Proteins also form vital substances such as enzymes and hormones that regulate body systems.

Minerals. Minerals help build tissues with very specific functions. The major minerals—calcium and phosphorus—give strength to bones and teeth. The trace element iron is a component of hemoglobin and binds oxygen for transport to cells.

Vitamins. Vitamins are complex molecules needed in very minute amounts but are essential in certain tissues. Vitamin C helps produce the intercellular ground substance that cements tissues together and prevents tissue bleeding. Vitamin A in the rods and cones of the eye is needed for vision in dim light.

Metabolic Regulation

Minerals. Minerals serve as cofactors in controlling cell metabolism. Iron controls the enzyme actions in the cell mitochondria that produce and store high-energy compounds.

Vitamins. Vitamins are components of cell enzyme systems and govern reactions that produce energy and synthesize important molecules. Thiamin helps control the release of energy to carry on the work of the cell.

Water. Water forms the blood, lymph, and intercellular fluids that transport nutrients to cells and remove waste. Water also functions as a regulatory agent, providing the fluid environment in which all metabolic reactions take place.

Nutrient Interrelationships

An important principle in nutrition is *nutrient interaction,* which includes the following two parts:

1. Individual nutrients participate in many different metabolic functions; in some functions a nutrient has a primary role, and in others, it has a supporting role.
2. No nutrient ever works alone.

BOX 1-2 USEFUL MEASUREMENTS IN EVALUATING NUTRITIONAL STATUS

Dietary Intake
- Where and when food is eaten
- Use of dietary or nutritional supplements
- Food resources
- Special diet, if any
- Facilities for cooking and storing food

Biochemical Measurements
- Blood protein levels
- Blood lipid levels
- Blood vitamin levels

Anthropometric Measurements
- Body weight for height (body mass index)
- Skinfold thicknesses
- Waist circumference

Clinical Evaluation
- Skin
- Hair
- Eyes

Intimate and ongoing metabolic relationships exist among all the nutrients and their metabolites. Although we separate the nutrients to simplify our study, they do not exist separately in the body. Nutrients are always working together as an integrated whole, providing energy, building and rebuilding tissue, and regulating metabolic activities. This synergy and interaction among nutrients is important in carrying out body functions and may be overlooked when we examine the effects of one nutrient at a time.[23]

Nutritional Status

The nutritional health of an individual is known as his or her *nutritional status* and describes how well nutrient needs are being met.[24] Nutritional status is influenced by living situation, available food, food choices, and state of health. A complete evaluation of nutritional status requires a combination of dietary, biochemical, anthropometric, and clinical measurements (Box 1-2). Knowing not only what an individual is eating, but also whether the body is absorbing and making use of those nutrients is important. Blood nutrient levels can help identify a nutrient deficiency or a nutrient excess brought about by overuse of highly fortified foods or supplements. Body weight for height and other anthropometric measurements provide estimates of body fat and muscle mass. (Nutrition assessment is discussed in greater detail in Chapter 16.)

Optimal Nutrition

Individuals with optimal nutritional status have neither a deficiency nor an excess of nutrients. Nutrient reserves are at the upper end of the normal range. Evidence of optimal nutrition includes appropriate weight for height (ratio of muscle mass to fat) and good muscle development and tone. The skin is

TABLE 1-1 CLINICAL SIGNS OF NUTRITIONAL STATUS

FEATURE(S)	GOOD NUTRITIONAL STATUS	POOR NUTRITIONAL STATUS
General appearance	Alert, responsive	Listless, apathetic, cachectic
Hair	Shiny, lustrous, healthy scalp	Stringy, dull, brittle, dry, depigmented
Neck glands	No enlargement	Thyroid enlarged
Skin—face, neck	Smooth, slightly moist	Greasy, scaly
Eyes	Bright, clear, no fatigue circles	Dryness, signs of infection, increased vascularity, glassiness, thickened conjunctivae
Lips	Good color, moist	Dry, scaly, swollen, angular lesions (stomatitis)
Tongue	Good pink color, surface papillae present, no lesions	Papillae atrophy, smooth appearance, swollen, red, beefy (glossitis)
Gums	Good pink color, no swelling or bleeding, firm	Marginal redness or swelling, receding, spongy
Teeth	Straight, no crowding, well-shaped jaw, no discoloration	Unfilled cavities, absent teeth, worn surfaces, mottled, malpositioned
Skin, general	Smooth, slightly moist	Rough, dry, scaly, irritated; petechiae, bruises
Abdomen	Flat	Swollen
Legs, feet	No tenderness, weakness, swelling	Edema, tender calf, tingling, weakness
Skeleton	No malformations	Bowlegs, chest deformity at the diaphragm, beaded ribs, prominent scapulas
Weight	Normal for height, age, body build	Overweight or underweight
Posture	Erect, arms and legs straight, abdomen in, chest out	Sagging shoulders, sunken chest, humped back
Muscles	Well developed, firm	Flaccid, poor tone, undeveloped, tender
Nervous control	Good attention span for age, does not cry easily, not irritable or restless	Inattentive, irritable
Gastrointestinal function	Good appetite and normal digestion, regular elimination	Anorexia, indigestion, constipation or diarrhea
General vitality	Endurance, energetic, sleeps well at night, vigorous	Easily fatigued, no energy, falls asleep in school, appears tired, apathetic

smooth, and the eyes are clear and bright. Appetite, digestion, and elimination are normal. Characteristics of good and poor nutritional status are listed in Table 1-1. Think about these signs and begin to look for them so you become a more skilled observer. Well-nourished persons are more likely to be alert, both mentally and physically. They not only meet their day-to-day needs, but they also maintain appropriate nutrient stores to resist disease and support body function in periods of stress.

Undernutrition

Undernutrition may take various forms ranging from marginal nutritional status to the famine victim with kwashiorkor or marasmus. Persons with *marginal nutritional status* are meeting their minimal day-to-day nutritional needs but lack the nutrient reserves to cope with any added physiologic or metabolic demand arising from injury or illness, the need to sustain a healthy pregnancy, or a childhood growth spurt. Marginal nutritional status results from poor eating habits, stressful environments, or insufficient resources to obtain appropriate types or amounts of food. Meals at fast-food restaurants, a matter of convenience for families with busy lifestyles, are associated with increased intakes of fat; reduced intakes of calcium, vitamins A and C, and fiber; and reduced intakes of vegetables.[25-26] Three food categories—(1) candy and baked desserts such as cakes and cookies, (2) soft drinks and sports drinks, and (3) alcoholic beverages—provide 21% of the kcalories in the diets of Americans but contain little or no protein, vitamins, or minerals.[27] Many of these kcalories come from added sugar, which, in the average person, accounts for 377 kcal per day.[28] Pastries and baked goods, candy, and

KEY TERMS

amino acid An acid containing the essential element nitrogen in the chemical group NH_2. Amino acids are the structural units of protein and the building blocks of body tissue.

synthesize The action of forming new compounds in the body for use in building tissues or carrying out metabolic or physiologic functions.

metabolites Any substance produced by metabolism or by a metabolic process.

anthropometric Measurement of the human body to determine height, weight, skinfold thickness, or other dimensions that can estimate the relative proportion of body fat and body muscle; such measurements are used to evaluate health status and chronic disease risk.

carbonated and other sweetened beverages are replacing nutrient-dense foods such as fruits, vegetables, whole-grain breads and cereals, and milk. Individuals with increased intakes of sugar have reduced intakes of vitamins and minerals.[29]

Public health nutritionists describe the American diet as energy rich but nutrient poor. Although persons with less-than-optimal intakes of micronutrients may not be undernourished, they are at greater risk of physical illness than those who are well nourished. The body can adapt to marginal nutrient intake, but any added physiologic stress that calls on nutrient reserves will lead to overt malnutrition.

Overt Malnutrition

When nutrient intake is not sufficient to meet day-to-day needs and nutrient reserves are depleted, signs of malnutrition begin to appear. Individuals and families with incomes below the poverty threshold often have diets lacking in both food quantity and quality. Approximately 12% of U.S. households (13.5 million) report some level of food insecurity.[30] Single-parent families, families with incomes below the poverty line, and African-American and Hispanic families are most at risk. Even if energy needs are met, foods high in micronutrients—fruits, vegetables, and whole grains—may not be accessible to limited-resource families based on the amount of food money available[31] or location of food outlets offering healthy food options.[32]

Hunger influences health among all ages and genders, but the most vulnerable are infants, children, pregnant women, and older adults. Prenatal care for women who are poor, young, or lack education is often inadequate, leading to poor pregnancy outcomes. Toddlers from families that are food insecure are more likely to have only fair or poor health, have greater risk of hospitalization for health problems, or show deficits in cognitive development compared with those from families that have an adequate food supply.[33] Children with chronically inadequate diets develop anemia, with reduced resistance to infection and impaired learning ability, and have low energy levels. Food pantries serving homeless and limited-resource families are often low in supplies of nutrient-dense items such as dairy foods, fruits, and vegetables.[34-35]

Malnutrition also exists among hospitalized patients and residents of long-term care facilities. Hypermetabolic diseases or prolonged illnesses in older persons lead to nutrient depletion and debilitating weight loss.[36] Both prescription and over-the-counter medications have adverse effects on nutritional status.

Overnutrition

Overnutrition can take various forms. Excessive energy intake coupled with low physical activity leads to unwanted weight gain. In contrast to colonial times when a portly appearance was a sign of prosperity, overweight and obesity are recognized as health risks that set the stage for development of type 2 diabetes and cardiovascular disease.[37] Overnutrition also occurs with excessive intakes of micronutrients. Inappropriate amounts of vitamin or mineral supplements can damage tissues and interfere with the absorption and metabolism of other essential nutrients. Herbal preparations, growing in popularity, carry the potential for harmful interactions with nutrients or medications.

NUTRITION POLICY AND NATIONAL HEALTH PROBLEMS

Diet, Health, and Public Policy

Public policy refers to the laws, regulations, and government programs pertaining to a certain topic. Nutrition policies are concerned with food guidance for the public, nutrition standards for government food programs, and the health and well-being of our population. In recent years, nutrition policy has focused on obesity and how we can reduce chronic disease. In future chapters, we will discuss food safety laws and nutrition labeling—other examples of public policy. As a health professional, you should stay informed and actively participate in public policy discussions that will influence services and resources for the populations you serve.

Development of Nutrition Policy

Until the mid-1900s, government policies and programs were intended to eradicate hunger and malnutrition. Deficiency diseases such as rickets and pellagra still existed in various parts of the United States, and a law passed in the 1930s mandated the addition of vitamin D to milk as a measure against rickets. The enrichment of grains with thiamin, riboflavin, niacin, and iron began sometime later to address the issues of pellagra and anemia. The development of the School Nutrition Program with policies for free or reduced-cost lunches responded to existing hunger among children and adolescents. By the 1980s, however, the focus had shifted to overnutrition as new research linked dietary habits to the growing prevalence of cardiovascular disease. Congressional committees began to discuss the role of government in setting dietary guidelines to improve health.

The first major policy report issued by the U.S. government linking nutrition and chronic disease was the *Surgeon General's Report on Nutrition and Health*[38] released in 1988. This report established the connection between the typical American diet high in fat and salt and both morbidity and early death from cardiovascular disease. The American people were urged to cut down on foods high in fat and salt and increase foods high in complex carbohydrates and fiber. In 1989 the Food and Nutrition Board of the Institute of Medicine issued its extensive report, *Diet and Health: Implications for Reducing Chronic Disease Risk.*[39] The report's dietary recommendations agreed with those of the Surgeon General and advised persons to (1) reduce total fat to 30% or less of total kcalories, (2) reduce saturated fat and cholesterol, (3) increase fiber and complex carbohydrates, (4) avoid excessive sodium and protein, and (5) maintain appropriate levels of calcium.

Healthy People 2020

In 1990 the U.S. Department of Health and Human Services (USDHHS) introduced the public health initiative *Healthy People 2000* that established science-based, national objectives for promoting health and preventing disease.[40] These objectives are updated every 10 years using a process that allows for input by both health professionals and consumers. The *Healthy People 2020* program now in development will focus on risks to health and wellness and prevention of chronic disease It will likely include goals relating to food intake, nutrition, physical activity, and weight management.[41–42]

NUTRITION GUIDES FOR FOOD SELECTION

For the last 100 years the government has been issuing food guides to help Americans meet their nutritional needs. The underlying assumptions in developing these guides were influenced by the growing body of nutrition science, as well as social, political, and economic events, including wars and national emergencies. Over time the focus of these guides also shifted from preventing undernutrition to controlling chronic diseases related to overnutrition. These guides are of three types: (1) nutrition standards, (2) dietary guidelines, and (3) food guides. Each has a different purpose and target audience.

Nutrition Standards

Dietary Reference Intakes

Most countries have standards for nutrient intakes of healthy persons according to age and gender. Professionals use these standards in making decisions about the nutritional health of individuals and groups. In the United States, these nutrient and energy standards are called the Dietary Reference Intakes (DRIs) and include several categories of recommendations.[43]

Each category within the DRIs is useful to the health professional:

- The Recommended Dietary Allowance (RDA) serves as an intake goal for all healthy people; RDAs have been set for protein and most vitamins and minerals.
- The Adequate Intake (AI) provides a dietary goal when research suggests a particular health benefit resulting from a certain intake. The current AIs for calcium and vitamin D were developed to support bone health.
- The Tolerable Upper Intake Level (UL) is an important guide for advising individuals on the use of dietary supplements.
- The Estimated Average Requirement (EAR) is used by nutrition researchers to evaluate the nutrient intakes of population groups.
- The Acceptable Macronutrient Distribution Range (AMDR) guides the division of kcalories among carbohydrate, fat, and protein in ranges supportive of health.

The DRIs for vitamins, minerals, and macronutrients are found on the inside front cover and first pages of this text. Note the two age categories for individuals over age 50, directing our attention to the changes in nutrient requirements as we age.

The first set of DRIs released in 1997 provided new standards for calcium, phosphorus, magnesium, and vitamin D and emphasized the role of these nutrients in bone health.[44] Since then, DRIs have been established for the B-complex vitamins (1998)[45]; antioxidant nutrients and carotenoids (2000)[46]; vitamins A and K and the trace minerals (2001)[47]; energy, the energy-yielding macronutrients, and fiber (2002)[22]; and electrolytes and water (2004).[48]

The nutrient standards of Canada and Great Britain are similar to those of the United States. Developing countries use standards set by the Food and Agriculture Organization (FAO) of the World Health Organization (WHO).

Dietary Guidelines

Dietary guidelines are the second type of nutrition guide. Dietary guidelines are intended for use by policymakers, health professionals, and nutrition educators and provide food guidance for healthy Americans 2 years of age and older. The Dietary Guidelines for Americans forms the basis for federal nutrition policy and nutrition education and gives direction to government programs involving food and nutrition, such as Head Start, school meals, and nutrition programs for older adults. The Dietary Guidelines are evidence-based, building on the most current scientific and medical research relating to nutrient requirements, public health, and the nutritional

KEY TERMS

anemia A condition of abnormally low blood hemoglobin level caused by too few red blood cells or red blood cells with low hemoglobin content.

Dietary Reference Intakes (DRIs) The framework of nutrient standards now in place in the United States that provide reference values for use in planning and evaluating diets for healthy people. The DRIs include the Recommended Dietary Allowance, the Adequate Intake, the Tolerable Upper Intake Level, and the Estimated Average Requirement.

Recommended Dietary Allowance (RDA) The average daily intake of a nutrient that will meet the requirement of nearly all (97% to 98%) healthy people of a given age and gender. RDAs were established and are reviewed periodically by an expert panel of nutrition scientists and based on new research findings are amended as needed. When planning diets, aiming for this level of intake is best.

Adequate Intake (AI) A suggested daily intake of a nutrient to meet body needs and support health that is used when available research is insufficient to develop an RDA. The AI serves as a guide for intake when planning diets.

Tolerable Upper Intake Level (UL) The highest amount of a nutrient that can be consumed safely with no risk of toxicity or adverse effects on health. The UL is used to evaluate dietary supplements or review total nutrient intake from food and supplements. Intakes exceeding the UL usually result from concentrated supplements, not food.

Estimated Average Requirement (EAR) The average daily intake of a nutrient that will meet the requirement of 50% of healthy people of a given age and gender. The EAR is used to plan and evaluate the nutrient intakes of groups rather than individuals.

Acceptable Macronutrient Distribution Range (AMDR) The suggested proportional distribution of kcalories across the macronutrients; carbohydrate should provide 45% to 65% of total kcalories, fat should provide 20% to 35% of total kcalories, and protein should provide 10% to 35% of total kcalories.

EVIDENCE-BASED PRACTICE: HOW DO I USE IT?

As a health professional, what information will you use to develop a plan of action for your patient or client? What you have learned in your clinical rotation? What has been the long-term protocol in your facility? What you have learned in your beginning nutrition class? Over time, new evidence becomes available and new practice standards are developed—how do you avoid being left behind?

The new paradigm in health care is evidence-based practice—making your decisions regarding patient care or appropriate community interventions based on current research and published findings. Successful evidence-based practice requires that you read the latest journals, keep up to date on practice standards, carry out planned protocols to evaluate methods of treatment, and share your treatment outcomes with others.

Evidence-based practice follows a five-step process, as follows:

- Develop the question that you need to answer.
- Search for studies in your professional journals that address this question.
- Evaluate the studies you find: How many patients or clients participated? What was the time period? What types of information did they collect? Were their participants and circumstances similar to yours?
- If studies are valid and treatment is acceptable, apply the recommendations in your practice.
- Assess the outcome: Was the treatment successful or not? Can you share this information with others at a local or state professional meeting?

Nutrition and medical experts have developed evaluation systems for grading research evidence according to its validity. Evidence may be rated as good, fair, limited, or supported only by opinion. These rating scales are being used in review articles published in professional journals and on reputable websites maintained by government agencies and professional societies. The article by Van Horn and colleagues published in the *Journal of the American Dietetic Association* and given in the references below uses the evidence-based approach for evaluating strategies to prevent and treat cardiovascular disease.

Visit the websites of the National Institutes of Health, Office of Dietary Supplements, at http://dietary-supplements.info.nih.gov/Health_Information/Botanical_Supplements.aspx and the Agency for Healthcare Research and Quality at http://ftp.ahrq.gov/clinic/epcquick.htm for other examples of evidence-based evaluations.

Begin to look for these evaluations and use them in your decision-making process.

BIBLIOGRAPHY

Gray GE, Gray LK, et al: Evidence-based medicine: applications in dietetic practice, *J Am Diet Assoc* 102:1263, 2002.

Laramee SH: Evidence-based practice: a core competency for dietetics, *J Am Diet Assoc* 105:333, 2005.

Vaughan LA, Manning CK: Meeting the challenges of dietetic practice with evidence-based decisions, *J Am Diet Assoc* 104:282, 2004.

Van Horn L, McCoin M, Kris-Etherton PM, et al: The evidence for dietary prevention and treatment of cardiovascular disease, *J Am Diet Assoc* 108:287, 2008.

status of the U.S. population. (See the *Evidence-Based Practice* box, "How Do I Use It?" to learn more about this concept.)

First published in 1980, the *Dietary Guidelines for Americans* reflects the growing health concerns of government agencies, health care providers, and professional groups. By law the *Guidelines* are updated every 5 years and represent a cooperative effort between the USDHHS, the federal agency concerned with health, and the U.S. Department of Agriculture (USDA), the federal agency concerned with food. An advisory panel of experts is appointed and charged with the responsibility of reviewing the current guidelines and identifying changes that are needed or new issues to be addressed.

HEALTH PROMOTION

Dietary Guidelines for Americans 2010

The report prepared by the 2010 Dietary Guidelines Advisory Committee (DGAC) differs from previous reports in two major ways: (1) it is directed toward a U.S. population that is now markedly overweight or obese yet lacking in various important nutrients, and (2) it focuses attention on the total diet and the practical and environmental issues that influence the successful implementation of dietary recommendations.[49-51] Based on the scientific literature available to them in the USDA Nutrition Evidence Library, the DGAC developed several broad recommendations that will form the basis for a new set of Dietary Guidelines to guide federal food programs and policies over the next 5 years. These recommendations are as follows:

- Reduce the incidence and prevalence of overweight and obesity by reducing overall calorie intake and increasing physical activity.
- Move toward a more plant-based diet that emphasizes vegetables, cooked dry peas and beans, fruits, whole grains, and nuts and seeds; increase the use of seafood and fat-free or low-fat milk products with only moderate use of lean meat, poultry, and eggs.
- Reduce the use of foods with added sugars, fat, and sodium, and especially refined grains with high levels of these ingredients.
- Meet the 2008 Physical Activity Guidelines for Americans.

The DGAC emphasizes the need to help youth and families develop skills for preparing and eating healthy meals at home and the need for financial support to help families with limited resources purchase healthy food. School programs, restaurants, and other food service organizations must be enlisted in the effort to provide appropriate amounts and types of food. Farmers must be assisted in developing environmentally sustainable production of fruit, vegetables, and whole grains.

The current *Dietary Guidelines for Americans* released in 2005 (Box 1-3) emphasize (1) smart choices from every food group, (2) a balance between food and activity, and (3) getting the most nutrition from calories.[52] They give helpful advice for choosing foods rich in important nutrients

BOX 1-3 2005 DIETARY GUIDELINES FOR AMERICANS—KEY RECOMMENDATIONS

Adequate Nutrients Within Calorie Needs

- Consume a variety of nutrient-dense foods and beverages within and among the basic food groups while choosing foods that limit the intake of saturated and *trans* fats, cholesterol, added sugars, salt, and alcohol.
- Meet recommended intakes within energy needs by adopting a balanced eating pattern, such as the USDA Food Guide (MyPyramid) or the Dietary Approaches to Stop Hypertension (DASH) Eating Plan.

Recommendations for Specific Population Groups

- *People over age 50.* Consume vitamin B_{12} in its crystalline form (i.e., fortified foods or supplements).
- *Women of child-bearing age who may become pregnant.* Eat foods high in heme-iron and/or consume iron-rich plant foods or iron-fortified foods with an enhancer of iron absorption, such as vitamin C–rich foods.
- *Women of child-bearing age who may become pregnant and those in the first trimester of pregnancy.* Consume adequate synthetic folic acid daily (from fortified food or supplements) in addition to food forms of folate from a varied diet.
- *Older adults, people with dark skin, and people exposed to insufficient ultraband radiation (i.e., sunlight).* Consume extra vitamin D from vitamin D–fortified foods and/or supplements.

Weight Management

- To maintain body weight in a healthy range, balance calories from foods and beverages with calories expended.
- To prevent gradual weight gain over time, make small decreases in food and beverage calories and increase physical activity.

Recommendations for Specific Population Groups

- *Persons who need to lose weight.* Aim for a slow, steady weight loss by decreasing calorie intake while maintaining an adequate nutrient intake and increasing physical activity.
- *Overweight children.* Reduce the rate of body weight gain while allowing growth and development. Consult a health care provider before placing a child on a weight-reduction diet.
- *Pregnant women.* Ensure appropriate weight gain as specified by a health care provider.
- *Breastfeeding women.* Moderate weight reduction is safe and does not compromise weight gain of the nursing infant.
- *Overweight adults and overweight children with chronic diseases and/or medication.* Consult a health care provider about weight loss strategies before starting a weight-reduction program to ensure appropriate management of other health conditions.

Physical Activity

- Engage in regular physical activity and reduce sedentary activities to promote health, psychological well-being, and a healthy body weight.
- To reduce the risk of chronic disease in adulthood, engage in at least 30 minutes of moderate-intensity physical activity, above the usual activity, at work or home on most days of the week.
- For most people, increased health benefits can be obtained by engaging in physical activity of more vigorous intensity or extended duration.
- To help manage body weight and prevent gradual, unhealthy body weight gain in adulthood, engage in approximately 60 minutes of moderate- to vigorous-intensity activity on most days of the week while not exceeding caloric intake requirements.
- To sustain weight loss in adulthood, participate in at least 60 to 90 minutes of daily moderate-intensity physical activity while not exceeding caloric intake requirements. Some people may need to consult with a health care provider before participating in this level of activity.
- Achieve physical fitness by including cardiovascular conditioning, stretching exercises for flexibility, and resistance exercises or calisthenics for muscle strength and endurance.

Recommendations for Specific Population Groups

- *Children and adolescents.* Engage in at least 60 minutes of physical activity on most, preferably all, days of the week.
- *Pregnant women.* In the absence of medical or obstetric complications, incorporate 30 minutes or more of moderate-intensity physical activity on most, if not all, days of the week. Avoid activities with a high risk of falling or abdominal trauma.
- *Breastfeeding women.* Be aware that neither acute nor regular exercise adversely affects the mother's ability to breastfeed successfully.
- *Older adults.* Participate in regular physical activity to reduce functional declines associated with aging and to achieve the other benefits of physical activity identified for all adults.

Food Groups to Encourage

- Consume a sufficient amount of fruits and vegetables while staying within energy needs. Two cups of fruit and 2½ cups of vegetables per day are recommended for a reference 2000-calorie intake, with higher or lower amounts depending on the calorie level.
- Choose a variety of fruits and vegetables each day. In particular, select from all five vegetable subgroups (dark-green, orange, legumes, starchy vegetables, and other vegetables) several times a week.
- Consume three or more ounce-equivalents of whole-grain products per day, with the rest of the recommended grains coming from enriched or whole-grain products. In general, at least one half the grains should come from whole grains.
- Consume 3 cups per day of fat-free or low-fat milk or equivalent milk products.

Recommendations for Specific Population Groups

- *Children and adolescents.* Consume whole-grain products often; at least one half the grains should be whole grains. Children 2 to 8 years of age should consume 2 cups per day of fat-free or low-fat milk or equivalent milk products. Children 9 years of age and older should consume 3 cups per day of fat-free or low-fat milk or equivalent milk products.

Fats

- Consume less than 10% of calories from saturated fatty acids and less than 300 mg/day of cholesterol, and keep *trans* fatty acid consumption as low as possible.
- Keep total fat intake between 20% and 35% of calories, with most fats coming from sources of polyunsaturated and monounsaturated fatty acids, such as fish, nuts, and vegetable oils.

Continued

BOX 1-3 2005 DIETARY GUIDELINES FOR AMERICANS—KEY RECOMMENDATIONS—cont'd

- When selecting and preparing meat, poultry, dry beans, and milk or milk products, make choices that are lean, low fat, or fat free.
- Limit intake of fats and oils high in saturated and/or *trans* fatty acids, and choose products low in such fats and oils.

Recommendations for Specific Population Groups

- *Children and adolescents.* Keep total fat intake between 30% and 35% of calories for children 2 to 3 years of age and between 25% and 35% of calories for children and adolescents 4 to 18 years of age, with most fats coming from sources of polyunsaturated and monounsaturated fatty acids such as fish, nuts, and vegetable oils.

Carbohydrates

- Choose fiber-rich fruits, vegetables, and whole grains often.
- Choose and prepare foods and beverages with little added sugars or caloric sweeteners, such as amounts suggested by the USDA Food Guide (MyPyramid) and the DASH Eating Plan.
- Reduce the incidence of dental caries by practicing good oral hygiene and consuming sugar- and starch-containing foods and beverages less frequently.

Sodium and Potassium

- Consume less than 2300 mg of sodium (approximately 1 tsp of salt) per day.
- Choose and prepare foods with little salt. At the same time, consume potassium-rich foods, such as fruits and vegetables.

Recommendations for Specific Population Groups

- *Individuals with hypertension, African Americans, and middle-aged and older adults.* Aim to consume no more than 1500 mg of sodium per day, and meet the potassium recommendation (4700 mg/day) with food.

Alcoholic Beverages

- Persons who choose to drink alcoholic beverages should do so sensibly and in moderation—defined as the consumption of up to one drink per day for women and up to two drinks per day for men.
- Alcoholic beverages should not be consumed by some individuals, including those who cannot restrict their alcohol intake, women of childbearing age who may become pregnant, pregnant and lactating women, children and adolescents, individuals taking medications that can interact with alcohol, and those with specific medical conditions.
- Alcoholic beverages should be avoided by individuals engaging in activities that require attention, skill, or coordination, such as driving or operating machinery.

Food Safety

- To avoid microbial foodborne illness, do the following:
  - Clean hands, food contact surfaces, and fruits and vegetables. Meat and poultry should *not* be washed or rinsed.
  - Separate raw, cooked, and ready-to-eat foods while shopping, preparing, or storing foods.
  - Cook foods to a safe temperature to kill microorganisms.
  - Chill (refrigerate) perishable food promptly, and defrost foods properly.
  - Avoid raw (unpasteurized) milk or any products made from unpasteurized milk, raw or partially cooked eggs or foods containing raw eggs, raw or undercooked meat and poultry, unpasteurized juices, and raw sprouts.

Recommendations for Specific Population Groups

- *Infants and young children, pregnant women, older adults, and persons who are immunocompromised.* Do not eat or drink raw (unpasteurized) milk or any products made from unpasteurized milk, raw or partially cooked eggs, raw or undercooked meat and poultry, raw or undercooked fish or shellfish, unpasteurized juices, and raw sprouts.
- *Pregnant women, older adults, and persons who are immunocompromised.* Only eat certain deli meats and frankfurters that have been reheated to steaming hot.

Note: For detailed information on food selection and food sources of specific nutrients, see the complete *Dietary Guidelines for Americans 2005,* available at *www.health.gov/DietaryGuidelines/.*

From U.S. Department of Health and Human Services, U.S. Department of Agriculture: *Dietary guidelines for Americans 2005,* ed 6, Washington, DC, 2005, U.S. Government Printing Office. See the Evolve website for the 2010 Dietary Guidelines when they become available.

but low in fat and sodium. Older, at-risk women who adhered to these Guidelines slowed the progression of their coronary artery disease.[53] (The 2005 Dietary Guidelines will remain in effect until the 2010 Guidelines are released. See the Evolve website for the new guidelines when they become available.)

Although the *Dietary Guidelines* provide positive goals for food selection, they do not include a daily food pattern that tells consumers the specific items of food they should eat and how much. Offering help with meal planning is the role of the third type of nutrition guide—the food guides.

Food Guides

Food guides are intended to help individuals with day-to-day meal planning. They give a practical interpretation of nutrition standards and dietary guidelines useful in daily food selection. Most food guides group foods based on their nutrient content and recommend a certain number of servings from each group. The most commonly used food group guides are the MyPyramid developed by the USDA and USDHHS and Choose Your Foods: Exchange List for Diabetes from the American Diabetes Association and the American Dietetic Association. These guides group foods differently and serve different needs.

USDA Food Guides

The USDA issued its first food guide in the 1940s, and, over time, food guides evolved to various shapes and formats. MyPyramid: Steps to a Healthier You, the current USDA food guidance system, provides *one-stop shopping* for advice on both food intake and physical activity.[54]

MyPyramid Food Guidance System

MyPyramid promotes a personalized approach to healthy eating and physical activity (Figure 1-4).[55] The pyramid symbol reminds consumers to make healthy food choices and be

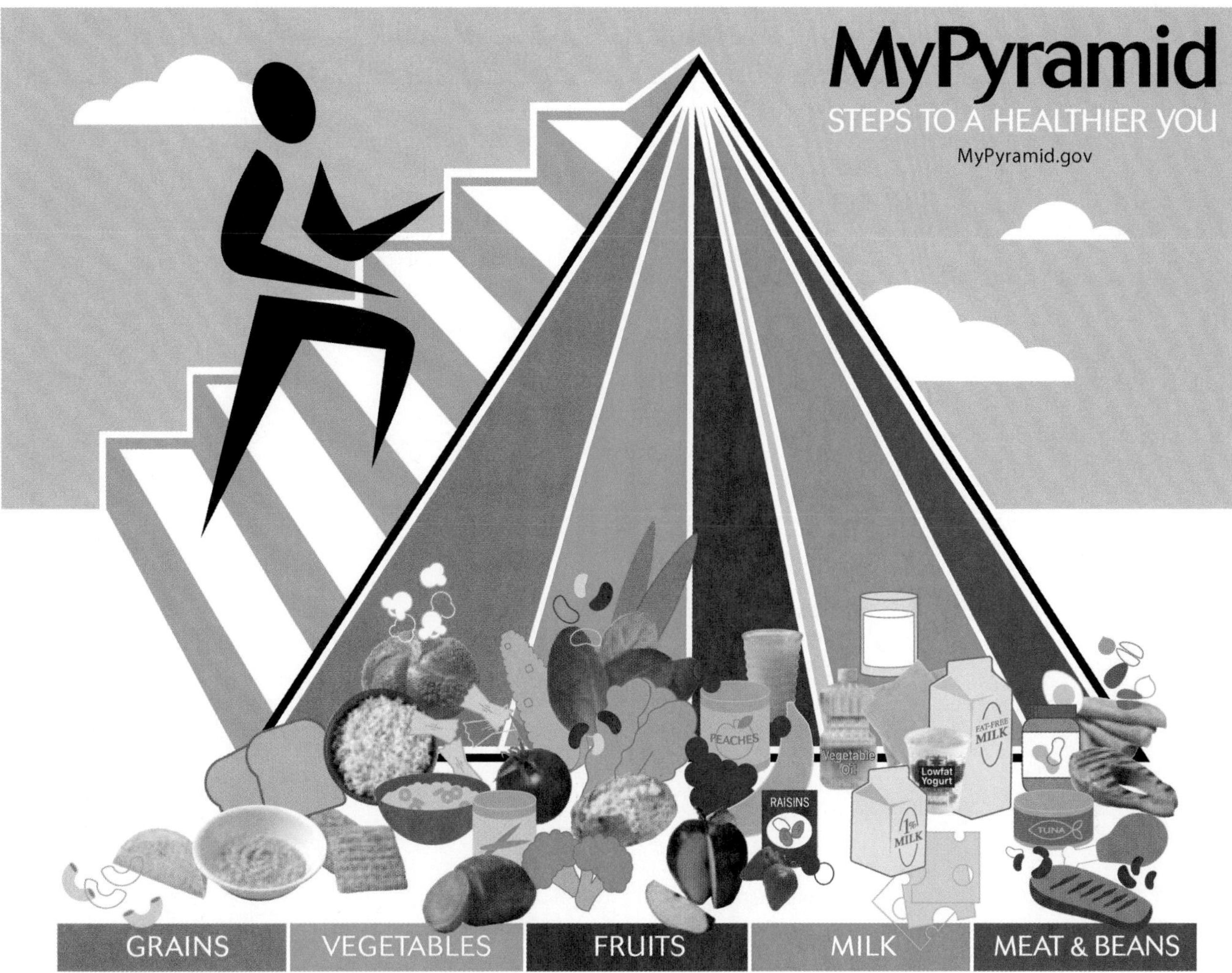

One size doesn't fit all

USDA's new MyPyramid symbolizes a personalized approach to healthy eating and physical activity. The symbol has been designed to be simple. It has been developed to remind consumers to make healthy food choices and to be active every day. The different parts of the symbol are described below.

Activity

Activity is represented by the steps and the person climbing them, as a reminder of the importance of daily physical activity.

Moderation

Moderation is represented by the narrowing of each food group from bottom to top. The wider base stands for foods with little or no solid fats or added sugars. These should be selected more often. The narrower top area stands for foods containing more added sugars and solid fats. The more active you are, the more of these foods can fit into your diet.

Personalization

Personalization is shown by the person on the steps, the slogan, and the URL. Find the kinds and amounts of food to eat each day at MyPyramid.gov.

Proportionality

Proportionality is shown by the different widths of the food group bands. The widths suggest how much food a person should choose from each group. The widths are just a general guide, not exact proportions. Check the Web site for how much is right for you.

Variety

Variety is symbolized by the 6 color bands representing the 5 food groups of the Pyramid and oils. This illustrates that foods from all groups are needed each day for good health.

Gradual Improvement

Gradual improvement is encouraged by the slogan. It suggests that individuals can benefit from taking small steps to improve their diet and lifestyle each day.

FIGURE 1-4 MyPyramid: Steps to a Healthier You. The MyPyramid graphic emphasizes activity, moderation, personalization, proportionality, variety, and gradual improvement. (From Center for Nutrition Policy and Promotion: *MyPyramid food guidance system mini-poster,* Washington, DC, 2005, U.S. Department of Agriculture. Retrieved July 29, 2009, from www.mypyramid.gov/downloads/MiniPoster.pdf.)

TABLE 1-2 MAJOR NUTRIENTS SUPPLIED BY THE MYPYRAMID FOOD GROUPS

FOOD GROUP	MAJOR NUTRIENTS*	SERVING EQUIVALENTS
Fruit group (color code red)	Vitamin C Folate Potassium Fiber	1 cup fruit or 1 cup 100% fruit juice or ½ cup dried fruit equals 1 cup from the fruit group
Vegetable group (color code green)	Vitamin A Vitamin C Vitamin E Vitamin B_6 Folate Potassium Fiber	1 cup raw or cooked vegetables or 1 cup vegetable juice or 2 cups raw leafy greens equal 1 cup from the vegetable group
Grains group (color code orange) Enriched grains	Thiamin Riboflavin Niacin Folate Iron	1 slice of bread, 1 cup ready-to-eat cereal, or ½ cup cooked rice, pasta, or cooked cereal equals 1 oz from the grains group
Whole grains	Zinc, magnesium and fiber in addition to the nutrients in enriched grains	
Meat, poultry, fish, eggs, beans, and nut group (color code purple)	Protein Thiamin Riboflavin Niacin Vitamin B_6 Vitamin B_{12}† Iron Zinc Vitamin E (nuts)	1 oz lean meat, poultry, or fish, 1 egg, 1 tbsp peanut butter, ¼ cup cooked dry beans, or ½ oz nuts or seeds equals 1 oz from the meat and beans group
Milk group (color code blue)	Protein Vitamin A Riboflavin Vitamin B_{12} Calcium Phosphorus Magnesium	1 cup milk, 1 cup yogurt, 1½ oz natural cheese or 2 oz processed cheese equals 1 cup from the milk group
Oils and soft margarine (color code yellow)	Vitamin E Linoleic acid‡ Alpha-linolenic acid	6 tsp

Modified from Dietary Guidelines Advisory Committee, 2005: *Report of the dietary guidelines advisory committee on the dietary guidelines for Americans 2005,* U.S. Department of Agriculture, Agricultural Research Service, Beltsville, Md, 2004 (August).

*Each of the MyPyramid food groups is a major source of the nutrients listed but also adds smaller amounts of other nutrients to the daily diet.

†Vitamin B_{12} is found only in animal foods.

‡Linoleic acid and alpha-linolenic acid are the essential fatty acids that we obtain from dietary fats.

physically active every day. The vertical food bands include grains, vegetables, fruits, milk, oils, and meat and beans. Consumers are reminded to eat servings from different categories of food that supply specific nutrients (Table 1-2), although, for the general public, food should remain the fundamental unit in nutrition.[56]

The MyPyramid interactive website[55] gives access to daily food plans ranging from 1000 kcal to 3200 kcal, intended for individuals age 2 and older (Table 1-3). Persons can view both the types and amounts of food needed for their age, gender, and activity level. Figure 1-5 displays the reference food intake pattern containing 2000 kcal. Attractive nutrition aids offer help with choices within each food group, learning to *vary your veggies,* and tracking the number of kcalories you eat each day. Each food plan defines the number of discretionary calories that can be used for solid fats, added sugars, alcohol, or added servings from any food group. However, for sedentary persons, discretionary calories are quite limited. Note that the 2000-kcal food plan allows only 267 discretionary calories—the equivalent of two chocolate chip cookies. The MyPyramid website has become an enormously popular resource for the public, registering over 600 million hits in its first 3 months of operation[57] and 5.7 billion hits since then.[58]

TABLE 1-3 MYPYRAMID FOOD INTAKE PATTERNS FOR DIFFERENT KCALORIE LEVELS

Daily Amount of Food from Each Group

CALORIE LEVEL[1]	1000	1200	1400	1600	1800	2000	2200	2400	2600	2800	3000	3200
Fruits[2]	1 cup	1 cup	1½cups	1½ cups	1½ cups	2 cups	2 cups	2 cups	2 cups	2½ cups	2½ cups	2½ cups
Vegetables[3]	1 cup	1½ cups	1½ cups	2 cups	2½ cups	2½ cups	3 cups	3 cups	3½ cups	3½ cups	4 cups	4 cups
Grains[4]	3 oz-eq	4 oz-eq	5 oz-eq	5 oz-eq	6 oz-eq	6 oz-eq	7 oz-eq	8 oz-eq	9 oz-eq	10 oz-eq	10 oz-eq	10 oz-eq
Whole grains	1.5	2	2.5	3	3	3	3.5	4	4.5	5	5	5
Other grains	1.5	2	2.5	2	3	3	3.5	4	4.5	5	5	5
Meat and beans[5]	2 oz-eq	3 oz-eq	4 oz-eq	5 oz-eq	5 oz-eq	5½ oz-eq	6 oz-eq	6½ oz-eq	6½ oz-eq	7 oz-eq	7 oz-eq	7 oz-eq
Milk[6]	2 cups	2 cups	2 cups	3 cups	3 cups	3 cups	3 cups	3 cups	3 cups	3 cups	3 cups	3 cups
Oil[7]	3 tsp	4 tsp	4 tsp	5 tsp	5 tsp	6 tsp	6 tsp	7 tsp	8 tsp	8 tsp	10 tsp	11 tsp
Discretionary calorie allowance[8]	165	171	171	132	195	267	290	362	410	426	512	648

1. **Calorie Levels** are set across a wide range to accommodate the needs of different individuals. Another table found on the MyPyramid website "Estimated Daily Calorie Needs," can be used to help assign individuals to a particular calorie level.
2. **Fruit Group** includes all fresh, frozen, canned, and dried fruits and fruit juices: 1 cup of fruit or 100% fruit juice, or ½ cup of dried fruit, can be considered as 1 cup from the fruit group.
3. **Vegetable Group** includes all fresh, frozen, canned, and dried vegetables and vegetable juices: 1 cup of raw or cooked vegetables or vegetable juice, or 2 cups of raw leafy greens, can be considered as 1 cup from the vegetable group.
4. **Grains Group** includes all foods made from wheat, rice, oats, cornmeal, or barley, such as bread, pasta, oatmeal, breakfast cereals, tortillas, and grits: 1 slice of bread, 1 cup of ready-to-eat cereal, or ½ cup of cooked rice, pasta, or cooked cereal can be considered as 1 ounce equivalent from the grains group. **At least one half of all grains consumed should be whole grains.**
5. **Meat and Beans Group** includes meat, poultry, fish, dry beans and peas, eggs, nuts and seeds: 1 ounce of lean meat, poultry, or fish, 1 egg, 1 tbsp peanut butter, ¼ cup cooked dry beans, or ½ ounce of nuts or seeds can be considered as 1 ounce equivalent from the meat and beans group.
6. **Milk Group** includes all fluid milk products and foods made from milk that retain their calcium content, such as yogurt and cheese. Foods made from milk that have little to no calcium, such as cream cheese, cream, and butter, are not part of the group. Most milk group choices should be fat free or low fat: 1 cup of milk or yogurt, 1½ ounces of natural cheese, or 2 ounces of processed cheese can be considered as 1 cup from the milk group.
7. **Oils** include fats from many different plants and from fish that are liquid at room temperature, such as canola, corn, olive, soybean, and sunflower oil. Some foods are naturally high in oils, such as nuts, olives, some fish, and avocados. Foods that are mainly oil include mayonnaise, certain salad dressings, and soft margarine.
8. **Discretionary Calorie Allowance** is the remaining amount of calories in a food intake pattern after accounting for the calories needed for all food groups—using forms of foods that are fat free or low fat and with no added sugars.

From Center for Nutrition Policy and Promotion: *MyPyramid food intake patterns,* Washington, DC, 2005, U.S. Department of Agriculture. Retrieved July 30, 2009, from *www.mypyramid.gov/downloads/MyPyramid_Food_Intake_Patterns.pdf.*
oz-eq, Ounce-equivalents.

GRAINS Make half your grains whole	VEGETABLES Vary your veggies	FRUITS Focus on fruits	MILK Get your calcium-rich foods	MEAT & BEANS Go lean with protein
Eat at least 3 oz. of whole-grain cereals, breads, crackers, rice, or pasta every day 1 oz. is about 1 slice of bread, about 1 cup of breakfast cereal, or ½ cup of cooked rice, cereal, or pasta	Eat more dark-green veggies like broccoli, spinach, and other dark leafy greens Eat more orange vegetables like carrots and sweetpotatoes Eat more dry beans and peas like pinto beans, kidney beans, and lentils	Eat a variety of fruit Choose fresh, frozen, canned, or dried fruit Go easy on fruit juices	Go low-fat or fat-free when you choose milk, yogurt, and other milk products If you don't or can't consume milk, choose lactose-free products or other calcium sources such as fortified foods and beverages	Choose low-fat or lean meats and poultry Bake it, broil it, or grill it Vary your protein routine – choose more fish, beans, peas, nuts, and seeds
For a 2,000-calorie diet, you need the amounts below from each food group. To find the amounts that are right for you, go to MyPyramid.gov.				
Eat 6 oz. every day	Eat 2½ cups every day	Eat 2 cups every day	Get 3 cups every day; for kids aged 2 to 8, it's 2	Eat 5½ oz. every day

Find your balance between food and physical activity

- Be sure to stay within your daily calorie needs.
- Be physically active for at least 30 minutes most days of the week.
- About 60 minutes a day of physical activity may be needed to prevent weight gain.
- For sustaining weight loss, at least 60 to 90 minutes a day of physical activity may be required.
- Children and teenagers should be physically active for 60 minutes every day, or most days.

Know the limits on fats, sugars, and salt (sodium)

- Make most of your fat sources from fish, nuts, and vegetable oils.
- Limit solid fats like butter, stick margarine, shortening, and lard, as well as foods that contain these.
- Check the Nutrition Facts label to keep saturated fats, *trans* fats, and sodium low.
- Choose food and beverages low in added sugars. Added sugars contribute calories with few, if any, nutrients.

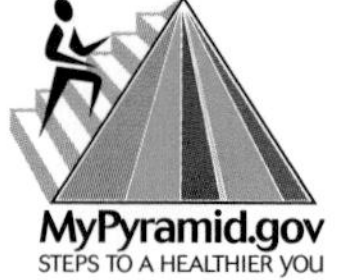

U.S. Department of Agriculture
Center for Nutrition Policy and Promotion
April 2005
CNPP-15

USDA is an equal opportunity provider and employer.

FIGURE 1-5 MyPyramid food intake pattern for a 2000-kcal diet. Consumers can access a food intake pattern based on their age, gender, and level of physical activity to assist them in daily food selection. (From Center for Nutrition Policy and Promotion: *MyPyramid food guidance system mini-poster,* Washington, DC, 2005, U.S. Department of Agriculture. Retrieved July 29, 2009, from www.mypyramid.gov/downloads/MiniPoster.pdf.)

Although MyPyramid is not intended to provide a therapeutic diet for any specific health condition, it is remarkably consistent with the Dietary Approaches to Stop Hypertension (DASH) diet pattern proposed by the National Heart, Lung and Blood Institute and the food patterns proposed by the American Heart Association and the American Cancer Society. However, individuals must select the appropriate kcalorie level and profile of foods within the choices provided to be compliant with these patterns.[59] We will explore the *MyPyramid for Kids* in Chapter 12.

Successful implementation of any food and activity plan requires an understanding of serving size and physical activity levels, but both concepts are poorly understood by the general public. Consumers often describe a serving size as "what I have on my plate,"[60] and this confusion has contributed to weight gain across all age groups.[61] MyPyramid gives food amounts in household measures and illustrations of various serving sizes. Advice is also offered on how to divide the ingredients of mixed dishes such as pizza into the appropriate food group portions. Consumers might be encouraged to measure their food servings for several meals at home to establish what standard serving sizes look like. Figure 1-6 presents a simple tool that can be carried in a wallet or school pack to help with serving size.

Estimating activity level—sedentary, low active, or active—is also difficult, given that most of us think we are more physically active than we really are. MyPyramid provides definitions and offers suggestions for increasing physical activity to at least 30 minutes on most days. As we see in Figure 1-5, 60 minutes of daily physical activity may be needed to prevent weight gain and more than 60 minutes daily to sustain weight loss. When using MyPyramid, think about the stepwise progression found on the graphic. *Steps to a Healthier You* supports the idea of small changes over time that will accumulate and positively affect health.

Despite the efforts of health and nutrition professionals to develop nutrition programs to assist individuals in planning their meals and snacks, intakes of healthy foods such as fruit and vegetables still fall far below optimal levels. Nutrition messages that are easy to understand, tailored to specific

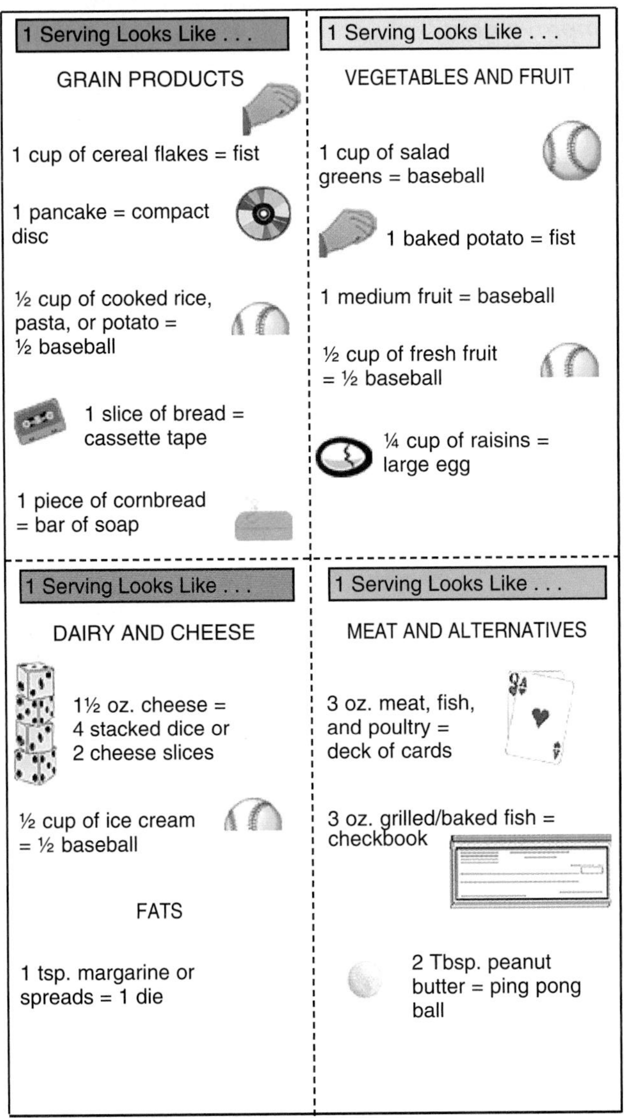

FIGURE 1-6 Serving size card. This pocket-sized guide can be useful when choosing serving sizes at home and away from home. (From U.S. Department of Health and Human Services, National Institutes of Health, National Heart, Lung and Blood Institute, Obesity Education Initiative: *Keep an eye on portion size,* Bethesda, Md, 2004, U.S. Department of Health and Human Services. Retrieved July 29, 2009, from http://hp2010.nhlbihin.net/portion/servingcard7.pdf.)

audiences, and make use of existing technology require the combined efforts of behavioral and communication experts working side by side with nutrition scientists. Government agencies and nutrition educators must join forces to produce practical materials in formats and languages appropriate to all segments of our society.[62–63]

Exchange Lists for Meal Planning

The *Exchange Lists for Meal Planning* was introduced in 1950 by the American Diabetes Association and the American Dietetic Association as a meal-planning tool for persons with diabetes. The *Exchange Lists* group foods based on macronutrient content and equivalent energy values, making this tool useful for planning any diet in which control of carbohydrate, fat, protein, and total kcalories is the goal. Because the foods in each list are equal to one another when eaten in the portions indicated, items can be freely interchanged within each list, and food values and kcalories remain constant. The freedom to exchange within groups promotes increased variety and satisfaction with meals and snacks.

The most recent edition of the *Choose Your Foods: Exchange List for Diabetes* is found in Appendix B.[64] Foods are arranged into the following three groups:

1. *Carbohydrates:* includes starches (grains, starchy vegetables, crackers, snacks, and legumes), fruits, milk, sweets, and nonstarchy vegetables
2. *Meat and meat substitutes:* includes animal protein foods arranged by fat content (lean, medium fat, and high fat) and plant-based proteins
3. *Fats:* includes both animal and plant fats arranged by degree of saturation—unsaturated (monounsaturated and polyunsaturated) and saturated

Serving sizes and macronutrient content for combination foods, fast foods, and free foods are also provided. Use of the *Exchange Lists* in helping persons with diabetes plan their carbohydrate intake is discussed in Chapter 22.

A SAFE AND HEALTHY FOOD SUPPLY

Prevalence and Causes of Foodborne Illness

When planning your nutrient intake, an equally important issue is the safety of the food that supplies those nutrients. Contamination can occur at any point as a food travels from the farm to the processor to the marketplace or food service worker and finally to the consumer, but it does not end there. How we store, prepare, or reheat food items after they enter our home also presents opportunities for food spoilage and foodborne illness. Between 250 million and 350 million Americans suffer acute gastroenteritis each year, and 25% to 30% are believed to result from foodborne illness.[65] Although most healthy individuals recover after a few hours or days of distress, 5000 people die. Foodborne illness within a household often goes unreported, whereas outbreaks involving large numbers of people within a community or related to a national supplier are highly publicized. Traditionally, protein foods—meat, milk, poultry, and eggs—were most likely the source of foodborne illness, and food safety education emphasized appropriate cooking and storage of these items. In recent years, however, national outbreaks of foodborne illness have been traced to bottled water, fruit, and salad greens, with contamination relating to processing and agricultural practices.

Groups particularly vulnerable to foodborne illness are elderly adults, children (especially those under the age of 5), pregnant women, and patients with compromised immune function as related to acquired immunodeficiency syndrome or cancer. Nursing homes and long-term care facilities; food programs in day care centers, schools, and senior centers; and meal delivery programs to homebound elderly persons must be especially vigilant.

Perspective on Food Safety

The goal of a safe food supply goes beyond the control of microorganisms that cause foodborne illness. Appropriate use of pesticides, the testing of genetically modified plants, the evaluation and approval of food additives before their use in human or animal foods, and the on-going monitoring of imported foods all play a role in ensuring the overall safety of the food we eat. In our study of foods and nutrition we will address the need for food inspection and safety education and the government agencies responsible for their implementation.

ASSESSING FOOD PATTERNS

Personal Perceptions of Food

Each of us develops ways of eating based on our ethnic background, cultural or religious beliefs, family habits, socioeconomic status, health status, geographic location, and personal likes and dislikes. However, the growing ethnic and cultural diversity in our society has brought about a greater intermingling of foods and ideas about food. How people perceive themselves in relation to food and food patterns also plays a role in their attitudes toward food and personal eating behavior.

A simple way to get an idea of your own food pattern (or that of a patient or client) is to look at what you actually eat. (See the *Perspectives in Practice* box, "My Personal Food Patterns—Do They Need Improvement?" for directions on keeping a food record.) Keeping a record of everything you eat and drink for a day noting the time, place, any related activity, and people with you gives insight to your true relationship with food. Most of us eat by habit, according to where we are and what is available, rather than by serious thought or plan. Evaluating food and beverage intake using the MyPyramid plan for the appropriate kcalorie intake increases awareness of personal food patterns and provides a rapid dietary assessment of those we counsel in community or health care settings.

PERSPECTIVES IN PRACTICE

My Personal Food Patterns—Do They Need Improvement?

Before we can help others make healthy food choices, we need to help ourselves. What do you usually eat? Do you eat regular meals or snack most of the time? Do you make an effort to choose nutritious foods or eat mostly whatever is around?

- Keep a detailed record of everything you eat and drink for 3 days: 2 weekdays and 1 weekend day. List the type and amount of food in household measures (e.g., cups or tablespoons), how it was prepared, and brand name, if applicable. Be specific: Was your milk nonfat, 1% fat, 2% fat, or whole? Include butter, margarine, salad dressings, condiments, and additions to coffee or tea.
- What social or emotional factors influenced your food choices? Where and when did you eat? Were you alone or with someone? How did you feel at the time?
- *Using MyPyramid,* compare what you ate with the number of servings and portion sizes recommended for your age, gender, and level of physical activity (see the MyPyramid website at *www.mypyramid.gov*). Did you have too many or too few servings from any of the food groups?
- *Using the Nutritrac software available on the Evolve website that accompanies this book,* evaluate your intakes of the macronutrients and micronutrients. Are your kcalories partitioned appropriately? How do your intakes compare with the DRIs for your age and gender?

Now that you have thought about it, how do you see yourself as an eater? Do you have food behaviors that you should modify to promote good health? Do you feel good about specific categories in which you are meeting current recommendations?

Nutritional Analysis by Nutrients and Energy Values

A comprehensive nutritional analysis of food intake is accomplished using a computer-assisted nutrient analysis program, as included on the Evolve website that accompanies this text. A computer-assisted program enables you to evaluate individual vitamins and minerals, specific fats, fiber, and energy as compared to the DRIs. Government agencies use such a nutritional analysis to evaluate dietary information obtained in national surveys and identify nutrition problems among various age, gender, or ethnic groups.

TO SUM UP

The role of nutrition in human health has evolved in response to our changing society and food supply. As the supply of available food increased and the physical activity required in daily living decreased, overweight and obesity emerged as major health problems in the United States and many parts of the world. Discoveries of new substances in food that are beneficial to health have attracted the attention of nutrition experts and food technologists and led to the definition of functional foods. Despite the accessibility of foods rich in vitamins and minerals, many Americans choose a diet high in sugar and fat compromising their nutritional status. Others are chronically undernourished as a result of illness or disease or inadequate resources for purchasing appropriate amounts or types of food, increasing their vulnerability to infection, poor growth, and nutrition-related disease. Resources developed by government scientists are available for use in planning and evaluating the diets of both individuals and population groups. The DRIs intended for use by health professionals provide the foundation for the *Dietary Guidelines for Americans* and MyPyramid that offer practical guidance for meal planning. Together, these materials build a framework for public policy that directs state and federal nutrition programs and health education messages reaching people of all ages.

QUESTIONS FOR REVIEW

1. Visit the U.S. Obesity Trends website of the Centers for Disease Control and Prevention at *www.cdc.gov/obesity/data/trends.html#State* and scroll down to the state maps and overweight/obesity statistics. What is the prevalence of obesity and overweight in your state as compared with the national average? How has it changed over the last 5 to 10 years?
2. What are the two major disciplines that provide the foundation for the study of nutrition? What is the contribution of each discipline toward our understanding of human nutrition needs?
3. What is the difference between the terms *nutrition* and *dietetics?* What are three work-related roles of professionals in human nutrition.
4. What are the differences between the four levels of nutritional status: optimal nutrition, marginal nutrition, malnutrition, and overnutrition? In what community or clinical situations might you expect to find individuals representing each of these conditions and what physical or clinical signs would you use to identify them?
5. What are the six major nutrient groups. What is the primary function of each?
6. What are the various categories within the DRIs. What is the purpose of each?
7. Compare nutrient standards, dietary guidelines, and food guides. What is (a) an example of each now in use, (b) the intended audience (professional or consumer), (c) the type of information included, and (d) a professional situation in which you would use it.
8. Visit the *Healthy People 2020* website at www.healthypeople.gov/. What are five measurable objectives that pertain to nutrition or food intake?
9. Visit your local library and research the food patterns of a cultural or ethnic group different from your own. Using MyPyramid *(www.mypyramid.gov/)*, develop a 1-day menu for a child or adult in that group using foods common to their daily pattern.

REFERENCES

1. Popkin BM: What can public health nutritionists do to curb the epidemic of nutrition-related noncommunicable disease? *Nutr Rev* 67(Suppl 1):S79, 2009.
2. Jeffery RW, Harnack LJ: Evidence implicating eating as a primary driver for the obesity epidemic, *Diabetes* 56:2673, 2007.
3. Ogden CL, Carroll MD, Curtin LR, et al: Prevalence of overweight and obesity in the United States, 1999-2004, *JAMA* 295:1549, 2006.
4. Ogden CL, Carroll MD, Flegal KM: High body mass index for age among US children and adolescents, 2003-2006, *JAMA* 299(20):2401, 2008.
5. Ogden CL, Yanovski SZ, Carroll MD, et al: The epidemiology of obesity, *Gastroenterology* 132:2087, 2007.
6. Ledikwe JH, Ello-Martin JA, Rolls BJ: Portion sizes and the obesity epidemic, *J Nutr* 135:905, 2005.
7. Jeffery RW, Rydell S, Dunn CL, et al: Effect of portion size on chronic energy intake, *Int J Behav Nutr Phys Act* 4:27, 2007.
8. Colapinto CK, Fitzgerald A, Taper LJ, et al: Children's preference for large portions: prevalence, determinants, and consequences, *J Am Diet Assoc* 107:1183, 2007.
9. Federal Interagency Forum on Aging-Related Statistics: *Older Americans 2008: Key indicators of well-being*, Washington, DC, March 2008, U.S. Government Printing Office.
10. United States Bureau of Census: *People, race and ethnicity: The face of our population, annual demographic supplement to the March 2002 Annual Population Survey*, Retrieved January 23, 2009, from http://factfinder.census.gov/jsp/saff/SAFFInfo.jsp?_pageId=tp9_race_ethnicity.
11. Yang EJ, Chung HK, Kim WY, et al: Chronic diseases and dietary changes in relation to Korean Americans' length of residence in the United States, *J Am Diet Assoc* 107:942, 2007.
12. Kumanyika S: Nutrition and chronic disease prevention, *Nutr Rev* 64(2):S9, 2006.
13. Mossavar-Rahmani Y: Applying motivational enhancement to diverse populations, *J Am Diet Assoc* 107:918, 2007.
14. Birt DF: Phytochemicals and cancer prevention: from epidemiology to mechanism of action, *J Am Diet Assoc* 106:20, 2006.
15. Engler MB, Engler MM: The emerging role of flavonoid-rich cocoa and chocolate in cardiovascular health and disease, *Nutr Rev* 64:109, 2006.
16. DeBusk RM, Fogarty CP, Ordovas JM, et al: Nutritional genomics in practice: where do we begin? *J Am Diet Assoc* 105:589, 2005.
17. Boehl T: Emerging science raises questions: What to tell your clients about nutritional genomics, *J Am Diet Assoc* 107:1094, 2007.
18. Ferguson LR: Nutrigenomics approaches to functional foods, *J Am Diet Assoc* 109:452, 2009.
19. Ordovas JM: Nutrigenetics, plasma lipids, and cardiovascular risk, *J Am Diet Assoc* 106:1074, 2006.
20. International Food Information Council Foundation: This for my heart and this for my bones: food conscious consumers are looking beyond basic nutrition. In *Food Insight*, 2007. Retrieved March 7, 2010, from www.foodinsight.org/Portals/0/pdf/novdecfi607.pdf.
21. American Dietetic Association: Position of the American Dietetic Association: the roles of registered dietitians and dietetic technicians, registered, in health promotion and disease prevention, *J Am Diet Assoc* 106:1875, 2006.
22. Food and Nutrition Board, Institute of Medicine: *Dietary Reference Intakes for energy, carbohydrate, fiber, fat, fatty acids, cholesterol, protein, and amino acids, (macronutrients)*, Washington, DC, 2002, National Academies Press.
23. Jacobs DR, Gross MD, Tapsell LC: Food synergy: an operational concept for understanding nutrition, *Am J Clin Nutr* 89(Suppl):1543S, 2009.
24. Mahan LK, Escott-Stump S, editors: *Krause's food and nutrition therapy*, ed 12, St Louis, 2008, Saunders.
25. Paeratakul S, Ferdinand DP, Champagne CM, et al: Fast-food consumption among U.S. adults and children: dietary and nutrient intake profile, *J Am Diet Assoc* 103:1332, 2003.
26. Jeffery RW, Baxter J, McGuire M, et al: Are fast food restaurants an environmental risk factor for obesity? *Int J Behav Nutr Phys Act* 3:2, 2006.

27. Bosire C, Reedy J, Krebs-Smith SM: *Sources of energy and selected nutrient intakes among the U.S. population, 2005-06*, A report prepared for the 2010 Dietary Guidelines Advisory Committee, April 22, 2009, U.S. Department of Health and Human Services, U.S. Department of Agriculture, Retrieved July 29, 2009, from www.cnpp.usda.gov/Publications/DietaryGuidelines/2010/Meeting3/AdditionalResources/Mtg3-SourcesofEnergyandSelectedNutrients.pdf.
28. Duffey KJ, Popkin BM: High-fructose corn syrup. Is this what's for dinner? *Am J Clin Nutr* 88(Suppl):1722S, 2008.
29. Bhargava A, Amialchuk A: Added sugars displaced the use of vital nutrients in the National Food Stamp Program Survey, *J Nutr* 137:453, 2007.
30. American Dietetic Association: Position of the American Dietetic Association: food insecurity and hunger in the United States, *J Am Diet Assoc* 106:446, 2006.
31. Zizza CA, Duffy PA, Gerrior SA: Food insecurity is not associated with lower energy intakes, *Obesity* 16:1908, 2008.
32. Baker EA, Schootman M, Barnidge E, et al: The role of race and poverty in access to foods that enable individuals to adhere to dietary guidelines, *Prev Chronic Dis* 3(3):A76, 2006. [on-line serial]. Retrieved November 21, 2008, from www.cdc.gov/pcd/issues/2006/jul/05_0217.htm.
33. Cook JT, Frank DA, Levenson SM, et al: Child food insecurity increases risks posed by household food insecurity to young children's health, *J Nutr* 136:1073, 2006.
34. Akobundu UO, Cohen NL, Laus MJ, et al: Vitamins A and C, calcium, fruit, and dairy products are limited in food pantries, *J Am Diet Assoc* 104:811, 2004.
35. Algert SJ, Agrawal A, Lewis DS: Disparities in access to fresh produce in low-income neighborhoods in Los Angeles, *Am J Prev Med* 30(5):365, 2006.
36. Morley JE, Thomas DR, Wilson MM: Cachexia: pathophysiology and clinical relevance, *Am J Clin Nutr* 83:735, 2006.
37. Mayer-Davis EJ: Type 2 diabetes in youth: epidemiology and current research toward prevention and treatment, *J Am Diet Assoc* 108:S45, 2008.
38. U.S. Department of Health and Human Services, Public Health Service: *The Surgeon General's report on nutrition and health*, PHS publication No. 88-50210, Washington, DC, 1988, U.S. Government Printing Office.
39. Food and Nutrition Board, Institute of Medicine: *Diet and health: implications for reducing chronic disease risk*, Washington, DC, 1989, National Academies Press.
40. U.S. Department of Health and Human Services, Public Health Service: *Healthy People 2000: national health promotion and disease prevention objectives*, Washington, DC, 1990, U.S. Government Printing Office.
41. U.S. Department of Health and Human Services: *Healthy People 2010: understanding and improving health*, Washington, DC, 2000, U.S. Government Printing Office (for full report, see *www.health.gov/healthypeople/*).
42. Brown DW: The dawn of Healthy People 2020: a brief look back at its beginnings, *Prev Med* 48:94, 2009.
43. Food and Nutrition Board, Institute of Medicine: *Dietary Reference Intakes [DRI]. The essential guide to nutrient requirements*, Washington, DC, 2006, National Academies Press.
44. Food and Nutrition Board, Institute of Medicine: *Dietary Reference Intakes for calcium, phosphorus, magnesium, vitamin D, and fluoride*, Washington, DC, 1997, National Academies Press.
45. Food and Nutrition Board, Institute of Medicine: *Dietary Reference Intakes for thiamin, riboflavin, niacin, vitamin B_6, folate, vitamin B_{12}, pantothenic acid, biotin, and choline*, Washington, DC, 1998, National Academies Press.
46. Food and Nutrition Board, Institute of Medicine: *Dietary Reference Intakes for vitamin C, vitamin E, selenium, and carotenoids*, Washington, DC, 2000, National Academies Press.
47. Food and Nutrition Board, Institute of Medicine: *Dietary Reference Intakes for vitamin A, vitamin K, arsenic, boron, chromium, copper, iodine, iron, manganese, molybdenum, nickel, silicon, vanadium, and zinc*, Washington, DC, 2001, National Academies Press.
48. Food and Nutrition Board, Institute of Medicine: *Dietary Reference Intakes for sodium, potassium, sulfur, chloride, and water*, Washington, DC, 2004, National Academies Press.
49. U.S. Department of Health and Human Services, U.S. Department of Agriculture: *Report of the Dietary Guidelines Advisory Committee on the Dietary Guidelines for Americans 2010*, Washington, DC, 2010, Center for Nutrition Policy and Promotion, U.S. Department of Agriculture. Retrieved July 28, 2010, from http://www.cnpp.usda.gov/DGAs2010-DGACReport.htm.
50. Dwyer J: Getting started on the Dietary Guidelines for Americans 2010, *Nutr Today* 43:178, 2008.
51. Bier DM, Derelian D, German JB, et al. Improving compliance with dietary recommendations. Time for new inventive approaches? *Nutr Today* 43:180, 2008.
52. U.S. Department of Health and Human Services, U.S. Department of Agriculture: *Dietary guidelines for Americans 2005*, ed 6, Washington, DC, 2005, U.S. Government Printing Office (www.healthierus.gov/dietaryguidelines).
53. Imamura F, Jacques PF, Herrington DM, et al: Adherence to 2005 Dietary Guidelines for Americans is associated with a reduced progression of coronary artery atherosclerosis in women with established coronary artery disease, *Am J Clin Nutr* 90:193, 2009.
54. McDermott AY: MyPyramid.gov, *Nutr Clin Care* 8:103, 2005.
55. U.S. Department of Agriculture, Center for Nutrition Policy and Promotion: *MyPyramid food guidance system*, Washington, DC, 2005, U.S. Government Printing Office (*www.mypyramid.gov/*).
56. Jacobs DR, Tapsell LC: Food, not nutrients, is the fundamental unit in nutrition, *Nutr Rev* 65(10):439, 2007.
57. Haven J, Britten P: MyPyramid—the complete guide, *Nutr Today* 41(6):253, 2006.
58. International Food Information Council Foundation: Promoting health at the Center for Nutrition Policy and Promotion: an interview with Brian Wansink, PhD. In *Food Insight*, Nov/Dec 2008. Retrieved March 7, 2010, from www.foodinsight.org/Portals/0/pdf/novdecfi608.pdf.
59. Krebs-Smith SM, Kris-Etherton P: How does MyPyramid compare to other population-based recommendations for controlling chronic disease? *J Am Diet Assoc* 107:830, 2007.
60. U.S. Department of Agriculture, Center for Nutrition Policy and Promotion: *MyPyramid—USDA's new food guidance system*, [peer-to-peer PowerPoint presentation], Washington, DC, 2005, U.S. Government Printing Office. Retrieved November 22, 2005, from www.mypyramid.gov/professionals/index.html.
61. Wansink B, van Ittersum K: Portion size me: downsizing our consumption norms, *J Am Diet Assoc* 107:1103, 2007.
62. Rowe S, Alexander N: Communicating Dietary Guidelines to a balking public, *Nutr Today* 44:81, 2009.
63. Rowe S, Alexander N: Miscommunicating science, *Nutr Today* 43:103, 2008.

64. American Dietetic Association, American Diabetes Association: *Choose your foods: exchange lists for diabetes*, New York, 2007, American Dietetic Association, American Diabetes Association.
65. McCabe-Sellers BJ, Beattie SE: Food safety: Emerging trends in food borne illness surveillance and prevention, *J Am Diet Assoc* 104:1708, 2004.

FURTHER READINGS AND RESOURCES

Readings

Baker EA, Schootman M, Barnidge E, et al: The role of race and poverty in access to foods that enable individuals to adhere to dietary guidelines, *Prev Chronic Dis* 3:1, 2006. Retrieved March 31, 2009, from www.cdc.gov/pcd/issues. *[These authors point out the need for social and community support systems to assist families in obtaining an adequate diet.]*

Cappellano KL: Web-based dietary advice for the public, *Nutr Today* 43:188, 2008.

Rowe S, Alexander N: Miscommunicating science, *Nutr Today* 43:103, 2008.

[These articles offer both advice and appropriate resources for sharing nutrition and health information with the general public.]

Jeffery RW, Harnack LJ: Evidence implicating eating as a primary driver for the obesity epidemic, *Diabetes* 56:2673, 2007. *[These authors give us their views on what has contributed to the obesity epidemic and how health professionals can help to solve this problem.]*

Krebs-Smith SM, Kris-Etherton P: How does MyPyramid compare to other population-based recommendations for controlling chronic disease? *J Am Diet Assoc* 107:830, 2007. *[These researchers offer insight on how the MyPyramid food system compares with food patterns suggested for chronic disease intervention.]*

Murphy SP, Barr SI: Food guides reflect similarities and differences in dietary guidance in three countries (Japan, Canada, and the United States), *Nutr Rev* 65:141, 2007. *[Cross-cultural differences are reflected in this comparison of the USDA MyPyramid food system with food guidance systems used in other countries.]*

Rydell SA, Harnack LJ, Oakes JM, et al: Why eat at fast-food restaurants: reported reasons among frequent consumers, *J Am Diet Assoc* 108:2066, 2008. *[Meals eaten away from home can lead to inappropriate increases in energy intake. These researchers explored the reasons why people eat at fast-food restaurants and found differences depending on age, gender, and various other consumer characteristics.]*

U.S. Department of Agriculture, Center for Nutrition Policy and Promotion: An evidence-based approach to reviewing the science on nutrition and health, Nutrition Insight, 38, Alexandria, VA, January, 2008, U.S. Government Printing Office. Retrieved on April 23, 2010 from www.cnpp.usda.gov/Publications/NutritionInsights/Insight38.pdf. *[This publication provides a helpful summary on why we need to apply an evidence-based approach to our practice and gives an example of the process.]*

Wansink B, van Ittersum K: Portion size me: downsizing our consumption norms, *J Am Diet Assoc* 107:1103, 2007. *[These authors offer suggestions on how we can approach the problem of portion size that is contributing to the growing obesity in both children and adults.]*

Websites of Interest

U.S. Department of Agriculture Nutrition Evidence Library. This website evaluates the scientific evidence reviewed by the 2010 Dietary Guidelines Advisory Committee in preparation of their report: http://www.cnpp.usda.gov/NEL.htm.

U.S. Department of Health and Human Services; 2008 Physical Activity Guidelines for Americans; this website presents science-based physical activity guidelines for both youth and adults along with helpful materials for both health professionals and consumers: http://www.health.gov/paguidelines/guidelines/default.aspx.

U.S. Centers for Disease Control and Prevention; this site provides an overview of nutrition and health problems in the United States, along with consumer health information and materials: www.cdc.gov.

U.S. Department of Agriculture, Agricultural Research Service, Food Surveys Research Group: Beltsville, MD; What We Eat In America: NHANES; this site is a source of data on the food and nutrient intakes of Americans, data are presented according to age, gender, race and ethnicity, and economic status, www.ars.usda.gov/Services/docs.htm?docid=15044.

U.S. Department of Health and Human Services, U.S. Department of Agriculture; the site of the Dietary Guidelines for Americans 2005 includes materials for both health professionals and consumers; www.health.gov/DietaryGuidelines/; progress reports on the development of the 2010 Dietary Guidelines can be found at www.cnpp.usda.gov/dietaryguidelines.htm.

U.S. Department of Agriculture, Center for Nutrition Policy and Promotion; the MyPyramid website offers materials for health professionals, as well as practical tips for consumers to use in planning their meals: www.mypyramid.gov/; a PowerPoint presentation titled MyPyramid—USDA's New Food Guidance System found at www.mypyramid.gov/professionals/index.html describes and pictures the changes in U.S. food guides over the years.

U.S. Department of Health and Human Services, National Heart, Lung and Blood Institute; Keep an Eye on Portion Distortion; this site offers consumer materials describing portion sizes and how they have changed over the years: http://hp2010.nhlbihin.net/portion/keep.htm.

CHAPTER

2

Digestion, Absorption, and Metabolism

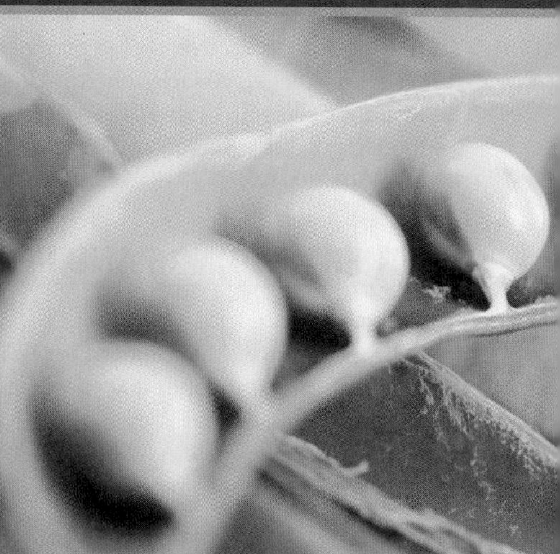

Eleanor D. Schlenker

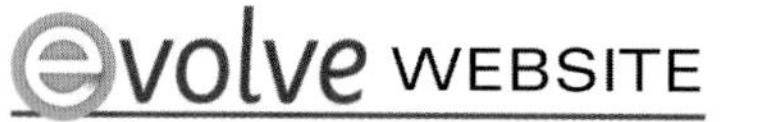

http://evolve.elsevier.com/Williams/essentials/

OUTLINE

We continue our study of nutrition by looking at what happens to food as it follows its path through the digestive system and is broken down into forms that the body can use to perform its work. We will review all the steps that must occur to convert the tuna sandwich we had at lunch into the energy-yielding nutrients—glucose, amino acids, and fatty acids. These steps are accomplished by an integrated system that receives the foods we take in and transforms them for our use.

The physiologic and biochemical process that turns the food we eat into energy and body tissue has three parts: digestion, absorption, and metabolism. We begin with a review of the gastrointestinal tract and then follow the path of the nutrients to the cells, where they nourish and protect us. We will see how all parts work together to accomplish this task.

HUMAN BODY: THE ROLE OF NUTRITION

FOOD: CHANGE AND TRANSFORMATION

The foods we eat contain the nutrients necessary for our survival, but these life-sustaining materials must first be released from other food components and transformed into units the body can use. Through a successive interrelated system, foods are broken down into simpler substances and then still simpler substances that can enter the metabolic pathways in cells. Each section of the gastrointestinal tract has a unique function, but together they form a continuous *whole.* A problem in one organ has clinical consequences for the entire system.

IMPORTANCE FOR HEALTH AND NUTRITION

Gastrointestinal function is a partner in nutritional well-being.[1] *Food,* as it occurs in nature and as we eat it, is not a single substance but a mixture of nutrients and other chemical matter. These substances must be separated so the body can handle each one as an individual unit. *Nutrients* released from food remain unavailable to the body until they cross the intestinal wall and enter the circulatory system for transport to tissues. Diseases affecting the organs of the gastrointestinal tract or the absorbing surface of the intestinal wall have adverse effects on nutritional status because nutrients are not made available in the amounts needed. At the same time, moderate to severe malnutrition lowers secretion of digestive enzymes and blunts the absorbing structures, further limiting digestion and nutrient passage. This vicious cycle results in rapid and progressive deterioration of nutritional status.[1]

The gastrointestinal tract is one of the many body systems with an output that is essential to the chemical work taking place in tissues and cells. The recognition of the human body as an integrated physiochemical organism is basic to understanding human nutrition in both health and disease. The internal control responsible for maintaining a constant

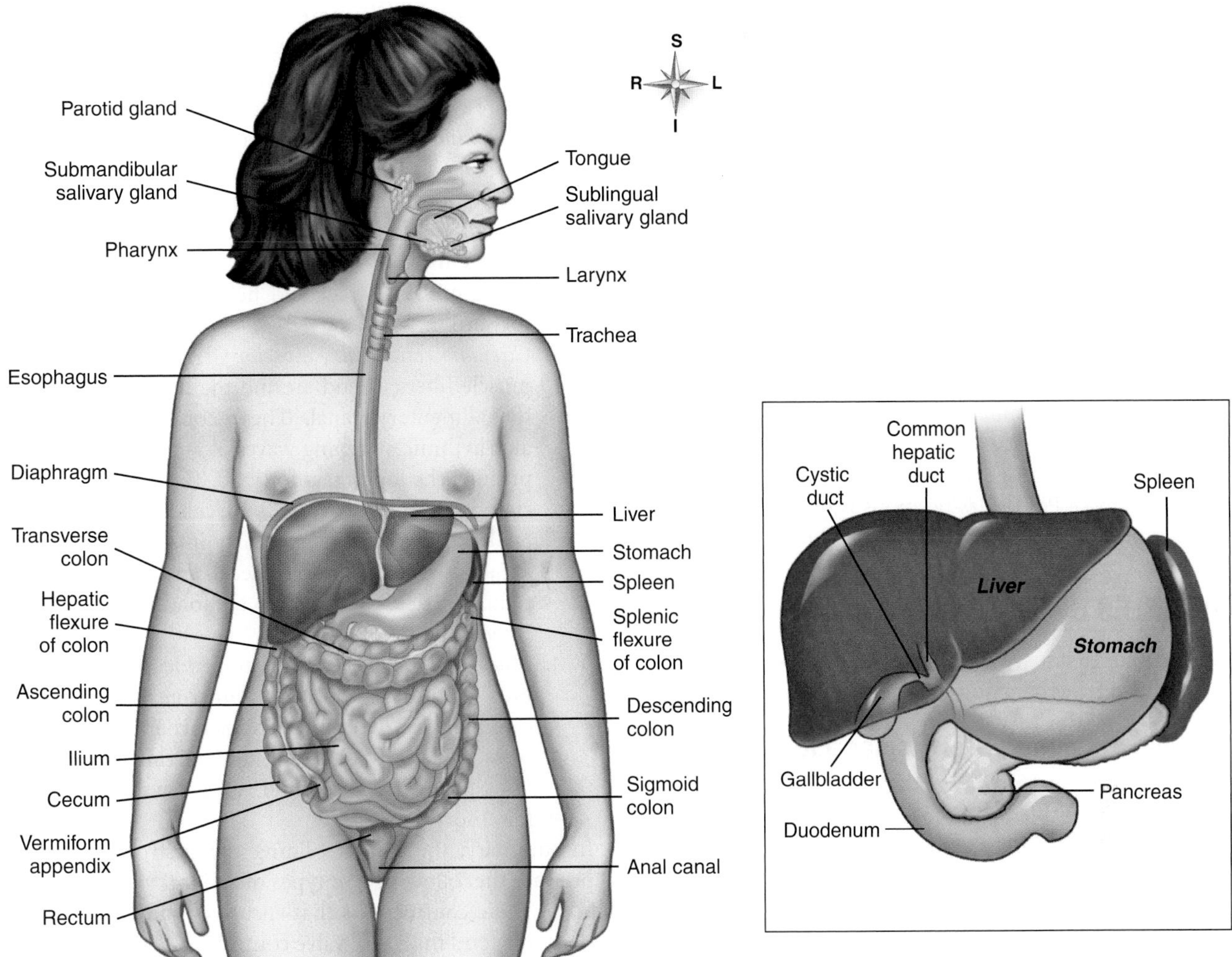

FIGURE 2-1 The gastrointestinal system. Throughout the successive parts of the gastrointestinal system, multiple activities of digestion liberate and reform food nutrients for our use. (From Thibodeau GA, Patton KT: *Anatomy and physiology,* ed 7, St. Louis, 2010, Mosby.)

chemical environment and keeping the many functional systems operating in harmony with one another is called **homeostasis.**[2]

THE GASTROINTESTINAL TRACT

Component Parts

The gastrointestinal tract, also called the *alimentary canal,* is a long hollow tube that begins at the mouth and ends at the anus. The specific parts that make up the tract are the mouth, esophagus, stomach, small intestine, large intestine or colon, and rectum. Other organs that lie outside the tract but support its work by secretion of important enzymes and digestive fluids are the pancreas, gallbladder, and liver. Look at the respective components of the gastrointestinal tract and their relative position to one another, as shown in Figure 2-1. These organs, working as a team, can break down and/or absorb several kilograms of carbohydrate, one half kilogram of fat, one half kilogram of protein, and 20 or more liters of water daily.[2] We will follow these food components as they travel *together* through the successive parts of the gastrointestinal tract.

General Functions

The gastrointestinal tract has the following four major functions:

1. *Receives food:* The mouth is the entrance to the gastrointestinal tract. From here the food is moved on to the stomach and other organs for digestion and absorption.
2. *Releases nutrients from food:* Digestion and the separation of nutrients from other food components take place in the stomach and small intestine.
3. *Delivers nutrients into the blood:* Absorbing structures called microvilli located in the small intestine transfer the nutrients into the portal blood (glucose and amino acids) or lymph (fatty acids). Water is absorbed later in the colon.
4. *Excretes nondigestible waste:* The fecal mass moves from the colon into the rectum, where it is stored until excreted.

Both physical and chemical actions accomplish these tasks.

KEY TERMS

homeostasis State of dynamic equilibrium within the body's internal environment; a balance achieved through the operation of many interrelated physiologic mechanisms.

Sensory Stimulation and Gastrointestinal Function

Both physiologic and psychologic stimuli influence the gastrointestinal tract. The physical presence of food in the mouth, stomach, or small intestine initiates a variety of responses that coordinate the muscular movements and chemical secretions necessary for digestion and absorption. Sensory stimuli—the sight, smell, or proximity to food—brings about the secretion of digestive juices and muscle motility.[2] Smelling cookies baking, hearing foods sizzle on an outdoor grill, or picking a fresh berry can evoke the physiologic process of digestion. Seeing a sign advertising your favorite food or even thinking about food stimulates the gastrointestinal tract. On the other hand, dread of an unpleasant-tasting medication or recalling the nausea brought on by chemotherapy can repress the desire for food. Positive associations with food and mealtime promote efficient digestion and absorption of nutrients.

PRINCIPLES OF DIGESTION

Digestion is the first step in preparing food for use by the body. It includes two types of actions: muscular and chemical.

Gastrointestinal Motility: Muscles and Movement

Digestion involves mechanical mixing and propulsive movements controlled by neuromuscular, self-regulating systems. These actions work together to move the food mass along the alimentary canal at the best rate for digestion and absorption.

Types of Muscles

Organized muscle layers in the gastrointestinal wall provide the motility needed for digestion (Figure 2-2). From the outer surface inward the layers are (1) the serosa, (2) a *longitudinal muscle layer,* (3) a *circular muscle layer,* (4) the *submucosa,* and (5) the mucosa. Embedded in the deeper layers of the mucosa are thin bundles of smooth-muscle fibers called the *muscularis mucosae.* The coordinated interaction of the following four smooth-muscle layers makes possible four different types of movement (Figure 2-3).

1. *Longitudinal muscles:* These long, smooth muscles arranged in fiber bundles extend lengthwise along the gastrointestinal tract and help propel the food mass forward.
2. *Circular contractile muscles:* The circular smooth-muscle fibers extend around the hollow tube forming the alimentary canal. These contractile rings initiate rhythmic sweeping waves along the digestive tract, pushing the food mass forward. These regularly occurring propulsive movements are called peristalsis.
3. *Sphincter muscles:* At strategic points, muscle sphincters act as valves—pyloric, ileocecal, and anal—to prevent reflux or backflow and keep the food mass moving in a forward direction.
4. *Mucosal muscles:* This thin embedded layer of smooth muscle produces *local constrictive contractions* every few centimeters. These contractions mix and chop the food mass, effectively churning and mixing it with secretions to form a semiliquid called chyme that is ready for absorption.

In summary, the muscles lining the gastrointestinal tract produce the following two types of action:

1. Tonic contractions that ensure continuous passage of the food mass and valve control
2. Periodic rhythmic contractions that mix and propel the food mass forward

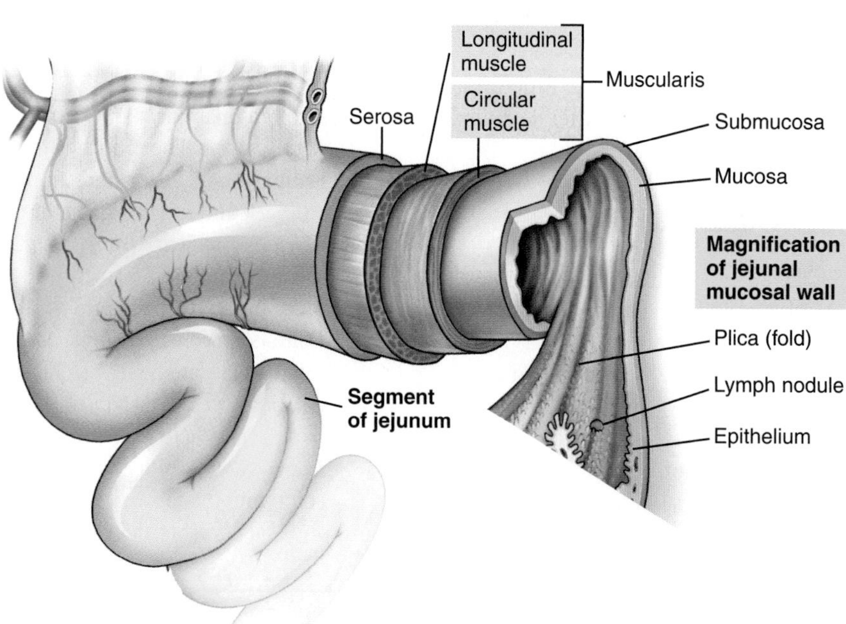

FIGURE 2-2 Muscle layers of the intestinal wall. Notice the five layers of muscle that produce the movements necessary for digestion and keeping the food mass going forward. (Modified from Thibodeau GA, Patton KT: *Anatomy and physiology,* ed 7, St. Louis, 2010, Mosby.)

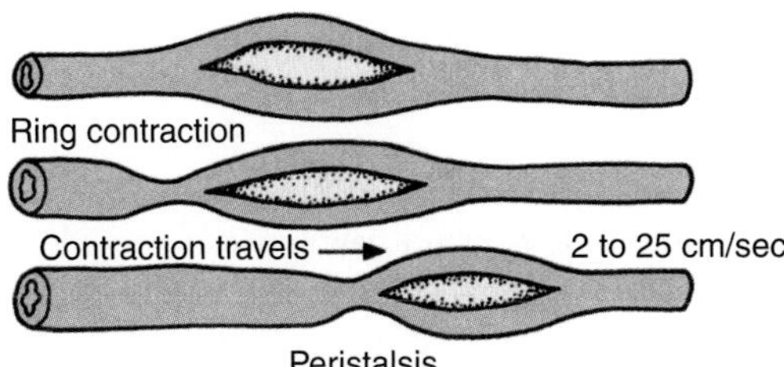

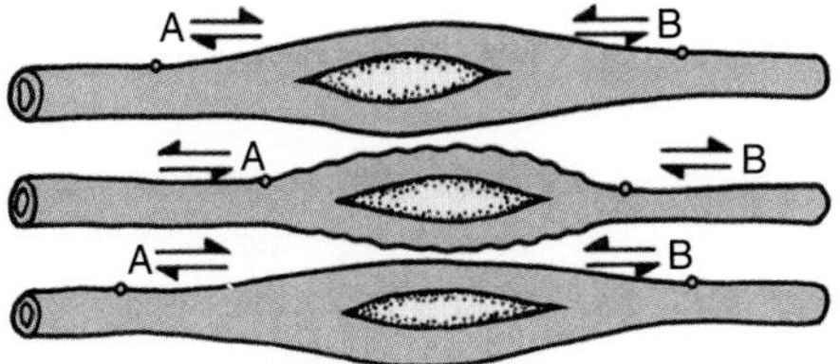

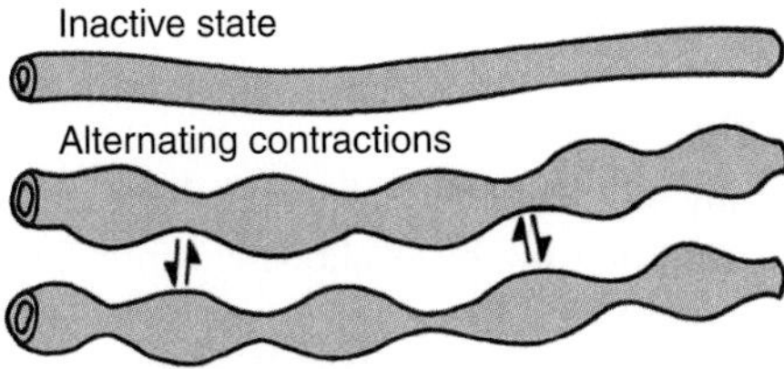

FIGURE 2-3 Types of movement produced by muscles of the intestine: peristaltic waves from contraction of deep circular muscle, pendular movements from small local muscles, and segmentation rings formed by alternate contraction and relaxation of circular muscle.

Alternating contraction and relaxation of these muscles moves the food contents along the tract and facilitates digestion and absorption.

Nervous System Control

Throughout the gastrointestinal tract, specific nerves regulate muscle action. An interrelated network of nerves within the gastrointestinal wall called the **intramural nerve plexus** (Figure 2-4) extends from the esophagus to the anus. This network of approximately 100 million nerve fibers regulates the rate and intensity of muscle contractions, controls the speed at which the food mass moves along the tract, and coordinates the digestive process, including the secretion of enzymes and digestive juices.[3]

KEY TERMS

digestion The process of breaking down food to release its nutrients for absorption and transport to the cells for use in body functions.

serosa Outer surface layer of the intestines interfacing with the blood vessels of the portal system going to the liver.

mucosa The mucous membrane forming the inner surface of the gastrointestinal tract with extensive nutrient absorption and transport functions.

peristalsis A wavelike progression of alternate contraction and relaxation of the muscle fibers of the gastrointestinal tract.

chyme Semifluid food mass in the gastrointestinal tract after gastric digestion.

tonic On-going low-level muscle contraction and relaxation.

intramural nerve plexus Network of nerves in the walls of the intestine that make up the intramural nervous system, controlling muscle action and secretions for digestion and absorption.

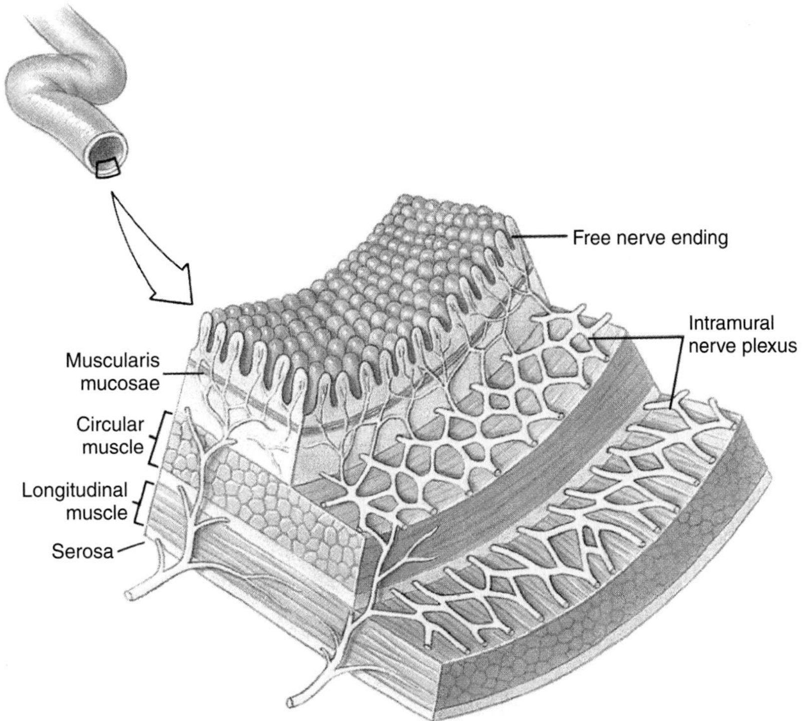

FIGURE 2-4 Innervation of the intestine by the intramural nerve plexus. A network of nerves controls and coordinates the movements of the intestinal muscles. (Courtesy Medical and Scientific Illustration.)

Gastrointestinal Secretions

Food is digested chemically through the combined action of several secretions. These secretions are of the following four types.

1. *Enzymes:* Certain enzymes attack designated chemical bonds within the structure of nutrient compounds, freeing their component parts.
2. *Hydrochloric acid and buffer ions:* These secretions produce the pH necessary for the activity of certain enzymes.
3. *Mucus:* This sticky, slippery fluid lubricates and protects the inner lining of the gastrointestinal tract and eases the passage of the food mass.
4. *Water and electrolytes:* These agents provide appropriate solutions in the amounts needed to circulate the substances released in the digestive process.

These secretions are produced by special cells in the mucosal lining of the gastrointestinal tract and in adjacent accessory organs, especially the pancreas. Their release is stimulated by (1) the presence of food in the gastrointestinal tract, (2) the sensory nerve network activated by the sight, taste, or smell of food, and (3) hormones specific to certain nutrients.

MOVEMENT OF FOOD THROUGH THE DIGESTIVE TRACT

Up to now, we looked at the integrated muscular and secretory functions that govern the overall operation of the gastrointestinal tract. Here, we begin to follow this process through its successive stages to see what happens to the food we eat.

MOUTH AND ESOPHAGUS: PREPARATION AND DELIVERY

Eating begins the physiologic process by which food is broken down into individual nutrients. The first step takes place in the mouth, where food is prepared for digestion and delivered to the stomach by way of the esophagus.

Taste and Smell

Much of our enjoyment of food comes from its unique flavors and aromas. Taste buds located on the tongue, roof of the mouth, and throat contain chemical receptors that respond to food and produce the four sensations of taste: *salty, sweet, sour,* and *bitter.* Some individuals have a stronger perception of one taste over another, and certain medications produce a bitter taste or loss of taste. Genetic-related differences in taste affecting our preference for one type of food over another (e.g., fatty foods, sweets, or vegetables) can influence what we eat and our risk for developing a particular disease or condition.[4] Patients on chemotherapy often have distorted taste (dysgeusia). Zinc deficiency causes a loss of taste (hypogeusia), and older people sometimes experience changes in taste as the number of taste buds decreases.[5]

Foods contain volatile components that move from the back of the mouth up into the nasal cavity, where they act on olfactory receptors to produce the pleasant odors we associate with particular foods. In fact, much of what we perceive as a food taste may actually be its odor. Radiation therapy of the head or neck, Parkinson's disease, and senile dementia of the Alzheimer type often lead to olfactory losses and reduced joy in eating.

Mastication

Biting and chewing break food into smaller particles. The incisors cut; the molars grind. Jaw muscles provide tremendous force: 55 lb of muscular pressure is applied through the incisors, and 200 lb is applied through the molars.[2] Digestive enzymes act only on the surface of food particles; therefore chewing to enlarge the surface area available for enzyme action is an important step in preparing food for digestion. Chewing produces fine particles that ease the passage of the food mass down the esophagus and into the stomach. Chewing is necessary to prepare fiber-containing foods—fruits, vegetables, and whole grains—for digestion. Decayed teeth, loss of teeth, or poorly fitting dentures make eating difficult. Gingivitis and other diseases of the gums and supporting structures of the teeth resulting in mouth pain, infection, or further loss of teeth restrict food intake and contribute to malnutrition.

Swallowing

Swallowing involves both the mouth and the pharynx. It is intricately controlled by the swallowing center in the brainstem,[2] and damage to these nerves through radiation therapy, aging, or disease makes swallowing difficult. The tongue initiates a swallow by pressing the food upward and backward against the palate. From this point on, swallowing proceeds as an involuntary reflex and, once begun, cannot be interrupted. Swallowing occurs rapidly, taking less than 1 second, but in that time (1) the larynx must close to prevent food from entering the trachea and moving into the lungs, and (2) the soft palate must rise to prevent food from entering the nasal cavity (Figure 2-5). Patients must never be fed in a supine position because it increases the risk of aspirating food into the lungs.

Esophagus

The esophagus is a muscular tube that connects the mouth and throat with the stomach and serves as a channel to carry the food mass into the body. Functionally, it has the following three parts[2]:

1. *Upper esophageal sphincter (UES):* The UES controls the entry of the food bolus into the esophagus. Between intakes the UES muscle is closed. Within 0.2 to 0.3 second after a swallow, nerve stimuli open the sphincter to receive the food mass.
2. *Esophageal body:* The mixed bolus of food passes immediately down the esophagus, moved along by peristaltic waves controlled by nerve reflexes. Changes in the muscles or nerves lower the intensity and frequency of the peristaltic waves, slowing passage down the channel. Diabetic neuropathy is one cause of such problems.[6] Pain and discomfort associated with these changes can add to anorexia and weight loss in older persons. Gravity aids the passage of food down the esophagus when the person eats in an upright position.
3. *Lower esophageal sphincter (LES):* The LES controls the movement of the food bolus from the esophagus into

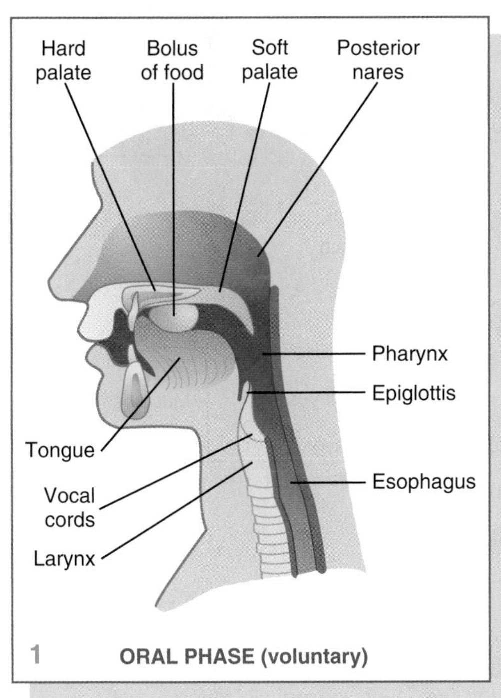

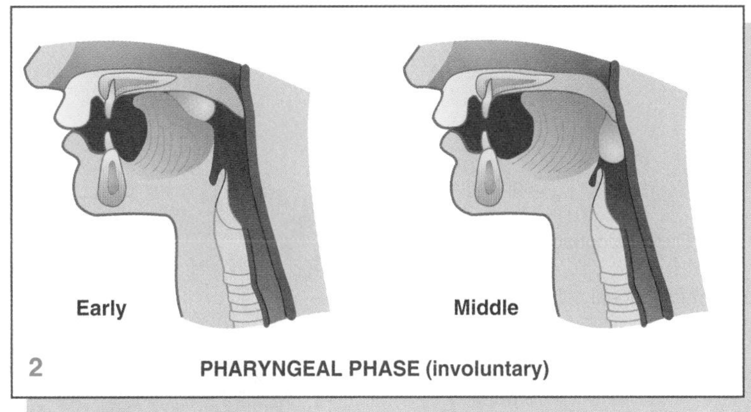

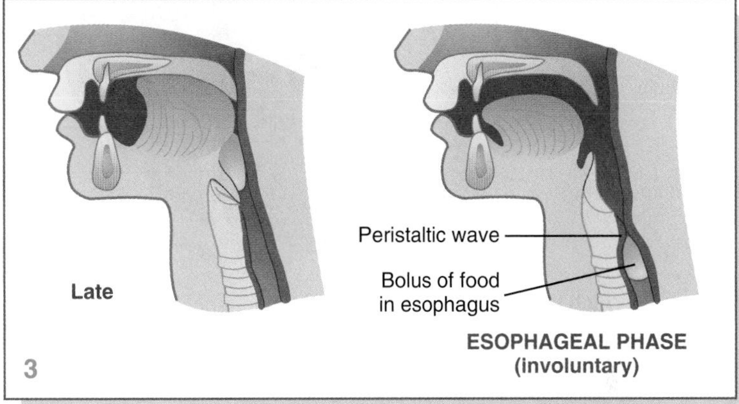

FIGURE 2-5 Swallowing is a highly coordinated task directed by a special nerve center in the hypothalamus. (From Mahan KL, Escott-Stump S, editors: *Krause's food, nutrition, and diet therapy,* ed 12, Philadelphia, 2008, Saunders.)

the stomach. When the LES muscles maintain excessively high muscle tone, they fail to open after a swallow, preventing the passage of food into the stomach. This condition is called *achalasia,* meaning unrelaxed muscle. (See Chapter 20 for a discussion of this condition.)

Entry into the Stomach

At the point of entry into the stomach the gastroesophageal constrictor muscle relaxes to allow the food to pass and then contracts quickly to prevent regurgitation or reflux of the acidic stomach contents back into the esophagus. When this mechanism fails and regurgitation occurs, one feels what is often called *heartburn.* The medical name for this condition is gastroesophageal reflux disease (GERD), and an estimated 25% of the population experience GERD on an occasional or chronic basis.[7] GERD damages the tissues of the esophagus which are unprotected against the destructive effects of gastric acid. (Mucus secreted by cells in the stomach wall protects those tissues against the harsh effects of gastric acid.) Obesity, overeating, physical inactivity, smoking, and certain medications contribute to this condition.[8–9] Increasing severity of GERD affects quality of life.[9]

Chemical Digestion

In the mouth, three pairs of salivary glands—(1) parotid, (2) submaxillary, and (3) sublingual—produce a watery fluid containing salivary amylase. This enzyme is specific for starch. The salivary glands also secrete mucus to lubricate and bind the food particles together. Sensory stimuli—and even thoughts of favorite or disliked foods—influence these secretions. As described in Table 2-1, large amounts of digestive fluids are secreted throughout the gastrointestinal tract. Saliva secretion ranges from 800 to 1500 mL a day, with a pH range of 6.0 to 7.4 (approximately neutral). Food remains in the mouth for only a short time, thus starch digestion here is brief. However, when salivary amylase binds to starch molecules, it becomes resistant to inactivation by gastric acid, thus breakdown of starch continues in the stomach.[3] A second digestive enzyme released in saliva is lingual lipase, which begins the digestion of fat. Cigarette smoke alters the composition of saliva even in passive smokers,[10] and this effect may contribute to the loss of taste associated with smoking, as well as the increased risk of oral cancer.[11]

Salivary secretions have other important functions in addition to initiating digestion. They (1) moisten the food particles so they bind together to form a bolus that moves easily down the esophagus, and (2) they lubricate and cleanse

> **KEY TERMS**
> **gingivitis** Red, swollen, bleeding gums, most often caused by accumulation of bacterial plaque on the teeth.
> **pharynx** Throat.
> **bolus** Rounded mass of food formed in the mouth and ready to be swallowed.

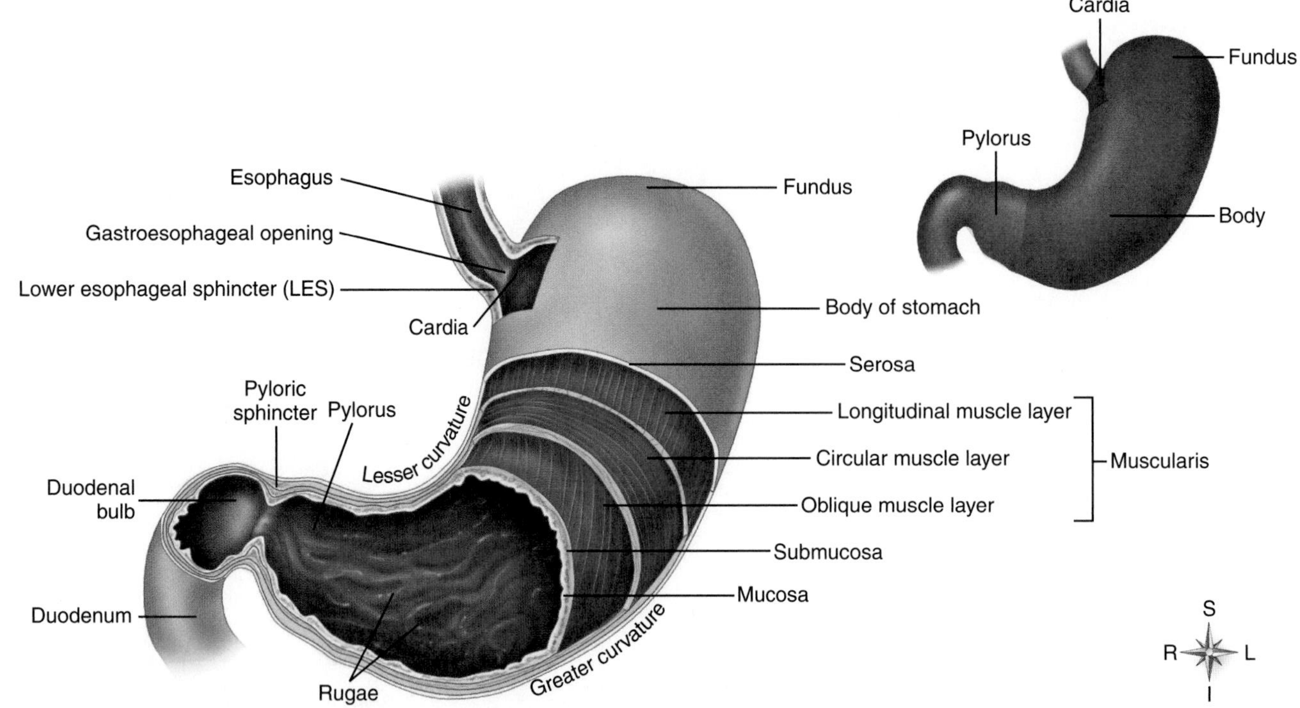

FIGURE 2-6 Stomach. The pyloric sphincter controls passage from the stomach into the duodenum, the upper section of the small intestine. See also the five layers of muscle found in the stomach wall. The mucosa lining the stomach forms folds called rugae. (From Thibodeau GA, Patton KT: *Anatomy & physiology*, ed 7, St. Louis, 2010, Mosby.)

TABLE 2-1 COMPARATIVE pH VALUES AND APPROXIMATE DAILY VOLUMES OF GASTROINTESTINAL SECRETIONS

SECRETION	pH	DAILY VOLUME (in mL)
Salivary	6.0-7.4	1000
Gastric	1.0-3.5	1500
Pancreatic	8.0-8.3	1000
Small intestinal	7.5-8.0	1800
Brunner gland (bicarbonate)	8.0-8.9	200
Bile	7.5-7.8	1000
Large intestinal	7.5-8.0	200
TOTAL		6700

Modified from Guyton AC, Hall JE: *Textbook of medical physiology*, ed 10, Philadelphia, 2000, Saunders.

the teeth and tissues of the mouth, destroying harmful bacteria and neutralizing toxic substances entering the mouth. Inadequate secretion leads to the condition known as *dry mouth*. Everyone experiences dry mouth now and then when nervous, upset, or under stress. However, when saliva production is drastically reduced and prolonged, it leads to swallowing problems because individual particles of food get separated in the esophagus. Infections and ulcers in the mouth along with tooth decay are other outcomes of extreme dry mouth, usually known as *xerostomia*. Radiation therapy causing damage to the salivary glands and diseases such as diabetes, Parkinson's disease, and autoimmune deficiency disease can lead to xerostomia. Various medications for the management of cardiac failure, hypertension, depression, or chronic pain contribute to dry mouth and are often associated with this condition in elderly adults.[12]

STOMACH: STORAGE AND INITIAL DIGESTION

Motility

The major parts of the stomach are shown in Figure 2-6. Muscles in the stomach wall have three motor functions: (1) storage, (2) mixing, and (3) controlled emptying. As the food mass enters the stomach it rests against the stomach walls, which stretch to store as much as 1 L of food and fluid. Local tonic muscle waves increase their kneading and mixing action to move the mass of food and secretions toward the pyloric valve at the distal end of the stomach. Waves of peristaltic contractions reduce the food mass to the semifluid chyme. Finally, with each wave, small amounts of chyme pass through the pyloric valve into the duodenum. The pyloric sphincter periodically constricts and relaxes to control the rate of emptying of the stomach contents. The highly acid chyme must be released slowly enough to allow it to be buffered by the alkaline secretions of the duodenum.

The caloric density of a meal, along with its volume and composition, influences the rate of stomach emptying. The speed at which food moves from the gastroesophageal sphincter to the distal end of the stomach and into the small intestine influences food intake, as messages to the brain signaling the arrival of food in the small intestine induce feelings of satiety.

EVIDENCE-BASED PRACTICE

Why Are Many Older Adults Deficient in Vitamin B_{12}?

Over the years, clinicians have frequently observed vitamin B_{12} deficiency among older adults despite their liberal intakes of meat and other animal foods containing vitamin B_{12}. Researchers found that some older individuals develop vitamin B_{12} deficiency because their stomach no longer produces intrinsic factor, a carrier required for absorption of this vitamin. To confirm this diagnosis the patients were given a labeled dose of vitamin B_{12}, and their ability to absorb this vitamin was evaluated by the appearance of labeled vitamin B_{12} in the urine. Much to the surprise of the physicians, many of these older adults were able to absorb the labeled test vitamin; so why were they deficient? Further studies revealed that the problem was an acid problem—older adults secrete smaller amounts of gastric hydrochloric acid, and a highly acid environment is required to activate pepsinogen to pepsin, the enzyme needed to break down protein. When animal proteins are not broken down to amino acids, their vitamin B_{12} is not released for absorption and is lost in the feces.

How Can We Solve this Problem?

Crystalline vitamin B_{12} as added to breads, cereals, or juices is not bound to protein and does not require an acid environment for absorption. This form of vitamin B_{12} found in fortified foods and supplements is well absorbed by older adults. Also, we have learned that vitamin B_{12} in milk and dairy products is fairly well absorbed even if gastric acid levels are low because these foods are more easily digested than tissues in meat, poultry, and fish.

Older adults should be encouraged to include a vitamin B_{12}-fortified food in their diet several times a week to ensure an adequate intake. Based on the vitamin B_{12} deficiency identified in many older age groups, some researchers are evaluating the need for mandatory vitamin B_{12} fortification of grains, as is now required for folic acid. (Folic acid fortification for the prevention of neural tube defects is discussed in Chapter 6.)

BIBLIOGRAPHY

Dharmarajan TS, Adiga GU, Norkus EP: Vitamin B_{12} deficiency: recognizing subtle symptoms in older adults, *Geriatrics* 58:30, 2003.

Russell RM, Baik H, Kehayias JJ: Older men and women efficiently absorb vitamin B-12 from milk and fortified bread, *J Nutr* 131:291, 2001.

Allen LH: How common is vitamin B-12 deficiency? *Am J Clin Nutr* 89(suppl):693S, 2009.

Green R: Is it time for vitamin B-12 fortification? What are the questions? *Am J Clin Nutr* 89(suppl):712S, 2009.

Chemical Digestion

Types of Secretions

Secretions produced in the stomach include acid, mucus, and enzymes, as follows:

- *Acid:* Hydrochloric acid creates the acidic environment necessary for certain digestive enzymes to work. For example, a pH of 1.8 to 3.5 is needed for the enzyme pepsin to act on protein; at a pH of 5.0 or above, little or no pepsin activity occurs.
- *Mucus:* This viscous secretion protects the stomach lining from the eroding effect of the acid. Mucus also binds and mixes the food mass and helps move it along.
- *Enzymes:* The major enzyme in the stomach is pepsin, which begins the breakdown of protein. Pepsin is secreted in the form of pepsinogen and activated by hydrochloric acid. The stomach also produces a small amount of gastric lipase (tributyrinase) that acts only on butterfat and has a relatively minor role in overall digestion. Children have a gastric enzyme called rennin (not to be confused with the renal enzyme renin) that aids in the coagulation of milk. Coagulation of the proteins in milk, changing them from a liquid to a semisolid (as occurs when egg white is heated), slows the rate of stomach emptying, ensuring gradual passage of material to the small intestine. Rennin is absent in adults.

Control of Secretions

Stimuli for the release of gastric secretions come from the following two sources:

1. *Nerve stimuli* are produced in response to the visual and chemical senses, the presence of food in the gastrointestinal tract, and emotional distress. Anger and hostility increase gastric secretions; fear and depression lower secretions and inhibit both blood flow to the region and gastric motility.
2. *Hormonal stimuli* are produced when food enters the stomach. Certain food components, especially caffeine, alcohol, and meat extracts, cause the mucosal cells of the antrum to release the local gastrointestinal hormone gastrin. Gastrin, in turn, stimulates the secretion of hydrochloric acid. When the pH falls below 3, a feedback mechanism halts the release of gastrin, preventing accumulation of excess acid.[3] A second gastrointestinal hormone, enterogastrone, produced in the mucosa of the duodenum, prevents excessive gastric activity by inhibiting secretion of hydrochloric acid and pepsin and slowing gastric motility. (See the *Evidence-Based Practice* box, "Why Are Many Older Adults Deficient in Vitamin B_{12}?" for an example of a problem related to inadequate secretion of gastric acid.)

KEY TERMS

distal Away from the point of origin.

duodenum The first section of the small intestine entered by food passing through the pyloric valve from the stomach.

viscous Sticky.

antrum Lower section of the stomach.

gastrin Hormone secreted by mucosal cells in the antrum of the stomach that stimulates the parietal cells to produce hydrochloric acid. Gastrin is released into the stomach in response to various stimulants, especially caffeine, alcohol, and meat extracts. When the gastric pH falls below 3, a feedback mechanism cuts off gastrin secretion to prevent excess acid formation.

enterogastrone Hormone produced in the mucous membrane of the duodenum that inhibits gastric acid secretion and motility.

SMALL INTESTINE: MAJOR DIGESTION, ABSORPTION, AND TRANSPORT

Motility

Intestinal Muscle Layers

Review the complex structure of the intestinal wall pictured in Figure 2-2. Coordination of intestinal motility is accomplished by three layers of muscle: (1) the thin layer of smooth muscle embedded in the mucosa (the muscularis mucosae) with fibers extending up into the villi, (2) the circular muscle layer, and (3) the longitudinal muscle lying next to the outer serosa.

Types of Intestinal Muscle Action

Under the control of the intramural nerve plexus, wall-stretch pressure from food or hormonal stimuli produces muscle action of the following two types:

1. *Propulsive movements:* Peristaltic waves from contractions of the deep circular muscles propel the food mass slowly forward. The presence of food or irritants brings about long sweeping waves over the entire intestine. A series of local segmental contractions also support the forward movement of the food bolus. Fiber and other indigestible materials from plant foods aid this process, providing bulk for the action of these muscles.
2. *Mixing movements:* Local constrictive contractions occurring every few centimeters mix and chop the food particles to form the semiliquid chyme.

The interaction of the muscles in the small intestine producing (1) general tonic contractions that ensure continuous passage and valve control and (2) periodic, rhythmic contractions that mix and propel the food mass forward facilitates ongoing digestion and future absorption.

Chemical Digestion

Major Role of the Small Intestine

In comparison to other sections of the gastrointestinal tract, the small intestine carries the major burden of chemical digestion. It secretes various enzymes, each specific for carbohydrate, fat, or protein, and is assisted by other enzymes entering from the pancreas. The small intestine acts as a regulatory center sensing the nutrient content, pH, and osmolarity of its contents and controls enzyme secretion accordingly.[3]

Types of Secretions

The following four types of digestive secretions complete this final stage of chemical breakdown:

1. *Enzymes:* Specific enzymes act on specific macronutrients to bring about their final breakdown to forms the body can absorb and use (review Table 2-2).
2. *Mucus:* Glands located at the entrance to the duodenum secrete large amounts of mucus. As in the stomach, mucus protects the intestinal mucosa from irritation and digestion by the highly acid chyme entering from the stomach. Other cells along the length of the inner intestinal wall secrete mucus when touched by the moving food mass, lubricating and protecting the mucosal tissues from abrasion.
3. *Hormones:* When signaled by the presence of acid in the food mass entering from the stomach, mucosal cells in the upper part of the small intestine produce the local gastrointestinal hormone secretin.[3] Secretin, in turn, stimulates the pancreas to send alkaline pancreatic juices into the duodenum to buffer the acidic chyme. The intestinal mucosa in the upper duodenum cannot withstand the high acid of the entering chyme without the neutralizing action of the bicarbonate-containing pancreatic juice.

TABLE 2-2 SUMMARY OF DIGESTIVE PROCESSES

NUTRIENT	MOUTH	STOMACH	SMALL INTESTINE
Carbohydrate	Salivary amylase breaks down starch to dextrins		Pancreatic amylase breaks down starch to disaccharides—lactose, sucrose, and maltose Disaccharides are broken down to monosaccharides Lactase breaks down lactose to glucose and galactose Sucrase breaks down sucrose to glucose and fructose Maltase breaks down maltose to form two molecules of glucose
Protein		Pepsin and HCl break down protein to polypeptides	Trypsin breaks down proteins and polypeptides to dipeptides Chymotrypsin breaks down proteins and polypeptides to dipeptides Carboxypeptidase breaks down polypeptides and dipeptides to amino acids Aminopeptidase breaks down polypeptides and dipeptides to amino acids Dipeptidase breaks down dipeptides to amino acids
Fat	Lingual lipase has a minor role in beginning fat digestion	Tributyrinase breaks down tributyrin (butterfat) to glycerol and fatty acids	Pancreatic lipase breaks down fat to glycerol, glycerides (diglycerides and monoglycerides), and fatty acids Bile emulsifies fat

HCl, Hydrochloric acid.

4. *Bile:* Bile emulsifies fat and facilitates its digestion. Bile is produced in the liver as a dilute watery solution and then is concentrated and stored by the gallbladder. When fat enters the duodenum, the local gastrointestinal hormone cholecystokinin (CCK) is secreted by glands in the intestinal mucosa and stimulates the gallbladder to contract and release bile. By means of the *enterohepatic circulation* (Figure 2-7), molecules of bile are reabsorbed and returned to the liver and gallbladder to be used over and over again. CCK also acts on the pancreas to stimulate the release of enzymes that break down fats, proteins, and carbohydrates.[3]

End Products of Digestion

When digestion of the macronutrients is complete, the simplified end products, summarized in Table 2-3, are ready for absorption. At times, undigested nutrients remain in the small intestine,[6] with accompanying discomfort or distress. When persons lack the digestive enzyme lactase, the disaccharide lactose remains in the small intestine, attracting large amounts of fluid and resulting in abdominal pain and diarrhea, nausea, or flatulence.[13] (This condition and its clinical management are discussed later in this chapter.)

Absorption

Surface Structures

Viewed from the outside, the small intestine appears smooth, but the inner surface is quite different. Note in Figure 2-8 the following three types of convolutions and projections that greatly expand the area of the absorbing surface:

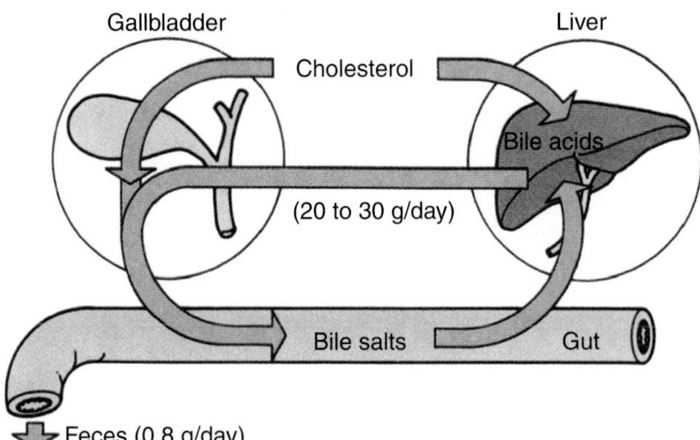

FIGURE 2-7 Enterohepatic circulation of bile salts. Bile salts are reabsorbed from the small intestine and returned to the liver and gallbladder to be used again and again.

TABLE 2-3 END PRODUCTS OF DIGESTION

MACRONUTRIENT	END PRODUCTS OF DIGESTION
Carbohydrate	Glucose, fructose, and galactose (monosaccharides)
Fat	Fatty acids, monoglycerides, diglycerides, and glycerol
Protein	Amino acids, dipeptides

1. *Mucosal folds:* Large folds similar to hills and valleys in a mountain range can be easily seen with the naked eye.
2. *Villi:* Finger-like projections on these folds called villi can be seen through a simple compound microscope.
3. *Microvilli:* These extremely small projections on each villus can be seen only with an electron microscope. The array of microvilli covering the edge of each villus is called the *brush border* because it resembles bristles on a brush. Each villus has an ample network of blood capillaries for the absorption of monosaccharides and amino acids and a central lymph vessel called a *lacteal* for the absorption of fatty acids.

The mucosa, villi, and microvilli together increase the inner surface area of the small intestine approximately 1000 times over that of the outside serosa.[2] These specialized structures, plus the contracted length of the small intestine—630 to 660 cm (21-22 feet)—produce a tremendously large surface area to capture and absorb nutrients. This absorbing surface, if stretched out flat, would be as large as a tennis or basketball court! The small intestine is one of the most highly developed organs in the body, making possible its tremendous absorptive capacity for food and fluid (Table 2-4).

Mechanisms of Absorption

Absorption of the nutrients dispersed in the water-based solution entering the small intestine involves several transport mechanisms. The particular transport used depends on the

KEY TERMS

osmolarity Number of millimoles of liquid or solid in a liter of solution.

mucus Viscous fluid secreted by mucous membranes and glands, consisting mainly of mucin (a glycoprotein), inorganic salts, and water. Mucus lubricates and protects the gastrointestinal mucosa and helps move the food mass along the digestive tract.

secretin Hormone produced in the mucous membrane of the duodenum in response to the entrance of acid contents from the stomach. Secretin in turn stimulates the flow of pancreatic juices, providing needed enzymes and the proper alkalinity for their action.

cholecystokinin (CCK) A peptide hormone secreted by the mucosa of the duodenum in response to the presence of fat. Cholecystokinin causes the gallbladder to contract and propel bile into the duodenum, where it is needed to emulsify the fat and prepare it for digestion and absorption.

absorption Transport of nutrients from the lumen of the intestine across the intestinal wall into the blood (glucose and amino acids) or the lymph (fatty acids).

villi Small protrusions from the surface of a membrane; fingerlike projections covering mucosal surfaces of the small intestine.

microvilli Minute vascular structures protruding from the villi covering the inner surface of the small intestine and forming a "brush border" that facilitates absorption of nutrients.

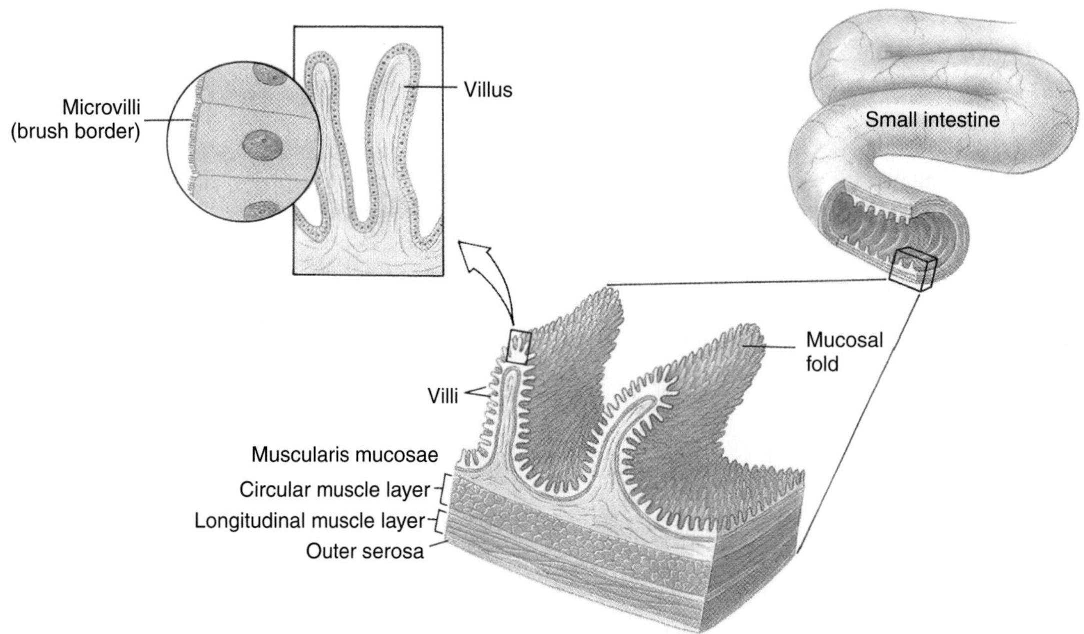

FIGURE 2-8 Absorbing structures of the intestine. Note the structures of the intestinal mucosa that increase the surface area for absorption: mucosal folds, villi, and microvilli. (Courtesy Medical and Scientific Illustration.)

TABLE 2-4 VOLUME OF NUTRIENTS ABSORBED DAILY BY THE GASTROINTESTINAL SYSTEM

SUBSTANCE	INTAKE (in L)	INTESTINAL ABSORPTION (in L)	ELIMINATION (in L)
Food ingested	1.5		
Gastrointestinal secretions	8.5		
TOTAL	10.0		
Fluid absorbed in small intestine		9.5	
Fluid absorbed in large intestine		0.4	
TOTAL		9.9	
Feces			0.1

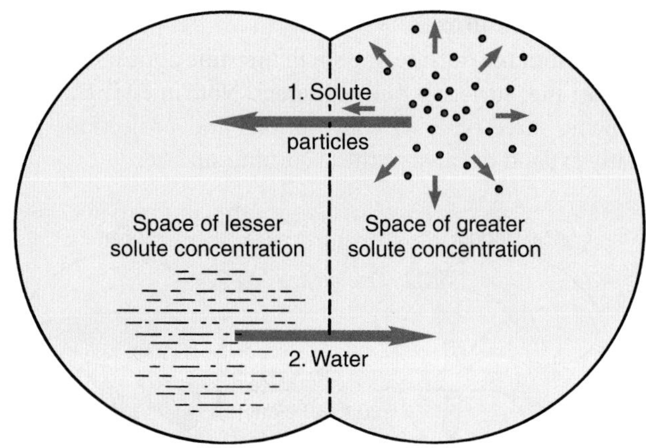

FIGURE 2-9 Movement of molecules, water, and solutes through osmosis and diffusion.

nutrient and the prevailing electrochemical fluid pressure gradient, as follows:

- *Passive diffusion and osmosis:* When no opposing fluid pressure is present, molecules small enough to pass through the capillary membranes diffuse easily into the villi (Figure 2-9). High concentrations of nutrients waiting to move into the capillaries where nutrient concentrations are low create an electrochemical gradient and osmotic pressure that promote absorption.[2]
- *Facilitated diffusion:* Even when the pressure gradient is favorable, some molecules may be too large to pass easily through the membrane pores and need assistance. Specific proteins located in the membrane facilitate passage by carrying the nutrient across the membrane.
- *Energy-dependent active transport:* Nutrients must cross the intestinal membrane to reach hungry cells even when the flow pressures are against them. Such active work requires extra energy along with a pumping mechanism. A special membrane protein carrier, coupled with the active transport of sodium, assists in the process. The energy-requiring, sodium-coupled transport of glucose is an example of this action. The enzyme *sodium/potassium-dependent adenosine triphosphatase* (Na^+/K^+-ATPase), in the cell membrane, supplies the energy for the pump.
- *Engulfing pinocytosis:* At times, fluid and nutrient molecules are absorbed by pinocytosis. When the nutrient

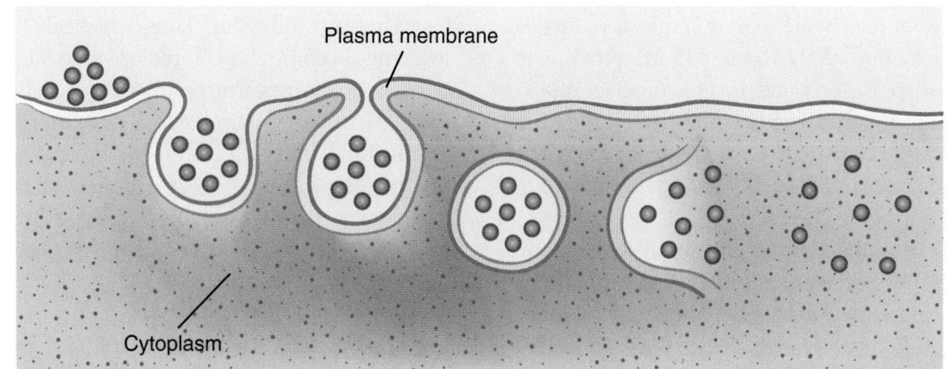

FIGURE 2-10 Pinocytosis—the engulfing of large molecules by the cell. (From Nix S: *Williams' basic nutrition and diet therapy,* ed 13, St. Louis, 2009, Mosby.)

particle touches the absorbing cell membrane, the membrane dips inward around the nutrient, surrounds it to form a vacuole, and then engulfs it. The nutrient is then conveyed through the cell cytoplasm and discharged into the circulation. Smaller whole proteins and neutral fat droplets can be absorbed through pinocytosis (Figure 2-10).

Routes of Absorption

After their absorption, the water-soluble monosaccharides and amino acids enter directly into the portal blood and travel to the liver and other tissues. Fat, which is not water soluble, follows a different route. Fats packaged in a bile complex called a *micelle* (to be described in more detail in Chapter 4) are carried into the cells of the intestinal wall, where they are processed into human lipid compounds and joined with protein as a carrier. These lipoproteins, called *chylomicrons,* flow into the lymph, empty into the cisterna chyli (the central abdominal collecting vessel of the lymphatic system), travel upward into the chest through the thoracic duct, and finally flow into the venous blood at the left subclavian vein. The chylomicrons are rapidly cleared from the blood by a special fat enzyme—lipoprotein lipase.

Exceptions to this route of fat absorption are the short-chain fatty acids with 10 or fewer carbons. Because these short-chain fatty acids are water soluble, they can be absorbed directly into the blood, as are carbohydrate and protein breakdown products. However, most dietary fats are made of long-chain fatty acids that are not water soluble and must take the lymphatic route.

COLON (LARGE INTESTINE): FINAL ABSORPTION AND WASTE ELIMINATION

Role in Absorption

Within a 24-hour period, approximately 1500 mL of the remaining food mass leaves the *ileum,* the last section of the small intestine, and enters the *cecum,* the pouch at the entrance to the colon. Passage is controlled by the *ileocecal valve.* Normally the valve remains closed, but each peristaltic wave relaxes the valve muscle, squirting a small amount of remaining chyme into the cecum. This action holds the food mass in the small intestine long enough to ensure maximal digestion and absorption. Nutrients and other materials, including electrolytes, minerals, vitamins, intestinal bacteria, and nondigestible residue, remain in the chyme delivered to the large intestine.

Water Absorption

The main task remaining for the colon is the absorption of water. The capacity of the colon to absorb water is vast, with

KEY TERMS

pinocytosis Means of nutrient absorption by which the molecule is engulfed by the cytoplasm of the receiving cell.

lipoprotein Noncovalent complexes of fat with protein. The lipoproteins function as major carriers of lipids in the plasma; this combination of fat surrounded by protein makes possible the transport of fatty substances in a water medium such as plasma.

cisterna chyli Cistern or receptacle of the chyle; a dilated sac at the origin of the thoracic duct, which is the common trunk that receives all the lymphatic vessels. The cisterna chyli lies in the abdomen between the second lumbar vertebra and the aorta. It receives the lymph from the intestinal trunk, the right and left lumbar lymphatic trunks, and two descending lymphatic trunks. The chyle, after passing through the cisterna chyli, is carried upward into the chest through the thoracic duct and empties into the venous blood at the point where the left subclavian vein joins the left internal jugular vein. This is the way absorbed fats enter the general circulation.

colon The large intestine extending from the cecum to the rectum.

a net daily maximum of 5 to 8 L.[2] Normally, from 1.0 to 1.5 L is received from the ileum, and 95% of that is absorbed (see Table 2-4).

Much of the water in the chyme (350-400 mL) is absorbed in the first half of the colon. Only 100 to 150 mL remains to form the feces.[2] Absorption of water in the colon is important in the regulation of water balance and the elimination of fecal waste. When the chyme first enters the colon, it is a semiliquid, but water absorption during passage changes it to the semisolid nature of normal feces.

The amount of water absorbed in the colon depends on motility and rate of passage. Poor motility and a slow passage rate, often related to low dietary fiber and low fecal mass, allow greater absorption of water, resulting in hard stools that are difficult to pass and constipation. Excess motility and too-rapid passage limit the absorption of water and important electrolytes, producing a high volume of loose, watery stool (diarrhea). Diarrhea can result from disease, microbial infection, as in foodborne illness, or large amounts of undigested sugar such as lactose that exert osmotic pressure and hold vast amounts of fluid. Severe or extended diarrhea leads to dehydration and serious loss of electrolytes.

Mineral Absorption

Sodium and other electrolytes are absorbed from the colon. Intestinal absorption exerts major control on body content of many minerals, and much of the dietary intake is unabsorbed and excreted in the feces. Up to 90% of the calcium and iron in the food we eat is not absorbed. The proportion of a mineral intake that is generally absorbed is an important aspect of nutrient balance and dietary evaluation.

Vitamin Absorption

Conditions in the gastrointestinal tract influence the absorption of vitamins. When gastric acid is lower than normal, vitamin B_{12} is not easily released from animal tissues and is lost in the feces (see the *Evidence-Based Practice* box). Conversely, colon bacteria synthesize vitamin K and biotin, which are actively absorbed and serve as a major source of the body's supply.

Role of Intestinal Bacteria

At birth the colon is sterile, but intestinal bacteria soon become established. More than 500 different species of bacteria are found in the normal gastrointestinal tract, and intestinal contents may contain as many as 1 billion bacteria per gram.[14] Various factors influence the composition of the microflora. Dietary intake of fiber or other nondigestible carbohydrates, immune responses favoring one group of bacteria over another, and the use of antibiotics affect the types and numbers of particular bacteria. Bacterial populations also differ along the length of the gastrointestinal tract based on differences in structure and pH.[15] Many bacteria ingested with food cannot survive the extreme acid environment in the stomach.

Intestinal bacteria make up approximately one third of fecal weight[2] and affect the color and odor of the stool. The customary brown color comes from bile pigments produced by colon bacteria from bilirubin. Thus, when bile flow is hindered, the feces may become clay colored or white. The characteristic odor of the stool comes from amines, especially *indole* and *skatole*, formed by the action of bacterial enzymes on amino acids.

Intestinal microflora have many roles. Particular microorganisms produce bothersome gas or increase the risk of gastrointestinal disease. Other species make positive contributions to health (Box 2-1).

Excessive Gas Production

Intestinal bacteria are the major contributors to gas production, including carbon dioxide (CO_2), molecular hydrogen (H_2), methane, and sometimes hydrogen sulfide. Gas formation is a normal occurrence and, though harmless, is distressful when it causes pain or embarrassment. Intestinal gas, or flatus, can be exaggerated as a result of specific foods or physiologic circumstances in the person eating them.

In general, gas is produced by the bacterial fermentation of undigested or incompletely absorbed carbohydrate. Humans lack the enzymes necessary to digest the oligosaccharides raffinose and stachyose in legumes that cause the intestinal gas associated with these foods. Certain starches and fibrous materials in whole grains, fruits, and vegetables are resistant to pancreatic amylase and are not broken down and absorbed. People should be encouraged to increase their intakes of fiber gradually to allow a more comfortable adjustment and prevent gastrointestinal distress.

Excessive gas has social implications. CO_2, H_2, and methane are odorless, but hydrogen sulfide carries a striking odor. Hydrogen sulfide most often arises from cruciferous vegetables (cabbage, cauliflower, or broccoli) or large amounts of beer, all high in sulfur. Various over-the-counter products claim to reduce the formation of gas or eliminate gaseous odors, but all of these products have limitations. Persons should check with their physician before using such preparations.[16] (See the *Complementary and Alternative Medicine [CAM]* box, "Bismuth and Certain Herbs: A Dangerous Combination" for cautions.)

Waste Elimination

Fully formed and ready for elimination, normal feces contain approximately 75% water and 25% solids.[2] The solids include

BOX 2-1 HEALTHFUL EFFECTS OF INTESTINAL BACTERIA

- Produce short-chain fatty acids that nourish the cells of the intestinal mucosa
- Assist in absorbing and activating phytochemicals
- Prevent harmful bacteria from growing and forming colonies
- Support immune cells that attack harmful body invaders
- Synthesize various vitamins such as biotin and vitamin K

COMPLEMENTARY AND ALTERNATIVE MEDICINE (CAM)

Bismuth and Certain Herbs: A Dangerous Combination

Bismuth-containing medications such as Pepto-Bismol are sometimes used to ease gas and bloating. Bismuth also binds with the odor-causing sulfur compounds in intestinal gas and helps reduce embarrassment. However, when combined with ginkgo, garlic, ginger, or ginseng, bismuth can have serious side effects. Working together bismuth and these herbs act as anticoagulants.

Bonci L: *American Dietetic Association guide to better digestion,* Hoboken, NJ, 2003, John Wiley & Sons.

fiber, bacteria, inorganic matter such as minerals, a small amount of fat and its derivatives, some mucus, and sloughed-off mucosal cells.

The mass of food residue now slows its passage. Approximately 4 hours after a meal is eaten, it enters the cecum, having traveled the entire length of the small intestine, 630 to 660 cm (21-22 feet). Approximately 8 hours later, it reaches the sigmoid colon, having traveled an additional 90 cm (3 feet) through the large intestine. In the sigmoid colon, the residue descends still more slowly toward its final destination, the rectum.

The rectum begins at the end of the large intestine immediately past the descending colon and ends at the anus. Feces are usually stored in the descending colon; however, when it becomes full, feces pass into the rectum, resulting in the urge to defecate. Anal sphincters under voluntary control regulate the elimination of feces from the body. As much as 25% of a meal may remain in the rectum for up to 72 hours.

GASTROINTESTINAL FUNCTION AND CLINICAL APPLICATIONS

Chronic Gastrointestinal Distress

Most of the time the gastrointestinal tract is a smoothly working system that allows us to enjoy the food we eat while effectively handling digestion, absorption, and the elimination of waste. However, for some people, abdominal pain, nausea, vomiting, or diarrhea is a regular occurrence, and no specific biochemical or structural explanation can be found.[17-18] Mental and emotional stress, depression, various prescription medications, foods eaten, and chronic disease all influence gastrointestinal function. Some populations appear to be particularly vulnerable to chronic gastrointestinal distress (see the *Focus on Culture* box, "Digestive Distress in African Americans and Hispanic Americans").

We need to listen carefully when people tell us about gastrointestinal problems that interfere with eating and their enjoyment of food.[19] Health education for self-care should point to the dangers of over-the-counter supplements such as food enzymes claiming to enhance digestion, inappropriate laxatives, or ill-advised procedures such as colonic irrigation. Chronic digestive problems demand medical assessment and intervention.

FOCUS ON CULTURE

Digestive Distress in African Americans and Hispanic Americans

Chronic digestive distress can influence food choices, nutrient intake, and general health. African Americans and Hispanic Americans may be at greater risk than other groups. When adults were asked to complete a questionnaire asking about abdominal pain and fullness, nausea, vomiting, or gastric reflux, almost one third of the participants indicated at least one of these problems.[1] The majority reporting problems were African Americans, and on follow-up, many were found to have previously undiagnosed gastric ulcers, duodenal ulcers, or damage to their esophagus. African Americans and Hispanic Americans are more likely than other groups to be infected with *Helicobacter pylori,* the microorganism known to have a role in development of ulcers, as well as other digestive disorders.[2-3] Infection with *H. pylori* relates to socioeconomic rather than genetic factors, and infection rates are higher than normal in both children and adults from families with lower incomes, reduced access to health care facilities, and living in a rural environment. This burden of infection may contribute to the increased prevalence of **dyspepsia** and digestive disease in these groups.

REFERENCES

1. Shaib Y, El-Serag HB: The prevalence and risk factors of functional dyspepsia in a multiethnic population in the United States, *Am J Gastroenterol* 99:2210, 2004.
2. Kruszon-Moran D, McQuillan GM: *Seroprevalence of six infectious diseases among adults in the United States by race/ethnicity: data from the third National Health and Nutrition Examination Survey, 1988-94, advance data, vital and health statistics,* No. 352, Hyattsville, Md, 2005, U.S. Department of Health and Human Services.
3. Malaty HM: Epidemiology of *Helicobacter pylori* infection, *Best Pract Res Clin Gastroenterol* 21(2):205, 2007.

Lactose Intolerance

Lactose intolerance is a digestive problem facing 70%[20] of the world's population—as many as 22% of Caucasians, 80% of African Americans and Latinos, and almost 100% of Asians.[13] Those with lactose intolerance may have symptoms after taking in as little as 6 g or as much as 12 to 18 g of lactose (1 cup of milk contains 12 g of lactose).[13] This problem stems

KEY TERMS

ileum The distal section of the small intestine that connects with the colon.

bilirubin A reddish bile pigment resulting from the degradation of heme by reticuloendothelial cells in the liver; a high level in the blood produces the yellow skin symptomatic of jaundice.

oligosaccharide Chain of 8 to 10 glucose units.

dyspepsia Gastric distress or indigestion involving nausea, pain, burning sensations, or excessive gas.

from a deficiency of lactase, the digestive enzyme in the microvilli of the small intestine that breaks lactose into its simple sugars—glucose and galactose. When undigested lactose remains in the small intestine and colon, it absorbs large amounts of water and is fermented by resident bacteria, producing diarrhea, bloating, and gas.

Congenital intolerance to lactose is rare; infants usually produce enough lactase to digest the large amounts of lactose in mother's milk. However, loss of lactase activity beyond early childhood is the normal physiologic pattern, with relatively few adults retaining their former capacity for lactose digestion. Before the domestication of cows, lactose was not present in the diet after weaning, therefore this enzyme was no longer needed. The introduction of a dairy-based culture in particular geographic regions 10,000 years ago likely contributed to the retention of lactase activity among certain European groups.[13] Most populations lose more than 70% of their lactase activity within 3 to 4 years of weaning, although Caucasians may retain high lactase activity through adolescence.[20]

Other conditions can cause or worsen symptoms after eating lactose-containing foods. Irritable bowel syndrome, celiac disease, cystic fibrosis, or other disorders that damages the intestinal mucosa can interfere with the digestion of lactose, and medical diagnosis is often needed to confirm the problem. Viral infections can cause temporary lactose intolerance.

Distinguishing between lactose maldigestion and lactose intolerance is important. Individuals with some degree of lactose maldigestion may not necessarily exhibit symptoms characteristic of lactose intolerance. When lactose maldigesters were given a lactose-containing beverage as compared with a similar beverage that looked and tasted the same but had the lactose removed, their responses were similar, suggesting that lactose is not a major cause of symptoms when consumed in the customary dietary portion of one cup of milk.[21] Most people with problems digesting lactose do not need to follow a totally lactose-free diet, although milk may be limited in favor of other dairy foods[20] or lactose-containing foods gradually added to the diet. Maldigesting lactose does not mean that you are allergic to milk or dairy foods. A true milk allergy is caused by the *protein* in milk, not the *lactose*.[16]

To increase their intakes of calcium and vitamin D, people with lactose maldigestion might begin to include dairy foods in their diet in the following ways[16]:

- *Add dairy foods gradually:* Begin with a small amount of one dairy food each day, one quarter cup of milk or one half ounce of cheese; include only one lactose-containing food per meal. (See Box 2-2 for food lactose content.)
- *Include lactose-containing foods with a meal or snack:* This combination slows the movement of lactose into the intestine and may reduce discomfort.
- *Choose dairy foods low in lactose:* Use lactose-free or lactose-reduced milk. *(Acidophilus milk is not lactose free.)* Add lactase enzyme drops (Lactaid or Dairy Ease) to milk to lower the lactose. Lactase tablets taken right before eating dairy foods can reduce discomfort. Aged cheeses such as cheddar or Swiss are lower in lactose than cheese spreads or other processed cheese.

Lactose is also found in nondairy foods that have milk as an ingredient. Breads and other baked products, some ready-to-eat breakfast cereals, pancake and cookie mixes, instant potatoes, cream soups, hot dogs, and luncheon meats may contain lactose. Read the Nutrition Facts label, and look for the word *milk* or *whey.* (See Chapter 7 for food sources of calcium for persons who cannot tolerate dairy foods.)

HEALTH PROMOTION

Prebiotics and Probiotics

Many people have the perception that all microbes are harmful, as we read reports of antibiotic-resistant virus, outbreaks of foodborne illness, or advertisements for antibacterial

BOX 2-2 FOOD SOURCES OF LACTOSE

0 to 2 g Lactose	5 to 8 g Lactose
1 to 2 oz Swiss or cheddar cheese	½ cup regular milk
1 oz American cheese	½ cup white sauce
½ cup cottage cheese	½ cup yogurt
½ cup lactase-treated milk	1 cup ice cream or ice milk
	2 tbsp powdered milk

Data from Bonci L: *American Dietetic Association guide to better digestion,* Hoboken, NJ, 2003, John Wiley & Sons.

soap. Nonetheless, in the nineteenth century, Elie Metchnikoff speculated that Bulgarian peasants enjoyed long lives because of their use of fermented milk that supplied microbes beneficial to colonic health. Today, we recognize that certain microbes found in the gastrointestinal tract contribute to human health and provide new tools for improving gastrointestinal function (see Box 2-1). These microbes and related food components have been termed *prebiotics* and *probiotics* based on their use and intestinal effects. Prebiotics are food ingredients that selectively stimulate the growth of one or more bacteria in the colon. Probiotics are live microorganisms that when administered in adequate amounts result in a health benefit to the host.[22]

Prebiotics

Prebiotics are indigestible carbohydrates, mostly polysaccharides, that promote the growth of the microbes *Lactobacilli* and *Bifidobacteria.* Any dietary component that reaches the colon intact is a potential prebiotic. Prebiotics used clinically include oligosaccharides (isolated from wheat, onions, bananas, garlic, soybeans, and artichokes), various fiber derivatives, and lactulose, a synthetic disaccharide.[22-23]

Increases in *Lactobacilli* and *Bifidobacteria* have various favorable actions, including:

- *Increase in mineral absorption:* Although most minerals are absorbed in the small intestine, the lower pH in the colon resulting from bacterial fermentation stimulates the absorption of zinc, calcium, magnesium, and iron still remaining in the food residue. These microbes break down phytate, an indigestible material found in plant foods that binds minerals and prevents their absorption.[23-24]
- *Promotion of normal laxation:* The fermenting action of bacteria on lactulose relieves constipation and helps avoid dependence on laxatives. Prebiotics can be added to tube feedings to prevent the common problem of diarrhea.[22-23]
- *Protection against colon cancer:* The fermentation products of healthful bacteria destroy cancer cells and toxic enzymes produced by harmful bacteria.[23]

Probiotics

The benefits of probiotics depend on the particular strain of bacteria and the active substances it produces. Lactic acid–producing bacteria have been used over the centuries to acidify and preserve foods. Common fermented foods include cultured milk and yogurt, cheese, distilled mash, pickled cabbages, and tempeh. Probiotic cultures are available from pharmaceutical companies for clinical use, although lactic acid–producing bacteria that survive the passage through the gastrointestinal tract and thrive in the colon can be obtained from commercially produced yogurt.[22]

Clinical applications of probiotics include the following:

- *Diarrhea:* Species of *Lactobacillus* are effective in treating infectious diarrhea in children and the diarrhea induced by antibiotics.[22] Loss of the normal microflora through antibiotics allows the growth of harmful bacteria, and the resulting diarrhea adds days to the usual hospital stay.[23]
- *Infant allergies:* Poi, a probiotic made from the taro plant of the Pacific Islands, can be fed to babies allergic to cereals. When given to expectant mothers with a family history of cereal allergy, only one half of their infants showed signs of potential allergy.[25]
- *Inflammatory bowel disease:* Patients with ulcerative colitis and Crohn's disease have abnormal patterns of intestinal bacteria that foster these diseases. Probiotics may assist in prevention or treatment.[22]
- *Inhibition of H. pylori:* This pathogenic bacterium attaches to the gastric mucosa and is implicated in the development of peptic ulcer, gastric cancer, and chronic gastritis. Probiotics seem to inhibit its growth and prevent it from burrowing into the stomach lining.[25]
- *Gastrointestinal immune response:* Probiotics support the immune cells in the gastrointestinal tract that provide the first line of defense against pathogens entering the body.[22]
- *Lactose intolerance*: Probiotics in the colon help break down lactose, preventing symptoms associated with lactase deficiency.[22]

Although lactic acid–producing bacteria have been used successfully in food and therapeutic preparations, new strains must be determined safe before being sold as a supplement. Individuals with compromised immune function should not use probiotics without medical supervision. Contamination of the probiotic with a pathogenic strain or the passage of a probiotic microorganism across the intestinal mucosa and into the blood could lead to sepsis in an infant or adult lacking normal immune response.[26] Currently, no legal definitions have been formulated for the terms *prebiotic* or *probiotic,* and as dietary supplements, their product labels are not reviewed for accuracy or efficacy by the U.S. Food and Drug Administration. Accurate information relating to the exact strain or species of bacteria, dosage required for effective intervention, safety of a particular product, or product shelf life can be difficult to obtain.[22]

Fermented dairy products are sources of both important nutrients and live bacteria, although the strain of microorganism and the level present may be unknown. Yogurt, cheese, and kefir (fermented milk prepared by adding kefir grains to cow's or goat's milk) all contain potentially beneficial live bacteria. Some yogurts currently sold in the United States contain not only starter cultures of bacteria, but also added *Lactobacillus* or *Bifidobacterium* to produce a probiotic effect, although label information as to the amount added is often limited. New commercial fermented milk and yogurt products marketed as functional foods containing known strains of bacteria at probiotic levels are also entering the market place.[22]

(See the *Perspectives in Practice* box, "Help Your Digestive System Work for You," for ideas on maintaining optimum digestive function.)

PERSPECTIVES IN PRACTICE

Help Your Digestive System Work for You

Our personal eating habits can either support or stress the normal function of the digestive tract. Positive practices will maximize our enjoyment of food and help regulate our food intake.

- Do not gulp your food; allow time for the vapors to enter your sinus cavity and contribute to your sensation of taste.
- Wait 15 to 20 minutes before taking second helpings; when food moves from your stomach into your small intestine, it triggers feelings of satiety, and you may find that you do not need that extra spoonful.[1]
- Try to concentrate on pleasant thoughts or conversation while eating; emotional distress—fear, anger, worry—depresses the secretion of digestive enzymes and slows peristalsis, leading to gastrointestinal discomfort or upset.
- Enjoy the sight, smells, and anticipation of food as you prepare or serve your meals; these responses promote enzyme secretion and digestive function.
- The cells lining the gastrointestinal tract derive most of their energy from the food passing through and require a constant supply of nutrients to meet their high metabolic demands; try to eat about the same amount of food every day; do not gorge one day and fast the next.

REFERENCE

[1]Rolls B, Barnett RA: *Volumetrics,* New York, 2000, HarperCollins.

METABOLISM

After their absorption, nutrients are transported to the cells to be used for energy or to produce substances and tissues needed to sustain life. Cell metabolism encompasses the total spectrum of chemical changes associated with the final use of the individual nutrients.

Carbohydrate Metabolism

Although glucose is an immediate energy source for all body cells, it is also the preferred energy source for the brain and nervous system. Because glucose is so critical to life, its level in the blood is carefully regulated.

Sources of Blood Glucose

Both carbohydrate and noncarbohydrate molecules are sources of blood glucose, described as follows:

- *Carbohydrate sources:* Three carbohydrate substances can be converted to glucose: (1) dietary starches and sugars, (2) glycogen stored in the liver and muscle, and (3) products of carbohydrate metabolism such as lactic acid and pyruvic acid.
- *Noncarbohydrate sources:* Both protein and fat are indirect sources of glucose. Certain amino acids are called *glucogenic amino acids* because they can form glucose after their amino group (NH_2^+) is removed. Approximately 58% of the protein in a mixed diet is made of glucogenic amino acids. Thus more than one half of dietary protein might ultimately be used for energy if sufficient carbohydrate and fat were not available. After fats are broken down into fatty acids and *glycerol,* the glycerol portion (approximately 10% of the fat) can be converted to glycogen in the liver and then to glucose as needed. The formation of glucose from protein, glycerol, and carbohydrate metabolites is called gluconeogenesis.

Uses of Blood Glucose

Blood glucose is maintained within a normal range of 70 to 140 mg/dL (3.9-7.8 mmol/L) but is in constant flux as absorbed glucose is transported to cells for immediate use or removed from the circulation and stored as glycogen or fat. Blood glucose is used in three different ways:

- *Energy production:* The primary function of glucose is to supply energy to meet the body's constant demand. An array of metabolic pathways requiring specific and successive enzymes accomplishes this task.
- *Energy storage:* Glucose is stored in two forms: (1) glycogen—held in limited amounts in liver and muscle, and (2) fat (adipose tissue)—the storage form for all excess glucose after energy demands have been met. Only a small supply of glycogen exists at any one time, and it turns over rapidly. Fat can be stored in unlimited amounts in adipose tissue and provides long-term energy stores.
- *Glucose products:* Small amounts of glucose are used to produce various carbohydrate compounds with important roles in body metabolism. Examples include deoxyribonucleic acid (DNA) and ribonucleic acid (RNA), galactose, and certain amino acids.

These sources and uses of glucose act as checks and balances to maintain normal blood glucose levels, adding or removing glucose as needed.

Hormonal Controls

Several hormones directly and indirectly influence glucose metabolism and regulate blood glucose levels.

- *Blood glucose–lowering hormone.* Only one hormone—insulin—lowers blood glucose. Insulin is produced by the beta cells in the pancreas. These cells are scattered in clusters, forming "islands" in the pancreas—giving rise to the name *islets of Langerhans* after the German scientist who first discovered them. Insulin lowers blood glucose by the following actions:
  - *Glycogenesis* stimulates the conversion of glucose to glycogen in the liver for energy reserve.
  - *Lipogenesis* stimulates the conversion of glucose to fat for storage in adipose tissue.
  - *Cell permeability* increases, allowing more glucose to enter the cell and be oxidized for energy.
- *Blood glucose–raising hormones.* The following hormones effectively raise blood glucose levels:
  - *Glucagon* produced by the alpha cells in the pancreas acts in opposition to insulin, increasing the breakdown of liver glycogen to glucose and maintaining blood glucose levels during fasting or sleep hours. (The hydrolysis of liver glycogen to yield glucose is called glycogenolysis.)
  - *Somatostatin,* produced in the delta cells of the pancreas and in the hypothalamus, suppresses insulin and glucagon and acts as a general modulator of related metabolic activities.

- *Steroid hormones,* secreted by the adrenal cortex, release glucose-forming carbon units from protein and oppose the actions of insulin.
- *Epinephrine,* originating from the adrenal medulla, stimulates the breakdown of liver glycogen and quick release of glucose.
- *Growth hormone (GH)* and *adrenocorticotropic hormone (ACTH),* released from the anterior pituitary gland, oppose the actions of insulin.
- *Thyroxine,* originating in the thyroid gland, increases the rate of insulin breakdown, increases glucose absorption from the small intestine, and liberates epinephrine.

Lipid Metabolism

Lipid Synthesis and Breakdown

Two organ tissues—(1) liver and (2) adipose tissue—form a balanced axis of lipid metabolism. Both tissues participate in lipid synthesis and breakdown. The fatty acids released from lipids are used by body cells as concentrated fuel for energy.

Lipoproteins

Lipid-protein complexes are the transport form of lipids in the blood. An excess of blood lipoproteins produces a clinical condition called *hyperlipoproteinemia.* Lipoproteins are produced (1) in the intestinal wall after the initial absorption of dietary lipids and (2) in the liver for constant recirculation to and from cells.

Hormonal Controls

Because lipid and carbohydrate metabolism are interrelated, the same hormones are involved, as follows:

- *GH, ACTH,* and *thyroid-stimulating hormone (TSH),* all from the pituitary gland, increase the release of free fatty acids from stored lipids when energy demands are imposed.
- *Cortisol* and *corticosterone,* from the adrenal gland, release free fatty acids.
- *Epinephrine* and *norepinephrine* stimulate the breakdown of lipids and release of free fatty acids.
- *Insulin* from the pancreas promotes lipid synthesis and storage, whereas *glucagon* has the opposite effect of breaking down lipid stores to release free fatty acids.
- *Thyroxine* from the thyroid gland stimulates release of free fatty acids and lowers blood cholesterol levels.

When fatty acids from the gastrointestinal tract are delivered to the liver and muscle in larger amounts than needed for immediate energy or synthesis of important molecules, the hormone insulin promotes the formation of triglycerides for storage in the adipose tissue. In situations of prolonged physical activity, starvation, physical stress, or other circumstances requiring energy beyond what can be supplied by available glycogen, these triglycerides are broken down and their fatty acids released. Free fatty acids are delivered to the liver to be packaged in lipoproteins for transport to cells for meeting energy needs or for redeposition in adipose tissue. Muscle cells, including the heart muscle, depend on free fatty acids for their ongoing energy needs.

Protein Metabolism

Anabolism (Tissue Building)

Protein metabolism centers on the critical balance between anabolism (tissue building) and catabolism (tissue breakdown). The process of anabolism builds tissue through the synthesis of new protein. The making of new protein is governed by a definite pattern or "blueprint" provided by DNA in the cell nucleus that calls for specific amino acids. Specific enzymes and coenzymes along with certain hormones—GH, gonadotropins, and thyroxine—control and stimulate the building of tissue protein.

Catabolism (Tissue Breakdown)

Amino acids released by tissue breakdown are reused for making new proteins or, if not needed for protein synthesis, are further broken down and used for other purposes. The breakdown of these amino acids yields two parts: (1) the nitrogen-containing group and (2) the remaining nonnitrogen residue, described as follows:

1. *Nitrogen group:* The nitrogen portion is split off first, a process called **deamination.** This nitrogen can be converted to ammonia and excreted in the urine or retained for use in making other nitrogen compounds.
2. *Nonnitrogen residue:* The nonnitrogen residues are called **keto acids.** They can be used to form either carbohydrates or fats. With the addition of a nitrogen group, they can form a new amino acid.

Cell enzymes and coenzymes along with hormones control tissue breakdown. In health, a dynamic equilibrium exists between anabolism and catabolism that sustains growth and maintains sound tissue.

Metabolic Interrelationships

Each of the chemical reactions in body metabolism is purposeful, and all are interdependent. They are designed to fill two essential needs: produce energy and support growth and maintenance of healthy tissue. The controlling agents necessary for these reactions to proceed in an orderly manner are the cell enzymes, their coenzymes (that often include vitamins and minerals), and special hormones. Overall, human metabolism is an exciting biochemical process designed to develop, sustain, and protect our most precious possession—life itself.

KEY TERMS

gluconeogenesis Production of glucose from keto acid carbon skeletons from deaminated amino acids and the glycerol portion of fatty acids.

glycogenolysis Specific term for conversion of glycogen into glucose in the liver; chemical process of enzymatic hydrolysis or breakdown by which this conversion is accomplished.

deamination Removal of an amino group (NH_2) from an amino acid.

keto acid Amino acid residue after deamination. The glycogenic keto acids are used to form carbohydrates.

TO SUM UP

The process of digestion breaks down food to release and convert the nutrients to simple forms that the body can use and ensures their passage across the intestinal wall and into the circulatory system for delivery to the tissues. Digestion involves two types of activities: mechanical and chemical. Muscle action breaks down food through mixing and churning motions and moves the food mass along the gastrointestinal tract. The chemical activity of gastrointestinal secretions breaks down food into smaller and smaller components for absorption. Nutrients move across the intestinal wall by the process of diffusion, facilitated diffusion, active transport, or pinocytosis. Monosaccharides and amino acids are water soluble and pass from the mucosal cells of the small intestine into the portal blood. Long-chain fatty acids must be packaged in lipid-protein complexes that enter the lymph and then pass through the thoracic duct into the general circulation. New research is helping us learn more about the important roles of intestinal bacteria and their overall contribution to gastrointestinal health. The day-to-day function of the gastrointestinal tract, often taken for granted, represents a highly coordinated and efficient body system. The breakdown products released through digestion—glucose, amino acids, and fatty acids—participate in multiple metabolic pathways under hormonal and enzymatic control that provide energy and produce substances and tissues necessary for life and well-being.

QUESTIONS FOR REVIEW

1. List the muscle types and their locations in the walls of the gastrointestinal tract. What types of motions or movements do they provide in each section of the tract? What is the role of the intramural nerve plexus in controlling gastrointestinal muscle function?
2. You are working with an older adult who suffered a stroke resulting in damage to the nerves in the swallowing center of the hypothalamus. What are the implications for his food intake and nutritional well-being?
3. Make a chart describing the chemical actions of digestion that occur in each section of the gastrointestinal tract. List across the top of the page the mouth, esophagus, stomach, small intestine, and colon. What are (a) the enzymes or fluids that act on the food mass in that location, (b) the sources of those enzymes or fluids, (c) the factors that stimulate their release, and (d) the factors that inhibit their activity?
4. Describe what happens in absorption. What are the four mechanisms by which nutrients are absorbed from the small intestine?
5. You have just eaten a lunch that included a hamburger on a whole-wheat bun, a glass of low-fat milk, and a bunch of grapes. Trace the digestion and final use of each of the macronutrients present in your lunch. What are (a) the enzymes, locations, and breakdown products formed in the complete digestion of these foods; (b) the routes taken by the breakdown products after absorption; and (c) one possible body use for each breakdown product?
6. Visit a local supermarket or drug store and examine three over-the-counter medications that claim to (a) reduce stomach acid or (b) alleviate intestinal gas. Make a table that includes each product and list the active ingredients on the product label. Visit the National Library of Medicine/National Institutes of Health *MedlinePlus* website at *www.nlm.nih.gov/medlineplus/druginformation.html* or other drug index to identify the specific actions of the active ingredients. What is the mechanism by which each active ingredient is believed to bring about the desired effect? What is the relative safety of this drug based on the possible side effects or contraindications?
7. How might long-term use of an antibiotic affect the overall function of the gastrointestinal tract? Explain.
8. Describe the complementary roles of insulin and glucagon in regulating blood glucose levels. What are the effects of these hormones over the course of a day for an individual who eats breakfast at 7:00 AM, lunch at 12:00 PM, and dinner at 6:00 PM with no snacks?

REFERENCES

1. Mason JB: Nutrition and gastroenterology: a mutually supportive partnership, *Nutr Clin Care* 7(3):91, 2004.
2. Guyton AC, Hall JE: *Textbook of medical physiology*, ed 10, Philadelphia, 2000, Saunders.
3. Klein S, Cohn SM, Alpers DH: The alimentary tract in nutrition. In Shils MA, Olson JA, Shike M, et al, editors: *Modern nutrition in health and disease*, ed 10, Baltimore, 2006, Lippincott Williams & Wilkins.
4. Duffy VB: Variation in oral sensation: implications for diet and health, *Curr Opin Gastroenterol* 23:171, 2007.
5. Hays NP, Roberts SB: The anorexia of aging in humans, *Physiol Behav* 88(3):257, 2006.
6. Avunduk C: *Manual of gastroenterology: diagnosis and therapy*, ed 4, Philadelphia, 2008, Lippincott Williams & Wilkins.
7. Modlin IM: GERD evaluation: time for a new paradigm? *J Clin Gastroenterol* 41:237, 2007.
8. American Gastroenterological Association, Institute Medical Position Panel: American Gastroenterological Association medical position statement on the management of gastroesophageal reflux disease, *Gastroenterology* 135:1383, 2008.
9. Eslick GD, Talley NJ: Gastroesophageal reflux disease (GERD): risk factors and impact on quality of life—a population-based study, *J Clin Gastroenterol* 43(2):111, 2009.

10. Avsar A, Darka Ö, Bodrumlu E, et al: Evaluation of the relationship between passive smoking and salivary electrolytes, protein, secretory IgA, sialic acid, and amylase in young children, *Arch Oral Biol* 54:457, 2009.
11. Nagler R, Dayan D: The dual role of saliva in oral carcinogenesis, *Oncology* 71(1–2):10, 2006.
12. Gonsalves WC, Wrightson AS, Henry RG: Common oral conditions in older persons, *Am Fam Phys* 78:845, 2008.
13. Harrington LK, Mayberry JF: A re-appraisal of lactose intolerance, *Int J Clin Pract* 62:1541, 2008.
14. Dubert-Ferrandon A, Newburg DS, Walker WA: Part 1, Prebiotics. New medicines for the colon, *Nutr Today* 43:245, 2008.
15. Turner NJ, Thomson BM, Shaw IC: Bioactive isoflavones in functional foods: the importance of gut microflora on bioavailability, *Nutr Rev* 61:204, 2003.
16. Bonci L: *American Dietetic Association guide to better digestion*, Hoboken, NJ, 2003, John Wiley & Sons.
17. Feinle-Bisset C, Vozzo R, Horowitz M, et al: Diet, food intake, and disturbed physiology in the pathogenesis of symptoms in functional dyspepsia, *Am J Gastroenterol* 99:170, 2004.
18. Holtmann G, Gapasin J: Failed therapy and directions for the future in dyspepsia, *Dig Dis* 26:218, 2008.
19. Beyer PL: Gastrointestinal disorders: roles of nutrition and the dietetics practitioner, *J Am Diet Assoc* 98:272, 1998.
20. Lomer MCE, Parkes GC, Sanderson JD: Review article: lactose intolerance in clinical practice—myths and realities, *Aliment Pharmacol Ther* 27:93, 2008.
21. Savaiano DA, Boushey CJ, McCabe GP: Lactose intolerance symptoms assessed by meta-analysis: a grain of truth that leads to exaggeration, *J Nutr* 136:1107, 2006.
22. Douglas LC, Sanders ME: Probiotics and prebiotics in dietetic practice, *J Am Diet Assoc* 108:510, 2008.
23. Broussard EK, Surawicz CM: Probiotics and prebiotics in clinical practice, *Nutr Clin Care* 7(3):104, 2004.
24. Scholz-Ahrens KE, Ade P, Marten B: Prebiotics, probiotics, and synbiotics affect mineral absorption, bone mineral content, and bone structure, *J Nutr* 137:838S, 2007.
25. Brown AC, Valiere A: Probiotics and medical nutrition therapy, *Nutr Clin Care* 7(2):56, 2004.
26. Boyle RJ, Robins-Browne RM, Tang MLK: Probiotic use in clinical practice: what are the risks? *Am J Clin Nutr* 83:1256, 2006.

FURTHER READINGS AND RESOURCES

Readings

Mattes RD: The chemical senses and nutrition in aging: challenging old assumptions, *J Am Diet Assoc* 102:192, 2002. *[This author tells us about the genetic factors that influence taste and their relationships to food preferences. Genetic differences in taste may influence one's preference for sweet, high-fat, or bitter foods.]*

Andrade AM, Greene GW, Melanson KJ: Eating slowly led to decreases in energy intake within meals in healthy women, *J Am Diet Assoc* 108:1186, 2008. *[This research gives us suggestions for helping individuals decrease their energy intake.]*

Melanson KJ: Food intake regulation in body weight management: a primer, *Nutr Today* 39:203, 2004. *[The growing obesity crisis worldwide has brought new attention to the internal and environmental influences that control our desire to eat and how much we eat. These researchers tell us more about what regulates our food intake.]*

Grabitske H, Slavin JL: Low-digestible carbohydrates in practice, *J Am Diet Assoc* 108:1677, 2008.

Douglas LC, Sanders ME: Probiotics and prebiotics in dietetic practice, *J Am Diet Assoc* 108:510, 2008.

Dubert-Ferrandon A, Newburg DS, Walker WA: Part 1: Prebiotics. New medicines for the colon, *Nutr Today* 43:245, 2008.

Boyle RJ, Robins-Browne RM, Tang MLK: Probiotic use in clinical practice: what are the risks? *Am J Clin Nutr* 83:1256, 2006.

[These four publications provide an overview of the uses, benefits, and risks of low-digestible plant materials and microorganisms in treating digestive disorders.]

Brown AC, Valiere A: The medicinal uses of poi, *Nutr Clin Care* 7:69, 2004. *[Poi is a tropical plant that is being used as a probiotic and provides an example of an alternative therapy in the treatment of medical conditions.]*

Bonci L: *American Dietetic Association guide to better digestion*, Hoboken, NJ, 2003, John Wiley & Sons. *[This book is a general reference on dietary interventions for digestive disorders.]*

Websites of Interest

National Institutes of Health, Information on the Digestive System; this site offers perspectives on causes and appropriate treatments of digestive medical problems: http://health.nihgov/search.asp/5.

National Institutes of Health, National Institute of Diabetes and Digestive and Kidney Diseases, Lactose Intolerance; this site offers specific information on causes and useful interventions for lactose maldigesters: http://health.nih.gov/result.asp/391/5.

National Institutes of Health, National Center for Alternative and Complementary Medicine; this site offers information on herbs sometimes recommended for digestive disorders: http://nccam.nih.gov/health/herbsataglance.htm.

CHAPTER

3

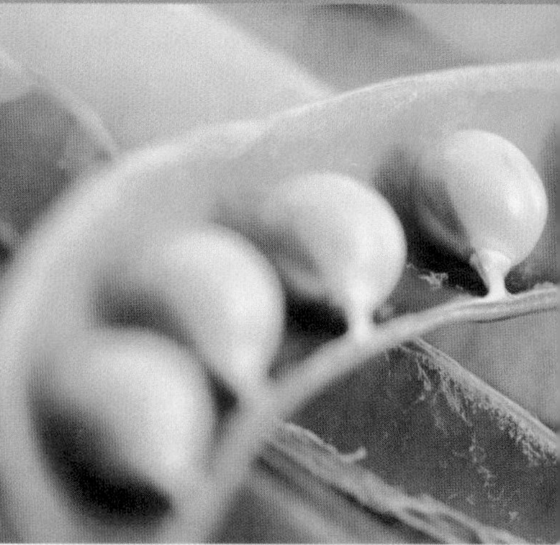

Carbohydrates

Eleanor D. Schlenker

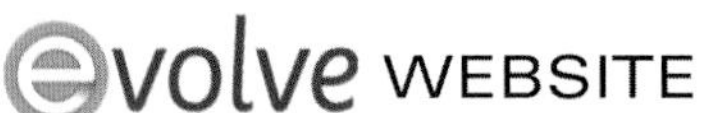

http://evolve.elsevier.com/Williams/essentials/

OUTLINE

With this chapter we begin a three-chapter sequence on the macronutrients—carbohydrates, fats, and proteins. These three nutrients share a unique characteristic, the ability to yield energy.

Carbohydrates are of prime importance in the human diet. Over the ages they have nurtured cultures throughout the world as the major source of energy to sustain work and growth. In recent years increasing attention has focused on the various forms of carbohydrate and their relationship to health and well-being. Nondigestible carbohydrates, usually referred to as fiber, cannot be broken down to provide energy but have important roles in maintaining the health of the gastrointestinal tract. In contrast, the increasing proportion of sugars in the American diet has been associated with poorer intakes of vitamins and minerals and the growing problem of obesity.

We look first at the nature of this macronutrient and then at its various functions, including that of primary body fuel.

THE NATURE OF CARBOHYDRATES

Basic Fuels: Starches and Sugars

Two forms of digestible carbohydrate occur naturally in plant foods: (1) starch and (2) sugars. Energy on planet Earth comes ultimately from the sun and its action on plants. Using their internal process of photosynthesis, plants transform the sun's energy into the stored fuel form of carbohydrate (Figure 3-1). By this process plants use carbon dioxide (CO_2) from the air and water from the soil—with the plant pigment chlorophyll as a chemical catalyst—to manufacture starch and sugars. The carbohydrates that plants store for their own energy needs become a source of fuel for humans who eat those plants. Because our bodies can rapidly break down starch and sugars, carbohydrates are often referred to as *quick energy foods.* They are our primary source of energy.

Dietary Importance

Carbohydrates comprise a major portion of the diets of people all over the world. Fruits, vegetables, cereals, grains, and dairy foods supply carbohydrate; in some countries fruits, vegetables, and grains make up 85% of the diet.[1] Rice is one of the world's most important sources of carbohydrate, feeding 3 billion people in the developing world.[2] In the typical American diet, close to one half of total kilocalories (kcalories or kcal) come from carbohydrates.[3] Carbohydrate foods are readily available, relatively low in cost, and easily stored. Compared with food items that require refrigeration or have a short shelf life, many carbohydrate foods can be kept in dry storage for fairly long periods without spoiling. Modern processing and packaging methods have extended the shelf life of carbohydrate products almost indefinitely.

CLASSIFICATION OF CARBOHYDRATES

The term *carbohydrate* comes from the chemical nature of these molecules. Carbohydrates contain the elements carbon, hydrogen, and oxygen, with the hydrogen/oxygen ratio usually that of water—CH_2O. Carbohydrates are classified according

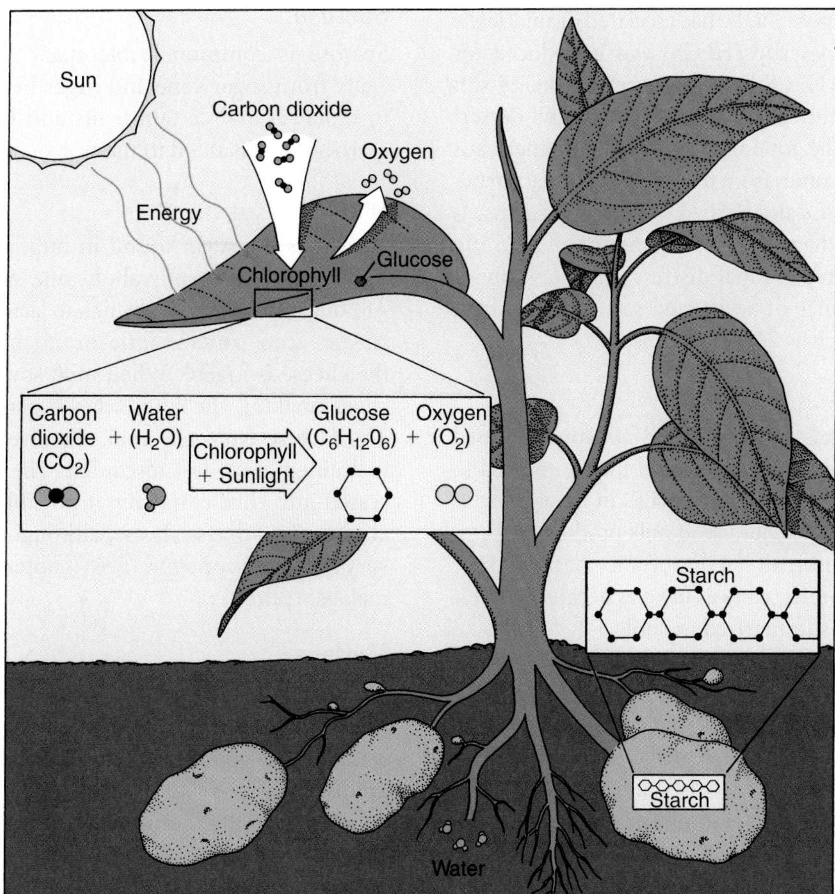

FIGURE 3-1 Photosynthesis. In the presence of sunlight and the green leaf pigment chlorophyll, green plants use water and carbon dioxide (CO_2) to produce glucose and starch by capturing the sun's energy and transforming it into chemical energy in the food products stored in their roots, stems, and leaves; through this process oxygen is returned to the atmosphere. (Courtesy Medical and Scientific Illustration.)

to the number of basic sugar or saccharide units that make up their structure. The monosaccharides and disaccharides are referred to as *simple carbohydrates* because of their relatively small size and structure. The polysaccharides, including starch and certain forms of fiber, are called *complex carbohydrates* based on their larger size and complicated structure.

Monosaccharides

The simplest form of carbohydrate is the monosaccharide, or single sugar. The three monosaccharides important in human nutrition are (1) glucose, (2) fructose, and (3) galactose.

Glucose

Glucose is a moderately sweet sugar found naturally in only a few foods, one being corn syrup. Glucose is the common body fuel oxidized by cells for energy. It is supplied to the body directly from the digestion of starch but is also obtained through the conversion of other simple sugars. Glucose (called by its older name, *dextrose,* in hospital intravenous solutions) is the form in which carbohydrates circulate in the blood.

Fructose

Fructose, the sweetest of the simple sugars, is found naturally in fruits and honey (see the *Focus on Food Safety* box,

FOCUS ON FOOD SAFETY

Honey

Honey is a natural sweetener but in fact contains no vitamins or minerals as is also true of table sugar. Honey should never be given to infants younger than 1 year old because it may contain small amounts of the bacteria spores that produce botulism, a form of food poisoning that is often fatal.

KEY TERMS

carbohydrate Compound made up of carbon, hydrogen, and oxygen; includes starches, sugars, and dietary fiber made and stored in plants; major energy source in the human diet; digestible carbohydrates yield 4 kcal/g.

photosynthesis Process by which plants containing chlorophyll are able to manufacture carbohydrate by combining CO_2 from air and water from soil with sunlight providing energy and chlorophyll as a catalyst.

$$6CO_2 + 6H_2O + \text{Energy} + \text{Chlorophyll} \Rightarrow C_6H_{12}O_6 + 6O_2$$

monosaccharide Simple sugar; a carbohydrate containing a single saccharide (sugar) unit. The most common monosaccharides are glucose, galactose, and fructose.

"Honey"); however, fructose intake has escalated dramatically since high-fructose corn syrup (HFCS) was introduced for use in food processing. HFCS is the sweetener in many soft drinks, fruit drinks, commercial baked products, and dessert mixes. About 10% of the total energy intake of Americans 2 years of age and older comes from fructose.[4] In humans fructose is converted to glucose and burned for energy. Fructose is absorbed less efficiently than glucose, and amounts of 25 to 50 g or more can cause gastrointestinal distress in some individuals.[5–6] (A 12-oz container of sweetened soft drink or fruit drink can supply as much as 22 g of fructose.[6])

Galactose

The simple sugar galactose is not found free in foods but is released in the digestion of lactose (milk sugar) and then converted to glucose in the liver. This reaction is reversible; in lactation, glucose is reconverted to galactose for use in milk production.

The physiologic and nutritional importance of the monosaccharides (sometimes referred to as *hexoses* because of their six-carbon structure) is summarized in Table 3-1.

Disaccharides

The disaccharides are double sugars made up of two monosaccharides linked together. The three disaccharides of physiologic importance are sucrose, lactose, and maltose. Their monosaccharide components are as follows:

Sucrose = one glucose + one fructose
Lactose = one glucose + one galactose
Maltose = one glucose + one glucose

Notice that glucose is found in each of the disaccharides.

TABLE 3-1 PHYSIOLOGIC AND NUTRITIONAL SIGNIFICANCE OF MONOSACCHARIDES

MONOSACCHARIDE	SOURCE	SIGNIFICANCE
D-Glucose*	Fruit juices; hydrolysis of starch, cane sugar, maltose, and lactose	Form of sugar used by the body for fuel; found in blood and tissue fluids
D-Fructose	Fruit, juices, honey; hydrolysis of sucrose from cane sugar	Changed to glucose in the liver and intestine to serve as body fuel
D-Galactose	Hydrolysis of lactose (milk sugar)	Changed to glucose in the liver to be used as body fuel; synthesized in the mammary glands to make lactose for milk; constituent of glycolipids and glycoproteins

*Monosaccharides can exist in D or L forms depending on the position of the hydroxyl group on the right (D) or left (L) side of a specific carbon. Digestive enzymes are stereospecific and act only on D sugars.

Sucrose

Sucrose is common "table sugar" and is made commercially from sugar cane and sugar beets. It is found naturally in molasses and certain fruits and vegetables (e.g., peaches, carrots) and is added to many processed foods.

Lactose

Lactose is the sugar found in milk and is the least sweet of the disaccharides, only about one sixth as sweet as sucrose. Although milk is relatively high in lactose, one of its products—cheese—can contain little or no lactose (because of how the cheese is made). When milk sours in the initial stage of cheese making, the liquid whey separates from the solid curd. The lactose from the milk dissolves into the whey, which is drained away and discarded. The remaining curd is processed into cheese, making it possible for many lactose malabsorbers to digest cheese, although particular cheeses may vary in lactose content.[7] (See Chapter 2 for a review of lactose malabsorption.)

Maltose

Maltose occurs naturally in relatively few foods but is formed in the body as an intermediate product in starch digestion. It is found in commercial malt products and germinating cereal grains.

The physiologic and nutritional significance of disaccharides is summarized in Table 3-2. Although sugars occur naturally in fruit and milk, the preponderance of sugar in the U.S. diet is added in food preparation or processing.[8] We add sugar when we pour syrup on pancakes or use table sugar to sweeten coffee, tea, or cereal. Various forms of sugar are added to pies, cakes, cookies, candy, soft drinks, fruit drinks, and breakfast cereals. Researchers from the U.S. Department of Agriculture (USDA) found that children consume about

TABLE 3-2 PHYSIOLOGIC AND NUTRITIONAL SIGNIFICANCE OF DISACCHARIDES

DISACCHARIDE	SOURCE	SIGNIFICANCE
Sucrose	Cane and beet sugar, sorghum cane, carrots, pineapples	Hydrolyzed to glucose and fructose, fuel source for cells
Lactose	Milk	Hydrolyzed to glucose and galactose, fuel source for cells, used in milk production in lactation
Maltose	Starch digestion by amylase or commercial hydrolysis; malt and germinating cereals	Hydrolyzed to glucose, fuel source for cells, can be fermented

24 tsp of added sugar every day and adults take in about 20 tsp.[9] Approximately 37% of added sugars consumed by Americans come from soft drinks; another 11% come from fruit drinks.[10] Unfortunately, the current nutrition label does not distinguish between naturally occurring and added sugars. (See Box 3-1 for examples of foods that contain sugar.)

Sugar Alcohols

Sugar alcohols (sometimes referred to as *polyols*) are other forms of carbohydrate with sweetening power. Sugar alcohols such as sorbitol, mannitol, and xylitol are found in nature but are also used in food processing. Under current labeling laws, processed foods in which sugar alcohols replace sugar can be labeled as *sugar free.* Sugar alcohols are poorly absorbed in the small intestine and add only 1.6 to 2.6 kcal/g to energy intake as compared with other sugars that add 4 kcal/g.[6] These sweeteners are used in foods such as candy, ice cream and other frozen desserts, and baked goods advertised as being artificially sweetened and lower in kcalories. They have also been used to replace sugar in products developed to meet the demand for low-carbohydrate foods by those adopting low-carbohydrate diets. Sugar alcohols are also attractive to consumers because the bacteria in the mouth that initiate dental caries do not attack them. These sweeteners offer an alternative for those with diabetes, because they do not require insulin for their metabolism; however, they do add kcalories. At high intakes, sugar alcohols can cause abdominal distress or exert a laxative effect; hence foods with these sweeteners are best used in moderation.[11]

Polysaccharides

Complex carbohydrates are called *polysaccharides* because they are made up of many (*poly*) single glucose (saccharide) units. Starch is the most important digestible polysaccharide; others are glycogen and dextrin. Nondigestible polysaccharides (discussed later in this chapter) such as cellulose provide important bulk to the diet and are categorized as dietary fiber. (Box 3-2 displays some common food sources of polysaccharides.)

Starch

Starch consists of many coiled and branching chains of single glucose units and yields only glucose on complete digestion. Cooking not only improves the flavor of starch but also softens and ruptures the starch cells, making digestion easier. Starch mixtures thicken when cooked because the substance encasing the starch granules has a gel-like quality that thickens mixtures in the same way as pectin causes jelly to set.

Resistant Starch

At one time we thought all starch was completely digested and absorbed in the small intestine. Now we know that some starch in particular foods such as whole grains, potatoes,

BOX 3-1 FOOD SOURCES OF SUGAR

Sources of Naturally Occurring Sugars*

- Orange juice
- Grape juice
- Peaches
- Apples
- Strawberries
- Grapes
- Bananas
- Fluid milk
- Powdered milk
- Some cheeses (cheeses vary in the amount of lactose they contain, depending on method of manufacture)

Sources of Added Sugars

- Pancake syrup
- Candy
- Fruit drinks
- Sports drinks
- Soft drinks
- Cookies
- Cake
- Ice cream
- Frozen desserts

*Fruit, fruit juices, and milk that contain naturally occurring sugars also supply other important nutrients; added sugars supply kcalories only.

KEY TERMS

disaccharides Class of sugars composed of two molecules of monosaccharide. The three most common disaccharides are sucrose, lactose, and maltose.

sugar alcohols Alcohol formed from a simple sugar; many sugar alcohols are used as sweetening agents by food manufacturers because they do not react with bacteria in the mouth to form dental caries; most sugar alcohols are poorly digested and absorbed and yield less than 4 kcal/g.

metabolism Sum of all the various biochemical and physiologic processes by which the body grows and maintains itself (anabolism), breaks down and reshapes tissue (catabolism), and transforms energy to do its work. Products of these various reactions are called *metabolites.*

glycogen A polysaccharide made up of many saccharide (glucose) units. Glycogen is the body storage form of carbohydrate (glucose) found mostly in the liver, with lesser amounts in the muscle.

dextrin Intermediate breakdown product in the digestion of starch.

dietary fiber Nondigestible carbohydrates and lignin found in plants; dietary fiber is eaten as an intact part of the plant in which it is found.

BOX 3-2 FOOD SOURCES OF COMPLEX CARBOHYDRATES

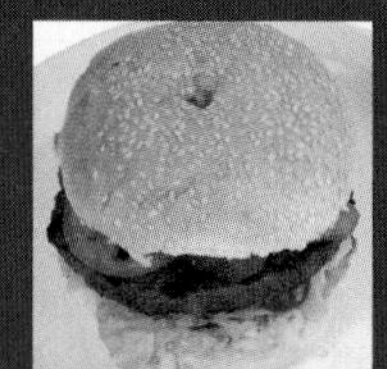
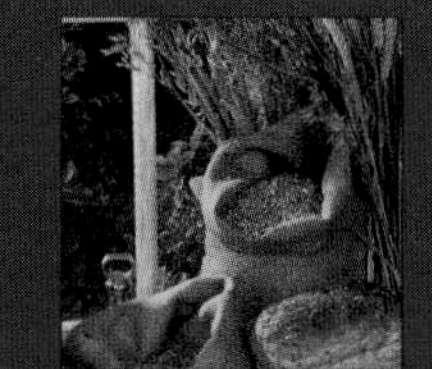
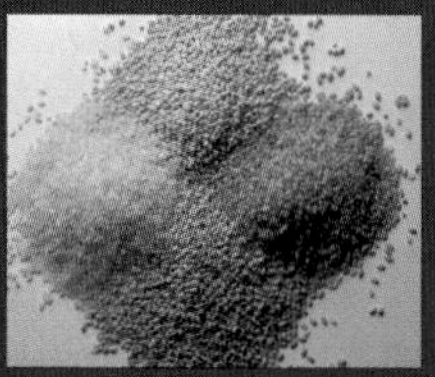
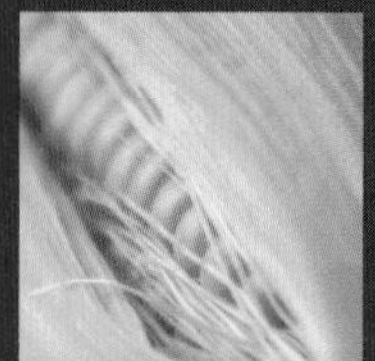
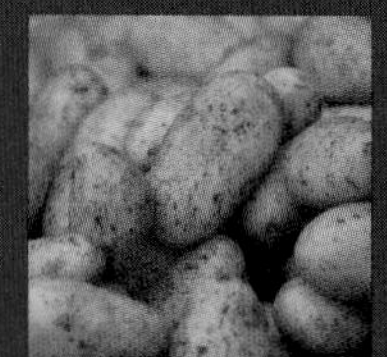
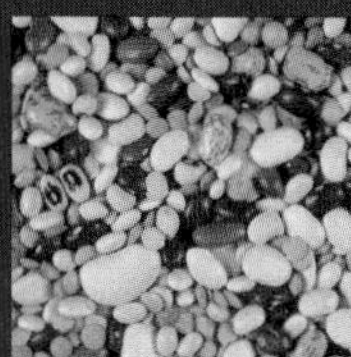

Hamburger buns
Whole wheat bread
Corn flakes
Baked potato with skin
Sweet potatoes
Corn
Peas
Oatmeal
Rice
Beans

- Grain foods such as bread, cereal, rice, and pasta; legumes; and certain vegetables such as potatoes contain large amounts of starch.
- Whole grain breads and cereals, legumes, vegetables, and whole fruits supply fiber.

bananas, and legumes escapes digestion and enters the large intestine generally intact.[12–13] This starch, called *resistant starch,* can make up as much as 8% by weight of a food high in starch.[13]

Undigested starch that moves into the colon plays an important role in health. Bacterial fermentation of resistant starch produces short-chain fatty acids such as butyric acid, the preferred energy source of the cells lining the colon. When butyric acid is not available, colonic diseases such as ulcerative colitis and colon cancer are more likely to occur.[14] Resistant starch has other health benefits similar to those of dietary fiber (discussed later). Based on its health-related properties, food researchers are looking for new ways of processing grain foods to maximize their content of resistant starch.

Glycogen

Glycogen is the storage form of carbohydrate in animals, whereas in plants it is starch. Glycogen is synthesized in liver cells and stored in small amounts in liver and muscle. Liver stores help sustain normal blood glucose levels during fasting periods such as sleep hours, and muscle glycogen provides immediate fuel for muscle action, especially during athletic activity. Athletes sometimes practice pregame "glycogen loading" to add fuel stores for athletic competition (see Chapter 14). Dietary carbohydrate is required to maintain normal glycogen stores and prevent the stress symptoms of low-carbohydrate intake—fatigue, dehydration, weakness, and light-headedness. When carbohydrate is not available in sufficient amounts, the body breaks down protein and converts the released amino acids to an energy form. A severe lack of carbohydrate to support energy needs leads to undesirable metabolic effects such as ketoacidosis (see Chapter 22).

Dextrins

Dextrins are polysaccharide compounds formed as intermediate products in the breakdown of starch (Box 3-3).

BOX 3-3 BREAKDOWN OF STARCH IN DIGESTION

Starch + Water ⇒ Soluble starch ⇒ Dextrins ⇒ Maltose ⇒ Glucose

Oligosaccharides

Oligosaccharides are small fragments of partially digested starch ranging in size from 3 to 10 glucose units. They are formed in digestion and are produced commercially by acid hydrolysis. These small starch molecules are used in special formulas for infants and others with gastrointestinal problems because they are so easy to digest. Oligosaccharides are also common in sports drinks in which they may contribute almost half of the total glucose (see Chapter 14).

Some naturally occurring oligosaccharides are formed with bonds that cannot be broken by human enzymes and therefore remain undigested. Two of these—(1) **stachyose** and (2) **raffinose**—are found in legumes such as beans, peas, and soybeans and provide a feast for bacteria in the colon, producing large amounts of gas that bring discomfort and embarrassment.

IMPORTANCE OF CARBOHYDRATES

Complex carbohydrate in the form of starch as found in vegetables, legumes, and grains should be the major dietary source of energy. On digestion, starch yields glucose—the favorite energy source of body cells. Fruit and dairy products supply energy-yielding carbohydrate in the form of natural sugars. All digestible carbohydrate supplies 4 kcal/g, making it a better choice than fat for weight management (fat supplies 9 kcal/g). Carbohydrate foods also supply other important nutrients in addition to their value as an energy source. Vegetables, legumes, fruits, and grains (especially whole grains) contain important vitamins, minerals, and fiber. Dairy products are a major source of calcium and protein in addition to other minerals and vitamins. The major food sources of starch in

PERSPECTIVES IN PRACTICE

Cutting Down on Sugar

A prudent goal for nutrition counseling is helping people reduce intake of added sugar. The MyPyramid food pattern (see Chapter 1) recommends that discretionary calories including added sugar not exceed 265 kcal on a 2000-kcal diet. The following suggestions can help lower added sugar:

- Use fresh fruit such as berries or sliced bananas or no-sugar-added applesauce rather than syrup to sweeten pancakes or waffles.
- Drink water, low-fat or skim milk, or fruit juice rather than soft drinks, fruit drinks, or sports drinks with added sugar.
- Choose fruit canned in water or juice rather than in heavy syrup.
- Select flavored yogurts, which are lower in added sugar, rather than yogurt with fruit preserves.
- When baking look for cake and cookie recipes that use fruit purees as sweeteners rather than sugar.

the current American diet are bread, potatoes, ready-to-eat cereals, pasta, and rice.[15] Nutrition educators need to encourage consumers to expand their variety of starchy vegetables to include other nutrient-rich items such as sweet potatoes and legumes. Choices of cereals, bread, and pasta should emphasize whole grains as good sources of fiber and other nutrients. In addition to their nutritional contribution, fruits add variety to the diet and can be a healthy dessert choice. Added sugars as found in processed foods supply kcalories but little else and should represent only a small fraction of carbohydrate intake. The *Dietary Guidelines Advisory Committee Report* issued in 2010 recommends that added sugar be limited to about 8 tsp (32 g or 128 kcal) or less per day.[16] (See Chapter 1 to review the *Dietary Guidelines for Americans.*) The *Perspectives in Practice* box, "Cutting Down on Sugar," offers suggestions for clients who need to lower sugar intake.

FUNCTIONS OF CARBOHYDRATES

Energy

The primary function of starches and sugars is to supply energy to cells, especially brain cells that depend on glucose. When carbohydrate is lacking, fats can be used as an energy source by most organ systems; however, to function most efficiently body tissues require a constant supply of glucose.

Body stores of carbohydrate are relatively small but still serve as an important energy reserve. An adult man has about 300 to 350 g of carbohydrate stored in his liver and muscle in the form of glycogen, and another 10 g of glucose is circulating in his blood (Table 3-3). Together, this glycogen and glucose will supply the energy for only a half day of moderate activity. To meet the body's constant demand, carbohydrate foods must be eaten regularly and at reasonably frequent intervals.

Special Functions

Carbohydrates have other specialized roles in overall body metabolism.

TABLE 3-3 CARBOHYDRATE STORAGE IN AN ADULT MAN (70 kg [154 lb])

	GLYCOGEN (in g)	GLUCOSE (in g)
Liver	72	
Muscles	245	
Extracellular fluids		10
Component totals	317	10
TOTAL STORAGE	327	

Glycogen—Carbohydrate Storage

Liver and muscle glycogen are in constant interchange with the body's overall energy system. These energy reserves protect cells, especially brain cells, from depressed metabolic function and injury and support urgent muscle responses.

Protein-Sparing Action

Carbohydrates help regulate protein metabolism. An adequate supply of carbohydrate to satisfy ongoing energy demands prevents the channeling of protein for energy. This protein-sparing action of carbohydrate allows protein to be reserved for tissue building and repair.

Antiketogenic Effect

Carbohydrates influence fat metabolism. The supply of carbohydrate determines how much fat must be broken down to meet energy needs, thereby controlling the formation and disposal of *ketones.* Ketones are intermediate products of fat metabolism that normally are produced in only small amounts as fats are oxidized. However, under extreme conditions when available carbohydrate is inadequate to meet energy needs, as in starvation or uncontrolled diabetes or on very low-carbohydrate diets, fat is oxidized at excessive rates. Sufficient amounts of dietary carbohydrates prevent any damaging excess of ketones.

Heart Action

Heart action is a life-sustaining muscular exercise. Although fatty acids are the preferred fuel for the heart, the glycogen stored in cardiac muscle is an important emergency source of contractile energy.

KEY TERMS

oligosaccharides Intermediate products of polysaccharide digestion that contain from 3 to 10 glucose units.

stachyose A colorless crystalline tetrasaccharide that cannot be broken down by human enzymes; stachyose is found in legumes and in the intestine and is fermented by bacteria, producing the gas associated with eating these foods.

raffinose A colorless crystalline trisaccharide composed of galactose and sucrose joined by bonds that human enzymes cannot break; raffinose is found in legumes and in the intestine and is fermented by bacteria, producing the gas associated with eating these foods.

FOCUS ON CULTURE

Cross-Cultural Competence: A Goal for the Health Professional

Consider the following situations:

- You are counseling pregnant mothers in a public health clinic and using MyPyramid to evaluate their food intake. A Hmong (Vietnamese) mother tells you that she never eats bread, and you express concern about her servings from the grains group.
- You are working with an older African-American man, and he mentions that his favorite meal is his daughter's homemade Brunswick stew. What foods are included?

As a nation we are becoming increasingly diverse. In another 10 to 15 years, one of every three Americans will be African American, Hispanic American, Asian American, Hmong American, Native American, or Pacific Islander American. To be effective educators we need to understand the food patterns of different ethnic, racial, and cultural groups, not just our own. We must acknowledge the health beliefs and values that influence an individual's food choices and nutritional status. The Hmong mother may not eat bread, but she is likely to have rice at every meal and more than meet her recommended servings of grains. However, she may be reluctant to take the vitamin and mineral supplements her physician recommended in the belief that they will cause her to have a large infant and difficult delivery. The African-American man obtains important vitamins, minerals, fiber, and protein from his Brunswick stew made with chicken, carrots, tomatoes, white beans, and greens.

Value Diversity

Our population includes people from different countries and cultures who have different customs. At one time we referred to our society as a *melting pot,* with newcomers expected to blend their customs and beliefs with the mainstream culture. Health care providers often imposed their beliefs and values on patients from other ethnic or cultural backgrounds. Today we strive to be a "salad bowl," with each person adding a special quality to the mix. Individual differences are important and enhance the lives of us all. As health professionals we must respect different customs and beliefs and provide counseling and support consistent with the values of the people we are helping.

Cross-Cultural Situations

Throughout our professional lives we will continue to experience cross-cultural situations in which we belong to a different race, culture, or ethnic group than our supervisors, our colleagues, or the individuals for whom we provide care.

We can begin to develop cross-cultural competence in various ways, as follows:

- *Learn about other cultures by reading, observing, and sharing experiences.* A potluck meal provides an opportunity to share foods and the cultural aspects surrounding food choices.

Central Nervous System

The brain and central nervous system (CNS) depend on carbohydrate for energy but have very low carbohydrate reserves—enough to last only 10 to 15 minutes. This makes them especially dependent on a minute-to-minute supply of glucose from the blood. Sustained *hypoglycemic* shock causes irreversible brain damage. Providing an adequate morning supply of glucose for brain function may help to explain why individuals who eat breakfast do better in school than those who skip breakfast.[17] Glucose increases the synthesis of acetylcholine, a neurotransmitter that acts on areas of the brain responsible for memory and cognitive function.[18]

RECOMMENDED INTAKE OF CARBOHYDRATES

Dietary Reference Intakes

The Recommended Dietary Allowance (RDA) for carbohydrate is the same for everyone older than 1 year. Children, adolescents, and adults need a minimum of 130 g/day,[14] the amount needed to supply the energy demands of the CNS for 1 day. Most people consume more than the minimum amount of carbohydrate to meet their overall energy requirement and keep fat and protein intakes at acceptable levels.

Acceptable Macronutrient Distribution Range

A diet rich in plant-based foods supplies important nutrients and fiber, but it is unwise to take in excessive amounts of carbohydrate, just as it is not prudent to severely limit carbohydrate. To provide guidance for developing dietary patterns, nutrition experts established the Acceptable Macronutrient Distribution Ranges (AMDRs) (Box 3-4) for allocating macronutrient intake as a proportion of total kcalorie intake. The adult AMDR for carbohydrate is 45% to 65% of total energy intake, with no more than 25% from added sugar.[14] This range allows for differences in cultural or ethnic food patterns or particular health needs. The AMDRs enable us to individualize diets to meet specific situations and encourage sound nutrition practices.

As we help persons make positive food choices for health and well-being, we need to consider their accustomed food patterns and recommend appropriate foods that are familiar to them. The *Focus on Culture* box, "Cross-Cultural Competence: A Goal for the Health Professional," presents some ideas on how to work effectively with individuals whose dietary patterns may differ from our own.

BOX 3-4 ACCEPTABLE MACRONUTRIENT DISTRIBUTION RANGES

Carbohydrate: 45% to 65% of total kcalories
Fat: 20% to 35% of total kcalories
Protein: 10% to 35% of total kcalories

Data from Institute of Medicine, National Academy of Sciences: *Dietary (DRI) reference intakes. The essential guide to nutrient requirements,* Washington, DC, 2006, National Academies Press.

FOCUS ON CULTURE

Cross-Cultural Competence: A Goal for the Health Professional—cont'd

- *Examine your own beliefs and feelings about other cultures.* Identify and resolve any stereotypes that you may hold about groups other than your own.
- *Assess how other cultures view you, and make an effort to present yourself in a positive light.* Develop verbal and nonverbal communication skills applicable to various cultural groups.
- *Value the differences among people.* Do away with the attitude that your way is best.
- *Consider language training as a means of preparing yourself to work with diverse population groups.* It is difficult to counsel through an interpreter who may not understand the implications of a particular food or food custom.

BIBLIOGRAPHY

Curry KR: Multicultural competence in dietetics and nutrition, *J Am Diet Assoc* 100:1142, 2000.

Diabetes Care and Education Dietetic Practice Group, Goody CM, Drago L, editors: *Cultural food practices*, Chicago, 2010, American Dietetic Association.

Kittler PG, Sucher KP: *Food and culture*, ed 4, Belmont, Calif, 2004, Brooks/Cole, a division of Thomson Learning.

McCaffree J: Language: a crucial part of cultural competency, *J Am Diet Assoc* 108:611, 2008.

OTHER RESOURCES

Diabetes Care and Education Dietetic Practice Group of the American Dietetic Association: *Ethnic and regional food practices: a series. Alaska native food practices, customs, and holidays*, Chicago/Alexandria, Va, 1998, American Dietetic Association/American Diabetes Association.

Diabetes Care and Education Dietetic Practice Group of the American Dietetic Association: *Ethnic and regional food practices: a series. Chinese American food practices, customs, and holidays*, Chicago/Alexandria, Va, 1998, American Dietetic Association/American Diabetes Association.

Diabetes Care and Education Dietetic Practice Group of the American Dietetic Association: *Ethnic and regional food practices: a series. Filipino American food practices, customs, and holidays*, Chicago/Alexandria, Va, 1994, American Dietetic Association/American Diabetes Association.

Diabetes Care and Education Dietetic Practice Group of the American Dietetic Association: *Ethnic and regional food practices: a series. Hmong American food practices, customs, and holidays*, Chicago/Alexandria, Va, 1999, American Dietetic Association/American Diabetes Association.

Diabetes Care and Education Dietetic Practice Group of the American Dietetic Association: *Ethnic and regional food practices: a series. Indian and Pakistani food practices, customs, and holidays*, ed 2, Chicago/Alexandria, Va, 2000, American Dietetic Association/American Diabetes Association.

Diabetes Care and Education Dietetic Practice Group of the American Dietetic Association: *Ethnic and regional food practices: a series. Jewish food practices, customs, and holidays*, Chicago/Alexandria, Va, 1998, American Dietetic Association/American Diabetes Association.

Diabetes Care and Education Dietetic Practice Group of the American Dietetic Association: *Ethnic and regional food practices: a series. Mexican American food practices, customs, and holidays*, Chicago/Alexandria, Va, 1998, American Dietetic Association/American Diabetes Association.

Diabetes Care and Education Dietetic Practice Group of the American Dietetic Association: *Ethnic and regional food practices: a series. Navajo food practices, customs, and holidays*, Chicago/Alexandria, Va, 1998, American Dietetic Association/American Diabetes Association.

Diabetes Care and Education Dietetic Practice Group of the American Dietetic Association: *Ethnic and regional food practices: a series. Soul and traditional southern food practices, customs, and holidays*, Chicago/Alexandria, Va, 1995, American Dietetic Association/American Diabetes Association.

Nonnutritive Sweeteners

Most of us have an inborn desire for foods that are sweet; however, we are faced with the dilemma of moderating our energy intakes to maintain a healthy weight. **Nonnutritive sweeteners** allow us to indulge our taste for sweets while limiting our kcalorie intake. Sweeteners are grouped as *nutritive* or *nonnutritive* depending on the kcalories they contain. Sucrose (table sugar) and other natural sugars yield 4 kcal/g. Nonnutritive sweeteners yield no energy or an insignificant amount of energy.[6] Because of their intense sweetening power, very small amounts are needed to produce the desired level of sweetness.

The U.S. Food and Drug Administration (FDA) has approved six nonnutritive sweeteners for use in the United States. They sweeten beverages, baked products, soft drinks, fruit drinks, and candy marketed as low or reduced calorie, and some are available for use in homemade products. The nonnutritive sweetener aspartame contains the amino acid phenylalanine, and aspartame-containing products must carry a label indicating that phenylalanine is present.[6] This protects persons with phenylketonuria, who lack the enzyme needed to metabolize phenylalanine and must eliminate it from their diets. Table 3-4 reviews the properties of nonnutritive sweeteners currently in use.

The two nonnutritive sweeteners most recently approved by the FDA are sucralose, marketed under the trade name of Splenda, and stevia. Sucralose is 600 times sweeter than sucrose and adds virtually no kcalories to food. Only 3.8 oz of sucralose has the sweetening power of 2 lb of sugar.[6] Sucralose

KEY TERMS

nonnutritive sweeteners Substances with sweetening power that are not efficiently absorbed by the body or cannot be metabolized to provide energy; these substances are used in small amounts, and the kcalories added to the food product are negligible.

EVIDENCE-BASED PRACTICE BOX

Do Nonnutritive Sweeteners Help You Lose Weight?

Since FDA first approved aspartame and acesulfame K as food additives in the early 1980s, the use of nonnutritive sweeteners has skyrocketed, with close to 90% of U.S. consumers reporting use of reduced-calorie products. With the growing prevalence of obesity among both children and adults and the high consumption of added sugar (these two trends do not necessarily reflect cause and effect), nonnutritive sweeteners that satisfy the palate without adding extra kcalories would seem to be a welcome alternative; however, the benefits associated with these products are still unclear. Although it might be expected that use of nonnutritive sweeteners would promote weight loss or at the very least reduce weight gain, experts on taste suggest that such intense sweeteners create neural responses that increase appetite and food intake. Existing evidence provides only limited support for either point of view.

Evaluations of body mass index (BMI) in users of nonnutritive sweeteners have been few. Over the short term of several weeks or months, results have been mixed; some individuals lost weight, whereas others gained weight. Persons with increased BMIs are more likely to use nonnutritive sweeteners, possibly in an effort to prevent further weight gain or bring about some degree of weight loss. Individuals of average weight may use nonnutritive sweetened foods to avoid gaining weight. For someone who consumes two 12-oz cans of sugar-sweetened carbonated beverages each day at a cost of 300 kcal (150 kcal/can), substitution of a calorie-free beverage could result in the loss of about 1 lb every 2 weeks. However, studies suggest that kcalories saved with use of calorie-free foods or beverages are often used to add other foods to the diet or enjoy larger portions of foods usually eaten. Unless the use of nonnutritive sweetened foods lowers overall kcalorie intake, weight loss will not occur; in several short term studies, overcompensation resulted in actual weight gain.

At present no compelling evidence indicates nonnutritive sweeteners increase food intake by an effect on appetite. On the other hand, sugar-sweetened foods are known to increase appetite, adding further to kcalorie intake.

How can health professionals use these findings?

TABLE 3-4 PROPERTIES AND APPLICATIONS OF COMMON NONNUTRITIVE SWEETENERS

NAME	SWEETENING POWER (COMPARED WITH SUCROSE)	EFFECT OF HEAT	TRADE NAMES	APPLICATIONS
Aspartame	160–220 times sweeter	Decomposes with high heat and loses sweetening power	NutraSweet, Equal, Sugar Twin (blue box)	Beverages, table sweetener, gelatin, pudding, chewing gum, cold breakfast cereal
Acesulfame-K	200 times sweeter	Not affected by heat	Sweet One, Sweet & Safe	Beverages, table sweetener, baked goods, all-purpose sweetener
Saccharin	200–700 times sweeter	Not affected by heat	Sweet'N Low, Sweet Twin, Necta Sweet, Sweet'N Low Brown	Beverages, table sweetener, chewing gum, baked goods, pudding
Sucralose	600 times sweeter	Not affected by heat	Splenda	Beverages, desserts, baked goods, candy, table sweetener, all-purpose sweetener
Neotame	8000 times sweeter	Not affected by heat	Neotame (not widely used in the United States)	Beverages, table sweetener, frozen desserts, chewing gum, candy, baked goods, sauces, cereals
Stevia	300 times sweeter	Not affected by heat	Truvia, Rebiana, PureVia, SweetLeaf	Beverages, table sweetener

Data from American Dietetic Association: Position of the American Dietetic Association: use of nutritive and nonnutritive sweeteners, *J Am Diet Assoc* 104:255, 2004; U.S. Food and Drug Administration: *2002 Approvals: food and color additive final rules, Washington, DC, Updated 2009.* Retrieved April 22, 2010 from www.fda.gov/Food/FoodIngredientsPackaging/FoodAdditives/ucm063065.htm; Voiland A: The zero-calorie sweetener stevia arrives, *U.S. News and World Report* website. Retrieved December 16, 2008, from www.usnews.com/health/family-health/articles/2008/07/28/the-zero-calorie-sweetener-stevia-arrives.html.

is poorly absorbed (only about 15% is absorbed). What is absorbed is excreted in the urine unchanged.[19] Because sucralose is heat stable and available in granular form, it has application for both commercial and home-prepared desserts. Stevia, extracted from a South American plant, was sold as a dietary supplement before being approved by FDA for use as a food additive. Yielding almost no kcalories, stevia is being marketed as a natural sweetener as compared with other nonnutritive sweeteners currently used in food processing.[20] (For a review of the current findings on this topic, see the *Evidence-Based Practice* box, "Do Nonnutritive Sweeteners Help You Lose Weight?")

EVIDENCE-BASED PRACTICE BOX

Do Nonnutritive Sweeteners Help You Lose Weight?—cont'd

- Recognize that use of nonnutritive sweeteners can assist in weight management, but for any benefit, overall kcalorie intake must be reduced. Kcalories "saved" on calorie-free foods cannot be added back in another form.
- Substitute calorie-free beverages for beverages high in kcalories. For persons who enjoy sweet drinks throughout the day, nonnutritive sweetened beverages will lower kcalorie intake and reduce the risk of dental caries. (A good transition may be one calorie-free sweetened beverage followed by one bottle of water.)
- Practice moderation. Include sweet items occasionally in the context of the total diet but emphasize nutrient-dense foods.
- Read food labels to evaluate content of added sugars, naturally occurring sugars, and nonnutritive sweeteners.

BIBLIOGRAPHY

American Dietetic Association: Position of the American Dietetic Association: use of nutritive and nonnutritive sweeteners, *J Am Diet Assoc* 104:255, 2004.

Bellisle F, Drewnowski A: Intense sweeteners, energy intake, and the control of body weight, *Eur J Clin Nutr* 61:691, 2007.

Mattes RD, Popkin BM: Nonnutritive sweetener consumption in humans: effects on appetite and food intake and their putative mechanisms, *Am J Clin Nutr* 89:1, 2009.

Vermunt SH, Pasman WJ, Schaafsma G, et al: Effects of sugar intake on body weight. A review, *Obes Rev* 4:91, 2003.

CARBOHYDRATES AND ORAL HEALTH

Oral health and nutrition have a synergistic relationship that goes in both directions. Malnutrition and nutrition-related diseases lead to deterioration of the teeth and supporting tissues of the mouth and gums, such that eating becomes difficult and nutrient intake is further compromised. Alternatively, infectious diseases of the mouth such as untreated and progressive periodontal disease result in systemic infections, worsen glucose control in diabetes, and increase inflammatory responses and cardiovascular risk.[21]

Dental caries is one of the most frequently occurring and preventable infectious diseases of the oral cavity and a major cause of tooth loss.[22] Oral hygiene, diet, and specific nutrients have been related to dental caries. Lack of exposure to fluoride in the form of fluoridated water or fluoride treatments results in tooth enamel that is less resistant to bacterial action and decay. Comparisons of individuals living in areas of fluoridation or nonfluoridation indicate an 18% difference in prevalence of dental caries.[23]

The amounts and types of carbohydrate in the diet and the conditions under which they are eaten influence the development of dental caries. Bacteria in the dental plaque ferment sugars (whether naturally occurring or added) and short-chain starch molecules to form acid. The resulting drop in pH favors the action of the streptococci strain of bacteria that initiates dental caries (Figure 3-2). Children and adolescents consuming increased amounts of added sugar have increased incidences of dental caries. Although naturally occurring sugars in fruit can also lead to tooth decay, citrus fruits with a high proportion of water, as well as other fruits containing citric acid that stimulates salivary secretion, rinse the teeth and help remove sugars from the surface of the enamel. The period of exposure to a sweet solution also affects its cariogenic potential. Continuous sipping of a sugar-sweetened soft drink, sports drink, or fruit drink throughout the day increases risk of tooth decay.

Finally, prevention of dental caries may be yet another reason to choose whole grain breads and cereals over highly processed and sugar-added grain foods. Unprocessed starch as a large molecule cannot pass through the dental plaque to attack the enamel, whereas shorter-chain oligosaccharides are easily broken down by salivary amylase to yield maltose—a choice substrate for plaque bacteria. Grain-sugar mixtures such as ready-to-eat breakfast cereals, cakes, and pastries, are especially cariogenic.[22]

Chronic disease increases an individual's vulnerability to dental caries and tooth loss. Age-related loss of calcium from the bones (or the more drastic bone loss occurring inosteoporosis) affects the alveolar bone, resulting in tooth loss. A reduction in salivary secretion associated with diabetes mellitus or particular prescription medications accelerates both tooth decay and damage to oral tissues.

IMBALANCES IN CARBOHYDRATE INTAKE

High-Carbohydrate Diets

The AMDR recommends that carbohydrate provide 45% to 65% of total energy;[14] however, individuals have adopted diets as high as 75% carbohydrate with the intent of lowering their intakes of fat and kcalories or achieving reductions in blood lipoproteins. When carbohydrate intake reaches 65% or more of total kcalories, fat intake may be disproportionately low, jeopardizing intakes of the essential fatty acids and vitamins and minerals associated with higher-fat foods. Such increases in dietary carbohydrate can trigger a rise in plasma triglycerides and low-density lipoprotein (LDL) cholesterol and a drop in high-density lipoprotein (HDL) cholesterol, increasing

KEY TERMS

cariogenic Promotes the development of dental caries or tooth decay.

low-density lipoprotein (LDL) cholesterol LDL cholesterol is a lipoprotein produced in the liver and transports fatty acids and cholesterol to the cells and tissues; this lipoprotein contains a high proportion of cholesterol, and inappropriately high blood levels increase the risk of heart disease.

high-density lipoprotein (HDL) cholesterol HDL cholesterol is a lipoprotein produced in the liver that carries cholesterol from the tissues back to the liver for degradation and elimination; appropriate blood levels of HDL cholesterol reduce the risk of heart disease.

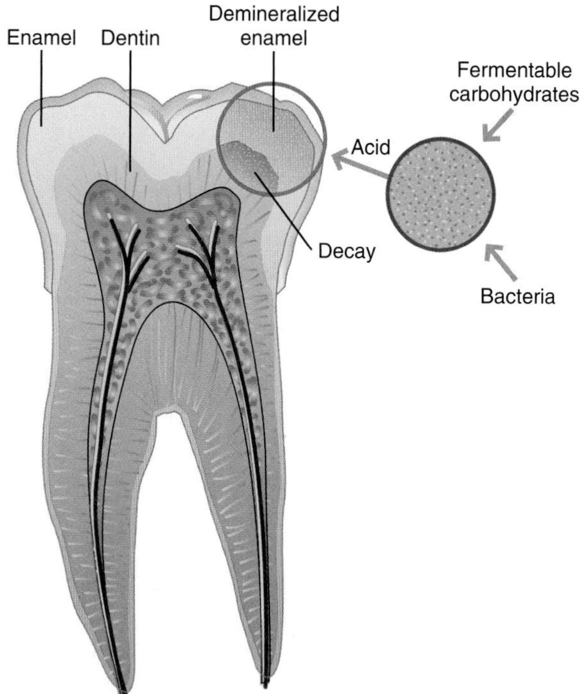

FIGURE 3-2 Dental caries can result from poor dental hygiene and continuous snacking and drinking of items high in added sugar or other refined carbohydrates. (From Mahan LK, Escott-Stump S: *Krause's food and nutrition therapy,* ed 12, St Louis, 2008, Saunders.)

cardiovascular risk.[14,24] Excessive carbohydrate intake, depending on the type of carbohydrate, causes rapid elevations in blood glucose, putting heavy demands on the beta cells of the pancreas for insulin production and release. Whole grain foods, legumes, or fruits and vegetables high in fiber rather than added sugars or other rapidly digested carbohydrates are better choices when increasing carbohydrate intake.[25]

Low-Carbohydrate Diets

Diets very low in carbohydrate have been popularized as efficient ways to lose weight. Such diets may restrict carbohydrate intake to 20% or less of total kcalories. These regimens result in weight loss over the short term *if* energy intake is sufficiently reduced; however, questions remain as to their appropriateness when extended for weeks or months.[26] Diets very low in carbohydrate are unlikely to contain the minimum daily servings of fruits, vegetables, and whole grains recommended by MyPyramid.[27] These plant-based carbohydrate foods supply health-promoting nutrients and fiber and assist in controlling blood pressure.[28] Low-carbohydrate diets often replace carbohydrate foods with high-fat foods and may provide as much as 46% of total kcalories as fat, adding to cardiovascular risk.[29] Low-carbohydrate diets that replace carbohydrate with protein exceeding AMDR levels increase the burden on the kidneys.

When comparing weight loss and related metabolic changes among individuals observing either low-carbohydrate diets (20% to 41% carbohydrate) or high-carbohydrate diets (20% to 63% carbohydrate) for at least 1 year, those observing the low-carbohydrate regimens lost the most weight, although weight loss was moderate (4.7 to 5.5 kg).[30-31] Despite their increased intakes of fat, the low-carbohydrate groups had improved serum triglyceride levels, HDL cholesterol levels, and systolic blood pressures. The increased amounts of protein included in the low-carbohydrate diets may have helped those individuals lower their energy intake because protein helps promote satiety. The apparent safety and effectiveness of low-carbohydrate diets with appropriate medical supervision reinforces the advantages of more than one dietary approach to weight loss adapted to individual preferences and metabolic needs.[31] Regardless, establishing a kcalorie deficit between energy intake and energy expenditure using a combination of foods that support nutritional well-being is the cornerstone of long-term weight management and health.

FIBER—THE NONDIGESTIBLE CARBOHYDRATE

Fiber is the nondigestible material found in whole grain cereals, fruits, vegetables, and legumes that our grandmothers referred to as *roughage.* Because humans lack the enzymes necessary to break down these complex carbohydrates into forms that can be absorbed, they travel the length of the gastrointestinal tract and are eliminated in the feces. Fiber's ability to promote regular bowel function has been recognized for generations. All types of fiber are beneficial to health, but different fibers have different physiologic effects; therefore we need a variety of foods supplying different types of fiber. Although most foods as found in nature contain more than one type of fiber, they likely have more of one type than they do of another.

At one time, fibers were classified as *soluble* or *insoluble,* based on their chemical properties in the laboratory that were believed to influence their behavior in the body as well. Now we know that characteristics of fiber other than solubility influence its role in the body, although these designations are still used on food labels.[32]

Two general categories of fiber exist: (1) dietary fiber and (2) functional fiber.[14]

Dietary Fiber

Dietary fiber includes the nondigestible carbohydrates and lignin that are intact in plant foods. Several dietary fibers important in human nutrition are described as follows:

- *Cellulose:* Cellulose is the material in plant cell walls that provides structure. We find it in the stems and leaves of vegetables, in the coverings of seeds and grains, and in skins and hulls. Because humans are unable to break down cellulose, it remains in the digestive tract and contributes bulk to the food mass.
- *Hemicellulose:* This polysaccharide is found in plant cell walls and often surrounds cellulose. Some hemicelluloses help regulate colon pressure by providing bulk for normal muscle action, whereas others are fermented by colonic bacteria.
- *Lignin:* Lignin is the only dietary fiber that is not a carbohydrate. It is a large molecule that forms the woody part

BOX 3-5 SOURCES OF DIETARY FIBER

Pectin, β-Glucans, Gums	Cellulose, Hemicellulose, Lignin
Oatmeal	Whole wheat bread
Oranges	Popcorn
Kidney beans	Baked beans
Carrots	Bananas
Apples	Pears

of plants and in the intestine combines with bile acids and prevents their reabsorption. Lignin contributes the sandy texture to pears and lima beans.

- *Pectin:* This fiber is found in plant cell walls. It forms a viscous, sticky gel that binds cholesterol and prevents its absorption. Pectin also helps to slow gastric emptying and extend feelings of satiety.
- *Gums:* Plants secrete gums in response to plant injury. In the intestine, gums bind cholesterol and prevent its absorption. Bacteria in the colon also ferment gums to form short-chain fatty acids that nourish colonic cells (this action was noted earlier for resistant starch).
- *β-Glucans:* These water-soluble fibers are found in oats and oat bran, foods that carry a health claim on the label indicating they can reduce the risk of heart disease. (β-Glucans interfere with the absorption of cholesterol.)

Box 3-5 gives examples of foods providing specific varieties of fiber.

Functional Fiber

Functional fibers are nondigestible polysaccharides that have been added to a food to increase its fiber content.[14] The term *functional fiber* is used to distinguish those fibers that are added to foods from those that are intact in plants and eaten in that form. Functional fibers can be isolated from plant foods or manufactured and are used as dietary supplements or added to processed foods to improve their nutritional quality. A particular fiber can be either a dietary fiber or a functional fiber depending on how it is eaten or used. The pectin in the apple you ate at lunch is considered a dietary fiber. On the other hand, pectin that was isolated from fruit sources and added to homemade or commercial jellies or used as a fiber ingredient in patient tube feedings is classed as a *functional fiber.*[33] Functional fibers added in food processing must be listed on the food label. Flaxseed and psyllium are two common functional fibers.

A person's **total fiber** intake includes both dietary and functional fiber. Food sources of dietary fiber and their energy content are listed in Table 3-5. Note that many foods high in fiber are low to moderate in kcalories.

TABLE 3-5 DIETARY FIBER AND ENERGY CONTENT OF SELECTED FOODS

FOOD GROUP	SERVING SIZE	DIETARY FIBER (in g)	ENERGY (in kcal)
Grains Group			
All bran	¾ cup	8.5	70
Bran buds	⅓ cup	7.9	75
Oatmeal	1 cup	2.5	144
Air-popped popcorn	1 cup	2.2	25
Whole wheat bread	1 slice	1.4	60
Vegetable Group			
Kidney beans	½ cup	7.3	110
Green peas	½ cup	3.6	55
Corn	½ cup	2.9	70
Potato, with skin	1 medium	2.5	95
Carrots	½ cup	2.3	25
Broccoli	½ cup	2.2	20
Lettuce, fresh	1 cup	0.8	7
Fruit Group			
Apple	1 medium	3.5	80
Raisins	¼ cup	3.1	110
Strawberries	1 cup	3.0	45
Orange	1 medium	2.6	60
Banana	1 medium	2.4	105

Nutrient data from USDA: *USDA National Nutrient Database for Standard Reference, Release 21,* Washington, DC, U.S. Department of Agriculture, 2009. Retrieved April 23, 2010 from www.ars.usda.gov/Services/docs.htm?docid=17477.

KEY TERMS

functional fiber Nondigestible carbohydrates isolated from plant foods or manufactured and added to foods to increase their fiber content.

total fiber Dietary fiber plus functional fiber; the total amount of fiber in an individual's diet from all sources.

HEALTH PROMOTION

Health Benefits of Fiber

Dietary fiber influences the food mix in the gastrointestinal tract and gastrointestinal function. Fiber helps promote satiety and is linked to lower body weights.[34] Populations that eat increased amounts of dietary fiber have less chronic disease. Fiber promotes appropriate gastrointestinal function and acts favorably on risk factors for various chronic conditions as follows:

- *Increases fecal mass and promotes laxation:* The capacity of dietary fibers to hold water and bacteria creates its bulk-forming and laxative effects. This added mass helps the food bolus move more rapidly through the small intestine, promoting normal bowel action and preventing or alleviating constipation. Dietary fiber has also been effective in treating diarrhea.[32] A larger food mass in the colon averts the development of diverticula, small pouches that protrude outward through the lining of the colon. When the food residue entering the colon is low in bulk, the muscles must contract more forcefully to move it forward, which over time contributes to the formation of diverticula with future risk of inflammation and infection.
- *Binds bile acids and cholesterol:* Fibers can lower blood cholesterol levels through their ability to bind both cholesterol and bile acids. When cholesterol is bound to fiber, it is not absorbed and is eliminated in the feces. Certain fibers also bind bile salts and prevent their reabsorption. When bile acids are lost, cholesterol must be removed from circulating blood lipoproteins to synthesize their replacements, with a resulting decrease in blood cholesterol levels.[32]
- *Promotes growth of beneficial colonic microflora:* Bacteria living in the colon ferment dietary fiber along with resistant starch. This action produces short-chain fatty acids that nourish the cells lining the colon and stimulate their growth.[14] Fiber has a positive effect on the growth of *Bifidobacterium* in the colon (see the discussion of prebiotic agents in Chapter 2) and has been used in the treatment of irritable bowel syndrome.
- *Slows rise in blood glucose and insulin levels:* Foods rich in fiber have a low glycemic index, meaning their glucose content is released slowly into the blood, preventing a rapid rise in blood glucose after eating. This blunting of blood glucose levels lessens the amount of insulin needed to move this glucose into muscle and fat cells, thereby reducing the work of the beta cells of the pancreas. Fiber intake at currently recommended levels assists in management of diabetes.[35]

Although we know that dietary fiber performs actions that support health, the research evidence associating fiber intake and chronic disease risk remains inconsistent. Large population studies suggest that mortality rates from cardiovascular disease and deaths from all causes are lower among persons who eat more fiber,[36] but this finding appears to relate to specific types of fiber.[37] Total fiber intake does not seem to protect against colorectal cancer, although increased use of whole grain cereals is associated with lower risk.[38] It may be that other dietary components associated with fiber—particular nutrients or phytochemicals—rather than the fiber itself confer resistance to chronic disease (we will discuss this again in our review of functional foods). The ability of fiber to slow gastric emptying and extend feelings of satiety may be helpful for weight loss.[32] In a national survey, individuals consuming more fiber in the form of beans had lower body weights and lower waist circumferences.[39]

Recommended Fiber Intake

The Adequate Intake (AI) for total fiber is based on the amount expected to lower the risk of coronary heart disease and type 2 diabetes. Men younger than 51 years old should consume 38 g/day; those age 51 and older need 30 g/day. The AIs for younger and older women are 25 g/day and 21 g/day, respectively.[14] Unfortunately, directives to consumers are inconsistent, because the nutrition label recommends a daily fiber intake of 25 g in a 2000-kcal diet, considerably lower than the current AI for men.

Fiber intake in the United States is barely half the Dietary Reference Intake (DRI). Median daily intake ranges from 16 to 18 g/day for men and 12 to 14 g/day for women.[14] The MyPyramid goal of 4½ cups of fruits and vegetables and three whole grain servings per day as part of a 2000-kcal diet provides about 31 g of fiber.[27]

FUNCTIONAL FOODS—SPECIAL CARBOHYDRATE FOODS

The discovery of food components conferring special benefits to health has renewed attention to carbohydrate foods. Fruits, vegetables, legumes, and grains contain tens of thousands of phytochemicals (from the Greek word *phyton* meaning plant) that have biologic effects. Plants produce phytochemicals to protect themselves against bacteria and viruses. When the plants are eaten, these substances are absorbed and act as protective factors for humans.[33] Foods containing these substances have been termed *functional foods,* meaning they provide health benefits beyond the basic roles of the nutrients they contain.[40] Functional foods include whole foods, as well as fortified, enriched, and enhanced foods. Tomatoes are an example of a functional food because the lycopene they contain has been associated with reduced risk of prostate cancer.[41] (Lycopene is a carotenoid that we will discuss in Chapter 6). Earlier in this chapter we learned about the positive effects of dietary and functional fiber on the microflora and health of the colon and control of blood cholesterol levels. Dairy foods and tree nuts are suggested to contain components that may assist in weight control.[42] The concept of functional foods or ingredients also includes new roles for familiar nutrients. Certain unsaturated fatty acids appear to reduce cardiovascular risk in addition to their well-known roles in maintaining skin integrity and providing energy. We will learn more about nonplant functional foods and their relation to particular health conditions in future chapters. (See Table 3-6 for some examples of functional foods and their bioactive ingredients.)

TABLE 3-6 SELECTED FUNCTIONAL FOODS AND THEIR PROPOSED HEALTH BENEFITS

FUNCTIONAL FOOD	FOOD COMPONENT OR FUNCTIONAL INGREDIENT	HEALTH BENEFIT
Whole grain oats	β-Glucans	Reduce the risk of heart disease*
Green tea	Catechins	Lower risk of certain cancers
Tomatoes	Lycopene	Lower risk of certain cancers
Fortified margarine	Plant sterols (added ingredient)	Reduce the risk of heart disease*
Tree nuts	Monounsaturated fatty acids/vitamin E	Reduce the risk of heart disease*
Psyllium	Soluble fiber	Reduce the risk of heart disease*
Soy	Protein	Reduce the risk of heart disease*

Adapted from American Dietetic Association: Position of the American Dietetic Association: functional foods, *J Am Diet Assoc* 109:735, 2009.
*When part of a diet low in saturated fat and cholesterol.

Various phytochemicals and other nonnutrient plant substances found to have positive effects on body function and health are being marketed as dietary supplements, apart from their original food source. Functional components—like nutrients—work best in combination with one another, so eating foods that contain a mixture of these substances offers the best protection against chronic disease.[43] In addition, phytochemicals are found in foods in very small amounts, and not much is known about the safety of using concentrated amounts as found in supplements. Phytochemicals and plant fibers are lost in food processing, so try to choose whole grain breads and cereals and eat fruits and vegetables without removing the skins or peels. Including a variety of fruits, vegetables, grains, legumes, and nuts in our daily diet provides an ample supply of these important substances.

DIGESTION-ABSORPTION-METABOLISM REVIEW

We discussed the digestion, absorption, and metabolism of the macronutrients in great detail in Chapter 2. This outline of the process for carbohydrate is intended as a brief review.

Digestion

Starches and sugars in carbohydrate foods must be converted to glucose for use by cells. This process begins in the mouth where salivary amylase (ptyalin) from the parotid gland acts on starch to begin its breakdown into dextrins and maltose. No specific enzyme in the stomach breaks down carbohydrate; however, before the food mass is completely mixed with gastric acid, as much as 20% to 30% of the starch is changed to maltose. Enzymes from two sources complete chemical digestion of carbohydrate: (1) the pancreas and (2) the small intestine, as follows:

- *Pancreatic secretions:* Pancreatic amylase entering the duodenum through the common bile duct completes the breakdown of starch to maltose.
- *Intestinal secretions:* Cells within the brush border of the small intestine secrete three disaccharidases, **sucrase**, **lactase**, and **maltase**, which act on their respective disaccharides to release the monosaccharides, glucose, galactose, and fructose. (See Table 2-2 for further review.)

Absorption and Metabolism

Glucose is absorbed by an active pumping system using sodium as a carrier. Of the total carbohydrate absorbed, 80% is in the form of glucose and the remaining 20% as galactose and fructose.[44] Via the capillaries in the villi, the products of carbohydrate digestion enter the **portal** blood circulation in route to the liver. Here, fructose and galactose are converted to glucose. Glucose not needed for immediate energy is converted to glycogen or adipose tissue for storage. In succeeding chapters we will learn how other macronutrients and micronutrients interact with carbohydrate to accomplish its tasks.

KEY TERMS

sucrase Enzyme that splits the disaccharide sucrose, releasing the monosaccharides glucose and fructose.

lactase Enzyme that splits the disaccharide lactose, releasing the monosaccharides glucose and galactose.

maltase Enzyme that splits the disaccharide maltose, releasing two units of the monosaccharide glucose.

portal An entryway, usually referring to the portal circulation of blood that delivers nutrients absorbed from the small intestine to the liver. Blood is brought into the liver via the portal vein and moves out via the hepatic vein.

TO SUM UP

Carbohydrates produced by photosynthesis in plants supply most of the world's population with its primary source of energy. Fruits, vegetables, grains, and most milk products supply dietary carbohydrate. Simple carbohydrates, the monosaccharides and disaccharides, are easily digested and provide quick energy. Starch, a digestible complex carbohydrate, requires increased breakdown to become available for use, but the final product in the digestion of both starches and sugars is glucose. Carbohydrates serve special functions through their ability to spare protein, prevent the build-up of ketones, and supply energy for the CNS. Fiber, the nondigestible carbohydrates found in the structural walls, hulls, seeds, leaves, and skins of fruits, vegetables, and whole grains, affect the digestion and absorption of food in ways that are beneficial to health. Carbohydrates should provide 45% to 65% of total kcalories. A healthy diet should emphasize foods containing complex carbohydrates and fiber, with a minimum of added sugar. Fruits, vegetables, and whole grains, rich in phytochemicals, are often referred to as *functional foods* because they contribute to health in ways beyond the actions of the nutrients they contain.

QUESTIONS FOR REVIEW

1. List the similarities and differences among monosaccharides, disaccharides, and polysaccharides. List two food sources of each.
2. What is resistant starch? Where is it found? Name two health benefits of resistant starch.
3. For breakfast you had a piece of whole grain bread with jelly, a banana, and a glass of low-fat milk. List both the digestible and the nondigestible forms of carbohydrate in this meal. Make a table of the digestible carbohydrates, indicating the site of digestion, the required enzymes, and the products formed.
4. Using the Nutritrac software found on this book's Evolve site, determine the daily energy need of a 25-year-old woman who is 5 feet 6 inches tall, weighs 125 lb, and is relatively sedentary. How many grams of carbohydrate should be included in her diet, and how many kcalories should it supply? What is her upper limit for grams of sugar? How much fiber does she need? Develop a 3-day menu that provides the appropriate amounts of carbohydrate and dietary fiber and does not exceed the limit for sugar.
5. Describe the clinical effects of fiber that may prevent or be useful in treating the following conditions: diverticular disease, hyperlipidemia, and type 2 diabetes.
6. Your client Mr. B wants to lose 20 lb before his high school reunion next month. He has decided to eat only meat and other fried foods for the next 4 weeks because he believes a very low-carbohydrate diet will help him lose weight. How would you respond—consider both the pros and the cons of this diet? How would you explain why he needs some carbohydrate?
7. Describe five special functions of carbohydrate in the body.
8. Visit your local grocery store and find two fruit juices, two fruit drinks, two carbonated beverages, and two sports drinks available in single-serving, easy-to-carry containers. Use the nutrition label to construct a table indicating the kcalories, total carbohydrate (g), sugar (g), vitamins, and minerals per 8-oz serving. Check the list of ingredients and indicate which products contain added sugar. Which are most appropriate for daily use? Which should be limited?
9. Define functional food. Choose one of the functional foods listed at the end of the question and research the following: (a) What are its important phytochemicals or functional components? (b) What effects do these components have on the body? (c) What is an appropriate portion size? Choose one: spinach, blueberries, apples, rolled oats.

REFERENCES

1. Englyst HN, Hudson GJ: Carbohydrates. In Garrow JS, James WPT, Ralph A, editors: *Human nutrition and dietetics*, ed 10, Edinburgh, 2000, Churchill Livingstone.
2. Mackey M, Montgomery J: Plant biotechnology can enhance food security and nutrition in the developing world, part 1, *Nutr Today* 39(2):52, 2004.
3. U.S. Department of Agriculture, Agricultural Research Service: *Nutrient intakes from food: mean amounts and percentages of calories from protein, carbohydrate, fat, and alcohol, one day, 2005–2006*, Washington, DC, 2008, U.S. Department of Agriculture. Retrieved December 20, 2008, from www.ars.usda.gov/ba/bhnrc/fsrg.
4. Vos MB, Kimmons JE, Gillespie C, et al: Dietary fructose consumption among U.S. children and adults, *Medscape J Med* 10(7):160, 2008.
5. Beyer PL, Caviar EM, McCallum RW: Fructose intake at current levels in the United States may cause gastrointestinal distress in normal adults, *J Am Diet Assoc* 105:1559, 2005.
6. American Dietetic Association: Position of the American Dietetic Association: use of nutritive and nonnutritive sweeteners, *J Am Diet Assoc* 104:255, 2004.
7. Lomer MCE, Parkes GC, Sanderson JD: Review article: lactose intolerance in clinical practice—myths and realities, *Aliment Pharmacol Ther* 27:93, 2008.
8. Duffey KJ, Popkin BM: High-fructose corn syrup: is this what's for dinner? *Am J Clin Nutr* 88(Suppl):1722S, 2008.
9. Sigman-Grant M, Morita J: Defining and interpreting intakes of sugars, *Am J Clin Nutr* 78(suppl):815S, 2003.
10. Bachman JL, Reedy J, Subar AF, et al: Sources of food group intakes among the U.S. population, *J Am Diet Assoc* 108:804, 2008.
11. International Food Information Council: *Sugar alcohols fact sheet*, Washington, DC, 2008, IFIC Foundation. Retrieved July 13, 2009, from www.ific.org/publications/factsheets/sugaralcoholsfs.cfm.
12. Grabitske HA, Slavin JL: Gastrointestinal effects of low-digestible carbohydrates, *Crit Rev Food Sci Nutr* 49:327, 2009.
13. Murphy MM, Douglass JS, Birkett A: Resistant starch intakes in the United States, *J Am Diet Assoc* 108:67, 2008.
14. Food and Nutrition Board, Institute of Medicine: *Dietary reference intakes for energy, carbohydrate, fiber, fat, fatty acids, cholesterol, protein, and amino acids, (macronutrients)*, Washington, DC, 2002, National Academies Press.

15. Cotton PA, Subar AF, Friday JE, et al: Dietary sources of nutrients among U.S. adults, *J Am Diet Assoc* 104:921, 2004.
16. U.S. Department of Health and Human Services, U.S. Department of Agriculture: *Report of the Dietary Guidelines Advisory Committee on the Dietary Guidelines for Americans 2010*, Washington, DC, 2010, Center for Nutrition Policy and Promotion, U.S. Department of Agriculture. Retrieved July 28, 2010, from http://www.cnpp.usda.gov/DGAs2010-DGACReport.htm.
17. Benton D, Maconie A, Williams C: The influence of the glycaemic load of breakfast on the behaviour of children in school, *Physiol Behav* 92:717, 2007.
18. Benton D, Nabb S: Carbohydrate, memory, and mood, *Nutr Rev* 61(5, part 2):S61, 2003.
19. Grotz VL, Munro IC: An overview of the safety of sucralose, *Regul Toxicol Pharmacol* 55(1):1-5, 2009.
20. Voiland A: *The zero-calorie sweetener stevia arrives, U.S. News and World Report* website. Retrieved December 16, 2008, from www.usnews.com/health/family-health/articles/2008/07/28/the-zero-calorie-sweetener-stevia-arrives.html.
21. American Dietetic Association: Position of the American Dietetic Association: oral health and nutrition, *J Am Diet Assoc* 107:1418, 2007.
22. DePaola DP, Faine MP, Palmer CA: Nutrition and dental medicine. In Shils MA, Olsen JA, Shike M, et al, editors: *Modern nutrition in health and disease*, ed 10, Baltimore, 2006, Lippincott Williams & Wilkins.
23. Food and Nutrition Board, Institute of Medicine: *Dietary reference intakes: the essential guide to nutrient requirements*, Washington, DC, 2006, National Academies Press.
24. Shin MJ, Blanche PJ, Rawlings RS, et al: Increased plasma concentrations of lipoprotein(a) during a low-fat, high-carbohydrate diet are associated with increased plasma concentrations of apolipoprotein C-III bound to apolipoprotein B-containing lipoproteins, *Am J Clin Nutr* 85:1527, 2007.
25. Ebbeling CB, Leidig MM, Feldman HA, et al: Effects of a low-glycemic load vs low-fat diet in obese young adults, *JAMA* 297:2092, 2007.
26. Astrup A, Larsen TM, Harper A: Atkins and other low-carbohydrate diets: hoax or an effective tool for weight loss? *Lancet* 364:897, 2004.
27. U.S. Department of Agriculture, Center for Nutrition Policy and Promotion: *MyPyramid food guidance system*, Washington, DC, 2005, U.S. Department of Agriculture. Retrieved December 20, 2008, from www.mypyramid.gov.
28. Champagne CM: Dietary interventions on blood pressure, the Dietary Approaches to Stop Hypertension (DASH) trials, *Nutr Rev* 64:S53, 2006.
29. Kennedy ET, Bowman SA, Spence JT, et al: Popular diets: correlation to health, nutrition, and obesity, *J Am Diet Assoc* 101(4):411, 2001.
30. Shai I, Schwarzfuchs D, Henkin Y, et al: Weight loss with a low-carbohydrate, Mediterranean, or low-fat diet, *N Engl J Med* 359:229, 2008.
31. Gardner CD, Kizand A, Alhassan S, et al: Comparison of the Atkins, Zone, Ornish, and LEARN diets for change in weight and related risk factors among overweight premenopausal women, *JAMA* 297:969, 2007.
32. American Dietetic Association: Position of the American Dietetic Association: health implications of dietary fiber, *J Am Diet Assoc* 108:1716, 2008.
33. Gropper SS, Smith JL, Groff JL: *Advanced nutrition and human metabolism*, ed 4, Belmont, CA, 2005, Thomson/Wadsworth.
34. Gaesser GA: Carbohydrate quantity and quality in relation to body mass index, *J Am Diet Assoc* 107:1768, 2007.
35. American Diabetes Association: Nutrition recommendations and interventions for diabetes—2006, *Diabetes Care* 29:2140, 2006.
36. Streppel MT, Ocké MC, Boshuizen HC, et al: Dietary fiber intake in relation to coronary heart disease and all-cause mortality over 40 y: the Zutphen Study, *Am J Clin Nutr* 88:1119, 2008.
37. Theuwissen E, Mensink RP: Water-soluble dietary fibers and cardiovascular disease, *Physiol Behav* 94:285, 2008.
38. Schatzkin A, Mouw T, Park Y, et al: Dietary fiber and whole-grain consumption in relation to colorectal cancer in the NIH-AARP Diet and Health Study, *Am J Clin Nutr* 85:1353, 2007.
39. Papanikolaou Y, Fulgoni VL: Bean consumption is associated with greater nutrient intake, reduced systolic blood pressure, lower body weight, and a smaller waist circumference in adults: results from the National Health and Nutrition Examination Survey 1999–2002, *J Am Coll Nutr* 27:569, 2008.
40. American Dietetic Association: Position of the American Dietetic Association: functional foods, *J Am Diet Assoc* 109:735, 2009.
41. Dwyer JT: Do functional components in foods have a role in helping to solve current health issues? *J Nutr* 137:2489S, 2007.
42. St-Onge M-P: Dietary fats, teas, dairy, and nuts: potential functional foods for weight control? *Am J Clin Nutr* 81:7, 2005.
43. Lila MA: From beans to berries and beyond: teamwork between plant chemicals for protection of optimal human health, *Ann N Y Acad Sci* 1114:372, 2007.
44. Marsh MN, Riley SA: Digestion and absorption of nutrients and vitamins. In Feldman M, Scharschmidt BF, Sleisenger MH, editors: *Gastrointestinal and liver disease*, ed 6, vol 2, Philadelphia, 1998, Saunders.

FURTHER READINGS AND RESOURCES

Readings

Mattes RD, Popkin BM: Nonnutritive sweetener consumption in humans: effects on appetite and food intake and their putative mechanisms, *Am J Clin Nutr* 89:1, 2009. *[These experts review the various actions of nonnutritive sweeteners on appetite and food intake and explain how we can apply this information in advising others.]*

Wang YC, Ludwig DS, Sonneville K, et al: Impact of change in sweetened caloric beverage consumption on energy intake among children and adolescents, *Arch Pediatr Adolesc Med* 163:336, 2009. *[These researchers share the results of an intervention program to reduce sugar and kcalorie intakes in children and adolescents. This project provides a model for interventions in other communities.]*

Grabitske HA, Slavin JL: Low-digestible carbohydrates in practice, *J Am Diet Assoc* 108:1677, 2008. *[These authors help us identify food sources of various low-digestible carbohydrates for use in nutrition counseling.]*

Grandjean AC, Fulgoni VL 3rd, Reimers KJ, et al: Popcorn consumption and dietary and physiological parameters of U.S. children and adults: analysis of the National Health and Nutrition Examination Survey (NHANES) 1999–2002 dietary survey data, *J Am Diet Assoc* 108:853, 2008.

Bachman JL, Reedy J, Subar AF, et al: Sources of food group intakes among the U.S. population, 2001–2002, *J Am Diet Assoc* 108:804, 2008.

Jones JM, Reicks M, Adams J, et al: Becoming proactive with the whole-grains message, *Nutr Today* 39(1):10, 2004.

[Whole grains are important sources of fiber and micronutrients but are used less often than refined grains in the American diet. These articles provide an overview of the effect of whole grains such as popcorn on physical well-being and sources of whole and refined grains chosen by consumers. Jones and colleagues provide suggestions for helping people raise their intake of whole grains.]

Websites of Interest

Centers for Disease Control and Prevention: *Nutrition for Everyone—Carbohydrates*; this site offers consumer information on the different types of carbohydrates including food sources, suggested intakes, descriptions of lesser-known whole grains, and label terms for added sugars: www.cdc.gov/nutrition/everyone/basics/carbs.html.

International Food Information Council Foundation; this site contains fact sheets and brochures for both consumers and health professionals describing functional foods and various carbohydrates occurring naturally in food and used in food processing: www.ific.org/.

Produce for Better Health Foundation; the Fruits & Veggies More Matters campaign encourages increased consumption of fruits and vegetables; this website offers games for children, recipes, and information on portion size, selection, safe handling, and cooking of fruits and vegetables: www.fruitsandveggiesmorematters.org/.

U.S. Department of Agriculture, Center for Nutrition Policy and Promotion; *MyPyramid food guidance system*; *MyPyramid* offers suggestions for increasing intakes of healthy carbohydrate foods: www.mypyramid.gov.

U.S. Department of Agriculture, Food and Nutrition Information Center; this site provides a bibliography of cultural and ethnic food and nutrition materials: www.nal.usda.gov/fnic/pubs/bibs/gen/ethnic.html#6.

U.S. Department of Health and Human Services, U.S. Department of Agriculture: *Dietary Guidelines for Americans 2005*; the *Dietary Guidelines for Americans 2005* provides guidance on increasing intakes of complex carbohydrates and decreasing intakes of sugar: www.health.gov/DietaryGuidelines/.

U.S. National Library of Medicine, U.S. National Institutes of Health: Medline Plus: *Trusted Health Information for You—Carbohydrates*; this website offers materials and information for health professionals and the general public on research news, facts about naturally occurring carbohydrates and artificial sweeteners, and choosing carbohydrate foods: www.nlm.nih.gov/medlineplus/carbohydrates.html.

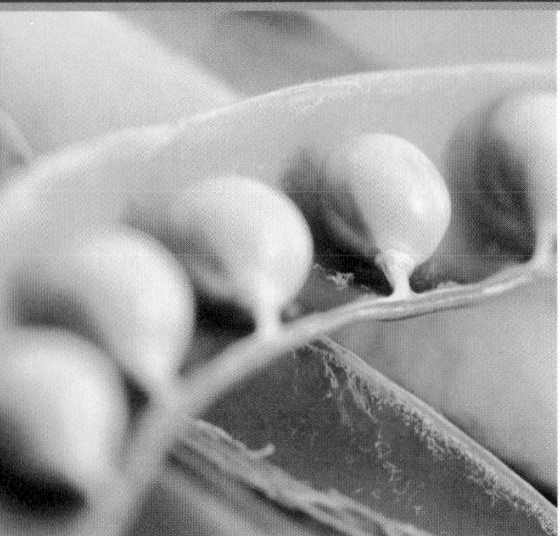

CHAPTER

4

Lipids

Eleanor D. Schlenker

evolve WEBSITE
http://evolve.elsevier.com/Williams/essentials/

OUTLINE

Lipids, the second of the energy-yielding macronutrients, carry mixed messages. Although we hear that a high-fat diet promotes the development of chronic disease, we also read about the health benefits of the Mediterranean diet that is moderately high in fat. When consumers were asked why they craved fast-food hamburgers, they gave such answers as, "Has a taste you can't duplicate," "Is warm and inviting," and "Fills that empty spot."[1] In large part these attributes come from fat. Fats add taste and pleasant mouth feel to our food and contribute to our "feeling full." Fat itself is an essential nutrient for the fatty acids it contains and has an important role in absorption of the fat-soluble vitamins.

Traditionally, fat held a prominent place in the American diet, providing the needed kilocalories (kcalories or kcal), for strenuous physical labor. Today we must assess not only how much fat we consume but also what type we eat, because different fats have different effects on our bodies and health. Fat is an important component of our total diet,[2] and a low-fat diet is not necessarily a nutritionally adequate diet. In our study of lipids, we will learn why we need fat and how to include it in diet planning.

LIPIDS IN NUTRITION AND HEALTH

Health Issues and Lipids

Lipids perform many essential functions in the body; however, questions exist regarding both the types and the amount of fat that we should eat.[3–5] You need what you need, but more than you need is not better. Health concerns related to dietary fat focus on two issues: (1) the high energy content of fat, and (2) the negative health effects of certain fatty acids. Although polyunsaturated and monounsaturated fatty acids have positive effects on body function, saturated and trans fats add to health risk.

Amount of Fat

Fat is energy dense, containing over twice as many kcalories per gram as protein or carbohydrate. Too much fat in the diet can supply more kcalories than required for immediate use, with the excess stored as adipose tissue. Over time such increases in body weight—or more precisely body fat—increase risk of type 2 diabetes, hypertension, and heart disease.[6–9] Watch for more discussion about increases in body fat and related health problems in later chapters.

KEY TERMS

lipids Chemical group name for fats and fat-related compounds such as cholesterol, lipoproteins, and phospholipids.

fatty acids The building blocks or structural components of fats.

saturated Term used for a substance that is united with the greatest possible number of other atoms or chemical groups. A fatty acid is saturated if all available chemical bonds on its carbon chain are filled with hydrogen. A fat is saturated if the majority of fatty acids making up its structure are saturated.

adipose Cells and tissues that store fat.

Type of Fat

Excessive amounts of saturated fat and cholesterol promote atherosclerosis, the buildup of fatty deposits on the interior walls of the major arteries that adds to risk of heart attack or stroke. Saturated fat is found primarily in animal sources, whereas cholesterol is found only in animal foods. Unsaturated fats, found mostly in vegetable oils and fatty fish, can modify blood lipid levels to lower the risk of cardiovascular disease.[4,6] Trans fats produced in the commercial processing of lipids are deleterious to health and best eliminated from the diet. Therefore it is important to help people recognize the different sources and types of fat and how they affect health.[10]

Functions of Lipids

Food Lipids

Dietary lipids support nutrition and health and add to the joy of eating. Following are descriptions of these important characteristics:

- *Provide energy:* Lipids are a concentrated source of fuel to store and use as needed. Food lipids yield 9 kcal/g when oxidized by the body as compared with carbohydrates and protein that yield only 4 kcal/g.
- *Supply essential fatty acids:* The essential fatty acids linoleic acid and α-linolenic acid must be obtained in food because they cannot be made by the body or cannot be made in the amounts needed.
- *Support absorption of the fat-soluble vitamins:* Lipid must be present in the food mix in the small intestine to provide a vehicle for absorption of the fat-soluble vitamins.
- *Add to food palatability:* Lipids add flavor and a pleasant mouth feel to food and heighten the pleasure that comes with eating. Our food choices are strongly influenced by tastes and textures from lipids that enhance our sensory response.
- *Promote satiety:* A meal containing lipids satisfies the appetite for a longer period than a meal containing only carbohydrate and protein. Particular brain cells respond to the mouth feel of fat and influence the region of the brain controlling satiety.[11] Fat contributes texture and body to food mixtures that slows their movement out of the stomach and helps prolong the feeling of fullness.

Body Lipids

Lipids are stored in the body as adipose tissue. This tissue performs many tasks essential to life, as follows:

- *Storage source of energy:* Lipids are an efficient fuel for all tissues except the brain and central nervous system (CNS). In fact, fatty acids are the preferred fuel of the heart muscle.
- *Thermal insulation:* The layer of lipid deposited directly beneath the skin helps maintain body temperature.
- *Protection of vital organs:* A weblike padding of adipose tissue surrounds vital organs such as the kidneys, protecting them from mechanical shock and providing structural support.
- *Transmission of nerve impulses:* Lipid layers surrounding nerve fibers provide electrical insulation and transmit nerve impulses.
- *Form membrane structure:* Lipids are structural components of cell membranes and help transport nutrients, metabolites, and waste products in and out of cells.
- *Carrier of fat-soluble materials:* Lipoproteins carry lipids to and from the liver and on to body tissues. Lipids transport the fat-soluble vitamins A, D, E, and K to the cells for metabolic use.
- *Precursors of other substances:* Lipids supply fatty acids and cholesterol for the synthesis of structural and metabolic compounds; brain tissue and the retina contain many fatty acids.

PHYSICAL AND CHEMICAL NATURE OF LIPIDS

Physical Characteristics

The chemical term *lipid* includes fats, oils, and related compounds that are insoluble in water and greasy to the touch. Some food lipids—butter, margarine, or cooking oil—are easily recognized as fats. Other foods that appear to be carbohydrate (bakery items or potato chips) or protein (beef patties) often contain significant amounts of fat.[12] We refer to this fat as *hidden fat.*

Chemical Characteristics

Lipids are organic compounds consisting of a carbon chain with hydrogen and oxygen atoms and other radicals or groups of elements attached. Fatty acids and their related compounds are the lipids important in human nutrition. Lipids have something in common with carbohydrates; the same chemical elements that make up carbohydrates—carbon, hydrogen, and oxygen—also make up fatty acids. However, carbohydrates and lipids have two important structural differences:

1. Lipids are more complex, with more carbon (C) and hydrogen (H) atoms and fewer oxygen (O) atoms.
2. The common structural units of lipids are fatty acids, whereas the common structural units of carbohydrates are simple sugars.

We will look first at the unique characteristics of fatty acids—their saturation, chain length, and essentiality—and then focus on the triglycerides built from fatty acids.

FATTY ACIDS AND TRIGLYCERIDES

Characteristics of Fatty Acids: Saturation

The saturation or unsaturation of a lipid governs its physical characteristics. Saturated fats are hard, less-saturated fats are soft, and unsaturated fats are liquid at room temperature (Box 4-1). These physical differences relate to the ratio of hydrogen atoms to carbon atoms in the fatty acids making up the lipid. If a fatty acid has a hydrogen atom attached at every available space, then it is completely saturated. If the fatty acid has some hydrogen spaces unfilled, then it is unsaturated. The following three terms are used to describe saturation in fats.

1. *Saturated:* Lipids composed mostly of saturated fatty acids are called *saturated fats.* The most saturated food fats are

two oils from plants: (1) coconut oil, which is 88% saturated, and (2) palm kernel oil, which is 80% saturated.[13] All other saturated fats are of animal origin as found in meat, butter, and whole milk dairy products.

2. *Monounsaturated:* Food lipids made up of fatty acids with one hydrogen space unfilled, creating one double bond, are called *monounsaturated fats.* These lipids are generally from plant sources. Canola oil (isolated from rapeseed) and olive oil are monounsaturated fats.
3. *Polyunsaturated:* When fatty acids have two or more spaces unfilled with hydrogen, creating two or more double bonds, they are called *polyunsaturated fats.* Many of these fats are from plant sources and include commonly used cooking oils such as corn oil and safflower oil. Polyunsaturated fatty acids with two or more double bonds are also classed as *n-3* or *n-6 fatty acids.* This number refers to the position in the carbon chain where the first double bond appears. An important n-6 fatty acid is linoleic acid, an essential fatty acid found in vegetable oils. The n-3 fatty acids in fatty fish have a role in cardiovascular health.[4,6]

Characteristics of Fatty Acids: Chain Length

A second characteristic of fatty acids important in human nutrition is the length of their carbon chain. Fatty acids in foods range from 4 to 22 carbons (Box 4-2). Chain length affects intestinal absorption. Long-chain fatty acids are more difficult to absorb and require a helping carrier to enter the lymph and then the blood. Short- and medium-chain fatty acids are soluble in water and are absorbed directly into the bloodstream. When intestinal diseases injure the absorbing surface of the small intestine, a commercial product called *medium-chain triglyceride* (MCT) oil (made of short- and medium-chain fatty acids) can replace ordinary vegetable oil in food preparation.

Essential Fatty Acids

Two different fatty acids—(1) **linoleic acid** (an n-6 fatty acid) and (2) **α-linolenic acid** (an n-3 fatty acid)—are **essential fatty acids** for humans. Arachidonic acid, another fatty acid important in human nutrition, can be made from linoleic acid. Two n-3 fatty acids associated with cardiovascular health—(1) **eicosapentaenoic acid** and (2) **docosahexaenoic acid**—can be made from α-linolenic acid (Figure 4-1), but dietary sources help ensure an adequate supply.

Linoleic acid and α-linolenic acid have the following roles in the body[14]:

- *Skin integrity:* The essential fatty acids strengthen cell membranes and prevent a harmful increase in skin permeability. Essential fatty acid deficiency causes breakdown in skin tissue, with characteristic eczema and skin lesions.

BOX 4-1 DEGREES OF SATURATION OF FOOD FATS

Highly Saturated Fat (solid at room temperature)
Stick margarine
Butter
Beef fat

Less-Saturated Fat (very soft at room temperature)
Tub margarine
Squeeze margarine

Unsaturated Fat (liquid at room temperature)
Salad oil

BOX 4-2 CHAIN LENGTH OF FATTY ACIDS

- Short-chain fatty acids have 4 to 6 carbons.
- Medium-chain fatty acids have 8, 10, or 12 carbons.
- Long-chain fatty acids have 14, 16, 18 or more carbons.

KEY TERMS

cholesterol A fat-related compound; a sterol ($C_{27}H_{45}OH$) that is normally found in bile and is a principal constituent of gallstones. Cholesterol is synthesized by the liver and is a precursor of various steroid hormones, such as estrogen and testosterone, and of the vitamin D molecule produced by the action of ultraviolet light on the skin. It is found in animal tissues such as meat, egg yolk, and milk fat.

lipoproteins Noncovalent complexes of fat with protein. The lipoproteins function as major carriers of lipids in the plasma; this combination of fat surrounded by protein makes possible the transport of fatty substances in a water medium such as plasma.

organic Carbon-based chemical compounds.

triglycerides Chemical name for fats that indicates the structure of three fatty acids attached to a glycerol base. A neutral fat synthesized from carbohydrate and stored in adipose tissue, it releases free fatty acids into the blood when needed for energy.

linoleic acid An essential fatty acid for humans; an n-6 polyunsaturated fatty acid.

α-linolenic acid An essential fatty acid for humans; an n-3 polyunsaturated fatty acid.

essential fatty acids Fatty acids that must be supplied in the diet because the body cannot make them or cannot make them in sufficient amounts.

eicosapentaenoic acid An n-3 polyunsaturated fatty acid that can be synthesized by the body in limited amounts from α-linolenic acid and can also be obtained from fish oil; this fatty acid helps lower the risk of heart attack or stroke.

docosahexaenoic acid An n-3 polyunsaturated fatty acid that can be synthesized by the body in limited amounts from α-linolenic acid and can also be obtained from fish oil; this fatty acid is important for brain and neural development in infants and helps lower the risk of heart attack or stroke.

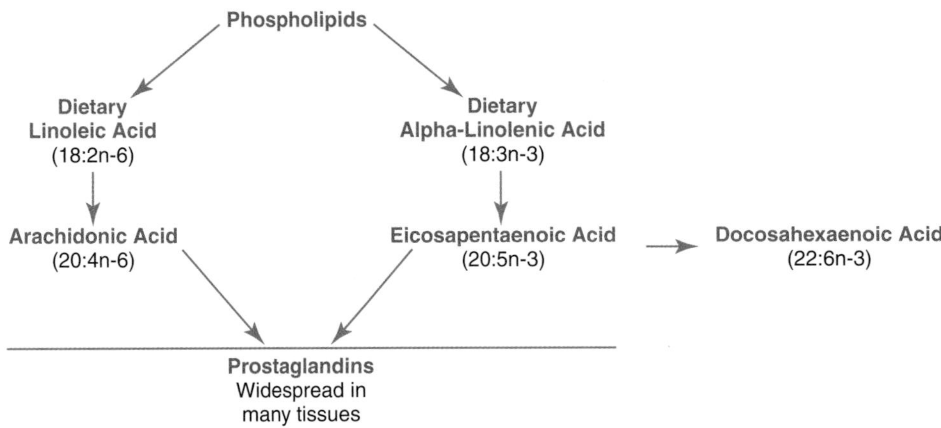

Control contraction of smooth muscle
Regulate blood pressure
Regulate secretion of gastric acid
Regulate body temperature
Regulate aggregation of blood platelets
Control inflammation and vascular permeability
Regulate immune function and resistance to harmful organisms

FIGURE 4-1 Various fatty acids and prostaglandins are made from each of the two essential fatty acids. Prostaglandins help regulate many important body functions.

- *Regulation of blood cholesterol:* These fatty acids participate in both transport and metabolism of cholesterol and help lower blood cholesterol levels.
- *Growth:* Normal growth requires an adequate supply of the essential fatty acids, and growth is impaired in essential fatty acid deficiency; α-linolenic acid is especially important for the development of brain tissue before and after birth.
- *Gene expression:* The essential fatty acids regulate the production of enzymes needed for synthesis of nonessential fatty acids.[15]
- *Immune function:* Persons with essential fatty acid deficiency have an increased rate of infection.[15]
- *Aggregation of blood platelets:* Eicosapentaenoic acid and docosahexaenoic acid, n-3 fatty acids made from α-linolenic acid, prevent unwanted aggregation of blood platelets that blocks the flow of blood in major arteries, causing heart attack or stroke.[16]
- *Synthesis of hormonelike agents:* Essential fatty acids are metabolic precursors of a group of physiologically and pharmacologically active compounds known as *prostaglandins* (see Figure 4-1). They were first identified in human semen and thought to originate in the prostate gland. Prostaglandins exist in virtually all body tissues and act as local hormones to direct and coordinate biologic functions. They influence blood pressure, blood clotting, and cardiovascular function.[16]

Dietary Reference Intakes

Adequate Intakes (AIs) have been established for both linoleic and α-linolenic acids. (See page 11 to review the various categories of the Dietary Reference Intakes [DRIs].) The AI for linoleic acid (an n-6 fatty acid) is 17 g/day for men and 12 g/day for women ages 19 to 50 years. Men ages 51 years and older should take in 14 g/day of linoleic acid, and women should take in 11 g/day. The AI for α-linolenic acid (an n-3 fatty acid) is 1.6 g/day for all adult men and 1.1 g/day for all adult women.[14]

Special Needs of Infants

Arachidonic acid and docosahexaenoic acid play a critical role in infant development and are found in breast milk in liberal amounts. Although the body can synthesize docosahexaenoic acid from α-linolenic acid, this reaction cannot proceed rapidly enough to supply the amount needed to ensure brain and neural development. Commercial infant formula sold in the United States is fortified with arachidonic and docosahexaenoic acids to the levels found in human milk.[17] Based on the important role of docosahexaenoic acid in both prenatal and postnatal development, some nutrition experts have proposed that both pregnant[18] and lactating women[17] be encouraged to eat one to two portions of oily, sea fish per week. It is important that selection be made from fish low in mercury and other contaminants. (See Chapter 9 for more information on this topic.)

Food Sources

The best sources of the two essential fatty acids are vegetable oils. Corn oil, safflower oil, soybean oil, cottonseed oil, sunflower oil, and peanut oil all contain linoleic acid (an n-6 acid). α-Linolenic acid (an n-3 acid) is found in canola oil, soy oil, linseed oil, rapeseed oil, and dark-green leafy vegetables. Although the body can make eicosapentaenoic acid and docosahexaenoic acid from α-linolenic acid, these fatty acids are also obtained from fish.[6] (Box 4-3 lists food sources that contain fatty acids.)

BOX 4-3 FOOD SOURCES OF FATTY ACIDS IMPORTANT TO HEALTH

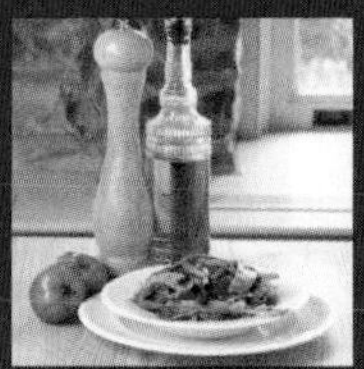
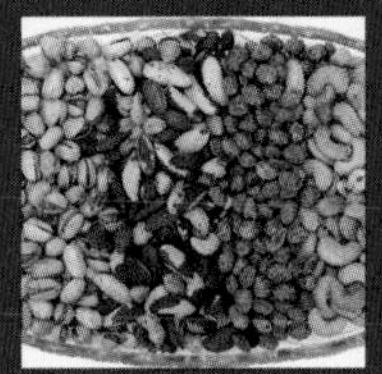
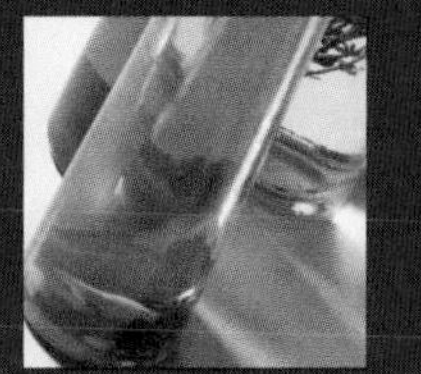
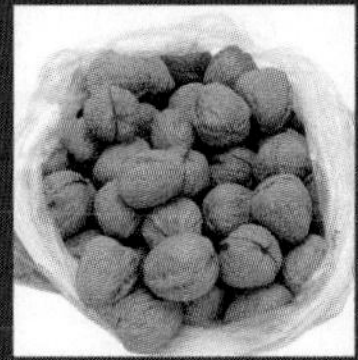
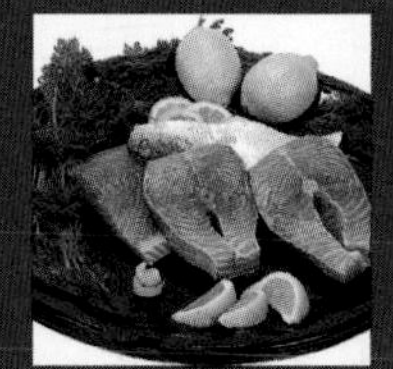
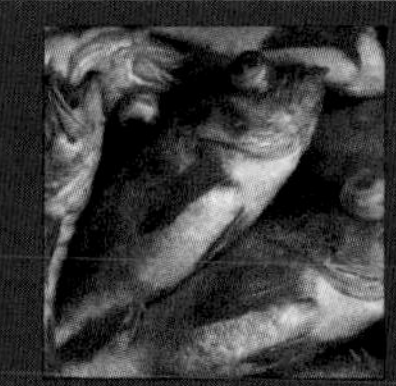

Linoleic Acid: n-6 Fatty Acid (essential)
- Safflower oil
- Corn oil
- Cottonseed oil
- Soybean oil
- Nuts
- Wheat germ

α-Linolenic Acid: n-3 Fatty Acid (essential)
- Soybean oil
- Flaxseed oil
- Canola oil
- Walnuts
- Wheat germ

Fatty Acids from Fish: n-3 Fatty Acids (can be synthesized by the body)

Eicosapentaenoic acid and docosahexaenoic acid
- Herring
- Mackerel
- Halibut
- Salmon
- Canned tuna

Use of Fish Oil Supplements

Nutrition experts recommend that children and adults consume two servings of fish a week to ensure an adequate intake of those fatty acids supplied in fish oils.[6,19] For people who require additional amounts of n-3 fatty acids as part of a therapeutic intervention and for vegans or other groups who do not consume fish, fortified foods and fatty acid–rich algae are useful supplements. However, inappropriately high intakes of these fatty acids lead to excessive bleeding and interfere with other aspects of fatty acid metabolism, so any use of supplements should be supervised by a health professional.[19] Food is always the best source of any nutrient.

Triglycerides

Structure

The body stores fatty acids in the form of triglycerides made from three fatty acids attached to a glycerol base. When glycerol is combined with one fatty acid it is called a *monoglyceride,* with two fatty acids it is a *diglyceride,* and with three fatty acids it is termed a *triglyceride.* Glycerides are found in food and also formed in the body. Most natural lipids from animal or plant sources are triglycerides. They appear in body cells as oily droplets and circulate in the water-based blood plasma encased in a covering of water-soluble protein (lipoproteins). Triglycerides serve multiple functions throughout the body.

FOOD LIPIDS AND HEALTH

Degree of Saturation

Food lipids contain a mixture of both saturated and unsaturated fats. Animal sources—meat, milk, and eggs—contain more saturated fats, whereas plant sources, primarily vegetable oils, are more unsaturated. The spectrum of food fats (from saturated to unsaturated) is illustrated in Figure 4-2. In general the saturated fats are solid at room temperature, and the plant lipids on the unsaturated end are free-flowing oils even at low temperatures; however, the *exceptions* to the usual pattern of saturation are important to human health. Coconut oil and palm kernel oil, highly saturated vegetable fats, are used extensively in nondairy creamers and baked goods because they are inexpensive.

The number of double bonds in a fatty acid influences its actions in the body. Certain saturated fats are harmful to health if eaten in large amounts, although fats with one double bond or more have the opposite effect (Table 4-1). Monounsaturated fatty acids with one double bond are associated with the healthful effects of the Mediterranean diet, a plant-based eating pattern rich in legumes, grains, seeds, and olive oil. Polyunsaturated fats with two or more double

KEY TERMS

prostaglandins Group of naturally occurring substances derived from long-chain fatty acids that have multiple local hormonelike actions; they regulate gastric acid secretion, blood platelet aggregation, body temperature, and tissue inflammation.

glycerol An alcohol that is esterified with fatty acids to produce triglycerides and released when fats are hydrolyzed; a colorless, odorless, syrupy sweet liquid.

glycerides Group name for fats; any of a group of esters obtained from glycerol by the replacement of one, two, or three hydroxyl (OH) groups with a fatty acid. Monoglycerides contain one fatty acid, diglycerides contain two fatty acids, and triglycerides contain three fatty acids. Glycerides are the structural units of adipose tissue and are found in animal and plant fats and oils.

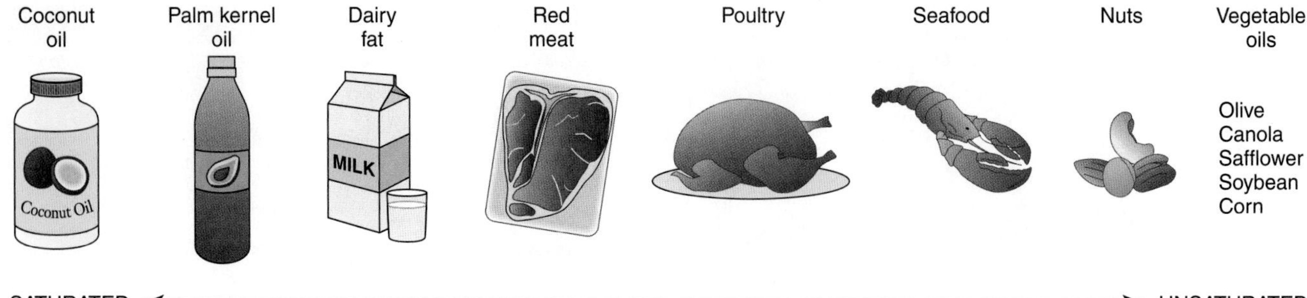

FIGURE 4-2 Spectrum of food fats according to degree of saturation. Note that the two food fats with the highest degree of saturation are plant fats, followed by various animal fats in decreasing order of saturation. In general, plant fats are less saturated.

TABLE 4-1 EFFECTS OF FATTY ACID SATURATION ON BLOOD LIPIDS

DEGREE OF SATURATION	NUMBER OF DOUBLE BONDS	PHYSIOLOGIC EFFECTS
Saturated fats	None	Raises blood levels of total cholesterol and low-density lipoprotein (LDL) cholesterol Encourages aggregation of blood platelets, increasing risk of unwanted clots
Monounsaturated fats	One	Decreases blood levels of total cholesterol and LDL cholesterol when substituted for saturated fat
Polyunsaturated fats (includes the essential fatty acids and fish oils)	Two or more	Decreases blood levels of total cholesterol and LDL cholesterol Discourages blood platelet aggregation decreasing risk of unwanted clots
Trans fats	One	Raises blood levels of total cholesterol and LDL cholesterol Decreases blood levels of high-density lipoprotein (HDL) cholesterol

Data from American Dietetic Association: Position of the American Dietetic Association and the Dietitians of Canada: dietary fatty acids, *J Am Diet Assoc* 107:1599, 2007.

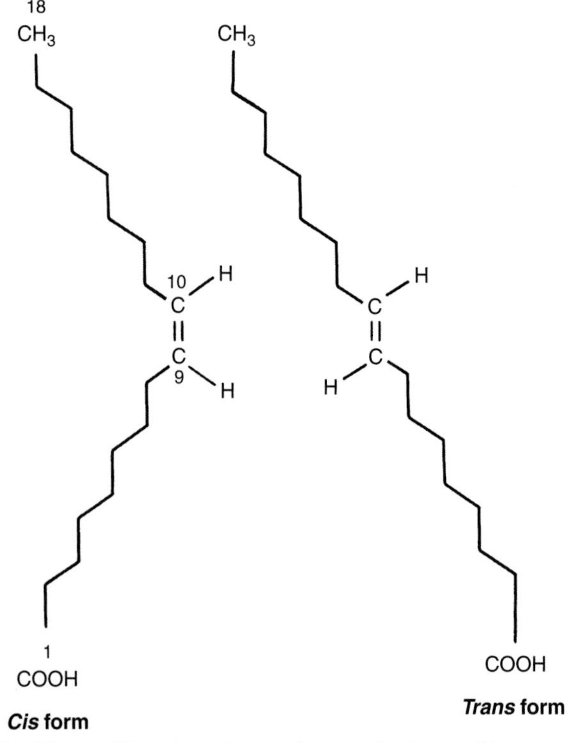

FIGURE 4-3 The *cis* and *trans* forms of a fatty acid.

bonds include the essential fatty acids and fish oils. Despite the positive effects of unsaturated fats, moderation should be the key.[4-5,19]

Cis versus *Trans* Fats

To meet the demand for inexpensive solid fats for use as table fats or food ingredients, the process of **hydrogenation** was developed. When unsaturated oils are surrounded with hydrogen gas, hydrogen ions attach at available sites, producing a more saturated (or solid) fat. This process makes unsaturated vegetable oils into margarine or vegetable shortenings. However, a particular type of unsaturated fatty acid that is formed, a *trans* fatty acid, is extremely detrimental to health.

In Figure 4-3 we compare the two possible structures of an unsaturated fatty acid. When double bonds occur in nature, the fatty acid chain bends in such a way that both parts are on the same side of the bond. In this case the fatty acid is called a *cis* fatty acid, meaning same side. Fatty acids in vegetable oils are in the *cis* form. However, when oils are partially hydrogenated, the normal bend can change with the two structural parts on opposite sides of the bend. This form is called a *trans* fatty acid, meaning opposite side. Commercially

BOX 4-4 VISIBLE AND HIDDEN FATS IN FOOD

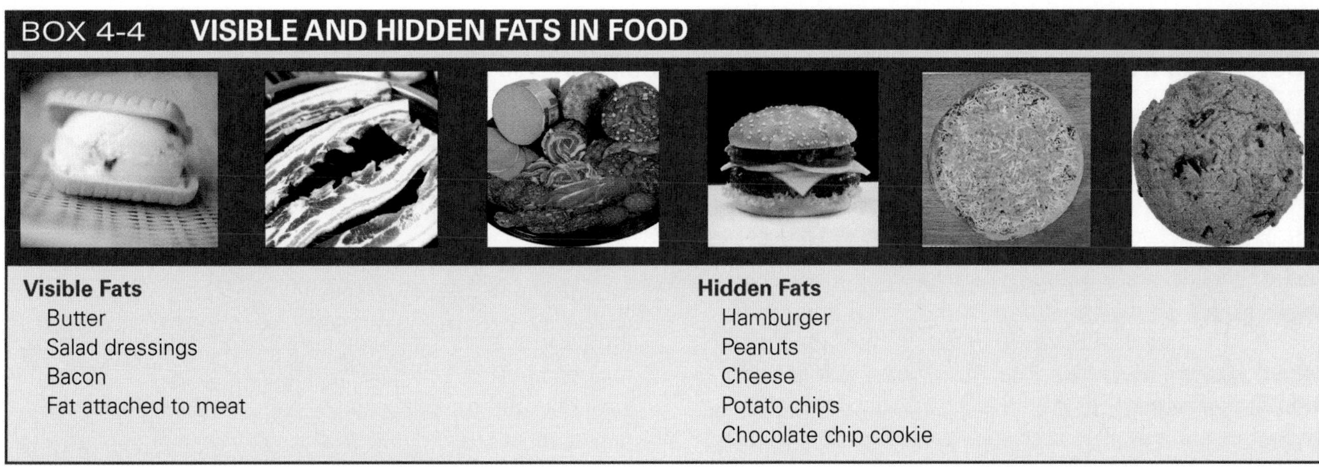

Visible Fats	Hidden Fats
Butter	Hamburger
Salad dressings	Peanuts
Bacon	Cheese
Fat attached to meat	Potato chips
	Chocolate chip cookie

hydrogenated lipids used in soft margarine and other food products often contained *trans* fatty acids.

Trans fatty acids have been implicated in the development of coronary artery disease.[20] In addition, they elevate the risk of type 2 diabetes,[21] as well as disrupt essential fatty acid functions in cells[14] (see Table 4-1 for specific actions of trans fatty acids). Before the required posting of trans fatty acid content on the nutrition label, it was estimated that trans fats provided 4% to 7% of total kcalories in the American diet.[22] These fatty acids were found in bread, cakes, cookies, crackers, margarine, frozen potato products, and oils used for frying at fast-food restaurants.[10] Based on the efforts of voluntary health organizations, public health departments, and health professionals, many fast-food restaurants and food manufacturers have voluntarily reduced their use of fats containing trans fatty acids. Several state and city governments including New York City have passed ordinances restricting use of trans fats in local restaurants.[23]

The nutrition label can help guide a consumer's intake of fats. Information given includes the grams per serving of total fat, saturated fat, unsaturated fat, and trans fat; however, confusion about portion size can add to intake. Packages assumed by the consumer to contain one serving are often labeled as containing two servings or more, with the result that actual fat intake is two or more times what was expected. As for trans fats, it is important for consumers to recognize the difference between the listing of none or zero trans fats. A label can indicate the content as zero if the amount of trans fat is 0.5 g or less per serving.[23] Eating several servings of such items adds significant amounts of trans fat to the diet. Added fats such as coconut oil and palm kernel oil can be found in the list of ingredients on the food label and can be identified as sources of saturated fat. Although we want to encourage people to avoid eating trans fats, it is important they understand that a food is not necessarily healthy just because it contains no trans fats.[10] Such a food may be high in total fat or saturated fat and still be best avoided or eaten in fairly limited amounts. Saturated fat may become an increased concern in the future if food manufacturers move to lard or other saturated fats to replace the trans fat–containing hydrogenated fats being discontinued.[24]

Visible and Hidden Fat

Fat enters the diet in many different forms and foods. Fats are quite visible in butter, margarine, vegetable oil, salad dressing, bacon, and similar added fats, which account for over 30% of the fat in the American diet.[12] However, less obvious are the fats in milk (unless it is nonfat), egg yolk, cheese, nuts, seeds, and olives—often referred to as *hidden fats*. Other major sources of hidden fats are bakery items, including cake, cookies, crackers, and muffins, or frozen entrees such as baked lasagna (Box 4-4). Meat and poultry have both visible and hidden fat. Even when visible fat has been trimmed away or the poultry skin removed, the remaining portion still contains some fat. Red meat, especially beef, is marbled with tiny fat deposits within the muscle tissue. When evaluating the nutrient intake of a cultural or ethnic group different from your own, it is important to consider potential sources of hidden fat in recipes or fats added in food preparation (see the *Focus on Culture* box, "Developing a Food Frequency Questionnaire for Culturally Diverse Groups").

Acceptable Macronutrient Distribution Range

The Acceptable Macronutrient Distribution Range (AMDR) for fat is 20% to 35% of total kcalories.[14] This range supports appropriate intake of the essential fatty acids and fat-containing foods that are rich sources of other important nutrients, yet helps control kcalories. The lower end of the

KEY TERMS

hydrogenation Process used to produce margarine and shortening from vegetable oil; when vegetable oils are exposed to hydrogen gas, hydrogen atoms are added at many of the double bonds of the polyunsaturated fatty acids, forming a solid fat.

FOCUS ON CULTURE

Developing a Food Frequency Questionnaire for Culturally Diverse Groups

Using a Food Frequency Questionnaire

Food frequency questionnaires (FFQs) are one way of learning what people eat; they provide a tool for evaluating an individual's diet and developing an intervention plan. An FFQ contains a list of common foods from all major food groups, and persons are asked how often they eat each food and the portion size usually eaten. The FFQ can be completed in writing or administered by interview. When collecting dietary information from individuals who do not speak or read English, it is necessary to translate the FFQ or hire an interviewer who is fluent in their language and familiar with their dietary patterns.

Developing a Food Frequency Questionnaire

To obtain an accurate response describing food intake, you must provide a comprehensive list of foods commonly eaten. The list of foods used by an East Indian or Chinese or Latino family who recently came to live in the United States will be very different from a list of foods used by a typical American family. Several researchers who developed an FFQ for use with Southeast Asian families have given us a framework that can be applied to any ethnic or cultural group.

Step 1

Talk with those who are doing the cooking about the types of foods they prepare for their family. Collect recipes for specific dishes to be sure that you understand what grains, fruits, vegetables, meats, and fats are included in each dish. Certain vegetables may be eaten only as components of mixed dishes and not eaten separately.[1] Check to see what ingredients are available in local shops and what substitutions the homemakers need to make when preparing their native dishes.

Step 2

Group foods together according to their nutrient content (e.g., put grain foods, protein foods, or calcium-rich foods together).

Step 3

Assign a food name that is familiar to your target group. For example, families from Southeast Asia may recognize broccoli by the name Chinese broccoli, Kai-lan, or Gai-lan.[2]

Step 4

Compile a database that includes the specific nutrient content of each food item that will appear on your FFQ. Many foods will likely be available in the USDA nutrient database used to calculate the nutrient content of diet records obtained in U.S. food surveys. Using these food values, calculate the nutrient content of mixed food dishes that are common to your target group.

Special Problems with Fats

Based on the high energy density of fat and its relationship to chronic disease, it is important that we obtain good estimates of the types and amounts of fat eaten regularly. Food preparation methods strongly influence fat intake and require particular attention. Food researchers found that Southeast Asian families obtained about 40% of their kcalories from fat, with much of it coming from oil-based curry sauces, whereas Chinese families took in only 34% of their total kcalories as fat—yet both added about the same amounts of oil to their stir-fried foods.[2] When the researchers looked at the actual foods being prepared, they found their answer. For the stir-fried foods, much of the fat remained in the pan when the food was served; with the thick curry sauces, most of the sauce was eaten along with the other ingredients. It may be helpful to visit a family at mealtime to fully appreciate their food intake patterns.

As groups become more health conscious, it is pertinent to include items on FFQs that are being marketed to them for their specific nutrient content. For example, health professionals developing an FFQ for African-American women trying to lower fat intake should include not only traditional foods these women enjoy but also any low-fat and modified-fat foods directed toward this particular audience.[3]

FFQs must be individualized for different ethnic or cultural groups. Think about your own group. If you were to develop an FFQ for them, then what foods would you include?

REFERENCES

1. Tseng M, Hernandez T: Comparison of intakes of U.S. Chinese women based on food frequency and 24-hour recall data, *J Am Diet Assoc* 105:1145, 2005.
2. Kelemen LE, Anand SS, Vuksan V, et al: Development and evaluation of cultural food frequency questionnaires for South Asians, Chinese, and Europeans in North America, *J Am Diet Assoc* 103:1178, 2003.
3. Schlundt DG, Hargreaves MK, Buchowski MS: The Eating Behavior Patterns Questionnaire predicts dietary fat intake in African American women, *J Am Diet Assoc* 103:338, 2003.

range can help with weight management or weight loss, whereas the upper level of 35% may promote weight gain in underweight individuals or ensure sufficient kcalories for an active lifestyle or growth. Fat intakes falling below 10% of total energy intake may not supply needed amounts of essential fatty acids.[14]

Appropriate Intakes of Fat and Carbohydrate

The AMDRs for fat (20% to 35% of total kcalories) and carbohydrate (45% to 65% of total kcalories) set a balance between these two energy sources.[14] Popular weight loss regimens often replace carbohydrate with fat and protein to the extent that fat supplies 46% or more of total kcalories.[25] Patients with type 2 diabetes were found to be consuming diets made up of 45% fat in an effort to lower their intakes of carbohydrates,[26] pointing to the need for nutrition counseling for this group. At the other extreme, when fat provides less than 20% of total kcalories, carbohydrate and protein levels can rise disproportionately. (Appropriate ranges for protein intake are discussed in Chapter 5.)

PERSPECTIVES IN PRACTICE

Lowering Your Fat Intake

A common problem for many of us is how to lower our intake of fats, especially unhealthy fats. Whether we are trying to reduce our kcalorie intake or improve our heart health, evaluating our current fat intake is a place to begin. As a nutrition counselor you want to encourage small changes that once begun will be continued. Even one change at a time can add up to measurable differences over weeks and months.

Following are some ways to get started:

1. Reduce the fat you add.
   - Use less butter or margarine on your toast.
   - Be stingy when adding salad dressing.
2. Reduce portion size.
   - Order the small rather than the "supersize" portion of French fries.
3. Eat a high-fat food less often.
   - Have ice cream as a snack or dessert only two or three times a week; choose fresh fruit on other days.
4. Choose a lower-fat version of a food.
   - Use low-fat milk or nonfat milk in place of whole milk.
   - Choose a broiled chicken breast with no skin rather than a fried chicken leg with skin.
   - Trim all visible fat from meats.
5. Substitute modified foods lower in fat.
   - Look for reduced-fat mayonnaise and salad dressings.
6. Eliminate fat when preparing foods.
   - Eat raw carrots without salad dressing.
   - Season cooked vegetables with lemon juice, orange juice, or chicken broth rather than margarine or butter.

HEALTH PROMOTION

Lowering Fat Intake

Despite public health campaigns urging Americans to limit their dietary fat, only small changes have occurred. Over the past 20 years, fat intake as a proportion of total kcalories dropped about 1% to 3% among Caucasian men and African-American men and women, but it rose slightly in Caucasian women. Despite this decrease in dietary fat, energy intake actually increased among all groups.[27] The perceived drop in kcalories from fat resulted from a rise in kcalories from carbohydrate,[28] not from an actual decrease in dietary fat. Fast-food adds to fat and kcalorie intake. On days when all meals were eaten at home or somewhere other than at a fast-food restaurant, men took in 33.6% of their kcalories as fat. On days including a fast-food meal, energy intake rose by 500 kcal, and fat intake reached 34.9% of total energy.[29] Women increased their energy intake by 220 kcal and their fat intake from 32.7% to 34.6% on days that included a fast-food meal. Carbohydrate intake also increased with fast-food meals.

Dietary fat can be lowered in various ways. Attempting to eliminate all foods high in fat not only lessens intakes of many important nutrients, such as iron, zinc, vitamin E, and essential fatty acids, but also is unlikely to be sustained over time. Alternatively, eating a mix of high-fat and modified-fat foods effectively lowers fat intake,[30–31] while maintaining appropriate levels of those nutrients found in higher-fat foods. Including a higher-fat food at mealtime adds to satiety and helps curb the urge to eat between meals. Limiting portion size is another effective way to reduce both fat and kcalories. Balancing the diet with a variety of both higher-fat and lower-fat foods is the best strategy for overall good health. (See the *Perspectives in Practice* box, "Lowering Your Fat Intake," for more ideas on moderating your intake of fats.)

Fat Replacers

Fats have many functions in food recipes and food preparation. In cooking and baking fats (1) absorb flavors from various ingredients and help to blend them throughout the food; (2) assist in heat transfer necessary for browning or crispiness; and (3) create a velvety mouth feel in foods such as ice cream, pudding, and cheese.[32] Fat replacers are ingredients that can fulfill these functions but are lower in kcalories than fat. Fruit purees made from apples or prunes are often used in home baking as fat replacers in cookies and moist cakes. Other fat replacers used as thickeners and emulsifiers have been developed for use in processed foods. In the United States, 79% of consumers buy foods containing fat replacers.[32]

Most fat replacers are carbohydrates—plant polysaccharides, celluloses, or gums—although protein and fat can help provide structure. Because they are poorly digested or absorbed, most add fewer kcalories than would fat (Table 4-2). One concern is their safety when used over time. Although studies reviewed by the U.S. Food and Drug Administration (FDA) indicate that fat replacers do not pose health risks for adults, little is known about their long-term effects in children. Olestra, a common fat replacer in snack foods, interferes with the absorption of fat-soluble vitamins, so olestra-containing products have added amounts of vitamins A, D, E, and K to compensate for any loss.[33] Although blood levels of vitamins A and E are maintained with vitamin supplements in users of olestra-containing foods, modest decreases occur in blood carotenoid concentrations.[34–35] (We will learn more about the importance of carotenoids to human health in Chapter 6.) Fat replacers that are not digested and remain in the stomach longer may add to satiety[36] and assist in appetite control.

Unfortunately the general public often assumes that baked goods, frozen desserts, and salad dressings made with fat replacers are lower in kcalories than those made with fat, but this is not always true. In fact, a food containing a fat replacer may contain the same number of kcalories or even more kcalories than its higher-fat counterpart if more sugar has been added to maintain flavor and mouth feel. People who

TABLE 4-2 FAT REPLACERS APPROVED FOR USE IN PROCESSED FOODS

TYPE	INGREDIENTS	ENERGY VALUE	TRADE NAMES	APPLICATIONS
Carbohydrate	Cellulose, pectin, gums, starches, dextrins, polydextrose, fruit-based fiber (dried plum or prune paste)	Typically only 1-2 kcal/g (cellulose or pectin contains 0 kcal/g)	Just Fiber, WonderSlim, Betatrim, Maltrin, Splendid, Litesse	Frozen desserts, salad dressings, baked goods, dry mixes, dairy foods, snack foods, cereal products, candy
Protein	Modified whey protein, milk and egg protein blends, microprotein particles, protein-starch mixtures	1-4 kcal/g (often usable in lower amounts than fat; 1 g can replace 3 g of fat in cream)	Simplesse, Dairy-Lo	Fat-free ice cream, frozen desserts; reduced-fat butter, sour cream, and cheese; baked goods; salad dressing; coffee creamers
Fat	Sucrose polyesters bonded with long-chain fatty acids, emulsifiers, triglycerides with short-chain fatty acids	0-9 kcal/g (those containing 9 kcal/g can be used in smaller amounts than fat)	Benefat (salatrim) contains 9 kcal/g; Olean (olestra) contains 0 kcal/g	Cake mixes, icing, dairy foods, fried snack foods

Data from American Dietetic Association: Position of the American Dietetic Association: fat replacers, *J Am Diet Assoc* 105:266, 2005.

presume they can eat a larger portion of an item made with a fat replacer may be taking in even more kcalories than they would with a smaller portion of the higher-fat food. Better to select snacks from fruit, whole grains, or low-fat dairy items that are not only lower in fat but also rich in nutrients.

LIPID-RELATED COMPOUNDS

Cholesterol

Structure

Although cholesterol is not a fat or a triglyceride, often it is discussed in connection with dietary lipids. Cholesterol belongs to a family of substances called steroids and travels in the blood attached to long-chain fatty acids. These cholesterol transport compounds are cholesterol esters. People sometimes confuse cholesterol with saturated fat because both substances are believed to promote atherosclerosis.

Functions

Cholesterol is required for normal body function[37] and is synthesized in the liver. If a person obtained no cholesterol whatsoever from food, the body would still have an adequate supply. Cholesterol has broad roles as follows:

- *Precursor to steroid hormones:* A cholesterol compound in the skin, 7-dehydrocholesterol, is converted to vitamin D when the ultraviolet rays of the sun pass into the skin; cholesterol is also a precursor of estrogen and testosterone.
- *Formation of bile acids:* Cholesterol is used to form bile acids, which emulsify fats and facilitate their digestion; bile acids serve as carriers in fat absorption.
- *Component of brain and nerve tissue:* The brain and nerves include cholesterol in their structure.
- *Component of cell membranes:* Cell membranes contain cholesterol.

Food Sources

Cholesterol is found in animal foods but not plant foods. Egg yolk, meat, whole and low-fat milk, cheese, and organ meats supply cholesterol. Animal fats (but *not* plant fats) are rich sources.

Suggested Cholesterol Intake

Because the body can synthesize cholesterol as needed, no DRI is required.[14] People are encouraged to limit their intake, keeping in mind that eliminating cholesterol entirely would also eliminate meat, eggs, and some dairy products that provide vitamins and minerals important to health. The American Heart Association recommends that dietary cholesterol be held to 300 mg/day or less, an intake associated with appropriate blood cholesterol levels.[6] By genetic selection the cholesterol content of eggs and meat has been lowered, reducing the cholesterol present in the food supply. Nevertheless, daily intake averages about 358 mg in men and 237 mg in women.[38] Eggs, beef, poultry, cheese, and milk add the most to cholesterol intake.[12] Certain plant sterols interfere with the absorption of cholesterol and help lower blood cholesterol levels. (See the *Evidence-Based Practice* box, "Plant Sterols: New Weapon for Lowering Blood Cholesterol Levels.")

Lipoproteins

Function

The liver is the body clearinghouse for fatty acids and cholesterol, whether supplied in food or produced in body tissues. When received by the liver, fatty acids and cholesterol are (1) packaged into lipoproteins and then (2) released into the circulation for transport to cells.[13]

Lipid Transport

Lipids are insoluble in water, which poses a problem when they need to be carried in a water-based circulatory system. The body solves this problem by producing lipoproteins, a complex of lipids and lipidlike substances surrounded

EVIDENCE-BASED PRACTICE

Plant Sterols: New Weapon for Lowering Blood Cholesterol Levels

Plant sterols, also known as *phytosterols or phytostanols,* are found in small amounts in vegetable oils and grains such as corn, rye, and wheat. The chemical structure of plant sterols is much like that of cholesterol; based on this similarity, plant sterols compete with cholesterol for absorption in the small intestine. For some time, nutrition researchers speculated that plant sterols would lower the amount of cholesterol absorbed and delivered to the liver. When less cholesterol is available, the liver produces fewer lipoproteins and blood levels of total cholesterol and LDL cholesterol drop.[1] Unfortunately, plant sterols occur naturally in food in very small amounts—too small to make a difference in cholesterol absorption. Food technologists have since found ways to incorporate plant sterols into food products to increase dietary intake. Table fats and orange juice with added plant sterols are two examples of new functional foods.

Clinical trials with patients having elevated blood cholesterol levels demonstrated the benefits of plant sterols in the prevention and treatment of cardiovascular disease. Adding 1.5 to 3 g of plant sterols to the daily diet lowered total cholesterol and LDL cholesterol levels by as much as 15%[1-2] and reduced the tendency of blood platelets to form unwanted blood clots.[3] This treatment was effective regardless of a patient's adherence to a low-fat diet (30% of total kcalories). Based on these results the FDA approved a health claim for sterol-containing foods, allowing a statement on the nutrition label that regular use along with a diet low in saturated fat and cholesterol may reduce the risk of heart disease.[4]

Although plant sterols support heart health, we must help people understand that these foods must replace the conventional item in their daily meal pattern, not add to total fat and kcalorie intake. An 8-oz serving of orange juice containing 1 g of plant sterols also provides 110 kcal but meets the MyPyramid equivalent of one serving of fruit. Additional fruit servings, however, should be selected from whole fruits that also add fiber to the diet. Table spreads containing about 0.7 g of plant sterols per tablespoon (1 tbsp being the recommended serving size) add 70 kcal and 8 g of fat per serving. Products advertised as "light" spreads usually contain about 50 kcal/tbsp and 5 g of fat. Two tablespoons per day are needed to reach the suggested intake of plant sterols.

Sterol-containing foods appear to be safe for use over long periods of time, although they may adversely affect the absorption of carotenoids and lower blood carotenoid levels.[5] Individuals using sterol-fortified foods should be encouraged to include generous servings of carotenoid-rich foods in their daily diet.[5]

REFERENCES

1. Castro IA, Barroso LP, Sinnecker P: Functional foods for coronary heart disease risk reduction: a meta-analysis using a multivariate approach, *Am J Clin Nutr* 82:32, 2005.
2. Castro Cabezas M, de Vries JH, Oostrom AJ, et al: Effects of a stanol-enriched diet on plasma cholesterol and triglycerides in patients treated with statins, *J Am Diet Assoc* 106:1564, 2006.
3. Kozlowska-Wojciechowska M, Jastrzebska M, Naruszewicz M, et al: Impact of margarine enriched with plant sterols on blood lipids, platelet function, and fibrinogen level in young men, *Metabolism* 52:1378, 2003.
4. U.S. Food and Drug Administration: Food labeling: Health claims; Plant sterol/stanol esters and coronary heart disease; Interim final rule, *Fed Regist* 65 (No. 175), FR 54685–FR 54739, Sept. 8, 2000, Rockville, Md, 2000, U.S. Department of Health and Human Services. Retrieved April 23, 2010, from www.fda.gov/Food/LabelingNutrition/LabelClaims/HealthClaimsMeetingSignificantScientificAgreementSSA/ucm074747.htm.
5. Van Horn L, McCoin M, Kris-Etherton PM, et al: The evidence for dietary prevention and treatment of cardiovascular disease, *J Am Diet Assoc* 108:287, 2008.

by water-soluble protein. Special compounds called **phospholipids** are important in the structure of lipoproteins. Phospholipids are molecules in which one of the three fatty acids attached to a glycerol base is replaced with a phosphate (PO_4^{-3}) group that is water soluble and assists in the transport of lipoproteins. Phospholipids in cell membranes help lipid molecules move from the circulatory system into the cell.

Lipoproteins contain fatty acids, triglycerides, cholesterol, phospholipids, and traces of fat-soluble vitamins and steroid hormones. They serve as the major vehicle for lipid transport in the blood.

Classes of Lipoproteins

Lipoproteins are classified according to their density, based on their relative content of lipid and protein. The more protein present, the greater the density. The amount of each lipoprotein in the blood is influenced by time since the last meal and the quantity and type of fat that a person consumes on a regular basis. The five lipoprotein classes are as follows:

KEY TERMS

steroids Group name for lipid-based sterols including hormones, bile acids, and cholesterol.

esters Compounds produced by the reaction between an acid and an alcohol with elimination of a molecule of water. This process is called *esterification.* A triglyceride is a glycerol ester, and cholesterol forms esters by combining with fatty acids.

bile A fluid secreted by the liver and transported to the gallbladder for concentration and storage. It is released into the duodenum on entry of fat and acts as an emulsifier to facilitate enzymatic fat digestion.

complex A chemical compound consisting of several atoms or molecules loosely connected and easily separated. The micelles formed in the lumen of the intestine, which carry fats into the intestinal wall, are bile-lipid complexes.

phospholipids A class of fat-related substances that contain phosphorus, fatty acids, and a nitrogen base. The phospholipids are important components of cell membranes, nerve tissues, and lipoproteins.

1. *Chylomicrons:* These relatively large particles are formed in the intestinal wall after a meal and carry the digested and absorbed fat to the liver for conversion to other lipoproteins.
2. *Very low-density lipoproteins (VLDLs):* The VLDLs are formed in the liver during the fasting interval between meals. When no food is in the digestive tract and chylomicrons are not entering the circulatory system, VLDLs transport endogenous triglycerides from the liver to tissue cells.
3. *Intermediate-density lipoproteins (IDLs):* IDLs are formed from VLDLs and continue the delivery of endogenous triglycerides to the cells.
4. *LDLs:* LDLs are formed from VLDLs and IDLs and carry primarily cholesterol, because most of the triglyceride has already moved into the cells.
5. *HDLs:* HDLs return cholesterol from the cells to the liver for breakdown and excretion.

Cholesterol, Lipoproteins, and Cardiovascular Risk

Of all the lipoproteins the two receiving the most attention in clinical practice are the LDLs and the HDLs. Both are primary carriers of cholesterol; thus their levels in the blood have important implications for health. The LDLs transport cholesterol from the liver to the tissues; in fact, about half of the cholesterol circulating in the blood is contained in the LDLs.[37] Conversely, the HDLs return cholesterol from the cells to the liver for excretion. Elevated blood cholesterol in the form of LDL cholesterol promotes *atherosclerosis,* the underlying pathologic condition in coronary heart disease. High LDL cholesterol levels cause a buildup of fatty plaque on the inner walls of the vessels supplying blood to the heart muscle. Over time, these plaques narrow the lumen of the coronary arteries, decreasing delivery of both oxygen and other nutrients. Interruption of blood to the heart, as a result of a blood clot or built-up plaque, causes a heart attack; a similar occurrence in an artery in the brain results in a stroke (cerebral hemorrhage). In contrast to LDLs, high HDLs slow or prevent the progression of atherosclerosis, lowering cardiovascular risk.

Although the types and amounts of dietary fat people consume affect LDL and HDL cholesterol levels, the situation is more complex. Some people absorb cholesterol more efficiently or synthesize increased amounts regardless of dietary intake. Genetic factors affect the production of HDLs and the rate at which cholesterol is eliminated from the body.[37] In Chapter 21 we will learn about dietary and lifestyle interventions and medications that help control blood lipoprotein levels.

DIGESTION-ABSORPTION-METABOLISM REVIEW

The digestion of the macronutrients was discussed in greater detail in Chapter 2. A brief summary of the chemical digestion and absorption process specific to lipids is provided here for review.

Digestion

Triglycerides in animal and plant foods must be broken down into individual fatty acids for absorption and later use.

TABLE 4-3 SUMMARY OF LIPID DIGESTION

ORGAN	ENZYME	ACTIVITY
Mouth	Lingual lipase (very limited)	Mechanical, mastication
Stomach	No major enzyme	Mechanical separation of fats as protein and starch are digested out
	Small amount of gastric lipase (tributyrinase)	Butterfat (tributyrin) to fatty acids and glycerol
Small intestine	Bile salts enter from gallbladder	Emulsifies fats
	Pancreatic lipase	Triglycerides to diglycerides and monoglycerides in turn; then fatty acids and glycerol

Mouth

Chemical breakdown in the mouth is limited, although lingual lipase from the salivary secretions begins the process of lipid digestion.

Stomach

The only gastric secretion specific to lipids is the enzyme gastric lipase (tributyrinase), which acts on emulsified butterfat. As gastric enzymes act on carbohydrates and proteins in the food mix, the lipids begin to separate out, making them more accessible to their own enzymes in the small intestine.

Small Intestine

The major breakdown of lipids begins in the small intestine. Digestive secretions come from three sources: (1) the biliary tract, (2) the pancreas, and (3) the small intestine, as follows:

1. *Bile from the liver and gallbladder:* The presence of fat in the upper duodenum triggers the release of cholecystokinin (CCK) from the intestinal mucosa, which in turn causes the gall bladder to contract, releasing a flow of bile. Bile acts as an emulsifier, preparing lipids for further digestion by (1) breaking them into smaller particles to increase the surface area accessible to enzyme action and (2) lowering the surface tension of the finely dispersed globules, enabling enzymes to penetrate more easily. Bile also provides the alkaline medium needed for the action of pancreatic lipase. When bile secretion is hindered, as much as 40% of dietary fat is lost in the feces.[13]
2. *Enzymes from the pancreas: Pancreatic lipase* breaks off one fatty acid at a time from the glycerol base of triglycerides. The initial action yields one fatty acid plus a diglyceride, and continuing action yields another fatty acid plus a monoglyceride. Each successive step becomes more difficult, with the result that less than one third of the fat in the food mass is broken down completely. The final products of lipid digestion ready to be absorbed are fatty acids, diglycerides, monoglycerides, and glycerol.
3. *Enzyme from the small intestine: Lecithinase* acts on lecithin, a *phospholipid,* to prepare it for absorption.

Table 4-3 summarizes lipid digestion.

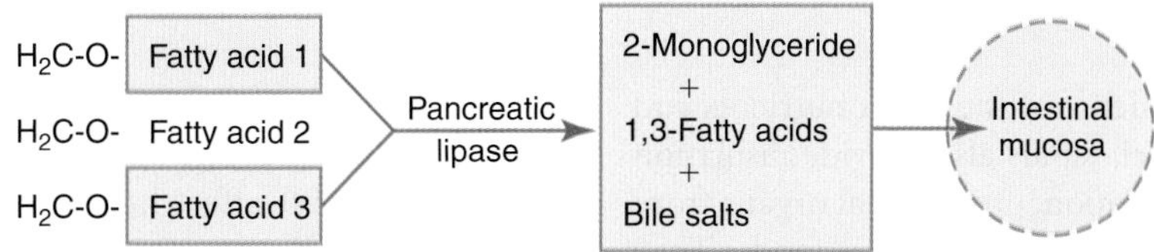

FIGURE 4-4 Micellar complex of fats and bile salts for transport into the intestinal wall. The fatty acid in the *2* position of the triglyceride is the most difficult to remove, and some fat is absorbed in the monoglyceride form.

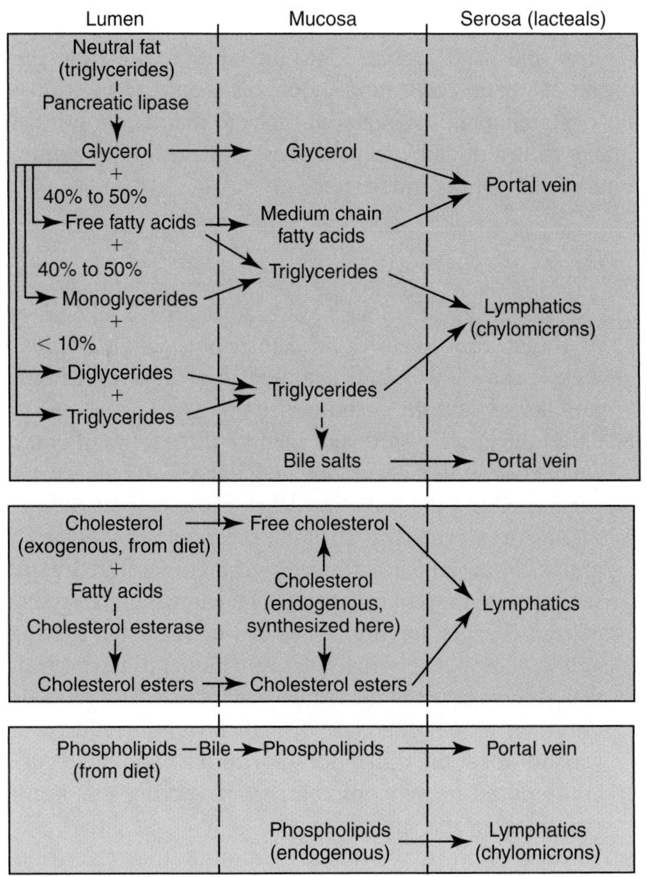

FIGURE 4-5 Absorption of fat, cholesterol, and phospholipids.

Absorption

The task of transporting lipids from the small intestine into the bloodstream takes place in three stages.

Stage I: Initial Lipid Absorption

In the small intestine, bile salts combine with the products of lipid digestion to form micelles, a bile-lipid complex. This carrier system (described in Figure 4-4) moves the lipid molecules from the lumen of the intestine into the intestinal wall.

Stage II: Absorption Within the Intestinal Wall

Once inside the wall of the small intestine the bile salts separate from the lipid complex, are absorbed, and return to the liver via the *enterohepatic circulation,* ready to carry out their task again. When the lipid products are released from the micellar complex, the following two actions take place:

1. *Enteric lipase digestion:* A lipase within the intestinal wall completes the digestion of any remaining diglycerides and monoglycerides, releasing fatty acids and glycerol.
2. *Triglyceride synthesis:* The available fatty acids and glycerol form new human triglycerides, ready for final absorption and transport.

Stage III: Final Absorption and Transport

The newly formed human triglycerides—along with any other lipid materials present—receive a protein covering to form the lipoproteins called *chylomicrons.* These lipid packages cross the cell membrane to enter the lymphatic system and drain into the portal blood. In the liver the lipids are converted into new lipoproteins for transport to body cells. Figure 4-5 illustrates lipid absorption through its three stages.

Metabolism

The metabolism of carbohydrates, proteins, and lipids are closely intertwined to effectively meet the body's constant demand for energy.

KEY TERMS

chylomicrons Lipoproteins formed in the intestinal wall after a meal that carry food fats into the lymph and then the general circulation for transport to the liver.

endogenous Originating from within the body; an example is endogenous cholesterol, which is produced by cells in the liver.

lipase Group of fat enzymes that cut the ester linkages between the fatty acids and glycerol in triglycerides (fats).

cholecystokinin (CCK) A peptide hormone secreted by the duodenal mucosa when fat is present. CCK causes the gallbladder to contract and propel bile into the duodenum, where it emulsifies fat and prepares it for digestion.

emulsifier An agent that breaks down large fat globules to smaller, uniformly distributed particles. This action is accomplished in the intestine by bile acids, which lower the surface tension of the fat particles. Emulsification increases the surface area of fat, expanding contact with digestive enzymes.

micelles Combinations of bile and fat that carry fat into the wall of the small intestine in preparation for the final stage of absorption into the lymph and general circulation.

portal An entryway, usually referring to the portal circulation of blood through the liver. Blood is brought into the liver via the portal vein and moves out via the hepatic vein.

TO SUM UP

Lipids are the most energy dense of the macronutrients and a concentrated source of fuel. Lipids also provide insulation to assist in temperature regulation, protect vital organs from damage, and contribute flavor and texture to foods. They have a role in neural transmission, structure of steroid hormones and cell membranes, and transport of the fat-soluble vitamins. The building blocks of lipids are fatty acids. Fatty acids are classified on the basis of chain length and degree of saturation. Two polyunsaturated fatty acids—(1) linoleic acid, an n-6 fatty acid, and (2) α-linolenic acid, an n-3 fatty acid—are essential and must be supplied in food. The essential fatty acids are important for skin integrity, growth (especially the development of brain and neural tissue), control of blood cholesterol levels, and immune function. Several n-3 fatty acids in fish control platelet aggregation and lower the risk of heart attack and stroke. Both the type and the amount of dietary lipids affect health. Inappropriately high intakes of fat, especially saturated fats and trans fats, increase cardiovascular risk. The AMDR for fat is 20% to 35% of total kcalories. When lipids provide less than 10% of total kcalories, supplies of the essential fatty acids may be inadequate. Consumers should consult the nutrition label and list of ingredients on processed foods to limit their intakes of total fat, trans fats, and saturated fats, including saturated vegetable fats. Nutrition education should focus on wise selection of fat-containing and fat-replaced foods to maintain a prudent intake of healthy fats, control energy intake, and maximize intakes of vitamins and minerals.

QUESTIONS FOR REVIEW

1. What is a lipid? Name several members of this nutrient class.
2. Describe the roles of fat in the body.
3. Compare saturated, monounsaturated, and polyunsaturated fatty acids based on their (a) chemical structure, (b) effects on health, and (c) usual food sources. Are plant fats always better?
4. Name the two essential fatty acids. Why are they considered essential? What happens when they are not available in the amounts needed? What foods supply the essential fatty acids?
5. You are counseling a patient who has been told that he should lose 10 to 15 lb. His usual fat intake is about 35% of his total energy intake. He has agreed to lower his intake of fat to 30% in an effort to reduce his daily kcalories. What are some strategies that might help him accomplish this? He and his co-workers eat their lunch at fast-food restaurants. Develop three fast-food lunch menus that limit fat and kcalories.
6. Two persons with strong family histories of cardiovascular disease are concerned about their heart health. Both lower their cholesterol intake and avoid eating butter. One person started to use a stick margarine made from corn oil and the other a soft tub corn oil margarine. Which person made the better choice? Why?
7. A woman runner has decided to remove all fat from her diet. If she is successful in doing this, then what health problems might she encounter?
8. Go to the grocery store and identify three types of crackers or cookies that offer both a regular and a "reduced-fat" version. Using the nutrition label, make a chart indicating the (a) serving size, (b) total kcalories per serving, (c) grams of total fat per serving, (d) grams of saturated fat per serving, (e) grams of unsaturated fat per serving, (f) grams of trans fat per serving, (g) grams of sugar per serving, and (h) cost per serving. What nutritional differences did you observe between the regular and reduced-fat versions? Was there a cost difference; if so, then was the reduced-fat version worth the difference in price? How do the regular and reduced-fat versions compare in serving size, kcalories, total fat, and sugar?
9. You are asked to provide a 10-minute update on trans fats to a citizens group that is concerned about public health. Develop an outline for your presentation including (a) examples of both processed and restaurant foods that contain trans fats and (b) use of the nutrition label to identify trans fats.

REFERENCES

1. Moskowitz H, Beckley J, Adams J: What makes people crave fast foods? *Nutr Today* 37:237, 2002.
2. American Dietetic Association: Position of the American Dietetic Association: total diet approach to communicating food and nutrition information, *J Am Diet Assoc* 107:1224, 2007.
3. Wahrburg U: What are the health effects of fat? *Eur J Nutr* 43(Suppl 1):I/6, 2004.
4. Van Horn L, McCoin M, Kris-Etherton PM, et al: The evidence for dietary prevention and treatment of cardiovascular disease, *J Am Diet Assoc* 108:287, 2008.
5. American Dietetic Association: Position of the American Dietetic Association and Dietitians of Canada: dietary fatty acids, *J Am Diet Assoc* 107:1599, 2007.
6. Lichtenstein AH, Appel LJ, Brands M, et al: Diet and lifestyle recommendations revision 2006: a scientific statement from the American Heart Association Nutrition Committee, *Circulation* 114:82, 2006.
7. American Diabetes Association: Nutrition recommendations and interventions for diabetes 2006, *Diabetes Care* 29:2140, 2006.
8. Bray GA, Wilson JK: In the clinic: obesity, *Ann Intern Med* 149(7):ITC4-1, 2008.
9. Bray GA, Bellanger T: Epidemiology, trends, and morbidities of obesity and the metabolic syndrome, *Endocrine* 29:109, 2006.
10. Eckel RH, Kris-Etherton P, Lichtenstein AH, et al: Americans' awareness, knowledge, and behaviors regarding fats: 2006–2007, *J Am Diet Assoc* 109:288, 2009.

11. Rolls ET: Sensory processing in the brain related to the control of food intake, *Proc Nutr Soc* 66:96, 2007.
12. Cotton PA, Subar AF, Friday JE, et al: Dietary sources of nutrients among U.S. adults, 1994 to 1996, *J Am Diet Assoc* 104:921, 2004.
13. Jones PJH, Kubow S: Lipids, sterols, and their metabolites. In Shils ME, Shike M, Olson J, et al, editors: *Modern nutrition in health and disease*, ed 10, Baltimore, 2006, Lippincott Williams & Wilkins.
14. Food and Nutrition Board, Institute of Medicine: *Dietary Reference Intakes for energy, carbohydrate, fiber, fat, fatty acids, cholesterol, protein, and amino acids (macronutrients)*, Washington, DC, 2002, National Academies Press.
15. Sampath H, Ntambi JM: Polyunsaturated fatty acid regulation of gene expression, *Nutr Rev* 62(9):333, 2004.
16. Riediger ND, Othman RA, Suh M, et al: A systematic review of the roles of n-3 fatty acids in health and disease, *J Am Diet Assoc* 109:668, 2009.
17. Makrides M: Outcomes for mothers and their babies: do n-3 long-chain polyunsaturated fatty acids and seafoods make a difference, *J Am Diet Assoc* 108:1622, 2008.
18. Carlson SE: Docosahexaenoic acid supplementation in pregnancy and lactation, *Am J Clin Nutr* 89(Suppl):678S, 2009.
19. Kris-Etherton PM, Hill AM: n-3 fatty acids: food or supplements, *J Am Diet Assoc* 108:1125, 2008.
20. Mozaffarian D, Katan MB, Ascherio A, et al: Trans fatty acids and cardiovascular disease, *N Engl J Med* 354:1601, 2006.
21. Riserus U, Willett WC, Hu FB, et al: Dietary fats and prevention of type 2 diabetes, *Prog Lipid Res* 48:44, 2009.
22. Elias SL, Innis SM: Bakery foods are the major dietary source of trans-fatty acids among pregnant women with diets providing 30% energy from fat, *J Am Diet Assoc* 102(1):46, 2002.
23. Borra S, Kris-Etherton PM, Dausch JG, et al: An update of *trans*-fat reduction in the American diet, *J Am Diet Assoc* 107:2048, 2007.
24. Eckel RH, Borra S, Lichtenstein AH, et al: Understanding the complexity of trans fatty acid reduction in the American diet, *Circulation* 115:2231, 2007.
25. Kennedy ET, Bowman SA, Spence JT, et al: Popular diets: correlation to health, nutrition, and obesity, *J Am Diet Assoc* 101(4):411, 2001.
26. Ma Y, Olendzki BC, Hafner AR, et al: Low-carbohydrate and high-fat intake among adult patients with poorly controlled type 2 diabetes mellitus, *Nutrition* 22:1129, 2006.
27. Kant AK, Graubard BI, Kumanyika SK: Trends in black-white differentials in dietary intakes of U.S. adults, 1971–2002, *Am J Prev Med* 32:264, 2007.
28. Chanmugam P, Guthrie JF, Cecilio S, et al: Did fat intake in the United States really decline between 1989–1991 and 1994–1996? *J Am Diet Assoc* 103:867, 2003.
29. Bowman SA, Vinyard BT: Fast food consumption of U.S. adults: impact on energy and nutrient intakes and overweight status, *J Am Coll Nutr* 23:163, 2004.
30. Sigman-Grant M, Warland R, Hsieh G: Selected lower-fat foods positively impact nutrient quality in diets of free-living Americans, *J Am Diet Assoc* 103:570, 2003.
31. Ledikwe JH, Blanck HM, Khan LK, et al: Low-energy-density diets are associated with high quality in adults in the United States, *J Am Diet Assoc* 106:1172, 2006.
32. American Dietetic Association: Position of the American Dietetic Association: fat replacers, *J Am Diet Assoc* 105:266, 2005.
33. Food and Drug Administration: Olestra labeling change, *FDA Consum* Nov-Dec 2003.
34. Neuhouser ML, Rock CL, Kristal AR, et al: Olestra is associated with slight reductions in serum carotenoids but does not markedly influence serum fat-soluble vitamin concentrations, *Am J Clin Nutr* 83:624, 2006.
35. Tulley RT, Vaidyanathan J, Wilson JB, et al: Daily intake of multivitamins during long-term intake of olestra in men prevents declines in serum vitamins A and E but not carotenoids, *J Nutr* 135:1456, 2005.
36. Bray GA, Lovejoy JC, Most-Windhauser M, et al: A 9-mo randomized clinical trial comparing fat-substituted and fat-reduced diets in healthy obese men: the Ole study, *Am J Clin Nutr* 76:928, 2002.
37. Grundy SM: Nutrition in the management of disorders of serum lipids and lipoproteins. In Shils ME, Shike M, Olson J, et al, editors: *Modern nutrition in health and disease*, ed 10, Baltimore, 2006, Lippincott Williams & Wilkins.
38. U.S. Department of Agriculture, Agricultural Research Service: *Nutrient intakes from food: mean amounts consumed per individual, one day, 2005–2006*, Washington, DC, U.S. Department of Agriculture. Retrieved July 18, 2009, from www.ars.usda.gov/ba/bhnrc/fsrg.

FURTHER READINGS AND RESOURCES

Readings

Whitfield Jacobsen PA, Prawitz AD, Lukaszuk JM: Long-haul truck drivers want healthful meal options at truck-stop restaurants, *J Am Diet Assoc* 107:2125, 2007.

Fitzgerald CM, Kannan S, Sheldon S, et al: Effect of a promotional campaign on heart-healthy menu choices in community restaurants, *J Am Diet Assoc* 104:429, 2004.

[These two articles discuss the need for community intervention programs in various types of food outlets. Restaurants should offer healthy choices to support individuals trying to make dietary changes.]

Kelley C, Krummel D, Gonzales EN, et al: Dietary intake of children at high risk for cardiovascular disease, *J Am Diet Assoc* 104:222, 2004. *[This article focuses on the cultural aspects of fat intake and the need to work with families as we develop diet intervention programs.]*

Borra S, Kris-Etherton PM, Dausch JG, et al: An update of trans-fat reduction in the American diet, *J Am Diet Assoc* 107:2048, 2007. *[This article reviews the changes in trans fat intake that has occurred in response to government and community interventions.]*

Hoy MK, Winters BL, Chlebowski RT, et al: Implementing a low-fat eating plan in the women's intervention nutrition study, *J Am Diet Assoc* 109:688, 2009. *[These authors provide a model for helping clients decrease their intakes of fat.]*

Johnson GH, Keast DR, Kris-Etherton PM: Dietary modeling shows that the substitution of canola oil for fats commonly used in the United States would increase compliance with dietary recommendations for fatty acids, *J Am Diet Assoc* 107:1726, 2007. *[Dr. Johnson and colleagues present an interesting perspective on how a change in choice of dietary fat could improve intake of healthy fatty acids.]*

Websites of Interest

American Heart Association: *Know Your Fats*; this reputable health organization provides information about healthy versus unhealthy fats and how to make good food choices; an animated program on "Meet the Fats" is applicable to youth audiences: www.americanheart.org/presenter.jhtml?identifier=532.

International Food Information Council Foundation; this site contains fact sheets and brochures for both consumers and health professionals on food fats and fat replacers: www.ific.org/.

National Heart, Lung, and Blood Institute, National Institutes of Health: *Information for … the Public*; this government agency provides tutorials on various aspects of heart disease, recipe books for good eating that include cultural and ethnic food patterns, and a menu planner to help monitor fat intake: www.nhlbi.nih.gov/health/index.htm.

National Heart, Lung, and Blood Institute, National Institutes of Health: *Tips for Dining Out on the TLC (Therapeutic Lifestyle Changes) Diet*; this publication offers insight for healthy choices in menu selection: www.nhlbi.nih.gov/chd/Tipsheets/diningout.htm.

New York City Department of Health: *The Regulation to Phase Out Artificial Trans Fat in New York City Food Service Establishments*; this document describes the public health campaign to remove trans fats: www.nyc.gov/html/doh/downloads/pdf/cardio/cardio-transfat-bro.pdf.

CHAPTER

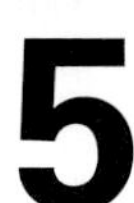

Proteins

Eleanor D. Schlenker

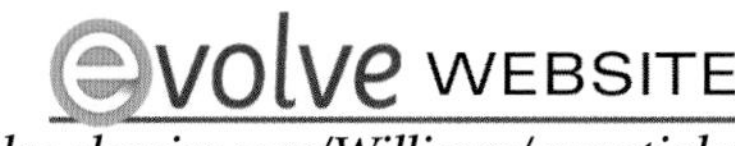

http://evolve.elsevier.com/Williams/essentials/

OUTLINE

This chapter describing protein completes our sequence on the macronutrients. Protein is quite different from its partners, carbohydrate and fat. First, it is the body's major source of nitrogen, the essential element of all living things. Second, its main task is forming body tissues using its individual building units, the amino acids. Protein is critical to growth and health, and protein deficiency associated with crop failure, poverty, or other food shortages has caused widespread malnutrition and death among infants, children, and adults in the developing world. In affluent societies, intakes of protein—especially animal protein—have escalated and for some individuals may be inappropriately high. Protein is a critical component in the rehabilitation and nutrition support of patients recovering from surgery, trauma, or serious illness. Our growing understanding of the health benefits of various plant proteins encourages their use in menu planning for all age groups.

PHYSICAL AND CHEMICAL NATURE OF PROTEINS

General Definition

In 1838 when Dutch chemist Johann Mulder first identified protein as a substance in all living things, it is unlikely he realized how far-reaching his work would become. Proteins shape our lives. Protein enzymes break down our food into nutrients the cells can use. As antibodies they shield us from disease. Peptide hormones carry messages that coordinate continuous body activity. In addition, they guide our growth in childhood and maintain our bodies thereafter; they make us each unique.

Chemical Nature

The proteins we eat do none of this work as proteins. Rather, their structural units—the amino acids—are the working currency of protein in body cells. Amino acids are composed of the elements carbon, hydrogen, oxygen, and nitrogen—the special element of all living matter. Protein is about 16% nitrogen. Several amino acids also contain sulfur.

The name *amino acid* tells us they have a dual nature. The word *amino* refers to a base or alkaline substance, so at once we have a contradiction. How can a chemical substance be both a base and an acid, and why is this important? Consider the significance of this fact as we learn more about amino acids and their roles in the body.

General Pattern and Structure

A common structural pattern holds for all amino acids. This pattern is built around a central α-carbon, with several attached chemical groups (Figure 5-1) as follows:

- *Amino (base, NH_2) group:* The amino group contains the essential element nitrogen and as an ion carries a positive charge.

KEY TERMS

amino acids Acids containing the essential element nitrogen within an amino group—NH_2. Amino acids are the structural units of protein.

amino group The monovalent radical, NH_2, an essential component of all amino acids.

- *Carboxyl (acid, COOH) group:* The carboxyl group is found in all acids and as an ion carries a negative charge.
- *An attached radical (R) group:* The *R* stands for *radical,* a general term referring to a group of elements attached to a chemical compound. In this case it refers to the attached side chains on amino acids, each one different. The distinctive side chain on an amino acid gives it a unique size, shape, and set of properties.[1–2] Compare the structure of the two simplest amino acids, glycine and alanine (Figure 5-2), with the larger and more complex amino acid arginine (Figure 5-3), with its extended carbon chain (R) and three additional amino groups.

Amino acids contain the same three elements—carbon, hydrogen, and oxygen—that make up carbohydrates and fats. However, amino acids and their proteins have the additional element—nitrogen—in the amino portion of their structure. Twenty different amino acids are used to build body proteins.[3] They all have the same core pattern, but each has a specific and different side group. The dual chemical structure of amino acids containing both acid and base groups gives

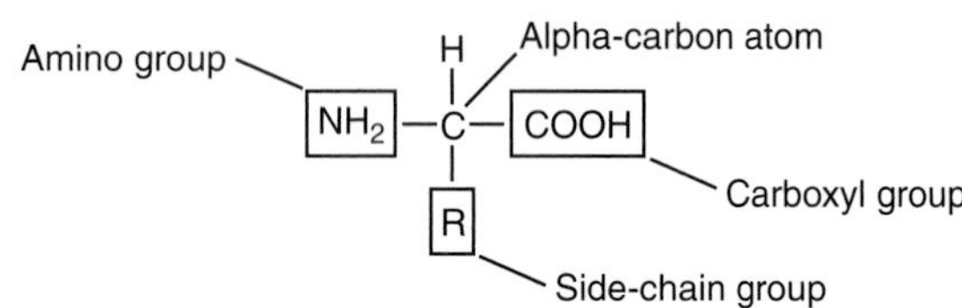

FIGURE 5-1 Basic structure of an amino acid.

BOX 5-1 CATEGORIES OF AMINO ACIDS

Indispensable (Essential)
- Histidine
- Isoleucine
- Leucine
- Lysine
- Methionine
- Phenylalanine
- Threonine
- Tryptophan
- Valine

Conditionally Indispensable (Essential)
- Arginine
- Cysteine
- Glutamine
- Glycine
- Proline
- Tyrosine

Dispensable (Nonessential)
- Alanine
- Aspartic acid
- Asparagine
- Glutamic acid
- Serine

Data from Food and Nutrition Board, Institute of Medicine: *Dietary Reference Intakes for energy, carbohydrate, fiber, fat, fatty acids, cholesterol, protein, and amino acids (macronutrients),* Washington, DC, 2002, National Academies Press.

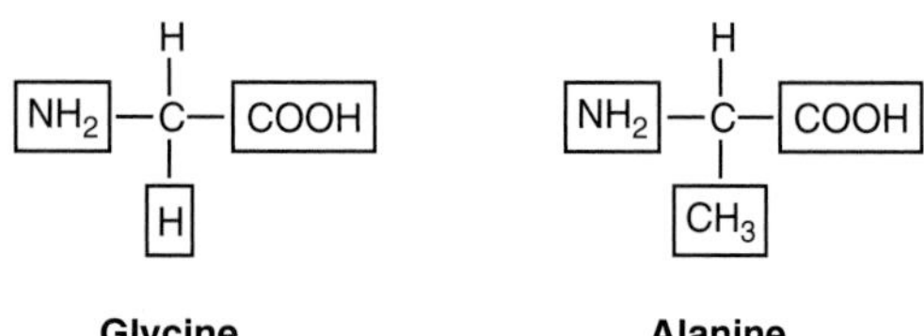

FIGURE 5-2 Structure of glycine and alanine.

them a unique amphoteric nature, meaning that an amino acid can behave as either an acid or a base, depending on the pH of the solution in which it is found. This makes it possible for amino acids to act as buffers, important in clinical care.

Essential Amino Acids

Of the 20 amino acids used to build body proteins, nine cannot be synthesized by the body and must be supplied in food. These nine amino acids are designated as indispensable (essential) amino acids. Another 5 of the 20 can be synthesized in adequate amounts and are termed *dispensable (nonessential) amino acids.* The remaining six fall in between and are known as *conditionally indispensable amino acids* (Box 5-1).[3] Although the body is able to synthesize the conditionally indispensable amino acids, it cannot meet the demand when tissue needs are elevated or the supply of necessary precursors is inadequate. Arginine is such an amino acid. The amount that can be produced in the liver is not sufficient to meet the needs of the newborn. The concept of *dietary* essentiality for the indispensable and conditionally indispensable amino acids is important when assessing protein quality.

THE BUILDING OF PROTEINS

Protein Structure

Peptide Bond

The dual chemical nature of amino acids—with a base group on one end and an acid group on the other—enables them to form the unique chain structure found in all proteins. The end amino group of one amino acid joins with the end carboxyl group of the amino acid next to it. This joining of amino acids is called a *peptide bond.* Specific amino acids are joined in a particular sequence to form long chains called *polypeptides,* and specific polypeptides come together to form proteins. Polypeptides vary in length from relatively short chains of 3 to 15 amino acids called *oligopeptides* to medium-sized polypeptides with chains of 21 to 30 amino acids such as insulin. Larger still are complex proteins made up of several hundred amino acids.

Large-Complex Proteins

New technology has helped us learn how protein chains fold and twist in space and interact with other body molecules.

Arginine

FIGURE 5-3 Structure of arginine.

To build a compact structure, long polypeptide chains coil or fold back in a spiral shape called a helix. Other proteins form a pleated sheet held together by strengthening cross-links of sulfur and hydrogen bonds. Learning more about the structure of body proteins helps medical researchers develop effective medications and understand how genes influence disease risk.

Types of Proteins

Proteins are a widely diverse group of compounds. They have important roles in body structure and metabolism made possible by their specific content and placement of amino acids. Consider the following examples.

Myosin

This fibrous protein found in muscle (Figure 5-4) is built from chains of 153 amino acids that coil and unfold as needed. Shaped into long rods, these fibers end in two-headed bundles so that they can change shape and bend, making it possible to tighten and contract muscles and then relax them.

Collagen

This structural protein contains three separate polypeptide chains that wind around each other to produce a triple helix (Figure 5-5). Thus reinforced, collagen is shaped into long rods and bundled into stiff fibers to do its job of strengthening bone, cartilage, and skin to maintain body form.

Hemoglobin

This globular protein (Figure 5-6) includes four globin polypeptide chains per molecule of hemoglobin. Each chain has several hundred amino acids conjugated with a nonprotein, the iron-containing pigment called *heme*. The globin wraps around the heme and forms protective pockets to secure the iron. The iron in heme has a special ability to bind oxygen and, as part of the red blood cell, delivers oxygen to the tissues.

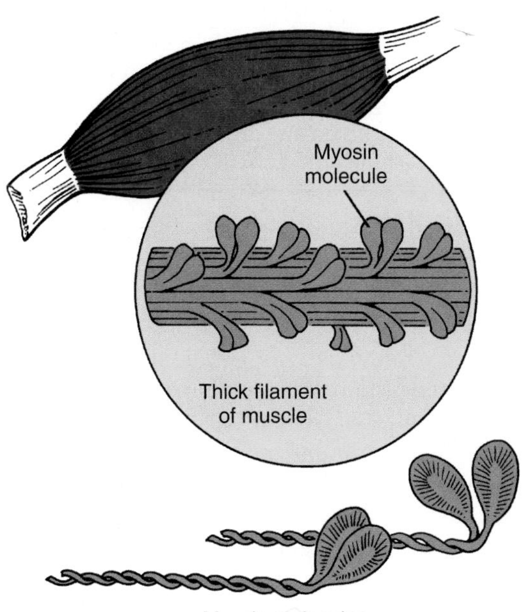

FIGURE 5-4 Myosin is a globular protein in muscle that combines with actin to form actomyosin, the fundamental contractile unit of muscle.

Albumin

Albumin is the major plasma protein and has a compact globular shape. It consists of a single polypeptide chain of 584 amino acids, twisted and coiled into helix structures held together by disulfide bridges.[4] Albumin is the most abundant plasma protein and serves as a carrier protein for drugs, hormones, enzymes, and trace elements. Albumin helps maintain fluid balance by exerting colloidal pressure in the capillaries that forces the flow of nutrients and fluids into the cells and the return of fluid and waste products out of the cells. In serious illness, albumin is broken down to supply amino acids for the synthesis of new proteins to meet the body emergency.

KEY TERMS

carboxyl group The monovalent radical, COOH, found in organic acids.

amphoteric Having opposite characteristics; capable of acting either as an acid or a base or combining with an acid or a base.

pH A scale ranging from 1 to 14 that describes the hydrogen ion concentration of a solution and its relative acidity or alkalinity; 7 is neutral, with lower numbers becoming progressively more acidic and higher numbers becoming progressively more alkaline.

buffers Mixtures of acid and alkaline components that, as part of a solution, protect against large changes in pH even if strong acids and bases are added. If an acid is added, then the alkaline partner reacts to counteract the acidic effect. If a base is added, then the acid partner reacts to counteract the alkalizing effect. This process keeps body fluids at the pH levels required for life.

indispensable (essential) amino acids Amino acids that the body cannot synthesize or cannot synthesize in sufficient amounts to meet body needs so must be supplied in the diet. The nine indispensable amino acids are histidine, isoleucine, leucine, lysine, methionine, phenylalanine, threonine, tryptophan, and valine. Six amino acids are conditionally indispensable because the body cannot synthesize sufficient amounts in situations of stress or increased need. These are arginine, cysteine, glutamine, glycine, proline, and tyrosine.

dispensable (nonessential) amino acids Amino acids that can be synthesized by the body from available precursors. The five dispensable amino acids are alanine, aspartic acid, asparagine, glutamic acid, and serine.

precursor A substance from which another substance is derived.

peptide bond The characteristic joining of amino acids to form proteins. Such a chain of amino acids is termed a *peptide*.

helix A coiled structure found in protein. Some are simple chain coils; others are made of several coils, as the triple helix.

synthesis The making of a substance or compound by the body.

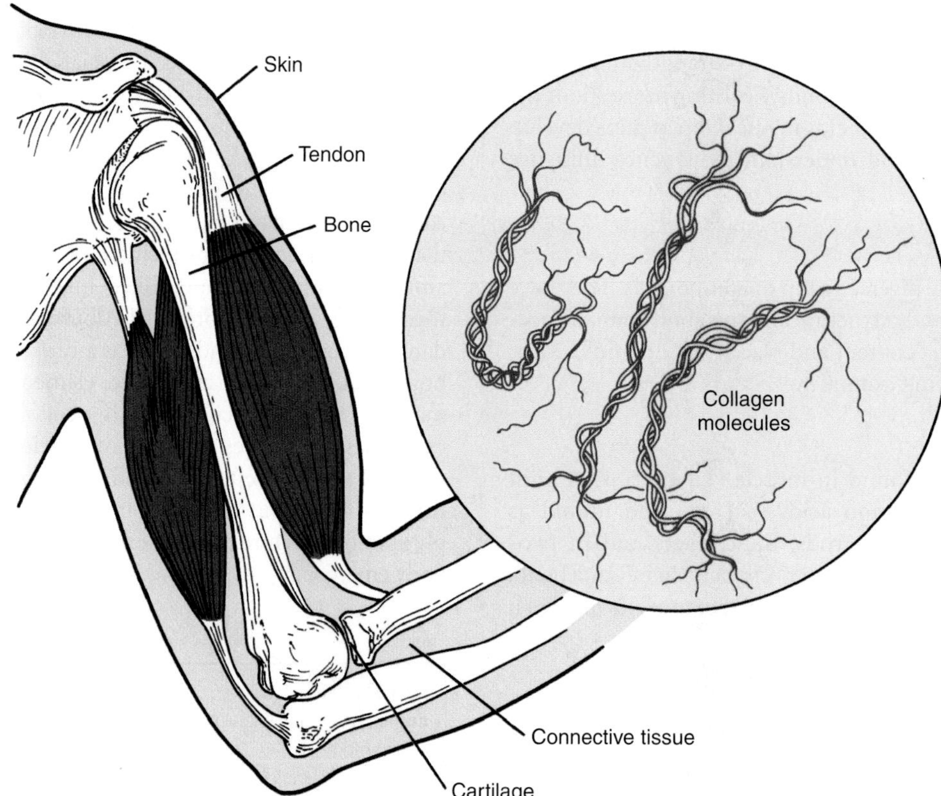

FIGURE 5-5 Tissues that contain collagen, a structural protein forming connective tissue.

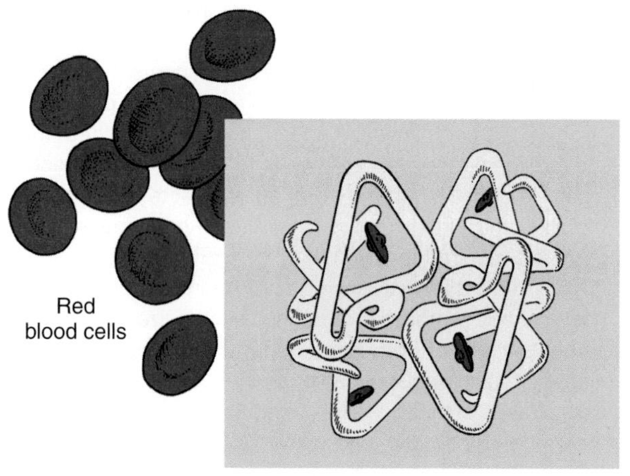

FIGURE 5-6 Hemoglobin is the iron-containing protein in red blood cells that carries oxygen to body cells and tissues.

Proteins with Special Roles

Other proteins with special structural or metabolic roles include the antibodies of the immune system and the blood protein fibrinogen, important in blood clotting. Hormones such as insulin and thyroxin and the enzymes that regulate our day-to-day metabolic activities such as digestion are proteins.[2]

FUNCTIONS OF PROTEIN

Growth, Tissue Building, and Maintenance

Dietary protein supplies the amino acid building material for the growth and maintenance of body tissues. It must furnish amino acids in the appropriate patterns and amounts for efficient synthesis of specific structural molecules. Dietary protein also supplies amino acids for making other nitrogen-containing substances such as the lipoproteins that transport fats in the blood and growth hormone that controls the growth of the long bones.

Physiologic Roles

All amino acids participate in tissue growth and maintenance. Some, however, have important metabolic roles of their own, as follows:

- *Form neurotransmitters for brain and nerve function*[5]*:* Methionine assists in the formation of choline, a precursor of acetylcholine, and tyrosine is used to synthesize the neurotransmitters dopamine and norepinephrine; tryptophan is the precursor of the neurotransmitter serotonin. Age-related decreases in the neurotransmitter dopamine are associated with Parkinson's disease, causing muscle tremors and rigidity.[6]
- *Form other amino acids:* Methionine is the precursor of the conditionally indispensable amino acid cysteine, as well as carnitine and taurine; carnitine transports long-chain fatty acids into the mitochondria for energy production

and taurine, found in bile salts, also regulates fluid pressure in the eyes.

- *Form hormones: Phenylalanine* is the precursor of the conditionally indispensable amino acid tyrosine needed to make thyroxin and epinephrine.
- *Support immune function:* Protein is needed to make antibodies for the immune system.
- *Maintain fluid balance:* Plasma proteins control the flow of fluids, nutrients, and waste products back and forth between the capillaries and the cells.

Role in Critical Care

Particular amino acids are beneficial in treating catabolic illness when breakdown and loss of skeletal muscle become critical. Leucine promotes protein synthesis and decreases muscle protein breakdown, improving recovery in patients with severe infection or after surgery or trauma. Branched chain amino acids—leucine, isoleucine, and valine—have positive effects in cancer patients for whom malnutrition is life threatening[7] and improve nitrogen retention and outcomes in liver disease.[8] These amino acids also increase the production of proteins that protect the mucosal lining of the intestine from invasion by harmful bacteria and contribute to the production of white blood cells, giving them special importance in critical care. Burn patients may have an increased need for arginine[1] and methionine[9] for tissue regeneration. Cysteine has an important role in protein synthesis and assists in recovery from protein-energy malnutrition (PEM).[10] Although we are learning how increased amounts of individual amino acids can improve patient status, self-medication with amino acid supplements is dangerous in both sickness and health.

Energy Source

Protein contributes to overall energy metabolism if needed, particularly during aerobic exercise.[11] Protein is seldom used for energy in the fed state, because glucose is readily available; however, it can be used in the fasting state. Before amino acids can be burned for energy, the nitrogen-containing amino group must be removed. The carbon skeleton that remains can be converted to either glucose or fat. In adults about 17 to 25 g of every 100 g of protein ingested are oxidized for energy.[3] Adequate carbohydrate spares protein for its primary purpose of tissue building.

PROTEIN AND NITROGEN BALANCE

Concept of Balance

Many interdependent checks and balances keep the body in working order. A constant ebb and flow exists, with tissue building and breaking down and body materials being stored and released. These coordinated activities enable the body to respond to any situation disturbing its normal function.

Protein Reserves

The average man contains about 11 kg of protein.[3] Forty percent is found in skeletal muscle, with the remainder in skin, blood, kidney, liver, brain, and other organs. Body distribution of protein changes with growth and development. The newborn has relatively little skeletal muscle, with proportionately more protein in the brain and visceral organs.

In contrast to the extensive fat reserves held by most people, body protein reserves are quite limited. What are referred to as the *labile protein reserves,* meaning they are easily broken down to meet immediate needs, make up only about 1% of total body protein; like glycogen, these reserves are sufficient to maintain body functions for only a short period of time.[3] The labile protein reserves are intended to provide amino acids for an emergency; if the condition continues, as in chronic illness or body wasting, then these reserves are rapidly depleted and skeletal muscle is broken down to furnish amino acids as needed. Muscle has an important role in overall body metabolism, and extreme loss of muscle mass is a predictor of mortality.[12]

Protein Balance

The concept of balance as related to protein balance refers to the steady state between protein synthesis (anabolism) and protein breakdown (catabolism). In periods of growth, synthesis exceeds breakdown, with a net gain of new tissue. When food intake is drastically reduced, as in famine or extreme voluntary food restriction or serious illness, tissue breakdown exceeds synthesis and body protein is lost.

Finely tuned mechanisms regulate protein synthesis and breakdown across all body tissues. When less protein is supplied in the diet, protein is conserved and protein losses are minimized. When fighting infection the body uses available protein reserves to obtain amino acids for making immune cells or other proteins necessary to preserve life. When more protein is available than is needed for body growth or repair, amino acids are broken down and used for energy or stored as fat. In healthy individuals, adjustments in protein balance on a day-to-day basis manage the daily variations in protein intake or short-term emergencies.

Various systems and protein compartments participate in this control of protein metabolism, as follows:

- *Protein turnover:* Protein turnover is the process by which body proteins are continuously broken down and the released amino acids made into new proteins.[3] New proteins are formed to replace worn-out proteins, and different proteins are formed to meet changing needs.

KEY TERMS

carnitine A naturally occurring amino acid ($C_{17}H_{15}NO_3$) formed from methionine and lysine; carnitine transports long-chain fatty acids into the mitochondria where they are oxidized for energy.

taurine A sulfur-containing amino acid, $NH_2(CH_2)_2 \bullet SO_2OH$, formed from the indispensable amino acid methionine. It is found in lung and muscle tissues and in bile and breast milk.

labile Easily changed or modified; unstable.

protein balance The balance between the building up (anabolism) and the breaking down (catabolism) of body tissues as necessary to maintain positive growth and maintenance.

anabolism Metabolic process for building body tissue.

catabolism Metabolic process for breaking down body tissue; the opposite of anabolism.

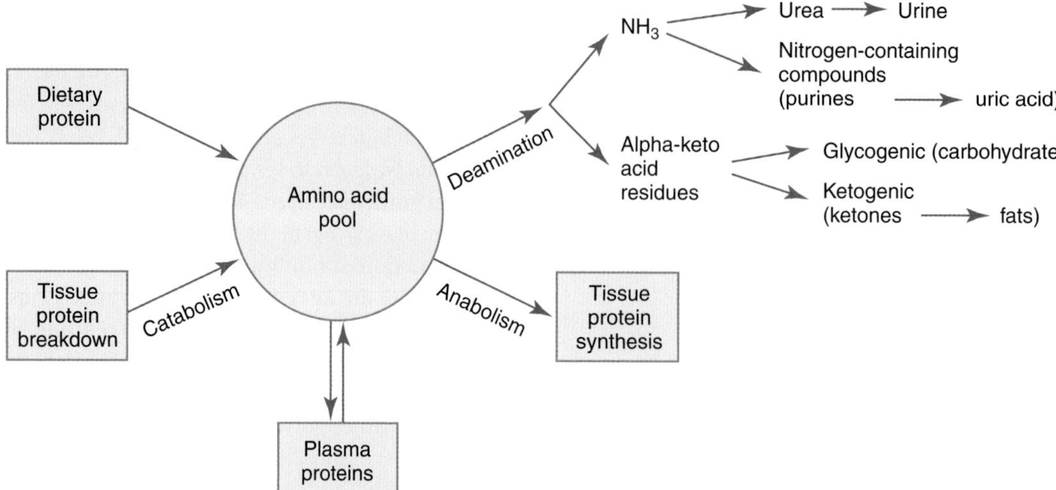

FIGURE 5-7 Flow between protein compartments and the amino acid pool. Amino acids are constantly entering and leaving the body's amino acid pool to form new proteins or other nitrogen-containing compounds, to be converted to carbohydrate and used for energy, or to be converted to fat for storage.

When an amino acid labeled with a radioactive carbon atom is incorporated into a protein food and eaten, it can be traced—that is, we can follow its journey through the body. By these studies we learned that amino acids are rapidly incorporated into body proteins and then, when these proteins are broken down, they are reused to form new proteins. Protein turnover varies among tissues. Turnover rates are increased in the intestinal mucosa, liver, pancreas, kidney, and plasma, tissues that are more metabolically active, and decreased in muscle, brain, and skin. Protein turnover is very slow in structural tissues such as collagen. Total body protein turnover is increased in infants and children who are growing rapidly and decreased in older adults.

- *Protein compartments:* Body protein is divided between two compartments—(1) tissue protein and (2) plasma protein. Protein from one compartment may be drawn to supply a need in the other. Muscle tissue becomes an important source of amino acids in periods of stress or low-protein intake. Plasma proteins such as prealbumin and albumin have very rapid turnover and are early indicators of protein catabolism brought on by inflammation, surgery, cancer, or other serious illness. Plasma protein levels identify patients at risk of nutritional deficiency or in need of nutrition intervention.[13–14] A low plasma albumin level is characteristic of children with kwashiorkor, the protein-energy deficiency disease seen in countries with food shortages. Plasma protein levels are restored to normal when the disease or catabolic stress has abated and protein and kilocalories (kcalories or kcal) have been made available.[13]
- *Metabolic amino acid pool:* Amino acids derived from tissue breakdown or supplied by dietary protein contribute to a common metabolic "pool." Amino acids from this pool are used to synthesize body proteins as needed. Figure 5-7 summarizes the many aspects of protein metabolism.

Nitrogen Balance

Protein balance is sometimes described as **nitrogen balance.** Total nitrogen balance involves all of the nitrogen in the body—protein nitrogen, as well as nonprotein nitrogen in such compounds as urea, uric acid, and ammonia. Nitrogen balance is the net result of nitrogen gain and loss across all body tissues. Negative nitrogen balance exists when body nitrogen loss exceeds the nitrogen input from food as occurs in long-term illness, hypermetabolic wasting disease, and inadequate protein intake.

PROTEIN QUALITY

Evaluating Food Proteins

The nutritional quality of a protein relates to its ability to sustain the growth and repair of body tissues and is based on the following two characteristics[15]:

1. *Protein digestibility:* To be of use to the body, amino acids must be released from other food components and made available for absorption. If nondigestible components prevent this breakdown, then the amino acids are lost in the feces.
2. *Amino acid composition:* All 20 amino acids used in making body proteins must be available at the same time for new tissues to be formed; therefore food proteins should

KEY TERMS

nitrogen balance The metabolic balance between nitrogen intake from dietary protein and nitrogen losses in urine, feces, sweat, and cells; dietary protein is 16% nitrogen (6.25 g dietary protein contains 1 g of nitrogen).

limiting amino acid The indispensable amino acid in a food present in the smallest amount as related to the reference amino acid pattern.

incomplete proteins Proteins with a lower amount of one or more of the indispensable amino acids as related to the reference amino acid pattern or missing an indispensable amino acid needed to form body proteins.

BOX 5-2 COMPLETE PROTEINS

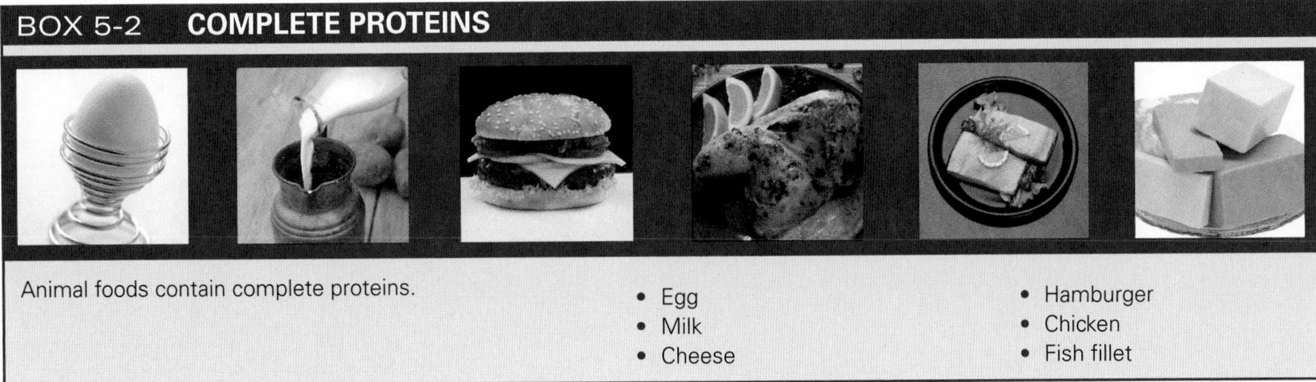

Animal foods contain complete proteins.

- Egg
- Milk
- Cheese
- Hamburger
- Chicken
- Fish fillet

supply each of the indispensable amino acids in the amount required. Other sources of amino (NH_2) groups in a food protein can be used to synthesize any dispensable amino acids needed.

Comparing Food Proteins

The nutritive value of a food protein is often expressed as its *amino acid score,* a value based on both its digestibility and amino acid composition. The Amino Acid Reference Pattern used to evaluate proteins is quite similar to the pattern of egg white, the reference protein often used in nutrition studies. When evaluating an amino acid score, it is important to identify the **limiting amino acid** (or acids). A limiting amino acid is any indispensable amino acid falling below the amount recommended in the Amino Acid Reference Pattern. For protein synthesis to take place, all indispensable amino acids must be available in the required amount. Thus the limiting amino acid "limits" or hinders the body from effectively using the other amino acids in that protein regardless of their adequacy. When one or two limiting amino acids are identified in a food protein having optimal levels of the other indispensable amino acids, that protein can be combined with another food protein that will supply the amino acid or acids needed.

Other methods have been used in animal studies to evaluate protein digestibility and composition:

- *Biologic value (BV)* is based on the ability of a protein to replace daily nitrogen losses or support growth.
- *Net protein utilization (NPU)* is based on BV and degree of digestibility.
- *Protein efficiency ratio (PER)* is based on weight gain of a growing test animal divided by its protein intake.

A comparison of the amino acid scores and digestibility of various protein foods is found in Table 5-1. In general, proteins from animal sources have higher scores than those from plant sources.

Amino Acid Content of Plant and Animal Foods

Plant and animal foods differ in their content of indispensable amino acids. Animal foods contain all of the indispensable amino acids in the amounts and ratio needed to support protein synthesis and are referred to as *complete proteins.* These foods include eggs, milk, cheese, meat, poultry, and fish (Box 5-2). Plant proteins vary in quality but are **incomplete proteins** (Box 5-3); either they supply less than the required amount

TABLE 5-1 COMPARATIVE PROTEIN QUALITY OF SELECTED FOODS ACCORDING TO AMINO ACID SCORE AND DIGESTIBILITY

FOOD	AMINO ACID SCORE	DIGESTIBILITY
Egg	100	100
Cow's milk	95	95
Beef	89	95
Soy flour	47	86
Peanuts	65	94
Polished rice	57	89
Whole wheat	53	87
Sesame seeds	42	90
Peas	37	88

Data from Committee on Amino Acids, Food and Nutrition Board: *Improvement of protein nutriture,* Washington, DC, 1974, National Academy of Sciences and Hopkins, DT: Effects of variation in protein digestibility. In Bodwell CE, Adkins JS, Hopkins DT, editors: *Protein quality in humans: assessment and in vitro estimation,* Westport, CN, 1981, Avi Publishing Company.

BOX 5-3 INCOMPLETE PROTEINS

Plant foods are incomplete proteins, but they can be combined to form a complete protein.

- Meat analogue
- Beans
- Peanuts
- Rice
- Tofu
- Sesame seeds

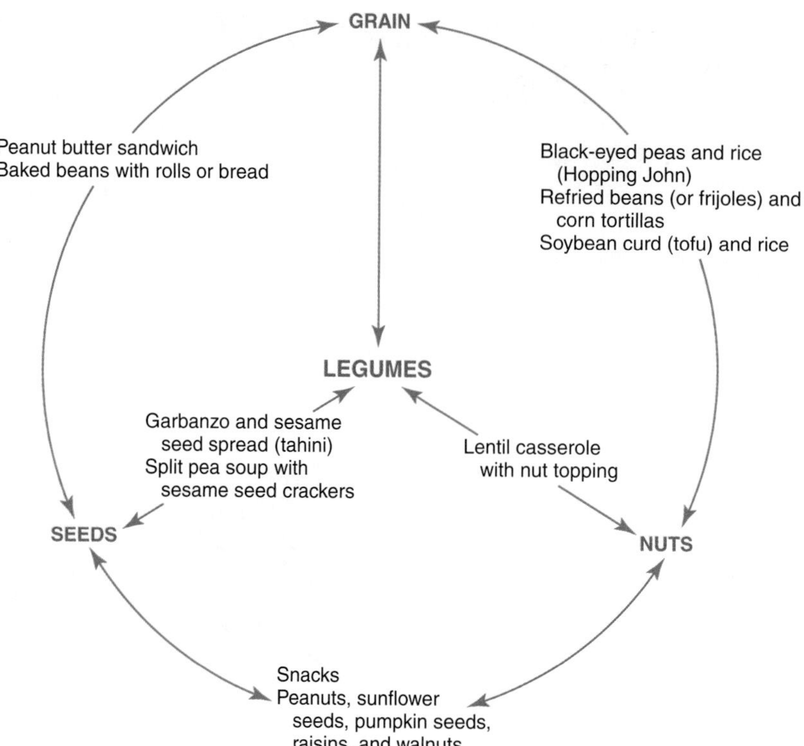

FIGURE 5-8 Complementary vegetable proteins. Examples of common plant foods that when eaten together supply the amounts of essential amino acids required for protein synthesis. (Redrawn from Stanfield PS, Hui YH: *Nutrition and diet therapy: self-instructional modules,* ed 4, Sudbury, Mass, 2003, Jones & Bartlett, with permission.)

of one or more indispensable amino acids or are missing an indispensable amino acid. However, several plant proteins eaten together or combined with a small amount of animal protein can supply the amino acids required to support tissue growth and repair.[3,16] This concept of complementary proteins, by which one protein helps meet the amino acid shortage in another, has been at work in the traditional food patterns of families worldwide (see Figure 5-8 for examples of complementary vegetable proteins). Soy protein, although lower in methionine than animal protein, meets the amino acid needs of adults. (See the *Focus on Culture* box, "Soy: A Protein Source for Thousands of Years," to learn more about this food.)

PROTEIN REQUIREMENTS

Factors Influencing Protein Requirements

Protein Quality

The quality of dietary protein and its amino acid composition influence the type and amount needed. Individuals who consume some animal protein along with plant protein will have an adequate supply of all amino acids. Those who eat no animal protein should emphasize a wide variety of complementary plant proteins to ensure appropriate amounts of the indispensable amino acids.

Protein Digestibility

Food preparation affects amino acid availability, because heat causes chemical bonding between some sugars and amino acids, forming compounds that cannot be digested. Protein digestion and amino acid absorption are influenced by the time interval between meals, with longer intervals lowering the competition for available enzymes and absorption sites.

Tissue Growth

Protein requirements reflect the growth patterns of infancy, childhood, and adolescence. Pregnancy and lactation increase protein needs.

Energy Content of the Diet

When carbohydrate intake is sufficient to meet energy needs, dietary protein can be used exclusively for tissue building (protein-sparing action of carbohydrate). Dietary carbohydrates also support protein synthesis by stimulating the release of insulin, which promotes the use of amino acids for tissue building.

Health Status

Conditions and diseases that increase the rate of protein turnover and tissue breakdown raise the protein requirement. After trauma or surgery, amino acids are needed for wound healing and formation of new tissue, as well as the production of infection-fighting immune factors. Serious burns with extensive tissue destruction substantially increase protein needs. In critically ill patients, protein requirements reach 1.5 to 2.0 g/kg of body weight.[17-18] Amino acid supplementation may help limit the loss of muscle protein that occurs with immobilization and bed rest.[19]

FOCUS ON CULTURE

Soy: A Protein Source for Thousands of Years

Populations throughout Asia have used soybeans for centuries. In China, Japan, Vietnam, Indonesia, the Philippines, Cambodia, and Laos, soybeans in various forms are a dietary staple and a major source of protein. In many geographic regions, population density and limited land for agriculture restricted the number of cattle, making meat or milk-based foods costly and relatively uncommon. Traditional soy foods such as tofu, tempeh, and soy milk were introduced to Americans by newcomers to the United States and over time have gained broad acceptance. Vegetarians, lactose malabsorbers, and others looking to expand their food horizons have adopted soy foods. A growing interest in Asian cooking and increasing availability of ethnic restaurants encourage more people to try these foods each year.

The most important soy-based protein foods are tofu and tempeh, as described following:

- *Tofu:* In Chinese *fu* means "riches," so tofu is usually served at New Year's celebrations to bring good luck. Tofu is made by a process similar to cheese making. A coagulating agent such as calcium sulfate, vinegar, or lemon juice is added to pureed soybeans. After the curd has formed, it is placed in molds to form cakes and the liquid whey is discarded. Tofu made with calcium sulfate has increased calcium content. Some types of tofu look much like farmer cheese, although they are very different in flavor. Although most cheeses have strong flavors, tofu is very bland and absorbs flavors from other foods. This makes it an excellent addition to cooked mixed dishes with a variety of seasonings or highly spiced ingredients. Tofu is available in two forms: (1) soft and (2) firm. Soft tofu can be mashed and used in recipes in place of ground beef or ricotta cheese; firm tofu can be grilled or stir-fried. Tofu has a limited shelf life, so consumers should check the expiration date on the package and be sure to keep it refrigerated.
- *Tempeh:* This soy food originated in Indonesia and is a mixture of soy and grain. When fermented, it becomes a firm mass that can be sliced or made into patties. Tempeh has more flavor than tofu and is a rich source of protein.

Soybeans are mixed with other ingredients to make sauces and seasonings used in Asian cooking, as follows:

- *Hoisin sauce:* Used in Chinese cooking, hoisin sauce is a combination of fermented soybeans, water, flour, sugar, and garlic.
- *Miso:* Miso originated in Japan and is a fermented mixture of soybeans and rice or barley. It is a pungent, salty paste used as a seasoning or soup base. Miso is very high in sodium, containing 900 mg of sodium or more per tablespoon.
- *Soy sauce:* This seasoning is a combination of steamed rice, roasted soybeans, and salt that is fermented. Based on its high sodium content, it should be used in moderation.

Tofu and tempeh are available in supermarkets and Asian food stores and add variety and nutrition to the meal pattern. If you have not tasted these foods, then look for an Asian cookbook in your local library or search the Internet for a good recipe.

BIBLIOGRAPHY

Diabetes Care and Education Dietetic Practice Group of the American Dietetic Association: *Ethnic and regional food practices: A series. Hmong American food practices, customs, and holidays,* Chicago/Alexandria, Va, 1999, American Dietetic Association/American Diabetes Association.

Kittler PG, Sucher KP: *Cultural foods: traditions and trends,* Belmont, Calif, 2000, Wadsworth/Thompson Learning.

Margen S, editor: *The wellness encyclopedia of food and nutrition,* New York, 1992, Health Letter Associates.

Muscle protein synthesis is influenced not only by the amount of protein available but also by the timeframe in which the protein is consumed. Older adults or others undergoing resistance training to build or maintain muscle mass may benefit from eating some high-quality protein during or immediately after the activity.[20–21]

Dietary Reference Intakes

Protein

The Recommended Dietary Allowance (RDA) for protein is 0.8 g/kg body weight or 56 g/day for men and 46 g/day for women.[3] This intake will maintain body tissues and replace daily nitrogen losses via the urine, feces, and sweat. An additional 25 g/day is needed for pregnancy and lactation. Protein requirements of infants and children vary according to age and growth.

A Tolerable Upper Intake Level (UL) has not been established for protein; however, the safety of protein intakes well in excess of the RDA is a concern. Protein waste products are excreted in the urine, and high protein intakes lead to dehydration if fluid intake is not adjusted accordingly. It is recommended that protein intake not exceed two times the RDA.[3]

Amino Acids

Individuals meeting the RDA who eat both animal and plant proteins will have an adequate supply of the indispensable amino acids. If no animal foods are consumed, then an intake of mixed plant proteins obtained from legumes (including soy), grains, nuts, seeds, and vegetables can supply amino acids in the pattern needed, although it is important to choose a wide variety of plant proteins.[3]

The specific amino acid requirements of particular age groups are described in reference 4, accessible on the web site of the National Academy of Sciences (see the Evolve web site that accompanies this text).

ULs have not been set for individual amino acids because amino acid imbalances and toxicity are not usually a hazard when amino acids are supplied in food. However, supplements that exaggerate the intake of one or more amino acids interfere with protein synthesis and can lead to toxicity.[3] Methionine, cysteine, and histidine supplements in particular can have adverse effects if taken over long periods.[22]

Acceptable Macronutrient Distribution Range

The Acceptable Macronutrient Distribution Range (AMDR) for protein is 10% to 35% of total kcalories.[3] Protein needs are generally met if protein makes up 10% of energy intake; however, if total energy intake is low, then it may be necessary to obtain more kcalories from protein to meet the RDA. The suggested calorie range for protein provides flexibility in balancing the suggested proportions of fat and carbohydrate to achieve a healthy diet pattern. Diets ranging from 15% to 27% protein that emphasized healthy fats, vegetables, moderate amounts of fruits and grains, and limited sweets had positive effects on risk factors for coronary heart disease.[23] (See Chapters 3 and 4 to review the AMDRs for carbohydrate and fat.)

PROTEIN INTAKE

Protein-Energy Malnutrition

Protein intake differs widely among population groups, with some getting far more and others far less than they need. PEM is a major health problem in many developing countries where protein intakes are low in both quantity and quality. More than 6 million children die each year from protein-related deficiencies.[3] PEM also contributes to the morbidity and mortality associated with infectious diseases such as malaria, respiratory tract infections, and gastroenteritis. Based on more than 13,000 hospital admissions during 5 years, it was estimated that malnutrition is the underlying cause of half of the inpatient morbidity and mortality rates of young children in rural Africa.[24]

Two forms of extreme malnutrition observed in persons of all ages when food supplies are insufficient are kwashiorkor and marasmus (Figure 5-9). Marasmus represents extreme starvation with a deficit of energy, protein, and micronutrients. These individuals have little or no body fat and exhibit extreme wasting. Rehabilitation must be initiated on a gradual basis to avoid refeeding syndrome, with severe complications or death. Kwashiorkor occurs in children or adults when diets are deficient in protein and likely limiting in energy and micronutrients as well. This form of PEM results in a characteristic edema, hypoalbuminemia, skin lesions, and fatty liver.[25] The primary cause of PEM is most often a lack of food or lack of food containing appropriate levels of nutrients; however, impaired digestion or absorption, diseases of the gastrointestinal tract, or chronic or acute vomiting or diarrhea are secondary causes or contributors to this condition.

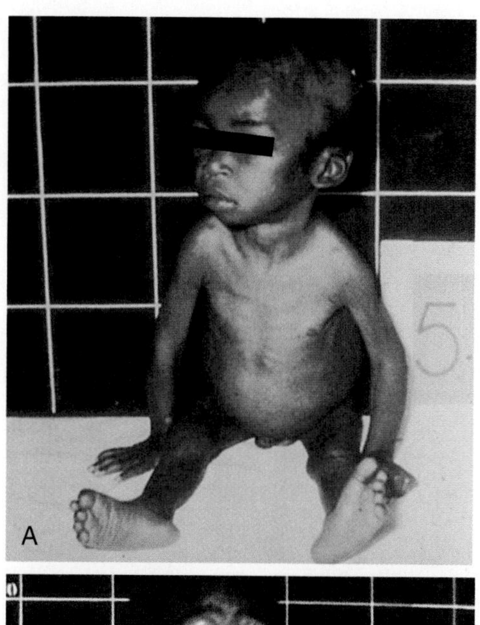

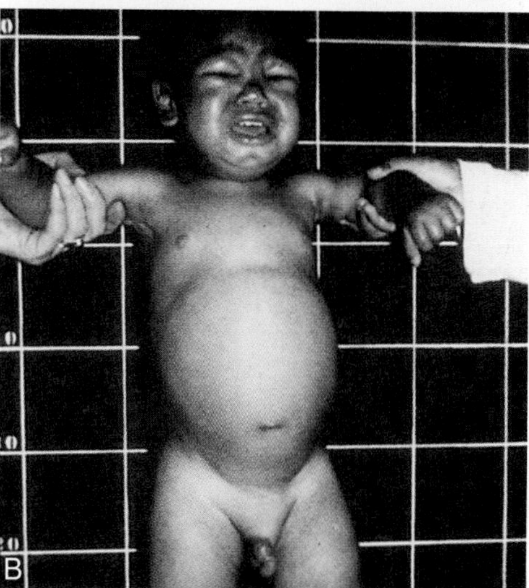

FIGURE 5-9 Protein-energy malnutrition (PEM). **A,** Marasmus results from starvation. **B,** Kwashiorkor results from a diet that may be sufficient in kcalories but is deficient in protein. Note the abdominal bloating typical of kwashiorkor. (From Thibodeau GA, Patton KT: *The human body in health & disease,* ed 5, St Louis, 2010, Mosby.)

Amounts and Types of Protein

Plant researchers are working to increase the indispensable amino acid content of grains such as rice[26] and vegetables such as sweet potatoes[27] that are dietary staples for millions of people around the world who take in little or no animal protein. At the other extreme, most persons in the United States meet or exceed their RDA for protein, with most coming from animal sources.[28] National surveys tell us that 95% of adult men reach at least 100% of their RDA and more than 25% are taking in at least twice the amount recommended.[29] About 10% of adult women older than 50 years fall below the RDA, whereas about 10% of women ages 19 to 30 have intakes at least two times their RDA. Protein intakes are also high among U.S. children. One half of the fast-food meals marketed to children contain 16 g of protein or more; this meal contains 123% of the daily protein allowance for 3 year olds and 84% of the day's needs for children ages 4 to 8.[30] Foods of animal origin make up 60% of the protein intake of U.S. adults, with 42% coming from meat, poultry, and fish; 15% from dairy foods; and 3% from eggs.[28]

Clinical Applications: Low and High Protein Intakes

Low-Protein Diets

We often associate low-protein diets with the severe PEM evident in famine-ravaged countries; however, degrees of malnutrition exist in all areas of the world, including the United

States. Children with chronic PEM have poor growth (low weight for height) and stunting (low height for age).[3] When protein status is marginal, immune function is impaired; this likely contributes to the chronic respiratory infections and diarrhea that trouble many poorly nourished children and adults. Low protein intake during pregnancy increases the risk of a low birth weight infant. Maintaining the recommended protein intake is also important in weight reduction; middle-aged and older women consuming less than 0.8 g/kg of protein each day lost more lean mass along with adipose tissue than women who met this level. Both groups lost about the same amount of body weight.[31]

In certain clinical situations, protein intake falls below the usual amount. When intake is reduced it is especially important to choose protein high in BV. The following serve as examples of situations when protein intake may be low:

- *Parkinson's disease:* Protein intake is usually controlled to prevent the build-up of excessive amino acids that compete with the treatment drug levodopa for passage across the blood-brain barrier.[6]
- *Chronic kidney disease (CKD):* When kidney function declines, protein intake is limited to minimize the burden of excreting urea and other nitrogen-containing waste.[32] Resistance training and regular exercise help preserve muscle mass in renal patients on protein-restricted diets.[33]
- *Vegan diets:* Individuals who consume no animal foods and must obtain all of their protein from plant sources can have marginal protein intakes based on the added bulk of plant protein foods. Protein may provide only 10% of total kcalories, the minimum AMDR.[3,16]

High-Protein Diets

High-protein diets moved into the spotlight when media attention became focused on weight loss regimens that restrict carbohydrate, with preference to protein and fat. Diets in which protein provides 25% or more of total kcalories support weight loss and effective energy regulation.[34] An added benefit of a weight loss diet that includes more protein is the satiety-producing effect of amino acids, which continues even as energy intake declines.[35] Protein also increases energy expenditure to a small degree as compared with carbohydrate and fat, based on the extra kcalories needed to convert protein for use as a fuel source; however, this alone is unlikely to produce significant weight loss. Increased protein intakes also appear to protect muscle mass during long-term weight reduction and maintenance and could help prevent sarcopenia, the age-related loss of muscle that contributes to frailty.[36] Nevertheless, reducing kcalorie intake and increasing energy expenditure are still key to weight loss, regardless of the proportion of specific macronutrients. Personal preferences, cultural food patterns, and metabolic considerations might form the basis for individual interventions.[37–39]

High-protein diets may have some advantages, but their long-term effects on renal function are uncertain. In persons with normal kidney function, intakes of animal protein in excess of 0.8 g/kg increase blood flow to the kidney and the glomerular filtration rate, although this is less evident with protein from vegetable sources. On the other hand, protein intakes higher than the RDA, whether animal or vegetable protein, accelerate the progression of even mild renal impairment,[40] and many adults in the early stages of chronic kidney disease are unaware of their condition. This points to the need for evaluation of older adults before protein supplementation. Attention to water needs should also be a part of dietary protein prescriptions.[41] Current nutrition standards for diabetes management recommend that protein intake not exceed 10% of total kcalories in those with impaired renal function.[32]

HEALTH PROMOTION

Health Benefits of Plant Protein Foods

Soy foods and other legumes supply good-quality protein along with an array of other important nutrients and have a role in preventing chronic disease.[16,42–43] Soy foods are sources of phytochemicals thought to have estrogen-like activity that may help prevent bone loss in older women.[44] Adults eating legumes at least four times a week had a lower risk of cardiovascular disease than those eating these foods less than once a week.[45] Vegetable protein foods are low in saturated fat, containing more monounsaturated and polyunsaturated fats. Soybeans and chickpeas are good sources of linoleic acid, an essential fatty acid. One cup of tofu or soybean curd supplies nearly 25% of the RDA (and one cup of chickpeas supplies 12% of the RDA) of linoleic acid for adult men.[3,46] Tree nuts and peanuts, often considered snack items rather than alternate sources of protein, are rich in antioxidants, trace minerals, essential fatty acids, and phytochemicals,[47] and they provide a rich protein source for sandwiches or stews. Beans and nuts are important foods in the Mediterranean diet and likely contribute to the healthful benefits attributed to that diet.[48] (See the *Evidence-Based Practice* box, "Effect of Soy on Cardiovascular Risk," to learn about these relationships.)

Nutritional Contributions of Animal Protein Foods

Proteins from animal sources—meat, fish, poultry, eggs, and milk—provide all of the indispensable amino acids in the appropriate amounts. Used alone or in combination with vegetable proteins, proteins from animal sources meet the amino acid needs of children and adults. Animal foods supply trace minerals such as iron and zinc that are difficult to obtain in sufficient amounts from plant foods, based on their lower content and interfering substances. Dairy foods are rich in calcium and riboflavin and provide preformed vitamin A. Vitamin B_{12} and vitamin D occur naturally in animal foods only.[49]

Mixing Animal and Plant Proteins

For persons choosing to eat animal foods, mixing plant and animal proteins can benefit overall nutrition and health. Calcium is well absorbed from dairy foods, and the vitamin D in milk and other fortified milk products supports calcium absorption and promotes bone density. Iron and zinc,

EVIDENCE-BASED PRACTICE

Effect of Soy on Cardiovascular Risk

In recent years soy has received increasing attention not only as an excellent source of plant protein but also for its special properties in reducing cardiovascular risk. In 1999 the Food and Drug Administration (FDA) approved the addition of a health claim to the nutrition label of soy-containing foods, indicating that soy was protective against heart disease. This was followed in 2000 by an advisory from the American Heart Association recommending the addition of soy protein to a diet low in saturated fat and cholesterol. Based on evidence available at the time, soy foods were believed to exert positive effects on low-density lipoprotein (LDL) cholesterol, high-density lipoprotein (HDL) cholesterol, serum triglycerides, and blood pressure.

Since then, additional research studies have looked at the effects of soy protein and the isoflavones (phytochemicals) it contains on cardiovascular risk. This new evidence has led to some differing conclusions regarding their effects on cardiovascular risk factors as described:

Blood lipoproteins: Critical evaluation of new evidence by the American Heart Association and the American Dietetic Association concluded that soy has no major effect on blood LDL cholesterol levels. In those with elevated LDL cholesterol levels, use of soy lowered levels by about 3%. No effect on blood HDL cholesterol levels was noted.

Blood pressure levels: Soy protein or isoflavones did not bring about any changes in blood pressure.

Therefore are soy products good foods to include in your diet? We do know that soy is not only a high-quality protein but also a rich source of vitamins, minerals, and polyunsaturated fats. When substituted for dairy or other animal foods high in saturated fat and cholesterol, soy contributes to dietary prevention of cardiovascular disease. However, early reports of its particular cholesterol-lowering ability, including those used to justify the health claim on the nutrition label have not been confirmed. This example reinforces the need for continuous review of the literature in our professional practice. New findings alert us to new roles of particular foods or, as in this case, provide us with a more realistic appraisal of a food or nutrient.

BIBLIOGRAPHY

Sacks FM, Lichtenstein A, Van Horn L, et al: Soy protein, isoflavones, and cardiovascular health. An American Heart Association Science Advisory for Professionals from the Nutrition Committee, *Circulation* 113:1034, 2006.

Van Horn L, McCoin M, Kris-Etherton PM, et al: The evidence for dietary prevention and treatment of cardiovascular disease, *J Am Diet Assoc* 108:287, 2008.

important for growth and body functions, are more easily absorbed from meats than plant foods. At the same time, plant protein foods such as legumes add important fiber and phytochemicals to the diet; nuts contribute essential fatty acids in addition to the amino acids they contain. Fortified soy milk is an important source of calcium and vitamin D for those avoiding dairy foods. Both types of protein should be included in a person's meal pattern as appropriate for that individual.

VEGETARIAN DIETS

Vegetarian diets existed in ancient times in early Greek culture. People choose to follow a plant-based diet and limit or exclude animal foods for many reasons (Box 5-4). Several major world religions, including Hinduism and Buddhism, advocate avoidance of meat and the preservation of animal life. Sustainability of the food supply and protection of the environment are growing concerns in many parts of the world. From the environmental perspective, production of nonvegetarian diets requires over three times the water, 13 times the fertilizer, and about 1.5 times the pesticides than production of vegetarian diets. The greatest contribution to this need for resources comes from production of beef.[50] Land requirements for producing meat protein are about 10 times greater than for producing plant protein.[51] With this in mind, some individuals have adopted a plant-based diet with the intent that direct consumption of grains will assist in reducing food shortages in various parts of the world.

Although diet patterns that emphasize plant foods are generally referred to as *vegetarian diets,* they differ according to the types of animal foods included, as follows:

- Ovolactovegetarian (includes all plant foods, dairy, and eggs)
- Lactovegetarian (includes all plant foods and dairy)
- Pescovegetarians (includes all plant foods, dairy, eggs, and fish)[52]
- Vegan (includes plant foods only)
- Flexitarian (includes predominantly plant foods with animal foods such as fish or poultry on occasion)[53]

About 5 million people (2.3% of the population) in the United States describe themselves as vegetarians and never eating meat, fish, or poultry; 1.4% are vegans.[16] Restaurants have responded to the interest in vegetarian diets, with 71% of chefs noting that vegetarian dishes are "perennial favorites" and fast-food restaurants are offering more meatless options. The U.S. market for vegetarian foods including meat analogues, nondairy milks, and vegetarian entrees has grown to

BOX 5-4 REASONS FOR FOLLOWING A PLANT-BASED DIET

- Religious preferences
- Cultural patterns
- Concern for animals
- Concern for the environment
- Health
- Extension of the world food supply

over $1.2 billion.[16] The availability of such foods in the marketplace has provided additional options for vegetarians in obtaining required nutrients.

Nutritional Implications of Vegetarian Diets

Vegetarian diets including vegan diets will support growth and well-being throughout the life cycle *if* they are well planned. Conversely, vegetarian and vegan diets, as well as diets that include all types of animal foods, will be inadequate if items high in fat and sugar and low in important nutrients are emphasized. In general the more restrictive the diet is, the more careful the planning must be to avoid nutrient deficiencies.

For those vegetarians who eat eggs and dairy foods, protein, calcium, vitamin D, and vitamin B_{12} are well supplied. Eggs also contain small amounts of n-3 fatty acids obtained from animal feeds. Vegans need to seek out fortified foods to obtain vitamin D and vitamin B_{12}. Some brands of soy milk and breakfast cereals are fortified with both of these vitamins; vegetarian formula yeast or vitamin supplements are other sources. Some of the meat analogues containing soy protein have added vitamin B_{12}. It is important that vegans read product labels to ensure their nutrition. The n-3 fatty acids can be obtained from flaxseed, canola, or soybean oils, as well as from walnuts.[15,54,55] Debate continues regarding the need for supplements of the n-3 fatty acids docosahexaenoic acid and eicosapentaenoic acid in vegetarians and vegans who do not eat fish.[55,56]

Although iron and zinc are found in many plant foods, phytates interfere with their absorption. A vitamin C source at the same meal facilitates iron absorption; soaking beans before cooking makes the iron more available for absorption. Fortified grains and cereals add iron and zinc to the diet. It may be that individuals can adapt to lower iron intakes with increased absorption, because iron deficiency anemia is no more prevalent among vegetarians than nonvegetarians.[16]

Calcium can be a problem for vegetarians avoiding dairy foods. Calcium is well absorbed from broccoli, cabbage, collards, kale, and bok choy (all vegetables low in oxalate). In fact, the calcium in these vegetables may be better absorbed than the calcium in tofu or fortified juices.[57] Spinach and Swiss chard, however, are poor sources of calcium based on their oxalate content, which interferes with calcium absorption. Fortified soy milk and fortified breakfast cereals supply calcium. Although calcium intakes of lactovegetarians are about the same as for nonvegetarians, vegans can have low intakes, increasing their risk of bone fractures.[58]

Planning Vegetarian Diets

In general, plant-based diets contain increased amounts of fiber, antioxidants, carotenoids, and phytochemicals and decreased amounts of saturated fat and cholesterol than the average diet, depending on the animal foods included. Vegetarians eat more fruits than nonvegetarians. In addition, they eat one and one half times more beans and two and one half times more nuts. Vegetarian diets are planned as any diet is planned, to include essential nutrients and sufficient kcalories for energy. A vegetarian food guide from the American Dietetic Association offers many alternative food sources of important nutrients, providing helpful advice for selecting nutritionally sound plant-based diets (Figure 5-10).[45] Portion sizes of equivalent protein-containing foods as described in Box 5-5 offer alternatives for variety in the daily meal plan. Use of complementary proteins to obtain a full set of essential amino acids is especially important when planning a vegan diet. Review Figure 5-8 and see the *Perspectives in Practice* box, "Increase Your Variety: Exploring Complementary Proteins," to consider food combinations that will meet amino acid needs; be sure to include the appropriate foods within the daily plan. Box 5-6 provides some general guidelines for helping vegetarians plan healthful meals.

Vegetarian Diets and Chronic Disease

In general, vegetarians have lower rates of coronary heart disease, lower prevalence of obesity, and likely lower risk of hypertension and diabetes. Blood levels of LDL cholesterol are lower in vegetarians, which helps to explain their resistance to heart disease. The influence of vegetarian diets on cancer risk is less well understood. Although vegetarians tend to have lower cancer rates than nonvegetarians living in the same community, the relationship of vegetarian food patterns to specific cancers requires more study. Rates of colorectal cancer tend to be lower in vegetarians and others who eat less meat; however, this is not the case among all groups of vegetarians. These differences may relate to the differences among vegetarians. As noted previously, eating patterns vary significantly among individuals who identify themselves as vegetarians, and future studies may need to track participants according to their specific food preferences.[52] Nevertheless, the emphasis on plant foods within a well-planned vegetarian diet ensures a generous intake of important micronutrients and phytochemicals, important to health. Appropriate diets for patients with renal disease, diabetes, or both can be developed within a vegetarian food plan.[16]

DIGESTION-ABSORPTION-METABOLISM REVIEW

Food proteins must be broken down into their building units—the amino acids—to meet body needs. A brief review of this process is outlined in the following sections. (See Chapter 2 for a detailed discussion of digestion, absorption, and metabolism.)

Digestion

Mouth

The only digestive action on protein taking place in the mouth is the mechanical effect of chewing, which breaks food into smaller particles for passage into the stomach.

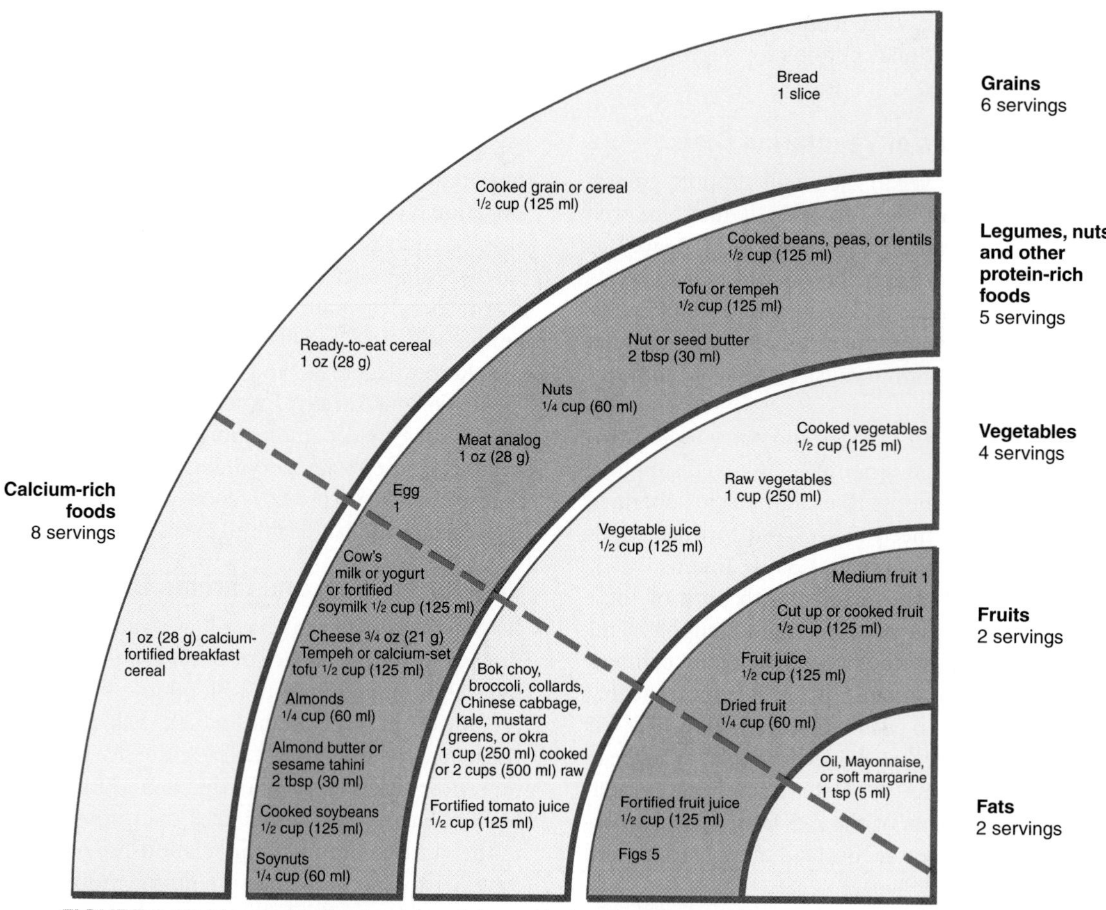

FIGURE 5-10 Vegetarian food guide rainbow. Notice the slice of the rainbow calling attention to the foods in each group that are good sources of calcium. (Redrawn from Messina V, Melina V, Mangels AR: A new food guide for North American vegetarians, *J Am Diet Assoc* 103:771, 2003; with permission from the American Dietetic Association.)

BOX 5-5 PLANT SOURCES OF PROTEIN

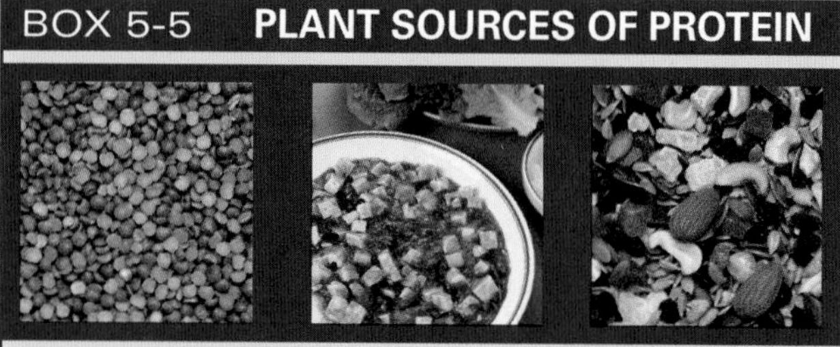

Each of the following servings provides at least 4 to 6g of protein:*

- Cooked beans, peas, or lentils: ½ cup
- Tofu or tempeh: ½ cup
- Nut butter: 2 tbsp
- Nuts: ¼ cup
- Tahini (sesame seed butter): 2 tbsp
- Meat (soy) analogue: 1 oz

Data from Messina V, Melina V, Mangels AR: A new food guide for North American vegetarians, *J Am Diet Assoc* 103:771, 2003. Images copyright 2006 JupiterImages Corporation.

*A plant protein can be combined with a small amount of animal protein to form a complete protein, or two different plant protein foods can be combined to form a complete protein (see Figure 5-8).

BOX 5-6 SUGGESTIONS FOR PLANNING VEGETARIAN MEALS

- Choose a variety of foods, including whole grains, vegetables, fruits, legumes, nuts, seeds, and if desired, dairy products and eggs.
- Minimize your intake of foods that have added sugar, are high in sodium, and are high in fat, especially saturated fats and trans fats.
- Choose a variety of fruits and vegetables.
- If animal foods such as dairy products and eggs are used, choose lower-fat dairy products and use both eggs and dairy products in moderation.
- Include a regular source of vitamin B_{12} and, if sunlight exposure is limited, then include a regular dietary source of vitamin D.

From American Dietetic Association: Position of the American Dietetic Association: vegetarian diets, *J Am Diet Assoc* 109:1266, 2009. Reprinted with permission.

PERSPECTIVES IN PRACTICE

Increase Your Variety: Exploring Complementary Proteins

Traditional diets the world over were plant based, emphasizing cereals, legumes, and vegetables. In many cultures the main dish is a stew containing a variety of plant foods; sometimes a small amount of animal protein is added. Exploring complementary proteins is a way to learn more about the food patterns of different cultural and ethnic groups. Try a new recipe and calculate the amounts of protein coming from animal and vegetable sources.

Some traditional plant-based meals follow:

- *Mexican:* Corn tortillas combined with beans and vegetables provide a complete protein, as do beans and rice. The addition of cheese to stews or tortillas complements the incomplete proteins of the grain foods. Eggs with beans are a favorite breakfast.
- *East Indian:* A stew containing rice, vegetables, and beans might be served with yogurt, cheese, and peanuts. Bread is made from wheat flour, often combined with flour from ground peas or beans.
- *Hmong (Vietnamese):* Rice mixed with green vegetables and small amounts of fish and peanuts are typical of this region. Rice rather than bread is the basic grain and is included in every meal, including breakfast.
- *Traditional American:* A peanut butter sandwich, a ready-to-eat cereal with milk, macaroni and cheese, pinto beans and corn bread, and "hoppin' John" (black-eyed peas and rice) illustrate complementary proteins.

BIBLIOGRAPHY

Diabetes Care and Education Dietetic Practice Group of the American Dietetic Association: *Ethnic and regional food practices: a series. Hmong American food practices, customs, and holidays*, Chicago/Alexandria, Va, 1999, American Dietetic Association/American Diabetes Association.

Diabetes Care and Education Dietetic Practice Group of the American Dietetic Association: *Ethnic and regional food practices: a series. Indian and Pakistani food practices, customs, and holidays*, ed 2, Chicago/Alexandria, Va, 2000, American Dietetic Association/American Diabetes Association.

Diabetes Care and Education Dietetic Practice Group of the American Dietetic Association: *Ethnic and regional food practices: a series. Mexican American food practices, customs, and holidays*, Chicago/Alexandria, Va, 1998, American Dietetic Association/American Diabetes Association.

Kittler PG, Sucher KP: *Cultural foods: traditions and trends*, Belmont, Calif, 2000, Wadsworth/Thompson Learning.

Stomach

The enzymatic breakdown of protein begins in the stomach. Three chemical agents in the gastric secretions help with this task: (1) pepsin, (2) hydrochloric acid, and (3) rennin.

- *Pepsin:* Pepsin is released by the chief cells in the stomach wall as the inactive proenzyme pepsinogen and requires hydrochloric acid to be transformed into the active enzyme pepsin. Pepsin splits the peptide linkages between amino acids, breaking large polypeptides into successively smaller peptides.
- *Hydrochloric acid:* This acid provides the acid medium needed to convert pepsinogen to pepsin.
- *Rennin:* This enzyme is present only in infancy and childhood. Rennin acts on casein, the major protein in milk, to produce a curd that slows the passage of food out of the infant's stomach.

Small Intestine

Protein digestion is completed in the small intestine assisted by enzymes secreted by the pancreas and glands in the intestinal wall. These include the following:

- Pancreatic secretions:
  1. Trypsin is secreted as inactive trypsinogen and activated by the hormone enterokinase produced in the duodenal wall. Trypsin acts on proteins and large polypeptides to yield smaller polypeptides and dipeptides.
  2. Chymotrypsin is secreted as chymotrypsinogen and activated by the trypsin already present. Chymotrypsin continues the same protein-splitting action of trypsin.
  3. Carboxypeptidase attacks the carboxyl (COOH) end of the peptide chain to produce smaller peptides and some free amino acids.
- Intestinal secretions:
  1. Aminopeptidase releases amino acids one at a time from the amino (NH_2) end of the peptide chain to produce smaller short-chain peptides and free amino acids.

KEY TERMS

pepsin A gastric enzyme that breaks large protein molecules into shorter-chain polypeptides. Gastric hydrochloric acid is necessary to activate pepsin.

proenzyme An inactive precursor converted to the active enzyme by the action of an acid or other enzyme.

trypsin A pancreatic enzyme secreted into the small intestine that acts on proteins and polypeptides to yield smaller peptides and dipeptides.

chymotrypsin A pancreatic enzyme secreted into the small intestine that breaks peptide linkages forming smaller polypeptides and dipeptides.

carboxypeptidase A protein-splitting enzyme secreted by the pancreas into the small intestine that splits the peptide bond at the carboxyl (COOH) end of the chain, producing smaller peptide chains and free amino acids.

aminopeptidase A protein-splitting enzyme secreted by the intestinal mucosa that releases amino acids one at a time from the amino (NH_2) end of the peptide chain to produce smaller short-chain peptides and free amino acids.

2. **Dipeptidase** breaks any remaining dipeptides into two free amino acids.

A summary of the steps in protein digestion can be reviewed in Table 2-2.

Absorption

Amino acids are absorbed by an energy-requiring, sodium-assisted transport system and enter the portal blood for passage to the liver. A few short-chain peptides and smaller intact proteins escape digestion and are absorbed in that form. Most are broken down as they cross the intestinal mucosa; however, those protein molecules that pass into the blood intact may play a part in the development of immunity and protein sensitivity. We know that antibodies in the mother's colostrum, the first milk secreted after birth, are passed on to her nursing infant. Inadvertent absorption of intact proteins has been implicated in the development of some food allergies.[59]

Metabolism

The construction sites for building tissue proteins are in the cells. Each cell, depending on its nature and function, requires a unique mix of amino acids to build the specific proteins needed. The metabolic activities of protein are interwoven with those of carbohydrate and fat, which provide the energy to drive on-going tissue building. We will continue to look at these interrelationships in our study of nutrition across the life cycle.

KEY TERMS

dipeptidase Final enzyme in the protein-splitting series that cleaves dipeptides to yield two free amino acids.

TO SUM UP

The primary function of dietary protein and its constituent amino acids is to build and repair body tissues and form the regulatory proteins that carry out important metabolic tasks. Of the 20 amino acids used to build proteins, nine cannot be synthesized by the body and are referred to as *indispensable* or *essential amino acids;* another six cannot be synthesized in adequate amounts under conditions of stress or accelerated growth and are considered conditionally indispensable. The remaining five amino acids are synthesized by the body and are termed the *dispensable* or *unessential amino acids.* Both indispensable and conditionally indispensable amino acids must be supplied in the diet. Animal proteins are considered complete proteins because they contain all the indispensable amino acids in the amounts and ratios needed for protein synthesis. Plant proteins or incomplete proteins are missing one or more indispensable amino acids or contain less than the amounts needed to make new proteins. Plant proteins can be mixed with animal proteins or with each other to provide the necessary proportions of all amino acids for body growth and maintenance. Protein requirements are influenced by growth, food protein quality, health status, and the availability of carbohydrate as an energy source. In many countries, protein shortages lead to malnutrition, with body wasting, stunted growth, chronic infection, and disease. In the United States, overconsumption rather than underconsumption of protein is receiving growing attention. Vegetarian diets emphasizing plant proteins can meet nutrient needs at all stages of the life cycle if well planned. Vegan diets excluding all animal foods require supplementation with vitamin D and vitamin B_{12} to meet nutritional needs.

QUESTIONS FOR REVIEW

1. What is the difference between an indispensable, a dispensable, and a conditionally indispensable amino acid? List the names of each.
2. What is meant by protein turnover, and how does it relate to nitrogen balance?
3. Distinguish between protein anabolism and protein catabolism. Describe a clinical situation in which protein anabolism exceeds protein catabolism and one in which the opposite is true.
4. Explain the term *protein-sparing effect.* Which nutrient has this effect?
5. Describe the factors that influence dietary protein needs.
6. Visit a grocery store or drugstore and examine five liquid protein supplements. Make a chart that includes (a) the number of grams of protein provided in the container, (b) the cost per container, and (c) the calculated cost for 8 g of protein. How does the cost of the protein supplement compare with the cost of 1 cup of milk or ½ cup of cooked kidney beans, which also provide about 8 g of good-quality protein? What are the better choices for supplying an individual's protein needs?
7. A pediatrician told a vegan couple that their 2-year-old daughter was falling behind in her growth rate. What dietary factor (or factors) is likely related to her poor growth? Using the various tools for developing vegetarian diets mentioned on pages 84 and 90 plan 1 day of meals for this child, indicating food amounts that would meet her protein and energy needs and respect the vegan food pattern.
8. Protein intakes two to three times the RDA are not uncommon in the United States. Using the food values found on the Evolve site that accompanies your

textbook, calculate the energy value and the number of grams of protein in a fast-food meal that includes one double-patty cheeseburger, a large serving of French fries, and a 12-oz milkshake. Compare the total grams of protein and the total kcalories with the protein and energy DRIs for a 16-year-old boy. What proportion of his daily protein and energy needs are provided in this one meal?

9. Describe the process of protein digestion and absorption including (a) the site in the gastrointestinal tract where each action occurs, (b) the secretions responsible and their source, and (c) the resulting products.

REFERENCES

1. Matthews DE: Proteins and amino acids. In Shils ME, Olsen JA, Shike M, et al, editors: *Modern nutrition in health and disease*, ed 10, Baltimore, 2006, Lippincott Williams & Wilkins.
2. Gropper SS, Smith JL, Groff JL: *Advanced nutrition and human metabolism*, ed 5, Belmont, Calif, 2008, Cengage Learning.
3. Food and Nutrition Board, Institute of Medicine: *Dietary Reference Intakes for energy, carbohydrate, fiber, fat, fatty acids, cholesterol, protein, and amino acids (macronutrients)*, Washington, DC, 2002, National Academies Press.
4. Guyton AC, Hall JE: *Textbook of medical physiology*, ed 10, Philadelphia, 2000, Saunders.
5. Pencharz PR, Young VR: Protein and amino acids. In Bowman BA, Russell RM, editors: *Present knowledge in nutrition*, ed 9, Washington, DC, 2006, International Life Sciences Institute.
6. Timiras PS: *Physiological basis of aging and geriatrics*, ed 4, New York, 2007, Taylor & Francis.
7. Choudry HA, Pan M, Karinch AM, et al: Branched-chain amino acid-enriched nutritional support in surgical and cancer patients, *J Nutr* 136:314S, 2006.
8. Khanna S, Gopalan S: Role of branched-chain amino acids in liver disease: the evidence for and against, *Curr Opin Clin Nutr Metab Care* 10:297, 2007.
9. Van de Poll MCG, Dejong CHC, Soeters PB: Adequate range for sulfur-containing amino acids and biomarkers for their excess: lessons from enteral and parenteral nutrition, *J Nutr* 136:1694S, 2006.
10. Jahoor F, Badaloo A, Reid M, et al: Sulfur amino acid metabolism in children with severe childhood undernutrition: methionine kinetics, *Am J Clin Nutr* 84:1400, 2006.
11. Williams MH: Sports nutrition. In Shils ME, Olsen JA, Shike M, et al, editors: *Modern nutrition in health and disease*, ed 10, Baltimore, 2006, Lippincott Williams & Wilkins.
12. Wolfe RR: The underappreciated role of muscle in health and disease, *Am J Clin Nutr* 84:475, 2006.
13. Fuhrman MP, Charney P, Mueller CM: Hepatic proteins and nutrition assessment, *J Am Diet Assoc* 104:1258, 2004.
14. Rambod M, Kovesdy CP, Bross R, et al: Association of serum prealbumin and its changes over time with clinical outcomes and survival in patients receiving hemodialysis, *Am J Clin Nutr* 88:1485, 2008.
15. Millward DJ, Layman DK, Tomé D, et al: Protein quality assessment: impact of expanding understanding of protein and amino acids for optimal health, *Am J Clin Nutr* 87(Suppl):1576S, 2008.
16. American Dietetic Association: Position of the American Dietetic Association: vegetarian diets, *J Am Diet Assoc* 109:1266, 2009.
17. Frankenfield D: Energy expenditure and protein requirements after traumatic injury, *Nutr Clin Prac* 21:430, 2006.
18. Stroud M: Protein and the critically ill: do we know what to give? *Proc Nutr Soc* 66:378, 2007.
19. Paddon-Jones D: Interplay of stress and physical activity on muscle loss, *J Nutr* 136:2123, 2006.
20. Beelen M, Koopman R, Gijsen AP, et al: Protein coingestion stimulates muscle protein synthesis during resistance-type exercise, *Am J Physiol Endocrinol Metab* 295:E70, 2008.
21. Brooks N, Cloutier GJ, Cadena SM, et al: Resistance training and timed essential amino acids protect against the loss of muscle mass and strength during 28 days of bed rest and energy deficit, *J Appl Physiol* 105:241, 2008.
22. Garlick PJ: The nature of human hazards associated with excessive intake of amino acids, *J Nutr* 134:1633S, 2004.
23. Swain JF, McCarron PB, Hamilton EF, et al: Characteristics of the diet patterns tested in the optimal macronutrient intake trial to prevent heart disease (OmniHeart): options for a heart-healthy diet, *J Am Diet Assoc* 108:257, 2008.
24. Bejon P, Mohammed S, Mwangi I, et al: Fraction of all hospital admissions and deaths attributable to malnutrition among children in rural Kenya, *Am J Clin Nutr* 88:1626, 2008.
25. Torun B: Protein-energy malnutrition. In Shils ME, Olsen JA, Shike M, et al, editors: *Modern nutrition in health and disease*, ed 10, Baltimore, 2006, Lippincott Williams & Wilkins.
26. Potrykus I: Nutritionally enhanced rice to combat malnutrition disorders of the poor, *Nutr Rev* 61(6,II):S101, 2003.
27. Santerre CR: Food biotechnology. In Bowman BA, Russell RM, editors: *Present knowledge in nutrition*, ed 9, Washington, DC, 2006, International Life Sciences Institute.
28. Cotton PA, Subar AF, Friday JE, et al: Dietary sources of nutrients among U.S. adults, 1994 to 1996, *J Am Diet Assoc* 104:921, 2004.
29. Fulgoni VL: Current protein intake in America: analysis of the National Health and Nutrition Examination Survey, 2003-2004, *Am J Clin Nutr* 87(Suppl):1554S, 2008.
30. O'Donnell SI, Hoerr SL, Mendoza JA, et al: Nutrient quality of fast food kids meals, *J Am Diet Assoc* 88:1388, 2008.
31. Bopp MJ, Houston DK, Lenchik L, et al: Lean mass loss is associated with low protein intake during dietary induced weight loss in postmenopausal women, *J Am Diet Assoc* 108:1216, 2008.
32. Burrowes JD: New recommendations for the management of diabetic kidney disease, *Nutr Today* 43:65, 2008.
33. Cupisti A, Licitra R, Chisari C, et al: Skeletal muscle and nutritional assessment in chronic renal failure patients on a protein-restricted diet, *J Intern Med* 255:115, 2004.
34. Kushner RF, Doerfler B: Low-carbohydrate, high-protein diets revisited, *Curr Opin Gastroenterol* 24:198, 2008.
35. Soenen S, Westerterp-Plantenga MS: Proteins and satiety: implications for weight management, *Curr Opin Clin Nutr Metab Care* 11:747, 2008.
36. Paddon-Jones D, Short KR, Campbell WW, et al: Role of dietary protein in the sarcopenia of aging, *Am J Clin Nutr* 87(Suppl):1562S, 2008.

37. Gardner CD, Kiazand A, Alhassan S, et al: Comparison of the Atkins, Zone, Ornish, and LEARN diets for change in weight and related risk factors among overweight premenopausal women, *JAMA* 297:969, 2007.
38. Shai I, Schwarzfuchs D, Henkin Y, et al: Weight loss with a low-carbohydrate, Mediterranean, or low-fat diet, *N Engl J Med* 359:229, 2008.
39. Sacks FM, Bray GA, Carey VJ, et al: Comparison of weight-loss diets with different compositions of fat, protein, and carbohydrates, *N Engl J Med* 360:859, 2009.
40. Bernstein AM, Treyzon L, Zhaoping LI: Are high-protein, vegetable-based diets safe for kidney function? A review of the literature, *J Am Diet Assoc* 107:644, 2007.
41. Martin WF, Cerundolo LH, Pikosky MA, et al: Effects of dietary protein intake on indexes of hydration, *J Am Diet Assoc* 106:587, 2006.
42. American Dietetic Association: Position of the American Dietetic Association: functional foods, *J Am Diet Assoc* 109:735, 2009.
43. Omoni AO, Aluko RE: Soybean foods and their benefits: potential mechanisms of action, *Nutr Rev* 63(8):272, 2005.
44. Xiao CW: Health effects of soy protein and isoflavones in humans, *J Nutr* 138:1244S, 2008.
45. Bazzano LA, He J, Ogden LG, et al: Legume consumption and risk of coronary heart disease in U.S. men and women: NHANES I epidemiologic follow-up study, *Arch Intern Med* 161:2573, 2001.
46. United States Department of Agriculture: *USDA National Nutrient Database for Standard Reference*, Release 21, Washington, DC, 2009, U.S. Department of Agriculture. Retrieved January 26, 2009, from http://www.ars.usda.gov/Services/docs.htm?docid=17477.
47. King JC, Blumberg J, Ingwersen L, et al: Tree nuts and peanuts as components of a healthy diet, *J Nutr* 138:1736S, 2008.
48. Giugliano D, Esposito K: Mediterranean diet and metabolic diseases, *Curr Opin Lipidol* 19:63, 2008.
49. Murphy SP, Allen LH: Nutritional importance of animal source foods, *J Nutr* 133:3932S, 2003.
50. Marlow HJ, Hayes WK, Soret S, et al: Diet and the environment: does what you eat matter? *Am J Clin Nutr* 89(Suppl):1699S, 2009.
51. Leitzmann C: Nutrition ecology: the contribution of vegetarian diets, *Am J Clin Nutr* 78(Suppl):657S, 2003.
52. Fraser GE: Vegetarian diets: what do we know of their effects on common chronic diseases? *Am J Clin Nutr* 89(Suppl):1607S, 2009.
53. Aronson D: Vegetarian nutrition: what every dietitian should know, *Today's Dietitian* 7(3):32, 2005. Retrieved from www.todaysdietitian.com/newarchives/td_0305p32.shtml.
54. Messina V, Melina V, Mangels AR: A new food guide for North American vegetarians, *J Am Diet Assoc* 103:771, 2003.
55. Kris-Etherton P, Hill AM: n-3 fatty acids: food or supplements? *J Am Diet Assoc* 108:1125, 2008.
56. Mangat I: Do vegetarians have to eat fish for optimal cardiovascular protection? *Am J Clin Nutr* 89(Suppl):1597, 2009.
57. American Dietetic Association: Position of the American Dietetic Association and Dietitians of Canada: vegetarian diets, *J Am Diet Assoc* 103:748, 2003.
58. Appleby P, Roddam A, Allen N, et al: Comparative fracture risk in vegetarians and nonvegetarians in EPIC-Oxford, *Eur J Clin Nutr* 61:1400, 2007.
59. Taylor SL, Hefle SL: Food allergy. In Bowman BA, Russell RM, editors: *Present knowledge in nutrition*, ed 8, Washington, DC, 2001, International Life Sciences Institute.

FURTHER READINGS AND RESOURCES

Readings

American Dietetic Association: Position of the American Dietetic Association: vegetarian diets, *J Am Diet Assoc* 109:1266, 2009.

Messina V, Melina V, Mangels AR: A new food guide for North American vegetarians, *J Am Diet Assoc* 103:771, 2003.

[These papers provide an overview of the development of a new vegetarian food guide that would meet nutritional requirements for all age and gender groups and current research evidence regarding the adequacy of vegetarian diets.]

Lupien J: Let's get our priorities straight in world nutrition, *Nutr Today* 39:227, 2004. *[Although obesity is a growing problem in many parts of the world, Dr. Lupien does not want us to lose sight of the food shortages and low nutrient intake among people in many developing countries.]*

Manninen AH: Are high-protein diets safe for kidney function, *J Am Diet Assoc* 107:1722, 2007. *[This author provides insight as to the effects of continued high-protein diets on renal health.]*

O'Donnell SI, Hoerr SL, Mendoza JA, et al: Nutrient quality of fast food kids meals, *J Am Diet Assoc* 88:1388, 2008. *[Does the average fast-food meal contain more protein than might be appropriate for a young child? These researchers tell us which nutrients are low and which are high in these meals.]*

Websites of Interest

National Institutes of Health, National Library of Medicine: Medline Plus: *Trusted Health Information for You*; this site provides links to many resources on vegetarianism including planning healthy diets, dangers of inadequate diets, and sources of problem nutrients; information provided in English and Spanish: www.nlm.nih.gov/medlineplus/vegetariandiet.html.

U.S. Department of Agriculture, Center for Nutrition Policy and Promotion: *MyPyramid food guidance system*; these websites describe healthy choices and portion sizes of animal and plant protein foods: www.mypyramid.gov/pyramid/meat.html, www.mypyramid.gov/pyramid/milk_tips.html, www.mypyramid.gov/tips_resources/vegetarian_diets.html.

U.S. Department of Agriculture, Food and Nutrition Information Center: *Vegetarian nutrition*; this site provides information and resource lists for vegetarian diets, general information for protein nutrition, and ideas for plant-based and vegetarian meal planning: www.nal.usda.gov/fnic/etext/000058.html.

CHAPTER

6

Vitamins

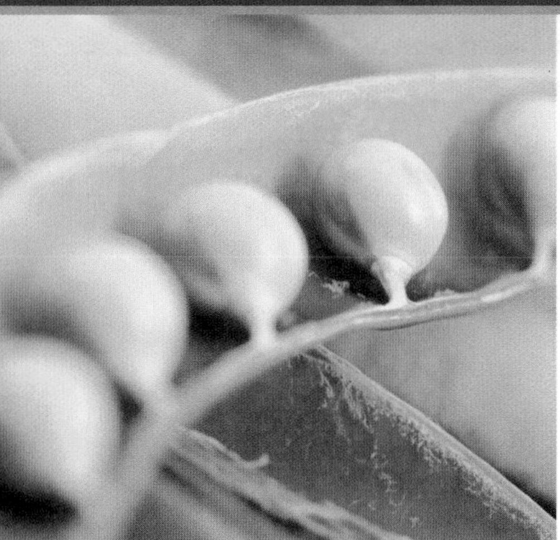

Eleanor D. Schlenker

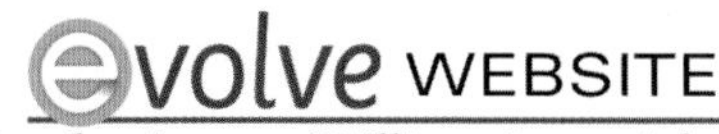

http://evolve.elsevier.com/Williams/essentials/

OUTLINE

Here we begin our study of the non–energy-yielding micronutrients: the vitamins and minerals. First, we look at the vitamins.

No other group of nutritional elements has so captured the interest of scientists, health professionals, and the general public as vitamins. Research journals and the popular press describe how vitamins help to prevent chronic disease and support well-being in ways beyond their generally accepted roles as nutrients. Opinions about vitamin needs vary widely, running the gamut from wise functional use to wild flagrant abuse. Scientists are intrigued with new plant chemicals identified in functional foods and trying to learn how these substances interact with known vitamins. In the future, we may identify new vitamins essential to human health.

In this chapter, we review fat-soluble and water-soluble vitamins. We focus on why we need them and how we obtain them.

VITAMINS: ESSENTIAL NUTRIENTS

General Nature and Classification

Scientists discovered most of the vitamins we know about today between 1900 and 1950. The name *vitamin* was adopted when one of the scientists working with a nitrogen-containing substance called an **amine** named his discovery *vitamine* ("vital amine"), thinking this was the common nature of all vitamins. At first, a letter designation was given to each vitamin as it was discovered. However, as the number grew this became confusing, and scientific names based on the structure or function of the vitamin were developed. Letter designations have been retained for the fat-soluble vitamins, because for each of these vitamins a number of closely related compounds exist that have similar metabolic activities and structures.[1]

What Is a Vitamin?

To be classified as a *vitamin,* a compound has to meet several criteria:

- It must be an organic dietary substance that is not energy producing, as are carbohydrate, fat, or protein.
- It is needed in very small quantities to perform a particular metabolic function and prevent an associated deficiency disease.
- The body cannot manufacture it, so must be supplied in food.

KEY TERMS
amine An organic compound containing nitrogen. Amino acids and pyridoxine are examples of amines.

These principles form the basis for establishing that a vitamin is essential. Over the years we have successfully identified the structure, chemistry, and metabolism of many vitamins. However, more must be learned about vitamin requirements, how vitamin needs can be met by the United States food supply, and current dietary habits influencing vitamin intake.[2] Other vitamin-like substances in food that appear to promote health and increase resistance to chronic diseases are also being identified, and in time new substances may be added to the list of essential vitamins.

Basic Principles

Over the years our understanding of the vitamins has expanded. Not only have we learned more about individual vitamins and their functions but also how they interact with other vitamins and other nutrients in carrying on their work. The following principles will guide our study of these nutrients:

- *Individual vitamins are multifunctional:* Most vitamins have multiple roles or actions in the body, sometimes working independently and sometimes working cooperatively with other nutrients. Although we associate vitamin A with its major role of helping us see in dim light, this vitamin also maintains the mucous membranes that protect against infection.
- *One vitamin cannot substitute for another vitamin:* All vitamins must be available in sufficient amounts for the body to function normally and for tissues to remain healthy. For example, an abundant supply of vitamin C cannot take the place of folate in preventing a neural tube defect (NTD).
- *Vitamins work together in carrying out body functions:* The formation and maturation of red blood cells require the actions of folate, pyridoxine, vitamin B_{12}, and ascorbic acid, along with several important minerals.
- *Vitamins function best when all are present in the appropriate proportions:* High-potency vitamin A supplements interfere with the action of vitamin D, decreasing calcium absorption and increasing the risk of hip fracture.

These functional truths underscore the importance of eating a variety of foods to obtain essential vitamins and other important substances that contribute to health. A supplement containing one vitamin will not take the place of fruits and vegetables that supply many different vitamins along with fiber and phytochemicals. When nutrients are obtained from food as part of a balanced diet, we are also unlikely to take in an excessive amount of any one vitamin that could interfere with the absorption or function of another.

Classification

As the vitamins were discovered, they were grouped according to their solubility in fat or water, and this classification has continued (Box 6-1).

Fat-Soluble Vitamins

The fat-soluble vitamins are A, D, E, and K. They are closely associated with body lipids and are easily stored. Their functions are usually related to structural activities with proteins.

BOX 6-1 CLASSIFICATION OF VITAMINS

Fat-Soluble Vitamins
- A
- D
- E
- K

Water-Soluble Vitamins
- Vitamin C (ascorbic acid)
- Thiamin
- Riboflavin
- Niacin
- Pantothenic acid
- Biotin
- Vitamin B_6 (pyridoxine)
- Folate
- Vitamin B_{12} (cobalamin)

Water-Soluble Vitamins

The water-soluble vitamins are vitamin C and the B-complex family. These vitamins are more easily absorbed and transported, but unlike the fat-soluble vitamins, they cannot be stored except in the general sense of tissue saturation. The B vitamins function mainly as coenzyme factors in cell metabolism. Vitamin C works with enzymes that support tissue building and maintenance.

Current Knowledge and Key Questions

In our study we will answer the following questions for each vitamin:

- *Chemical and physical nature:* What is the general structure of the vitamin?
- *Absorption, transport, and storage:* How does the body handle this particular vitamin?
- *Function:* What does this vitamin do?
- *Related deficiency symptoms or disease:* What happens when this vitamin is absent or not available in sufficient amounts?
- *Clinical role in health:* Does this vitamin prevent or ameliorate a chronic disease?
- *Recommended intake and possible toxicity:* How much of this vitamin do we need, and how much is too much? What are the consequences of excessive intake?
- *Food sources:* How do we obtain this vitamin?

In the following sections we will review the four fat-soluble vitamins and the nine water-soluble vitamins.

FAT-SOLUBLE VITAMINS

VITAMIN A

Chemical and Physical Nature

Vitamin A is the generic name for a group of compounds with similar biologic activity: retinol, retinal, and retinoic acid. The term *retinoids* refers to the natural forms of vitamin A and its synthetic copies. Retinol, an alcohol of high molecular weight ($C_{20}H_{29}OH$), was given its name based on its specific function in the retina of the eye. It is soluble in fat and ordinary fat solvents. Because retinol is insoluble in water, it is fairly stable in cooking.

BOX 6-2 SOURCES OF PREFORMED AND PROVITAMIN A

Preformed Vitamin A	**Provitamin A**
2% Milk	Broccoli
Cheese	Carrots
Egg yolk	Spinach
Liver	Cantaloupe
	Tomato juice
	Apricots

Forms

There are two dietary forms of vitamin A: (1) preformed vitamin A and (2) provitamin A (Box 6-2), as described following:

1. *Preformed vitamin A (retinol):* This is the natural form of vitamin A found only in animal foods and usually associated with fat. Vitamin A compounds are deposited primarily in the liver but also in small amounts in the kidneys, lungs, and adipose tissue, so organ meats are a rich source. Other dietary sources are the fat portion of dairy foods, egg yolk, and fish.
2. *Provitamin A or β-carotene:* Plants cannot synthesize vitamin A but instead produce a family of compounds called carotenoids. These substances in plants are eaten by animals and then converted to vitamin A. Thus humans can obtain their vitamin A directly by eating animal tissues or by converting carotenoids obtained from plant foods. The carotenoids were so named because β-carotene ($C_{40}H_{56}$) was found in the yellow and orange pigment in carrots and other vegetables and fruits. Examples of other carotenoids found in plant foods include β-cryptoxanthin, lutein, and zeaxanthin, but not all of these can be converted to vitamin A.

The carotenoids have an important role in human nutrition. β-Carotene, converted to vitamin A in the body, provides about 21% of the total vitamin A intake in the United States.[3] Enzymes that split the carotenoid molecule to yield retinol are found in the mucosal cells of the small intestine and in the liver. The yellow and red carotenoid pigments in many fruits and vegetables and in red palm oil are the major food sources of vitamin A in most developing countries. Unfortunately, the conversion of carotenes to retinol is much less efficient than we thought, raising concerns about how plant foods can provide an adequate supply of vitamin A in regions of the world where animal foods are scarce (Table 6-1).[4]

Absorption, Transport, and Storage

Substances Needed for Absorption

Whether vitamin A enters the body as preformed vitamin A or as the precursor β-carotene, various materials are needed for its absorption, as follows:

TABLE 6-1 CONVERSION OF CAROTENOIDS TO VITAMIN A

AMOUNT IN THE DIET	AMOUNT AVAILABLE TO THE BODY
1 mcg retinol	1 mcg retinol
12 mcg β-carotene	1 mcg retinol
24 mcg α-carotene or β-cryptoxanthin	1 mcg retinol

NOTE: Although these carotenoids can be converted to retinol (vitamin A) to help meet body needs, increased amounts of these molecules are required to produce 1 molecule of vitamin A.

- *Bile salts:* Vitamin A joins with fat, other fat-related compounds, and bile salts in the small intestine to form micelles, a bile-lipid complex. Bile salts are needed to carry fats and fat-soluble materials into the intestinal wall for further breakdown. Clinical conditions affecting the biliary system such as obstruction of the bile duct, infectious hepatitis, or liver cirrhosis that interfere with production or release of bile salts hinder vitamin A absorption.

KEY TERMS

coenzyme A substance that is a necessary partner with a cell enzyme in carrying out a chemical reaction; vitamins are important coenzymes in energy, lipid, and protein metabolism.

retinol Chemical name for vitamin A derived from its function in the retina of the eye producing light-dark adaptation.

retinal The aldehyde form of retinol (vitamin A) derived from the enzymatic splitting of β-carotene in the intestinal wall. In the retina of the eye, retinal combines with opsin to form visual pigments. In the rods it forms rhodopsin (visual purple), and in the cones it forms the pigments responsible for color vision.

carotenoids A group of yellow-red pigments widely distributed in plants that act as antioxidants and may have additional health-promoting properties; some carotenoids such as β-carotene can be converted to retinal in the intestinal wall.

precursor A substance from which another substance is derived.

micelle The bile-lipid complex that carries digested lipids and fat-soluble vitamins into the cells of the intestinal mucosa for absorption.

- *Pancreatic lipase:* This fat-splitting enzyme released into the upper small intestine carries out the hydrolysis of fat emulsions containing vitamin A. Water-based preparations of retinol are used when lipase secretion and absorption of fat is curtailed, as in cystic fibrosis or pancreatitis.[3]
- *Dietary fat:* Absorption of vitamin A requires fat to stimulate the release of bile salts and form micelles. Absorption is most efficient when fat intake is at least 10 g/day.[5]

Conversion of β-Carotene

β-Carotene can be absorbed and used by the body in its original form or be converted to vitamin A. Although at one time we believed that carotenoids were biologically important only as precursors to vitamin A, we have since learned that as members of that broad category of phytochemicals active in functional foods, they have roles in human health unrelated to the actions of vitamin A.

Transport and Storage

The route of absorption of vitamin A and the carotenoids parallels that of fat. In the intestinal mucosa, retinol—whether from preformed animal sources or converted from carotenes—along with intact plant carotenoids are incorporated into the chylomicrons. In this form they enter the bloodstream via the lymphatic system and are carried to the liver for storage or distribution to tissues. Age is a factor in absorption. Newborns, especially premature infants, absorb vitamin A poorly. Persons using mineral oil as a laxative reduce their absorption of vitamin A.

The liver, an efficient storage organ for vitamin A, contains up to 85% of the body's total supply. Liver stores are usually sufficient to prevent deficiency for about 6 to 12 months and in some individuals for as long as 4 years. The capacity of the liver to store a substantial amount of vitamin A has special significance in parts of the world where vitamin A–containing foods are in short supply, because a prophylactic dose of vitamin A administered every 6 months can prevent mortality and blindness and support normal growth in infants and young children.[6] Measles is a killer disease of malnourished children and a target for vitamin A supplementation.

Functions of Vitamin A

The role of vitamin A in vision is best known, but vitamin A also influences the integrity of body coverings and linings (epithelial tissues), growth, immunity, and reproductive function.

Vitamin A Deficiency and Clinical Applications

Vision

The ability of the eye to adapt to changes in light depends on a light-sensitive pigment, rhodopsin, located in the rods of the retina (Figure 6-1). Rhodopsin—commonly known

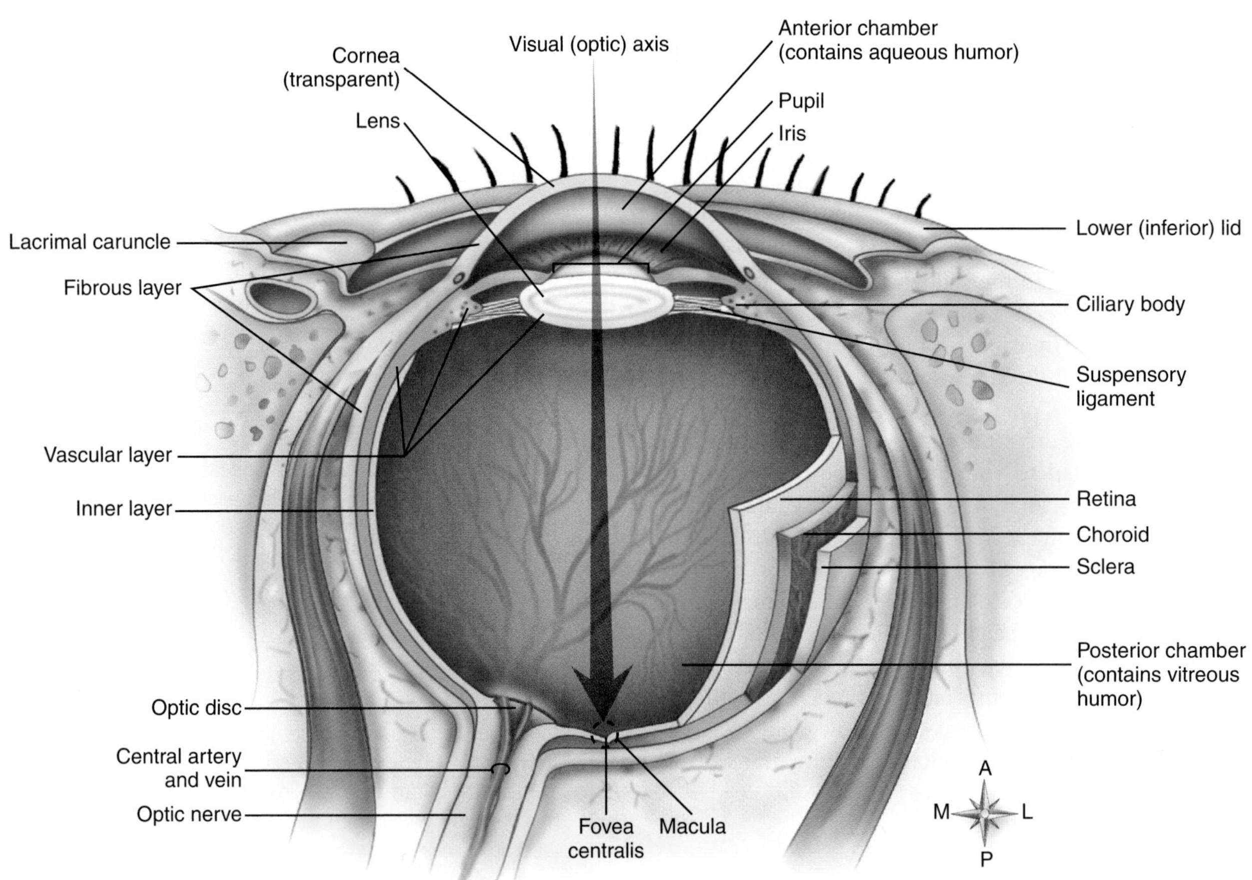

FIGURE 6-1 Structure of the eye as viewed from the side. (From Thibodeau GA, Patton KT: *Anatomy & physiology,* ed 7, St Louis, 2010, Mosby.)

as *visual purple*—is made up of the vitamin A compound retinal and the protein opsin (Figure 6-2). When the body lacks vitamin A, normal rhodopsin cannot be formed and the rods and cones of the retina become increasingly sensitive to changes in light, causing **night blindness.** This condition is reversed with an injection of vitamin A (retinol), which is readily converted to retinal and then rhodopsin.

Cell Differentiation

Vitamin A controls the differentiation of cells, or in other words, the types of specialized cells that are formed from basic stem cells. Vitamin A is needed to develop and maintain healthy epithelial tissue, which provides our primary barrier to infection. The epithelium includes both the outer skin and the mucous membranes that line many body structures. Without vitamin A we form cells that are dry and flat rather than soft and moist. These dry, flat cells gradually harden to form keratin, a process called **keratinization.** Keratin is a protein that creates dry, scaly tissue, normal for nails and hair but abnormal for skin and mucous membranes. In vitamin A deficiency, such abnormal tissue changes occur in many body systems, as follows:

- *Eye:* The cornea dries and hardens, a condition called *xerophthalmia* (Figure 6-3). The tear ducts become dry, robbing the eye of its cleansing and lubricating fluid, and infection follows quickly. In extreme deficiency the keratinization progresses to blindness. Blindness related to vitamin A deficiency is a world public health problem, because each year more than 350,000 preschool children lose their sight and about half die within 1 year of becoming blind.[7]

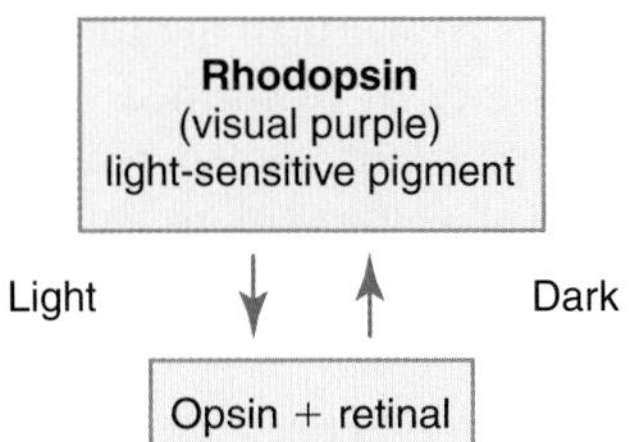

FIGURE 6-2 The vision cycle: light-dark adaptation role of vitamin A.

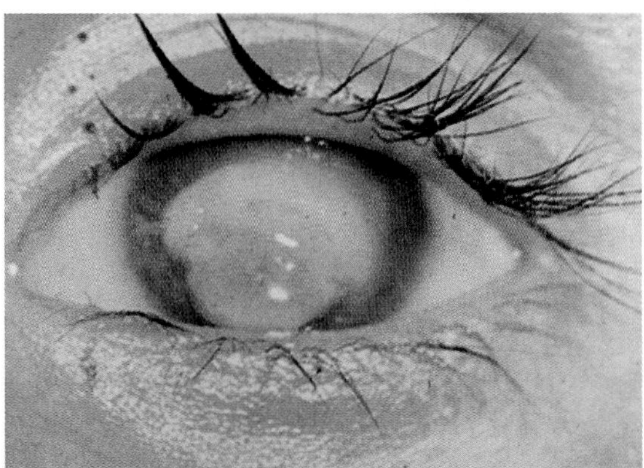

FIGURE 6-3 Xerophthalmia. (From McLaren DS: *A colour atlas and text of diet-related disorders,* ed 2, London, 1992, Mosby-Year Book Europe Limited.)

- *Respiratory tract:* The ciliated epithelium in the nasal passages dry and the cilia are lost, removing a barrier to infectious organisms. Nasal secretions that trap invading particles and remove them from the body become absent.
- *Gastrointestinal tract:* The salivary glands dry, and the mouth becomes dry and cracked, open to invading bacteria. Mucosal secretions decrease throughout the digestive tract, and tissues dry and slough off, affecting digestion and absorption.
- *Genitourinary tract:* When epithelial tissue begins to break down, problems such as vaginal infections, urinary tract infections, and formation of calculi increase.
- *Skin:* As skin becomes dry and scaly, small pustules (hardened, pigmented, papular eruptions) appear around hair follicles, a condition known as *follicular hyperkeratosis* (Figure 6-4).
- *Tooth formation:* Certain epithelial cells surrounding tooth buds in fetal gum tissue that normally become specialized cup-shaped organs called *ameloblasts* do not develop properly. These little organs form the enamel of the developing tooth.

Growth

Vitamin A is essential for the growth of bones and soft tissues. Vitamin A controls protein synthesis and *mitosis* (cell division) and stabilizes cell membranes. The growth and maintenance of bone require constant remodeling, reshaping, and expansion. Vitamin A participates in the important job of tunneling out old bone to make way for new bone; then the tunnels are filled in to accommodate growth according to the embryonic cartilage model. Although an inadequate supply of vitamin A is detrimental to bone health, so are excessive intakes that cause old bone to be lost more rapidly than new bone can be formed. Among postmenopausal women,

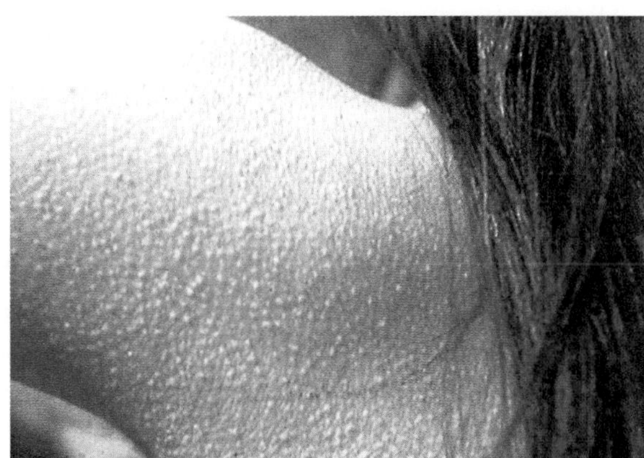

FIGURE 6-4 Follicular hyperkeratosis caused by vitamin A deficiency. (From McLaren DS: *A colour atlas and text of diet-related disorders,* ed 2, London, 1992, Mosby-Year Book Europe Limited.)

KEY TERMS

night blindness Inability to see well in diminished light; caused by vitamin A deficiency.

keratinization The process of creating the protein keratin, a principal constituent of skin, hair, nails, and the matrix forming tooth enamel.

intakes of preformed vitamin A in excess of the Dietary Reference Intake (DRI) are associated with lower bone mass and increased risk of hip fracture.[8] β-Carotene, the precursor of vitamin A supplied by fruits and vegetables, does not lead to excessive body levels of vitamin A or bone loss.

Based on its role in cell growth and differentiation, vitamin A supplements should be part of intervention and treatment of protein-energy malnutrition (PEM).[6] The action of vitamin A in controlling cell division has led researchers to consider a possible role for vitamin A in cancer prevention or treatment.[9]

Reproduction

Vitamin A is needed for normal sexual maturation and function. It participates in gene expression and plays an important role in fetal development, including the central nervous system (CNS).[3] A sufficient intake is required for successful lactation.

Immunity

Poor vitamin A status lowers resistance to infection in several ways. First, changes in epithelial and mucosal tissue allow disease organisms to enter the body more easily. Second, vitamin A has a direct effect on immune function, and both cell-mediated and antibody-mediated immunity are impaired when intake is low. Measles is more likely to be fatal in vitamin A–deficient children in developing countries. Immune response returns to normal quite rapidly when vitamin A is restored.[10]

Vitamin A Requirement

Influencing Factors

A number of variables modify the vitamin A needs of a given individual. These include the following:

- *Liver stores:* High vitamin A stores can supply body needs for an extended period; those with low body stores must depend on day-to-day intakes.
- *Intake of preformed versus provitamin A:* Increased amounts of carotenoids are required to meet the DRI for vitamin A.
- *Illness and infection:* Needs increase to support the production of immune cells and body defenses.
- *Gastrointestinal or hepatic defects:* Gallbladder or liver disease interfering with production of bile limits fat absorption and in turn the absorption of vitamin A and carotenoids.

Causes of Vitamin A Deficiency

In the United States the primary cause of vitamin A deficiency is inadequate dietary intake, usually the result of poor food selection rather than unavailability. The growing popularity of fast-food restaurants has influenced vitamin A status, because "kids meals" based on a burger or chicken sandwich with fries and a sweetened beverage rather than fruit and milk do not meet one third of the DRI for vitamin A.[11] Vitamin A deficiency occurs as a result of poor absorption based on a lack of bile or dietary fat, inadequate conversion of β-carotene, or liver or intestinal disease. A high intake of alcohol results in loss of vitamin A from the liver even if liver function remains normal.[3]

BOX 6-3 SIGNS OF VITAMIN A TOXICITY

- Vomiting
- Headache
- Joint pain
- Thickening of the long bones
- Hair loss
- Jaundice
- Liver injury and ascites (if the condition continues)

Dietary Reference Intake

The Recommended Dietary Allowance (RDA) for vitamin A is the amount required to maintain optimum liver stores. It is presented as micrograms (mcg) of retinol,[3] and the term retinol activity equivalent (RAE) takes into account the ratios for converting carotenoids to vitamin A. Early on, vitamin A was measured in international units (IU), and some food composition tables still use those units. Many of these older tables overestimate the amount of vitamin A available from carotenoid-containing foods, such that intakes are calculated to be greater than is true. The RDA for men ages 19 and older is set at 900 mcg, and the RDA for women of this age is 700 mcg. To ensure sufficient vitamin A to support a successful pregnancy and appropriate vitamin A content in breast milk, the RDA increases to 770 mcg in pregnancy and 1300 mcg in lactation.

Vitamin A Toxicity

Hypervitaminosis A

Because the liver can store very large amounts of vitamin A, persons taking high-potency supplements can develop toxicity. Characteristic signs of hypervitaminosis A are listed in Box 6-3. Daily intakes greater than the Tolerable Upper Intake Level (UL) of 3000 mcg of preformed vitamin A are especially dangerous for pregnant women, resulting in lower birth weights[12] or congenital malformations,[10] depending on intake. Increasing use of vitamin supplements and fortified foods are adding up to disturbing intakes of preformed vitamin A among some age-groups. Supplements often contain as much as two times the RDA and, if combined with highly fortified food items, bring children and adults dangerously close to the UL.[13]

Food Sources of Vitamin A

Animal sources of preformed vitamin A include liver, milk, cheese, butter, egg yolk, and fish. Nonfat and low-fat milk and some soy milks are fortified with vitamin A to the level found naturally in whole milk. Non-animal products such as margarine, ready-to-eat cereals, and cereal bars are often fortified with vitamin A. Dark-yellow, orange, red, and green vegetables and fruits contain a variety of carotenoids and help meet the vitamin A requirement. Cooked vegetables can be better dietary sources of carotenoids than raw vegetables, because cooking helps to release these substances from their plant sources, making them more available for absorption. The vitamin A content of selected foods is listed in Box 6-4. (The *Focus on Culture* box, "Acculturation: Effect on Food Patterns," points to problems with low intakes of fruits and vegetables.)

BOX 6-4 FOOD SOURCES OF VITAMIN A

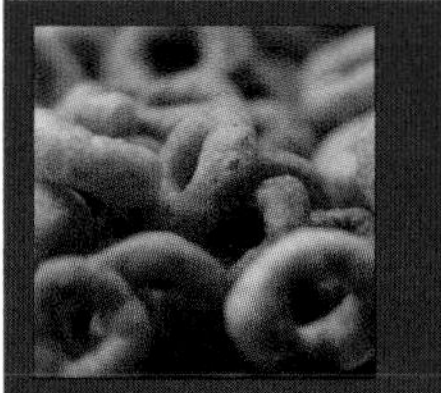
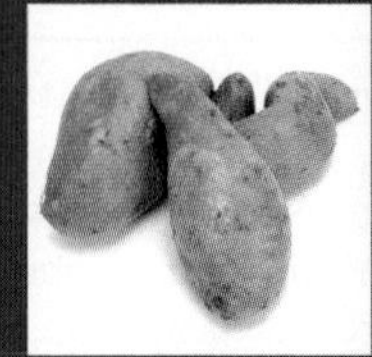
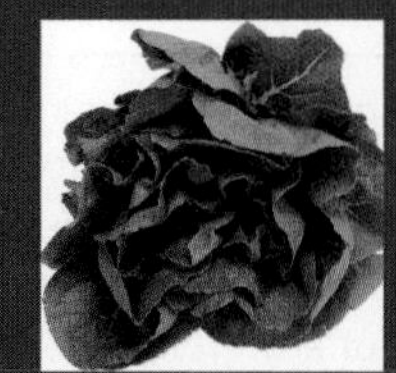
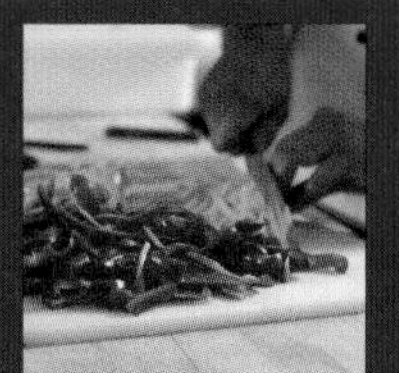
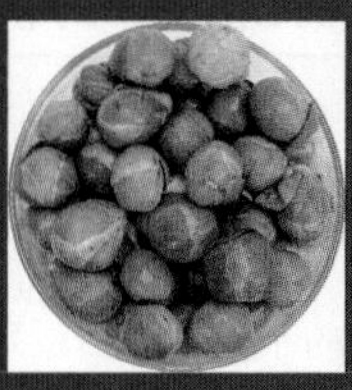
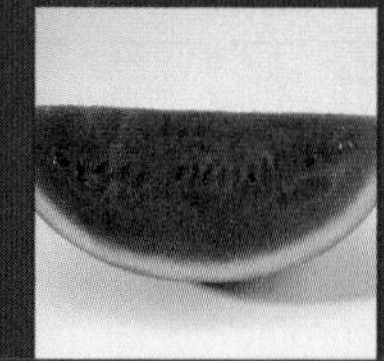

FOOD SOURCE	QUANTITY	VITAMIN A (in mcg RAE)*
Grains Group		
Fortified ready-to-eat cereals		
Instant oatmeal	1 packet	329
Special K	1 cup	230
Cheerios	1 cup	260
Wheaties	1 cup	150
Vegetable Group		
Sweet potato, baked in skin	1 medium	1403
Pumpkin, canned	½ cup	953
Spinach, frozen, cooked	½ cup	572
Collard greens, frozen, cooked	½ cup	488
Carrot, raw	1 medium	601
Chinese cabbage (bok choy), cooked	1 cup	360
Lettuce, dark green	1 cup	207
Peppers, sweet, chopped	½ cup	116
Broccoli, raw	6 flowerets	96
Brussels sprouts, cooked	1 cup	71
Fruit Group		
Cantaloupe	⅛ melon	117
Apricots, canned in juice	½ cup	104
Watermelon	1 wedge (4 × 8 inch)	80
Meat, Beans, Eggs, and Nuts Group		
Chicken livers, cooked	1	780
Clams, canned	3 oz	153
Milk Group		
Milk, skim, fortified	1 cup	148
Milk, low fat, fortified	1 cup	142
Soy milk, unfortified	1 cup	0
Cheddar cheese	1 oz	75
Milk, whole, unfortified	1 cup	68
Fats, Oils, and Sugars Group		
Margarine	1 tbsp	115
Butter	1 tbsp	97

Recommended Dietary Allowances (RDAs) for adults: women, 700 mcg RAE; men, 900 mcg RAE.
*1 RAE (retinol activity equivalent) = 1 mcg retinol.
Nutrient data from USDA: *USDA National Nutrient Database for Standard Reference, Release 21,* Washington, DC, U.S. Department of Agriculture, 2009. Retrieved April 23, 2010 from http://www.ars.usda.gov/Services/docs.htm?docid=17477.

VITAMIN D

Chemical and Physical Nature

When first discovered, vitamin D was classified as a *vitamin,* although it is now clear that vitamin D is actually a **prohormone,** and in its active form functions as a hormone. Chemically, vitamin D is a sterol and its precursor found in

KEY TERMS

retinol activity equivalent (RAE) Unit of measure for dietary sources of vitamin A, including preformed retinol and the precursor provitamins β-carotene, α-carotene, and β-cryptoxanthin.

prohormone A substance that when converted to its active form acts as a hormone; vitamin D obtained from food or synthesized in the skin is a prohormone, and its active hormonal form is named *calcitriol.*

FOCUS ON CULTURE

Acculturation: Effect on Food Patterns

The term *acculturation* refers to the adoption of local customs and practices by persons entering a new country, and such changes often influence disease risk. Individuals who move from one part of the world to another begin to develop the chronic diseases of their host country, based on the changes in their diet and environment. For example, those who move from Mexico to the United States are more likely to develop cardiovascular disease than their counterparts who remain in Mexico.[1] Latinos taking up residence in the United States increase their intakes of fat, sugars, and sweetened beverages but decrease their use of fruits and vegetables, including beans, lowering their intakes of fiber, provitamin A, and the B-complex vitamins. The more time these subjects spend in the United States, the more their intakes of these foods decrease.[2,3]

The availability of fruits and vegetables in their new neighborhoods as compared with their former neighborhoods may contribute to these changes. Latino homemakers accustomed to purchasing fresh produce at local street markets in Mexico or Puerto Rico must adjust to different marketing environments and likely higher prices in urban settings. Some shoppers commented that fruits and vegetables purchased in the United States tasted different from those obtained in their home country, which could relate to degree of ripeness, cultivar, or how one remembers the food "at home."[3]

The language spoken in the home and in the country of birth also predict acculturation and food patterns.[4] When foods eaten by women born in the United States and women born in Mexico were compared on the basis of language generally spoken, English or Spanish, those using Spanish had higher intakes of fruits, vegetables, and beans than those speaking English, regardless of birthplace. Women born in the United States who spoke predominantly English had the lowest use of fruits, green leafy vegetables, and beans, and the highest use of fried potatoes of any group. They used only two thirds as many beans as their counterparts born in the United States who spoke predominantly Spanish and less than half as many beans as women born in Mexico who still spoke predominantly Spanish. This research suggests that changes in food patterns proceed more slowly when language holds ties to a native culture. Health professionals working with populations new to a host country must recognize the role of language in the acculturation process.

REFERENCES

1. Neuhouser ML, Thompson B, Coronado GD, et al: Higher fat intake and lower fruit and vegetables intakes are associated with greater acculturation among Mexicans living in Washington State, *J Am Diet Assoc* 104:51, 2004.
2. Kittler PG, Sucher KP: *Cultural foods: traditions and trends*, Belmont, Calif, 2000, Wadsworth/Thomson Learning.
3. Ayala GX, Baquero B, Klinger S: A systematic review of the relationship between acculturation and diet among Latinos in the United States: implications for future research, *J Am Diet Assoc* 108(8):1330, 2008.
4. Montez JK, Eschbach K: Country of birth and language are uniquely associated with intakes of fat, fiber, and fruits and vegetables among Mexican-American women in the United States, *J Am Diet Assoc* 108:473, 2008.

human skin is the lipid molecule **7-dehydrocholesterol.** All compounds with vitamin D activity are soluble in fat but not water and are heat stable.

Forms

The body can use two forms of vitamin D: (1) ergocalciferol (vitamin D_2) and (2) **cholecalciferol** (vitamin D_3). Vitamin D_2 is formed by irradiating ergosterol found in ergot (a fungus growing on rye and other cereal grains) and yeast. The more important form is vitamin D_3, made by the action of ultraviolet light from the sun on the 7-dehydrocholesterol in the skin and found naturally in fish liver oils. Vitamin D_3 is also the form used in the fortification of milk and other dairy products, cereals, and juice.

Absorption, Transport, and Storage

Absorption

Vitamin D is absorbed in the small intestine as part of the micelles, as are all fat-soluble vitamins. Malabsorption diseases such as celiac disease, cystic fibrosis, and Crohn's disease or pancreatic insufficiency hinder vitamin D absorption.

Active Hormone Synthesis

The active hormone form of vitamin D is 1,25-dihydroxycholecalciferol [1,25$(OH)_2D_3$], given the chemical name **calcitriol.** Calcitriol is produced by the combined action of the skin, liver, and kidneys, an overall process referred to as the *vitamin D endocrine system.*

We will look at each of the following three steps in this process (Figure 6-5):

1. *Skin:* When 7-dehydrocholesterol, the vitamin D precursor in the skin, is exposed to the ultraviolet rays of the sun, it is converted into vitamin D_3. The amount produced depends on the length and intensity of sun exposure and skin pigment. For those living in northern climates, sun exposure is not sufficient to supply all of their vitamin D needs, especially in the winter months.[14] People who are confined indoors and those residing in crowded city areas with high air pollution do not receive adequate ultraviolet exposure to synthesize vitamin D. Heavy skin pigment prevents ultraviolet rays from reaching the deep layer in the skin where synthesis of vitamin D_3 occurs. The use of sunscreen with a sun protection factor of 8 lowers vitamin D production by as much as 95%.[14] Obesity influences available vitamin D levels because body vitamin D is sequestered in body fat.[15]
2. *Liver:* Vitamin D, whether produced in the skin or absorbed from dietary sources, is transported to the liver where it is converted to **25-hydroxycholecalciferol [25$(OH)D_3$].** This intermediate product goes on to the kidneys for final activation.

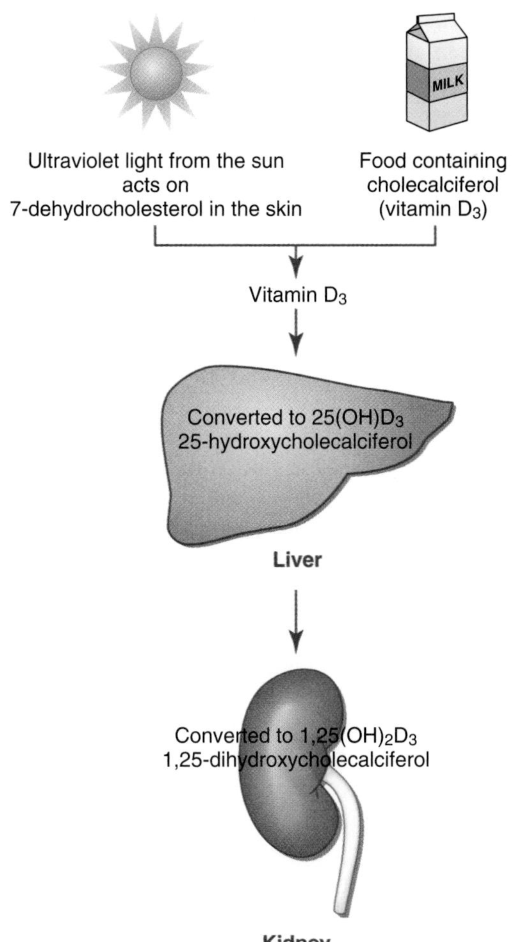

FIGURE 6-5 Formation of the active vitamin D hormone. Vitamin D undergoes a conversion in the liver and then a second conversion in the kidneys to form the vitamin D hormone calcitriol. Notice that vitamin D is handled in the same way whether it was synthesized in the skin or obtained from dietary sources.

3. *Kidneys:* In the kidneys a special enzyme completes the last step in forming the physiologically active vitamin D hormone 1,25-dihydroxycholecalciferol [$1,25(OH)_2D_3$], or calcitriol. Individuals with kidney disease are often unable to convert vitamin D to its active form.

Functions of Vitamin D

Vitamin D has been predominantly associated with calcium and phosphorus absorption and deposition in bone, but we continue to learn of other functions important to health.

Control of Calcium and Phosphorus Levels in Bone and Blood

The vitamin D endocrine system in cooperation with parathyroid hormone and calcitonin (1) stimulates the active transport of calcium and phosphorus in the small intestine, (2) promotes bone mineralization, and (3) maintains blood calcium at the normal level. Each hormone—calcitriol, parathyroid hormone, and calcitonin—has a specific role in controlling bone and blood calcium levels. Vitamin D acts primarily on the intestine to stimulate calcium and phosphorus absorption and facilitate their deposition in bone tissue. Parathyroid hormone and calcitonin are responsible for keeping blood calcium and phosphorus levels in the normal ranges.

Blood calcium is maintained within very narrow limits to ensure proper function of the heart and nervous system. If blood calcium begins to fall, then parathyroid hormone stimulates calcium withdrawal from the bone and excretion of phosphorus in the urine to restore the calcium/phosphorus ratio to normal. If blood calcium levels rise, then calcitonin increases calcium excretion to lower blood calcium. Parathyroid hormone and calcitonin are constantly present at low levels to prevent rapid fluctuations in blood calcium.

Optimum calcium intake and an adequate supply of vitamin D ensure the absorption of sufficient amounts of calcium to maintain normal blood calcium and phosphorus levels and prevent a rise in parathyroid hormone and mobilization of bone calcium. Limited hours in the sun and use of sun screen, lower milk intake, and higher body weights have had a detrimental effect on vitamin D status in all age-groups, including adolescents in peak bone growth.[16]

New Roles for Vitamin D

New research tells us that vitamin D acts on many tissues throughout the body and may have a role in preventing various chronic conditions. Vitamin D acts in the following ways:

- *Cell growth:* The rate of cell division in tissues, such as the colon, prostate, and breast, is controlled by vitamin D. This ability to prevent abnormal cell proliferation assists in cancer prevention and is the basis for using vitamin D analogues to treat the skin disorder psoriasis.[16]
- *Muscle strength:* Vitamin D participates in muscle metabolism and influences muscle strength and contraction. Individuals lacking in vitamin D are more likely to experience muscle weakness, including weakness of the heart muscle. Falls are more frequent among older persons with poor vitamin D status.[17]

KEY TERMS

7-dehydrocholesterol A precursor cholesterol compound in the skin that is irradiated by sunlight to produce cholecalciferol (D_3).

cholecalciferol Chemical name for vitamin D in its inactive form. When cholecalciferol is consumed in food or synthesized in the skin, its first activation step occurs in the liver; the final activation step is completed in the kidneys to form the active vitamin D hormone calcitriol.

calcitriol Activated hormone form of vitamin D [$1,25(OH)_2D_3$]-1,25-dihydroxycholecalciferol.

25-hydroxycholecalciferol [$25(OH)D_3$] Intermediate product formed in the liver in the process of forming the active vitamin D hormone.

calcitonin A polypeptide hormone secreted by connective tissue cells in the thyroid gland that promotes calcium excretion when blood calcium levels rise beyond normal.

- *Immune function:* Inappropriate autoimmune responses contribute to the incidence of type 1 diabetes, multiple sclerosis, and inflammatory bowel disease. Vitamin D helps to control immune response.
- *Insulin levels:* The beta cells of the pancreas require vitamin D for normal secretion of insulin.[18]
- *Hypertension and cardiovascular disease:* Vitamin D assists in regulation of the renin-angiotensin-aldosterone system that controls sodium and water retention by the kidney and thus influences blood pressure.[16]

Vitamin D Deficiency and Clinical Applications

Bone Disease

Without sufficient vitamin D, the body cannot build or maintain normal bones. In children the vitamin D deficiency disease is called *rickets* and results in a malformed skeleton (Figure 6-6). Vitamin D–deficient adults develop osteomalacia in which previously deposited bone mineral is mobilized, leading to bone pain and weak, brittle bones. Osteomalacia occurs in women of childbearing age who have little exposure to sunlight, diets low in calcium and vitamin D, and frequent pregnancies followed by periods of lactation. Older adults who use aluminum-containing antacids are at risk of osteomalacia because aluminum binds phosphorus and causes it to be excreted along with calcium. Osteomalacia sometimes accompanies osteoporosis, another bone disease common in older men and women and treated with vitamin D (see Chapter 7).

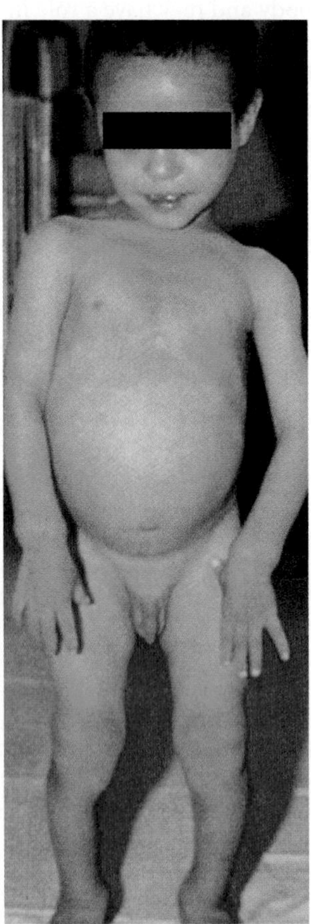

FIGURE 6-6 Bowlegs in rickets. (From McLaren DS: *A colour atlas and text of diet-related disorders,* ed 2, London, 1992, Mosby-Year Book Europe Limited.)

The widespread use of vitamin D–fortified milk and other foods had nearly eliminated rickets in the United States, but it is making a comeback among breast-fed infants not receiving vitamin D supplements.[19] Breast milk is generally low in vitamin D—especially so among mothers with poor vitamin D status. It is recommended that infants in northern climates and all African-American infants regardless of location be given vitamin D supplements. The vitamin D needs of breast-fed infants will be discussed in greater detail in Chapter 12.

Because of the active regulatory role of vitamin D in balancing bone mineral absorption and deposition, it has been used to treat the bone disease renal osteodystrophy. This condition is secondary to renal failure and results in defective bone formation.

Vitamin D Requirement

Influencing Factors

Setting dietary recommendations for vitamin D is complicated by differing degrees of sun exposure and skin synthesis. Those working in offices must obtain more of their vitamin D from dietary sources than people who work outdoors. Individuals residing in northern latitudes are more vulnerable to vitamin D deficiency. Older adults are less able to synthesize vitamin D regardless of sun exposure because of aging changes in the skin.[14]

Dietary Reference Intake

The current Adequate Intake (AI) estimates the amount of dietary vitamin D required to sustain appropriate blood levels in the absence of sun exposure. The AI for persons between 6 months and 50 years of age is 5 mcg (200 IU). For adults ages 51 to 70, the AI rises to 10 mcg (400 IU); for those 71 and older it increases to 15 mcg (600 IU),[18] based on their diminishing skin synthesis of vitamin D. Infant needs pose special problems. Vitamin D–fortified formula and cereal provide the current AI (5 mcg or 200 IU) for this age-group; however, as noted previously, breast-fed infants may require supplements. The DRI for vitamin D continues to be controversial, with experts citing the need for intakes of at least 25 mcg (1000 IU) per day to avoid deficiency.[20]

Vitamin D Toxicity

Vitamin D is stored in the adipose tissue and released slowly, so toxic amounts can accumulate when intake is inappropriately high. Toxic levels arise from self-administered doses of vitamin D supplements, not from fortified foods or long-term sun exposure. Adults taking daily megadoses of 1000 mcg (40,000 IU) or more develop signs of severe intoxication, including progressive weakness, bone pain, and hypercalcemia. Symptoms of toxicity in young children include failure to thrive and calcium deposits in soft tissues such as the kidneys. The UL is set at 50 mcg.[18] Note that the proposed increase in daily intake to 25 mcg falls well below the current UL.

HEALTH PROMOTION

Implications of Vitamin D Deficiency

Public health leaders continue to call attention to the broad spectrum of individuals who are vitamin D–deficient. Medical advice for reducing skin cancer encourages people to use sunscreen. Frail older people seldom venture outdoors. Youth are more likely to entertain themselves with video games or the Internet than outdoor activities. In a study of 382 healthy children and adolescents, nearly one half had vitamin D intakes less than 200 IU/day; more than half had low blood vitamin D levels, putting them at risk of poor calcium absorption at a time when bone mineral deposition should be reaching its peak.[21] Older adults with poor vitamin D status experience more falls,[17] and vitamin D deficiency can cause musculoskeletal pain.[22] A majority of Americans do not obtain sufficient amounts of dietary vitamin D.[23] Intakes including both food and supplements were lowest in girls ages 9 to 18 and highest in women older than age 50. African Americans and Mexican Americans had lower intakes than Caucasians at all ages. All of these groups are at risk of poor bone health, falls, and related chronic disease.

Food Sources of Vitamin D

Natural sources of vitamin D are few. Vitamin D_2 is found only in yeast, and vitamin D_3 occurs mostly in fish liver oils. Fatty fish such as mackerel or salmon contain reasonable amounts of vitamin D, and a small amount is found in egg yolk. Major dietary sources are fortified foods. Milk was selected as a practical carrier more than 50 years ago because it contained calcium and phosphorus and was commonly used by children. The vitamin D content of milk is standardized at 10 mcg (400 IU)/qt, and selected other dairy foods such as yogurt often have vitamin D added. Fortification of milk was credited with eradicating rickets in the United States in the 1930s; however, less use of milk in preference to soft drinks and fruit drinks has lowered intakes of calcium and vitamin D. Margarine is fortified with 37.5 mcg (1500 IU)/lb to serve as a butter substitute, and various ready-to-eat cereals have vitamin D added. Juices fortified with calcium and vitamin D to the level usually found in milk are potential sources for the lactose intolerant, and both nutrients are well absorbed from this food. Based on the need to increase vitamin D intake across the general population, one nutrition expert proposed that it be added to the mandatory enrichment standards for grain and cereal products.[24] Good food sources of Vitamin D are displayed in Box 6-5.

VITAMIN E

Chemical and Physical Nature

Vitamin E was first discovered by researchers studying reproduction in laboratory animals. Because of its association with reproduction and its chemical structure as an alcohol, it was named tocopherol from the Greek word *tokos,* meaning childbirth. Vitamin E came to be known as the *antisterility vitamin,* although this has been demonstrated only in laboratory animals and not in humans.

Forms

Vitamin E is the generic name given to a group of eight compounds having to some extent the biologic activity of α-tocopherol. Vitamin E is a pale yellow oil, stable to acids and heat, and insoluble in water. It oxidizes very slowly, which gives it an important role as an antioxidant. As an antioxidant it inactivates free cell radicals that attack cell tissues and prevents the oxidation of unsaturated fatty acids.[18]

BOX 6-5 FOOD SOURCES OF VITAMIN D

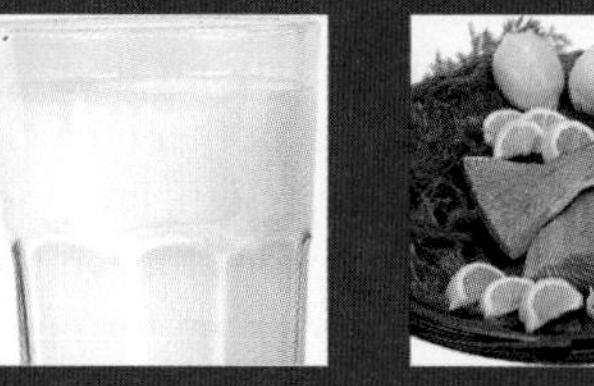
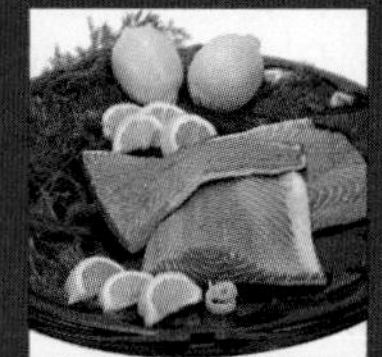
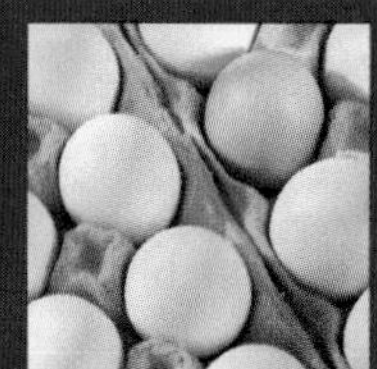

Vitamin D occurs naturally in eggs and fish. Fortified dairy foods, soy milk, juices, and cereals are other good sources for persons with limited exposure to sunlight.

FOOD SOURCE	QUANTITY	VITAMIN D (in mcg)
Grains Group		
Fortified ready-to-eat cereal	¾ cup	1.0
Fruit Group		
Orange juice, fortified*	1 cup	2.5
Meat, Beans, Eggs, and Nuts Group		
Tuna fish, canned in oil	3 oz	5.7
Egg yolk	1	0.5
Milk Group		
Milk, fluid, fortified†	1 cup	2.9
Soy milk, fortified*	1 cup	2.5

Adequate Intake (AI) for adults: ages 19-50, 5 mcg; 51-70, 10 mcg; ≥71, 15 mcg.

*Consumers should check the nutrition label to ensure the brand they select is fortified with vitamin D.

†With few exceptions, commercially marketed fluid, dried, and evaporated milk sold in the United States is fortified with vitamin D; amount added may vary.

Nutrient data from USDA: *USDA National Nutrient Database for Standard Reference, Release* 22, Washington, DC, U.S. Department of Agriculture, 2009. Retrieved August 29, 2010, from http://www.ars.usda.gov/ba/bhnrc/ndl.

KEY TERMS

osteoporosis Abnormal loss of bone mineral and matrix leading to porous, fragile bone with enlarged spaces that is prone to fracture or deformity; common disease of aging in older men and women.

osteodystrophy Defective bone formation.

megadoses Doses greatly exceeding what is recommended.

tocopherol Chemical name for vitamin E; it functions as an antioxidant to preserve structural membranes and other tissues with a high content of polyunsaturated fatty acids.

antioxidant A substance that prevents the formation and destructive actions of free radicals in the cells.

Absorption, Transport, and Storage

Vitamin E is absorbed in the micelles with the aid of bile. Along with other lipids in the chylomicrons, it is transported out of the intestinal wall, into the lymph, and then into the general circulation. Vitamin E is stored in the liver and adipose tissue, where it is held in bulk liquid droplets. The mobilization of α-tocopherol from these storage sites is slow.

Functions of Vitamin E

Antioxidant Activity

As we study the vitamins, we will continue to hear the term *antioxidant* and the role such nutrients play in destroying molecules called *free radicals.* Free radicals have an unpaired electron and are constantly on the lookout for another molecule with an unpaired electron with which they can join. Free radicals are highly active, and the oxidation reactions they initiate are very damaging to body tissues. Free radicals are formed as by-products of normal cell metabolism but also are found in tobacco smoke, car exhaust fumes, and other air pollutants.

Polyunsaturated fatty acids with several double bonds and the tissues where they are found are especially vulnerable to attack. Cell membranes contain a high proportion of polyunsaturated fatty acids, and oxidation by free radicals alters their structure and destroys their ability to recognize harmful substances and prevent them from entering the cell. Brain cells and nerve fibers are high in unsaturated fatty acids. Deoxyribonucleic acid (DNA) and other proteins in the cell nucleus can be modified by unwanted oxidation reactions and produce molecules that are ineffective in carrying out body functions. Oxidation reactions may promote the development of various chronic conditions. Antioxidants such as vitamin E join with the unpaired electron of free radicals and interrupt the chain of oxidation reactions across tissues. Vitamin E is nature's most potent antioxidant, although particular tocopherol compounds differ in their degree of antioxidant activity.

Partnership with Selenium

Despite an adequate supply of vitamin E, a second line of defense against free radical damage may be needed. This added defense is an enzyme containing selenium, a trace mineral. Selenium can spare vitamin E and reduce the vitamin E requirement. In this partnership role, vitamin E can also reduce the selenium requirement.

New Roles for Vitamin E

Researchers continue to evaluate potential therapeutic roles for vitamin E in preventing age-related changes and chronic disease. Many such changes are related to oxidative damage; however, evidence pointing to the ability of vitamin E to prevent these changes is not convincing. In large-scale trials, vitamin E supplements did not protect against the progression of atherosclerosis[25] or the occurrence of cardiovascular incidents in either men or women,[26-28] suggesting that the general public would be better served by adopting interventions of proven benefit such as a healthy diet, walking regularly, or smoking cessation.[28] Vitamin E alone does not lower the incidence or progression of age-related cataracts or macular degeneration, major causes of blindness among older adults, although several carotenoids such as lutein, found in fruits and vegetables, appear to have a preventive effect.[29] Vitamin E has been used clinically to ameliorate disturbing side effects and toxicity associated with chemotherapy and may have application in helping patients extend their period of treatment.[30]

Vitamin E Deficiency and Clinical Applications

Premature Infants

Inadequate vitamin E has disastrous effects on red blood cells. When polyunsaturated fatty acids in the lipid membranes of red blood cells are exposed to oxidation, the membranes break, the cell contents are lost, and the cell is destroyed. Continued loss of red blood cells leads to anemia; this vitamin E deficiency disease is called hemolytic anemia. Premature infants are especially vulnerable to hemolytic anemia because they miss the last month or two of fetal life when vitamin E stores are normally built up. This condition responds positively to vitamin E therapy[31] and is prevented with vitamin E supplementation at birth. Adequate intake during pregnancy can help ensure optimum vitamin E stores in the full-term infant.

Children and Adults

In older children and adults, vitamin E deficiency presents a different set of symptoms associated with the nervous system.[31] The nerves affected are (1) the spinal cord fibers that control physical movement such as walking and (2) the retina of the eye. Such problems were recognized in children with defective absorption of fat and fat-soluble vitamins related to cystic fibrosis and pancreatic insufficiency. Vitamin E deficiency disrupts the making of myelin, the protective lipid covering of the nerve cell axons that helps pass messages along to muscles. Lack of vitamin E also causes degeneration of the pigment in the rods and cones of the retina that depend on vitamin E to prevent oxidation damage. Optimum intakes of vitamin E and other antioxidants may be especially important for cystic fibrosis patients who have high tissue oxidation related to their disease.[32] Regular vitamin E replacement therapy is needed for those with fat malabsorption syndromes.

Vitamin E Requirement

Dietary Reference Intake

The RDA for vitamin E is expressed in milligrams of α-tocopherol because other forms of tocopherol are less effective. About 80% of the vitamin E from dietary sources including fortified foods is α-tocopherol, and about 20% is other forms. The RDA is 15 mg for both males and females age 14 and older,[18] but actual intake falls much below this level. In the United States, adult men averaged 8.6 mg/day of α-tocopherol and adult women averaged 6.5 mg/day of α-tocopherol.[33] Even the meal plans presented in MyPyramid and the Dietary Approaches to Stop Hypertension (DASH) diet do not meet the RDA for vitamin E.[34]

Vitamin E Toxicity

Vitamin E is the only fat-soluble vitamin for which a toxicity syndrome has not been identified. Daily intakes up to 3200 mg of α-tocopherol did not produce adverse effects but were short term—continued for only a few weeks or months; therefore potential harm from such intakes over long periods is unknown.

EVIDENCE-BASED PRACTICE

Food or Supplements: Do They Both Produce the Same Results?

The physiologic functions of the carotenoids, the substances that form the rich yellow, orange, green, and red pigments in fruits and vegetables, are not well understood but are distinct from those of the essential vitamins. Because the general public is paying closer attention to nutrition and its relation to lifelong health, sellers of dietary supplements are offering new combinations of both nutrients and nonnutrients to meet this demand. Several of the better known carotenoids such as β-carotene, lycopene, and cryptoxanthin have been isolated from their natural sources and are being marketed in supplement form. These supplements are touted as beneficial for life and health. However, what does the research tell us? Will we receive the same benefit if we shop in the supplement section and forget about eating fruits and vegetables?

Long-term studies monitoring individuals over periods of years have recorded fewer incidents of heart attack or stroke or cancer deaths among men and women who consumed more servings of fruits and vegetables each day. At the same time, supplements containing various carotenoids or antioxidant nutrients, such as ascorbic acid and vitamin E, did not offer similar protection against chronic disease.

Researchers have speculated as to why these dietary components must be eaten in their food form to convey their important benefits. One reason could be that fruits and vegetables contain a mixture of these chemical substances that work together to bring about important effects on health. To achieve this important **synergy,** these active substances (also called **synergistic** *substances*) must be present in the natural combinations found in fruits and vegetables. Another explanation might be that the health benefits associated with certain foods are provided by active substances that we have not yet identified. Finally, we do not know how much of an individual carotenoid is needed to support health, and the amounts provided in supplements may not be helpful, or at worst, could be harmful.

Although ascorbic acid, vitamin E, and various carotenoids act as antioxidants, they might also act in other ways to prevent chronic disease. Individuals who have higher blood carotenoid levels have a lower risk of death from all causes and fewer diagnoses of heart disease, cancer, macular degeneration, and cataract. Supplements containing vitamins A, C, and E will not take the place of plant foods in providing this protection. Last but not least, fruits and vegetables add variety and taste to our meals—qualities that pills cannot provide. Therefore we should all head to the fruit and vegetable sections of our local grocery stores, or better yet, start a garden and grow our own produce.

BIBLIOGRAPHY

Buijsse B, Feskens EJ, Schlettwein-Gsell D, et al: Plasma carotene and alpha-tocopherol in relation to 10-y all-cause and cause-specific mortality in European elderly: the Survey in Europe on Nutrition and the Elderly, a Concerted Action (SENECA), *Am J Clin Nutr* 82:879, 2005.

Dauchet L, Amouyel P, Hercberg S, et al: Fruit and vegetable consumption and risk of coronary heart disease: a meta-analysis of cohort studies, *J Nutr* 136:2588, 2006.

Food and Nutrition Board, Institute of Medicine: *Dietary Reference Intakes for vitamin C, vitamin E, selenium, and carotenoids,* Washington, DC, 2000, National Academies Press.

Lila MA: From beans to berries and beyond: teamwork between plant chemicals for protection of optimal human health, *Ann N Y Acad Sci* 1114:372, 2007.

Liu S, Manson JE, Lee I-M, et al: Fruit and vegetable intake and risk of cardiovascular disease: the Women's Health Study, *Am J Clin Nutr* 72:922, 2000.

Mares-Perlman JA, Millen AE, Ficek TL, et al: The body of evidence to support a protective role for lutein and zeaxanthin in delaying chronic disease, *J Nutr* 132:518S, 2002.

Neuhouser ML, Wassertheil-Smoller S, Thomson C, et al: Multivitamin use and risk of cancer and cardiovascular disease in the Women's Health Initiative cohorts, *Arch Intern Med* 169:294, 2009.

Sesso HD, Buring JE, Christen WG, et al: Vitamins E and C in the prevention of cardiovascular disease in men. The Physicians' Health Study II randomized controlled trial, *JAMA* 300:2123, 2008.

Voutilainen S, Nurmi T, Mursu J, et al: Carotenoids and cardiovascular health, *Am J Clin Nutr* 83:1265, 2006.

The UL for vitamin E is 1000 mg of α-tocopherol.[18] Intakes exceeding the UL could interfere with blood platelet aggregation and prevent normal blood clotting. This is particularly important information for persons with low intakes of vitamin K or patients using anti-clotting medications.

Food Sources of Vitamin E

Vegetable oils are rich dietary sources of vitamin E. Sunflower, safflower, and canola oil contain the highest amounts, followed by corn oil and olive oil.[35] As might be expected, these oils are also rich sources of polyunsaturated fatty acids, which vitamin E protects from oxidation. Other vitamin E sources include peanut butter, nuts, and certain vegetables and fruits, especially tomatoes. Fortified ready-to-eat cereals contribute significantly to intake, and the vitamin is well absorbed from these foods.[36] Box 6-6 lists major food sources of vitamin E. For reasons why we should obtain our vitamin E from food, see the *Evidence-Based Practice* box, "Food or Supplements: Do They Both Produce the Same Results?"

KEY TERMS

macular degeneration Destructive changes in the macula, a small spot in the center of the retina required for relay of the visual image; this condition is a major cause of blindness in older adults.

anemia Condition of abnormally low blood hemoglobin levels caused by too few red blood cells or red blood cells with an abnormally low hemoglobin content.

hemolytic anemia An anemia caused by breakdown of the outer membrane of red blood cells and loss of their hemoglobin; occurs in vitamin E deficiency.

myelin Substance made of fat and protein that forms a fatty sheath around the nerve axons; this covering protects and insulates the nerves and facilitates the transmission of neuromuscular impulses.

synergy (synergistic) The joint action of separate agents in which the total effect of their combined action is greater than the sum of their separate actions.

BOX 6-6 **FOOD SOURCES OF VITAMIN E**

FOOD SOURCE	QUANTITY	VITAMIN E (in mg)
Grains Group		
Fortified ready-to-eat cereal	¾-1 cup	13.5
Vegetable Group		
Spaghetti sauce, tomato	1 cup	6.0
Spinach, frozen, cooked	½ cup	3.3
Meat, Beans, Eggs, and Nuts Group		
Dry-roasted sunflower seeds	¼ cup	8.3
Peanut butter, creamy	2 tbsp	2.9
Sardines, canned	3 oz	1.7
Red kidney beans, canned	1 cup	0.05
Fats, Oils, and Sugars Group		
Corn oil	1 tbsp	1.9

Recommended Dietary Allowance (RDA) for adults: 15 mg.
Nutrient data from USDA: *USDA National Nutrient Database for Standard Reference, Release 21,* Washington, DC, U.S. Department of Agriculture, 2009. Retrieved April 23, 2010 from http://www.ars.usda.gov/Services/docs.htm?docid=17477.

VITAMIN K

Chemical and Physical Nature

The studies of Henrik Dam, a biochemist at the University of Copenhagen working on a hemorrhagic disease in chicks, led to the discovery of vitamin K. Because of its blood-clotting function, he called it the *koagulations vitamin,* or vitamin K. For this discovery he received the Nobel Prize in physiology and medicine.

Chemical Nature

The form of vitamin K found in plants is named phylloquinone for its chemical structure. Phylloquinone is the major dietary form and is widely distributed in both animal and plant foods. Menaquinone is synthesized by intestinal bacteria, but either form can be used by the body to meet its need for vitamin K. A water-soluble analogue of vitamin K, menadione, can be absorbed directly into the portal blood,[37] making it an important source for individuals with fat malabsorption.

Absorption, Transport, and Storage

Both naturally occurring forms of vitamin K, phylloquinone and menaquinone, require pancreatic lipase and bile salts for absorption as do the other fat-soluble vitamins.[3] After entering the intestinal wall via the micelles, they are packaged into chylomicrons and travel by means of the lymphatic system and then the portal blood to the liver. In the liver, vitamin K is stored in small amounts but excreted rapidly after administration of therapeutic doses.

Functional Roles of Vitamin K

Blood Clotting

The major function of vitamin K is to initiate liver synthesis of four necessary blood-clotting factors.[18] Each clotting factor is in the form of an inactive precursor that depends on vitamin K for activation. This activation step converts the precursor protein prothrombin to thrombin, which in turn acts on the precursor fibrinogen to form fibrin and complete the clotting process. Calcium ions and vitamin K are needed for normal blood clotting.

Vitamin K requires a functioning liver to carry out its tasks. When liver damage is the cause of low prothrombin levels and hemorrhage, vitamin K is ineffective as a therapeutic agent. Vitamin K also controls the liver synthesis of other proteins that regulate the speed and duration of coagulation. These regulatory proteins prevent the development of dangerous, unwanted blood clots or thromboses.[3,37]

Bone Metabolism

Vitamin K stimulates the synthesis of osteocalcin and other proteins important to bone health.[37,38] Bone is constantly being remodeled, and vitamin K–dependent proteins are necessary for the formation of bone matrix and mineral deposition. Children with higher vitamin K intakes appear to have improved bone mineral content; however, we do not know if increasing vitamin K will protect against bone loss in later life.[38]

COMPLEMENTARY AND ALTERNATIVE MEDICINE

Vitamin K, Vitamin E, and Anticoagulant Drugs

Patients using medications such as Coumadin (warfarin), Plavix (clopidogrel), or Aggrenox (dipyridamole and aspirin) to prevent unwanted blood clots should monitor their intakes of vitamin K and vitamin E. Too much vitamin K will counter the effect of the drug and reduce its effect. Several herbs used in cooking such as parsley, coriander, and mint contain vitamin K but are usually present in recipes in small amounts. At the other extreme, concentrated amounts of vitamin E oppose the action of vitamin K and extend the anticoagulant action of these drugs, increasing the risk of bleeding. Vitamin E supplements should be avoided by patients on anticoagulant therapy without the advice of a physician.

Data from Herr SM: *Herb-drug interaction handbook*, ed 2, Nassau, NY, 2002, Church Street Books.

Vitamin K Deficiency and Clinical Applications

Neonatology

The sterile intestinal tract of the newborn cannot supply vitamin K during the first few days of life until normal bacterial flora develop. During this immediate postnatal period, hemorrhage could occur. To prevent this a prophylactic dose of vitamin K is usually given soon after birth.

Malabsorption Problems

Any defect in fat absorption impairs vitamin K absorption, resulting in prolonged blood-clotting time. Thus several clinical situations exist for which supplemental vitamin K is required. Patients with bile duct obstruction are usually given vitamin K before surgery. Children with cystic fibrosis can become deficient, because frequent use of antibiotics interferes with bacterial synthesis of this vitamin.[32]

Drug Therapy

Several drug-nutrient interactions involve vitamin K. Anti-clotting drugs such as Coumadin (warfarin), Plavix (clopidogrel), or Aggrenox (dipyridamole and aspirin) act as **antimetabolites**, preventing the synthesis of blood-clotting factors in the liver and therefore inhibiting the action of vitamin K (see the *Complementary and Alternative Medicine* [CAM] box, "Vitamin K, Vitamin E, and Anticoagulant Drugs"). When these drugs are used to prevent unwanted clots in the lungs or blood vessels, dietary intake of vitamin K must be closely monitored. Too much vitamin K will oppose the action of the drug and neutralize its effect; too little vitamin K could lead to serious hemorrhage.[39,40] Dark-green leafy vegetables are rich in naturally occurring vitamin K, but other sources also need to be monitored. Snack foods made with Olestra, a noncaloric fat substitute, are fortified with 80 mcg of vitamin K per 1-oz serving, and vitamin K is added to many multivitamin supplements. With extended use of antibiotics much of the intestinal bacterial flora is lost, eliminating one of the body's main sources of vitamin K, and supplements may be required.

BOX 6-7 FOOD SOURCES OF VITAMIN K

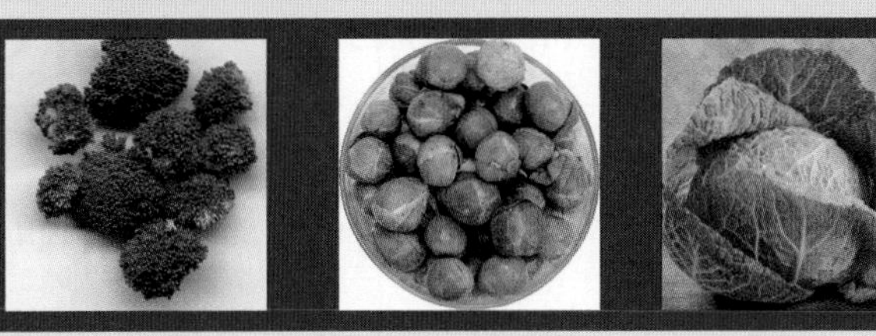

Spinach	Cabbage
Brussels sprouts	Canned tuna (packed in oil)
Broccoli	Spaghetti sauce
Lettuce	

Adequate Intake (AI) for adults: women, 90 mcg; men, 120 mcg.
Nutrient data from USDA: *USDA National Nutrient Database for Standard Reference, Release 21,* Washington, DC, U.S. Department of Agriculture, 2009. Retrieved April 23, 2010 from http://www.ars.usda.gov/Services/docs.htm?docid=17477.
Images copyright 2006 JupiterImages Corporation.

Vitamin K Requirement

Dietary Reference Intake

It is difficult to set a DRI for vitamin K because part of the requirement can be met by intestinal bacterial synthesis. Moreover, reliable information is lacking as to the vitamin K content of many foods or its bioavailability. With this in mind the expert committee established an AI rather than an RDA. The AI for men age 19 and older is 120 mcg/day, and the AI for women is 90 mcg/day.[3] These values represent the median intakes of nearly 20,000 men and women participating in national nutrition and health surveys between 1988 and 1994. This amount is adequate to preserve blood clotting, but the correct intake needed for optimum bone health is unknown. Toxicity has not been reported.

Food Sources of Vitamin K

Phylloquinone is found in many vegetables but is highest in dark-green vegetables and liver. Menaquinones occur in milk, meat, and certain cheeses.[37] A list of good food sources can be found in Box 6-7.

Table 6-2 provides a complete summary of the fat-soluble vitamins.

KEY TERMS

phylloquinone A fat-soluble vitamin of the K group found in green plants or prepared synthetically.

menaquinone Form of vitamin K synthesized by intestinal bacteria.

menadione A water-soluble analogue of vitamin K.

prothrombin Blood-clotting factor synthesized in the liver and activated by vitamin K.

antimetabolites Substances bearing a close structural resemblance to those required for normal physiologic function that interfere with the use of the essential nutrient or metabolite.

TABLE 6-2 SUMMARY OF FAT-SOLUBLE VITAMINS

VITAMIN	PHYSIOLOGIC FUNCTIONS	RESULTS OF DEFICIENCY	DIETARY REFERENCE INTAKE	FOOD SOURCES
Vitamin A				
Provitamin: β-carotene Vitamin: retinol	Production of rhodopsin and other light receptor pigments Formation and maintenance of epithelial tissue Growth Reproduction Toxic in large amounts	Poor dark adaptation, night blindness, xerosis, xerophthalmia Keratinization of epithelium Growth failure Reproductive failure	Adults: men ages ≥19: 900 mcg RAE; women ages ≥19: 700 mcg RAE Pregnancy: ages ≥19: 770 mcg RAE Lactation: ages ≥19: 1300 mcg RAE	Butter, fortified margarine Whole, fortified low-fat, and fortified nonfat cow's milk Fortified soy milk Dark-green, deep-yellow, and orange vegetables Yellow and orange fruits
Vitamin D				
Provitamins: ergosterol (plants), 7-dehydro-cholesterol (skin) Vitamins: D_2 (ergocalciferol) and D_3 (cholecalciferol, used in food fortification)	Calcium and phosphorus absorption Calcitriol is major hormone regulator of bone mineral metabolism Possible roles in muscle function and control of cell growth Toxic in large amounts	Faulty bone growth, rickets (in children and youth), osteomalacia (in adults)	Adults: men/women ages 19-50: 5 mcg; ages 51-70: 10 mcg; ages ≥71: 15 mcg Pregnancy: all ages 5 mcg Lactation: all ages 5 mcg	Fortified cow's milk Fortified soy milk Fortified orange juice Fortified margarine Oily fish (e.g., salmon, tuna) Egg yolk Sunlight on the skin
Vitamin E				
Tocopherols (most active form is α-tocopherol)	Antioxidant Protects cell membranes including red blood cell membranes Partners with selenium in antioxidant function	Anemia in premature infants Increased risk of oxidative damage to body tissues	Adults: men/women ages ≥19: 15 mg Pregnancy: all ages 15 mg Lactation: all ages 19 mg	Vegetable oils Fortified ready-to-eat cereals Nuts Dark-green leafy vegetables Spaghetti sauce
Vitamin K				
K_1 (phylloquinone) K_2 (menaquinone) Analogue: K_3 (menadione)	Activates blood-clotting factors (e.g., converts prothrombin to thrombin) Participates in bone formation and remodeling (synthesis of osteocalcin) Interferes with anticoagulant therapy	Hemorrhagic disease of the newborn Defective blood clotting Deficiency symptoms produced by anticoagulant and antibiotic therapy	Adults: men ages ≥19: 120 mcg; women ages ≥19: 90 mcg Pregnancy: ages ≥19: 90 mcg Lactation: ages ≥19: 90 mcg	Green leafy vegetables Canned tuna Spaghetti sauce Synthesized by intestinal bacteria

WATER-SOLUBLE VITAMINS

VITAMIN C (ASCORBIC ACID)

Chemical and Physical Nature

The discovery of vitamin C is associated with the ancient hemorrhagic disease scurvy. Early observations of British sailors led to the discovery of an acid in lemon juice that could prevent or cure this disease. Its chemical name, *ascorbic acid,* is based on its antiscorbutic properties. The structure of vitamin C is similar to glucose, and most animals can convert glucose to ascorbic acid. Humans, however, lack this enzyme. Therefore human scurvy could be called a *disease of distant genetic origin,* an inherited metabolic defect.

Vitamin C is an unstable, easily oxidized acid. It is destroyed by oxygen, alkali, and heat.

Absorption, Transport, and Storage

Vitamin C is easily absorbed from the small intestine but requires an acidic environment. When gastric hydrochloric acid is lacking, absorption is hindered. In contrast to vitamin A, vitamin C is not stored in a single site but rather generally distributed throughout the body, maintaining limited tissue saturation. Any excess is excreted in the urine. The total body pool in adults varies from about 2 g to as little as 0.3 g, depending on intake.[18] Optimum tissue saturation can meet day-to-day needs for as long as 3 months when intake is lacking. This explains why generally healthy people in isolated living situations could survive the winter without eating fresh fruits and vegetables.

Breast milk provides sufficient vitamin C for early infancy if the mother is eating a good diet. Cow's milk contains very little vitamin C, as would be expected, because these animals have the enzymes to make their own vitamin C from glucose. Human infant formulas made from cow's milk are supplemented with ascorbic acid.

Functions of Vitamin C

Antioxidant Capacity

Vitamin C, along with vitamin E, is a powerful antioxidant. Vitamin C takes up free oxygen arising from cell metabolism, making it unavailable to fuel the destructive actions of free radicals.

Formation of Intercellular Cement

Vitamin C helps build and maintain many body tissues including bone matrix, cartilage, dentin, collagen, and connective tissue. Collagen is a protein found in the white fibers of connective tissue. When vitamin C is absent, an important ground substance is not formed and collagen fibers are defective and weak.[41] Blood vessels require this cementing substance to form firm capillary walls. In vitamin C deficiency, capillaries are fragile and easily ruptured by blood pressure or trauma, and small hemorrhages occur in the skin and other tissues. When vitamin C is restored, the formation of normal collagen follows quickly.[41] Box 6-8 lists common signs of vitamin C deficiency.

Support of General Body Metabolism

Vitamin C is found in greater amounts in metabolically active tissues such as the adrenal and pituitary glands, brain, eyes, and leukocytes. The multiplying tissues of children contain more vitamin C than the resting tissues of adults. Vitamin C helps in the formation of hemoglobin and the development of red blood cells by (1) promoting iron absorption and (2) assisting in the removal of iron from the protein-iron complex, called *ferritin,* in which it is stored.

Vitamin C participates in other functions of metabolic importance, as described following:

- Assists the synthesis of carnitine, an amino acid that transports long-chain fatty acids into cell mitochondria where they are burned for energy
- Assists the synthesis of peptide hormones such as norepinephrine and receptors for the neurotransmitter acetylcholine
- Supports the action of the mixed-function oxidase system that metabolizes drugs and breaks down carcinogens and other foreign molecules (This system sequesters lead and other heavy metals and neutralizes their effects.)

BOX 6-8 SIGNS OF VITAMIN C DEFICIENCY

- Easy bruising
- Pinpoint hemorrhages of the skin (petechiae)
- Weak bones that fracture easily
- Poor wound healing
- Bleeding gums (often termed *gingivitis*)
- Anemia

Clinical Applications

- *Wound healing:* The role of vitamin C in forming the cement for building supporting tissues creates added demands for the vitamin in traumatic injury or surgery when extensive tissue regeneration is required. Formulas for parenteral feeding generally provide 100 mg/day of vitamin C. Protocols for burn patients with elevated needs for tissue growth and defense against infection call for 1000 mg/day.[42]
- *Fever and infection:* The body's response to infection depletes tissue vitamin C stores. Fever adds to losses because it accompanies infection and produces a catabolic effect.
- *Growth:* Additional vitamin C is required during periods of rapid growth in infants and children. An adequate supply is critical in pregnancy to support fetal development and expansion of maternal tissues. Pregnant women who smoke may have elevated needs.[43]
- *Stress and body response:* Body stress arising from injury, illness, debilitating disease, or emotional upset calls on vitamin C stores. The adrenal glands, which have a primary role in stress response, contain large amounts of vitamin C.
- *Chronic disease prevention:* As an antioxidant, vitamin C has been studied as a possible factor in the prevention of chronic disease. Individuals with higher intakes of fruits and vegetables have higher intakes and plasma levels of vitamin C and lower incidence of age-related cataract,[44] type 2 diabetes,[45] and cardiovascular mortality[46,47]; although, other nutrients or phytochemicals in fruits and vegetables along with ascorbic acid may have contributed to these effects. Vitamin C supplements, on the other hand, do not prevent cardiovascular disease[27] or cancer.[48] It may be that vitamin C must work cooperatively with other food components to prevent chronic disease. High doses of antioxidant supplements such as vitamin C or E may actually damage tissues and interfere with normal processes.[49]

Vitamin C Requirement

Dietary Reference Intake

In the past the RDA for vitamin C was set at the level required to maintain tissue saturation and prevent symptoms of deficiency; however, the current DRI takes into account the need for antioxidant protection of body tissues. For men the RDA is 90 mg.[18] Based on their smaller body size and lean mass, the RDA for women is 75 mg. Cigarette smokers require an additional 35 mg. Vitamin C needs increase in pregnancy, lactation, and periods of growth.

KEY TERMS

scurvy A hemorrhagic disease caused by lack of vitamin C; physical changes include diffuse tissue bleeding, painful and swollen limbs and joints, swollen and bleeding gums, loosening of teeth, and poor wound healing.

collagen The protein substance of the white fibers of skin, tendon, bone, cartilage, and all other connective tissue.

parenteral A mode of feeding that does not use the gastrointestinal tract but instead provides nutrition by intravenous delivery of nutrient solutions.

BOX 6-9 FOOD PREPARATION METHODS TO PRESERVE VITAMIN CONTENT

Vitamins can be destroyed by heat, light, or the action of oxygen in the air. Water-soluble vitamins, especially vitamin C, are particularly susceptible to such loss. The following practices will help consumers store and prepare their vegetables and fruits to retain the maximum vitamin content:

- Store cut-up fruits and vegetables in the refrigerator in tightly covered containers to protect them from light and oxygen; when preparing fresh fruit or vegetables for salads or cooking, try to minimize the length of time they are exposed to the air.
- Avoid cutting fruits and vegetables into very small pieces because this increases the surface area for nutrient loss.
- As a general rule, cook vegetables for a *limited* amount of time in a *limited* amount of water in a tightly covered pan to retain nutrients, flavor, color, and texture. (Vegetables should be tender but still retain their shapes.)
- Steam vegetables using a steamer basket with the water below to prevent the dissolving of nutrients into the water; vegetables need not be covered with water because the steam in a covered container will soften the food.
- Use the microwave to reduce the time and amount of water needed for cooking, but avoid overcooking. Remember that foods continue to cook for several minutes after being removed from the microwave.
- Stir-fry vegetables in a small amount of fat to conserve nutrients and food quality.
- Remember that fruits and vegetables add color and variety to your meals, along with important nutrients. Include both raw and cooked vegetables to add interest to your menus.

Vitamin C Toxicity

Vitamin C intakes far exceeding the recommended level have been promoted as effective in curing the common cold, protecting against degenerative disease, or delaying the signs of aging. Daily intakes of 1 g or more are not uncommon in the general population. A survey of nearly 3000 breast cancer survivors found that 24% were taking daily supplements of 1000 mg or more.[50] Supplement use should be monitored to prevent potential interactions with ongoing drug therapy or chemotherapy. The UL is set at 2 g; gastrointestinal symptoms and diarrhea are known to occur at higher levels.[18]

Food Sources of Vitamin C

The best known sources of vitamin C are citrus fruits and tomatoes. Broccoli, salad greens, strawberries, watermelon, cabbage, and sweet potatoes are other good sources. (For tips on the proper handling of fresh fruits and vegetables, see the *Focus on Food Safety* box, "Did You Wash That Orange?") Vitamin C is easily oxidized when exposed to the air or heated, so storage, preparation, and cooking methods must be chosen carefully to preserve vitamin content (Box 6-9). Vitamin C is quite stable in acid solutions, so citrus and tomato products remain good sources even if heated. Box 6-10 lists the vitamin C content of various food sources. A summary of vitamin C functions and requirements is found in Table 6-3.

FOCUS ON FOOD SAFETY

Did You Wash That Orange?

Fresh fruits and vegetables are good sources of vitamin C, folate, pyridoxine, provitamin A, and many other carotenoids. Oranges, apples, pears, grapes, bananas, and tiny raw carrots are healthy snacks and travel well in a backpack or school bag. Fresh produce should be washed before you eat or cook it to remove any remaining pesticides, soil particles, and bacteria that accumulated as it was picked, shipped, and handled in the store. Fruits and vegetables to be peeled still need to be washed. If your hands touch the banana peel that has not been washed, then you will transfer those bacteria to the fruit as you peel it. It is also a good idea to wash all "prewashed" vegetables and salad greens to be sure that all soil particles have been removed.

THE B VITAMINS

DEFICIENCY DISEASES AND VITAMIN DISCOVERIES

The discovery of the B vitamins is a story of persons dying of a puzzling, age-old disease for which no cure existed. Eventually it was learned that common, everyday food held the answer. The paralyzing disease was **beriberi,** which plagued East Asia for centuries (Figure 6-7). It was named by the native words, *I can't, I can't,* which described its crippling effects. The "vitamine" connection was established when an American chemist, R.R. Williams, used extracts of rice polishings to cure the epidemic infantile beriberi. The food factor that brought the cure was labeled *water-soluble B,* because it was thought to be a single vitamin. Now we know several vitamins exist in the B group, all water soluble but with unique metabolic functions. Each of the B vitamins has been given a specific chemical name.

COENZYME ROLE

The B vitamins have important metabolic roles as coenzyme partners with cell enzymes that control energy metabolism and build tissues. Eight vitamins are in this group. First we consider the three associated with classic deficiency diseases (thiamin, riboflavin, and niacin); then the more recently discovered coenzyme factors (**pantothenic acid,** biotin, and pyridoxine [vitamin B_6]); and, finally, the important blood-forming factors (folate and vitamin B_{12} [cobalamin]).

THIAMIN

The search for the cause of beriberi was successfully concluded with the identification of thiamin. Its nature and metabolic role were clarified in the early 1930s.

Chemical and Physical Nature

Thiamin is a water-soluble and fairly stable vitamin, although it is destroyed in alkaline solutions. Its name comes from its chemical ring-like structure.

BOX 6-10 FOOD SOURCES OF VITAMIN C

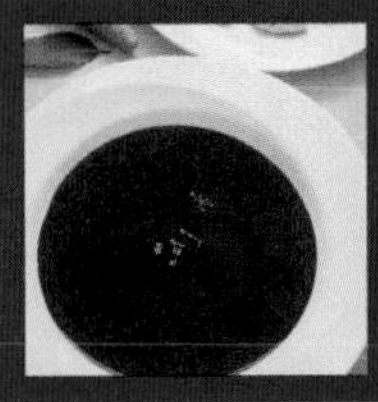
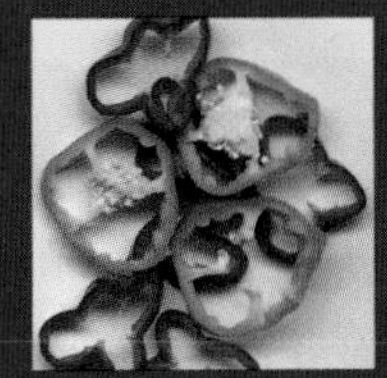
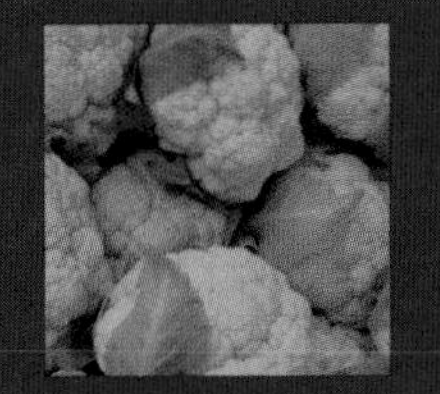
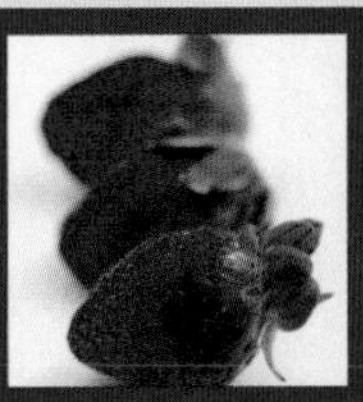
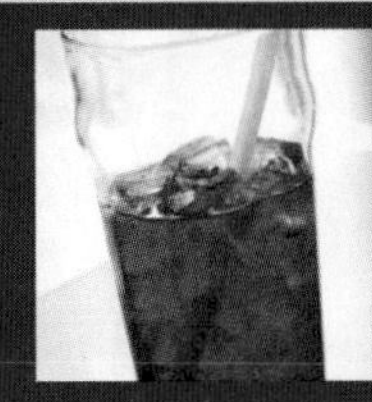
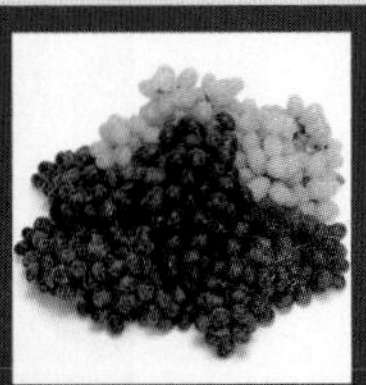

FOOD SOURCE	AMOUNT	VITAMIN C (in mg)
Vegetable Group		
Tomato juice	1 cup	44
Vegetable juice cocktail	1 cup	67
Pepper, chili, red	1	65
Peppers, sweet, green, chopped	½ cup	60
Peppers, sweet, red, chopped	½ cup	95
Broccoli, cooked	½ cup	51
Cole slaw, homemade	1 cup	39
Sweet potato, canned, cooked	½ cup	34
Cauliflower, frozen, cooked	½ cup	28
Fruit Group		
Strawberries	1 cup	98
Orange juice, frozen, reconstituted	1 cup	97
Grape juice, fortified	1 cup	60
Orange	1 medium	70
Cantaloupe	⅛ melon	25
Watermelon	1 wedge (4 × 8 inch)	23
Fats, Oils, and Sugars Group		
Fruit punch, fortified	1 cup	73

Recommended Dietary Allowances (RDAs) for adults: women, 75 mg; men, 90 mg.
Nutrient data from USDA: *USDA National Nutrient Database for Standard Reference, Release 21,* Washington, DC, U.S. Department of Agriculture, 2009. Retrieved April 23, 2010 from http://www.ars.usda.gov/Services/docs.htm?docid=17477.

TABLE 6-3 SUMMARY OF VITAMIN C (ASCORBIC ACID)

PHYSIOLOGIC FUNCTIONS	CLINICAL APPLICATIONS	DIETARY REFERENCE INTAKE	FOOD SOURCES
Antioxidant activity Collagen synthesis General metabolism Makes iron available for hemoglobin synthesis Controls the conversion of the amino acid phenylalanine to tyrosine	Wound healing Tissue formation Fevers and infections Stress reactions Growth Scurvy (classic deficiency disease)	Adults: men ages ≥19: 90 mg; women ages ≥19: 75 mg Pregnancy: ages ≥19: 85 mg Lactation: ages ≥19: 120 mg	Citrus fruits and berries Vegetables: broccoli, cabbage, chili peppers, potatoes, tomatoes

Absorption, Transport, and Storage

Thiamin is absorbed most efficiently in the acid environment of the upper duodenum before the food mass is buffered by the alkaline fluids entering from the pancreas. Thiamin is not stored in large amounts, so a continuous dietary supply is needed.[51] Tissue thiamin responds rapidly to increased metabolic demand as occurs in fever, high muscular activity, pregnancy, and lactation. Tissue stores depend on both thiamin intake and general diet composition. Carbohydrate increases the need for thiamin, whereas fat and protein spare thiamin. When the tissues are saturated, unused thiamin is excreted in the urine.

KEY TERMS

beriberi A disease of the peripheral nerves caused by thiamin deficiency; characteristics include pain (neuritis), paralysis of the extremities, cardiovascular changes, and edema.

pantothenic acid A member of the B vitamin complex widely distributed in nature and throughout body tissues; it functions as a part of coenzyme A (CoA), important in lipid and carbohydrate metabolism.

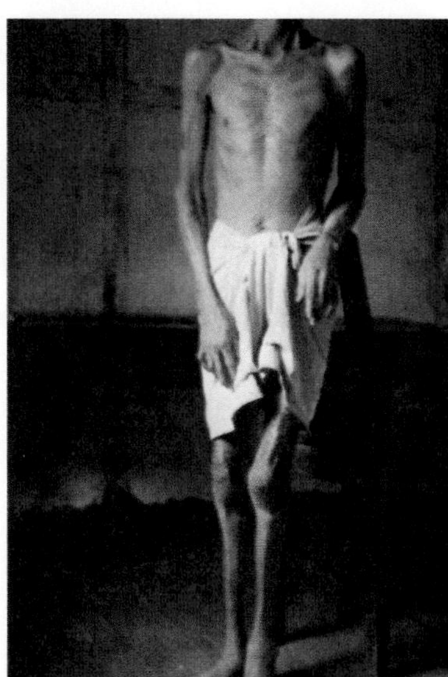

FIGURE 6-7 Beriberi is a thiamin deficiency disease characterized by extreme weakness, paralysis, anemia, and wasting away (e.g., decreased metabolic function in the liver). (From McLaren DS: *A colour atlas and text of diet-related disorders,* ed 2, London, 1992, Mosby-Year Book Europe Limited.)

Function of Thiamin

Coenzyme Role

Thiamin functions as a control agent in energy metabolism. When combined with phosphorus to form **thiamin pyrophosphate (TPP),** it serves as a coenzyme in reactions involving glucose. About 90% of body thiamin is in the coenzyme form.[52] The symptoms of beriberi, as we will see following, can be traced to the loss of energy usually provided by glucose metabolism.

Thiamin Deficiency and Clinical Applications

When thiamin levels are insufficient to support cellular energy metabolism, clinical effects become apparent, as follows:

- *Gastrointestinal system:* Anorexia, constipation, gastric atony, and poor hydrochloric acid secretion develop as the deficiency continues. When the cells of the smooth muscles and the secretory glands do not receive enough energy from the metabolism of glucose, they cannot perform the digestive work needed to supply still more glucose to meet body needs. This vicious cycle accelerates as the deficiency continues.
- *Nervous system:* The CNS depends on glucose to do its work. Without sufficient thiamin to provide this constant fuel, nerve activity is impaired, alertness and reflex responses are diminished, and general apathy and fatigue take over. If the deficiency continues, then lipogenesis is hindered, followed by damage to the myelin sheaths—the lipid tissue covering the nerve fibers. This causes increasing nerve irritation, pain, and prickly or deadening sensations. If unchecked, then paralysis will result as in the classic deficiency disease beriberi.
- *Cardiovascular system:* The heart muscle weakens, leading to cardiac failure and edema of the lower extremities.
- *Musculoskeletal system:* Inadequate TPP in muscle tissue results in widespread chronic pain that responds to thiamin therapy.

Thiamin status is evaluated by the activity of a TPP-dependent enzyme transketolase found in red blood cells.[52] This is a common test to determine whether a clinical observation is related to thiamin deficiency or another cause.

Thiamin Requirement

Dietary Reference Intake

The thiamin requirement is based on energy intake with a minimum of 0.3 mg of thiamin/1000 kcal. To provide a margin of safety the RDA is set at 1.2 mg for men and 1.1 mg for women.[51] Additional thiamin is needed during pregnancy and lactation. Because the kidneys excrete excess thiamin, no reports exist of toxicity from oral doses up to 50 mg. No UL has been established.

Clinical Applications

Several conditions influence thiamin needs:

- *Alcohol abuse:* Thiamin is important when planning medical nutrition therapy for those with alcohol problems.[51] Both a primary deficiency (an inadequate diet) and a conditioned deficiency (the effect of alcohol) contribute to thiamin malnutrition and, over time, serious neurologic disorders. Alcohol interferes with the active absorption of thiamin across the intestinal wall, resulting in rapid depletion of tissue stores.
- *Acute illness or disease:* Fever and infection increase energy requirements and the need for thiamin. Patients on hemodialysis lose thiamin and require supplementation to prevent deficiency.
- *Normal growth and development:* Thiamin needs increase in pregnancy and lactation to meet the demands of rapid fetal growth, the elevated metabolic rate of pregnancy, and the production of milk. Continuing growth throughout infancy, childhood, and adolescence requires attention to thiamin intake. At any point in the life cycle, the larger the body and its tissue mass are, the greater are the cellular energy requirements and need for thiamin.
- *Use of diuretics:* Some diuretics used to manage hypertension and cardiac failure increase urinary losses of thiamin. If thiamin intake is low, then these patients can develop a thiamin deficiency that worsens their cardiac symptoms.[53]
- *Gastric bypass surgery:* Thiamin supplementation is likely to be necessary after gastric bypass surgery because energy intake is drastically reduced and absorption less efficient.[54]

Food Sources of Thiamin

Thiamin is widespread in plant and animal foods, although the amount found in individual foods is usually small. As a result, intakes can be low when kilocalories (kcalories or kcal) are markedly curtailed. Major sources in the American diet are whole and enriched breads, ready-to-eat cereals, and legumes, although lean pork and beef are also good sources. Thiamin is extremely water soluble and readily lost in cooking water (review Box 6-9). Box 6-11 lists food sources of thiamin.

BOX 6-11 FOOD SOURCES OF THIAMIN

FOOD SOURCE	AMOUNT	THIAMIN (in mg)
Grains Group		
Ready-to-eat cereals		
Product 19	1 cup	1.50
Total Raisin Bran	1 cup	1.50
Rice Krispies	1¼ cup	0.60
Wheaties	1 cup	0.75
Corn flakes	1 cup	0.60
Instant oatmeal	1 packet	0.46
Rice, parboiled, cooked	1 cup	0.37
Waffles	2	0.39
Bagel	3½ in	0.38
Macaroni/spaghetti	1 cup	0.38
Hamburger roll	1	0.17
Bread, enriched	1 slice	0.11
Vegetable Group		
Green peas, frozen, cooked	½ cup	0.23
Potatoes, mashed	½ cup	0.14
Tomato juice	1 cup	0.11
Fruit Group		
Orange juice	1 cup	0.20
Grapes	1 cup	0.11
Meat, Beans, Eggs, and Nuts Group		
Pork, roasted	3 oz	0.62
Ham, sliced, lean	3 oz	0.58
Kidney beans, cooked	1 cup	0.28
Baked beans, canned	1 cup	0.24
Milk Group		
Milk, whole, skim, low fat	1 cup	0.11

Recommended Dietary Allowances (RDAs) for adults: women, 1.1 mg; men, 1.2 mg.
Nutrient data from USDA: *USDA National Nutrient Database for Standard Reference, Release 21,* Washington, DC, U.S. Department of Agriculture, 2009. Retrieved April 23, 2010 from http://www.ars.usda.gov/Services/docs.htm?docid=17477.

RIBOFLAVIN

Discovery

In 1897 a London chemist observed in milk whey a water-soluble pigment with a peculiar yellow-green fluorescence. However, it was not until 1932 that researchers in Germany actually discovered riboflavin.[55] The vitamin was given the chemical name *flavin* from the Latin word for yellow. Later, when it was found to contain a sugar called *ribose,* the name *riboflavin* was officially adopted.

Chemical and Physical Nature

Riboflavin is a yellow-green fluorescent pigment that forms yellowish-brown, needlelike crystals. It is water soluble and relatively heat stable but easily destroyed by light and irradiation.

Absorption, Transport, and Storage

Riboflavin is easily absorbed in the upper section of the small intestine. Bulk fiber supplements such as psyllium, especially when taken with milk or near meals, can hinder riboflavin absorption and contribute to deficiency. Body stores are limited, although small amounts are found in the liver and kidney. Day-to-day tissue needs must be supplied by the diet.

KEY TERMS

thiamin pyrophosphate (TPP) Activating coenzyme form of thiamin that is key in carbohydrate metabolism.

BOX 6-12 SIGNS OF RIBOFLAVIN DEFICIENCY

- Lips become swollen and cracked; characteristic cracks develop at the corners of the mouth (cheilosis).
- Nasal angles develop cracks and irritation.
- Tongue becomes swollen and reddened (glossitis; see Figure 6-8).
- Extra blood vessels develop in the cornea (corneal vascularization).
- Eyes burn, itch, and tear.
- Skin becomes greasy and scaly (seborrheic dermatitis), especially in skinfolds.

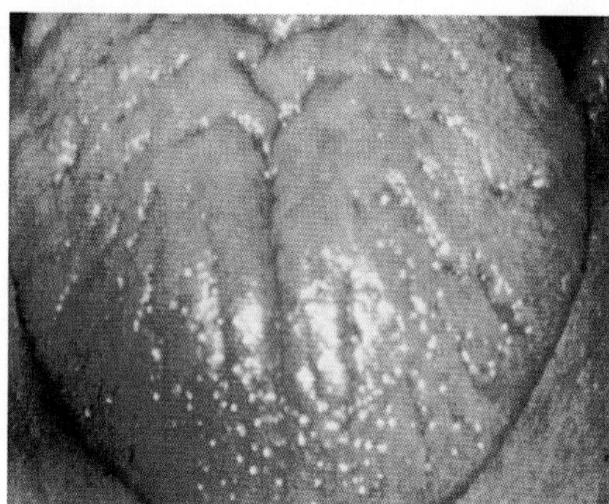

FIGURE 6-8 Glossitis resulting from riboflavin deficiency. (From McLaren DS: *A colour atlas and text of diet-related disorders*, ed 2, London, 1992, Mosby-Year Book Europe Limited.)

Functions of Riboflavin

Coenzyme Role

Riboflavin is a part of the cell enzymes called *flavoproteins*. These enzymes—flavin mononucleotide (FMN) and flavin adenine dinucleotide (FAD)—are integral to both energy metabolism and deamination. *Deamination* is the removal of a nitrogen-containing amino group from an existing amino acid so that a new amino acid can be formed. Accordingly, riboflavin is active in both energy production and tissue building.

Riboflavin Deficiency and Clinical Applications

Riboflavin deficiency leads to the condition termed ariboflavinosis. This includes a combination of clinical signs that center on tissue inflammation and breakdown and poor healing of even minor injuries (Box 6-12 and Figure 6-8). Tissues subject to persistent abrasion that require continual replacement, such as the cells in the corners of the mouth, are affected first. Riboflavin deficiency seldom occurs alone; it is most likely to develop in combination with other B vitamin deficits. Because riboflavin is light sensitive, infants with elevated blood levels of bilirubin who are treated with phototherapy may require additional riboflavin.

Riboflavin Requirement

Dietary Reference Intake

The RDA for riboflavin is based on the amount needed to sustain optimal levels of the flavoprotein enzymes. Recommended intakes are 1.3 mg/day for adolescent and adult men and 1.1 mg/day for adolescent and adult women.[51] The higher level for men relates to their higher kcalorie intakes and larger body size. No UL has been set for riboflavin, but supplements exceeding the RDA still carry risk.

Populations at Risk

Certain groups need additional riboflavin. Patients on hemodialysis must replace riboflavin lost in the dialysate fluids.[51] Pregnant and lactating women and infants and children are at risk of riboflavin deficiency based on their rapid growth and high energy and protein metabolism. People who engage in regular physical activity seem to have a greater need for riboflavin, likely related to increased energy expenditure and muscle maintenance and repair.[56] Milk supplies nearly 15% of riboflavin intake across population groups[57]; thus individuals who are lactose intolerant may not reach optimum levels unless they include fortified soy milk or lower lactose dairy products such as cheese or yogurt.

Food Sources of Riboflavin

Major sources of riboflavin are milk and cheese. One quart of cow's milk or fortified soy milk contains 2 mg of riboflavin, more than the daily requirement; however, the replacement of milk with soft drinks or juice drinks by children and youth has lowered intake.[58] Because riboflavin is destroyed by exposure to light, milk is usually packaged in cardboard or opaque plastic containers. Nursing mothers who store breast milk need to be reminded of potential riboflavin losses from glass containers. Other good sources of riboflavin are meat, whole or enriched grains and ready-to-eat cereals, and vegetables. Riboflavin is stable to heat and not easily destroyed with proper cooking. Box 6-13 describes some food sources of riboflavin.

NIACIN

The age-old disease related to niacin is pellagra. It is characterized by a typical dermatitis and eventually causes fatal effects in the nervous system.[59] Pellagra was first observed in eighteenth-century Europe and was common in the southern region of the United States in the early 1900s among families whose diet was largely based on corn. The American physician Goldberger noticed that children who did not have pellagra had higher intakes of meat and milk. His investigation established that pellagra was related to a food factor, not an infectious organism. However, it was not until 1937 that a researcher at the University of Wisconsin associated niacin with pellagra by using it to cure a related disease—black tongue—in dogs.

Chemical and Physical Nature

Two forms of niacin exist: (1) nicotinic acid and (2) nicotinamide. Nicotinic acid is easily converted to nicotinamide, which is water soluble, stable to acid and heat, and forms a white powder when crystallized.

Niacin also bears a close connection to the essential amino acid tryptophan, as described following:

- *Precursor role of tryptophan:* Curious observations by early researchers raised puzzling questions. Why was

BOX 6-13 FOOD SOURCES OF RIBOFLAVIN

FOOD SOURCE	AMOUNT	RIBOFLAVIN (in mg)
Grains Group		
Ready-to-eat cereals		
Product 19	1 cup	1.70
Wheaties	1 cup	0.85
Rice Krispies	1¼ cup	0.73
Corn flakes	1 cup	0.74
Instant oatmeal	1 packet	0.38
Waffle	1	0.26
Bagel	3½ in	0.20
Rice, parboiled, cooked	1 cup	0.03
Bread, enriched, white	1 slice	0.08
Vegetable Group		
Spinach, frozen, cooked	½ cup	0.17
Broccoli, frozen, cooked	½ cup	0.10
Meat, Beans, Eggs, and Nuts Group		
Pork, braised	3 oz	0.30
Egg	1	0.27
Turkey, dark meat, roasted	3 oz	0.21
Kidney beans, cooked, canned	1 cup	0.23
Baked beans, canned, no meat	1 cup	0.10
Milk Group		
Yogurt, flavored	1 cup	0.49
Milk, whole, skim, low fat	1 cup	0.45
Pudding	½ cup	0.25
Cottage cheese	½ cup	0.21

Recommended Dietary Allowances (RDAs) for adults: women, 1.1 mg; men, 1.3 mg.
Nutrient data from USDA: *USDA National Nutrient Database for Standard Reference, Release 21,* Washington, DC, U.S. Department of Agriculture, 2009. Retrieved April 23, 2010 from http://www.ars.usda.gov/Services/docs.htm?docid=17477.

pellagra rare in some populations whose diets were low in niacin but common in others whose diets were higher in niacin? Why did milk, which is low in niacin, cure or prevent pellagra? Why was pellagra so common in families subsisting on diets high in corn? Then came the key discovery—tryptophan can be used by the body to make niacin. In other words, tryptophan is a precursor of niacin. Milk prevents pellagra because it is high in tryptophan. A corn-based diet results in pellagra because it is low in both tryptophan and niacin, but this depends on how the corn is prepared. In the American South, where corn was eaten as a vegetable or made into corn bread or corn meal, the bound niacin present in corn could not be released and absorbed. In Mexican families who soaked corn in lime (alkali) when preparing tortillas, pellagra was rare because the lime treatment released the bound niacin so that it was able to be absorbed.[59] Others with diets low in niacin escaped pellagra because they had adequate amounts of tryptophan from animal protein.

KEY TERMS

ariboflavinosis Group of clinical manifestations of riboflavin deficiency.

cheilosis Cracks and scaly lesions on the lips and mouth resulting from riboflavin deficiency.

glossitis Swollen, reddened tongue; symptom of riboflavin deficiency.

seborrheic dermatitis Greasy scales and crusts that appear on the skin in riboflavin deficiency; they are most likely to occur in the moist folds of the body.

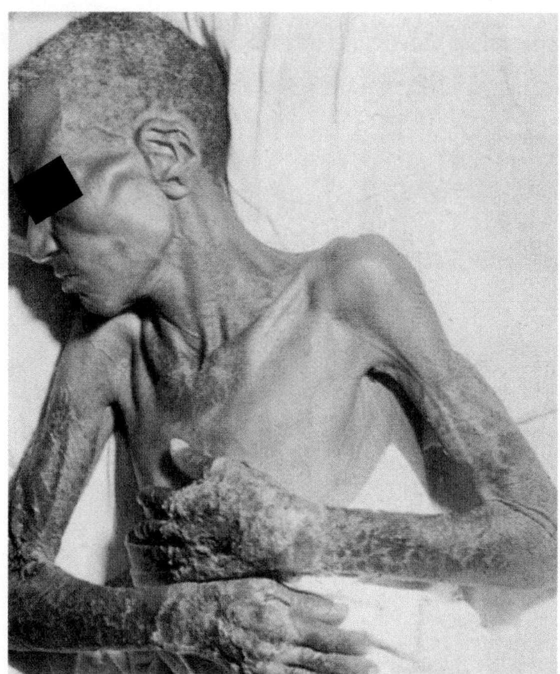

FIGURE 6-9 Pellagra is caused by niacin deficiency. (From McLaren DS: *A colour atlas and text of diet-related disorders*, ed 2, London, 1992, Mosby-Year Book Europe Limited.)

- *Niacin equivalent (NE):* The tryptophan-niacin relation led to the development of the unit of measure called an *NE*. In general, 60 mg of tryptophan can produce 1 mg of niacin, the amount designated as the *NE*. This is the unit used in the DRI for niacin.[51]

Functions of Niacin

Coenzyme Role

Niacin has two coenzyme forms: (1) nicotinamide-adenine dinucleotide (NAD) and (2) nicotinamide-adenine dinucleotide phosphate (NADP). In these forms, niacin partners with riboflavin in the cellular enzyme systems that convert amino acids and glycerol to glucose and then oxidize the glucose to release energy. (Glycerol is obtained from the hydrolysis of triglycerides.)

Use as a Drug

Pharmacologic doses of nicotinic acid have been prescribed for cardiovascular patients in an effort to raise blood high-density lipoprotein (HDL) cholesterol levels and lower low-density lipoprotein (LDL) cholesterol and triglyceride levels. However, at intake levels of 1000 to 2000 mg (the RDA is 14 to 16 mg) nicotinic acid acts as a vasodilator, causing skin flushing and itching. Harmful side effects can include gastrointestinal upset, hyperglycemia, and liver damage, so patients treated with these doses require constant medical supervision (see Chapter 21).[59,60]

Niacin Deficiency and Clinical Applications

Niacin deficiency and pellagra result in muscle weakness, anorexia, and indigestion. More specific symptoms involve the skin and nervous system, and skin areas exposed to sunlight develop a dark, scaly dermatitis (Figure 6-9). If the deficiency continues, then deterioration of the CNS leads to confusion, disorientation, neuritis, and finally death.

Niacin Requirement

Dietary Reference Intake

The current RDAs are 16 mg NE/day for adolescent and adult men and 14 mg NE/day for adolescent and adult women.[51] These recommendations allow for differences in energy intake and body size, as well as the availability and relative efficiency of converting tryptophan to niacin. Rapid growth, pregnancy, lactation, physical activity, or the need to replace tissues after surgery or trauma increases the need for niacin.

Food Sources of Niacin

Meat and dairy products are major sources of niacin and also high in tryptophan. Other foods include peanuts, dried beans and peas, and whole grain or enriched breads and cereals. Corn and rice are relatively poor sources because they are low in tryptophan. Box 6-14 lists some comparative food sources of niacin.

PANTOTHENIC ACID

Discovery

Pantothenic acid is found in all living things and participates in many body functions.[51] Intestinal bacteria synthesize considerable amounts. This source, along with its occurrence in a wide variety of foods, makes pantothenic acid deficiency unlikely.

Chemical and Physical Nature

Pantothenic acid is a white crystalline compound. It is readily absorbed in the small intestine and combines with phosphorus to make the active molecule acetyl coenzyme A (CoA). In this form, pantothenic acid has broad metabolic presence and use throughout the body. No known toxicity or natural deficiency exists.

Functions of Pantothenic Acid

As an essential constituent of CoA, pantothenic acid controls metabolic reactions involving carbohydrate, fat, and protein.[51]

Pantothenic Acid Requirements

The AI of 5 mg/day for all adults will replace the pantothenic acid lost daily in the urine. No UL exists for this nutrient.[51]

Food Sources of Pantothenic Acid

Pantothenic acid is found in both plant and animal foods. Good sources include egg yolk, milk, and broccoli.

BIOTIN

General Nature of Biotin

Biotin is a sulfur-containing vitamin, and the minute traces in the body perform multiple metabolic tasks. Natural deficiency is unknown; however, induced deficiencies have

BOX 6-14 FOOD SOURCES OF NIACIN

FOOD SOURCE	AMOUNT	NIACIN (in mg NE)*
Grains Group		
Ready-to-eat cereals		
Product 19	1 cup	20.0
Wheaties	1 cup	9.9
Rice Krispies	1¼ cup	7.1
Corn flakes	1 cup	6.8
Instant oatmeal	1 packet	5.3
Bagel	3½ in	2.4
Spaghetti	1 cup	2.3
Bread, enriched	1 slice	1.1
Vegetable Group		
Spaghetti sauce, no meat	1 cup	9.8
Potato, baked, with skin	1 medium	2.1
Sweet potato, baked	1 medium	2.1
Meat, Beans, Eggs, and Nuts Group		
Chicken breast	½	11.8
Tuna, canned in water	3 oz	11.2
Haddock, baked	3 oz	3.9
Beef, ground meat patty	3 oz	4.3
Peanuts, roasted	1 oz	3.9

Recommended Dietary Allowances (RDAs) for adults: women, 14 mg NE; men, 16 mg NE.
*1 mg niacin equivalent (NE) = 1 mg niacin or 60 mg tryptophan.
Nutrient data from USDA: *USDA National Nutrient Database for Standard Reference, Release 21,* Washington, DC, U.S. Department of Agriculture, 2009. Retrieved April 23, 2010 from http://www.ars.usda.gov/Services/docs.htm?docid=17477.

occurred in patients on long-term parenteral nutrition that omitted biotin. The protein avidin found in raw egg white binds biotin and, if consumed regularly, induces biotin deficiency. Cooking denatures this protein and destroys its ability to combine with biotin. (Raw eggs also carry the risk of foodborne illness that can be fatal to young children, older adults, or those with compromised immune function.) No known toxicity exists for biotin.

Functions of Biotin

Biotin functions as a partner with CoA in reactions that transfer carbon dioxide (CO_2) from one compound to another. Examples of this cofactor at work include (1) the synthesis of fatty acids, (2) the synthesis of amino acids, and (3) CO_2 fixation to form purines used in making genetic material.

Biotin Requirement

Because the amount of biotin needed is so small, the AI for this nutrient is 30 mcg/day for all adults.[51] Intestinal bacterial synthesis adds to the body's supply.

Food Sources of Biotin

Biotin is found in many foods, but its bioavailability varies greatly. The biotin in corn and soy is well absorbed, whereas the biotin in wheat is almost completely unavailable. Excellent food sources include egg yolk, liver, tomatoes, and yeast.

VITAMIN B_6 (PYRIDOXINE)

Chemical and Physical Nature

The chemical structure of vitamin B_6 is a pyridine ring, which accounts for its name. It is water soluble and heat stable but sensitive to light and alkaline solutions.

Forms

Vitamin B_6 is the generic term for the three forms of this vitamin found in nature: (1) pyridoxine, (2) pyridoxal,

KEY TERMS

niacin equivalent (NE) A measure of the total dietary sources of niacin; 1 NE equals 1 mg of niacin or 60 mg of tryptophan.

and (3) pyridoxamine. All three forms are equally active as precursors of the coenzyme pyridoxal phosphate (B_6-PO_4), or PLP.[51]

Absorption, Transport, and Storage

Vitamin B_6 is well absorbed in the upper segment of the small intestine. It is stored in muscle but found in tissues throughout the body, evidence of its many metabolic activities involving protein.

Functions of Vitamin B_6

Coenzyme in Protein Metabolism

In its active phosphate form (PLP), vitamin B_6 is a coenzyme in more than 100 amino acid reactions involving the synthesis of important proteins. Examples include the following:

- *Neurotransmitters:* PLP is needed to convert the essential amino acid tryptophan to serotonin, which carries messages across the cells in the brain; it helps to form γ-aminobutyric acid (GABA) found in the gray matter of the brain.
- *Amino group transfer:* PLP transfers nitrogen-containing amino groups from amino acids to form new amino acids and release carbon residues for energy.
- *Niacin:* PLP controls formation of niacin from tryptophan.
- *Hemoglobin:* PLP incorporates amino acids into heme, the nonprotein core of hemoglobin.
- *Immune function:* PLP participates in the production and release of antibodies and immune cells.

Coenzyme in Fat Metabolism

PLP converts the essential fatty acid linoleic acid to arachidonic acid.

Vitamin B_6 Deficiency and Clinical Applications

Vitamin B_6 is key in a number of clinical situations:

- *Anemia:* A lack of vitamin B_6 interrupts heme formation, resulting in a hypochromic anemia. This occurs despite a ready supply of iron and is reversed when vitamin B_6 is restored.
- *CNS changes:* Vitamin B_6 controls brain function through its role in the formation of serotonin and GABA. When a batch of commercial infant formula was mistakenly heated to a very high temperature, destroying the vitamin B_6, babies fed this formula experienced increasing irritability progressing to convulsions. Immediate supplementation with vitamin B_6 restored their normal function.
- *Physiologic demands in pregnancy:* Vitamin B_6 deficiency has been identified in mothers with preeclampsia (hypertension with edema and proteinuria) and eclampsia (convulsions).[51] Growth of the fetus along with rising metabolic needs of the mother increase the need for this vitamin. Vitamin B_6 supplements have been found to relieve severe nausea and vomiting in some pregnant mothers.[61]
- *Blood homocysteine levels:* Vitamin B_6 may help prevent a rise in blood homocysteine, believed to contribute to arterial disease, or lower cardiovascular risk in a way unrelated to blood homocysteine.[62–64] In any case optimum vitamin B_6 status appears to offer some protection against metabolic changes associated with cardiovascular disease.[63] Older women with rheumatoid arthritis (RA) had higher plasma homocysteine levels and poorer vitamin B_6 status than women of similar age not suffering with RA who had comparable vitamin B_6 intakes. It may be that older women with RA have a higher need for vitamin B_6.[65] (Plasma homocysteine and its clinical implications are discussed in more detail later in this chapter.)
- *Medications:* The drug isoniazid (isonicotinic acid hydrazide [INH]) used to treat tuberculosis is a vitamin B_6 **antagonist**; vitamin B_6 intakes of 50 to 100 mg/day are needed to overcome this effect. Levodopa, a medication for Parkinson's disease, lowers blood PLP levels.[51] Both current and former oral contraceptive users have low PLP levels despite intakes equal to or exceeding the RDA.[66]

Vitamin B_6 Requirement

Dietary Reference Intake

The RDA is expected to maintain optimum blood PLP levels,[51] although relatively high protein intakes increase the need for vitamin B_6. Men and women ages 19 to 50 should take in 1.3 mg/day. Older adults require higher amounts, and older men need more than older women. The RDA for men older than 50 is 1.7 mg/day; for women of this age it is 1.5 mg/day. Smokers may require higher amounts than nonsmokers.[66]

Vitamin B_6 Toxicity

Vitamin B_6 toxicity was reported in women taking supplements 1000-times the RDA in the belief that such a dose would alleviate premenstrual syndrome. Such intakes interfere with muscle coordination and over time damage the nervous system.[51] Luckily, the symptoms gradually disappeared after the supplements were discontinued. The UL for vitamin B_6 is 100 mg/day.

Food Sources of Vitamin B_6

Vitamin B_6 is found in many foods but usually in rather small amounts. Good sources include whole grains, legumes, meat, poultry, bananas, and potatoes. The highest contributor of vitamin B_6 in the diets of U.S. adults is ready-to-eat cereals.[57] Box 6-15 displays some food sources of this vitamin.

FOLATE

Discovery

The folate group was first extracted from dark leafy vegetables and given the name *folic acid* from the Latin word for *leaf.* Studies investigating anemia among poor pregnant Indian women led to the discovery of this vitamin group.[51]

Chemical and Physical Nature

Folic acid, a yellow crystal, has the chemical name of *pteroylmonoglutamic acid* based on its structure. Folic acid is seldom found naturally but is the form used in supplements and fortified foods. Naturally occurring folate or food folate is the

BOX 6-15 FOOD SOURCES OF VITAMIN B_6 (PYRIDOXINE)

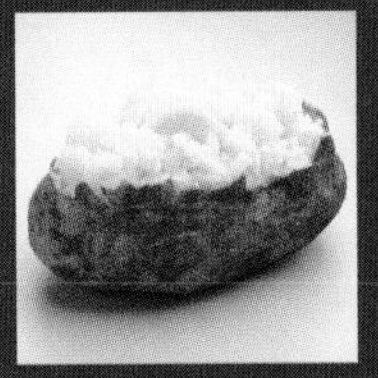
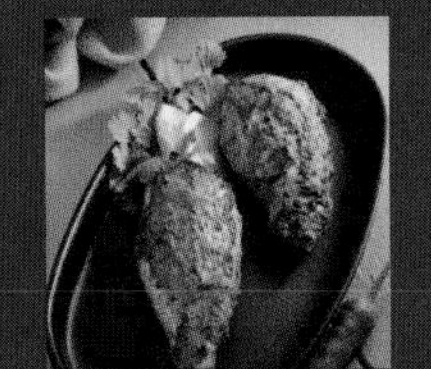
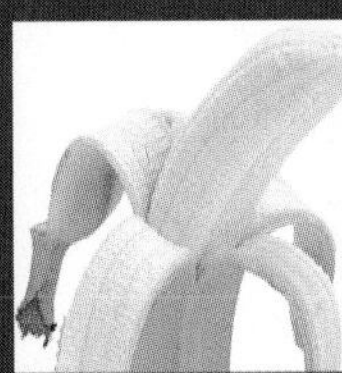

Vitamin B_6 (pyridoxine) is found in both plant and animal foods, although the milk group is low in this nutrient. Ready-to-eat cereals, potatoes, and poultry are especially good sources.

FOOD SOURCE	AMOUNT	VITAMIN B_6 (in mg)
Grains Group		
Corn flakes	1 cup	0.96
Instant oatmeal	1 packet	0.51
Vegetable Group		
Potato, baked, with skin	1 medium	0.63
Spaghetti sauce, tomato	1 cup	0.43
Fruit Group		
Banana	1	0.43
Meat, Beans, Eggs, and Nuts Group		
Chicken breast	½	0.52
Tuna, canned, packed in water	3 oz	0.30

Recommended Dietary Allowances (RDAs) for adults: men and women, ages 19-50, 1.3 mg; women, ages ≥51, 1.5 mg; men, ages ≥51, 1.7 mg. Nutrient data from USDA: *USDA National Nutrient Database for Standard Reference, Release 21,* Washington, DC, U.S. Department of Agriculture, 2009. Retrieved April 23, 2010 from http://www.ars.usda.gov/Services/docs.htm?docid=17477.

compound pteroylpolyglutamate, which contains additional glutamic acid molecules.[51] Both forms are well used by the body.

Absorption, Transport, and Storage

The absorption of folate depends on its source. About 50% of the folate occurring naturally in plant foods (food folate) is absorbed, compared with 85% of the folic acid added to fortified foods. Conversion factors have been developed for calculating folate intake (Box 6-16).[67]

Functions of Folate

Coenzyme Role

Folate is the coenzyme with the task of attaching single carbons to metabolic compounds. Several key molecules provide examples, as follows:

- *Purines:* Nitrogen-containing compounds in genetic material that participate in cell division and the transmission of inherited traits

BOX 6-16 CALCULATING DIETARY FOLATE EQUIVALENTS

- 1 mcg of food folate (folate occurring naturally in a food) = 1 dietary folate equivalent (DFE)
- 1 mcg folic acid (added in food fortification) = 1.7 mcg DFE (Folic acid added to foods is absorbed more efficiently than naturally occurring food folate.)

To estimate the DFEs in foods such as fortified breakfast cereals in which most or all of the folate is added folic acid, use the percent daily value listed on the food label:

% Daily value × 400 mcg (the daily value for folic acid) × 1.7 = DFEs per serving

Data from Suitor CW, Bailey LB: Dietary folate equivalents: interpretation and application, *J Am Diet Assoc* 100:88, 2000.

- *Thymine:* A component of DNA, the material in the cell nucleus that controls and transmits genetic characteristics
- *Hemoglobin:* Heme is the iron-containing nonprotein portion of hemoglobin that transports oxygen and CO_2 in the blood

Folate Deficiency and Clinical Applications

Anemia

A nutritional megaloblastic anemia often occurs in simple folate deficiency. Because folate needs are high during periods of rapid growth, folate deficiency anemia is most likely to occur in pregnant women, growing infants, and young children. Adolescent girls who severely limit their food intake are also at risk.

Presence of Gastric Acid

An acid environment is required to release folate from its food source and enable its absorption. Low hydrochloric acid secretion in the stomach, a common problem in older people, or use of medications that raise the pH in the gastrointestinal tract can adversely affect folate status.[68]

Medications

The drug amethopterin (methotrexate) used in cancer treatment is a folate antagonist and prevents the synthesis of DNA and purines, thereby preventing the growth of the cancer. High intakes of folate interfere with the action of phenobarbital used to control epilepsy.[51]

Folate and Birth Defects

NTDs, a worldwide vitamin-related problem, are congenital abnormalities that occur when the spinal cord and its coverings fail to develop normally. If part of the brain fails to

KEY TERMS

antagonist A substance that acts in opposition to another physiologic substance preventing its normal action; vitamin antagonists prevent the usual action of the vitamin.

megaloblastic anemia Anemia characterized by abnormally large immature red blood cells; occurs in vitamin B_{12} or folate deficiency.

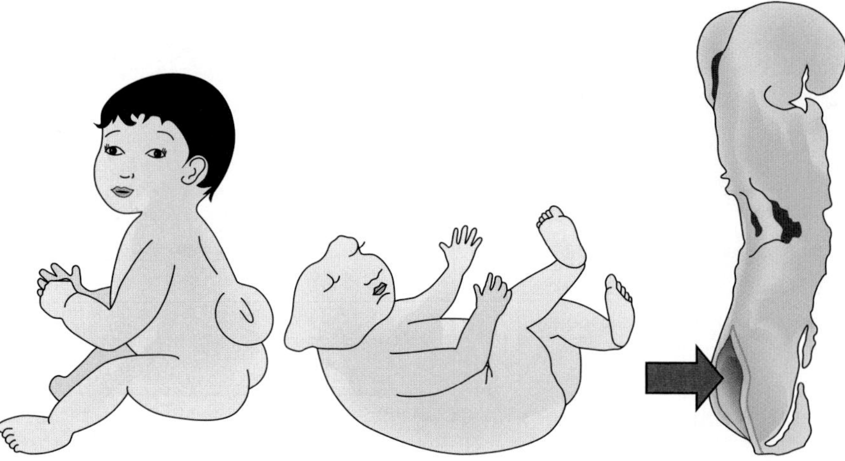

FIGURE 6-10 Neural tube defects (NTDs) include spina bifida and anencephaly. They result from a lack of folate needed to close the neural tube that becomes the spinal cord in the developing fetus. (Redrawn from http://www.cdc.gov/ncbddd/birthdefects/Anencephaly.htm and http://www.cdc.gov/ncbddd/birthdefects/SpinaBifida.htm, Centers for Disease Control and Prevention, Atlanta, Ga.)

develop (anencephaly), then the infant is likely to die shortly after birth. The more common NTD is spina bifida, in which the neural tube fails to close during embryonic development and the spinal cord remains on the outside of the body (Figure 6-10). In less severe cases a child may live a productive life if surgical and medical intervention is effective; but for many a normal life cannot be achieved.

Folate is essential for the formation and closure of the neural tube in the early weeks of fetal development, between day 21 and day 28 of gestation, before a woman is even aware that she might be pregnant. Therefore it is critical that a mother be in good folate status before conception occurs. It is estimated that 70% of NTDs can be prevented with adequate folate.[69] To combat this problem the U.S. Food and Drug Administration (FDA) in 1998 instituted a mandatory folate fortification program requiring the addition of 140 mcg of folic acid per 100 g of flour or uncooked grain. In practical terms, one slice of fortified bread and one serving of fortified pasta provides 136 mcg, or about one third of the RDA.[51] Many ready-to-eat cereals provide 400 mcg of folate per serving or 100% of the RDA.

Although the incidence of NTDs has declined, the fortification program remains controversial.[70-72] As we learn later in this chapter, excessive folate intake can mask a vitamin B_{12} deficiency, allowing the neural damage resulting from the B_{12} deficiency to continue. More recently it has been reported that high intakes of folate-fortified foods can promote the growth of existing tumors in the colon.[71] An unsolved problem is how we encourage appropriate folate intakes among women of child-bearing age while preventing any negative effects on men and older adults who may be eating numerous servings of grain products in addition to using folate supplements. A recent national survey indicated that only about 8% of women of child-bearing age are meeting the recommended amount of folate.[69]

Folate and Chronic Disease

When folate is in short supply, the conversion of methionine to cysteine cannot be completed and homocysteine (the intermediate product) accumulates in the blood. Elevated plasma homocysteine levels have been implicated in the worsening of various chronic conditions including cardiovascular disease, osteoporosis, and age-related cognitive impairment. Intervention trials have demonstrated that supplementation of folic acid along with other B vitamins (vitamin B_{12}, vitamin B_6, or both) brings about a significant decrease in blood homocysteine levels; however, contrary to what was expected, this drop in blood homocysteine did not have positive effects on bone turnover[73,74] or reduce cardiovascular incidents or mortality in men[75-77] or women.[78] It also appears that this combination of vitamins does not slow cognitive decline in patients with mild-to-moderate Alzheimer's disease.[79] The relationship between the B vitamins, blood homocysteine levels, and chronic disease remains elusive.

Folate Requirement

Dietary Reference Intake

The RDA for adolescents and adults is 400 mcg/day and increases to 600 mcg/day in pregnancy.[51] The mandatory fortification of flour and grain foods has increased average intake by as much as 200 mcg of folic acid a day and is credited with the decrease in NTD-affected births.[69]

Folate Toxicity

The UL for folate is 1000 mcg/day,[51] and supplements exceeding the recommended intake of 400 mcg are best avoided. The basis for concern is the relationship between folate and vitamin B_{12}. If vitamin B_{12} levels are low but folate levels are high, then folate can substitute for vitamin B_{12} in formation of red blood cells and prevent the development of a megaloblastic anemia. However, vitamin B_{12} also has a critical role in maintaining nerve tissue, and folate cannot meet that need. The appearance

BOX 6-17 **FOOD SOURCES OF FOLATE**

FOOD SOURCE	AMOUNT	FOLATE (in mcg DFE)*
Grains Group		
Fortified ready-to-eat cereals		
Product 19	1 cup	676
Wheaties	1 cup	336
Corn flakes	1 cup	222
Instant oatmeal	1 packet	138
Rice, parboiled, cooked	1 cup	238
Spaghetti, cooked	1 cup	167
Hamburger roll	1	73
Bread, white, enriched	1 slice	43
Vegetable Group		
Spinach, frozen, cooked	½ cup	115
Broccoli, frozen, cooked	½ cup	84
Lettuce, dark green (romaine or similar)	1 cup	76
Tomato juice	1 cup	49
Fruit Group		
Orange juice	1 cup	74
Strawberries	1 cup	40
Meat, Beans, Eggs, and Nuts Group		
Kidney beans, canned	1 cup	51

Recommended Dietary Allowances (RDAs) for adults: 400 mcg.
*1 mcg dietary folate equivalent (DFE) = 1 mcg food folate.
Nutrient data from USDA: *USDA National Nutrient Database for Standard Reference, Release 21,* Washington, DC, U.S. Department of Agriculture, 2009. Retrieved April 23, 2010 from http://www.ars.usda.gov/Services/docs.htm?docid=17477.

of a megaloblastic anemia is often the first alert to vitamin B_{12} deficiency. If high intakes of folate "mask" this effect, then damage to the nervous system continues unabated.

Food Sources of Folate

Folate is widely distributed in plant foods. Good sources include dark green leafy vegetables, citrus fruits, tomatoes, cantaloupe, and legumes, as well as fortified grains. Ready-to-eat cereal is a major contributor of folic acid in the U.S. diet.[57] Box 6-17 summarizes food sources of folate.

VITAMIN B_{12} (COBALAMIN)

Discovery

The discovery of vitamin B_{12} coincided with the search for a cure for pernicious anemia.[80] In 1948 workers crystallized a red compound from liver, which controlled both the blood-forming defect and the nerve involvement in pernicious anemia. This molecule was numbered *vitamin B_{12}* and later named *cobalamin,* based on the single red atom of the trace element cobalt at its center.

Chemical and Physical Nature

Vitamin B_{12} is a complex red crystal of high molecular weight. It occurs as a protein complex in animal foods only. The source of vitamin B_{12} is the synthesizing bacteria in the intestinal tract of herbivorous animals, although some bacterial synthesis also takes place in the human intestine.

Absorption, Transport, and Storage

Vitamin B_{12} is split from its protein complex by the hydrochloric acid in the stomach and then bound to a specific glycoprotein called *intrinsic factor,* secreted by the mucosal cells lining the stomach. This vitamin B_{12}-intrinsic factor complex then moves into the intestine, where special receptors

KEY TERMS

pernicious anemia A macrocytic anemia caused by the absence of the intrinsic factor necessary for absorption of vitamin B_{12} (cobalamin); this condition is fatal unless treated with intramuscular injections of vitamin B_{12}.

in the wall of the ileum absorb it. The loss of gastric acid or failure of the gastric mucosa to secrete intrinsic factor will impair absorption and result in vitamin B_{12} deficiency.

Approximately 50% of body vitamin B_{12} is stored in the liver, with the remainder distributed among active tissues. The amounts are minute but held tenaciously and only slowly depleted. Vitamin B_{12} deficiency does not become apparent for 3 to 5 years after a gastrectomy and loss of required secretions.

Functions of Vitamin B_{12}

Basic Coenzyme Role

Vitamin B_{12} participates in amino acid metabolism and formation of the heme portion of hemoglobin. It has a role in the synthesis of important lipids and proteins that form the myelin sheath covering the nerves of the brain and spinal cord.

Vitamin B_{12} Deficiency and Clinical Applications

Vitamin B_{12} deficiency disrupts blood formation and affects cognitive function:

- *Pernicious anemia:* The megaloblastic anemia arising from vitamin B_{12} deficiency took on the name *pernicious* anemia because it is fatal if left untreated. When this vitamin is lacking, the production of red blood cells is halted because (1) the heme portion of the hemoglobin molecule cannot be synthesized and (2) the activated form of folate needed to assist in the process cannot be formed. The root cause of pernicious anemia is the lack of intrinsic factor required for the absorption of vitamin B_{12} from the small intestine, so another way must be found to supply this vitamin. A monthly intramuscular injection of 1000 mcg controls the blood-forming disorder and prevents the degenerative effects on the nervous system.[81]
- *Cognitive function:* Vitamin B_{12} deficiency causes fatigue, lassitude, and a decline in cognitive function as damage to the nervous system continues. Even in the absence of overt deficiency, older adults with low blood vitamin B_{12} levels are more likely to experience cognitive decline than those with normal levels.[82,83] Excessively high blood folate levels appear to exacerbate the cognitive losses associated with vitamin B_{12} deficiency (see previous section).[84]
- *Low gastric acid secretion*: As many as 30% of people older than 50 have low gastric acid levels,[84] putting them at risk of vitamin B_{12} deficiency; Latino older adults appear to be especially vulnerable.[85] Crystalline vitamin B_{12} used in food fortification and vitamin supplements does not require gastric acid for effective absorption, and use of vitamin B_{12}–fortified foods several times each week can supply the amount needed. Based on the growing numbers of older adults and increased intakes of folic acid as a result of mandatory folic acid fortification of grains, researchers have proposed that mandatory vitamin B_{12} fortification of flour also be considered.[86]

Vitamin B_{12} Requirement

The amount of vitamin B_{12} required for normal metabolism is minute. The RDA is 2.4 mcg for both younger and older adults.[51]

Food Sources of Vitamin B_{12}

In nature, vitamin B_{12} is found only in animal foods; rich sources include lean meat, fish, poultry, milk, eggs, and cheese. For individuals consuming any animal foods, the recommended intake is easily obtained. Vegans and individuals with low gastric acid levels can obtain the amount needed from fortified grains, cereals, juices, and soy milk or vitamin B_{12} supplements. Box 6-18 lists some good sources.

A summary of the water-soluble B vitamins is presented in Table 6-4.

As we conclude our discussion of this important micronutrient group, consider your own vitamin intake and review the *Perspectives in Practice* box, "Do I Need a Vitamin-Mineral Supplement?"

BOX 6-18 FOOD SOURCES OF VITAMIN B_{12} (COBALAMIN)

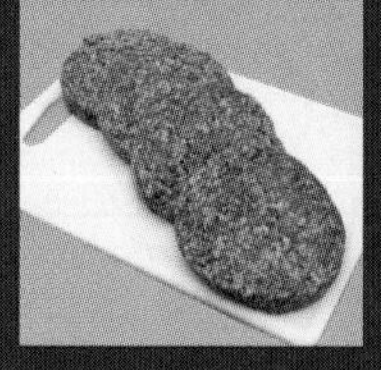
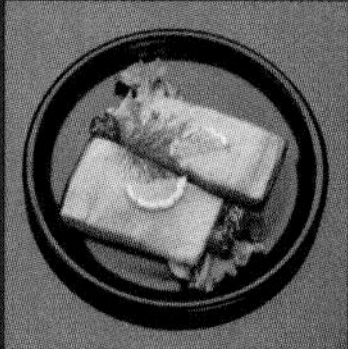
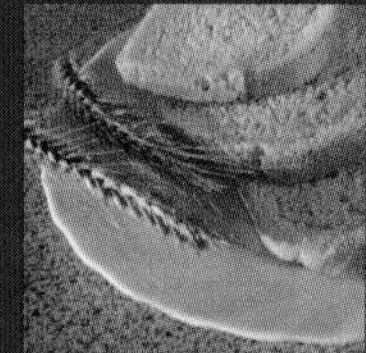

Vitamin B_{12} (cobalamin) is found naturally in animal foods only, but various grain foods and juices are fortified with this vitamin. Vegans who consume no animal foods and older persons with reduced gastric acid levels should check the nutrition label to identify products with added vitamin B_{12}.

Naturally Occurring Sources of Vitamin B_{12}

Meat patty
Chicken leg
Fish serving
Milk
Cheese

Examples of Non-Animal Foods Sometimes Fortified with Vitamin B_{12}

Ready-to-eat cereal
Bread
Orange juice

Recommended Dietary Allowances (RDAs) for adults: 2.4 mcg.

TABLE 6-4 SUMMARY OF B-COMPLEX VITAMINS

VITAMIN	COENZYME: PHYSIOLOGIC FUNCTIONS	CLINICAL APPLICATIONS	DIETARY REFERENCE INTAKE	FOOD SOURCES
Thiamin	Carbohydrate metabolism Thiamin pyrophosphate (TPP): oxidative decarboxylation	Beriberi (deficiency) Neuropathy Wernicke-Korsakoff syndrome (alcoholism) Depressed muscular and secretory functions	Adults: men ages ≥19: 1.2 mg; women ages ≥19: 1.1 mg Pregnancy: all ages 1.4 mg Lactation: all ages 1.4 mg	Pork, beef, organ meats Whole or enriched grains and cereals Legumes
Riboflavin	General metabolism Flavin mononucleotide (FMN) Flavin adenine dinucleotide (FAD)	Cheilosis, glossitis, seborrheic dermatitis	Adults: men ages ≥19: 1.3 mg; women ages ≥19: 1.1 mg Pregnancy: all ages 1.4 mg Lactation: all ages 1.6 mg	Milk products, organ meats Enriched grains and cereals
Niacin (nicotinic acid, nicotinamide)	General metabolism Nicotinamide adenine dinucleotide (NAD) Nicotinamide adenine dinucleotide phosphate (NADP)	Pellagra (deficiency) Weakness, anorexia Scaly dermatitis Neuritis	Adults: men ages ≥19: 16 mg NE; women ages ≥19: 14 mg NE Pregnancy: all ages 18 mg NE Lactation: all ages 17 mg NE	Meat, dairy foods containing tryptophan Peanuts Enriched grains and cereals
Vitamin B_6 (pyridoxine, pyridoxal, pyridoxamine)	General metabolism Pyridoxal phosphate (PLP): transamination and decarboxylation	Reduced serum levels associated with pregnancy and use of certain oral contraceptives Antagonized by isoniazid, penicillamine, various other drugs	Adults: men ages 19-50: 1.3 mg; ages ≥51: 1.7 mg Adults: women ages 19-50: 1.3 mg; ages ≥51: 1.5 mg Pregnancy: all ages 1.9 mg Lactation: all ages 2.0 mg	Meat, organ meats Whole grains and cereals Legumes Bananas
Pantothenic acid	General metabolism Coenzyme A (CoA): acetylation	Many roles through acyl transfer reactions (e.g., lipogenesis, amino acid activation; formation of cholesterol, steroid hormones, heme)	Adults: men/women ages ≥19: 5 mg Pregnancy: all ages: 6 mg Lactation: all ages 7 mg	Egg, milk, liver
Biotin	General metabolism Carbon dioxide (CO_2) transfer reactions	Deficiency induced by avidin (a protein in raw egg white) and by antibiotics	Adults: men/women ages ≥19: 30 mcg Pregnancy: all ages 30 mcg Lactation: all ages 35 mcg	Egg yolk, liver Synthesized by intestinal microorganisms
Folate (folic acid, folacin)	General metabolism Single carbon transfer reactions (e.g., purine nucleotide, thymine, heme synthesis)	Megaloblastic anemia Elevated blood homocysteine levels Neural tube defect (NTD)-affected pregnancy	Adults: men/women ages ≥19: 400 mcg Pregnancy: all ages 600 mcg Lactation: all ages 500 mcg	Green leafy vegetables Oranges, orange juice, tomatoes Liver and organ meats Fortified breads and cereals
Vitamin B_{12} (cobalamin)	General metabolism Methylcobalamin: methylation reactions (e.g., synthesis of amino acids, heme)	Pernicious anemia induced by lack of intrinsic factor for B_{12} absorption Megaloblastic anemia Peripheral neuropathy Changes in cognitive function (occurs on a vegan diet with no animal foods and no B_{12} supplements or fortified foods) Deficiency can also result from low gastric acid secretion hindering absorption	Adults: men/women ages ≥19: 2.4 mcg Pregnancy: all ages 2.6 mcg Lactation: all ages 2.8 mcg	Meat, milk, cheese, egg, liver (all animal foods) Fortified cereals, juices, and soy milk

NE, Niacin equivalent.

PERSPECTIVES IN PRACTICE

Do I Need a Vitamin-Mineral Supplement?

We are constantly barraged by advertisements urging us to purchase a vitamin or mineral supplement to prevent or cure real or imagined nutrient deficiencies. Sales of dietary supplements now exceed $23.7 billion[1] and is one of the world's fastest growing industries.[2] The U.S. Food and Drug Administration (FDA) estimates more than 29,000 supplements are currently on the market, including nutritional, herbal, botanical, and sports products.[3]

The best strategy for obtaining appropriate amounts of vitamins and minerals is to choose a variety of foods.[1] Fortified foods such as breakfast cereals or juices can provide additional vitamins or minerals. Nevertheless, some individuals may need supplements to meet their dietary reference intake (DRI) for particular nutrients, as follows[1,3,4-5]:

- Older adults with low levels of gastric acid are less able to absorb vitamin B_{12} from animal protein foods. Vegans who eat no animal foods require a vitamin B_{12} supplement or fortified plant food.
- Women of childbearing age who may become pregnant require 400 mcg of folate daily to help prevent neural tube defects (NTDs).
- Pregnant women whose DRI for iron is 27 mg are unlikely to obtain this amount from food, even including fortified foods.
- Youth and adults who cannot tolerate milk or do not drink milk may need a supplement to reach their calcium goal for the day.
- Older adults with low energy needs who eat very limited amounts of food and others who restrict their intake of kcalories may benefit from a multivitamin-mineral supplement. Energy intakes less than 1500 to 1600 kcal are unlikely to contain all vitamins and minerals in required amounts.
- Individuals confined indoors, vegans, and those whose skin pigment makes it difficult to synthesize vitamin D will need vitamin D–fortified foods or a supplement.

Recommendations regarding the use of vitamin-mineral supplements must be individualized; no one piece of advice fits all. The following guidelines offer suggestions for selecting a supplement when indicated:

- Use supplements in addition to, not in place of, real food. A poor diet with added supplements is still a poor diet.
- Avoid multivitamin-mineral supplements or single-nutrient supplements that exceed 100% of the DRI for any nutrient. Individuals using highly fortified foods might aim for no more than 50% of the DRI in a supplement or consider whether a supplement is really necessary. Intake should not exceed the Tolerable Upper Intake Level (UL) for any vitamin or mineral.
- Check with your physician first if you use prescription or nonprescription medications or regularly eat a fortified cereal supplying 100% of the DRI for most minerals and vitamins.
- Take the supplement with meals to enhance nutrient absorption.

REFERENCES

1. American Dietetic Association: Position of the American Dietetic Association: nutrient supplementation, *J Am Diet Assoc* 109:2073, 2009.
2. Foote JA, Murphy SP, Wilkens LR, et al: Factors associated with dietary supplement use among healthy adults of five ethnicities, *Am J Epidemiol* 157:888, 2003.
3. American Dietetic Association: Position of the American Dietetic Association: fortification and nutritional supplements, *J Am Diet Assoc* 105:1300, 2005.
4. Hunt JR: Tailoring advice on dietary supplements, *J Am Diet Assoc* 102:1754, 2002.
5. Sheth A, Khurana R, Khurana V: Potential liver damage associated with over-the-counter vitamin supplements, *J Am Diet Assoc* 108:1536, 2008.

TO SUM UP

A vitamin is an organic, non–energy-yielding substance that is (1) required in very small amounts; (2) participates in specific metabolic functions, often as a coenzyme; and (3) must be supplied by diet. The metabolic tasks of the fat-soluble vitamins, A, D, E, and K, involve the synthesis of important proteins related to vision, blood clotting, and bone health. Vitamins A and D influence the differentiation of cells and tissues, and vitamin E, a powerful antioxidant, protects membranes and other structures made up of polyunsaturated fatty acids. The fat-soluble vitamins are absorbed and transported with lipids and easily stored; thus excessive intake can lead to toxicity.

The water-soluble vitamins including ascorbic acid and the B-complex vitamins are synthesized by plants and (with the exception of vitamin B_{12}) supplied in both plant and animal foods. They function as coenzymes in cell metabolism and protein synthesis and must be consumed regularly because body stores are limited. Excess intake is excreted in the urine. Ascorbic acid functions as an antioxidant and is important for tissue integrity. Folate and vitamins B_6 and B_{12} have important roles in formation of red blood cells and development of nerve structures and function. Vitamin B_6 and ascorbic acid have shown evidence of toxicity with excessive supplement use. Water-soluble vitamins, especially vitamin C and folate, are easily oxidized, and appropriate cooking and storage practices are required to prevent losses from food sources.

QUESTIONS FOR REVIEW

1. Explain how the absorption and storage of a vitamin influence the risk of deficiency and toxicity. Provide several examples to illustrate this concept.
2. List and describe three health problems resulting from a vitamin A deficiency. Give three causes of a vitamin A deficiency.
3. What organ systems participate in the formation of the vitamin D hormone calcitriol, and what are their roles? Who is at risk for vitamin D deficiency? Why?
4. What is an antioxidant, and how does it protect body tissues? A woman tells you that she is taking 1000 mg of vitamin E to prevent signs of aging. How would you advise her?
5. You have a client who is taking a prescription anticoagulant. What do you need to tell him about (1) food choices and (2) use of other supplements?
6. You are working with a child who has cystic fibrosis. What should you be telling her caregivers about her vitamin needs? Does she require a vitamin supplement? Why?
7. What three characteristics are shared by most water-soluble vitamins? Identify an exception to each and explain the reason.
8. Define the term *coenzyme* as applied to the role of the water-soluble vitamins. Give several examples.
9. A patient tells you that he is taking multiple vitamin supplements including 1000 mg of ascorbic acid, 5 mg of thiamin, 10 mg of riboflavin, and 50 mg of vitamin B_6. How would you evaluate this vitamin regimen? What advice would you give him and why? Develop menus for 2 days that include good food sources of these vitamins.
10. Name the B vitamins involved in blood formation. Describe their roles and interactions.
11. Visit a grocery store and, from the food label, record the folate content per serving of (1) three different breads, (2) three different ready-to-eat cereals, (3) three types of rice or rice-containing dishes, and (4) three types of pasta or pasta-containing dishes. Rice and pasta dishes may be dry mixes or frozen entrees. Using these foods, develop menus for 3 days that include a daily minimum of six servings from the grains group and provide at least 400 mcg of folate.
12. You have been asked to speak at a senior citizens' center on the topic of carotenoids. Outline your presentation, including the following: (1) What is a carotenoid? (2) Why are carotenoids important? (3) What are some good food sources of carotenoids? The senior center director has given you some money for groceries to provide taste treats to serve with your program. What foods or recipes will you prepare?

REFERENCES

1. Carpenter KJ, Harper AE: Evolution of knowledge of essential nutrients. In Shils ME, Shike M, Olson J, et al, editors: *Modern nutrition in health and disease*, ed 10, Baltimore, 2006, Lippincott Williams & Wilkins.
2. Russell RM: Current framework for DRI development: what are the pros and cons? *Nutr Rev* 66(8):455, 2008.
3. Food and Nutrition Board, Institute of Medicine: *Dietary Reference Intakes for vitamin A, vitamin K, arsenic, boron, chromium, copper, iodine, iron, manganese, molybdenum, nickel, silicon, vanadium, and zinc*, Washington, DC, 2001, National Academies Press.
4. de Pee S, Bioem MW: The bioavailability of (pro) vitamin A carotenoids and maximizing the contribution of homestead food production to combating vitamin A deficiency, *Int J Vitam Nutr Res* 77:182, 2007.
5. Olson JA, Loveridge N, Duthie GG, et al: Fat-soluble vitamins. In Garrow GS, James WPT, Ralph A, editors: *Human nutrition and dietetics*, ed 10, Edinburgh, 2000, Churchill Livingstone.
6. Solomons NW: Vitamin A. In Bowman BA, Russell RM, editors: *Present knowledge in nutrition*, ed 9, vol I, Washington, DC, 2006, International Life Sciences Institute.
7. Kraemer K, Waelti M, de Pee S, et al: Are low tolerable upper intake levels for vitamin A undermining effective food fortification efforts? *Nutr Rev* 66:517, 2008.
8. Ribaya-Mercado JD, Blumberg JB: Vitamin A: is it a risk factor for osteoporosis and bone fracture? *Nutr Rev* 65:425, 2007.
9. Davis CD, Ross SA: Evidence for dietary regulation of microRNA expression in cancer cells, *Nutr Rev* 66:477, 2008.
10. Ross AC: Vitamin A and carotenoids. In Shils ME, Shike M, Olson J, et al: *Modern nutrition in health and disease*, ed 10, Baltimore, 2006, Lippincott Williams & Wilkins.
11. O'Donnell SI, Hoerr SL, Mendoza JA, et al: Nutrient quality of fast food kids meals, *Am J Clin Nutr* 88:1388, 2008.
12. Thorsdottir I, Birgisdottir BE, Halidorsdottir S, et al: Association of fish and fish liver oil intake in pregnancy with infant size at birth among women of normal weight before pregnancy in a fishing community, *Am J Epidemiol* 160:460, 2004.
13. Penniston KL, Tanumihardjo SA: Vitamin A in dietary supplements and fortified foods: too much of a good thing, *J Am Diet Assoc* 103:1185, 2003.
14. Holick MF, Chen TC, Lu Z, et al: Vitamin D and skin physiology: a D-lightful story, *J Bone Miner Res* 22(Suppl 2):V27, 2007.
15. Looker AC, Pfeiffer CM, Lacker DA, et al: Serum 25-hydroxyvitamin D status of the US population: 1988-1994 compared with 2000-2004, *Am J Clin Nutr* 88:1519, 2008.
16. Holick MF: The vitamin D deficiency pandemic and consequences for nonskeletal health: mechanisms of action, *Mol Aspects Med* 29:361, 2008.
17. Bischoff-Ferrari HA, Dawson-Hughes B, Willett WC, et al: Effect of vitamin D on falls: a meta-analysis, *JAMA* 291:1999, 2004.
18. Food and Nutrition Board, Institute of Medicine: *Dietary Reference Intakes. The essential guide to nutrient requirements*, Washington, DC, 2006, National Academies Press.
19. Taylor SN, Wagner CL, Hollis BW: Vitamin D supplementation during lactation to support infant and mother, *J Am Coll Nutr* 27:690, 2008.

20. Yetley EA, Brule D, Cheney MC, et al: Dietary Reference Intakes for vitamin D: justification for a review of the 1997 values, *Am J Clin Nutr* 89:719, 2009.
21. Weng FL, Shults J, Leonard MB, et al: Risk factors for low serum 25-hydroxyvitamin D concentrations in otherwise healthy children and adolescents, *Am J Clin Nutr* 86:150, 2007.
22. Mouyis M, Ostor AJ, Crisp AJ, et al: Hypovitaminosis D among rheumatology outpatients in clinical practice, *Rheumatology* 47:1348, 2008.
23. Yetley EA: Assessing the vitamin D status of the US population, *Am J Clin Nutr* 88(Suppl):558S, 2008.
24. Newmark HL, Heaney RP, LaChance PA: Should calcium and vitamin D be added to the current enrichment program for cereal-grain products? *Am J Clin Nutr* 80:264, 2004.
25. Bleys J, Miller ER 3rd, Pastor-Barriuso R, et al: Vitamin-mineral supplementation and the progression of atherosclerosis: a meta-analysis of randomized controlled trials, *Am J Clin Nutr* 84:880, 2006.
26. Lee I-M, Cook NR, Gaziano JM, et al: Vitamin E in the primary prevention of cardiovascular disease and cancer. The Women's Health Study: a randomized controlled trial, *JAMA* 294:56, 2005.
27. Sesso HD, Buring JE, Christen WG, et al: Vitamins E and C in the prevention of cardiovascular disease in men. The Physicians' Health Study II randomized controlled trial, *JAMA* 300:2123, 2008.
28. Redberg RF: Vitamin E and cardiovascular health, *JAMA* 294:107, 2005.
29. Seddon JM: Multivitamin-multimineral supplements and eye disease: age-related macular degeneration and cataract, *Am J Clin Nutr* 85(Suppl):304S, 2007.
30. Block KI, Koch AC, Mead MN, et al: Impact of antioxidant supplementation on chemotherapeutic toxicity: a systematic review of the evidence from randomized controlled trials, *Int J Cancer* 123:1227, 2008.
31. Traber MG: Vitamin E. In Shils ME, Shike M, Olson J, et al, editors: *Modern nutrition in health and disease*, ed 10, Baltimore, 2006, Lippincott Williams & Wilkins.
32. Maqbool A, Stallings VA: Update on fat-soluble vitamins in cystic fibrosis, *Curr Opin Pulm Med* 14:574, 2008.
33. U.S. Department of Agriculture, Agricultural Research Service: *Nutrient intakes from food: mean amounts consumed per individual, one day, 2005-2006*, Washington, DC, 2008, U.S. Department of Agriculture. Retrieved May 1, 2010 from http://www.ars.usda.gov/SP2UserFiles/Place/12355000/pdf/0506/Table_1_NIF_05.pdf.
34. Reedy J, Krebs-Smith SM: A comparison of food-based recommendations and nutrient values of three food guides: USDA's MyPyramid, NHLBI's dietary approaches to stop hypertension eating plan, and Harvard's healthy eating pyramid, *J Am Diet Assoc* 108:522, 2008.
35. U.S. Department of Agriculture, Agricultural Research Service: *USDA National Nutrient Database for Standard Reference, Release 21*, Washington, DC, 2009, U.S. Department of Agriculture. Retrieved April 23, 2010 from http://www.ars.usda.gov/Services/docs.htm?docid=17477.
36. Leonard SW, Good CK, Gugger ET, et al: Vitamin E bioavailability from fortified breakfast cereal is greater than that from encapsulated supplements, *Am J Clin Nutr* 79:86, 2004.
37. Suttie JW: Vitamin K. In Shils ME, Shike M, Olson J, et al, editors: *Modern nutrition in health and disease*, ed 10, Baltimore, 2006, Lippincott Williams & Wilkins.
38. Cashman KD, O'Connor E: Does vitamin K_1 intake protect against bone loss in later life? *Nutr Rev* 66:532, 2008.
39. Rohde LE, Silva de Assis MC, Rabelo ER: Dietary vitamin K intake and anticoagulation in elderly patients, *Curr Opin Clin Nutr Metab Care* 10:1, 2007.
40. Marcason W: Vitamin K: What are the current dietary recommendations for patients taking Coumadin? *J Am Diet Assoc* 107:2022, 2007.
41. Guyton AC, Hall JE: *Textbook of medical physiology*, ed 10, Philadelphia, 2000, Saunders.
42. Winkler MA, Manchester S: Medical nutrition therapy for metabolic stress, sepsis, trauma, burns, and surgery. In Mahan KL, Escott-Stump S, editors: *Krause's food, nutrition, & diet therapy*, ed 12, Philadelphia, 2007, Saunders.
43. Cogswell ME, Weisberg P, Spong C: Cigarette smoking, alcohol use and adverse pregnancy outcomes: implications for micronutrient supplementation, *J Nutr* 133:1722S, 2003.
44. Tan AG, Mitchell P, Flood VM, et al: Antioxidant nutrient intake and the long-term incidence of age-related cataract: the Blue Mountains Eye Study, *Am J Clin Nutr* 87:1899, 2008.
45. Harding A-H, Wareham NJ, Bingham SA, et al: Plasma vitamin C level, fruit and vegetable consumption, and the risk of new-onset type 2 diabetes mellitus, *Arch Intern Med* 168:1493, 2008.
46. Khaw KT, Wareham N, Bingham S, et al: Combined impact of health behaviours and mortality in men and women: The EPIC-Norfolk Prospective Population Study, *PLoS Med* 5(1):e12, 2008.
47. Myint PK, Luben RN, Welch AA, et al: Plasma vitamin C concentrations predict risk of incident stroke over 10 y in 20,649 participants of the European Prospective Investigation into Cancer—Norfolk prospective population study, *Am J Clin Nutr* 87:64, 2008.
48. Li Y, Schellhorn HE: New developments and novel therapeutic perspectives for vitamin C, *J Nutr* 137:2171, 2007.
49. Greenwald P, Anderson D, Nelson SA, et al: Clinical trials of vitamin and mineral supplements for cancer prevention, *Am J Clin Nutr* 85(1):314S, 2007.
50. Rock CL, Newman VA, Neuhouser ML, et al: Antioxidant supplement use in cancer survivors and the general population, *J Nutr* 134:3194S, 2004.
51. Food and Nutrition Board, Institute of Medicine: *Dietary Reference Intakes for thiamin, riboflavin, niacin, vitamin* B_6, *folate, vitamin* B_{12}, *pantothenic acid, biotin, and choline*, Washington, DC, 1998, National Academies Press.
52. Thurnham DI, Bender DA, Scott J, et al: Water-soluble vitamins. In Garrow GS, James WPT, Ralph A, editors: *Human nutrition and dietetics*, ed 10, Edinburgh, 2000, Churchill Livingstone.
53. Wooley JA: Characteristics of thiamin and its relevance to the management of heart failure, *Nutr Clin Pract* 23:487, 2008.
54. Gasteyger C, Suter M, Gaillard RC, et al: Nutritional deficiencies after Roux-en-Y gastric bypass for morbid obesity often cannot be prevented by standard multivitamin supplementation, *Am J Clin Nutr* 87:1128, 2008.
55. McCormick DB: Riboflavin. In Shils ME, Shike M, Olson J, et al, editors: *Modern nutrition in health and disease*, ed 10, Baltimore, 2006, Lippincott Williams & Wilkins.

56. Powers HJ: Riboflavin (vitamin B-2) and health, *Am J Clin Nutr* 77:1352, 2003.
57. Cotton PA, Subar AF, Friday JE, et al: Dietary sources of nutrients among U.S. adults, 1994-1996, *J Am Diet Assoc* 104:921, 2004. Additional tables retrieved November 3, 2004, from www.eatright.org.
58. LaRowe TL, Moeller SM, Adams AK: Beverage patterns, diet quality, and body mass index of US preschool and school-aged children, *J Am Diet Assoc* 107:1124, 2007.
59. Bourgeois C, Cervantes-Laurean D, Moss J: Niacin. In Shils ME, Shike M, Olson J, et al: *Modern nutrition in health and disease*, ed 10, Baltimore, 2006, Lippincott Williams & Wilkins.
60. Guyton JR, Bays HE: Safety considerations with niacin therapy, *Am J Cardiol* 99(Suppl):22C, 2007.
61. Koren G, Maltepe C: Pre-emptive therapy for severe nausea and vomiting of pregnancy and hyperemesis gravidarum, *J Obstet Gynaecol* 24:530, 2004.
62. McCully KS: Homocysteine, vitamins and vascular disease prevention, *Am J Clin Nutr* 86(Suppl):1563S, 2007.
63. Shen J, Lai CQ, Mattei J, et al: Association of vitamin B-6 status with inflammation, oxidative stress, and chronic inflammatory conditions: the Boston Puerto Rican Health Study, *Am J Clin Nutr* 91:337, 2010.
64. Toole JF, Malinow MR, Chambless LE, et al: Lowering homocysteine in patients with ischemic stroke to prevent recurrent stroke, myocardial infarction, and death: the Vitamin Intervention for Stroke Prevention (VISP) randomized trial, *JAMA* 291(5):565, 2004.
65. Woolf K, Manore MM: Elevated plasma homocysteine and low vitamin B-6 status in nonsupplementing older women with rheumatoid arthritis, *J Am Diet Assoc* 108:443, 2008.
66. Morris MS, Picciano MF, Jacques PF, et al: Plasma pyridoxal 5'-phosphate in the US population: the National Health and Nutrition Examination Survey, 2003-2004, *Am J Clin Nutr* 87:1446, 2008.
67. Suitor CD, Bailey LB: Dietary folate equivalents: interpretation and application, *J Am Diet Assoc* 100(1):81, 2000.
68. Gregory JF: Case study: folate bioavailability, *J Nutr* 131:1376S, 2001.
69. Yang Q-H, Carter HK, Mulinare J, et al: Race-ethnicity differences in folic acid intake in women of childbearing age in the United States after folic acid fortification: findings from the National Health and Nutrition Examination Survey, 2001-2002, *Am J Clin Nutr* 85:1409, 2007.
70. Kim Y-I: Folic acid fortification and supplementation—good for some but not so good for others, *Nutr Rev* 65:504, 2007.
71. Solomons NW: Food fortification with folic acid: has the other shoe dropped? *Nutr Rev* 65:512, 2007.
72. Heseker HB, Mason JB, Selhub J, et al: Not all cases of neural-tube defect can be prevented by increasing the intake of folic acid, *Br J Nutr* 102(2):173, 2009.
73. Green TJ, McMahon JA, Skeaff CM, et al: Lowering homocysteine with B vitamins has no effect on biomarkers of bone turnover in older persons: a 2-yr randomized controlled trial, *Am J Clin Nutr* 85:460, 2007.
74. McLean RR, Hannan MT: B vitamins, homocysteine, and bone disease: epidemiology and pathophysiology, *Curr Osteoporos Rep* 5:112, 2007.
75. Ebbing M, Bleie Ø, Ueland PM, et al: Mortality and cardiovascular events in patients treated with homocysteine-lowering B vitamins after coronary angiography: a randomized controlled trial, *JAMA* 300:795, 2008.
76. Jamison RL, Hartigan P, Kaufman JS, et al: Effect of homocysteine lowering on mortality and vascular disease in advanced chronic kidney disease and end-stage renal disease. A randomized controlled trial, *JAMA* 298:1163, 2007.
77. Lonn E: Homocysteine-lowering B vitamin therapy in cardiovascular prevention—wrong again? *JAMA* 299:2086, 2008.
78. Albert CM, Cook NR, Gaziano JM, et al: Effect of folic acid and B vitamins on risk of cardiovascular events and total mortality among women at high risk for cardiovascular disease. A randomized trial, *JAMA* 299:2027, 2008.
79. Aisen PS, Schneider LS, Sano M, et al: High-dose B vitamin supplementation and cognitive decline in Alzheimer disease: a randomized controlled trial, *JAMA* 300:1774, 2008.
80. Carmel R: Cobalamin (Vitamin B_{12}). In Shils ME, Shike M, Olson J, et al: *Modern nutrition in health and disease*, ed 10, Baltimore, 2006, Lippincott Williams & Wilkins.
81. Carmel R: How I treat cobalamin (vitamin B_{12} deficiency), *Blood* 112:2214, 2008.
82. Haan MN, Miller JW, Aiello AE, et al: Homocysteine, B vitamins, and the incidence of dementia and cognitive impairment: results from the Sacramento Area Latino Study on Aging, *Am J Clin Nutr* 85:511, 2007.
83. Morris MS, Jacques PF, Rosenberg IH, et al: Folate and vitamin B-12 status in relation to anemia, macrocytosis, and cognitive impairment in older Americans in the age of folic acid fortification, *Am J Clin Nutr* 85:193, 2007.
84. Johnson MA: If high folic acid aggravates vitamin B_{12} deficiency, what should be done about it? *Nutr Rev* 65:451, 2007.
85. Campbell AK, Miller JW, Green R, et al: Plasma vitamin B_{12} concentrations in an elderly Latino population are predicted by serum gastrin concentrations and crystalline vitamin B_{12} intake, *J Nutr* 133:2770, 2003.
86. Green R: Is it time for vitamin B_{12} fortification? What are the questions? *Am J Clin Nutr* 89(Suppl):712S, 2009.

FURTHER READINGS AND RESOURCES

Readings

Olson BH, Keast DR, Song WO, et al: Effectiveness and safety of folic acid fortification, *Nutr Today* 39(4):169, 2004. *[This article provides insight as to the value and the concerns pertaining to folate fortification of grain foods.]*

Sheth A, Khurana R, Khurana V: Potential liver damage associated with over-the-counter vitamin supplements, *J Am Diet Assoc* 108:1536, 2008. *[Over-the-counter supplements are often perceived by the general public as carrying no risk; these authors point to the dangers of unsupervised self-medication.]*

The following four articles point to community nutrition practice and fruit and vegetable intake:

Akobundu UO, Cohen NL, Laus MJ, et al: Vitamins A and C, calcium, fruit, and dairy products are limited in food pantries, *J Am Diet Assoc* 104:811, 2004. *[Food pantries are a source of emergency foods for many women, children, and families. We need to consider how we can improve the nutrient quality of foods available to them.]*

Boyington JE, Schoster B, Remmes Martin K, et al: Perceptions of individual and community environmental influences on fruit and vegetable intake, North Carolina, 2004, *Prev Chronic Dis* 6:1, 2009. Retrieved July 24, 2009, from www.cdc.gov/pcd/issues/2009/jan/07_0168.htm. *[These authors help us understand how many factors influence fruit and vegetable intake.]*

Robinson-O'Brien R, Storey M, Heim S: Impact of garden-based youth nutrition intervention programs: a review, *J Am Diet Assoc* 109:273, 2009. *[Community gardens not only provide fresh vegetables to families who may otherwise not be able to obtain them but also encourage children to eat what they have helped to grow.]*

Wansink B, Lee K: Cooking habits provide a key to 5 a day success, *J Am Diet Assoc* 104:1648, 2004. *[This author tells us how cooking skills can influence the use of fruits and vegetables.]*

Websites of Interest

National Institutes of Health, National Heart, Lung and Blood Institute: Healthy Eating: *The DASH Eating Plan*. The DASH diet provides advice for selecting fruits and vegetables and helpful recipes for their preparation: http://www.nhlbi.nih.gov/hbp/prevent/h_eating/h_eating.htm.

National Institutes of Health, Office of Dietary Supplements. This site provides fact sheets on all types of dietary supplements including botanicals, vitamins, and minerals, noting functions, strength of related research, food sources, known requirements, contraindications, and potentially harmful drug, nutrient, or herbal interactions: http://ods.od.nih.gov/health_information/health_information.aspx.

Produce for Better Health Foundation. This site provides nutrition education materials and recipes to help consumers eat the recommended five to nine fruits and vegetables each day: http://www.fruitsandveggiesmorematters.org/.

U.S. Department of Agriculture, Center for Nutrition Policy and Promotion: *MyPyramid food guidance system*. These websites describe healthy choices and portion sizes of fruits and vegetables: http://www.mypyramid.gov/.

United States Department of Agriculture, United States Department of Health and Human Services: *Dietary Guidelines for Americans*, 2005, ed 6. The *Dietary Guidelines for Americans* provides important information on choosing fruits and vegetables for good health: http://www.cnpp.usda.gov/dietaryguidelines.htm.

CHAPTER

7

Minerals

Eleanor D. Schlenker

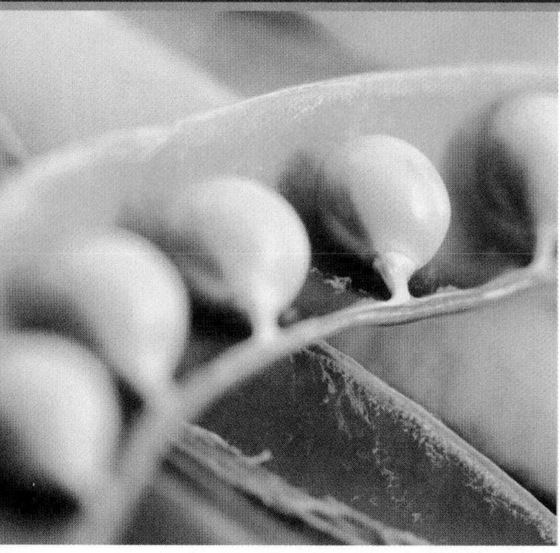

evolve WEBSITE

http://evolve.elsevier.com/Williams/essentials/

CHAPTER OUTLINE

In this chapter we complete our review of the two remaining classes of nutrients—the micronutrient minerals and water. As individual elements, minerals seem simple in comparison with the complex structures of vitamins, but they fulfill equally important roles. New technologies making it possible to measure extremely small quantities of trace minerals in body tissues have opened new opportunities to study the roles of these nutrients and how they may interact with vitamins in maintaining body functions and preventing disease. In time we may identify additional minerals essential to human health.

Minerals having a requirement greater than 100 mg/day are called major minerals, not because they are more important but because more of them are found in the body. Those needed in smaller amounts are called trace elements, and a few required in only minute amounts are referred to as ultratrace elements.

As with the vitamins we will focus on why we need them and how we obtain them.

MINERALS IN HUMAN NUTRITION

Comparison of Vitamins and Minerals

The two classes of micronutrients, vitamins and minerals, have similarities and differences (Table 7-1). Vitamins are complex organic molecules that serve primarily as coenzymes or regulators of body metabolism, especially energy metabolism. Minerals, on the other hand, are simple elements with important roles in both structure and function. As was true for the vitamins, an excess of one mineral cannot remedy a deficit of another, so we need to eat a variety of foods.

Cycle of Minerals

On Earth we live within a vast slow-motion cycle of minerals essential to life. Elements present in water find their way into rocks and soil; through plants they find their way to animals and humans.[1] Until recent times our access to these elements depended on luck—where we happened to live—because

TABLE 7-1 MINERAL AND VITAMIN COMPARISON

CHARACTERISTIC	MINERALS	VITAMINS
Similarities		
Essentiality	Must be obtained in food	Must be obtained in food
Unique role	One cannot take the place of another	One cannot take the place of another
Interactions	Can interfere with another if present in inappropriate amounts	Can interfere with another if present in inappropriate amounts
Impact on chronic disease	May have a role in prevention of chronic disease	May have a role in prevention of chronic disease
Differences		
Structure	Simple organic elements	Complex organic structures
Absorption	Absorption hindered by interfering or binding substances in foods	More easily absorbed
Classification	Based on amount needed by the body	Based on solubility in water or lipid
Roles in body	Structural and metabolic	Primarily metabolic
Relative amount needed	Varies depending on the mineral	Needed in very minute amounts
Stability	Seldom lost in cooking	Easily lost in cooking

most people obtained all of their food from nearby farms. However, with expanding knowledge of how these elements are incorporated into foods, plus the fact that much of the food we eat is grown outside of our immediate community, people living in all parts of the world have the potential to receive adequate mineral nutrition.

Metabolic Roles

Differing Functions

The roles of minerals are as varied as the elements themselves. They participate in an impressive array of structural and metabolic activities:

- *Structural:* Calcium and phosphorus give strength to bones and body frame. Iron provides the core for the *heme* in hemoglobin that carries oxygen to the tissues. Red cobalt is the atom at the center of the vitamin B_{12} molecule.
- *Metabolic:* Ionized sodium and potassium exercise control over body water. Iodine is a necessary constituent of the thyroid hormones that set the rate of metabolism in the cells. Iron is a coenzyme in the mitochondrial oxidase system that supplies our bodies with energy.

Some minerals such as iron contribute to structure and function. Far from being static and inert, minerals are active participants in many systems that support life.

Differing Amounts

Minerals differ from vitamins in the amounts needed to complete their tasks. Vitamins are required in very small amounts, but minerals vary depending on function. A man weighing 150 lb has nearly 3 lb of calcium in his body, most of which is in the skeleton. This same adult contains only about 3 g (1⁄10 oz) of iron, found mainly in the hemoglobin of red blood cells.

Concept of Bioavailability

In general, minerals are absorbed less efficiently than vitamins. The amount of mineral in a food as determined by laboratory analysis may not be the amount that can be absorbed. The term bioavailability refers to the proportion of a food nutrient that can be absorbed successfully and used in body functions.[2] Bioavailability is influenced by the food source and the recipient, as follows:

- *Binding substances:* In some plants, minerals are bound in chemical complexes and not easily released. Oxalates in green leafy vegetables and phytates in grains bind minerals and prevent their absorption.
- *Gastric acidity:* Most minerals are better absorbed in an acidic environment.
- *Chemical form:* Iron cannot be absorbed in the ferric form; it must first be reduced to ferrous iron for absorption to take place.
- *Other foods in the meal:* Some foods such as tea contain substances that interfere with the absorption of certain minerals.
- *Body need:* Various minerals such as iron are absorbed at higher rates in periods of active growth, pregnancy, and lactation.

Bioavailability issues make it difficult to set dietary recommendations for minerals.

Classification

The essential minerals are organized into two groups: (1) major minerals and (2) trace elements.

Major Minerals

The seven minerals present in the body in large amounts, the major minerals, are (1) calcium, (2) phosphorus, (3) magnesium, (4) sodium, (5) potassium, (6) sulfur, and (7) chloride.

Trace Elements

Trace elements are present in the body in very small amounts, and ten are essential for human body function and health. Various other trace elements have been identified as necessary for animals but at this time are not known to be required for humans.

BOX 7-1 ESSENTIAL MAJOR MINERALS AND TRACE ELEMENTS

Major Minerals (Required Intake ≥100 mg/day)

Calcium (Ca)	Potassium (K)
Phosphorus (P)	Chloride (Cl)
Magnesium (Mg)	Sulfur (S)
Sodium (Na)	

Trace Elements (Required Intake <100 mg/day)

Iron (Fe)	Chromium (Cr)
Iodine (I)	Cobalt (Co)
Zinc (Zn)	Selenium (Se)
Copper (Cu)	Molybdenum (Mo)
Manganese (Mn)	Fluoride (F)

The minerals (and their chemical symbols) are listed in Box 7-1. We will review five areas related to these minerals: (1) regulation of absorption, (2) physiologic function, (3) clinical applications, (4) daily requirement, and (5) food sources.

MAJOR MINERALS

CALCIUM

Of all the minerals in the body, calcium is present in the largest amount. The adult woman contains about 1000 g (2.2 lb) of calcium, and the adult man contains about 1200 g (2.6 lb). Total body calcium reflects the constant interchange of calcium supplied in food or supplements, calcium stores in the skeleton, and urinary calcium loss. Calcium balance is applied at three levels: (1) the intake-absorption-excretion balance, (2) the bone-blood balance, and (3) the calcium-phosphorus blood serum balance.

Intake-Absorption-Excretion Balance

Calcium Intake

National surveys indicate that barely 1 in 4 Americans takes in the suggested amounts of calcium, and women and girls have lower intakes than men and boys.[3] Young adult women consume about 784 mg/day, and young adult men about 1098 mg (the Adequate Intake [AI] for these groups is 1000 mg).[3] Milk, cheese, and bread with added nonfat milk powder contribute the most calcium in the typical U.S. diet.[4] Mexican Americans and African Americans are less likely to meet their calcium needs with food and are less likely to take supplements.[5]

Skeletal growth in childhood and adolescence creates a tremendous demand for calcium,[6–8] because 40% of lifetime bone mass is developed in the 3 to 4 years of the adolescent growth spurt.[6] During these periods of maximal bone growth, calcium needs may actually exceed the AI.[7] Boys have an increased need for calcium based on their larger body size and appear to be more efficient in absorption and retention.[8] If calcium intake is low or primary sources have low bioavailability, then bone growth is compromised. This has lifelong effects for some women: Caucasian women reporting low milk intake as children and adolescents had lower bone mass and were more likely to experience hip fractures in later life, although in African-American women early intake appeared to have less influence.[9]

Calcium Absorption

Calcium absorption ranges from 20% to 60% of intake but decreases with age.[10] Absorption takes place in the small intestine, chiefly the duodenum. Here the gastric acidity is still effective, but as the food mass moves along the intestine, it is buffered by pancreatic juices and becomes more alkaline, limiting calcium absorption.

Factors Increasing Calcium Absorption. The following factors increase calcium absorption:

- *Vitamin D hormone:* Vitamin D is necessary for the active transport of calcium. Calcitriol, the vitamin D hormone, controls the synthesis of a calcium-binding protein that carries the mineral across the mucosal cell and into the blood.[10]
- *Body need:* Physiologic conditions over the life cycle—growth, pregnancy, lactation, and older age—strongly influence the rate of absorption. Absorption is higher in times of greatest need, such as the adolescent growth spurt. Calcium absorption is greatly reduced in older persons.[11]
- *Dietary protein and carbohydrate:* Optimal protein intake supports bone health and increases calcium absorption.[12] High intakes of meat protein and the related acid production in the kidneys were thought to increase urinary calcium, but this remains controversial. Soy protein is proposed to have a favorable effect on calcium balance through the action of its phytoestrogens with estrogen-like activity.[13] Lactose enhances calcium absorption through the action of the intestinal bacteria *Lactobacilli*, which produce lactic acid and lower intestinal pH.
- *Acidic environment:* Lower pH or a more acidic environment favors the solubility of calcium and enhances absorption.

Factors Decreasing Calcium Absorption. The following factors decrease calcium absorption:

- *Vitamin D deficiency:* A lack of vitamin D or inability to form the active vitamin D hormone calcitriol depresses absorption.
- *Fat malabsorption*: Excessive amounts of fatty acids remaining in the small intestine combine with calcium to form insoluble soaps that cannot be absorbed.
- *Fiber and other binding agents:* Dietary fiber can bind calcium and hinder its absorption. Other binding agents include *oxalic acid* and *phytic acid.* Oxalic acid is found in varying amounts in green leafy vegetables, so some are better sources of calcium than others. The outer hull of many cereal grains, especially wheat, contains phytates.
- *Alkaline environment:* Calcium is insoluble at a high pH (alkaline medium) and poorly absorbed.

KEY TERMS

hemoglobin Oxygen-carrying pigment in red blood cells.

bioavailability Amount of a nutrient in a food that is absorbed and available to the body for metabolic use.

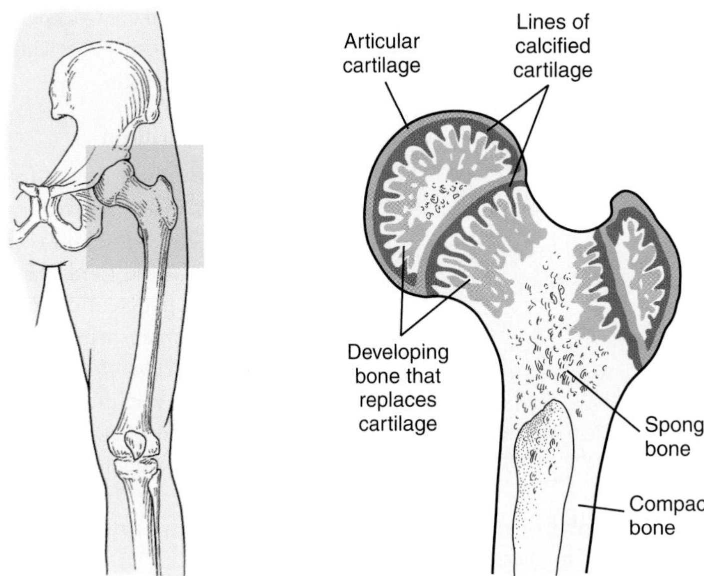

FIGURE 7-1 Bone and cartilage development.

Calcium Excretion

Calcium balance is controlled primarily at the point of absorption, as is the case for various minerals. A large proportion of dietary calcium—50% to 90% depending on body need—remains unabsorbed and is eliminated in the feces. A small amount of calcium, about 200 mg/day, is excreted in the urine to maintain normal levels in body fluids.

Bone-Blood Balance

Calcium in the Bones

The skeleton is the major site of calcium storage. Bones and teeth contain about 99% of body calcium, but these tissues are not static. Bone is constantly being built and reshaped according to period of growth and hormonal influences (Figure 7-1). As much as 700 mg of calcium enters and leaves the bones each day. Under certain conditions withdrawals exceed deposits. Immobility from a body cast or the bone disease osteoporosis results in excessive calcium withdrawal and loss.

Calcium in the Blood

The small amount of body calcium that is not in bone—about 1%—circulates in the blood and other body fluids. Blood calcium exists in two forms:

1. *Bound calcium:* About 40% of the calcium in the blood is bound to plasma proteins and not *diffusible,* that is, not able to move into cells or enter into other activities.
2. *Free ionized calcium:* Free calcium carrying an electrical charge moves about unhindered and diffuses through membranes to control body functions. Free calcium accomplishes a great deal of metabolic work because it is in an activated form.

Calcium-Phosphorus Serum Balance

The final level of calcium balance is the calcium-phosphorus balance in the blood. These two minerals maintain a defined relationship based on their relative solubility. The calcium-phosphorus serum balance is the solubility product of calcium and phosphorus expressed in milligrams per deciliter (mg/dL). Normal calcium serum levels are 10 mg/dL in children and adults. For phosphorus, normal levels are 4 mg/dL in adults and 5 mg/dL in children. Thus the normal serum calcium-phosphorus solubility products are $10 \times 4 = 40$ in adults and $10 \times 5 = 50$ in children. Any situation that increases the serum phosphorus level will decrease the serum calcium level to keep the calcium-phosphorus solubility product constant. A drop in serum calcium interferes with important functions such as muscle contraction.

The three hormones that work together to maintain calcium balance are parathyroid hormone (PTH), the vitamin D hormone calcitriol, and the hormone calcitonin. The cooperative action of these three hormones is an example of the synergism among metabolic control agents:

1. *Parathyroid hormone (PTH):* The parathyroid glands lying adjacent to the thyroid glands are particularly sensitive to changes in the blood level of free ionized calcium. When ionized calcium levels begin to fall, PTH is released and restores the levels to normal by the following actions:
   - Stimulates the intestinal mucosa to absorb more calcium
   - Rapidly withdraws calcium from bone
   - Increases calcium reabsorption and phosphorus excretion by the kidneys
2. *Vitamin D hormone (calcitriol):* Calcitriol cooperates with PTH to control the absorption of calcium in the small intestine and regulate the deposit of calcium and phosphorus in bone. Calcitriol exerts more control on calcium absorption and its deposit in bone, and PTH exerts more control on calcium withdrawal from bone and kidney excretion of phosphorus.
3. *Calcitonin:* Calcitonin is produced by special C cells in the thyroid gland. It prevents an abnormal rise in serum calcium by modulating the release of bone calcium. Thus

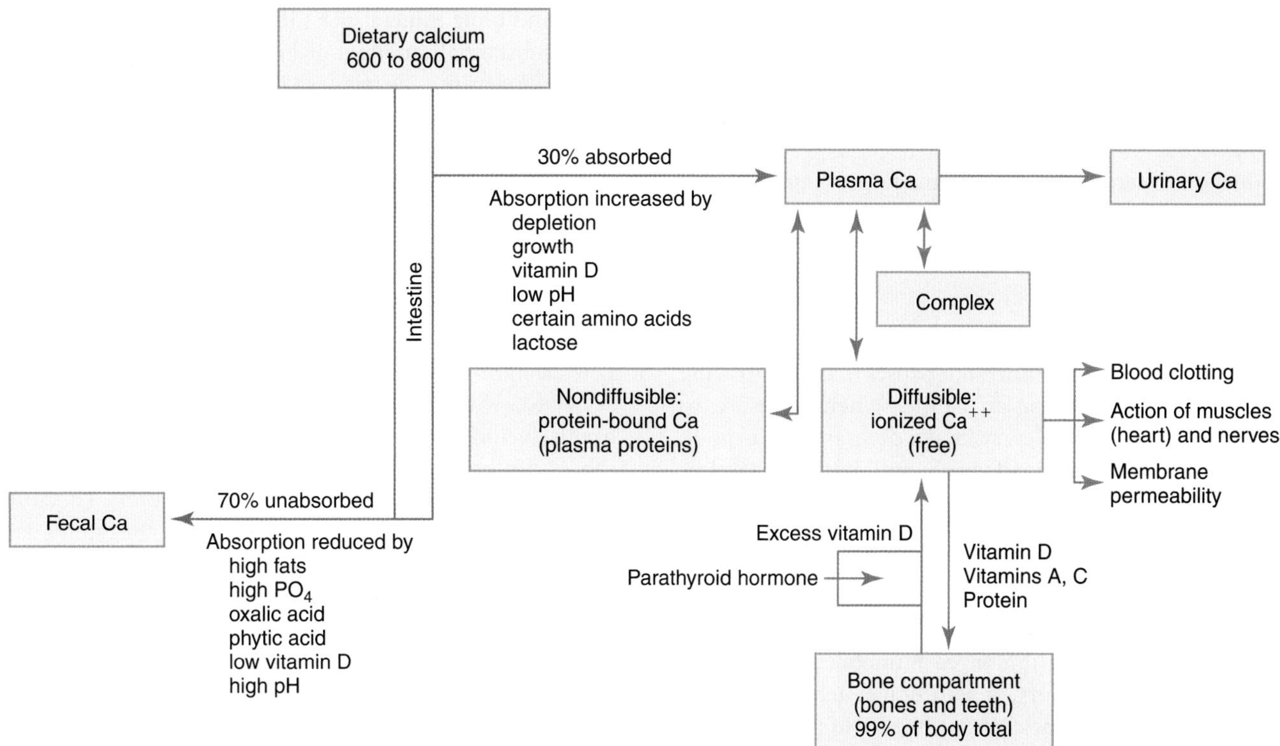

FIGURE 7-2 Calcium metabolism. Note the relative distribution of calcium in the body.

its action counterbalances that of PTH to keep serum calcium at normal levels. The overall relationship of the factors involved in calcium balance and regulation is illustrated in Figure 7-2.

Physiologic Functions of Calcium

Bone Formation

Calcium, along with phosphorus, provides strength and rigidity to the skeleton. Building and maintaining bone mass is accomplished through the action of specialized cells that handle the deposit and withdrawal of bone calcium.

Tooth Formation

Special organs in the gums deposit calcium to form teeth, and this mineral exchange continues as in bone. Calcium deposit and withdrawal occur mainly in the dentin and cementum. Very little exchange occurs in the enamel once the tooth is formed.

General Metabolic Functions

The relatively small amount of body calcium in blood and body fluids has an amazing number of physiologic roles:

- *Blood clotting:* Serum calcium ions are required for the cross-linking of fibrin, giving stability to the fibrin threads.
- *Nerve transmission:* A current of calcium ions triggers the flow of signals from one nerve cell to another. Calcium ions in cells of the cardiac muscle direct the nerve signals to these fibers.
- *Muscle contraction and relaxation:* Ionized serum calcium initiates the contraction of muscle fibers and controls their return to steady state. Calcium ions released into the cytoplasm of the muscle cell create the attractive forces between actin and myosin that result in the contraction of the muscle fiber. This action of calcium is particularly critical to the constant contraction-relaxation cycle of the heart muscle. Calcium channel blockers slow heart action by preventing this release of calcium.
- *Cell membrane permeability:* Ionized calcium controls the passage of fluids and solutes across cell membranes by its effect on the intercellular membrane cement.
- *Enzyme activation:* Calcium ions activate certain cell enzymes, particularly those that release energy for muscle contraction. They have a similar role with protein-splitting enzymes and the lipase enzyme that digests fat.

KEY TERMS

osteoporosis The abnormal loss of bone mineral and matrix leading to porous, fragile bone tissue with enlarged spaces that is prone to fracture or deformity; common disease of aging in both men and women.

calcitonin A polypeptide hormone secreted by the C cells in the thyroid gland in response to hypercalcemia, which lowers calcium and phosphate levels in the blood.

synergism The joint action of two or more agents in which the total effect of their combined action is greater than the sum of their individual actions (adjective: synergistic).

solutes Particles of a substance in solution; a solution consists of a solute and a dissolving medium (solvent), usually a liquid.

Clinical Applications

Disruption of the physiologic and metabolic functions of calcium is associated with several clinical problems.

Tetany

A reduction in serum ionized calcium causes *tetany*, marked by severe, intermittent spastic muscle contractions and muscular pain. Seizures and convulsions ensue if the situation is not corrected.

Rickets and Osteomalacia

A deficiency of vitamin D hormone causes *rickets* in growing children and *osteomalacia* in adults. When exposure to sunlight is limited and dietary intake of vitamin D is poor, calcium absorption is inadequate and bone mineral is lost. (See Chapter 6 to review vitamin D and its deficiency diseases.)

Resorptive Hypercalciuria and Renal Calculi

Resorption of calcium from bone and its excretion in the urine accelerates during prolonged immobilization. A full-body cast, spinal cord injury, or body brace after a back injury decreases the normal muscle tension needed to preserve bone. The subsequent rise in urinary calcium increases the risk of renal stones.

Calcium and Health

Bone Disease

A calcium-related condition increasing in prevalence in the United States is osteoporosis, estimated to affect 4 to 6 million women and 1 to 2 million men. With advancing age and loss of bone mineral, bones become progressively more fragile, with increasing risk of fractures, physical disability, mortality, and enormous costs.[14] Loss of the steroid hormones estrogen and testosterone bring about alterations in calcium balance and changes in bone structure (Figure 7-3).[14–16] In women, bone loss accelerates after menopause; in men, testosterone levels and bone mineral mass decline gradually in later life. Once substantial amounts of bone are lost, treatment with drug regimens may be required to lower the risk of fracture.[14] Nutrition education of parents and caregivers promoting adequate intake of calcium need to begin in infancy and continued through childhood and adolescence as bones are being formed and mineralized.[6,17] Low calcium intake with poor bone mineral deposition in youth has implications for bone health in later life.

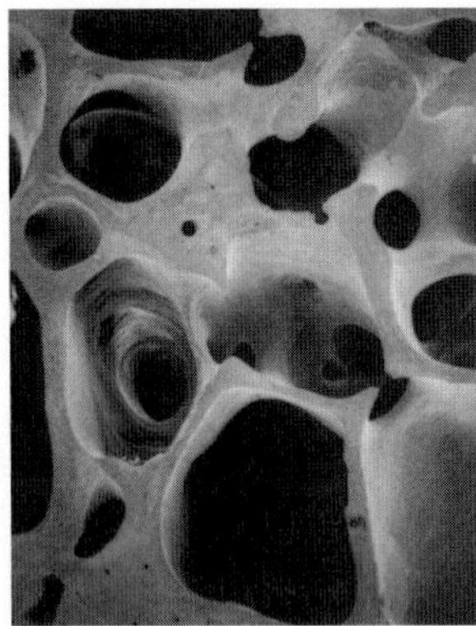
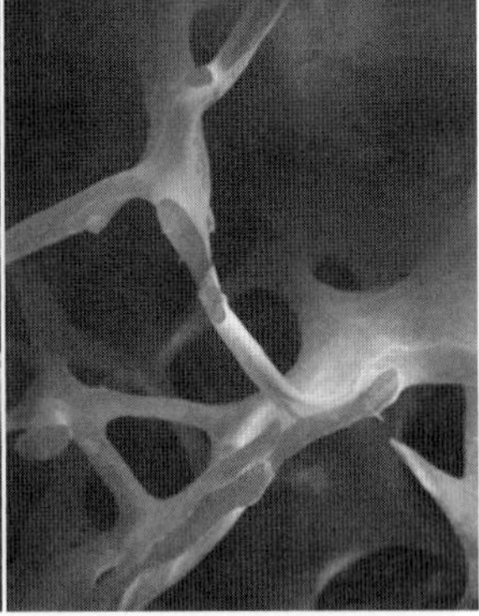

Normal bone — Bone with osteoporosis

FIGURE 7-3 Comparison of normal and osteoporotic spongy bone. Scanning electron micrograph (SEM) of **A,** normal bone, and **B,** bone with osteoporosis. Note the loss of trabeculae and appearance of enlarged pores in the osteoporotic bone. (From Kumar V, Abbas A, Fausto N: *Robbins basic pathology,* ed 7, Philadelphia, 2002, Saunders.)

Metabolic Disease

Low calcium intake or limited use of dairy foods has been associated with other chronic problems unrelated to bone health, including obesity, hypertension, and certain types of cancer. Unfortunately, conflicting evidence exists regarding the role of calcium in preventing these conditions. The source of calcium (supplements versus dairy foods), the type of dairy food (high-fat or low-fat milk, yogurt, or cheese), and other nutrients found in dairy foods such as magnesium, potassium, or vitamin D, as well as unknown nutritional factors could contribute to this lack of agreement.[18,19]

- *Weight gain/body fatness:* The capacity of calcium or calcium-containing foods to assist in weight management appears to vary according to gender and ethnicity.[18–20] Women taking calcium and vitamin D supplements were less likely to gain weight than men,[18] and African-American adults benefited more from use of dairy foods than Caucasian adults.[19] Weight reduction regimens can lead to serious bone loss if optimum calcium intakes are not maintained.[21,22]
- *Hypertension:* Calcium has a role in controlling blood pressure but likely does not work alone. More servings of dairy foods[23] resulting in higher intakes of calcium and potassium[24] are associated with modest reductions in blood pressure.
- *Cancer:* Researchers are continuing to examine the relationship between calcium and cancer and the possible role of vitamin D.[25] Risk of all cancers was lower in postmenopausal women,[26] and colorectal cancer risk was lower in middle-aged men,[27] with higher intakes of calcium.

Overall evidence points to potential benefits from calcium intakes approaching the suggested level. Public health initiatives directed toward availability and selection of calcium-rich foods could affect the future health care costs of our aging population.

Calcium Requirement

Dietary Reference Intake

Increasing concerns about the calcium required for lifetime maintenance of healthy bones led to the current Dietary Reference Intake (DRI).[11] For youth ages 9 to 18, the AI of 1300 mg/day ensures maximum deposition of bone calcium. Men and women ages 19 to 50 should take in 1000 mg/day to maintain positive calcium balance; in those older than age 50, 1200 mg of calcium per day is needed to support bone health and prevent bone loss. Intakes greater than the Tolerable Upper Intake Level (UL) of 2500 mg/day can inhibit the absorption of other important minerals or lead to kidney insufficiency and milk alkali syndrome.

Food Sources of Calcium

Calcium is present in a highly available form in dairy products, making these foods ideal sources. One quart of cow's milk supplies 1200 mg of calcium along with 10 mg (400 IU) of vitamin D. Most commercial yogurt also has vitamin D added. Green leafy vegetables, broccoli, legumes, nuts, and grains contain calcium, but oxalic acid and phytates can compromise bioavailability. Calcium-fortified soy milk, juices, and cereals can meet calcium needs of the lactose intolerant. Aged cheeses such as cheddar or Swiss, also good sources of calcium, are low in lactose. (See Box 7-2 for food servings equivalent in calcium to 8 oz of milk.) It is important to emphasize low-calorie, low-fat, or nonfat dairy foods to young women for whom weight gain is a major concern.[28] Box 7-3 suggests more food sources of calcium.

BOX 7-2 COMPARISON OF CALCIUM FOOD SOURCES

Each of the following foods supplies approximately 300 mg of calcium. Those who are lactose intolerant can obtain their calcium from sources other than milk or dairy foods.

- Milk (8 oz)
- Yogurt (8 oz)
- Cheddar cheese (1½ oz)
- Calcium-fortified soy milk (8 oz)
- Calcium-fortified orange juice (8 oz)
- Frozen cooked spinach (1 cup)
- Cooked white beans (1½ cups)
- Tofu (5 oz)

BOX 7-3 FOOD SOURCES OF CALCIUM

FOOD SOURCE	QUANTITY	CALCIUM (in mg)
Grains Group		
Fortified ready-to-eat cereals		
Total	¾ cup	1000
All Bran	½ cup	117
Cheerios	1 cup	122
Bread, white	1 slice	38
Vegetable Group		
Vegetable juice, fortified	8 fl oz	300
Collard greens, boiled	1 cup	266
Potato, baked, with 2 tbsp shredded cheese	1 medium	132
Kale, frozen, boiled	1 cup	179
Broccoli, raw	1 cup	61
Fruit Group		
Orange juice, fortified	8 fl oz	300
Figs, dried	2	62
Meat, Beans, Eggs, and Nuts Group		
Soybeans, boiled	1 cup	175
Almonds, roasted	1 oz	75
Milk Group		
Yogurt, whole milk	8 fl oz	275
Milk, skim, low fat, whole	8 fl oz	302
Soy milk, fortified with calcium	8 fl oz	300
Fats, Oils, and Sugars Group		
These foods do not supply calcium.		

Adequate Intake (AI) for adults: ages 19 to 50, 1000 mg; ages ≥51, 1200 mg.
Nutrient data from USDA: *USDA National Nutrient Database for Standard Reference, Release 21,* Washington, DC, U.S. Department of Agriculture, 2009. Retrieved April 23, 2010 from http://www.ars.usda.gov/Services/docs.htm?docid=17477.

TABLE 7-2 CHOOSING A CALCIUM SUPPLEMENT

CHARACTERISTIC	RECOMMENDATION
Amount of elemental calcium present	Calcium compounds contain different amounts of elemental calcium. Calcium carbonate is 40% calcium by weight, but calcium citrate is only 21% calcium; you would need twice as many tablets of calcium citrate to get the same amount of calcium.
Absorption	Calcium carbonate, calcium citrate, and calcium citrate malate (the form found in fortified juices) are all well absorbed; calcium citrate is better absorbed than calcium carbonate when gastric acid is low.
Purity	Do not use supplements made from bone meal, oyster shell, or dolomite because they may contain lead or other toxic elements; coral calcium may contain lead and mercury. Look for a well-known brand of pharmaceuticals or check for the USP *(United States Pharmacopeia)* symbol or the word *purified.*
Dose	Calcium is absorbed best when taken in doses of 500 mg or less; depending on need, take divided doses of 500 mg each rather than one dose of 1000 mg.
When best taken	Calcium carbonate is best absorbed with food; calcium citrate can be taken anytime.
Combination products	Some calcium supplements are combined with other nutrients such as phosphorus, magnesium, or vitamin D; phosphorus is readily available in the U.S. diet and not needed in supplements. Unless vitamin D is being provided in another supplement, it could be included here.
Potential interactions	Calcium can decrease the absorption of various medications including digoxin, phenytoin, and tetracycline, and it interacts with thiazide and similar diuretics. Medications to be taken on an empty stomach should not be taken with a calcium supplement. Persons on prescription or over-the-counter medications should check with their physician or pharmacist before adding a supplement.
Form	Calcium supplements are available as tablets, gel capsules, liquids, and chewables; liquids and chewables might be helpful for those with difficulty in swallowing.
Ability to dissolve in the stomach	Chewables and liquids are broken down before they enter the stomach. To test a tablet, place one in warm water for 30 minutes and stir occasionally; if it has not dissolved in this time, then it likely will not dissolve in the stomach.

Data from National Institute of Arthritis and Musculoskeletal and Skin Diseases: *Calcium supplements: what to look for,* Washington, DC, 2005, National Institutes of Health, U.S. Department of Health and Human Services. Retrieved August 18, 2009, from *www.niams.nih.gov/bone/hi/calcium_supp.htm;* Office of Dietary Supplements: *Dietary supplement fact sheet: calcium,* Washington, DC, 2005, National Institutes of Health, U.S. Department of Health and Human Services. Retrieved August 18, 2009, from *www.ods.od.nih.gov/factsheets/calcium.asp;* Blumberg S: Is coral calcium a safe and effective supplement? *J Am Diet Assoc* 104:1335, 2004.

Calcium Supplements

Many persons cannot or will not consume enough calcium-rich foods to meet their requirements and need supplements. Table 7-2 proposes criteria to be considered in the selection of a calcium supplement and suggestions for use. To help meet all dietary requirements, it is best to obtain at least half your daily calcium from food that will supply other important nutrients in addition to calcium. (For more discussion on calcium and bone health see the *Evidence-Based Practice* box, "Restoring Lost Bone: Are Drugs Always Needed?")

PHOSPHORUS

Phosphorus is closely associated with body calcium, although it has some unique characteristics and functions of its own. The adult human body contains about 850 g (1.9 lb) of phosphorus, with 85% in the skeleton, 14% in the soft tissues, and the remaining 1% in extracellular fluids (ECFs) and cell membranes. Phosphorus makes up about 1% of body weight.

Absorption-Excretion Balance

Absorption

Free phosphate is absorbed along the entire length of the small intestine. Absorption is regulated by the vitamin D hormone calcitriol and phosphate carrier proteins.[29] Phosphorus exists in food as a phosphate compound joined with calcium and must be split off as a free mineral to be absorbed. An excess of other minerals such as aluminum or iron or calcium depresses phosphorus absorption. Phytates in whole grains prevent its absorption.

Excretion

Phosphorus is excreted via the kidneys, which help regulate serum phosphorus levels. Usually 85% to 95% of the plasma phosphate filtered by the renal glomeruli is reabsorbed along with calcium under the influence of vitamin D hormone. However, when phosphate must be excreted to preserve the normal serum calcium-phosphorus balance, PTH overrides vitamin D hormone and increases excretion.

Bone-Blood-Cell Balance

Bone

About 80% to 90% of body phosphorus is in the skeleton and teeth combined with calcium. Bone phosphorus is in constant interchange with the phosphorus in blood and other body fluids.

Blood

The normal range for serum phosphorus in adults is 3.0 mg/dL to 4.5 mg/dL; levels less than 2.5 mg/dL or greater than 5.0 mg/dL demand immediate medical attention.[29] High phosphorus intakes leading to elevated serum levels stimulate PTH

EVIDENCE-BASED PRACTICE

Restoring Lost Bone: Are Drugs Always Needed?

The aging of our population has brought new attention to age-related bone loss and the financial and human cost of osteoporosis and bone fracture. Hip fractures are the most serious injuries, leading to loss of independence in 10% to 20% of patients and increasing risk of death. Bone health has moved into the forefront as a current public health problem, and new drugs have been introduced to treat bone loss. However, are there alternatives to these treatments?

Although it would seem that increasing daily intakes of calcium would stem the loss of bone mineral mass, the answer has not been that simple. Increases in the Adequate Intake (AI) for calcium attempted to address this problem, but the evidence for improved bone health has been mixed. Other factors such as adequate vitamin D to enable calcium absorption and compliance with suggested calcium intake have likely added to the differing results. Researchers have also looked at the responses of both women and men; men in their eighth and ninth decades become increasingly vulnerable to bone fracture.

Postmenopausal women and older men given 1000 to 1200 mg of calcium daily in the form of a well-absorbed supplement were monitored for 1 to 5 years, and their bone mineral mass was compared with that of individuals of similar age who were given a **placebo**. Participants receiving the calcium had an increase in bone mass of 1% to 2% at the wrist, vertebrae, and hip, whereas those given the placebo showed no gain in bone calcium and in most cases decreased in bone mineral density. Although any gain in bone mineral mass would forestall reaching the lower threshold where bone fracture is likely to occur, calcium supplementation was more effective in reducing forearm and vertebral fractures than hip fractures. However, Prince and colleagues carried their evaluation one step further—they separated out the findings from the women who consumed at least 80% of their calcium supplements from those who were less compliant, and the outcomes were different. The group who took their supplements regularly had about one third fewer hip fractures than those who did not. Supplements of vitamin D also affected outcome. Older adults who took a vitamin D supplement along with their calcium supplement were less likely to suffer a hip fracture; however, vitamin D was not effective in preventing fractures unless given along with calcium.

In summary, calcium intakes meeting the AI for older adults (1200 mg/day) *when consumed regularly* along with the recommended level of vitamin D appear to slow bone loss and reduce fracture risk. Increasing calcium intake affects bone health in several ways. First, more available calcium entering the blood effectively lowers parathyroid hormone (PTH) levels and the resorption of bone calcium. Overall bone turnover slows, less bone is lost, and less calcium is excreted in the urine. Adequate vitamin D not only ensures the absorption of dietary calcium but also exerts a direct effect on bone, increasing deposition and decreasing loss.

So what advice do we give to those we care for?

- Maintain a consistent intake of 1200 mg calcium each day. If you use supplements, then put them in a prominent place and establish a regular schedule for when you take them.
- Maintain an intake of 600 to 800 IU of vitamin D each day; choose fortified foods or calcium supplements that also supply vitamin D.
- Ask your physician for help in choosing calcium and vitamin D supplements.
- Try to maintain the highest level of physical activity possible; calcium supplements were found to be more effective in those with regular physical activity.
- Have a bone scan on a regular basis to monitor bone status before a fracture occurs.

For those individuals who have already lost significant bone mass and are at immediate risk of bone fracture, drug intervention may be required. Meeting target intakes of calcium and vitamin D during adulthood may help prevent such losses.

BIBLIOGRAPHY

Bischoff-Ferrari HA, Dawson-Hughes B, Baron JA, et al: Calcium intake and hip fracture risk in men and women: a meta-analysis of prospective cohort studies and randomized controlled trials, *Am J Clin Nutr* 86:1780, 2007.

Boonen S, Lips P, Bouillon R, et al: Need for additional calcium to reduce the risk of hip fracture with vitamin D supplementation: evidence from a comparative meta-analysis of randomized control trials, *J Clin Endocrinol Metab* 92:1415, 2007.

Prince RL, Devine A, Dhaliwal SS, et al: Effects of calcium supplementation on clinical fracture and bone structure: results of a 5-year, double-blind, placebo-controlled trial in elderly women, *Arch Intern Med* 166:869, 2006.

Reid IR, Mason B, Horne A, et al: Randomized controlled trial of calcium in healthy older women, *Am J Med* 119:777, 2006.

Reid IR, Ames R, Mason B, et al: Randomized controlled trial of calcium supplementation in healthy, nonosteoporotic, older men, *Arch Intern Med* 168:2276, 2008.

Zhu K, Devine A, Dick IM, et al: Effects of calcium and vitamin D supplementation on hip bone mineral density and calcium-related analytes in elderly ambulatory Australian women: a five-year randomized controlled trial, *J Clin Endocrinol Metab* 93:743, 2008.

release and mobilization of bone calcium to restore the serum calcium-phosphorus balance to normal. Aluminum-containing antacids bind phosphorus and lower serum levels.[29]

Cells

In its active phosphate form, phosphorus works with proteins, lipids, and carbohydrates to produce energy, build and repair tissues, and act as a buffer to maintain appropriate pH.

KEY TERMS

placebo An inert and nonharmful substance such as sugar used in clinical studies testing the effects of particular drugs, nutrients, herbs, or other substances on body function and well-being. Comparisons of the group receiving the active substance with the group receiving the placebo helps control for any psychologic or unrelated effects that might have influenced the study outcomes.

Hormonal Controls

Because calcium and phosphorus work closely together, phosphorus balance is under the control of two hormones that also control calcium balance—(1) vitamin D hormone and (2) PTH. Phosphate depletion results from (1) low intake; (2) poor absorption, usually caused by an interfering substance such as phytate or aluminum; or (3) excessive wasting by the kidney.

Physiologic Functions

Bone and Tooth Formation

Phosphorus helps build bones and teeth. As a component of calcium phosphate, it is constantly deposited and resorbed in the continuing process of bone formation and remodeling.

General Metabolic Activities

Phosphorus is found in every living cell, where it participates in overall metabolism. Several specific activities are described below:

- *Absorption of glucose and glycerol:* Phosphorus combines with these molecules to assist their absorption from the intestine. Phosphorus also promotes the reabsorption of glucose in the renal tubules.
- *Transport of fatty acids:* Phospholipids transport fats in the blood.
- *Energy metabolism:* Phosphorus-containing compounds such as adenosine triphosphate (ATP) are high-energy storage molecules that meet instant demands for energy.
- *Buffer system:* The buffer system of phosphoric acid and phosphate helps maintain blood acid-base balance.

Clinical Applications

Changes in the normal serum phosphorus level occur under various circumstances, as follows:

- *Recovery from diabetic acidosis:* Active carbohydrate absorption and metabolism place a high demand on serum phosphorus, causing temporary hypophosphatemia. (Phosphate is combined with glucose in the formation of glycogen.)
- *Growth:* Children have higher serum phosphate levels related to their high levels of growth hormone.
- *Hypophosphatemia:* Low serum phosphorus levels occur with intestinal diseases such as sprue and celiac disease that hinder phosphorus absorption. Excessive secretion of PTH (primary hyperparathyroidism) causes inappropriate excretion of phosphorus and hypophosphatemia. Low serum phosphorus may accompany the refeeding syndrome often seen in the first days of nutritional repletion of a severely wasted patient, when glycogen stores are being rapidly replenished. One symptom of hypophosphatemia is muscle weakness, because cells are deprived of the phosphorus needed for energy metabolism. If left untreated, then it will lead to metabolic acidosis, heart failure, and sudden death.[30]
- *Hyperphosphatemia:* In renal failure and hypoparathyroidism, excess phosphate accumulates in the serum. This causes the serum calcium level to drop, resulting in tetany.

Phosphorus Requirement

Dietary Reference Intake

The Recommended Dietary Allowance (RDA) for phosphorus is 1250 mg/day for those ages 9 to 18 years and 700 mg/day for all adults over age 18. At one time the relative intake of calcium to phosphorus was considered important in building and remodeling bone. Higher intakes of phosphorus than calcium were believed to hinder bone mineral deposition. More recently we learned that sufficient amounts of both nutrients is more important than their ratio to each other.[11] Because both minerals are found in many of the same foods, meeting calcium needs will likely provide adequate phosphorus.

Food Sources of Phosphorus

Milk and milk products contain significant amounts of phosphorus. Because phosphorus is important in muscle metabolism, lean meats are a good source. Phosphorus-containing food additives and the high phosphorus content of soft drinks add this mineral to the American diet.

SODIUM

Sodium, the major cation in the ECF, is one of the most plentiful minerals in the body. The average adult contains approximately 100 g (3.5 oz) of sodium. About half circulates in the ECF as free ionized sodium, 40% is found in bone, and 10% resides inside the cell.

Absorption-Excretion Balance

Absorption

Sodium is easily absorbed in the small intestine; usually no more than 2% remains to be excreted in the feces.

Excretion

The major route of excretion is through the kidneys under the control of **aldosterone,** the sodium-conserving hormone produced in the adrenal cortex. For individuals in temperate climates with a steady state of fluid and sodium balance, urinary sodium excretion is about equal to intake. Sodium is lost in sweat during exercise or in hot environments.

Physiologic Functions of Sodium

Water Balance

Ionized sodium is the major guardian of the body water outside the cells. Differences in the sodium concentrations of body

KEY TERMS

aldosterone Hormone from the cortex of the adrenal glands that acts on the distal renal tubule to reabsorb sodium in exchange for potassium; the aldosterone mechanism conserves sodium and also water, because water absorption follows sodium reabsorption.

fluids largely determine the distribution of water via osmosis from one area to another.

Acid-Base Balance

In cooperation with chloride and bicarbonate ions, ionized sodium helps regulate acid-base balance.

Cell Permeability

The sodium pump located in all cell membranes controls the passage of materials in and out of the cell. Potassium is moved into the cell, and sodium is moved out of the cell. Glucose also moves into the cell via this active transport system.

Muscle Action

Sodium ions help transmit electrochemical impulses along nerve and muscle membranes. Potassium and sodium ions work together to balance the response of nerves to stimulation and control the flow of nerve impulses to muscles and contraction of muscle fibers.

Sodium Requirement

Dietary Reference Intake

The body can adjust to a wide range of sodium intakes. When intake is low, the body conserves sodium by reducing output in urine and sweat. At high intakes, excretion equals intake. The AI for sodium covers short-term sweat losses from physical activity or exposure to high environmental temperatures. Those with exceptionally high losses, such as endurance runners, will require more sodium.[31] For young adults the AI is 1500 mg of sodium or 3800 mg of table salt. (Sodium chloride or table salt is 40% sodium by weight.) The suggested intake drops to 1300 mg of sodium (about 3300 mg of table salt) for those ages 51 to 70; it drops to 1200 mg (about 3000 mg of table salt) for those ages 71 and older, based on their lower energy intakes. The UL is 2300 mg of sodium or 5800 mg of table salt.[31]

HEALTH PROMOTION

Sodium and Blood Pressure

Excessive sodium raises blood pressure in certain individuals, and the high levels of sodium in the U.S. diet could be contributing to the growing prevalence of hypertension among various groups of youth and adults. Although the UL is 2300 mg/day, the average woman takes in about 3000 mg/day and the average man about 4000 mg/day.[3] Reducing dietary sodium is known to be effective in lowering systolic blood pressure in certain high-risk and "salt-sensitive" groups, including older adults; African Americans; and those with hypertension, kidney disease, or diabetes.[32] However, the benefits of sodium reduction across the general population is still in question. In some individuals low sodium intakes lead to responses in the renin-angiotensin system that increase rather than decrease cardiovascular risk.[33] (As we will learn later in this chapter, the renin-angiotensin system influences blood pressure by controlling sodium reabsorption in the kidneys.) Holding sodium intake to the UL limit of 2300 mg offers a prudent choice.

The Dietary Approaches to Stop Hypertension (DASH) food study took a broad view of diet and blood pressure; looking beyond sodium intake, it encouraged volunteers to eat at least nine servings of fruits and vegetables and three servings of low-fat dairy foods every day. This food plan high in fiber, calcium, magnesium, potassium, vitamins, and phytochemicals[34] brought about a significant decline in systolic blood pressure in the study participants.[35] When adults following the DASH diet also limited their sodium intake to the UL (2300 mg per day), systolic blood pressures fell even more than with the DASH diet alone.[36] About 25% of adults in the United States have hypertension. Experts estimate that a decrease in systolic blood pressure of 5 mm Hg across the population could reduce mortality from stroke by 14% and mortality from coronary heart disease by 9%.[31] (To learn more about dietary intervention for hypertension among African Americans see the *Focus on Culture* box, "Low Mineral Intake: Does It Have an Effect on Blood Pressure Among African Americans?")

FOCUS ON CULTURE

Low Mineral Intake: Does It Have an Effect on Blood Pressure Among African Americans?

African Americans are especially at risk for hypertension. For some individuals, this relates to salt sensitivity.[1] However, evidence indicates that not only sodium but also other minerals—calcium, potassium, and magnesium—have a role in regulating blood pressure. The Dietary Approaches to Stop Hypertension (DASH) food pattern rich in potassium, calcium, and magnesium successfully assisted persons with lowering their blood pressure. The DASH food plan provides the following intakes[2]:

- Potassium: 4706 mg (Dietary Reference Intake [DRI] = 4700 mg for those age 51 and older)
- Magnesium: 500 mg (DRI = 310 mg for those age 51 and older)
- Calcium: 1619 mg (DRI = 1200 mg for those age 51 and older)
- Sodium: DASH diet does not exceed the Tolerable Upper Intake Level (UL) of 2300 mg set for all adults

In a recent National Health and Nutrition Examination Survey, potassium and calcium intakes were more predictive of elevated systolic blood pressure than were sodium intakes.[3] For many African Americans, intakes of several nutrients important to blood pressure control were barely half the recommended amounts, with potassium intake reaching only 2408 mg and calcium intake only 612 mg. Magnesium intake was 230 mg, about two thirds the suggested amount.[4]

Why are intakes of calcium and potassium comparatively low in this group, and what can we do to raise them? Many African Americans are lactose intolerant and avoid dairy foods. Other items that could supply calcium include fortified cereals or orange juice. We might also encourage the use of aged cheese,

Continued

FOCUS ON CULTURE

Low Mineral Intake: Does It Have an Effect on Blood Pressure Among African Americans?—cont'd

which is lower in lactose than milk and may be tolerable. Various vegetables, including broccoli, collard greens, spinach, and kale are good sources of calcium, as well as potassium. Legumes add both calcium and potassium to the diet. (Refer to Boxes 7-2, 7-3, 7-5, and 7-6 to find good sources of these nutrients.)

All population groups can benefit from lowering sodium intake. Cutting down on the use of processed luncheon meats and salty snacks or choosing frozen or no salt added canned vegetables is a way to begin. Avoiding frozen dinners and canned soups unless labeled *low sodium* reduces sodium intakes (see Box 7-4). Unfortunately, processed foods with reduced sodium often cost more, putting them out of reach for families with limited resources.

Intervention for elevated blood pressure must be two pronged. Lowering sodium intake to the extent possible is one step, but equally important is the need to help African Americans raise their intakes of calcium, potassium, and magnesium.

REFERENCES

1. U.S. Department of Health and Human Services: *The seventh report of the Joint National Committee on Prevention, Detection, Evaluation, and Treatment of High Blood Pressure*, NIH Pub No 03-5230, Washington, DC, 2003, U.S. Government Printing Office.
2. U.S. Department of Health and Human Services, U.S. Department of Agriculture: *Dietary guidelines for Americans 2005*, ed 6, Washington, DC, 2005, U.S. Government Printing Office. Available at http://www.health.gov/dietaryguidelines/.
3. Townsend MS, Fulgoni VL 3rd, Stern JS, et al: Low mineral intake is associated with high systolic blood pressure in the third and fourth National Health and Nutrition Examination Surveys: could we all be right? *Am J Hypertens* 18:261, 2005.
4. Champagne CM, Bogle ML, McGee BB, et al: Dietary intake in the lower Mississippi delta region: results from the Foods of Our Delta Study, *J Am Diet Assoc* 104:199, 2004.

Unfortunately, adults with hypertension appear to have increased rather than decreased their intakes of sodium over the past 15 years.[37] When individuals are accustomed to liberal use of salt as a seasoning, adjusting to a reduced level of sodium can be difficult. The limited number of sodium-reduced products in the food supply is also a barrier to change,[38] and the reduced-sodium foods that are available tend to be higher in cost. Adjusting to a diet within the UL for sodium may be easier if foods naturally lower in sodium are substituted for foods higher in sodium, rather than relying on customary foods with less sodium added.[38]

Sodium Intake

About 95% of men and 75% of women in the United States consume more than 2300 mg/day of sodium.[32] Mean sodium intakes in all age categories beginning at age 2 exceed their UL, although intakes decline somewhat in older adults.[3] Boys and girls ages 6 to 11 consume about 3000 mg of sodium daily (the ULs for this age range are 1900 mg to 2200 mg), and males ages 12 to 19 are taking in almost 4300 mg. Females in this age range have intakes of 2950 mg. Snack items such as crackers and chips along with hot dogs and other processed meats contribute 25% of the sodium in the U.S. diet,[4] and such foods are popular among children and teenagers. The median sodium content of fast-food restaurant kids' meals is 810 mg, and 10% of the meals evaluated contained more than 1250 mg.[39] Sodium intakes are highest in the southern region of the United States—which also has the highest average systolic blood pressure—and lowest in the western region, which has the lowest average systolic blood pressure.[40]

Controlling Sodium Intake

The primary source of sodium for most people is processed food. As described in Figure 7-4, only 12% of the sodium in our diet occurs naturally in food, whereas 77% is added in food processing.[32] Varying amounts of sodium are added in home cooking or at the table, but it is usually less than that consumed in processed foods or when dining in restaurants. A few vegetables, such as spinach and celery, are fairly high in sodium. Food additives containing sodium serve a variety of functions as flavorings, leavening agents, and preservatives (Table 7-3), and they add to the high sodium content of many processed items. Compare the sodium in natural and processed foods in Box 7-4. In Chapter 9 we will learn to use the nutrition label to check the sodium content of foods we buy.

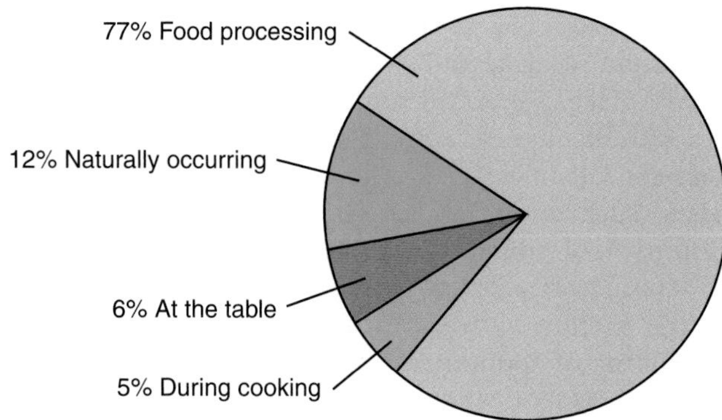

FIGURE 7-4 Sources of dietary sodium. Most of our dietary sodium comes from processed food. (Redrawn from U.S. Department of Health and Human Services, U.S. Department of Agriculture: *Dietary guidelines for Americans 2005,* ed 6, Washington, DC, 2005, U.S. Government Printing Office.)

POTASSIUM

Potassium is about twice as plentiful in the body as sodium. An adult contains about 270 g (9.5 oz) or 4000 mEq (milliequivalents). Most body potassium is inside cells, where it guards intracellular water; however, the relatively small amount of

TABLE 7-3 SODIUM-CONTAINING ADDITIVES COMMONLY USED IN FOOD PROCESSING

ADDITIVE	PURPOSE	WHERE USED
Sodium chloride (table salt)	Flavoring	Condiments (ketchup, soy sauce, onion salt, bouillon cubes, Worcestershire sauce); food mixtures; heat-and-serve entrees; snack foods
	Dough conditioner	Yeast breads
	Preservative	Fermented products (pickles), luncheon meats and frankfurters, canned vegetables, smoked fish
Sodium citrate	Texture agent	Frozen foods
Sodium bicarbonate	Leavening agent	Muffins, biscuits, cakes
Sodium aluminum phosphate	Leavening agent	Muffins, biscuits, cakes
Sodium benzoate	Preservative	Many processed items
Sodium bisulfate	Preservative	Many processed items
Sodium nitrite	Preservative	Luncheon meats, frankfurters

potassium in ECF is important for muscle activity, especially heart muscle activity. Plasma potassium levels are maintained within very narrow limits of 3.5 to 5.0 mEq/L.

Absorption-Excretion Balance

Absorption

Dietary potassium is readily absorbed in the small intestine, and potassium circulating in the gastrointestinal secretions is also reabsorbed. Prolonged vomiting or diarrhea results in serious losses.

Excretion

The principal route of potassium excretion is the urine. Because plasma potassium levels are critical to heart muscle action, the kidneys guard potassium carefully. At least 70% of the potassium filtered by the kidneys is reabsorbed. Aldosterone, the hormone that acts on the kidneys to conserve sodium, also regulates plasma potassium because potassium is lost in exchange for sodium. Elevated plasma potassium levels stimulate the release of aldosterone. The normal obligatory potassium loss is about 160 mg/day, although certain diuretic drugs cause excessive losses.

Physiologic Functions of Potassium

Water Balance

The potassium inside the cells balances with sodium outside the cells to maintain normal osmotic pressures and water distribution.

Muscle Activity

Potassium is needed for the action of cardiac and skeletal muscles. Together with sodium and calcium, potassium regulates neuromuscular stimulation, transmission of electrochemical impulses, and contraction of muscle fibers. Low plasma potassium leads to muscle irritability and paralysis. This effect is particularly notable for the heart muscle, which develops a gallop rhythm ending in cardiac arrest. Even small variations in plasma potassium are reflected in electrocardiograms (ECGs).

Carbohydrate Metabolism

When glucose is converted to glycogen, 0.36 mmol of potassium is stored in each gram of glycogen. When a patient in diabetic acidosis is treated with insulin and glucose, the ensuing rapid production of glycogen draws potassium from the plasma. Serious **hypokalemia** will result if adequate potassium replacement does not accompany treatment. Even moderate potassium deficiency without overt hypokalemia can aggravate existing glucose intolerance.

Protein Synthesis

Potassium is required for the storage of nitrogen as muscle protein or other cell protein. When tissue is broken down, potassium is lost along with nitrogen. Amino acid replacement in rehabilitation includes potassium to ensure nitrogen retention.

Control of Blood Pressure

Potassium helps control blood pressure by offsetting the pressor effect of sodium that raises blood pressure, such that persons with higher potassium intakes have lower pressures.[31,35] Potassium also increases the excretion of sodium through the action of aldosterone.

Acid-Base Balance

Potassium helps protect bone mass and lowers loss of calcium in the urine. Potassium along with other bicarbonate-yielding compounds in fruits and vegetables helps to neutralize sulfur-containing acids produced by the metabolism of meat and other animal protein foods.[41] When potassium and bicarbonate buffers are not available in sufficient amounts, these acids act on bone, releasing bone calcium and reducing bone mass.

KEY TERMS

hypokalemia A lower than normal level of potassium in the blood (usually defined as <3.5 mEq/L).

BOX 7-4 **SODIUM CONTENT OF PROCESSED VERSUS UNPROCESSED FOODS***

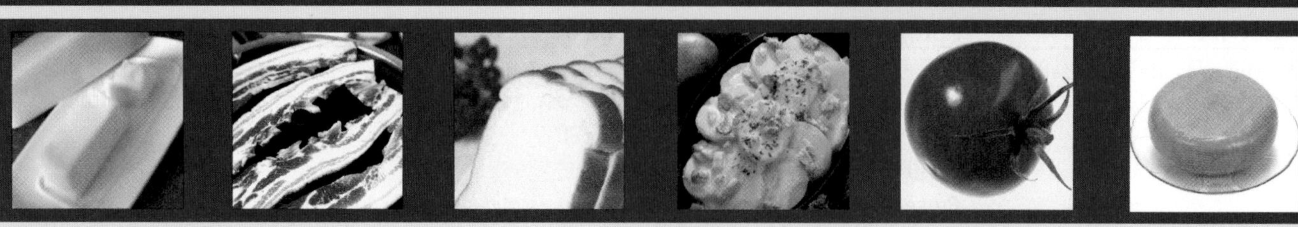

FOOD SOURCE	QUANTITY	SODIUM (in mg)
Grains Group		
Ready-to-Eat Cereals		
Cheerios	1 cup	200
Total	¾ cup	192
All Bran	½ cup	73
Shredded Wheat, no salt added	2 biscuits	3
Bread, white	1 slice	170
Vegetable Group		
Potato salad, homemade	1 cup	1324
Stewed tomatoes, canned	1 cup	564
Broccoli, frozen with cheese sauce	½ cup	402
Potato, baked, with skin	1 med	20
Broccoli, boiled with no salt	½ cup	32
Tomato, raw	1 med	6
Meat, Beans, Eggs, and Nuts Group		
Ham, canned, lean	3 oz	908
Baked beans, canned	½ cup	436
Bacon, broiled or fried	3 med pieces	439
Tuna, light, canned in water with salt	3 oz	287
Peanut butter, creamy with salt	1 tbsp	73
Ground beef, regular, broiled	3 oz	66
Beef top round, lean, broiled	3 oz	48
Halibut, baked	3 oz	59
Black-eyed peas, boiled without salt	1 cup	6
Peanut butter, creamy, unsalted	1 tbsp	3
Milk Group		
Cottage cheese, creamed	1 cup	764
Cheddar cheese	1 oz	176
Milk, whole, low fat, or skim	8 fl oz	103
Swiss cheese	1 oz	54
Processed cheese, sliced and individually wrapped	1 oz	422
Fats, Oils, and Sugar Group		
Margarine, stick, corn oil, salted	1 tbsp	112
Butter, salted	1 tbsp	82
Butter, unsalted	1 tbsp	2
Margarine, stick corn oil, unsalted	1 tbsp	14

Adequate Intake (AI) for adults: ages 19-50, 1500 mg; ages 51-70, 1300 mg; ages ≥71, 1200 mg; Tolerable Upper Intake Level (UL) for adults: 2300 mg.
*Sodium is added to foods in home food preparation and in food industry processing.
Nutrient data from USDA: *USDA National Nutrient Database for Standard Reference, Release 21,* Washington, DC, U.S. Department of Agriculture, 2009. Retrieved April 23, 2010 from http://www.ars.usda.gov/Services/docs.htm?docid=17477.

Potassium Requirement

Dietary Reference Intake

The AI for potassium is 4700 mg/day for all adults.[31] This intake is expected to lower blood pressure and reduce bone loss, but less than 10% of men and 5% of women reach this goal.[3] African-American men and women meet less than half

KEY TERMS
hyperkalemia A higher than normal level of potassium in the blood (usually defined as >5.0 mEq/L).

PERSPECTIVES IN PRACTICE

Potassium—The Other Side of the Blood Pressure Equation

Health experts encourage us to limit our sodium intake to prevent an inappropriate rise in blood pressure. However, what about the other piece of advice—increasing our intake of potassium, which helps lower our blood pressure? Fruits and vegetables are major sources of potassium along with meat and dairy foods. MyPyramid suggests that we eat 2½ cups of vegetables and 2 cups of fruit each day to take in the potassium we need. Currently, Americans fall short of this daily goal by about 1 cup of vegetables and 1 cup of fruit. So how do we get five to nine servings each day from this group?

Begin gradually by adding another fruit or vegetable to every meal. Start with a goal of five servings a day and move up from there. Try to vary your colors to ensure a variety of fruits and vegetables that will add not only potassium but also other important nutrients to your diet.

See the following suggestions for adding fruits and vegetables throughout the day:*

- Breakfast
  - Cereal with fruit (fresh banana, raisins, berries, or canned fruit out of season)
  - Juice (orange, cranberry, apple, or grapefruit*)
- Lunch
  - Chicken or tuna salad sandwich with lettuce or salad greens
  - Baby carrots, celery sticks, serving of tossed salad or potato salad
  - Fresh fruit (apple, orange, grapes, or berries)
- Dinner
  - Spaghetti or meat loaf with tomato sauce
  - Green salad or bean salad
  - Cooked vegetable (string beans, broccoli, lima beans, cauliflower, green peas)
  - Fruit dessert (fresh or canned fruit, apple crisp, berries with ice cream)
- Snacks
  - Fresh fruit, raisins, or melon cup
  - Baby carrots
  - Juice (apple, grape, cranberry, if omitted at breakfast)

*Menu ideas adapted from reference 3; grapefruit or grapefruit juice is contraindicated for persons on certain medications.

1. U.S. Department of Agriculture, Center for Nutrition Policy and Promotion: *MyPyramid food guidance system,* Washington, DC, 2005, U.S. Department of Agriculture. Available at *www.mypyramid.gov/.*

2. U.S. Department of Health and Human Services, U.S. Department of Agriculture: *Dietary guidelines for Americans 2005,* ed 6, Washington, DC, 2005, U.S. Government Printing Office. Available at http://www.health.gov/dietaryguidelines/.

3. U.S. Department of Health and Human Services, National Heart, Lung, and Blood Institute: *Your guide to lowering your blood pressure with DASH,* NIH Pub No. 06-4082, Bethesda, Md, 2006, U.S. Department of Health and Human Services. Available at *http://www.nhlbi.nih.gov/health/public/heart/hbp/dash/new_dash.pdf.*

of the AI,[42] likely related to fewer servings of milk, fruits, and vegetables. In light of the age-related increase in blood pressure and loss of bone that occurs in both genders and all population groups, increased servings of high-potassium foods would be a cost-effective health intervention.

Clinical Implications of Excessive Intake

When kidney function is normal, potassium is easily excreted; thus no UL exists for this nutrient. Nevertheless, potassium supplements can be dangerous, regardless of kidney status. Hyperkalemia with serious cardiac arrhythmias can occur in apparently healthy individuals who accidentally or intentionally take potassium supplements. Potassium-containing salt substitutes can be unrecognized sources of potassium. Individuals with diabetes, renal impairment, or heart failure have increased risk of hyperkalemia. Certain medications impair potassium excretion.[31]

Food Sources of Potassium

Potassium as a component of all living cells is found in many foods. Legumes, whole grains, fruits such as oranges and bananas, leafy green vegetables, broccoli, potatoes, meats, and milk supply considerable amounts (Box 7-5). Persons who eat many servings of fruits and vegetables have potassium intakes of about 8 to 11 g/day.[31] It is important to note that potassium toxicity does not occur from high intakes of potassium-containing foods but rather from potassium supplements. (For ideas on how to add more potassium to your diet in the form of fruits and vegetables see the *Perspectives*

BOX 7-5 FOOD SOURCES OF POTASSIUM

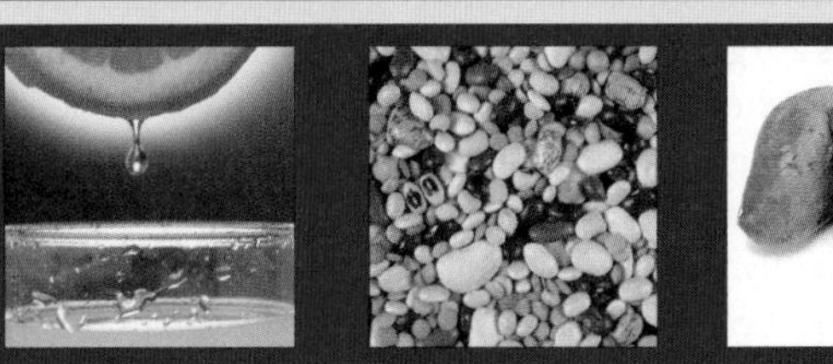

FOOD SOURCE	QUANTITY	POTASSIUM (in mg)
Vegetable Group		
Potato, baked	1	610
Sweet potato	½ cup	397
Fruit Group		
Orange juice	1 cup	473
Banana	1	422
Meat, Beans, Eggs, and Nuts Group		
Lima beans, dried	½ cup	478
Milk Group		
Milk, low fat	8 oz	366
Cottage cheese, low fat	8 oz	194
Other		
Spaghetti sauce	½ cup	395

Adequate Intake (AI) for adults: 4700 mg.

Nutrient data from USDA: *USDA National Nutrient Database for Standard Reference, Release 21,* Washington, DC, U.S. Department of Agriculture, 2009. Retrieved April 23, 2010 from http://www.ars.usda.gov/Services/docs.htm?docid=17477.

in Practice box, "Potassium – The Other Side of the Blood Pressure Equation.")

Based on their body content, three additional minerals—magnesium, chloride, and sulfur—are assigned to the major minerals group.

MAGNESIUM

An adult body contains about 25 g of magnesium, a little less than 1 oz. Most is combined with calcium and phosphorus in bone, with the remainder distributed in muscle, other tissues, and fluids. Magnesium activates enzymes for energy production and tissue building and has a role in normal muscle action. Magnesium is receiving new attention as a possible contributor to the positive health effects associated with the DASH diet.[43] Older individuals with magnesium intakes at least 80% of the RDA were less likely to develop metabolic syndrome.[44] The relatively high magnesium content in whole grains may help to bring about their positive effect in lowering chronic disease risk.[45,46]

Magnesium Requirement

The RDA for magnesium is 400 mg for younger men and 310 mg for younger women. To compensate for age-related changes in the kidneys that lead to greater losses, the RDA for persons older than age 50 increases to 420 mg and 320 mg in men and women, respectively.[11]

Food Sources

Magnesium is widespread in nature and unprocessed foods. Whole grains are good sources, but more than 80% of the magnesium is lost when the germ and bran layers of the kernel are removed. Although milk contains only a modest amount of magnesium, it is a major source in the U.S. diet because it is consumed frequently.[4] Other foods include nuts, soybeans, cocoa, seafood, dried beans and peas, and green vegetables. Except for bananas, fruits are relatively poor sources, as are meat and fish. Diets rich in vegetables and unrefined grains are higher in magnesium than diets based on highly processed foods and meat. Box 7-6 lists some good sources of magnesium.

BOX 7-6 FOOD SOURCES OF MAGNESIUM

FOOD SOURCE	QUANTITY	MAGNESIUM (in mg)
Grains Group		
Bite-Size Shredded Wheat cereal	1 cup	48
Vegetable Group		
Spinach	½ cup	81
Meat, Beans, Eggs, and Nuts Group		
Baked beans	1 cup	66
Peanuts	1 oz	50
Milk Group		
Soy milk	1 cup	61
Cow's milk	1 cup	27

Recommended Dietary Allowance (RDA) for adults: women ages 19-50, 310 mg; women ages ≥51, 320 mg; men ages 19-50, 400 mg; men ages ≥51, 420 mg.

Nutrient data from USDA: *USDA National Nutrient Database for Standard Reference, Release 21,* Washington, DC, U.S. Department of Agriculture, 2009. Retrieved April 23, 2010 from http://www.ars.usda.gov/Services/docs.htm?docid=17477.

CHLORIDE

Chlorine appears in the body as the chloride ion (Cl^-). Chloride accounts for about 3% of body mineral content, and most is found in the ECF where it helps control water balance and acid-base balance. Spinal fluid has the highest concentration. A fair amount of ionized chloride is found in the gastrointestinal secretions as a component of gastric hydrochloric acid (HCl). Uncontrolled vomiting and diarrhea with continuing loss of gastric fluids can lead to chloride deficiency with muscle cramps and disturbed acid-base balance.

SULFUR

Sulfur is found in all body cells as a constituent of cell protein. Elemental sulfur forms sulfate compounds with sodium, potassium, and magnesium. Other forms of sulfur include (1) sulfur-containing amino acids such as methionine and cysteine; (2) glycoproteins in cartilage, tendons, and bone matrix; (3) detoxification products formed by intestinal bacteria; (4) organic molecules such as heparin, insulin, coenzyme A (CoA), thiamin, and biotin; and (5) keratin in hair and nails.

The major minerals are summarized in Table 7-4.

ESSENTIAL TRACE ELEMENTS

TRACE ELEMENTS: THE CONCEPT OF ESSENTIALITY

By the simplest definition an essential element is one required to sustain life and that, if absent, brings death. For major elements found in relatively large amounts in the body, such a determination is fairly easy based on the quantity available for study. It is more difficult to establish the essentiality of the trace elements because we seem to need so little of them. Trace elements have a required intake of less than 100 mg/day, yet some of them exist in fairly large amounts in our diet and our environment.

Trace elements have two major functions: (1) to catalyze chemical reactions and (2) to serve as structural components

TABLE 7-4 SUMMARY OF MAJOR MINERALS

MINERAL	METABOLISM	PHYSIOLOGIC FUNCTIONS	CLINICAL APPLICATIONS	DIETARY REFERENCE INTAKE	FOOD SOURCES
Calcium (Ca)	Absorption according to body need; requires Ca-binding protein and regulated by vitamin D, parathyroid hormone (PTH), and calcitonin; absorption favored by protein and acidity Excretion chiefly in feces: 50%-90% of amount ingested Deposition-mobilization in bone tissue is regulated by vitamin D and PTH	Constituent of bones and teeth Participates in blood clotting, nerve transmission, muscle action, cell membrane permeability, enzyme activation	Tetany (decrease in serum Ca) Rickets, osteomalacia Osteoporosis Hyperparathyroidism and hypoparathyroidism	Adults: men/women ages 19-50: 1000 mg; ages ≥51:1200 mg Pregnancy: ages ≤18: 1300 mg; ages ≥19: 1000 mg Lactation: ages ≤18: 1300 mg; ages ≥19: 1000 mg	Milk, cheese, yogurt Green leafy vegetables Whole grains Legumes, nuts Fortified soy foods Fortified fruit juice
Phosphorus (P)	Absorption with Ca aided by vitamin D and PTH; hindered by binding agents Excretion chiefly by kidney according to serum level, regulated by PTH Deposition-mobilization in bone compartment is constant	Constituent of bones and teeth, adenosine triphosphate (ATP), phosphorylated intermediary metabolites Participates in absorption of glucose and glycerol, transport of fatty acids, energy metabolism, and buffer system	Growth Recovery from diabetic acidosis Hypophosphatemia: bone disease, malabsorption syndromes, primary hyperparathyroidism Hyperphosphatemia: renal insufficiency, hypoparathyroidism, tetany	Adults: men/women ages ≥19: 700 mg Pregnancy: ages ≤18:1250 mg; ages ≥19: 700 mg Lactation: ages ≤18:1250 mg; ages ≥19: 700 mg	Milk, cheese Meat, egg yolk Whole grains Legumes, nuts Soft drinks
Magnesium (Mg)	Absorption according to intake load; hindered by excess fat, phosphate, calcium, protein Excretion regulated by kidney	Constituent of bones and teeth Coenzyme in general metabolism, smooth muscle action, neuromuscular irritability Cation in intracellular fluid (ICF)	Low serum level after gastrointestinal losses Tremor, spasm in deficiency induced by malnutrition, alcoholism	Adults: men ages 19-50: 400 mg; ages ≥51: 420 mg Adults: women ages 19-50: 310 mg; women ages ≥51: 320 mg Pregnancy: ages ≤18: 400 mg; ages 19-30: 350 mg; ages 31-50: 360 mg Lactation: ages ≤18: 360 mg; ages 19-30: 310 mg; ages 31-50: 320 mg	Milk, cheese Meat, seafood Whole grains Legumes, nuts

Continued

TABLE 7-4 SUMMARY OF MAJOR MINERALS—cont'd

MINERAL	METABOLISM	PHYSIOLOGIC FUNCTIONS	CLINICAL APPLICATIONS	DIETARY REFERENCE INTAKE	FOOD SOURCES
Sodium (Na)	Readily absorbed Excretion chiefly by kidney, controlled by aldosterone	Major cation in extracellular fluid (ECF), water balance, acid-base balance Cell membrane permeability, absorption of glucose Normal muscle irritability	Losses in gastrointestinal disorders, diarrhea Fluid-electrolyte and acid-base balance problems Muscle action	Adults: men/women ages 19-50: 1500 mg; ages 51-70: 1300 mg; ages ≥71: 1200 mg UL for all adults: 2300 mg Pregnancy: all ages 1500 mg Lactation: all ages 1500 mg	Salt Sodium compounds used in baking and food processing Milk, cheese, carrots, spinach, beets, celery
Potassium (K)	Readily absorbed Secreted and reabsorbed in gastrointestinal circulation Excretion chiefly by kidney, regulated by aldosterone	Major cation in ICF, water balance, acid-base balance Normal muscle irritability Glycogen formation Protein synthesis	Losses in gastrointestinal disorders, diarrhea Fluid-electrolyte and acid-base balance problems Muscle action, especially heart muscle Losses in tissue catabolism Treatment of diabetic acidosis: rapid glycogen production lowers serum potassium levels Losses with diuretic therapy	Adults: men/women all ages 4700 mg Pregnancy: all ages 4700 mg Lactation: all ages 5100 mg	Fruits Vegetables Legumes, nuts Whole grains Meat
Chloride (Cl)	Readily absorbed Excretion controlled by kidney	Major anion in ECF, water balance, acid-base balance, chloride-bicarbonate shift Gastric hydrochloric acid (HCl)—digestion	Losses in gastrointestinal disorders, vomiting, diarrhea, tube drainage Hypochloremic alkalosis	Adults: men/women ages 19-50: 2300 mg; ages 51-70: 2000 mg; ages ≥71: 1800 mg Pregnancy: all ages 2300 mg Lactation: all ages 2300 mg	Salt
Sulfur (S)	Elemental form absorbed as such; split from amino acid sources (methionine and cysteine) in digestion and absorbed into portal circulation Excreted by kidney in relation to protein intake and tissue catabolism	Essential constituent of protein structure Detoxification reactions Enzyme activity and energy metabolism through free sulfhydryl group (–SH)	Cystine renal calculi Cystinuria	Adults: no specific recommendation; diets adequate in sulfur-containing amino acids are adequate in sulfur	Meat, eggs Milk, cheese Legumes, nuts

of larger molecules. They can be separated into two groups: (1) those that are known to be essential and (2) those for which additional research is needed.

Ten trace elements are considered essential in human nutrition based on defined function and need (see Box 7-1).

Various other trace elements are thought to be essential for animals, but researchers have yet to demonstrate a role for them in *human* health.[32] As we develop better techniques of tissue analysis and functional tests appropriate for human studies, we will learn more about these trace elements and the dietary needs related to them.

IRON

Of all the micronutrients, iron has the longest history; the body mechanisms regulating its absorption and use are well understood.

Forms of Iron in the Body

The average adult body contains about 3 to 4 g of iron. This iron is distributed in the following forms, each with a specific metabolic function:

- *Transport iron:* A trace of iron, 0.05 to 0.18 mg/dL, is found in blood plasma bound to the transport carrier protein transferrin.
- *Hemoglobin and myoglobin:* Most body iron, about 70%, resides in the red blood cells as part of the heme portion of the hemoglobin molecule that delivers oxygen to body cells. Another 5% helps form myoglobin, the oxygen-carrying molecule found in the heart and skeletal muscles. Skeletal muscles continuing contraction over extended periods of time, as for marathon runners or cyclists, require an ongoing supply of oxygen from myoglobin. (We will learn more about energy metabolism in skeletal muscle in Chapter 14.)
- *Storage iron:* About 20% of body iron is stored as the protein-iron compound **ferritin** in the liver, spleen, and bone marrow. Excess iron is held in the body as **hemosiderin** and exchanges with ferritin as needed.
- *Cellular iron:* The remaining 5% is distributed across all body cells as an enzyme cofactor in oxidative enzyme systems that produce energy.

Absorption-Transport-Storage-Excretion Balance

Iron is regulated differently from most other nutrients. Generally, urinary excretion, which rids the body of any excess that has accumulated, controls plasma and tissue levels. For iron, control is exerted at the points of absorption, transport, and storage. The body has no system for excreting iron.

Absorption

Major control of iron balance takes place at the site of absorption in the small intestine. Two forms of dietary iron are found in food: (1) **heme iron** and (2) **nonheme iron** (Table 7-5). The larger portion by far is nonheme iron, which includes all plant sources plus 60% of animal sources.[47] Nonheme iron is absorbed at a much slower rate than the smaller heme molecule because it is tightly bound to organic components in the form of ferric iron (Fe^{3+}). In the acid medium of the stomach, ferric iron must be separated and reduced to the more soluble ferrous form (Fe^{2+}) before it can be absorbed. If too little gastric acid is available to accomplish this conversion, then the ferric iron will be lost in the feces.

TABLE 7-5 CHARACTERISTICS OF HEME AND NONHEME DIETARY IRON

	DIETARY IRON	
	HEME (SMALLER PORTION)	NONHEME (LARGER PORTION)
Food sources	None in plant sources, 40% of iron in animal sources	All plant sources, 60% of iron in animal sources
Absorption rate	Rapid, transported and absorbed intact	Slow, tightly bound in organic molecules

Iron distribution and transfer within the absorbing cells of the intestinal mucosa involve several carrier substances. Iron never travels unescorted. First, a protein carrier in the mucosal cell binds the ferrous iron. This protein carrier leaves behind enough iron to serve the needs of the energy-producing mitochondria of the absorbing cell and then delivers specific amounts to waiting carriers that control its destination. These carriers are (1) apoferritin, a protein receptor that combines with iron to form the iron-holding compound ferritin for storage in the cell, and (2) apotransferrin, the protein receptor that combines with iron to form the iron-carrier compound serum transferrin, which circulates in the blood.

The proportion of dietary iron that is absorbed or rejected is determined by the amount of ferritin already present in the intestinal mucosal cells. When all available apoferritin has joined with iron to form ferritin, any additional iron arriving at the binding site is rejected and returned to the lumen of the intestine for excretion in the feces. Approximately 1% to 15% of nonheme iron is absorbed compared with 15% to 45% of heme iron.[48] Most absorption takes place in the upper small intestine.

Three factors favor absorption:

1. *Body need:* In iron deficiency or increased demand (e.g., in periods of growth, pregnancy, or weight training), more iron is absorbed.[47] When tissue reserves are ample or saturated, iron is rejected and excreted.

KEY TERMS

ferritin Protein-iron compound for storing iron in tissues.

hemosiderin Insoluble iron oxide-protein compound for storing iron in the liver when the amount of iron in the blood exceeds the storage capacity of ferritin.

heme iron Form of dietary iron found only in animal sources coming from the heme portion of hemoglobin in red blood cells. Heme iron is more easily absorbed than nonheme iron but supplies the smaller portion of the body's total iron intake.

nonheme iron The larger portion of dietary iron that includes all plant food sources and 60% of animal food sources. This form of iron is not part of a heme complex and is less easily absorbed.

2. *Ascorbic acid (vitamin C) or other acids:* An acidic environment increases iron absorption.[49] Acid reduces ferric iron to ferrous iron, the soluble form that is absorbed. Adding 50 mg of ascorbic acid to a meal by including orange juice or similar acid source can triple the absorption of nonheme iron.[47] Gastric HCl provides the optimal acid medium to prepare iron for absorption.
3. *Animal tissues:* Heme iron improves the absorption of nonheme iron eaten at the same meal.[50] Peptides released in digestion of meat, fish, and poultry enhance iron absorption from other food sources.[51]

Five factors hinder iron absorption:

1. *Binding agents:* Phosphates, phytates, and oxalates bind iron and prevent its absorption. Certain vegetable proteins including soy protein decrease iron absorption independent of their phytate content.[52] Substances in tea and coffee decrease absorption of nonheme iron.
2. *Low gastric acid:* Surgical removal of a portion of the stomach reduces the number of acid-secreting cells and decreases iron absorption. Iron supplements are likely to be necessary after bariatric surgery.[53] Persons who abuse antacids will have trouble absorbing nonheme iron.[49]
3. *Infection:* Severe infection depresses iron absorption, because the body attempts to suppress the supply of iron to the infectious microorganisms.
4. *Gastrointestinal disease:* Malabsorption syndromes such as celiac disease or steatorrhea hinder iron absorption.
5. *Calcium:* Large amounts of calcium may inhibit the absorption of both heme and nonheme iron consumed at the same meal. This interaction could affect the iron status of those taking concentrated calcium supplements, although the addition of 300 mg of calcium (the equivalent of one glass of milk) did not affect iron absorption from several test meals.[54] Adding calcium at the levels normally found in food might be the best approach for optimum absorption of all nutrients.

Transport

After absorption, iron is bound with the protein transferrin for transport to storage sites or body cells. Normally only 20% to 35% of the iron-binding capacity of transferrin is filled. The remainder serves as a reserve for handling any emergency or variance in iron intake.

Storage

Bound to transferrin, iron is delivered to storage sites in the bone marrow and liver. Here it is recombined with apoferritin to form ferritin, an exchangeable storage form that can release iron as needed. The second, less soluble storage form, hemosiderin, provides reserve storage in the liver. From these sites, iron is mobilized for hemoglobin synthesis and production of red blood cells or other body cells. Adults use 20 to 25 mg of iron per day for hemoglobin synthesis, but much of this represents iron that was conserved and recycled when old red blood cells were destroyed. The average life span of a red blood cell is about 120 days. These interrelationships of body iron absorption-transport-storage are diagrammed in Figure 7-5.

Excretion

Because iron regulation occurs at the point of absorption, only minute amounts are lost through the kidneys. The body also loses iron by the normal sloughing off of skin cells and gastrointestinal cells, as well as through normal gastrointestinal and menstrual blood loss. Heavy menstrual flow, childbirth, surgery, acute and chronic hemorrhage, gastrointestinal disease, or parasitic infestation causes exceptional iron loss and depletes body stores.

Physiologic Functions of Iron

Oxygen Transport

Iron is "pocketed" within the heme molecule, the nonprotein portion of hemoglobin in the red blood cell, and carries oxygen to the cells for respiration and metabolism. Iron has a similar role in myoglobin, which delivers oxygen within the muscle cell.

Cellular Oxidation

Iron is a component of cell enzyme systems that oxidize glucose and other energy-yielding nutrients to produce energy.

Immune Function

Iron is needed for the production of immune cells and cytokines that attack foreign bacteria invading the body.

Growth Needs

Positive iron balance is imperative for growth. At birth an infant has a 4- to 6-month supply of iron stored in its liver. Breast-fed infants obtain some iron in breast milk, and iron is added to commercial infant formulas. Supplementary iron-rich and iron-fortified foods are introduced to an infant's diet at 4 to 6 months of age to prevent milk anemia.[55] Throughout childhood, iron is needed for continued growth and to build reserves for the physiologic stress of adolescence—muscle development in boys and the onset of menses in girls. The need for iron escalates during pregnancy to produce red blood cells for the expanding blood volume and build iron reserves in the developing fetal liver. Normal blood loss in childbirth draws on iron stores.

Brain and Cognitive Function

Iron is important for brain development and the synthesis and breakdown of neurotransmitters. Iron deficiency in the critical periods of gestation and early lactation can have long-lasting effects on the child's development of motor skills and ability to explore and interact with the environment.[56] Iron status influenced cognitive function and time to complete mental tasks in young women, with improved performance after treatment for iron deficiency.[57]

Clinical Applications

Clinical abnormalities result from either a deficiency or an excess of iron.

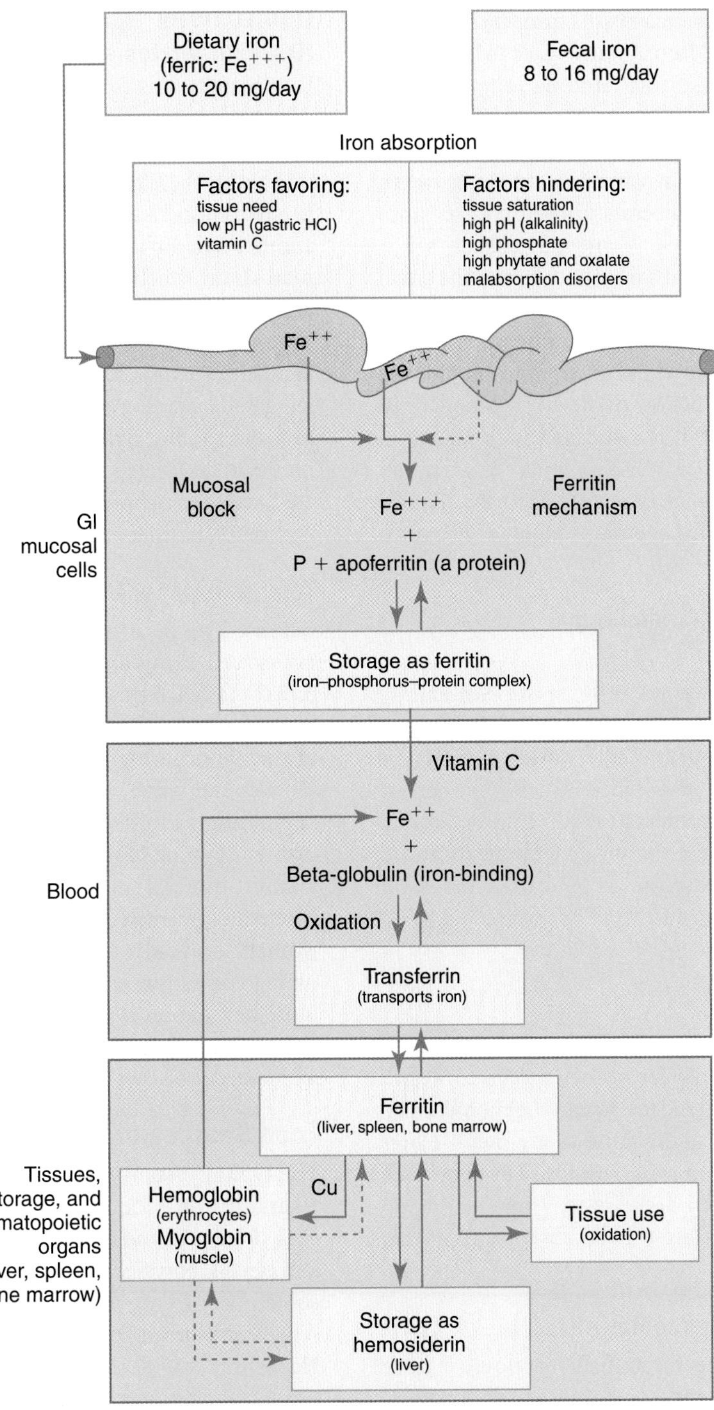

FIGURE 7-5 Summary of iron metabolism, showing its absorption, transport, use in hemoglobin formation, and storage forms (ferritin and hemosiderin).

Iron Deficiency Anemia

Iron deficiency is a worldwide public health problem and leads to a hypochromic microcytic anemia. Iron deficiency may have various causes, as described following:

- *Low iron intake:* Nutritional anemia develops when iron or other nutrients needed for hemoglobin synthesis and red blood cell production are not available in adequate amounts. The role of hemoglobin in carrying oxygen to the cells is important in understanding the symptoms of iron deficiency anemia (Box 7-7).

BOX 7-7 SIGNS OF IRON DEFICIENCY

- Fatigue
- Muscle weakness
- Pale color
- Decreased resistance to infection
- Spoon nails
- Angular stomatitis

- *Blood loss:* Hemorrhagic anemia results from excessive loss of blood and its associated iron. Aspirin leads to blood loss through the gastrointestinal tract, and its long-term use for pain relief can lower body stores. Severe hemorrhoids cause blood loss.
- *Gastrectomy:* Postgastrectomy anemia develops when gastric acid is insufficient to liberate iron for absorption.
- *Malabsorption:* Iron deficiency anemia ensues when mucosal lesions damage the absorbing surface of the small intestine.
- *Chronic disease:* An anemia of chronic disease is related to irregularities in the recycling of iron from old red blood cells and the production of new red blood cells, not iron deficiency per se. It is associated with infection, inflammatory disorders, heart disease, renal disease, and connective tissue diseases such as osteoarthritis. Found mostly in older persons, this anemia is highly resistant to treatment.

Worldwide Problem of Iron Deficiency Anemia

Iron deficiency anemia is second only to protein-energy malnutrition as the most prevalent nutritional deficiency in the world. More than one fourth of the world's population is believed to be anemic or iron deficient, with women of childbearing age and children most at risk.[58] Iron deficiency anemia respects neither social class nor geographic location; iron balance in developing countries is precarious based on low intakes of bioavailable iron and iron loss through parasitic infections.

Iron Requirement

Dietary Reference Intake

The RDAs for iron are 18 mg/day for women ages 19 to 50 and 8 mg/day for men ages 19 and older.[47] When the menses have ceased, the RDA for women is the same as for men—8 mg/day. Pregnancy has a "high iron cost," and the daily allowance rises to 27 mg/day. Iron needs decrease to 9 mg/day during lactation because the menses are usually absent during this period.[47]

Special Considerations for Vegetarians

Individuals who do not eat meat, fish, or poultry have increased risk of iron deficiency. Not only is the bioavailability of iron lower in plant foods but also heme iron is unavailable to enhance its absorption. As a result, overall iron absorption from plant foods is estimated to be only 10% as compared with 18% for the typical American diet. With this in mind it is recommended that vegetarian men take in 14 mg of iron per day and vegetarian premenopausal women take in 33 mg/day. Vegetarian adolescent girls need 26 mg/day.[47] Note that these recommendations are nearly twice those for persons of comparable age and gender who consume a mixed diet, so individual counseling regarding iron sources and supplements is warranted.[47] (See Chapter 5 for a review of plant-based diets.)

Iron Toxicity

Hemochromatosis

Iron toxicity was first identified in a population in Southern Africa who cooked their food in iron vessels and also had a genetic tendency to absorb and store abnormally high amounts of iron. In the United States, accidental iron poisoning occurs in children and adults who overuse iron supplements. However, another cause of iron overload is the genetic disease **hemochromatosis**, in which iron continues to be absorbed at a high rate despite elevated liver stores. It is estimated that 1 of every 385 Americans has this genetic mutation, although not all develop hemochromatosis.[59] Excessive body iron is associated with increased oxidation and initiation of free radicals and is believed to foster cardiac arrhythmias, liver disease, and diabetes. Even moderately elevated iron stores, much lower than those associated with hemochromatosis, appear to increase the risk of type 2 diabetes in otherwise healthy persons.[60,61]

Tolerable Upper Intake Level

Because iron becomes toxic at high levels, iron intake should not exceed 45 mg/day.[47] Although it would seem unlikely that one could reach this level from food alone, current iron fortification policies developed to meet the iron needs of women in the childbearing years add significant amounts of iron to the diet. Individuals who eat more than one serving of a cereal containing 15 to 18 mg of iron per serving, along with other iron-containing foods and possibly an iron-containing multivitamin-mineral supplement, can approach or exceed the UL. Moderately elevated iron stores were found in middle-age women[61] and older adults who ate large amounts of meat supplying heme iron and took iron supplements[62] or used alcoholic beverages on a regular basis.[63] (Alcohol increases iron absorption.) Iron supplements should always be approved and supervised by a physician.

Food Sources of Iron

The typical Western diet contains about 5 to 7 mg of iron per 1000 kcal. Iron is found in highest amounts in meat, fish, poultry, eggs, dried peas and beans, and whole grain and fortified breads and cereals. Fortified grain products such as breakfast bars may contain from 1 mg to 24 mg of iron per serving. Ready-to-eat cereals and bread add the most to the iron intake of adults.[4] Heme iron provides less than 10% of the iron intake of girls and women and less than 12% of the iron intake of boys and men.[47] Box 7-8 lists some comparative food sources of iron.

IODINE

Iodine has been of interest worldwide, based on the need to identify the cause of goiter and other disorders found to relate to iodine deficiency. Iodine is a component of the hormone thyroxine, produced in the thyroid gland, which controls the rate of energy metabolism in cells. The body contains only 15 to 20 mg of iodine, and most of this (70% to 80%) is in the thyroid gland. This gland has a remarkable ability to concentrate iodine.

BOX 7-8 FOOD SOURCES OF IRON

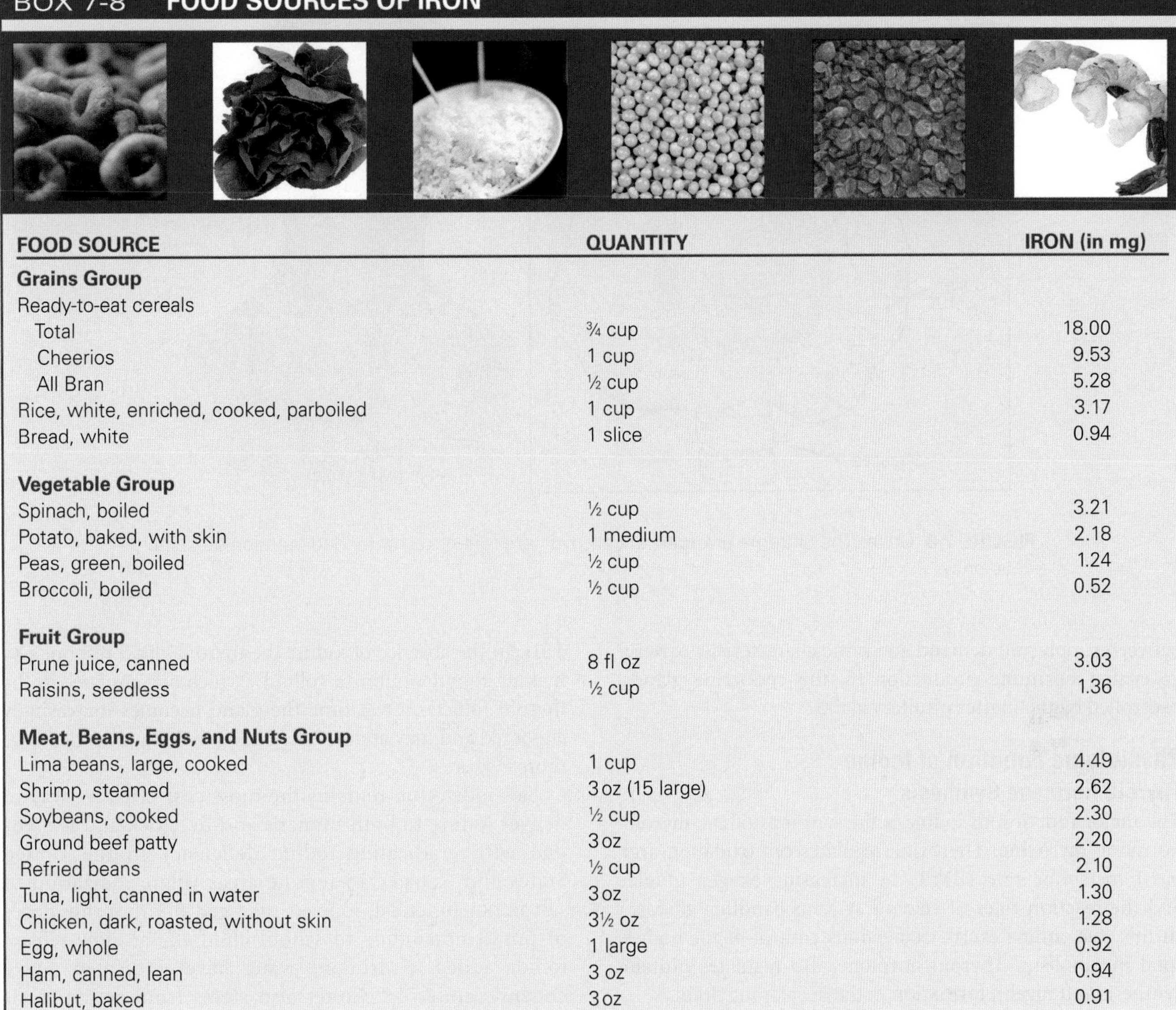

FOOD SOURCE	QUANTITY	IRON (in mg)
Grains Group		
Ready-to-eat cereals		
Total	¾ cup	18.00
Cheerios	1 cup	9.53
All Bran	½ cup	5.28
Rice, white, enriched, cooked, parboiled	1 cup	3.17
Bread, white	1 slice	0.94
Vegetable Group		
Spinach, boiled	½ cup	3.21
Potato, baked, with skin	1 medium	2.18
Peas, green, boiled	½ cup	1.24
Broccoli, boiled	½ cup	0.52
Fruit Group		
Prune juice, canned	8 fl oz	3.03
Raisins, seedless	½ cup	1.36
Meat, Beans, Eggs, and Nuts Group		
Lima beans, large, cooked	1 cup	4.49
Shrimp, steamed	3 oz (15 large)	2.62
Soybeans, cooked	½ cup	2.30
Ground beef patty	3 oz	2.20
Refried beans	½ cup	2.10
Tuna, light, canned in water	3 oz	1.30
Chicken, dark, roasted, without skin	3½ oz	1.28
Egg, whole	1 large	0.92
Ham, canned, lean	3 oz	0.94
Halibut, baked	3 oz	0.91

Recommended Dietary Allowance (RDA) for adults: women ages 19-50, 18 mg; women ages ≥51, 8 mg; men, 8 mg.
Nutrient data from USDA: *USDA National Nutrient Database for Standard Reference, Release 21,* Washington, DC, U.S. Department of Agriculture, 2009. Retrieved April 23, 2010 from http://www.ars.usda.gov/Services/docs.htm?docid=17477.

Absorption-Excretion Balance

Absorption

Iodine is absorbed in the form of iodides. Iodides are then loosely bound to proteins and carried by the blood to the thyroid gland, which takes up as much as it needs for hormone synthesis. About one third of the available iodide is used to produce active thyroid hormone, with the remainder used to form hormone precursors for later use.

Excretion

Absorbed iodide not needed by the thyroid gland is excreted in the urine. More than 90% of the iodine taken into the body appears in the urine.

Hormonal Control

Thyroid-stimulating hormone (TSH) from the anterior lobe of the pituitary gland directs the uptake of iodine by thyroid cells in response to plasma thyroid hormone levels. When plasma levels are high, less thyroid hormone is produced. When plasma levels are low, the thyroid cells are stimulated to take up more iodine and produce more hormone. This feedback mechanism maintains a healthy circular balance

KEY TERMS

goiter Enlargement of the thyroid gland caused by lack of available iodine to produce the thyroid hormone thyroxine.

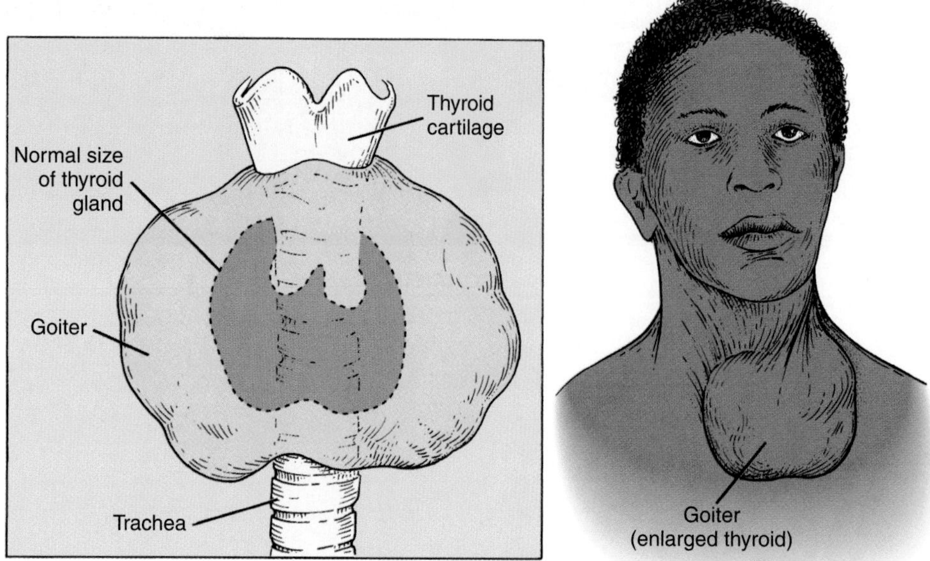

FIGURE 7-6 Goiter. The extreme enlargement shown here reflects an extended duration of iodine deficiency.

between supply and demand and is the characteristic pattern governing hormone production by the endocrine glands controlled by the master pituitary gland.

Physiologic Function of Iodine

Thyroid Hormone Synthesis

The major function of iodine is the synthesis of the thyroid hormone thyroxine. Thyroxine regulates cell oxidation and basal metabolic rate (BMR) by increasing oxygen uptake and the reaction rates of enzyme systems handling glucose. In this role, iodine exerts tremendous control of the body's total metabolism. Thyroid hormone also regulates protein synthesis and myelin formation in the developing brain.[64]

Plasma Thyroxine

Thyroxine is secreted into the bloodstream bound to plasma protein for transport to the cells. After completing its work, the hormone is degraded in the liver and the iodine excreted in the bile.

Clinical Applications

Hyperthyroidism and hypothyroidism affect the rate of thyroxine production and the body's overall metabolic rate.

Iodine Deficiency Disorder: Goiter

Endemic goiter, visible as a great enlargement of the thyroid gland, is a problem in geographic areas where water and soil, and in turn locally grown foods, contain little iodine. Up to 2 billion people live in iodine-deficient areas, including one third of all school children.[64] Africa, Southeast Asia, the Eastern Mediterranean, and parts of Europe have widespread iodine deficiency. When iodine is unavailable the thyroid gland cannot produce a normal quantity of thyroxine, and low plasma thyroxine levels signal the pituitary to release TSH. In the absence of iodine the thyroid gland responds by making thyroglobulin (a colloid), which accumulates in the thyroid follicles. Over time the gland becomes increasingly engorged and may attain a size of 500 to 700 g (1 to 1½ lb) or more (Figure 7-6).

Salt iodization remains the most cost-effective way to deliver iodine to both humans and livestock and is credited with eradicating iodine deficiency in the United States and Canada. In remote areas where iodization of salt is not practical, iodized rapeseed oil, monthly doses of potassium iodide to school children, or slow-release iodide added to drinking water have eradicated severe endemic goiter.[64–66] Goiter also stems from eating foods containing substances that inhibit the synthesis of thyroxine. Pearl millet, a cereal grain used in the Sudan region of Africa, can cause goiter.

Iodine Deficiency Disorder: Cretinism

Iodine deficiency has been referred to as *the most common cause of preventable mental impairment in the world*,[64] and pregnant and lactating women and their infants are especially at risk. When iodine deficiency is severe in fetal and infant periods of critical brain development, the outcome is **cretinism**, with irreversible mental retardation and disability. Salt fortification programs appear to provide sufficient iodine to support the elevated needs of pregnancy and the production of breast milk with appropriate iodine content.[65]

Iodine Overload

Food production and processing methods add to iodine intake. Dairy farms use iodophors, iodine-containing chemicals, for sanitizing milking machines and milk tanks. Other iodine-containing compounds finding their way into the human food supply are the iodates used as dough conditioners in breads, erythrosine, a food coloring, and derivatives of iodine supplements added to animal feeds. Case reports of iodine toxicity indicate that iodine-containing dietary supplements or topical medications, when added to the iodine contributed by food, result in intakes that exceed by many times the RDA.

Iodine Requirement

Dietary Reference Intake

The RDA for men and women is 150 mcg/day.[47] To meet the needs of mother and developing fetus, the RDA in pregnancy increases to 220 mcg/day and in lactation to 290 mcg/day. Because of increased demand for iodine during accelerated growth, the allowance for youth ages 14 to 18 is the same as for adults.

Food Sources of Iodine

Seafood is rich in iodine. Other foods vary widely, depending on the iodine content of the soil and the iodine compounds used in processing. Iodized table salt fortified at the level of 1 mg of iodine per 10 g of salt is a major dietary source in the United States. Calcium and potassium iodates are common additives in commercially produced bread. Avoidance of salt for health reasons could help explain the decrease in iodine intakes in the United States occurring over the past 30 years.[64]

ZINC

Zinc is a component of over 100 different enzymes and a factor in growth.[47] Total body zinc ranges from 1.5 g in women to 2.5 g in men. It is present in minute quantities in all body organs, tissues, and fluids. Although zinc is vital throughout life, it is particularly important in growth periods such as pregnancy and lactation, infancy and childhood, and adolescence.[47,67] Zinc is closely involved with deoxyribonucleic acid (DNA) and ribonucleic acid (RNA) metabolism and protein synthesis. It is necessary for tissue growth to progress at normal rates.

Clinical Applications

Several clinical problems stem from zinc deficiency, as follows:

- *Hypogonadism:* Dwarfism with arrested development and function of the gonads results from pronounced zinc deficiency in childhood and adolescence. Sexual maturation is delayed in male adolescents deprived of zinc.
- *Loss in taste and smell:* Hypogeusia (diminished taste) and hyposmia (diminished smell) are associated with severe zinc deficiency but improve when zinc is restored.
- *Wound healing:* Healing of wounds or tissue injuries from trauma, surgery, or physiologic stress is retarded in those who are zinc deficient. Older adults with pressure sores may benefit from zinc supplementation.
- *Growth, development, and life cycle needs:* Rapid growth in infants, children, and adolescents carries special needs for zinc. When zinc is inadequate, proteins necessary for the linear growth of the long bones are not produced and growth is stunted.[47] Poor zinc intake in pregnancy can result in congenital malformations and low infant birth weight.
- *Immune function:* Zinc promotes optimum immune function. Older individuals with normal serum zinc levels had greater resistance to infections and less need for antibiotics than those with low serum zinc.[68]
- *Malabsorption:* Malabsorption diseases such as Crohn's disease lead to zinc deficiency. Dietary restrictions imposed in the treatment of these conditions can further limit zinc availability.

Zinc Requirement

Dietary Reference Intake

The RDA for zinc is 11 mg for men and 8 mg for women.[47] Women's needs are lower because of their generally smaller body size. National surveys tell us that adolescent girls and older adults are most likely to have intakes less than recommended levels,[3] but young children may also be at risk. Less than half of the sack lunches preschool children brought to a day care center met 33% of the DRI for zinc[69]; the omission of milk in many of those lunches likely contributed to the low zinc content.[70] Beef is a major zinc source in the United States accounting for nearly 25% of total intake, followed by ready-to-eat cereals, milk, and poultry. Zinc can be a problem for vegetarians because phytates in plant foods interfere with absorption.[71]

Food Sources of Zinc

Good sources of dietary zinc are seafood (especially oysters), meat, and eggs. Legumes and whole grains contain zinc, but bioavailability can be a problem. Box 7-9 lists some comparative foods containing zinc.

COPPER

Copper and iron have many characteristics in common, as listed below:

- Both are components of cell enzymes.
- Both are involved in energy production.
- Both participate in hemoglobin synthesis.

Copper is found in many foods, but deficiency has been reported in patients on total parenteral nutrition (TPN) that excluded copper. Persons using concentrated zinc supplements that interfere with copper absorption can develop copper deficiency as can premature infants fed only cow's milk, which is low in copper.[47]

The RDA for copper is 900 mcg/day (0.9 mg/day), but it appears that many adults do not reach this level.[47] Copper, like

KEY TERMS

cretinism A congenital disease resulting from a lack of iodine and thyroxin secretion, characterized by physical deformity, dwarfism, mental retardation, and often goiters.

many trace elements, is lost in food processing. The richest sources are liver, seafood (particularly oysters), nuts, and seeds, with smaller amounts in whole grains and legumes. The *Focus on Food Safety* box, "Minerals from Cooking Utensils: What Is Safe and What Is Harmful?" discusses how copper and other minerals can enter our food in cooking.

BOX 7-9 FOOD SOURCES OF ZINC

FOOD SOURCE	QUANTITY	ZINC (in mg)
Grains Group		
Bite-Size Shredded Wheat cereal	1 cup	1.50
Oat bran muffin	1	1.05
Vegetable Group		
Peas, green	1 cup	1.07
Meat, Beans, Eggs, and Nuts Group		
Oysters, cooked	3 oz	74.06
Ground-beef patty	3 oz	5.26
Baked beans	1 cup	5.79
Peanut butter	2 tbsp	0.94
Milk Group		
Milk, low-fat	8 oz	1.02
Cheddar cheese	1 oz	0.88

Recommended Dietary Allowance (RDA) for adults: women, 8 mg; men, 11 mg.
Nutrient data from USDA: *USDA National Nutrient Database for Standard Reference, Release 21,* Washington, DC, U.S. Department of Agriculture, 2009. Retrieved April 23, 2010 from http://www.ars.usda.gov/Services/docs.htm?docid=17477.

MANGANESE

The adult body contains about 20 mg of manganese distributed in the liver, bones, pancreas, and pituitary gland.[47] Like other trace elements, manganese is a part of important cell enzymes. Manganese deficiency has been reported in patients with pancreatic insufficiency and protein-energy malnutrition. Although a dietary essential, manganese is toxic at high levels, as when miners or other workers have prolonged exposure to manganese dust. Excess manganese accumulates in the liver and central nervous system (CNS), producing psychiatric disturbances and neuromuscular symptoms resembling those of Parkinson's disease. The AI for manganese is 2.3 mg/day for men and 1.8 mg/day for women.[47] The typical American diet supplies manganese at a level of 1.6 mg/1000 kcal. The best sources are plant foods—grains, legumes, seeds, nuts, leafy vegetables, tea, and coffee.

CHROMIUM

Chromium is found in minute amounts in liver, soft tissues, and bone, although the precise amount in the body is not known. Chromium is part of a protein complex that potentiates insulin activity and assists in moving glucose into cells. Through its role with insulin, chromium influences carbohydrate, protein, and fat metabolism. Chromium picolinate is widely advertised as a body-building and weight-loss supplement, despite the fact that no research evidence supports these claims and, indeed, existing evidence even contradicts these claims. (See Chapter 14 for more discussion of chromium picolinate.)

The AI for chromium is 35 mcg/day for men and 25 mcg/day for women ages 19 to 50. Based on their lower energy intakes, the AIs for those older than age 50 decrease to 30 mcg and 20 mcg, respectively.[47] Information about the chromium content of common foods is sparse. Brewer's yeast is a rich source. Other food sources include liver, cheddar cheese, wheat germ, and whole grains.

FOCUS ON FOOD SAFETY

Minerals from Cooking Utensils: What Is Safe and What Is Harmful?

Some dishes and containers intended to be decorative are lined with copper or enhanced with lead-containing glazes. Copper and lead are easily dissolved by acid—this includes acids in food. It is dangerous to cook or serve foods in copper-lined or lead-glazed utensils because harmful amounts of these minerals can dissolve and enter your food. The body requires copper in very minute amounts, but higher levels become toxic. Lead exposure is harmful for all age-groups but especially for children. The Food Code developed by the U.S. Food and Drug Administration (FDA), which sets standards for safe food handling in restaurants, institutions, and other food service operations forbids any use of such containers. It is well known that very small amounts of iron from cast iron cooking utensils enter the food during cooking, especially when cooking acid-containing foods. For most people this is not a problem and may actually be helpful in raising iron intake levels. In general, cookware bought in reputable retail stores will not pose any health risk, but consumers should use caution when buying cookware from other sources. Persons with hemochromatosis, who absorb iron in exceptionally large amounts, must avoid all cast iron utensils.

Data from U.S. Food and Drug Administration: *Food Code: 2005,* Washington, DC, 2005, U.S. Government Printing Office.
Duyff RL: *American Dietetic Association complete food and nutrition guide,* ed 3, Hoboken, NJ, 2006, John Wiley & Sons.
U.S. National Library of Medicine, U.S. National Institutes of Health: Medline Plus, Trusted Health Information for You: *Cooking utensils and nutrition,* updated August 2009. Retrieved August 18, 2009, from http://www.nlm.nih.gov/medlineplus/ency/article/002461.htm - Recommendations.

COBALT

Cobalt is found in minute traces in body tissues, with storage in the liver. As part of vitamin B_{12} (cobalamin), the known functions of cobalt are associated with red blood cell formation and support of the myelin sheath surrounding nerve fibers in the CNS. Cobalt is provided in the human diet only in the form of vitamin B_{12}.

SELENIUM

Selenium is deposited in all body tissues except adipose tissue. Concentrations are highest in liver, kidney, heart, and spleen. Selenium is an integral part of an antioxidant enzyme that protects cells and lipid membranes from oxidative damage. Selenium partners with vitamin E, each sparing the other. Highly bioavailable selenium compounds are found in breast milk, suggesting an important role for this element in early life.[72] The RDA for all adults is 55 mcg/day.[73] Foods vary in selenium based on the content of the soil in which they were grown. In general, good sources include seafood, legumes, whole grains, lean meats, and dairy products; vegetables have the smallest amounts.

MOLYBDENUM

Molybdenum is an enzyme cofactor in reactions that move hydroxyl (OH^-) groups.[47] The RDA is set at 45 mcg/day for all adults. The amount of molybdenum in foods varies according to the soil content. The richest sources generally include legumes, whole grains, and nuts. Animal products, fruit, and most vegetables are poor sources.

FLUORIDE

Fluoride accumulates in the calcified tissues and protects bones and teeth from mineral loss. If fluoride is present when calcium-phosphorus crystals are being formed, then a fluoride ion (F^-) replaces a hydroxyl ion (OH^-) in the crystal, resulting in a material that is more resistant to resorption. Fluoride-containing crystals are also more resistant to the erosive effect of bacterial acids formed by microorganisms that feed on fermentable carbohydrates adhering to the teeth and initiate tooth decay.[74]

The AI for fluoride is expected to protect against dental caries. Intake is set at 4 mg/day for men and 3 mg/day for women.[11] Fish, fish products, and tea contain the highest amounts. Fluoridated dental products also contribute to fluoride intake. Adding fluoride to public water supplies in the amount of 1 part per million (ppm) reduces dental caries in those communities. Cooking with fluoridated water increases the level in many foods.

The roles of the essential trace elements are summarized in Table 7-6.

OTHER TRACE ELEMENTS

The metabolic functions or need for five other trace elements, arsenic, boron, vanadium, nickel, and silicon, are not understood. Although they appear to have beneficial roles in various animal species, evidence of their nutritional importance, essentiality, or role in human health is lacking.[32] At this time, insufficient research data are available to set an RDA or AI for these nutrients. Based on the potential for toxicity as observed in animal experiments, a UL has been established for boron, nickel, and vanadium.[32]

WATER-ELECTROLYTE BALANCE

Hydration status is fundamental to health and a vital part of patient care. In this section we will look at the three interdependent factors that control fluid balance: (1) the water itself (the solvent base for solutions), (2) the various particles (solutes) in the water, and (3) the separating membranes that control flow from one **compartment** to another.

BODY WATER DISTRIBUTION

If you are a woman, your body is about 50% to 55% water; if you are a man, then it is about 55% to 60% water. Men have higher water content because they have proportionately more muscle and less fat. Muscle contains more water than any other tissue except blood. Women have proportionately less muscle and more fat, which is low in water content compared with muscle.

FUNCTIONS OF WATER

Body water has many roles (Box 7-10). Much of our body form comes from the *turgor* water provides for tissues. Cell water furnishes the fluid environment for the vast array of chemical reactions that sustain life. Medications are dissolved in body fluids. The evaporation of water from the skin is an important means of controlling body temperature.

OVERALL WATER BALANCE: INPUT AND OUTPUT

The average adult processes 2.5 to 3 L of water per day. Water enters and leaves the body by various routes, controlled by the thirst mechanism and regulatory hormones (Table 7-7).

Water enters the body in three forms:

1. As preformed water taken in as water or in other beverages
2. As preformed water in food
3. As metabolic water produced by cell oxidation

It is estimated that 81% of fluid intake comes from water and beverages and 19% comes from food.[30] Plain water contributes about a third of the total and other beverages about half.[75] Many common foods contain large amounts of water (Table 7-8). Metabolic water contributes less to total

KEY TERMS

compartment The collective quantity of material of a given type in the body. The four body compartments are (1) lean body mass (muscle and vital organs), (2) bone, (3) fat, and (4) water.

TABLE 7-6 SUMMARY OF TRACE ELEMENTS

ELEMENT	METABOLISM	PHYSIOLOGIC FUNCTIONS	CLINICAL APPLICATIONS	DIETARY REFERENCE INTAKE	FOOD SOURCES
Iron (Fe)	Absorption controls body supply; favored by body need, acidity, and reduction agents such as vitamin C; hindered by binding agents, reduced gastric acid, infection, gastrointestinal losses Transported as transferrin, stored as ferritin or hemosiderin Excreted in sloughed cells, bleeding	Hemoglobin synthesis, oxygen transport Cell oxidation, heme enzymes	Anemia (hypochromic, microcytic) Excess: hemosiderosis, hemochromatosis Growth and pregnancy needs	Adults: men ages ≥19: 8 mg; women ages 19-50: 18 mg; women ages ≥51: 8 mg Pregnancy: all ages 27 mg Lactation: ages ≤18: 10 mg; ages ≥19: 9 mg	Meat, eggs, liver Whole grain and enriched breads and cereals Dark-green vegetables Legumes, nuts, acidic foods cooked in iron utensils
Iodine (I)	Absorbed as iodides, taken up by thyroid gland under control of thyroid-stimulating hormone (TSH) Excretion by kidney	Synthesis of thyroxin, which regulates cell metabolism, basal metabolic rate (BMR)	Endemic colloid goiter, cretinism Hypothyroidism and hyperthyroidism	Adults: men/women ages ≥19: 150 mcg Pregnancy: all ages 220 mcg Lactation: all ages 290 mcg	Iodized salt Seafood
Zinc (Zn)	Absorbed in small intestine Transported in blood by albumin Stored in many sites Excretion largely intestinal	Essential coenzyme constituent: carbonic anhydrase, carboxypeptidase, lactic dehydrogenase	Growth: hypogonadism Sensory impairment: taste and smell Wound healing Malabsorption disease	Adults: men ages ≥19: 11 mg; women ages ≥19: 8 mg Pregnancy: ages ≤18: 12 mg; ages ≥19: 11 mg Lactation: ages ≤18: 13 mg; ages ≥19: 12 mg	Beef and other meats, liver Oysters, seafood Milk, cheese, eggs Whole grains Widely distributed in food
Copper (Cu)	Absorbed in small intestine Transported in blood by histidine and albumin Stored in many tissues	Associated with iron in enzyme systems, hemoglobin synthesis, metalloproteinases	Hypocupremia: nephrosis and malabsorption Wilson's disease, excess copper storage	Adults: men/women ages ≥19: 900 mcg Pregnancy: all ages 1000 mcg Lactation: all ages 1300 mcg	Meat, liver, seafood Whole grains Legumes, nuts Widely distributed in food

Manganese (Mn)	Absorbed poorly Excretion mainly by intestine	Enzyme component in general metabolism	Low serum levels in protein-energy malnutrition Inhalation toxicity	Adults: men ages ≥19: 2.3 mg; women ages ≥19: 1.8 mg Pregnancy: all ages 2.0 mg Lactation: all ages 2.6 mg	Whole grains and cereals Legumes, soybeans Green leafy vegetables
Chromium (Cr)	Absorbed in association with zinc Excretion mainly by kidneys	Associated with glucose metabolism	Potentiates action of insulin	Adults: men ages 19-50: 35 mcg; ages ≥51: 30 mcg Adults: women ages 19-50: 25 mcg; ages ≥51: 20 mcg Pregnancy: ages ≤18: 29 mcg; ages ≥19: 30 mcg Lactation: ages ≤18: 44 mcg; ages ≥19: 45 mcg	Whole grains and cereals Brewer's yeast Animal protein foods
Cobalt (Co)	Absorbed as component of vitamin B_{12} Stored in liver	Constituent of vitamin B_{12}, functions with vitamin	Deficiency associated only with deficiency of vitamin B_{12}	Unknown (usually consumed as part of the vitamin B_{12} molecule)	Animal foods containing vitamin B_{12}
Selenium (Se)	Absorption depends on solubility of compound form Excreted mainly by kidneys	Constituent of enzyme glutathione peroxidase Synergistic antioxidant with vitamin E	Marginal deficiency when soil content is low Deficiency secondary to total parenteral nutrition (TPN) or malnutrition Toxicity observed in livestock	Adults: men/women ages ≥19: 55 mcg Pregnancy: all ages 60 mcg Lactation: all ages 70 mcg	Seafood Legumes Whole grains Vegetables Low-fat meats and dairy foods Varies with soil content
Molybdenum (Mo)	Readily absorbed Excreted rapidly by kidneys Small amount excreted in bile	Constituent of oxidase enzymes, xanthine oxidase	Deficiency unknown in humans	Adults: men/women ages ≥19: 45 mcg Pregnancy: all ages 50 mcg Lactation: all ages 50 mcg	Legumes Whole grains Milk Organ meats Leafy vegetables
Fluoride (F)	Absorbed in small intestine, little known of bioavailability Excreted by kidneys—80%	Accumulates in bones and teeth, increases hardness	Inhibits dental caries Osteoporosis: may reduce bone loss Excess: dental fluorosis	Adults: men ages ≥19: 4 mg; women ages ≥19: 3 mg Pregnancy: all ages 3 mg Lactation: all ages 3 mg	Fish and fish products Tea Drinking water if fluoridated Foods cooked in fluoridated water

TABLE 7-7 APPROXIMATE DAILY ADULT WATER INTAKE AND OUTPUT

	INTAKE (REPLACEMENT) (in mL/day)		OUTPUT (LOSS) (in mL/day) OBLIGATORY (INSENSIBLE) (in mL/day)	ADDITIONAL (ACCORDING TO NEED) (in mL/day)
Preformed in liquids	1200-1500	Lungs	350	
In foods	700-1000	Skin diffusion	350	
Metabolism (oxidation of food)	200-300	Sweat	100	≈250
		Kidneys	900	≈500
		Feces	150	
TOTAL	2100-2800 (≈2600 mL/day)	TOTAL	1850	750
			(≈2600 mL/day)	

BOX 7-10 FUNCTIONS OF BODY WATER

- Gives form and structure
- Provides environment for chemical reactions to take place
- Dissolves important substances in tissues and cells
- Transports nutrients and waste
- Controls body temperature
- Dissolves medications

TABLE 7-8 WATER CONTENT OF SELECTED FOODS AND BEVERAGES

FOOD	PERCENT (%)
Coffee, milk, sports drinks, watermelon, broccoli, lettuce	91-100
Soda, fruit drinks, fruit juice, apples, oranges, grapes	80-90
Peas, frozen desserts, bananas, casseroles	70-79
Meat, fish, poultry	60-69
Bread, pasta	30-40
Cereals, nuts	<5

Data from Campbell S: Dietary Reference Intakes: water, potassium, sodium, chloride, and sulfate, *Nutr MD* 30(6):13, 2004.

TABLE 7-9 ADEQUATE INTAKES OF FLUID*

AGE (YEARS)	MALES	FEMALES
1-3	4 cups	4 cups
4-8	5 cups	5 cups
9-13	8 cups	7 cups
14-18	11 cups	8 cups
≥19	13 cups	9 cups

Data from Food and Nutrition Board, Institute of Medicine: *Dietary Reference Intakes for water, potassium, sodium, chloride, and sulfate,* Washington, DC, 2004, National Academies Press.
*Expressed as cups of beverages/drinking water, with additional fluid to be supplied in food.

water entering the body than do beverages or food. However, all water entering the body, regardless of source, is of equal value in meeting fluid needs.

Water leaves the body via the kidneys, skin, and lungs, as well as by fecal elimination (see Table 7-7). Vomiting and diarrhea bring abnormal losses of fluid and serious clinical problems if prolonged. Extensive loss of body fluid is especially dangerous for infants and children, whose bodies contain a greater proportion of water; in addition, more of this water is outside the cells and easily lost. Water retention associated with heart failure or electrolyte disturbances requires immediate medical attention. Intake and output must remain in balance to sustain normal hydration levels.

WATER REQUIREMENTS

For years we were told to drink eight glasses of water a day, although it is difficult to find documentation on the origin of this advice.[76,77] References to hydration in the popular press and advertisements for bottled water promote deliberate water consumption. Nutrition experts emphasize that for most individuals fluid needs are adequately met by drinking when thirsty.[31,78]

Dietary Reference Intake

The AIs for fluid (Table 7-9) are based on the median water intake reported by participants in recent national surveys[31]; thus half of the people in each age and gender category drank more and half drank less. Note, however, that these guidelines are intended for healthy individuals who are relatively sedentary and live in temperate climates. Athletes engaging in vigorous physical activity of long duration, the critically ill, persons in very hot environments, or those doing strenuous physical work require special attention.[31,79]

Over the years researchers have put forth conflicting opinions as to the value of caffeinated beverages in meeting fluid needs. It was commonly held that water from caffeine-containing beverages such as coffee or soft drinks was lost to the body. It has since been learned that people accustomed to drinking caffeinated beverages have no increase in urine output,[80] and such beverages contribute to meeting fluid needs.[81–82] Alcoholic beverages do bring about water loss shortly after drinking, but the effect is transient, with no appreciable loss over a 24-hour period.[31]

Special Clinical Applications

The following clinical situations influence water needs:

- *Uncontrolled diabetes mellitus:* Patients losing excessive amounts of water through the osmotic effect of large amounts of glucose in the urine need additional fluid.
- *Cystic fibrosis:* Children and adults with this disease have increased fluid needs.
- *High fiber intake:* As dietary fiber increases, so do fluid requirements. Adequate fluid is needed to replace the water absorbed by the fiber in the gastrointestinal tract.
- *High protein intake:* Protein metabolism produces urea and other nitrogenous wastes that must be excreted via the kidneys. Providing an appropriate level of fluid is important for patients given high-protein supplements.
- *Intense physical activity:* Exercise of high intensity or duration such as marathon runs or strenuous physical work requires a consistent fluid intake to replace water lost in sweat and enable this cooling mechanism to continue. A lack of fluid in such situations can lead to heat stroke and death (see Chapter 14).
- *Impaired thirst in older adults:* Some older persons, particularly frail older adults in poor health or taking numerous medications, do not become thirsty when they should, based on aging changes in the thirst center of the hypothalamus. In such cases it is prudent to monitor fluid intake.[83]
- *Medications:* Diuretics increase fluid output, as do certain analgesics and decongestants.

Water Compartments

Body water is divided into two major compartments: (1) the water outside the cells, the *ECF (extracellular fluid) compartment,* and (2) the water inside the cells, the *ICF (intracellular fluid) compartment* (Figure 7-7). We describe these following:

- *ECF:* The water outside the cells makes up about 20% of total body weight. It has four sections: (1) blood plasma, which accounts for about 5% of body weight; (2) **interstitial fluid,** the water surrounding the cells; (3) secretory fluid, the water circulating in transit; and (4) dense tissue fluid, water in deep connective tissue, cartilage, and bone.
- *ICF:* The water inside the cells makes up about 40% to 45% of total body weight. All of the metabolic activity of organs and tissues takes place within cells, so it could be expected that the amount of water inside the cells would be greater than the amount outside the cells (intracellular water is about twice that of extracellular water).

FORCES CONTROLLING WATER DISTRIBUTION

Two forces control the distribution of body water: (1) the number of solutes or particles in solution and (2) the membranes that separate water compartments. We will look at the properties of each.

Solutes

A variety of particles are found in body water in differing concentrations. Two types control water balance: electrolytes and plasma proteins.

Electrolytes

Several minerals serve as major electrolytes in controlling body fluid compartments. In this role they are called *electrolytes* because they are free in solution and carry an electrical charge. Free, charged chemical forms are also called *ions,* a term that refers to atoms, elements, or groups of atoms that in solution carry either a positive or negative electrical charge. An ion carrying a positive charge is called a *cation:* examples are sodium (Na^+), the major cation in extracellular water; potassium (K^+), the major cation in intracellular water; calcium (Ca^{+2}); and magnesium (Mg^{+2}). An ion carrying a negative charge is called an *anion:* examples are chloride (Cl^-), bicarbonate (HCO_3^-), phosphate (HPO_4^{-2}), and sulfate (SO_4^{-2}). By virtue of their small size, these ions or electrolytes can diffuse freely across cell membranes and create forces that control the movement of water within the body.

Plasma Proteins

Albumin and globulin, plasma proteins of large molecular size, influence the movement of water in and out of capillaries. In this function these plasma proteins are called *colloids* (from the Greek word *kolla* for "glue") and form colloidal solutions. Because of their large size, plasma proteins cannot pass through the capillary membrane into the interstitial fluid. Instead they remain in the blood vessels, where they exert **colloidal osmotic pressure (COP)** to maintain vascular blood volume. We will learn more about this process a bit later.

Organic Compounds of Small Molecular Size

Other organic compounds small in size such as glucose, urea, and amino acids diffuse freely in and out of the various fluid compartments but do not influence shifts of water unless they are present in abnormally large concentrations. Such a situation occurs in patients with uncontrolled diabetes mellitus, when large amounts of glucose being excreted in the urine cause an abnormal osmotic diuresis or excess water output.

KEY TERMS

electrolyte A chemical element or compound that, in solution, forms ions carrying a positive (e.g., H^+, Na^+, K^+, Ca^{+2}, and Mg^{+2}) or negative (e.g., Cl^-, HCO_3^-, HPO_4^{-2}, and SO_4^{-2}) charge. Electrolytes control fluid balances within the body.

interstitial fluid The fluid situated between parts or in the interspaces of a tissue.

colloidal osmotic pressure (COP) Pressure produced by the protein molecules in the plasma and in the cell. Because proteins are large molecules, they do not pass through the separating membranes of the capillary cells but exert a constant osmotic pull that protects vital plasma and cell fluid volumes in both compartments.

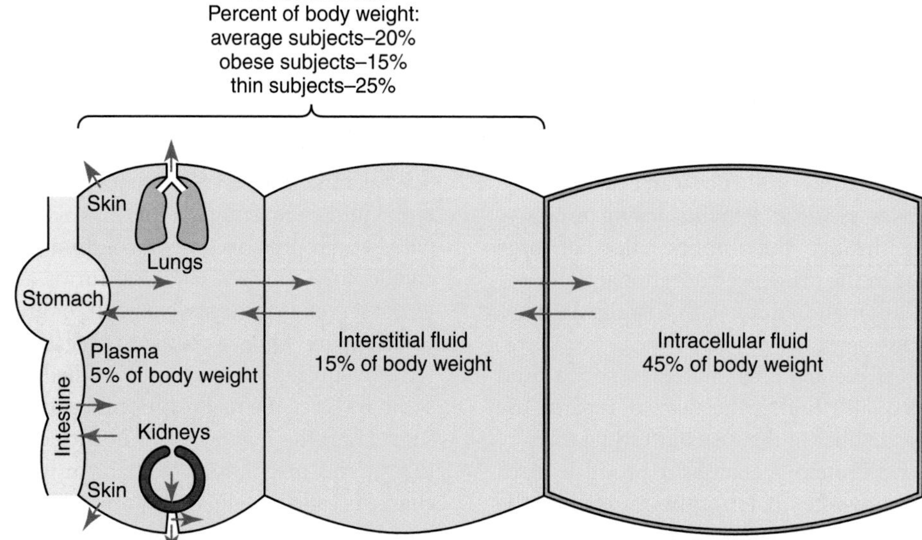

FIGURE 7-7 Body fluid compartments. Note the relative amounts of water in the intracellular compartment and extracellular compartment. (Data from Gamble JL: *Chemical anatomy, physiology, and pathology of extracellular fluid,* Cambridge, Mass, 1964, Harvard University Press.)

Membranes

Water and solutes move across the separating membranes according to the physiologic mechanisms that handle fluid shifts. These mechanisms include osmosis, diffusion, filtration, active transport, and pinocytosis. We learned about these mechanisms in Chapter 2 (see page 34).

INFLUENCE OF ELECTROLYTES ON WATER BALANCE

Measurement of Electrolytes

The concentration of electrolytes or particles in a given solution determines the chemical activity of that solution. It is the *number* of particles, not the *size* of the particles, which determines chemical combining power, so electrolytes are measured according to the total number of particles in solution. Each particle contributes chemical combining power according to its valence, not its total weight. The unit of measure commonly used is the *equivalent.* Because we are usually talking about very small amounts, these measurements are expressed in *milliequivalents (mEq),* or thousandths of an equivalent. This term refers to the number of ions—cations and anions—in solution in a given volume of body fluid. It is expressed as the number of *milliequivalents per liter (mEq/L).*

Electrolyte Balance

Electrolytes are distributed in body water compartments in a definite pattern. According to biochemical and electrochemical laws, a stable solution must have equal numbers of positive and negative particles. This means it must be electrically neutral. When shifts or losses occur, compensating shifts and gains must follow to maintain this balance of *essential* electrochemical neutrality.

Electrolyte Control of Body Hydration

Ionized sodium is the chief cation of ECF, and ionized potassium is the chief cation of ICF. These two electrolytes control the amount of water retained in each compartment. Shifts in water from one compartment to the other reflect changes in the ECF concentration of these electrolytes. The terms *hypertonic* and *hypotonic* refer to the electrolyte concentration of the water outside the cell. When surrounded by a hypertonic solution, water flows out of the cell and the cell becomes dehydrated and shrinks in size. When the cell is surrounded by a hypotonic solution, water flows into the cell, causing it to swell and eventually burst if the situation is not corrected.

KEY TERMS

capillary fluid shift mechanism Process that controls the movement of water and small molecules (electrolytes, nutrients) between the blood in the capillary and the surrounding interstitial area. Shifts in balance between the intracapillary hydrostatic blood pressure and the colloidal osmotic pressure exerted by the plasma proteins accomplish filtration of water and solutes out of the capillary at the arteriole end and reabsorption at the venule end.

renin-angiotensin-aldosterone system Three-stage system of sodium conservation and control of water loss; in response to diminished filtration pressure in the kidney nephrons—(1) the kidneys secrete the enzyme renin, which combines with and activates angiotensinogen from the liver; (2) active angiotensin stimulates the adjacent adrenal gland to release the hormone aldosterone; and (3) aldosterone causes reabsorption of sodium in the kidney nephrons and water follows.

INFLUENCE OF PLASMA PROTEINS ON WATER BALANCE

Capillary Fluid Shift Mechanism

Water is constantly circulating throughout the body in the blood vessels; fluid must move out of the vessels to service the tissues and then be drawn back into the vessels to maintain normal transport flow. Two opposing pressures—(1) the hydrostatic pressure (blood pressure) of the capillary blood flow and (2) the COP from plasma proteins (mainly albumin)—control the movement of water and solute across capillary membranes. The flow of water, nutrients, and waste to and from the cells occurs by the shifting balance of these two pressures. It works as a filtration process driven by the differences in osmotic pressure on either side of the capillary membrane.

When blood first enters the capillary system, the existing blood pressure forces water and small solutes such as glucose out into the tissues to bathe and nourish the cells. The plasma proteins, however, are too large to pass through the pores of the capillary membrane and now exert the greater COP that draws fluid and waste materials back into the capillary circulation. This process is called the **capillary fluid shift mechanism.** It is one of the most important homeostatic mechanisms in the body for maintaining water balance, without which cells would die.

Cell Fluid Control

Just as plasma proteins provide COP to maintain the volume of the ECF, cell protein provides the osmotic pressure that maintains the volume of the ICF. Electrolytes also play a role, with ionized potassium guarding water within the cell and ionized sodium guarding water outside the cell. This balance supports the sustaining flow of water, nutrients, metabolites, and waste in and out of cells.

HORMONES CONTROLLING WATER BALANCE

Antidiuretic Hormone

The posterior lobe of the pituitary gland secretes the antidiuretic hormone (ADH), also called *vasopressin.* It controls the reabsorption of water by the kidneys according to body need, acting as a water-conserving mechanism. In times of threatened or actual loss of body water, this hormone is released to retain precious fluid.

Aldosterone

Aldosterone is a sodium-conserving hormone associated with the **renin-angiotensin-aldosterone system,** but it also exerts secondary control over body water. Renin, an enzyme secreted by the kidney, and angiotensin, a product of the liver, trigger the release of aldosterone from the adrenal cortex. Aldosterone acts on the kidney to reabsorb sodium, but in the process water is also reabsorbed. Both aldosterone and ADH are activated by injury, surgery, or other physiologic stress.

TO SUM UP

Minerals are inorganic substances widely distributed in nature. They build body tissues; activate, regulate, and control metabolic processes; and help transmit messages across nerve fibers. Minerals are classified as (1) *major minerals* and (2) *trace elements.* Major minerals are required in larger amounts and make up 60% to 80% of all the inorganic material in the body. Trace elements, measured in amounts as small as a microgram (mcg), make up less than 1% of the body's inorganic matter. Seven major minerals and 10 trace elements are known to be essential in human nutrition; another eight trace elements may be essential, but their roles remain to be defined. The major minerals include calcium and phosphorus, with roles in bone health, energy metabolism, and nerve transmission, and magnesium, a participant in many metabolic reactions. Sodium and potassium exert opposing effects on blood pressure, and increased potassium intake may help to moderate the pressor effect of sodium. The trace mineral iron (as a part of hemoglobin) transports oxygen to the cells and, along with iodine and zinc, regulates growth and body metabolism. Other trace minerals as enzyme partners regulate day-to-day metabolic activities. Sodium, potassium, and chloride particles in body fluids, along with plasma proteins, control water balance and the distribution of fluids inside (ICF) and outside (ECF) the cells. Maintenance of appropriate fluid compartments and hydration status are crucial components in clinical care.

QUESTIONS FOR REVIEW

1. List the seven major minerals and describe their (a) physiologic function, (b) problems related to deficiency or excess, and (c) dietary sources.
2. List the 10 trace elements with proven essentiality for humans. Why has it been difficult to establish DRIs for these nutrients?
3. The AI for calcium for persons older than 50 years is 1200 mg/day. Develop a menu for a frail 83-year-old woman that will provide this level of calcium within an energy intake of 1500 kcal/day.
4. You are working with a teenager who eats no red meat or fish but likes chicken. She is concerned about her weight

and follows the diet pattern of MyPyramid that provides an intake of 1600 kcal/day. List the foods with portion sizes that you would select to reach her iron RDA of 18 mg. When making your selections, consider other factors in the diet that will enhance or impede the absorption of the iron provided.

5. What causes the edema in protein-energy malnutrition?
6. Why does prolonged diarrhea lead to potassium depletion?
7. Visit the website of a chain fast-food or family restaurant in your locality and look for the nutrient content of their menu. To the extent possible, select a meal that will supply one third of the RDA or AI for (a) calcium, (b) iron, and (c) zinc, but not exceed one third of the MyPyramid energy recommendation for a sedentary 25-year-old man or woman. Were you able to accomplish this? If not, then what problems did you encounter? What might be the effect on an individual's nutritional status if he or she had a daily meal at this food outlet?
8. Go to a nearby grocery store or drug store that sells mineral supplements. Check three multimineral supplements marketed for children (use the DRI of the age-group noted on the label) and three marketed for adults. Prepare a table that lists each brand and include (a) the percent of the DRI provided for each mineral and (b) the cost of a 1-day supply of the supplement. Did any of the supplements you examined exceed the UL for any nutrient? If so, then what is the danger of toxicity? Based on cost and content, would an individual be better advised to spend that extra amount of money for food? What specific foods would you recommend?
9. You are working with a 37-year-old man who is beginning to experience a gradual increase in his blood pressure and has been advised to increase his intakes of potassium and calcium and lower his intake of sodium. When his work takes him on the road, he has lunch at a fast-food restaurant; on other days he takes a sandwich from home to eat at his desk. Develop a menu for a fast-food lunch and a packed lunch that will provide 33% of the DRI for potassium and calcium and no more than 33% of the UL for sodium.

REFERENCES

1. Weaver CM, Heaney RP: Calcium. In Shils ME, Shike M, Olson J, et al, editors: *Modern nutrition in health and disease*, ed 10, Baltimore, 2006, Lippincott Williams & Wilkins.
2. Hurrell RF: Influence of vegetable protein sources on trace element and mineral bioavailability, *J Nutr* 133:2973S, 2003.
3. U.S. Department of Agriculture, Agricultural Research Service: *Nutrient intakes from food: mean amounts consumed per individual, one day, 2005-2006, 2008*. Retrieved May 7, 2010, from http://www.ars.usda.gov/Services/docs.htm?docid=18349.
4. Cotton PA, Subar AF, Friday JE, et al: Dietary sources of nutrients among U.S. adults, 1994-1996, *J Am Diet Assoc* 104:921, 2004. Additional tables retrieved November 3, 2004, from www.eatright.org.
5. Ma J, Johns RA, Stafford RS: Americans are not meeting current calcium recommendations, *Am J Clin Nutr* 85:1361, 2007.
6. Greer FR, Krebs NF: Committee on Nutrition: Optimizing bone health and calcium intakes of infants, children, and adolescents, *Pediatrics* 117:578, 2006.
7. Vatanparast H, Whiting SJ: Calcium supplementation trials and bone mass development in children, adolescents, and young adults, *Nutr Rev* 64:204, 2006.
8. Whiting SJ, Vatanparast H, Baxter-Jones A, et al: Factors that affect bone mineral accrual in the adolescent growth spurt, *J Nutr* 134:696S, 2004.
9. Vatanparast H, Whiting SJ: Early milk intake, later bone health: results from using the milk history questionnaire, *Nutr Rev* 62:256, 2004.
10. Heaney RP: Vitamin D and calcium interactions: functional outcomes, *Am J Clin Nutr* 88(Suppl):541S, 2008.
11. Food and Nutrition Board, Institute of Medicine: *Dietary Reference Intakes for calcium, phosphorus, magnesium, vitamin D, and fluoride*, Washington, DC, 1997, National Academies Press.
12. Heaney RP, Layman DK: Amount and type of protein influences bone health, *Am J Clin Nutr* 87(Suppl):1567S, 2008.
13. Poulsen RC, Kruger MC: Soy phytoestrogens: impact on postmenopausal bone loss and mechanisms of action, *Nutr Rev* 66(7):359, 2008.
14. Canalis E, Giustina A, Bilezikian JP: Mechanisms of anabolic therapies for osteoporosis, *N Engl J Med* 357:905, 2007.
15. Bischoff-Ferrari HA, Orav EJ, Dawson-Hughes B: Additive benefit of higher testosterone levels and vitamin D plus calcium supplementation in regard to fall risk reduction among older men and women, *Osteoporosis Int* 19:1307, 2008.
16. Ebeling PR: Osteoporosis in men, *N Engl J Med* 358:1474, 2008.
17. Weaver CM: Back to basics: have milk with meals, *J Am Diet Assoc* 106:1756, 2006.
18. Astrup A: The role of calcium in energy balance and obesity: the search for mechanisms, *Am J Clin Nutr* 88:873, 2008.
19. Beydoun MA, Gary TL, Caballero BH, et al: Ethnic differences in dairy and related nutrient consumption among U.S. adults and their association with obesity, central obesity, and the metabolic syndrome, *Am J Clin Nutr* 87:1914, 2008.
20. Heaney RP: Low calcium intake among African Americans: effects on bones and body weight, *J Nutr* 136:1095, 2006.
21. Thorpe MP, Jacobsen EH, Layman DK, et al: A diet high in protein, dairy, and calcium attenuates bone loss over twelve months of weight loss and maintenance relative to a conventional high-carbohydrate diet in adults, *J Nutr* 138:1096, 2008.
22. Riedt CS, Schlussel Y, von Thun N, et al: Premenopausal overweight women do not lose bone during moderate weight loss with adequate or higher calcium intake, *Am J Clin Nutr* 85:972, 2007.
23. Snijder MB, van der Heijden AA, van Dam RM, et al: Is higher dairy consumption associated with lower body weight and fewer metabolic disturbances? The Hoorn Study, *Am J Clin Nutr* 85:989, 2007.
24. McCarron DA, Heaney RP: Estimated healthcare savings associated with adequate dairy food intake, *Am J Hypertens* 17:88, 2004.
25. Chia V, Newcomb PA: Calcium and colorectal cancer: some questions remain, *Nutr Rev* 62(3):115, 2004.
26. Lappe JM, Travers-Gustafson D, Davies KM, et al: Vitamin D and calcium supplementation reduces cancer risk: results of a randomized trial, *Am J Clin Nutr* 85:1586, 2007.

27. Ishihara J, Inoue M, Iwasaki M, et al: Dietary calcium, vitamin D, and the risk of colorectal cancer, *Am J Clin Nutr* 88:1576, 2008.
28. Poddar KH, Hosig KW, Nickols-Richardson SM, et al: Low-fat dairy intake and body weight and composition changes in college students, *J Am Diet Assoc* 109:1433, 2009.
29. Knochel JP: Phosphorus. In Shils ME, Shike M, Olson J, et al, editors: *Modern nutrition in health and disease*, ed 10, Baltimore, 2006, Lippincott Williams & Wilkins.
30. Marinella MA: Refeeding syndrome in cancer patients, *Int J Clin Pract* 62:460, 2008.
31. Food and Nutrition Board, Institute of Medicine: *Dietary Reference Intakes for water, potassium, sodium, chloride, and sulfate*, Washington, DC, 2004, National Academies Press.
32. Food and Nutrition Board, Institute of Medicine: *Dietary Reference Intakes (DRI). The essential guide to nutrient requirements*, Washington, DC, 2006, National Academies Press.
33. Lomangino K: Is salt getting a fair shake? *Clinical Nutrition Insight* 34(5):1, 2008.
34. Most MM: Estimated phytochemical content of the Dietary Approaches to Stop Hypertension (DASH) diet is higher than in the control study diet, *J Am Diet Assoc* 104:1725, 2004.
35. Sacks FM, Svetkey LP, Vollmer WM, et al: Effects on blood pressure of reduced dietary sodium and the Dietary Approaches to Stop Hypertension (DASH) diet, *N Engl J Med* 344:3, 2001.
36. Bray GA, Vollmer WM, Sacks FM, et al: A further subgroup analysis of the effects of the DASH diet and three dietary sodium levels on blood pressure: results of the DASH-Sodium Trial, *Am J Cardiol* 94:222, 2004.
37. Mellen PB, Gao SK, Vitolins MZ, et al: Deteriorating dietary habits among adults with hypertension. DASH dietary accordance, NHANES 1988-1994 and 1999-2004, *Arch Intern Med* 168:308, 2008.
38. Karanja N, Lancaster KJ, Vollmer WM, et al: Acceptability of sodium-reduced research diets, including the Dietary Approaches to Stop Hypertension diet, among adults with prehypertension and stage 1 hypertension, *J Am Diet Assoc* 107:1530, 2007.
39. O'Donnell SI, Hoerr SL, Mendoza JA, et al: Nutrient quality of fast food kids meals, *Am J Clin Nutr* 88:1388, 2008.
40. Hajjar I, Kotchen T: Regional variations of blood pressure in the United States are associated with regional variations in dietary intakes: the NHANES-III data, *J Nutr* 133:211, 2003.
41. Lanham-New SA: The balance of bone health: tipping the scales in favor of potassium-rich, bicarbonate-rich foods, *J Nutr* 138:172S, 2008.
42. U.S. Department of Agriculture, Agricultural Research Service: *Nutrient intakes from food: mean amounts consumed per individual, by race/ethnicity and age, one day, 2005-2006*, Washington, DC, 2008, U.S. Department of Agriculture. Retrieved May 7, 2010, from http://www.ars.usda.gov/Services/docs.htm?docid=18349.
43. Doyle L, Cashman KD: The DASH diet may have beneficial effects on bone health, *Nutr Rev* 62(5):215, 2004.
44. McKeown NM, Jacques PF, Zhang XL, et al: Dietary magnesium intake is related to metabolic syndrome in older Americans, *Eur J Nutr* 47:210, 2008.
45. Newby PK, Maras J, Bakun P, et al: Intake of whole grains, refined grains, and cereal fiber measured with 7-d diet records and associations with risk factors for chronic disease, *Am J Clin Nutr* 86:1745, 2007.
46. Sahyoun NR, Jacques PF, Zhang XL, et al: Whole-grain intake is inversely associated with the metabolic syndrome and mortality in older adults, *Am J Clin Nutr* 83:124, 2006.
47. Food and Nutrition Board, Institute of Medicine: *Dietary Reference Intakes for vitamin A, vitamin K, arsenic, boron, chromium, copper, iodine, iron, manganese, molybdenum, nickel, silicon, vanadium, and zinc*, Washington, DC, 2001, National Academies Press.
48. Hunt JR, Roughead ZK: Adaptation of iron absorption in men consuming diets with high or low iron availability, *Am J Clin Nutr* 71:94, 2000.
49. Alleyne M, Horne McDK, Miller JL: Individualized treatment for iron-deficiency anemia in adults, *Am J Med* 121:943, 2008.
50. Wells AM, Haub MD, Fluckey J, et al: Comparisons of vegetarian and beef-containing diets on hematological indexes and iron stores during a period of resistive training in older men, *J Am Diet Assoc* 103:594, 2003.
51. Hoppe M, Hulthen L, Hallberg L: The importance of bioavailability of dietary iron in relation to the expected effect from iron fortification, *Eur J Clin Nutr* 62(6):761, 2008.
52. Hunt JR: Bioavailability of iron, zinc, and other trace minerals from vegetarian diets, *Am J Clin Nutr* 78(Suppl):633S, 2003.
53. Gasteyger C, Suter M, Gaillard RC, et al: Nutritional deficiencies after Roux-en-Y gastric bypass for morbid obesity often cannot be prevented by standard multivitamin supplementation, *Am J Clin Nutr* 87:1128, 2008.
54. Grinder-Pedersen L, Bukhave K, Jensen M, et al: Calcium from milk or calcium-fortified foods does not inhibit nonheme-iron absorption from a whole diet consumed over a 4-day period, *Am J Clin Nutr* 80:404, 2004.
55. AAP Committee on Nutrition: In Kleinman RE, editor: *Pediatric nutrition handbook*, ed 6, Elk Grove Village, Ill, 2008, American Academy of Pediatrics.
56. Beard JL: Why iron deficiency is important in infant development, *J Nutr* 138:2534, 2008.
57. Murray-Kolb LE, Beard JL: Iron treatment normalizes cognitive functioning in young women, *Am J Clin Nutr* 85:778, 2007.
58. McLean E, Cogswell M, Egli I, et al: Worldwide prevalence of anaemia, WHO vitamin and mineral nutrition information system, 1993-2005, *Public Health Nutr* 12:444, 2009.
59. Heath ALM, Fairweather-Tait SJ: Health implications of iron overload: the role of diet and genotype, *Nutr Rev* 61(2):45, 2003.
60. Rajpathak SN, Wylie-Rosett J, Gunter MJ, et al: Biomarkers of body iron stores and risk of developing type 2 diabetes, *Diabetes Obes Metab* 11:472, 2009.
61. Jiang R, Manson JE, Meigs JB, et al: Body iron stores in relation to risk of type 2 diabetes in apparently healthy women, *JAMA* 291:711, 2004.
62. Beard J: Dietary iron intakes and elevated iron stores in the elderly: is it time to abandon the set-point hypothesis of regulation of iron absorption? *Am J Clin Nutr* 76:1189, 2002.
63. Liu JM, Hankinson SE, Stampfer MJ, et al: Body iron stores and their determinants in healthy postmenopausal U.S. women, *Am J Clin Nutr* 78:1160, 2003.
64. Zimmerman MB: Iodine requirements and the risks and benefits of correcting iodine deficiency in populations, *J Trace Elem Med Biol* 22:81, 2008.
65. Zimmerman MB: The impact of iodised salt or iodine supplements on iodine status during pregnancy, lactation and infancy, *Public Health Nutr* 10:1584, 2007.
66. Solomons NW: Slow-release iodine in local water supplies reverses iodine deficiency disorders: is it worth its salt? *Nutr Rev* 56:280, 1998.

67. Georgieff M: Nutrition and the developing brain: nutrient priorities and measurement, *Am J Clin Nutr* 85(Suppl):614S, 2007.
68. Meydani SN, Barnett JB, Dallal GB, et al: Serum zinc and pneumonia in nursing home elderly, *Am J Clin Nutr* 86:1167, 2007.
69. Sweitzer SJ, Briley ME, Robert-Gray C: Do sack lunches provided by parents meet the nutritional needs of young children who attend child care? *J Am Diet Assoc* 109:141, 2009.
70. LaRowe TL, Moeller SM, Adams AK: Beverage patterns, diet quality, and body mass index of U.S. preschool and school-aged children, *J Am Diet Assoc* 107:1124, 2007.
71. Hambidge KM, Miller LV, Westcott JE, et al: Dietary Reference Intakes for zinc may require adjustment for phytate intake based upon model predictions, *J Nutr* 138:2363, 2008.
72. Burk RF, Levander OA: Selenium. In Shils ME, Shike M, Olson J, et al: *Modern nutrition in health and disease*, ed 10, Baltimore, 2006, Lippincott Williams & Wilkins.
73. Food and Nutrition Board, Institute of Medicine: *Dietary Reference Intakes for vitamin C, vitamin E, selenium, and carotenoids*, Washington, DC, 2000, National Academies Press.
74. American Dietetic Association: Position of the American Dietetic Association: the impact of fluoride on health, *J Am Diet Assoc* 105:1620, 2005.
75. Kant AK, Graubard BI, Atchison EA: Intakes of plain water, moisture in foods and beverages, and total water in the adult U.S. population—nutritional, meal pattern, and body weight correlates: National Health and Nutrition Examination Surveys 1999-2006, *Am J Clin Nutr* 90:655, 2009.
76. Valtin H: "Drink at least eight glasses of water a day." Really? Is there scientific evidence for "8 × 8"? *Am J Physiol Regul Integr Comp Physiol* 283(5):R993, 2002.
77. Grandjean AC, Reimers KJ, Buyckx ME: Hydration: issues for the 21st century, *Nutr Rev* 61(8):261, 2003.
78. Weinheimer EM, Martin BR, Weaver CM, et al: The effect of exercise on water balance in premenopausal physically active women, *J Am Diet Assoc* 108:1662, 2008.
79. Kenefick RW, Sawka MN: Hydration at the work site, *J Am Coll Nutr* 26:597S, 2007.
80. Grandjean AC, Reimers KJ, Bannick KE, et al: The effect of caffeinated, non-caffeinated, caloric and non-caloric beverages on hydration, *J Am Coll Nutr* 19:591, 2000.
81. Armstrong LE, Casa DJ, Maresh CM, et al: Caffeine, fluid-electrolyte balance, temperature regulation, and exercise-heat tolerance, *Exerc Sport Sci Rev* 35:135, 2007.
82. Marcason W: Is caffeine considered a diuretic and should my clients increase their fluid intake to compensate for this effect? *J Am Diet Assoc* 108:908, 2008.
83. Lichtenstein AH, Rasmussen H, Yu WW, et al: Modified MyPyramid for older adults, *J Nutr* 138:5, 2008.

FURTHER READINGS AND RESOURCES

Readings

Caulfield LE: Maternal zinc deficiency and maternal and child health in Peru, *Nutr Today* 39:78, 2004. *[Dr. Caulfield describes interventions to improve maternal and child health in developing countries and the consequences when not enough zinc is available in the diet.]*

Florentino RF: Hydration and human health: critical issues update, *Nutr Today* 44:6, 2009. *[This article discusses new research pertaining to hydration in exercise and the effects of caffeinated beverages.]*

Gasteyger C, Suter M, Gaillard RC, et al: Nutritional deficiencies after Roux-en-Y gastric bypass for morbid obesity often cannot be prevented by standard multivitamin supplementation, *Am J Clin Nutr* 87:1128, 2008. *[As the number of patients opting for bariatric surgery continues to grow, we need to be aware of the effects of this surgery on mineral absorption and mineral status.]*

LaRowe TL, Moeller SM, Adams AK: Beverage patterns, diet quality, and body mass index of US preschool and school-aged children, *J Am Diet Assoc* 107:1124, 2007.

O'Donnell SI, Hoerr SL, Mendoza JA, et al: Nutrient quality of fast food kids meals, *Am J Clin Nutr* 88:1388, 2008.

[These articles describe the effect of milk versus other beverages on nutrient and energy intakes in children.]

Weaver CM: Back to basics: have milk with meals, *J Am Diet Assoc* 106:1756, 2006. *[Dr. Weaver shares her experiences in helping her own children meet their calcium requirements.]*

U.S. Department of Health and Human Services, National Heart, Lung and Blood Institute: *Your guide to lowering your blood pressure with DASH*, NIH Pub No 06-4082, Bethesda, MD, 2006, U.S. Department of Health and Human Services. *[This colorful booklet provides menu plans, recipes, and general tips for lowering your intake of sodium and increasing your intakes of potassium, magnesium, and calcium. Available at http://www.nhlbi.nih.gov/health/public/hear/hbp/dash/new_dash.pdf.]*

Websites of Interest

Three government sites provide comprehensive information on dietary supplements, what they are or what they include, guidelines for their use, and their interactions with prescription and over-the-counter medications:

National Institutes of Health, National Library of Medicine: Medline Plus, Trusted Health Information for You: *Dietary supplements*: www.nlm.nih.gov/medlineplus/dietarysupplements.html.

National Institutes of Health, Office of Dietary Supplements: www.dietary-supplements.info.nih.gov/.

U.S. Food and Drug Administration, Center for Food Safety and Applied Nutrition, Office of Nutritional Products, Labeling, and Dietary Supplements: http://www.fda.gov/food/DietarySupplements/default.htm.

National Institutes of Health. This site provides information on calcium and bone health: http://www.nlm.nih.gov/medlineplus/calcium.html.

National Institutes of Health. This site provides information on sodium and blood pressure: http://www.nlm.nih.gov/medlineplus/dietarysodium.html.

U.S. Department of Health and Human Services, U.S. Department of Agriculture: *Dietary guidelines for Americans 2005*. This site provides tips for healthy eating with special attention to sodium and potassium: http://www.health.gov/dietaryguidelines/.

U.S. Department of Agriculture, Center for Nutrition Policy and Promotion: *MyPyramid food guidance system*. This website describes healthy food choices and portion sizes: www.mypyramid.gov/.

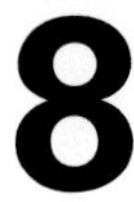

Energy Balance

Eleanor D. Schlenker

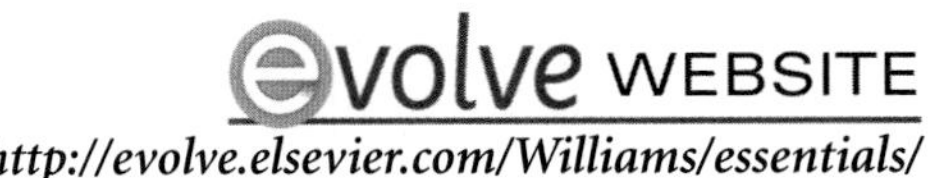

http://evolve.elsevier.com/Williams/essentials/

CHAPTER OUTLINE

Thus far we reviewed the three energy-yielding nutrients—carbohydrate, fat, and protein—and the micronutrients—vitamins and minerals—needed to catalyze the chemical reactions that convert food to energy. In this chapter we look at the relationship between energy intake and energy expenditure and their combined effect on body composition and body weight.

Energy balance is not a simple matter. Energy needs vary under different circumstances and for different body types. Each of us is unique, and our varying body weights and propensity to gain or lose weight reflect this. Physiologic, psychologic, environmental, metabolic, and genetic influences add to the complexities of energy balance. Modern conveniences supporting a sedentary lifestyle, coupled with an abundance of food, put people of all ages at risk of unwanted weight gain. At the other extreme, an obsession with thinness or unintentional weight loss stemming from debilitating disease leads to life-threatening malnutrition.[1] Healthy eating and regular physical activity are key to appropriate weight management.

THE HUMAN ENERGY SYSTEM

Energy Cycles and Energy Transformation

Forms of Human Energy

In our physical world, energy, like matter, is neither created nor destroyed. When we speak of energy being produced, what we really mean is energy being *transformed.* Energy constantly changes in form as it moves through various systems. In the human body, metabolic reactions convert the stored chemical energy in food to other forms of energy that carry out body work. The ultimate source of energy is the sun, with its vast reservoir of heat and light (Figure 8-1). Through the process of photosynthesis (review Figure 3-1), plants use water and carbon dioxide (CO_2) to transform the sun's energy into carbohydrate, a storage form of chemical energy. In the body these food fuels are converted to glucose, the energy unit that together with fatty acids is metabolized to release energy for use by body systems. The end products of body energy metabolism are water and CO_2, which enable plants to carry out the process once again.

Transformation of Energy

When food with its stored chemical energy is taken into the body, it undergoes many changes that convert it to other storage forms of chemical energy. This chemical energy is then further changed as work is performed. Our bodies use four forms of energy: (1) chemical, (2) electrical, (3) mechanical, and (4) thermal. In the brain, chemical energy is changed to electrical energy for transmitting nerve impulses and carrying out brain activities. Chemical energy is changed to mechanical energy when muscles contract; it is changed to thermal energy in the regulation of body temperature. Chemical

KEY TERMS

energy The capacity of a system for doing work; energy is manifest in various forms—motion, position, light, heat, and sound. Energy is interchangeable among these various forms and is constantly being transformed and transferred among them.

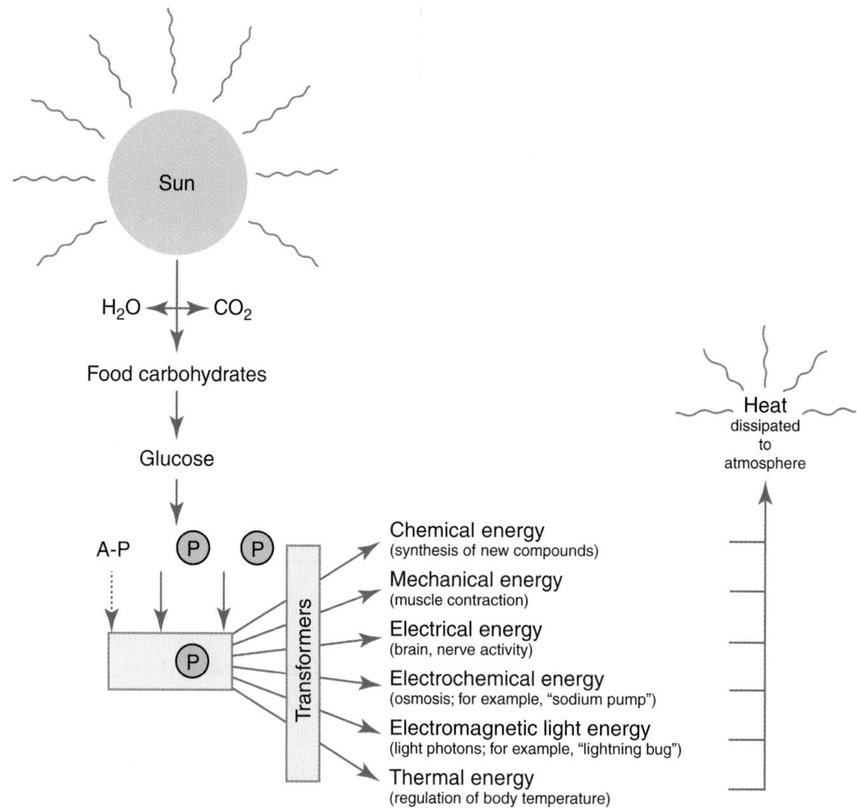

FIGURE 8-1 Transformation of energy from its primary source (the sun) to the forms needed for biologic work by means of metabolic processes ("transformers").

energy is used to form new tissues and proteins for growth and metabolism. Through all of this work, heat is given off to the surrounding atmosphere and larger biosphere.

In the human body, energy is present as either *free energy* or *potential energy.* Free energy is the energy being used at any given moment in the performance of a task. It is unbound and in motion. Potential energy is energy that is stored or bound in a chemical compound and can be converted to free energy when needed. For example, the energy stored in sugar is potential energy. When we eat it and it is metabolized, energy is released for body work such as contraction of the muscles. As work is completed, this energy, now in the form of heat or thermal energy, is given off into the air. This makes it possible for us to express body energy consumption in kilocalories (kcalories or kcals) or units of heat.

Energy Balance: Input and Output

A constant supply of energy is needed to sustain the activities essential to life. Energy is required to support internal needs along with the added expectations of physical activity. Whether the energy used is electrical, mechanical, thermal, or chemical, the supply of free energy and the reservoir of potential energy decrease as the metabolic and physical work of the body continues. Therefore the system must be constantly refueled from an outside source. For the human energy system, this outside fuel source is food.

Energy Control in Human Metabolism

If the energy produced in the body through its many chemical reactions were "exploded" all at once, it would damage tissues and systems. Therefore a mechanism must exist by which energy release can be controlled so that it may support life and not destroy it. Two means of control—(1) chemical bonding and (2) controlled reaction rates—make this possible.

Chemical Bonding

The primary mechanism controlling energy release in the human system is chemical bonding. The chemical bonds that hold the elements in compounds together are energy bonds. As long as the compound stays intact, energy is being exerted to maintain it. When the compound is broken into its parts, this energy is released and becomes available for work.

The following three types of chemical bonds transfer energy in the body:

1. *Covalent bonds:* These bonds are based on the relative valence of the elements making up a compound. The carbon atoms in organic compounds such as glucose are held together by covalent bonds.
2. *Hydrogen bonds:* Although weaker than covalent bonds, hydrogen bonds are nonetheless significant because large numbers of them exist. In addition, the very fact that they are less strong and more easily broken makes them important because they can transfer energy readily

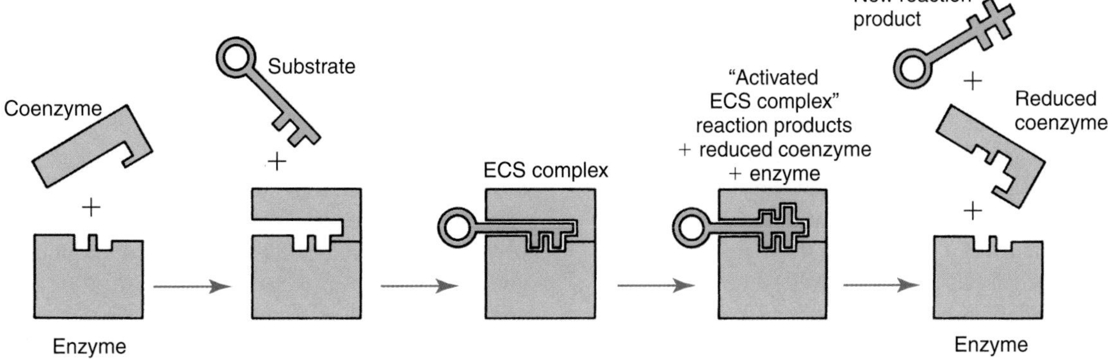

FIGURE 8-2 Lock-and-key concept of the actions of enzyme, coenzyme, and substrate to produce a new reaction product.

from one substance to another. The hydrogen attached to the oxygen molecule in the carboxyl group ($COOH^-$) of amino acids and fatty acids is an example of this type of bond.

3. *High-energy phosphate bonds:* The high-energy phosphate bonds in the compound adenosine triphosphate (ATP) are the major energy source for carrying out body functions. Working like storage batteries for electrical energy, these bonds are the controlling force of energy metabolism in the human cell.

Controlled Reaction Rates

The chemical reactions making up the body's energy system must have controls. Some reactions that break down protein, if left alone (as in the sterile decomposition of plants), would span several years. If such reactions were not accelerated, then getting needed energy from the food in a meal could take years. At the same time, chemical reactions must be prevented from occurring too rapidly, releasing destructive bursts of energy. Enzymes, coenzymes, and hormones regulate energy reactions in cells as follows:

- *Enzymes:* Enzymes are proteins produced in the cell under the direction of individual genes. One gene controls the making of one enzyme, and thousands of enzymes exist in each cell. Each enzyme acts on one particular substance, called its substrate. The enzyme and its substrate lock together to produce a new reaction product; however, the enzyme itself remains unchanged, ready to do its work over and over again (Figure 8-2).
- *Coenzymes and cofactors:* Many enzymes require partners to assist in completing their work. These coenzyme partners are often vitamins, especially B-complex vitamins. Various minerals also participate in enzyme reactions and in this role are referred to as *cofactors.* It may be helpful to think of coenzymes and cofactors as another substrate, because in receiving the material being transferred, they are changed or reduced.
- *Hormones:* In energy metabolism, hormones act as messengers to trigger or control enzyme action. The rate of oxidation reactions in the tissues—the body's metabolic rate—is controlled by thyroxin (T_4) from the thyroid gland. Another example is the controlling action of insulin on glucose utilization in the tissues. Various steroid hormones regulate the cell's ability to synthesize energy-related enzymes.

KEY TERMS

chemical bonding Process of linking elements or groups of elements in a chemical compound.

valence The combining power of an element or group of elements based on its number of unfilled electrons; an element with a valence of (−1) can combine with one atom of hydrogen with a valence of (+1); an element or group of elements with a valence of (−2) can combine with two atoms of hydrogen or one atom of an element with a valence of (+2). When these bonds are broken, energy is released for body work.

adenosine triphosphate (ATP) A high-energy phosphate compound important in energy exchange within the cell. ATP is formed from the nucleotide adenosine with three attached phosphoric acid groups. The splitting off of the terminal phosphate group (PO_4) to produce adenosine diphosphate (ADP) releases bound energy that is transformed to free energy and available for body work. ATP is then re-formed as an energy store for use when needed.

enzymes Complex proteins produced by living cells that act as catalysts to speed the rate of chemical reactions. Enzymes facilitate chemical changes in other substances without themselves being changed in the process. Digestive enzymes act on food substances to break them down into simpler compounds. An enzyme is usually named according to the substance (substrate) on which it acts, with the common suffix *-ase*; for example, sucrase is the enzyme that breaks down sucrose to glucose and fructose.

catalyst A chemical or compound that speeds up a chemical reaction but is not changed in the process. In the body, enzymes act as catalysts.

hormones Internally secreted substances from the endocrine glands that are carried in the blood to another organ or tissue on which they act to stimulate functional activity or secretion. This tissue or organ is called its *target tissue.*

substrate The specific organic substance on which a particular enzyme acts to produce a new metabolic product.

Types of Metabolic Reactions

Two types of reactions occur constantly in the body: (1) anabolic reactions and (2) catabolic reactions. Each of these reactions requires energy. The process of *anabolism* synthesizes new and more complex substances as in body growth and repair. The process of *catabolism* breaks down complex substances to more simple ones, as when worn-out proteins are broken down and their released amino acids are used to re-form new proteins. Both activities release free energy, but the work performed also uses up some free energy. This creates a constant energy deficit that must be met by food.

Sources of Stored Energy

When a person is not taking in food, as in fasting or starvation, the body must draw on its own stores for energy. Sources of stored energy can meet short-term or long-term needs, as follows:

- *Glycogen:* Only a 12-hour to 36-hour reserve of glycogen exists in liver and muscle and is quickly depleted.
- *Muscle mass:* Energy stores in the form of muscle protein exist in limited amounts but in greater volume than glycogen stores. Breakdown of muscle protein for energy should be a last resort after glycogen and adipose stores are depleted.
- *Adipose (fat) tissue:* Although fat stores are generally the largest resource of stored energy, the supply varies from person to person.

Measurement of Energy Balance

Kilocalorie

Because the release of energy and work performed by the body produces heat, energy expenditure can be measured in heat equivalents. This measure of heat is the **calorie.** To avoid having to calculate very large numbers, nutritionists use the **kilocalorie** to describe energy needs. The kilocalorie is equal to 1000 calories; this is the amount of heat required to raise 1 kg of water 1° C.

Joule

The international (*Système International d'Unités* [SI]) unit of energy measurement is the **joule.** It equals the amount of energy expended when 1 kg of a substance is moved 1 m by a force of 1 newton (N). It was named for James Prescott Joule, a nineteenth century English physicist who discovered the first law of thermodynamics. The conversion factor for changing kcalories to kilojoules (kJ) is 4.184 (1 kcal = 4.184 kJ). Because the energy contents of diets given in kilojoules are very large numbers, the more common term is the *megajoule (MJ);* 1 MJ equals 239 kcal. Some nutrition research journals use kilojoules rather than kcalories to describe energy intakes; therefore these conversion factors should be kept in reference.

Food Energy Measurement

When helping people develop a food pattern appropriate to their energy needs, it is necessary to know the energy content of individual foods. The energy value of particular foods can be determined by two methods: (1) direct **calorimetry** or (2) calculation of approximate composition.

Calorimetry

The kcalorie values of foods given in food tables were determined by the method called *direct calorimetry.*[2] This method uses a metal container called a *bomb calorimeter*, named from its long tubular shape. A weighed amount of food is placed inside and the bomb calorimeter is immersed in water. The food is then ignited by an electric spark in the presence of oxygen and burned to ash. The increase in the temperature of the surrounding water indicates the number of kcalories given off by the complete oxidation of the food sample. When you use food tables, remember that these values represent averages from a number of samples of the given food, thus the kcalorie value of a particular serving will vary around that average. Examples of food tables can be found in the Nutritrac program on the Evolve website that accompanies your text.

Approximate Composition

An alternative method of estimating the energy value of a food is calculating the kcalories contributed by the carbohydrate, fat, and protein content as listed in food tables. These calculations are based on the kcalorie value per gram of each of the energy-yielding macronutrients, values known as their **fuel factors** (Table 8-1). Note that 1 g of fat contains more than twice the number of kcalories as 1 g of carbohydrate or protein. The fuel factor for alcohol (7 kcal/g) falls about midway between fat and carbohydrate and protein. Using the method of approximate composition to calculate kcalorie content, a food containing 12 g of carbohydrate, 8 g of protein, and 5 g of fat would contain 125 kcal. (Calculation: carbohydrate: 12 g × 4 kcal/g = 48 kcal; protein: 8 g × 4 kcal/g = 32 kcal; fat: 5 g × 9 kcal/g = 45 kcal; 48 + 32 + 45 kcal = 125 kcal.) Did you recognize this food as a 1-cup serving of 2% milk?

TOTAL ENERGY REQUIREMENT

The total energy expended by an individual stems from three energy needs: (1) basal metabolism, (2) food intake effect, and (3) physical activity. Physical size and **body composition,** as well as level of physical activity, influence the energy needs of a given individual.

Basal Metabolic Needs

Basal Metabolic Rate

The **basal metabolic rate (BMR)** is a measure of the energy required to maintain the body at rest. This is the sum of all chemical activities going on in the body plus the energy needed to fuel the brain, heart, lungs, kidneys, and other

TABLE 8-1 FUEL FACTORS

ENERGY SOURCE	KCALORIES PER GRAM
Carbohydrate	4
Protein	4
Fat	9
Alcohol	7

vital organs that must continue to work even when the body rests.[3] Certain small but vitally active tissues—brain, liver, gastrointestinal tract, heart, and kidneys—make up less than 5% of total body weight but add up to about 60% of basal metabolic activity. The BMR is the largest of the energy needs of most people, accounting for 60% to 70% of the daily energy expenditure.[4] The physical characteristics of an individual and the pretesting environment influence the BMR (Box 8-1).[3] In practice, the BMR is seldom measured because of the many practical problems involved. Rather, the resting metabolic rate (RMR) is more commonly used because it does not require the individual to have fasted. However, note that the RMR may be as much as 10% to 20% higher than the BMR because of energy being expended in the digestion, absorption, or metabolism of food, as well as the delayed effect of recent physical activity.[3]

Measuring Basal Metabolic Rate

The BMR can be measured by direct and indirect methods of calorimetry, as follows:

- *Direct calorimetry:* By the direct method a person is placed in an enclosed chamber having the capacity to measure the body's heat production while the person is at rest. This instrument is large and costly and usually found only in research facilities.[2]
- *Indirect calorimetry:* With the indirect method a portable instrument called a *respirometer* is brought to the side of the bed or chair. This complete apparatus is often referred to as the *metabolic cart.* As the person breathes through a mouthpiece or ventilated hood, the exchange of gases in respiration, the *respiratory quotient* (CO_2/O_2), is measured. Because more than 95% of the body's energy comes from oxidation (oxygen-related) reactions,[5] the BMR can be calculated from the amount of oxygen consumed in a given period. The amount of oxygen used is equivalent to the amount of heat released; this can be converted to kcalories released by use of standardized equations.
- *Indirect laboratory tests:* The BMR is regulated by the thyroid hormone thyroxin (T_4); thus thyroid function tests can provide indirect measures of BMR and thyroid activity. These tests include measurements of serum thyroid-stimulating hormone (TSH) from the anterior pituitary gland, as well as triiodothyronine (T_3) and T_4 levels. T_3 and T_4 are produced in the final stages of thyroid hormone synthesis and reflect the levels of hormones influencing the BMR. Thyroid hormone levels within the normal range indicate that cell metabolism is occurring at normal rates but cannot be used to calculate BMR.

BOX 8-1 REQUIRED CONDITIONS FOR MEASURING BASAL METABOLIC RATE

- Overnight fast (no food for 12 to 14 hours)
- Comfortably resting in a supine position
- Relaxed state (no activity up to 1 hour prior)
- Awake but motionless
- Normal body temperature
- Comfortable room temperature (neither hot nor cold)

Factors Influencing Basal Metabolic Rate

Body size and composition, growth, fever and chronic disease, climate, and genetic makeup all influence the BMR of an individual, as explained following:

- *Body size and body composition:* Fat-free mass (FFM) is the body compartment made up of muscle and vital organs. It is the major factor influencing BMR because of the high metabolic activity of these tissues compared with the less active tissues of fat and bone. Differences in basal energy requirements between women and men with the same body weight relate to their differences in body composition. Compared with men, women have decreased muscle mass and increased body fat, resulting in lower BMRs.

KEY TERMS

calorie The amount of heat energy needed to raise the temperature of 1 g of water from 14° C to 15° C. Because this is a small unit, nutritionists use the term *kilocalorie,* which is 1000 small calories. A kilocalorie is the amount of heat required to raise the temperature of 1 kg of water 1° C (see also joule).

kilocalorie The general term *calorie* refers to a unit of heat measure and is used alone to designate the *small calorie.* The *large calorie,* 1000 calories or kilocalorie, is used in the study of metabolism to avoid the use of very large numbers in calculations.

joule A unit of energy. The International System of Units uses joules in place of calories to refer to food energy, and most nutrition journals use joules instead of calories (1 kcal = 4.184 kilojoules [kJ], often rounded to 4.2 kJ for ease in calculation). A 1000-kcal diet would be equivalent to a 4200 kJ or 4.2 megajoule (MJ) diet.

calorimetry Measurement of amount of heat absorbed or given off. *Direct method:* measurement of the heat produced by a subject enclosed in a small chamber. *Indirect method:* measurement of heat produced by a subject based on the quantity of oxygen (O_2) taken in and carbon dioxide (CO_2) exhaled.

fuel factors Kilocalorie values (energy potential) of food nutrients; the number of kcalories that 1 g of the nutrient yields when completely oxidized. The kilocalorie fuel factor is 4 for carbohydrate and protein, 9 for fat, and 7 for alcohol. Fuel factors are used in computing the energy values of foods and diets (e.g., 10 g of fat yields 90 kcal).

body composition The relative sizes of the four tissue compartments that make up the total body: lean body mass (LBM) (muscles and organs), fat, water, and mineral.

basal metabolic rate (BMR) Amount of energy required to maintain the body at rest after an overnight fast with the subject awake. See also resting metabolic rate (RMR).

resting metabolic rate (RMR) Amount of energy required to maintain the body at rest when in a comfortable environmental temperature and awake. Because of differences in measuring techniques, an individual's RMR and BMR (basal metabolic rate) differ slightly. Based on ease of measurement, RMR is often used in clinical practice.

supine Lying down.

As humans age, the loss of muscle tissue, and to a lesser extent organ tissue, lowers the BMR in older adults.[3]

- *Growth:* The increased anabolic work supported by growth hormone adds to the BMR in childhood, adolescence, pregnancy, and lactation.
- *Fever and disease:* With fever the BMR increases 7% for each 1° F (0.83° C) rise in body temperature. Diseases that increase cell activity such as cancer, cardiac failure, and chronic obstructive pulmonary disease increase BMR.[6] Diabetes[7] and renal disease[8] may increase the metabolic work of the body and the BMR. The involuntary muscle tremors of Parkinson's disease increase energy needs. Standard prediction equations may underestimate the BMR of children with cystic fibrosis.[9] Conversely, starvation and protein-energy malnutrition lower BMR as cell metabolism slows in response to the drop in energy intake and loss of FFM.
- *Climate:* BMR rises in response to lower environmental temperatures as the body takes action to increase heat production and minimize heat loss. Opposite reactions that reduce heat production and increase heat loss as environmental temperatures rise also increase the BMR. Unless weather conditions are extreme, these changes in BMR are temporary while the individual adapts to the new environment.
- *Genetics:* Race and ethnicity may influence BMR. African Americans appear to have a lower BMR per unit of FFM than Caucasians, possibly related to differences in tissue composition.[10] Commonly used prediction equations overestimate BMR in Chinese adults who appear to have a higher proportion of body fat than would be expected.[11] Studies of the human genome indicate that intrafamily differences in RMR may contribute to higher weight gain and development of metabolic syndrome.[12]

Food Intake Effect (Thermic Effect of Food)

Taking in food stimulates body metabolism as energy is needed to digest, absorb, metabolize, and store nutrients. The kcalories needed to perform these tasks is called the **thermic effect of food (TEF).** On average about 10% of the kcalories in a meal or snack are used to process and metabolize that food, although this varies depending on the food composition. Macronutrients differ in their TEFs. The TEF for fat is 0% to 5%, because fatty acids are easily burned for energy or stored in the form in which they enter the body; therefore few kcalories are used in their processing or storage. For carbohydrate the TEF is 5% to 10% of its kcalories; for protein the TEF is 20% to 30%. The TEF for alcohol is 10% to 30%.[3] The energy required to metabolize amino acids and synthesize new proteins raises the TEF of this nutrient and may explain why a high-protein diet helps with weight management.[13] The very low TEF of fat, along with its high fuel factor (9 kcal/g), accelerates weight gain on a high-fat diet.

Physical Activity Needs

Physical activity related to employment, housekeeping, recreation, organized sports, or physical training produces wide variations in individual energy requirements. For sedentary individuals the kcalories expended in physical activity may be less than one half their BMR, as compared with very active persons whose physical activity kcalories may be twice their BMR.[3] Table 8-2 describes the energy expended in common activities by a person weighing 154 lb, and additional activities can be found on the Evolve website. Remember that the energy cost of weight-bearing movements such as walking is proportional to body weight. Thus such an activity will require more kcalories for those whose body weight is average and fewer kcalories for those whose body weight is less than average (Figure 8-3). Obese adolescents can have the same activity energy expenditure as their nonobese counterparts, despite less body movement, based on their higher body weight.[14]

The speed at which a person moves also influences the number of kcalories required. Walking at a speed of 2 mph requires fewer kcalories than walking at 4 mph, regardless of body weight (see Figure 8-3).[3] Running requires 30% more energy than walking for the same distance.[15] Regular physical

TABLE 8-2 ENERGY EXPENDED IN SELECTED PHYSICAL ACTIVITIES

ACTIVITY	APPROXIMATE CALORIES PER HOUR (FOR PERSON WEIGHING 154 lb)*†
Moderate Intensity	
Hiking	370
Light gardening/yard work	330
Dancing	330
Golf (walking and carrying clubs)	330
Bicycling (<10 mph)	290
Walking (3.5 mph)	280
Weight lifting (general light workout)	220
Stretching	180
Vigorous Intensity	
Running/jogging (5 mph)	590
Bicycling (>10 mph)	590
Swimming (slow freestyle laps)	510
Aerobics	480
Walking (4.5 mph)	460
Heavy yard work (chopping wood)	440
Weight lifting (vigorous effort)	440
Basketball (vigorous)	440

From U.S. Department of Health and Human Services, U.S. Department of Agriculture: *Dietary guidelines for Americans 2005,* ed 6, Washington, DC, 2005, U.S. Government Printing Office. Available at http://www.health.gov/dietaryguidelines/dga2005/document/default.htm.

*Calories burned per hour will be increased for persons who weigh more than 154 lb (70 kg) and decreased for persons who weigh less.

†This caloric expenditure includes resting metabolic rate (RMR) calories and activity calories. Some of these activities can be either moderate-intensity or vigorous-intensity depending on the speed at which they are carried out (as for walking and bicycling).

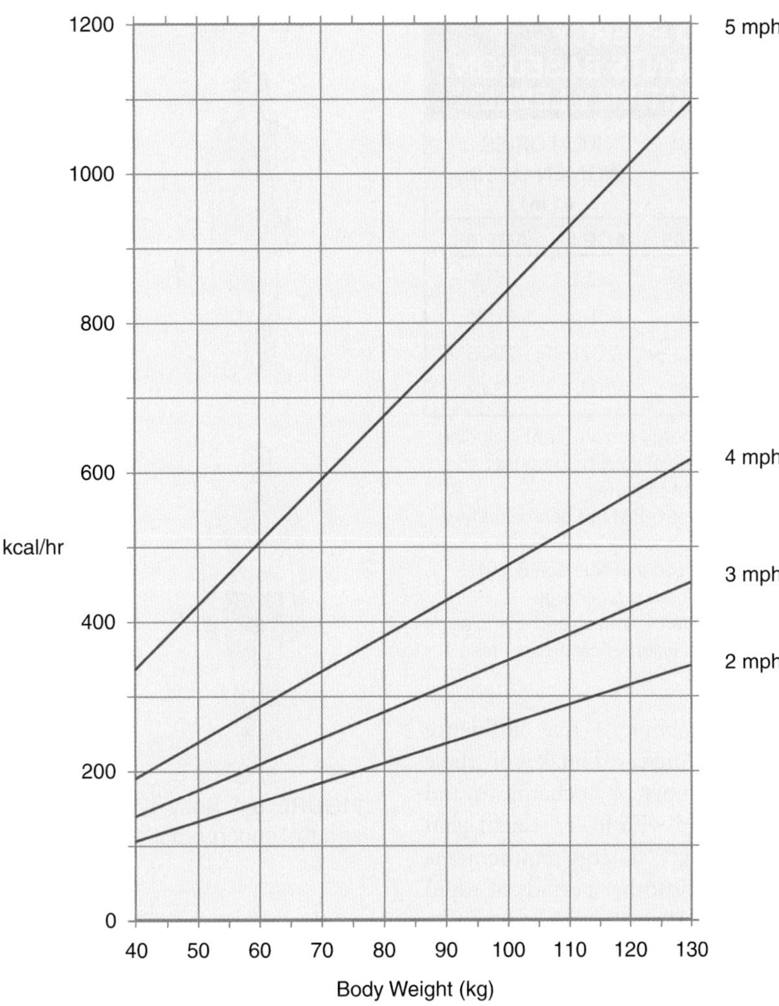

FIGURE 8-3 Effect of body weight on energy expended walking at different speeds. Body weight and walking speed influence the kcalories burned. Persons with a higher body weight use more kcalories in weight-bearing activities than persons with a lower body weight; the faster you walk the more kcalories you will use. (Redrawn with permission from Food and Nutrition Board, Institute of Medicine: *Dietary reference intakes for energy, carbohydrate, fiber, fat, fatty acids, cholesterol, protein, and amino acids (macronutrients),* Washington, DC, 2002, National Academies Press.)

activity not only supports energy balance but also reduces risk of chronic disease. (Note how pedometers help people increase their physical activity.)[16,17]

Another factor that may contribute to total energy expenditure is *nonshivering thermogenesis.* This is a response to cold that occurs in special tissue called *brown fat* and increases the BMR to produce more heat. Brown fat has a role in temperature regulation in infants but until recently was thought to have little significance in adults. New research suggests it can affect long-term energy balance through its action on BMR and may influence body weight.[18]

Estimating Energy Requirements

Estimating the total energy requirement for a given individual is difficult. An expert panel defined the Estimated Energy Requirement (EER) as the energy intake that will maintain energy balance in a healthy adult of a certain age, gender, weight, height, and level of physical activity and be consistent with good health.[3] Typical ranges for energy expenditure at rest are 0.8 to 1.0 kcal/min for women and 1.1 to 1.3 kcal/min for men (1 kcal/min is about equal to the heat released by a burning candle or 75-watt bulb over the course of a minute).[3] Differences in body dimensions and the proportion of body fat versus muscle influence the EER. Individuals with a greater amount of body fat and a lesser proportion of muscle will likely need fewer kcalories. Table 8-3 describes how age and physical activity influence the EER. Both genders have the same body weight and height, although older adults will have lost lean body mass (LBM) and gained body fat.

KEY TERMS

thermic effect of food (TEF) The amount of energy required to digest and absorb food and transport nutrients to the cells. This work accounts for about 10% of the day's total energy (kcalorie) requirement.

TABLE 8-3 ESTIMATED ENERGY REQUIREMENTS BASED ON AGE AND ACTIVITY LEVEL*

	KCALORIES MEN (178 lb, 71 in†)		KCALORIES WOMEN (132 lb, 61 in†)	
ACTIVITY LEVEL	AGE 25	AGE 65	AGE 25	AGE 65
Sedentary	2685	2285	1869	1589
Low active	2934	2534	2072	1792
Active	3250	2850	2325	2045
Very active	3770	3370	2628	2348

*These estimates represent the total energy requirement including basal needs, the effect of food, and physical activity; note that age and physical activity influence energy expenditure.
†These individuals have a body mass index (BMI) of approximately 25 kg/m^2.
Calculations based on data presented in Food and Nutrition Board, Institute of Medicine: *Dietary Reference Intakes for energy, carbohydrate, fiber, fat, fatty acids, cholesterol, protein, and amino acids (macronutrients)*, Washington, DC, 2002, National Academies Press.

Particular foods or their components may influence long-term energy balance favorably. Increased intakes of whole grains, fruits, and vegetables rich in fiber, phytochemicals, and trace minerals have been associated with lower weight gain among middle-age and older adults.[19,20] Energy requirements rise during pregnancy, lactation, and other periods of rapid growth and elevated metabolism. (We will learn to estimate energy requirements using specific equations that adjust for height, weight, and age in Chapter 19.)

BODY COMPOSITION: FATNESS AND LEANNESS

A person's body composition reflects his or her total lifetime nutrient and energy balance.[21] Individuals have different body shapes and sizes depending on their age, gender, genes, state of health, and body type. Ectomorphs have a body type that is generally slender and fragile, mesomorphs have prominent muscle and bone development, and endomorphs have a soft, round physique with some accumulation of body fat (Figure 8-4). Although each person's body type has a genetic base, dietary intake and physical activity influence how that body type is expressed. Some body types are associated with better health, whereas others carry increased risk of chronic disease. We need to be sensitive to different body types when developing strategies to improve body composition and health.

Body Weight and Body Fat

Overweight Versus Overfat

Because height and weight are easily measured, they are commonly used to assess health status. It is important to know what these measurements do and do not tell us. The terms *overweight* and *obesity* have different meanings as related to body composition, and these distinctions have implications for health. A football player in peak physical condition can be markedly "overweight" according to standard height-weight charts. That is, the player weighs more than an average person of similar height, but the player's body tissues are likely to be very different than expected. A sedentary man of more than average weight likely has an excess amount of body fat that is adding to his total body weight; however, an athlete above-average weight is likely to have an exceptionally large amount of muscle. In fact, the overweight athlete may have a lower proportion of body fat than a sedentary individual of average weight. When overweight is the result of excessive body fat rather than enhanced muscle or skeletal tissue, *overfat* or *obese* is the appropriate term.

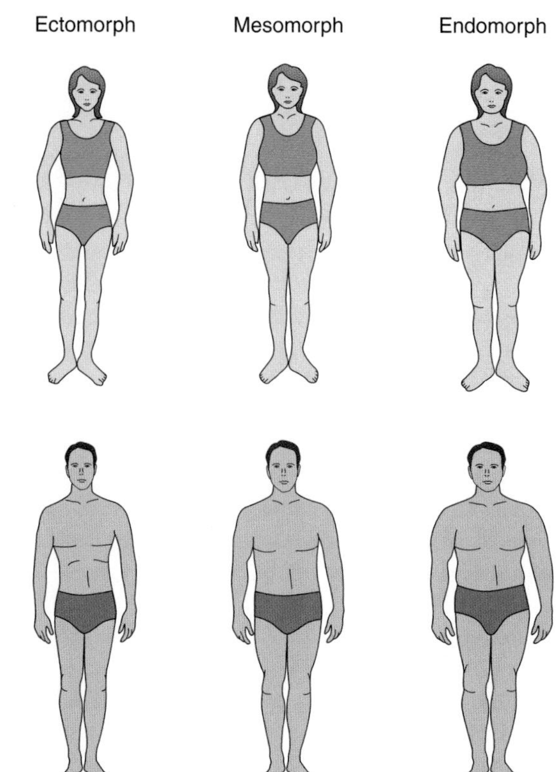

FIGURE 8-4 Body types: the ectomorph, the mesomorph, and the endomorph.

Body Compartments

The critical element when evaluating body build and health is body composition. What we really need to know is how much of a person's body weight is fat and how much is FFM. It is more precise to think in terms of *fatness* and *leanness* rather than body weight or overweight. When speaking of body weight, we need to consider the individual, his or her lifestyle and weight history, and the measures used.

Body compartments are defined on the basis of their comparative size and metabolic activity. Various methods exist for expressing the relative amounts of specific body tissues, and sometimes tissues overlap among compartments. The four-compartment model for evaluating body composition includes LBM, body fat, body water, and mineral mass, as defined following:

1. *LBM:* This compartment, made up of active cells from muscle and vital organs, largely determines the BMR and

related nutrient needs. In sedentary individuals it accounts for almost the entire energy requirement. LBM includes not only cell protein but also a large amount of water, because muscle cells are about 65% water. This compartment also contains a very small amount of fatty acids, found in the membranes of muscle and organ cells. LBM changes in size across the life cycle, with steady growth through young adulthood and gradual loss in later years. In adults it makes up 30% to 65% of total body weight. Most weight reduction diets result in a loss of body fat and LBM. Physical activity and weight-bearing exercise can help maintain muscle mass as people age.

2. *Body fat:* Total body fat reflects the number and size of the fat cells (adipocytes) that form the adipose tissue. In an adult man of normal weight, fat comprises 13% to 21% of body weight. In a woman of normal weight, the range is 23% to 31%. These amounts vary with age, body type, exercise, and fitness, and many people have body fat levels markedly greater than or less than these ranges. About one half of all body fat is located in the subcutaneous fat layers under the skin, where it serves as insulation. In children and young adults, the subcutaneous fat provides a useful measure for estimating body fat. Skinfold thicknesses measured at various locations on the body such as the triceps, subscapular region, or waist can be applied to existing standards to assess relative leanness or fatness. As individuals grow older, body fat is deposited on the trunk rather than the extremities, therefore waist circumference or waist-to-hip ratio becomes a useful tool to evaluate body fatness and health risk.[22–24]
3. *Body water:* Total body water includes both intracellular and extracellular water. Total body water varies with relative leanness or fatness, age, hydration status, and health status. Generally water makes up about 50% to 65% of body weight. Muscle tissue has high water content, whereas adipose tissue has low water content; thus men have a higher proportion of body water than women. Infants have a relatively high proportion of body water, which drops to adult levels by age 2.[9]
4. *Mineral mass:* Body mineral, found largely in the skeleton, accounts for only 4% to 6% of body weight. Major minerals are calcium and phosphorus located in bone and other body cells and fluids. Sodium is the major mineral in extracellular fluid (ECF), and potassium is the major mineral in intracellular fluid (ICF).

The following factors influence the relative sizes of the body compartments[25]:

- *Gender:* Women have more adipose tissue, and men have more lean tissue, particularly muscle.
- *Age:* Young adults have more LBM and less fat than older adults.
- *Physical activity:* Persons who are physically active have less fat and more LBM than persons who are sedentary.
- *Race:* African Americans have greater bone mineral than Caucasians or Hispanics.
- *Climate:* Individuals living in very cold climates develop more subcutaneous fat to insulate against heat loss.

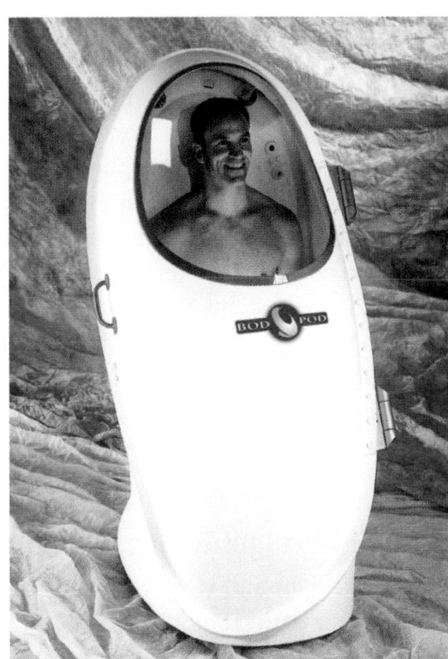

FIGURE 8-5 A pod for measuring body composition. The BOD POD uses air displacement technology to measure body composition. (Courtesy Life Measurement, Inc, Concord, Calif.)

Importance of Body Fat

Although excessive body fat is detrimental to health, some body fat is necessary for life. In human starvation, victims die from fat loss, not protein depletion. For mere survival, men require about 3% body fat and women require about 12%; however, for reproductive capacity women require a body fat of about 20%. The initiation of menstruation or menarche occurs when the female body attains a certain size or, more precisely, the critical proportion of body fat. Body fat gained during pregnancy serves as an important energy reserve for lactation, and the production of breast milk, with its high energy cost, usually brings about a gradual loss of these fat stores. Ill-advised dieting during pregnancy in an attempt to avoid normal weight gain interferes with fetal development and can result in a low-birth-weight infant with associated health risks.

Measuring Body Compartments

Specialized Methods

An estimate of the relative proportions of body fat and LBM is useful in evaluating health status. The classic method for determining body composition is hydrostatic weighing following Archimedes' principle. The individual is first weighed in air and then weighed completely submerged in water. The volume of water displaced is measured and, using standardized equations, the relative amounts of LBM and body fat can be calculated. In a new application of this principle, the individual is weighed in air and then introduced to an air-controlled chamber, referred to as a *pod,* in which the air displaced by the volume of the body can be measured (Figure 8-5).[26]

KEY TERMS

obesity Fatness; an excessive accumulation of fat in the body.
adipocyte A fat cell.
menarche The first menstruation with the onset of puberty.

Both methods take advantage of the fact that body fat and lean tissue differ in density, and standard calculations can be applied. The air displacement method offers an opportunity for measuring individuals who cannot be weighed under water. Dual-energy x-ray absorptiometry (DEXA) is an advanced form of radiographic technology that can differentiate among muscle, fat, and bone; this method is used to measure bone mineral density and age-related bone loss. Bioelectrical impedance systems that pass a very small current of electricity through the body can distinguish water, fat, and bone; these systems are applicable to clinical settings. (Use of body circumferences and skinfold thicknesses to estimate body muscle and body fat is discussed in more detail in Chapter 16.)

Reference Height-Weight Tables

In many situations, height and weight are the only measurements available for estimating body composition. These measurements can be compared with reference tables that suggest an appropriate body weight for a person of a given height and gender.

The Metropolitan Life Insurance Company, using information obtained from their life insurance policyholders, mostly Caucasian middle-aged men, constructed the first height-weight tables in the 1930s. Desirable weights were based on the body weights of the policyholders who lived the longest. Early height-weight tables also presented adult reference weights according to age, based on the assumption that weight gain continued throughout adult life. In recent years several new concepts have emerged regarding height-weight tables: (1) body weight (and body fat) should not increase as individuals move into middle and older ages, and (2) body build and body fat patterns differ across racial and ethnic groups, such that height-weight tables based on Caucasian populations may not be appropriate for African Americans, Hispanics, or Asians.[27-30] (See the *Focus on Culture* box, "Evaluating Body Compartments: One Size Really Doesn't Fit All," to explore this issue further.)

FOCUS ON CULTURE

Evaluating Body Compartments: One Size Really Doesn't Fit All

When assessing an individual's nutritional status, an important piece of information is the relative size of each body compartment. LBM gives us an estimate of body protein and muscle, and bone mass can tell us if a person is at risk for bone fracture. The proportion of body fat suggests risk of such conditions as diabetes, heart disease, or metabolic syndrome. Although researchers have developed sensitive equipment and standards for physical measurements, the relationships on which they are based were derived mostly from Caucasian populations.

We have learned that diverse groups differ in body composition and disease risk. African Americans have higher bone mineral per unit of body weight than Caucasians. The amount of total body potassium, a marker of LBM, is also at the greatest level for a given height in African Americans (followed by Caucasians and Hispanics). Asians have the lowest amount of bone mineral and body potassium for their size. Based on these differences, standard equations used to calculate LBM or body mineral must be adjusted accordingly.

Total body fat and abdominal fat also vary according to age, gender, and ethnicity, but these differences are not always apparent with simple measurements. Women have a higher percentage of total body fat, but men have a higher proportion of abdominal fat. Although all gender and ethnic groups increase their body fat in later years, abdominal fat increases to the greatest extent in African American men and Hispanic and Asian women, which may contribute to chronic disease prevalence in these groups.

Body mass index (BMI) and waist circumference (WC) are inexpensive methods for estimating body fat, but they are less reliable when evaluating various ethnic and racial groups. Compared with more sophisticated methods, BMI underestimated percent body fat in overweight Hispanic-American women and overestimated percent body fat in overweight Caucasian women. Results were less certain in men, although it appeared that Asian men and women with BMI measurements similar to Caucasians of the same age actually had higher amounts of total fat and abdominal fat.

The disease risk associated with certain BMI and WC measurements also differs depending on genetic background. Even slight increases in body weight and body fat carry greater health risks for Chinese men and women than for other groups. Cardiovascular mortality was higher among Chinese women whose waist-to-hip ratio (Figure 8-6) was more than 0.8, although their BMI was in the healthy weight range (<25 kg/m^2). Health experts have suggested that a cutoff of 23 kg/m^2 rather than 25 kg/m^2 to define overweight, and a level of 25 kg/m^2 rather than 30 kg/m^2 to designate obesity, may be more appropriate for Asian populations.

Common standards now used to evaluate body fat are not equally appropriate for all groups. Populations differ in their genetically determined amounts and locations of body fat. Differing relationships among body compartments may interfere with interpretation of standard measurements. As the population becomes more diverse, we must develop individualized assessment standards that will accurately target disease risk and early intervention.

BIBLIOGRAPHY

Chung S, Song M-Y, Shin HD, et al: Korean and Caucasian overweight premenopausal women have different relationship of body mass index to percent body fat with age, *J Appl Physiol* 99:103, 2005.

Fernandez JR, Heo M, Heymsfield SB, et al: Is percentage of body fat differentially related to body mass index in Hispanic Americans, African-Americans, and European Americans? *Am J Clin Nutr* 77:71, 2003.

He Q, Heo M, Heshka S, et al: Total body potassium differs by sex and race across the adult age span, *Am J Clin Nutr* 78:72, 2003.

Lear SA, Humphries KH, Kohli S, et al: Visceral adipose tissue accumulation differs according to ethnic background: results of the Multicultural Community Health Assessment Trial (M-CHAT), *Am J Clin Nutr* 86:353, 2007.

Sun AJ, Heshka S, Heymsfield SB, et al: Is there an association between skeletal muscle mass and bone mineral density among African-American, Asian-American, and European-American women? *Acta Diabetol* 40:S309, 2003.

Wu C-H, Heshka S, Wang J, et al: Truncal fat in relation to total body fat: influences of age, sex, ethnicity, and fatness, *Int J Obes* 31:1384, 2007.

Zhang X, Shu XO, Yang G, et al: Abdominal adiposity and mortality in Chinese women, *Arch Intern Med* 167:886, 2007.

Reference Tables From Government Agencies

Nutrition and health professionals from the U.S. Department of Health and Human Services and the U.S. Department of Agriculture have developed reference standards to define the terms *overweight* and *obesity.*[3,31,32] Appropriate ranges of body weight for adults of a given height, developed for use by clinicians, were adapted and included in the *Dietary Guidelines for Americans 2005* (see Table 8-4 and Appendix A).[32] Americans are becoming taller and heavier, but body weights have been rising at a faster rate than body heights.[33,34] Since 1960 average body weight in women increased by 24 lb (from 140 lb to 164 lb), although body height increased less than 1 inch. Men increased in average weight from 166 lb to 191 lb (a gain of 25 lb), with about an inch increase in height. On a positive note it appears the proportion of U.S. adults who are obese has stabilized, after doubling in number between 1980 and 2004.[35] Age becomes a factor when evaluating the risk associated with a rise in body weight.[23,36–38] Moderate obesity has a drastic effect on mortality risk in younger men, but overweight does not add to mortality risk in older age; even moderate obesity in older adults creates only a modest increase in risk.[38]

Body Mass Index

In 1871, Quetelet developed the BMI, which has replaced body weight as the medical standard used to define obesity. Although calculated using body weight and body height, BMI provides a better assessment of body fat than simple height-weight tables and correlates well with estimates of body fat obtained by underwater weighing. Nevertheless, BMI does not provide a quantitative measure of body fat and does not distinguish between excess body fat and increased muscle mass in persons of greater body weight. Differences in stature influence body composition because taller people have greater bone mass, adding to their body weight. Thus individuals with the same BMI may not have an identical body composition.[39] Despite these limitations, BMI is a useful tool relating the rise in health risk with excessive body fat, and it provides a basis for intervention when more sophisticated equipment is not available. The formula for calculating BMI is as follows:

$$\text{BMI} = \text{weight (kg) divided by height (m)}^2$$

$$\text{Weight: } 1\text{ kg} = 2.2\text{ lb}$$

$$\text{Height: } 1\text{ m} = 39.37\text{ inches}$$

TABLE 8-4 ADULT BODY MASS INDEX CHART

To determine body mass index (BMI), select the height of interest in the left-most column and read across the row for that height to the weight of interest. Follow the column of the weight up to the top row that lists the BMI.

BMI of 18.5 to 24.9 = healthy weight range

BMI of 25.0 to 29.9 = overweight range

BMI of ≥30 = obese range

BMI	19	20	21	22	23	24	25	26	27	28	29	30	31	32	33	34	35
HEIGHT									**WEIGHT IN POUNDS**								
4 ft 10 in	91	96	100	105	110	115	119	124	129	134	138	143	148	153	158	162	167
4 ft 11 in	94	99	104	109	114	119	124	128	133	138	143	148	153	158	163	168	173
5 ft 0 in	97	102	107	112	118	123	128	133	138	143	148	153	158	163	158	174	179
5 ft 1 in	100	106	111	116	122	127	132	137	143	148	153	158	164	169	174	180	185
5 ft 2 in	104	109	115	120	126	131	136	142	147	153	158	164	169	175	180	186	191
5 ft 3 in	107	113	118	124	130	135	141	146	152	158	163	169	175	180	186	191	197
5 ft 4 in	110	116	122	128	134	140	145	151	157	163	169	174	180	186	192	197	204
5 ft 5 in	114	120	126	132	138	144	150	156	162	168	174	180	186	192	198	204	210
5 ft 6 in	118	124	130	136	142	148	155	161	167	173	179	186	192	198	204	210	216
5 ft 7 in	121	127	134	140	146	153	159	166	172	178	185	191	198	204	211	217	223
5 ft 8 in	125	131	138	144	151	158	164	171	177	184	190	197	203	210	216	223	230
5 ft 9 in	128	135	142	149	155	162	169	176	182	189	196	203	209	216	223	230	236
5 ft 10 in	132	139	146	153	160	167	174	181	188	195	202	209	216	222	229	236	243
5 ft 11 in	136	143	150	157	165	172	179	186	193	200	208	215	222	229	236	243	250
6 ft 0 in	140	147	154	162	169	177	184	191	199	206	213	221	228	235	242	250	258
6 ft 1 in	144	151	159	166	174	182	189	197	204	212	219	227	235	242	250	257	265
6 ft 2 in	148	155	163	171	179	186	194	202	210	218	225	233	241	249	256	264	272
6 ft 3 in	152	160	168	176	184	192	200	208	216	224	232	240	248	256	264	272	279
			Healthy Weight						***Overweight***					***Obese***			

From U.S. Department of Health and Human Services, U.S. Department of Agriculture: *Dietary guidelines for Americans 2005,* ed 6, Washington, DC, 2005, U.S. Government Printing Office. Available at http://www.health.gov/dietaryguidelines/dga2005/document/default.htm.

Source: National Institutes of Health, National Heart, Lung, and Blood Institute: *Evidence report of clinical guidelines on the identification, evaluation, and treatment of overweight and obesity in adults,* Bethesda, Md, 1998, National Institutes of Health.

Height and weight equivalents for BMI levels beyond 35 can be found in Appendix A.

TABLE 8-5 CLASSIFICATION OF BODY WEIGHT ACCORDING TO BODY MASS INDEX

BMI (in kg/m²)	BODY WEIGHT STATUS
<18.5	Underweight
18.5-24.9	Normal
25-29.9	Overweight
30-34.9	Obese (class I)
35-39.9	Obese (class II)
≥40	Extreme obesity (class III)

Data from National Heart, Lung, and Blood Institute/National Institute of Diabetes and Digestive and Kidney Diseases: *Clinical guidelines on the identification, evaluation, and treatment of overweight and obesity in adults: the evidence report,* NIH Pub No 98-4083, Bethesda, Md, 1998, National Institutes of Health.
BMI, Body mass index.

The desirable BMI range for adults is 18.5 to 24.9 kg/m². Health risks associated with overweight begin at 25 kg/m² and become apparent at 30 kg/m². Values beyond 35 kg/m² indicate severe obesity (Table 8-5).[3]

Waist-to-Hip Ratio

Not only the amount of body fat but also where it is positioned on the body influences health and mortality. Figure 8-6 describes the *apple* shape versus the *pear* shape. The pear shape, with a smaller waist and larger hip (gynoid shape), is characteristic of women and controlled to some extent by the female sex hormone estrogen. The apple shape, with more fat around the abdomen (android shape), is common in men and postmenopausal women. Because abdominal (**visceral**) fat contributes to increased blood lipid levels and raises the risk of cardiovascular disease, extra weight around one's middle carries greater risk for most people than does extra weight on the hips or thighs. An appropriate ratio is 0.9 or less (indicating a smaller waist and larger hip measurement) for men and 0.8 or less for women. A ratio ≥1.0 falls in the danger zone.[31] Waist circumference is also a tool for evaluating an individual's abdominal fat and health status.[40] (See the *Perspectives in Practice* box, "Assessing Energy Expenditure and Body Weight," to estimate your energy requirements and evaluate your body weight status.)

HEALTH PROMOTION

Finding a Healthy Weight

The problem with the concept of normal body weight is that for many people it cannot be defined.[41] In the traditional sense, overweight (or an excess of body fat) represents an energy imbalance coming from a surplus in energy input (fuel from food) over energy output (total energy expenditure). However, it is not that simple. Our genetic makeup influences weight gain and the amount and position of body fat.

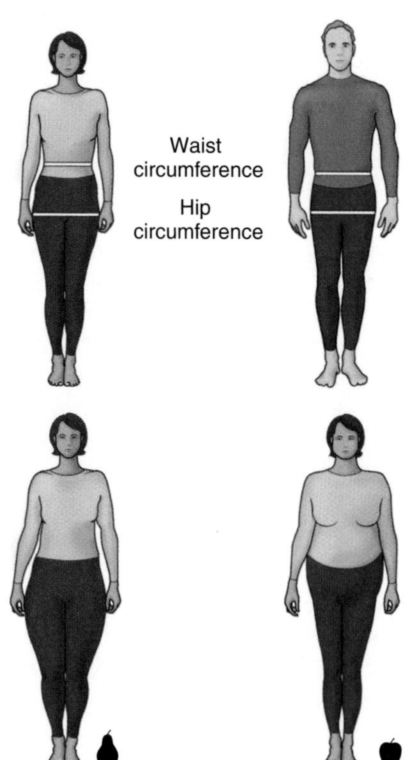

FIGURE 8-6 The pear shape versus the apple shape. Those with an apple shape and more abdominal fat have a greater risk of chronic disease than those with a pear shape and less abdominal fat. In women the waist-to-hip ratio should not exceed 0.8; in men it should not exceed 0.9. (From Grodner M, Long S, DeYoung S: *Foundations and clinical applications of nutrition: a nursing approach,* ed 3, St Louis, 2004, Mosby.)

Certain individuals have an exceptionally low RMR and high metabolic efficiency caused by an inherited obesity gene,[3,12] which adds to their risk of unwanted weight gain. Fidgeting increases energy expenditure and helps some people resist weight gain even if overfed.[42]

Just as weight gain results from a surplus of kcalories, weight loss should follow a kcalorie deficit. A deficit of 3500 kcal is expected to bring about the loss of 1 lb of body fat. However, body mechanisms designed to preserve body mass may act to decrease spontaneous activity (e.g., fidgeting) or lower BMR, making weight loss more difficult. For some individuals the weight loss required to move them into a more appropriate weight range is not possible. Therefore what should be our approach to a healthy weight?

Developing a Healthy Lifestyle

The goals of weight management go well beyond numbers on a scale, even if weight change is one of the objectives.[1] Successful weight management requires a lifelong

KEY TERMS
visceral Referring to the organs in the abdominal cavity.

PERSPECTIVES IN PRACTICE

Assessing Energy Expenditure and Body Weight

In your professional role you will be helping clients define their energy needs and assess their body weight and body fat. This exercise will give you experience in this process as you assess your own energy expenditure and weight status.

A. Calculate Your Total Energy Output per Day

Your total energy output in kcalories per day is the sum of your body's three uses of energy:

1. Resting metabolic rate (RMR)
2. Thermic effect of food (TEF)
3. Physical activity

1. Resting Metabolic Rate

Calculate your RMR using the following formula[1]:

a. Select one of the following:
   Women: 0.9 kcal/kg/hr
   Men: 1.0 kcal/kg/hr

b. Convert your body weight (lb) to kg: 1 kg = 2.2 lb Body weight (lb) ÷ 2.2 = ______ kg

c. RMR (kcalories) = 0.9 or 1.0 × kg body weight × 24 (hours in day) = ______

2. Thermic Effect of Food

The TEF is the energy the body uses in digesting and absorbing the food we eat. TEF equals about 10% of our kcalorie intake. The factors we will use to estimate the energy expended in physical activity include the kcalories required for the TEF, but you need to be aware of this component as part of your total energy expenditure.

3. Physical Activity

Energy expended in physical activity varies with the time and intensity of the activity. Two methods can be used to estimate these kcalories. You can keep a 24-hour activity record or approximate your activity kcalories from your RMR.

Calculating Your Physical Activity Kcalories Using an Activity Record

Recording your physical activity during a 24-hour period is much like recording your food intake. Prepare a chart that allows you to record the time you start and stop each activity and the type of activity. Review the activity expenditure database on the Evolve website so you can be sure to include the appropriate amount of detail when keeping your record. Carry a notebook with you as you did when recording your food intake for the day (see Chapter 1). Using the energy expenditures assigned to your body weight (in pounds), calculate your total energy expenditure over a 24-hour period. Keep in mind that the energy expenditures given in the activities database indicate the kcalories used per hour and include the total kcalories expended for RMR needs, TEF needs, and physical activity needs for the given period; thus you must sum only the time-corrected values from that table to estimate your total energy expenditure for the day.

Approximating Your Physical Activity Kcalories Using Your RMR

Because your RMR is based on your body weight, your energy expenditure in physical activity can be calculated using a factor that estimates your level of activity. Nutrition experts have defined several levels of physical activity and developed factors that estimate the kcalories required.[1] Look at the following definitions and see which meets your general level of activity. If your only physical activity for the day involves the casual walking and activities we all perform as part of our daily living, then your pattern is sedentary. Additional activity in the form of walking at a brisk pace, running, sports, dancing, or use of fitness equipment is needed for the higher categories of activity.

USUAL ACTIVITY PATTERN	DEFINITION	PHYSICAL ACTIVITY FACTOR*
Sedentary	Normal activities required for independent living	0.2
Low active	Normal activities required for independent living plus at least 30 to 60 minutes of moderately intensive activity	0.5
Active	Normal activities required for independent living plus *more* than 60 minutes of moderately intensive activity or a mix of moderately intensive and vigorous activity	0.7
Very active	Normal activities required for independent living plus 2 hours or more of vigorous activity	1.2

See the list of General Physical Activities Defined by Level of Intensity found on the website of the Centers for Disease Control and Prevention (CDC) for numerous examples of moderately intensive and vigorously intensive activities: *www.cdc.gov/physicalactivity/everyone/measuring/index.html.*

Calculate the energy cost of your physical activity using the activity factor that best fits your current activity level.

Physical activity kcalories = RMR × physical activity factor = ________

For example, if you are sedentary, then you would multiply your RMR by 0.2, as follows:

Physical activity kcalories = (RMR) × 0.2 = ________

4. Calculate Your Total Energy Expenditure

Total energy expenditure (kcalories) = RMR + physical activity kcalories (calculated using an activity factor listed previously) = ________

Refer to the dietary intake record that you completed as part of the *Perspectives in Practice* box in Chapter 1, and consider the following questions:

- How does your energy intake compare with your estimated total energy expenditure just completed? Are you taking in more kcalories, fewer kcalories, or about the same number of kcalories as you are using each day?
- What will be the effect on your body weight if you continue this pattern? What will be the effect on your health status?

Continued

PERSPECTIVES IN PRACTICE

Assessing Energy Expenditure and Body Weight—cont'd

B. Evaluate Your Body Weight Using the Body Mass Index

1. Calculate Your Body Mass Index

Body mass index (BMI) is usually calculated in metric terms as follows:

BMI = weight (kg) ÷ height (m)^2

BMI can also be calculated using weight in pounds and height in inches, as follows:

Step 1: body weight (lb) × 705 = _______

Step 2: result from step 1 ÷ height (inches) = _______

Step 3: result from step 2 ÷ height (inches) = _____BMI

You can also determine your BMI using Table 8-4 or Appendix A.

Health risks associated with overweight begin at a BMI of 25, and individuals with a BMI of 30 or greater have growing levels of risk (Table 8-5).[2]

- What is your assessment of your weight status using the BMI? Are you underweight, overweight, or in the healthy range?
- If you are not in the healthy range, how might you begin to improve your health status? (Consider being underweight to be as needful of attention as being overweight.)

C. Evaluate Your Health Status Using Waist Circumference

Measure your waist circumference using a nonstretch tape.

If you are a woman, then your waist circumference should not exceed 88 cm (35 inches); if you are a man, then it should not exceed 102 cm (40 inches).[2]

- What is your assessment of your chronic disease risk based on your waist circumference?
- If you are not in the healthful range, how might you begin to improve your health status?

REFERENCES

1. Food and Nutrition Board, Institute of Medicine: *Dietary Reference Intakes for energy, carbohydrate, fiber, fat, fatty acids, cholesterol, protein, and amino acids (macronutrients)*, Washington, DC, 2002, National Academies Press.
2. National Heart, Lung, and Blood Institute/National Institute of Diabetes and Digestive and Kidney Diseases: *Clinical guidelines on the identification, evaluation, and treatment of overweight and obesity in adults: the evidence report*, NIH Pub No 98-4083, Bethesda, Md, 1998, National Institutes of Health.

*The physical activity factors used in this assignment represent the midpoint of the range given for each activity level.

commitment to positive lifestyle behaviors emphasizing sustainable and enjoyable eating habits and daily physical activity.[43] A healthy food and activity pattern is a more appropriate goal than weight loss at any cost. The loss of even 10% of body weight can bring about functional improvements in blood glucose levels and blood pressure.[1] A meal plan low to moderate in fat and rich in fruits, vegetables, whole grains, and fiber at an energy level that prevents further weight gain adds to well-being regardless of weight loss. A stable weight, even if greater than the recommended weight, maintained with a healthy diet plan and regular physical activity is preferred over regular cycles of weight loss followed by even greater weight gain.

At the same time it is important to help our clients recognize the long-term consequences of continuing weight gain. A Science Advisory from the American Heart Association[44] points to the misperception created by the emphasis on body weight and mortality. Studies receiving widespread publicity have reported that body weights in the overweight or moderately obese range will not contribute to an earlier death, at least not in some population groups.[36–38] But even small increases in body weight can add to risk of diabetes, high blood pressure, and cardiovascular disease that over time adversely affect quality of life. (Review Chapter 1 for examples of sound eating plans.)

The *Dietary Guidelines for Americans* recommends that all adults obtain at least 30 minutes of physical activity most days of the week, and 60 minutes or more may be necessary to achieve or maintain weight loss.[32] Walking for even 10 minutes a day and gradually increasing to longer periods is a safe way to get started. Dividing physical activity across the day may work better for some people. Walking at a speed of 3 to 4 mph for 30 minutes or more at least 5 days each week meets current recommendations for improving health.[45] Regular activity lowered the risk of heart attack by 20% even when individuals remained obese.[46] An added benefit of physical activity is the increase in energy expenditure that can continue up to 15 hours after the activity is completed.[3] (For more discussion on the benefits of walking, see the *Evidence-Based Practice* box, "Is There a Role for Walking in Weight Management?") (See the *Focus on Food Safety* box, "Safe Snacking," for items to carry with you on hikes or bicycle trips.)

EVIDENCE-BASED PRACTICE

Is There a Role for Walking in Weight Management?

Health educators worldwide are encouraging people to increase their physical activity. Walking has many advantages as a form of exercise—it requires no special training, no special equipment other than a good pair of walking shoes, does not cost money, and has a relatively low risk of injury. However, does walking really count as an effective form of physical activity for weight management?

Current Recommendations

Adults are encouraged to have at least 30 minutes of moderate-intensity exercise on most days of the week, and walking at a speed of 3 to 4 mph (≥100 steps/minute) meets this standard. These steps are expected to be beyond the walking required to perform the general activities of independent living.

EVIDENCE-BASED PRACTICE

Is There a Role for Walking in Weight Management?—cont'd

Although the 30 minutes of walking can be spread throughout the day, each bout should extend for at least 10 minutes to meet the expectation for moderate-intensity activity.

Walking and Weight Management

Lean sedentary individuals tend to walk more as part of their day-to-day routine than obese sedentary individuals. Levine and colleagues, studying individuals fitted with locomotion detection devices, noted that both lean and obese subjects had the same number of walking bouts (46 to 47) over the course of the day; however, the lean subjects took more steps with each bout, thus their daily distance walked was about 3.5 miles greater as compared with the obese subjects. Other studies have looked at dog owners in regard to their walking habits and body weight. Within similar neighborhoods, dog owners who walk their dogs regularly are less likely to be obese than dog owners who do not walk their dogs or those without dogs. We do not know if obese individuals always walked less, which may have contributed to their obesity, or if they walked less after becoming obese, based on physical discomfort or other difficulty. Participants in walking intervention studies that used pedometers and set step goals walked an additional 2200 steps per day and improved their BMI.

Walking may be key to halting the increase in body weight occurring within the U.S. population. Gordon-Larsen and co-workers, who observed nearly 5000 young adults for 15 years, documented kcalorie intake, weight gain, and hours of walking. In general, individuals gained more than 2 lb per year; the average BMI rose from the healthy weight range (<25) to greater than 29 in women and 28 in men. Kcalorie intake changed very little over the 15-year span; hours of walking per week made the difference in the amount of weight gained or lost. Women walking 4 hours each week gained about 11 lb as compared with a gain of 29 lb by those with no leisure walking time. Among men the differences were 15 lb gained for leisure time walkers versus 24 lb for the others. For women 30 minutes of daily walking reduced weight gain by about 18 lb. Walking also has a dose effect: 2 hours per week are better than none, and 4 hours per week are better than 2 hours.

Weight gain over adulthood can result from a subtle increase in kcalorie intake, a reduction in physical activity, or the slow but incremental reduction in basal metabolism associated with age-related loss of LBM. An excess of only 50 kcal/day can lead to a weight gain of 5 to 6 lb per year. Adding 1000 to 2000 steps per day, accomplished in a 20-minute walk, could prevent such a gain. Walking as a public health intervention has been shown to lower blood pressure, improve glycemic control in type 2 diabetes, and prevent the progression from prediabetes to diabetes.

Walking as a positive force for health must be supported at the community level by neighborhood planning for safe walking. Modifying the built environment to establish favorable conditions for walking could pay long-term dividends in lowering health care costs.

BIBLIOGRAPHY

Berke EM, Koepsell TD, Moudon AV, et al: Association of the built environment with physical activity and obesity in older persons, *Am J Public Health* 97:486, 2007.

Bravata DM, Smith-Spangler C, Sundaram V, et al: Using pedometers to increase physical activity and improve health. A systematic review, *JAMA* 298:2296, 2007.

Coleman KJ, Rosenberg DE, Conway TL, et al: Physical activity, weight status, and neighborhood characteristics of dog walkers, *Prev Med* 47:309, 2008.

Gordon-Larsen P, Hou N, Sidney S, et al: Fifteen-year longitudinal trends in walking patterns and their impact on weight change, *Am J Clin Nutr* 89:19, 2009.

Lee I-M, Buchner DM: The importance of walking to public health, *Med Sci Sports Exerc* 40:S512, 2008.

Levine JA, McCrady SK, Lanningham-Foster LM, et al: The role of free-living daily walking in human weight gain and obesity, *Diabetes* 57:548, 2008.

Nelson ME, Folta SC: Further evidence for the benefits of walking, *Am J Clin Nutr* 89:15, 2009.

Tudor-Locke C, Hatano Y, Pangrazi RP, et al: Revisiting "how many steps are enough", *Med Sci Sports Exerc* 40(Suppl 7):S537, 2008.

FATNESS, THINNESS, AND HEALTH

Rise in Obesity

Attitudes toward obesity have undergone many changes over the years. In colonial times, obesity was a sign of economic well-being and identified a family that was prosperous. Although we have come to recognize the health risks associated with obesity, the number of persons either overweight or obese has been rising. Only 34% of U.S. adults ages 20 and older have a BMI less than 25.[47] African-American and Mexican-American women are more likely to be obese,[35] as are limited-resource families with poor diets, poor living conditions, and limited access to health care.

FOCUS ON FOOD SAFETY

Safe Snacking

Hiking, a bicycle trip, a game of soccer, or a 1-hour walk around your neighborhood can make you hungry. It is a good idea to take along a snack to provide the quick energy you need, but be sure to choose foods that can be carried safely in a backpack or gym bag. Bottled or boxed juices; fruit such as oranges, apples, or bananas; and pretzels or crackers with peanut butter contain carbohydrate that will replenish your energy supply and do not need to be kept cold. Trail or granola mix supplies energy but can be high in fat. Do not take a chance on spoiling your outing with an attack of foodborne illness. Always read the label on a packaged food to be sure that it does not require refrigeration.

Obesity and Health

Weight-related health problems can be divided into four categories: (1) metabolic, (2) degenerative, (3) neoplastic, and (4) anatomic:

- *Metabolic:* Type 2 diabetes, hypertension, and elevated blood lipids often accompany obesity. Regardless of total body fat, abdominal fat increases the risk of metabolic disorders.[40]
- *Degenerative:* Obesity and physical disability are strongly linked.[48] Osteoarthritis and joint problems, atherosclerotic changes, and pulmonary diseases are more serious in obese persons.[43]
- *Neoplastic:* Many forms of cancer including colorectal, breast, prostate, esophageal, and ovarian cancer are more frequent in increased weight categories.
- *Anatomic:* Individuals exceeding a healthy weight have a greater risk of gastroesophageal reflux disease (GERD) and obstructive sleep apnea.

Elevated body weight also contributes to health care costs in middle age and beyond. Cumulative Medicare expenditures for treating diabetes and related complications were more than doubled in women with a BMI greater than 34 as compared with those with a BMI less than 25.[49] The rise in obesity-related type 2 diabetes in children who will require lifetime care for this dangerous disease will heavily affect future health care costs. (Chapter 15 focuses on the environmental factors in our society that favor the development of obesity and discusses appropriate interventions.)

Obsession with Thinness

A trend opposite to obesity but equally harmful to health is the model of extreme thinness. Fueled by advertising dollars, an image of thinness drives the marketing of clothes, cosmetics, and food to teenagers and young adults. Social pressures have created an abnormally thin and unrealistic ideal to the point that even fashion models express dissatisfaction with their overall body shapes.[50] Boys and girls as young as age 7 perceive their mother's encouragement to remain thin and develop restrained eating and dissatisfaction with their body.[51] When parents restrict food intake to prevent weight gain, children may react by overeating when those restricted foods are available in another setting.[52,53] Guilt feelings after eating certain foods and distorted perceptions of body size often form the basis for serious eating disorders that threaten nutritional and physical health. School programs, voluntary community programs, and sports programs that build self-esteem offer primary prevention for disordered eating.

The ongoing quest for the perfect body has given rise to the chronic dieter who constantly tries to restrict food intake. Although restrained eating is often seen in women trying to lose weight, dieting is also a concern among boys and girls. The family setting plays a role in helping youth develop positive attitudes toward food. Adolescent girls who ate at least five meals a week with their family were less likely to engage in extreme weight control behaviors such as use of laxatives or diuretics, forced vomiting, fasting, or chronic dieting.[54] Teens participating in weight-related sports are especially vulnerable to unhealthy weight control practices, and preventive efforts targeting parents, coaches, and students are urgently needed.[55]

Eating Disorders: A High Price for Thinness

The total number of individuals affected by eating disorders is unknown. These conditions can exist for some time before diagnosis; based on their secretive nature, they often go unreported.[56] Eating disorders are most prevalent among young women ages 18 to 30 and are estimated to affect about 3% of this population; however, they also occur in men and older adults. As many as 10% to 20% of male and female athletes are believed to have an eating disorder.[56] Eating disorders are considered to be medical illnesses and lead to nutritional deficiencies, medical complications, and in the extreme, disability and death. We associate eating disorders with our society's emphasis on thinness, but physicians in Great Britain and France described anorexia nervosa in the 1800s.

Causes of Eating Disorders

Biologic, psychologic, and social forces all play a part in producing the behavior that we associate with eating disorders.[57] In some cases, hormonal changes associated with puberty and resulting changes in body shape lead to problems in self-image. Social pressures and perceived difficulty in meeting expectations of family or others may be a cause. Stressful life events such as the serious illness of a family member or parents' divorce or separation can initiate such behavior.[58] A history of substance abuse or physical abuse is also a risk factor for disordered eating.

Biologic factors can influence the development of eating disorders. Genetic predisposition and alterations in central nervous system (CNS) activity can directly affect food behavior. Levels of serotonin and other neurotransmitters can result in psychologic conditions such as depression that indirectly influence the development of eating disorders.[56] For every individual who develops an eating disorder, a particular factor may be more or less important. Eating disorders are found in all social classes and demographic groups. Although female adolescents are especially vulnerable to eating disorders, the incidence of such disorders among male adolescents is increasing. The male adolescents often have a history of obesity, leading them to begin dieting.[59]

The growing interest in athletics among children and youth can either increase risk of eating disorders or assist in prevention. Those participating in activities in which thinness is expected, such as gymnastics or dance, are more likely to develop an eating disorder. Students who take part in school or recreational sports that do not require a thin body are at lower risk. Self-esteem and activities that help young people feel good about themselves and their accomplishments help protect against eating disorders.

The general characteristics of eating disorders include the following[60]:

- A disturbed body image in which an individual perceives herself or himself as fat, even if body weight is normal or less than normal

- An intense fear of gaining weight
- An unrelenting desire to be thinner

Individuals with eating disorders may suffer from other psychiatric disorders that add to the complexity of their treatment.[56]

Types of Eating Disorders

The three types of eating disorders recognized by the American Psychiatric Association are (1) anorexia nervosa, (2) bulimia nervosa, and (3) eating disorders not otherwise specified (EDNOS).[59] Each has distinctive diagnostic criteria and symptoms.

The term *anorexia nervosa* means appetite loss from nervous disease. Anorexia nervosa is a form of starvation with excessive weight loss self-imposed at great physical and psychologic cost. Although these patients may have a body weight only 85% of average or a BMI of less than 17.5, they never see themselves as underweight and emaciated but always as fat.[56] This distorted body image often persists during recovery. Low bone mass is a frequent complication because amenorrhea usually accompanies this condition. Sudden death can result from cardiac arrest. Only about one half of anorexia nervosa patients fully recover, with others having a poor to moderate outcome.[53] Individuals with a higher percentage of body fat at the time of hospital discharge are more likely to have a positive long-term outcome.[61]

Bulimia nervosa, meaning "ox-hunger," describes the massive amounts of food consumed by patients with this condition. Because this individual is eating, body weight is usually normal or even above normal. Bulimia nervosa is often associated with depression or difficulty in meeting social or role expectations, and patients are consumed with guilt about their food behavior. Eating episodes are followed by purging through self-induced vomiting, use of laxatives or diuretics, enemas, or excessive exercise and may occur twice a week or more. Repeated vomiting of the highly acidic stomach contents can be harmful to the teeth and tissues of the mouth. This condition is sometimes referred to as the *binge and purge syndrome.*

About one half of those with eating disorders fall under the EDNOS category. If their problems remain untreated, then these individuals may progress over time to anorexia nervosa or bulimia nervosa. **Binge-eating disorder** includes binge-eating episodes without the purging behavior of bulimia nervosa. Binge eating may occur in response to stress or anxiety or to soothe or relieve painful feelings. Many of these patients are overweight and have the same medical problems as obese individuals who do not binge eat.

Prevention and Treatment

Identification of individuals at risk for an eating disorder can prompt early intervention and prevent the development of medical disorders and malnutrition. Health professionals and school personnel working with adolescents and athletes should watch for behavioral and clinical signs that indicate risk for disordered eating (Box 8-2). Parents need to be alerted to the behavioral and health characteristics of eating

BOX 8-2 SIGNS ASSOCIATED WITH DEVELOPMENT OF EATING DISORDERS IN ADOLESCENTS

Behavioral Signs
- Obsession with dieting
- Extreme level of exercise
- Dissatisfaction with body size or shape
- Higher level of perfectionism than seen in peers
- Extreme depression and anxiety
- Overestimation of their kcalorie intake (anorexia nervosa)

Clinical Signs (Anorexia Nervosa)
- Arrested growth and maturation
- Underweight (body mass index [BMI] <17.5 or body weight <85% of expected weight for height and gender)
- Poor concentration
- Dry and yellowish skin
- Growth of fine hair over body (e.g., lanugo)
- Brittle hair and nails
- Muscle weakness and lethargy
- Drop in internal body temperature, causing the person to feel cold all the time
- Severe constipation
- Low blood pressure, slowed breathing and pulse

Clinical Signs (Bulimia Nervosa)
- Growth status is generally normal
- Poor concentration
- Chronically inflamed and sore throat
- Swollen glands in the neck and below the jaw from chronic vomiting
- Worn tooth enamel and increasingly sensitive and decaying teeth as a result of exposure to stomach acids
- Intestinal distress and irritation from laxative abuse
- Severe dehydration from purging of fluids
- Gastroesophageal reflux disorder

Adapted from American Dietetic Association: Position of the American Dietetic Association: nutrition intervention in the treatment of anorexia nervosa, bulimia nervosa, and other eating disorders, *J Am Diet Assoc* 106:2073, 2006; U.S. Department of Health and Human Services, National Institute of Mental Health: *Eating disorders,* NIH Pub No 07-4901, Bethesda, Md, 2007, National Institute of Mental Health.

KEY TERMS

neoplastic Describing abnormal growth of tissue, usually associated with the formation of tumors.

anorexia nervosa Extreme psychophysiologic aversion to food resulting in life-threatening weight loss. An eating disorder caused by a morbid fear of fat in which a distorted body image is reflected as fat when the body is actually malnourished and thin from self-starvation.

bulimia nervosa An eating disorder in which cycles of gorging on large quantities of food are followed by self-induced vomiting and use of diuretics or laxatives to avoid weight gain.

binge-eating disorder An eating disorder in which individuals consume large amounts of food in a short period of time, but without the purging behavior of bulimia nervosa.

disorders and watch for such behaviors in their children. Individuals with anorexia nervosa will demonstrate characteristic signs of protein-energy malnutrition as the condition continues. Those with bulimia nervosa are less likely to be underweight. Regular family meals may help to prevent the development of eating disorders.[54]

Treatment of eating disorders requires medical nutrition therapy and psychotherapy. These conditions exert a high toll on physical and psychologic health and require individualized care. The best chance for success lies with an experienced team of health professionals including a physician, nurse, dietitian, clinical psychologist or psychiatrist, and dentist. Outpatient services may provide the care needed in less advanced cases, but for life-threatening anorexia nervosa intense inpatient therapy is essential.

The care plan for disordered eating patients should include nutritional, medical, and cognitive intervention. A meal plan that provides a framework for meals, snacks, and food choices must be implemented on a gradual basis to address the underweight or overweight. Medical complications arising from severe malnutrition, dehydration, habitual vomiting, or excessive use of diuretics or laxatives require immediate attention. The psychologist or psychiatrist on the health care team can address the personal or social issues that first led to the problem and help develop healthy behavior patterns that will sustain the nutritional and medical recovery. Unfortunately, many cases of eating disorders go undetected, delaying or preventing the intervention so urgently needed.[56]

The Problem of Underweight

Thus far we have discussed the problem of excessive body weight and body fat and situations in which individuals deliberately limit their food intake. Now we consider the causes and effects of underweight as related to lack of food or debilitating illness.

Definition

Extreme underweight is associated with serious health problems in all age-groups.[62,63] *Underweight,* defined as a BMI of less than 18.5, is relatively uncommon in the United States. A national survey identified only 2.2% of adults as underweight,[36] but nearly 5% of low-income children between the ages of 2 and 4 were classified as *low weight for height.*[64] Underweight springs from poverty, poor living conditions, long-term illness, or physiologic dysfunction. Infants, young children, and older adults are at greatest risk. Low weight for age is associated with more than 50% of child deaths in developing countries,[63] and those who do survive can experience long-term growth retardation. Resistance to infection is lower, general health is poorer, and physical strength is decreased in seriously underweight individuals.

General Causes

Conditions that lead to general malnutrition contribute to underweight. These fall into three categories: (1) those that decrease food intake, (2) those that increase energy requirements, and (3) those that prevent optimum utilization of food intake (Box 8-3):

1. *Poor food intake:* Lack of sufficient and appropriate food results in failure to thrive in children and older adults. Anorexia and nausea are common side effects of digoxin and chemotherapeutic agents and contribute to the devastating weight loss referred to as cachexia. Older people in poverty who live alone and lack transportation to a food store risk unwanted weight loss. Federal guidelines require monitoring of body weight in skilled nursing facilities where a patient's inability to self-feed can lead to significant weight loss. Self-imposed food restriction as in anorexia nervosa results in life-threatening underweight.
2. *Increase in energy requirements:* Long-term hypermetabolic conditions such as cancer, acquired immunodeficiency syndrome (AIDS), advanced heart disease, or infection impose energy demands that drain the body's resources. Hyperthyroidism increases caloric requirements. Extensive physical activity without a sufficient increase in energy intake will over time bring about inappropriate weight loss in the normal weight individual.
3. *Poor utilization of available nutrients:* Malabsorption associated with prolonged diarrhea, gastrointestinal disease, or laxative abuse depletes nutrient stores. Cytokines produced by the immune system in response to chronic conditions such as cancer, chronic kidney disease, congestive heart failure, and AIDS accelerate the breakdown of body protein and fat. Cytokines can also prevent the effective utilization of added nutrients, making it difficult to reverse the patient's deteriorating condition.[62]

BOX 8-3 CAUSES OF UNDERWEIGHT

- Lack of sufficient amounts or quality of food (limited resources to purchase food)
- Loss of appetite (aging changes, certain medications)
- Premature feeling of fullness
- Physical disability (problems with food shopping, meal preparation, or self-feeding)
- Long-term illness
- Cancer
- Cardiac failure
- Chronic obstructive pulmonary disease
- Sepsis
- Chronic renal disease
- Autoimmune deficiency disease
- Cystic fibrosis
- Hyperthyroidism

KEY TERMS

cachexia A wasting condition marked by weakness, extreme weight loss, and malnutrition.

hypermetabolic Increased rate of body metabolism usually occurring as a result of infection, trauma, or disease.

Nutritional Care

Underweight persons require special nutrition intervention to rebuild body tissues and nutrient stores. Food plans must be adapted to the individual's personal preferences, financial situation, and household concerns, along with any existing disease. The dietary recommendation should be (1) high in kcalories, at least 50% beyond standard needs; (2) high in protein to rebuild tissue; (3) high in carbohydrate to provide a primary energy source in an easily digested form; (4) moderate in unsaturated fats to add kcalories but not exceed recommended limits; and (5) optimum in vitamins and minerals, including supplements when deficiencies require them. A wide variety of food that is well prepared and seasoned and attractively presented helps revive a lagging appetite and the desire to eat. Meals and snacks spread throughout the day that include favorite foods increase interest in eating and promote optimal utilization of nutrients. Seasonings such as margarine, butter, or sauces, and liquid nutritional supplements add kcalories and key nutrients. In extreme cases, tube feeding or total parenteral nutrition (TPN) may be necessary (see Chapter 19).

The rehabilitation process requires creative counseling with the individual and caregivers, with attention to underlying socioeconomic and disease conditions. Practical guidance and ongoing support are needed to counteract the root causes of the malnutrition and build food patterns that will be continued when the person has returned to health.

TO SUM UP

Food provides the energy that enables the body to continue its life-sustaining physical and metabolic work. Through a series of ongoing metabolic reactions, the chemical energy in food is converted to thermal, electrical, and mechanical energy. All body work produces heat commonly expressed in kcalories, which serves as a measure of energy taken in through food and expended. One's total energy requirement is the sum of (1) basal metabolic needs, (2) the food intake effect (i.e., TEF), and (3) physical activity. Physical activity is the most variable component, adding relatively few kcalories to the total energy expenditure of sedentary persons but making up one half or more of the total energy requirement of highly active people. Both energy intake and physical activity influence the size of the four major body compartments: (1) LBM, (2) body fat, (3) body water, and (4) mineral mass. The total amount of body fat, as well as its position on the body influence disease risk, with inappropriate levels of abdominal fat carrying greater risk than overall body fat. Interventions focusing on positive food and activity behaviors are of greater value in addressing overweight and obesity than programs emphasizing weight loss only. At the other extreme, eating disorders with self-imposed food restriction lead to poor health and even death in adolescents and adults, and the prognosis for intervention can be poor. Poverty, chronic disease, and medications also contribute to underweight through low food intake, poor food utilization, or increased energy requirements A nutrient- and energy-rich diet combined with ongoing counseling to support the rehabilitation process can restore an underweight individual to a healthy weight.

QUESTIONS FOR REVIEW

1. Define the term *fuel factor.* What is the fuel value of each of the four energy sources found in food and beverages?
2. List the three components contributing to the total energy requirement. What is the BMR, and what factors influence it? Which body tissues contribute most to basal metabolic needs? Which is the most variable component of the total energy requirement and why?
3. What is the difference between the BMR and the RMR? Which is most often used in clinical practice? Why?
4. Name the four body compartments and describe the tissues found in each. How are they measured?
5. You are performing a nutritional assessment of a man who is 6 feet 2 inches tall and weighs 248 lb. What is his BMI? Is he overweight, overfat, or do you know? Explain.
6. Describe various eating disorders defined by the American Psychiatric Association. What social factors contribute to disordered eating? What are some preventive strategies?
7. You are working with a single mother and her 3-year-old daughter who are both underweight. They live in a small apartment in a dilapidated building in the inner city. Their electricity was disconnected, thus they have no working equipment for cooking and no refrigeration. They receive a noon and supper meal at a nearby food program for the homeless. Plan a breakfast and snacks throughout the day that could increase their kcalorie and nutrient intake. (Remember, all foods you suggest must be safely stored at room temperature.)
8. An adolescent girl wants to increase her energy expenditure by 250 kcal a day. Develop an activity plan that would mesh with her after-school hours and social time with friends.
9. Visit your local library, and review the magazines directed toward young adults. Look for three articles that suggest regimens for weight management for either male or female subjects. Evaluate each protocol in terms of (a) nutritional adequacy as compared with the MyPyramid eating pattern, (b) development of sustainable food patterns, (c) reliance on commercial weight loss products, and (d) safety for long-term use.

REFERENCES

1. American Dietetic Association: Position of the American Dietetic Association: weight management, *J Am Diet Assoc* 109:330, 2009.
2. Brody T: *Nutritional biochemistry*, ed 2, New York, 1999, Academic Press.
3. Food and Nutrition Board, Institute of Medicine: *Dietary Reference Intakes for energy, carbohydrate, fiber, fat, fatty acids, cholesterol, protein, and amino acids (macronutrients)*, Washington, DC, 2002, National Academies Press.
4. Das SK, Roberts SB: Energy metabolism. In Bowman BA, Russell RM, editors: *Present knowledge in nutrition*, ed 9, vol 1, Washington, DC, 2006, International Life Sciences Institute, pp. 45–55.
5. Guyton AC, Hall JE: *Textbook of medical physiology*, ed 10, Philadelphia, 2000, Saunders.
6. Kulstad R, Schoeller DA: The energetics of wasting diseases, *Curr Opin Clin Nutr Metab Care* 10:488, 2007.
7. Nawata K, Sohmiya M, Kawaguchi M, et al: Increased resting metabolic rate in patients with type 2 diabetes mellitus accompanied by advanced diabetic nephropathy, *Metabolism* 53:1395, 2004.
8. Haugen HA, Chan L-N, Li F: Indirect calorimetry: a practical guide for clinicians, *Nutr Clin Prac* 22:377, 2007.
9. AAP Committee on Nutrition, Kleinman RE, editors: *Pediatric nutrition handbook*, ed 6, Elk Grove Village, Ill, 2008, American Academy of Pediatrics.
10. Jones A, Shen W, St-Onge M-P, et al: Body composition differences between African American and white women: relation to resting energy requirements, *Am J Clin Nutr* 79:780, 2004.
11. Shetty P: Energy requirements of adults, *Public Health Nutr* 8(7A):994, 2005.
12. Jacobson P, Rankinen T, Tremblay A, et al: Resting metabolic rate and respiratory quotient: results from a genome-wide scan in the Quebec Family Study, *Am J Clin Nutr* 84:1527, 2006.
13. Paddon-Jones D, Westman E, Mattes RD, et al: Protein, weight management, and satiety, *Am J Clin Nutr* 87(Suppl):1558S, 2008.
14. Westerterp KR: Physical activity as determinant of daily energy expenditure, *Physiol Behav* 93:1039, 2008.
15. Hall C, Figueroa A, Fernhall BO, et al: Energy expenditure of walking and running: comparison with prediction equations, *Med Sci Sports Exerc* 36:2128, 2004.
16. Bravata DM, Smith-Spangler C, Sundaram V, et al: Using pedometers to increase physical activity and improve health. A systematic review, *JAMA* 298:2296, 2007.
17. Woolf K, Reese CE, Mason MP, et al: Physical activity is associated with risk factors for chronic disease across adult women's life cycle, *J Am Diet Assoc* 108:948, 2008.
18. Wijers SLJ, Saris WHM, van Marken Lichtenbelt WD: Recent advances in adaptive thermogenesis: potential implications for the treatment of obesity, *Obes Rev* 10:218, 2009.
19. Koh-Banerjee P, Franz M, Sampson L, et al: Changes in whole-grain, bran, and cereal fiber consumption in relation to 8-y weight gain among men, *Am J Clin Nutr* 80:1237, 2004.
20. Bes-Rastrollo M, Martinez-Gonzalez MA, Sanchez-Villegas A, et al: Association of fiber intake and fruit/vegetable consumption with weight gain in a Mediterranean population, *Nutrition* 22:504, 2006.
21. Heymsfield SB, Baumgartner RN: Body composition and anthropometry. In Shils ME, Shike M, Olson J, et al, editors: *Modern nutrition in health and disease*, ed 10, Baltimore, 2006, Lippincott Williams & Wilkins, pp. 751–770.
22. Zhu SK, Wang ZM, Heshka S, et al: Waist circumference and obesity-associated risk factors among whites in the Third National Health and Nutrition Examination Survey: clinical action thresholds, *Am J Clin Nutr* 76:743, 2002.
23. Price GM, Uauy R, Breeze E, et al: Weight, shape, and mortality risk in older persons: elevated waist-hip ratio, not high body mass index, is associated with a greater risk of death, *Am J Clin Nutr* 84:449, 2006.
24. Zhang C, Rexrode KM, van Dam RM, et al: Abdominal obesity and the risk of all-cause, cardiovascular, and cancer mortality. Sixteen years of follow-up in U.S. women, *Circulation* 117:1658, 2008.
25. Wells JCK: Lessons from body composition analysis. In Bowman BA, Russell RM, editors: *Present knowledge in nutrition*, ed 9, vol 1, Washington, DC, 2006, International Life Sciences Institute, pp. 23–33.
26. Fields DA, Goran MI, McCrory MA: Body composition assessment via air-displacement plethysmography in adults and children: a review, *Am J Clin Nutr* 75:453, 2002.
27. Wildman RP, Gu D, Reynolds K, et al: Appropriate body mass index and waist circumference cutoffs for categorization of overweight and central adiposity among Chinese adults, *Am J Clin Nutr* 80:1129, 2004.
28. Wu C-H, Heshka S, Wang J, et al: Truncal fat in relation to total body fat: influences of age, sex, ethnicity and fatness, *Int J Obes* 31:1384, 2007.
29. Obisesan TO, Aliyu MH, Bond V, et al: Ethnic and age-related fat free mass loss in older Americans: the Third National Health and Nutrition Examination Survey (NHANES III), *BMC Public Health* 5:41, 2005. Available at http://www.ncbi.nlm.nih.gov/pmc/articles/PMC1097739/.
30. World Health Organization Expert Consultation: Appropriate body-mass index for Asian populations and its implications for policy and intervention strategies, *Lancet* 363:157, 2004.
31. National Heart, Lung, and Blood Institute/North American Association for the Study of Obesity: *The practical guide: identification, evaluation, and treatment of overweight and obesity in adults*, NIH Pub No 00-4084, Bethesda, Md, 2000, National Institutes of Health. Available at http://www.nhlbi.nih.gov/guidelines/obesity/prctgd_c.pdf.
32. U.S. Department of Health and Human Services, U.S. Department of Agriculture: *Dietary guidelines for Americans 2005*, ed 6, Washington, DC, 2005, U.S. Government Printing Office. Available at www.health.gov/dietaryguidelines/.
33. Ogden CL, Fryar CD, Carroll MD, et al: *Mean body weight, height, and body mass index, United States 1960-2002: advance data, vital and health statistics*, No 347, Washington, DC, 2004, U.S. Department of Health and Human Services.
34. Hedley AA, Ogden CL, Johnson CL, et al: Prevalence of overweight and obesity among U.S. children, adolescents, and adults, 1999-2002, *JAMA* 291:2847, 2004.
35. Ogden CL, Carroll MD, McDowell MA, et al: *Obesity among adults in the United States—no statistically significant change since 2003-2004*, NCHS Data Brief No 1, Hyattsville, Md, 2007, National Center for Health Statistics.
36. Flegal KM, Graubard BI, Williamson DF, et al: Excess deaths associated with underweight, overweight, and obesity, *JAMA* 293:1861, 2005.

37. Adams KF, Schatzkin A, Harris TB, et al: Overweight, obesity and mortality in a large prospective cohort of persons 50 to 71 years old, *N Engl J Med* 355:763, 2006.
38. Janssen I, Mark AE: Elevated body mass index and mortality risk in the elderly, *Obes Rev* 8:41, 2007.
39. Heymsfield SB, Gallagher D, Mayer L, et al: Scaling of human body composition to stature: new insights into body mass index, *Am J Clin Nutr* 86:82, 2007.
40. Klein S, Allison DB, Heymsfield SB, et al: Waist circumference and cardiometabolic risk: a consensus statement from Shaping America's Health: Association for Weight Management and Obesity Prevention; NAASO, the Obesity Society; the American Society for Nutrition; and the American Diabetes Association, *Am J Clin Nutr* 85:1197, 2007.
41. Flegal KM, Shepherd JA, Looker AC, et al: Comparisons of percentage body fat, body mass index, waist circumference, and waist-stature ratio in adults, *Am J Clin Nutr* 89:500, 2009.
42. Levine JA: Non-exercise activity thermogenesis (NEAT), *Nutr Rev* 62(7, pt 2):S82, 2004.
43. American Dietetic Association: Position of the American Dietetic Association: weight management, *J Am Diet Assoc* 102:1145, 2002.
44. Lewis CE, McTigue KM, Burke LE, et al: Mortality, health outcomes, and body mass index in the overweight range. A science advisory from the American Heart Association, *Circulation* 119:3263, 2009.
45. Haskell WL, Lee IM, Pate RR, et al: Physical activity and public health: updated recommendation for adults from the American College of Sports Medicine and the American Heart Association, *Med Sci Sports Exerc* 39:1423, 2007.
46. Wessel TR, Arant CB, Olson MB, et al: Relationship of physical fitness vs body mass index with coronary artery disease and cardiovascular events in women, *JAMA* 292:1179, 2004.
47. Ogden CL, Carroll MD, Curtin LR, et al: Prevalence of overweight and obesity in the United States, 1999-2004, *JAMA* 295:1549, 2006.
48. Reuser M, Bonneux LG, Willekens FJ: Smoking kills, obesity disables: a multistate approach of the U.S. Health and Retirement Survey, *Obesity* 17:783, 2009.
49. Daviglus ML, Liu K, Yan LL, et al: Relation of body mass index in young adulthood and middle age to Medicare expenditures in older age, *JAMA* 292:2743, 2004.
50. Grivetti L: Psychology and cultural aspects of energy, *Nutr Rev* 59:S5, 2001.
51. Anschutz DJ, Kanters LJ, Van Strien T, et al: Maternal behaviors and restrained eating and body dissatisfaction in young children, *Int J Eat Disord* 42:54, 2009.
52. Birch LL, Fisher JO, Davison KK: Learning to overeat: maternal use of restrictive feeding practices promotes girls' eating in the absence of hunger, *Am J Clin Nutr* 78:215, 2003.
53. Shunk JA, Birch LL: Girls at risk for overweight at age 5 are at risk for dietary restraint, disinhibited overeating, weight concerns, and greater weight gain from 5 to 9 years, *J Am Diet Assoc* 104:1120, 2004.
54. Neumark-Sztainer D, Eisenberg ME, Fulkerson JA, et al: Family meals and disordered eating in adolescents. Longitudinal findings from Project EAT, *Arch Pediatr Adolesc Med* 162:17, 2008.
55. Vertalino M, Eisenberg ME, Story M, et al: Participation in weight-related sports is associated with higher use of unhealthful weight-control behaviors and steroid use, *J Am Diet Assoc* 107:434, 2007.
56. American Dietetic Association: Position of the American Dietetic Association: nutrition intervention in the treatment of anorexia nervosa, bulimia nervosa, and other eating disorders, *J Am Diet Assoc* 106:2073, 2006.
57. Polivy J, Herman PC: Causes of eating disorders, *Annu Rev Psychol* 53:187, 2002.
58. Loth K, van den Berg P, Eisenberg ME, et al: Stressful life events and disordered eating behaviors: findings from Project EAT, *J Adolesc Health* 43:514, 2008.
59. Rees L, Clark-Stone S: Can collaboration between education and health professionals improve the identification and referral of young people with eating disorders in schools? A pilot study, *J Adolesc* 29(1):137, 2006.
60. American Psychiatric Association: *Diagnostic and statistical manual of mental disorders, ed 4, text revision*, Washington, DC, 2000, American Psychiatric Association.
61. Mayer LE, Roberto CA, Glasofer DR, et al: Does percent body fat predict outcome in anorexia nervosa? *Am J Psychiatry* 164:970, 2007.
62. Morley JE, Thomas DR, Wilson MM: Cachexia: pathophysiology and clinical relevance, *Am J Clin Nutr* 83:735, 2006.
63. Caulfield LE, de Onis M, Blossner M, et al: Undernutrition as an underlying cause of child deaths associated with diarrhea, pneumonia, malaria, and measles, *Am J Clin Nutr* 80:193, 2004.
64. Sherry B, Mei Z, Scanlon KS, et al: Trends in state-specific prevalence of overweight and underweight in 2- through 4-year-old children from low-income families from 1989 through 2000, *Arch Pediatr Adolesc Med* 158:1116, 2004.

FURTHER READINGS AND RESOURCES

Readings

Alley DE, Chang VW: The changing relationship of obesity and disability, 1988-2004, *JAMA* 298:2020, 2007.

Ogden CL, Carroll MD, McDowell MA, et al: *Obesity among adults in the United States—no statistically significant change since 2003-2004*, NCHS Data Brief No 1, Hyattsville, Md, 2007, National Center for Health Statistics. Available at http://www.cdc.gov/nchs/data/databriefs/db01.pdf.

[These articles review the current obesity prevalence in the U.S. and implications for the future as more obese individuals live to older ages.]

American Dietetic Association: Position of the American Dietetic Association: nutrition intervention in the treatment of anorexia nervosa, bulimia nervosa, and other eating disorders, *J Am Diet Assoc* 106:2073, 2006. *[This article provides a comprehensive review of the prevalence, causes, symptoms, and treatment of eating disorders.]*

Fenton M: Battling America's epidemic of physical inactivity: building more walkable, livable communities, *J Nutr Educ Behav* 37(Suppl 2):S115, 2005.

McCrady SK, Levine JA: Sedentariness at work: how much do we really sit, *Obesity (Silver Spring)* 17(11):2103, 2009.

Woolf K, Reese CE, Mason MP, et al: Physical activity is associated with risk factors for chronic disease across adult women's life cycle, *J Am Diet Assoc* 108:948, 2008.

[These authors focus on physical activity and prevention of chronic disease and suggest how we can encourage walking as a safe and effective activity.]

Grivetti L: Psychology and cultural aspects of energy, *Nutr Rev* 59(1, pt 2):S5, 2001.

Provencher V, Polivy J, Herman CP: Perceived healthiness of food. If it is healthy you can eat more! *Appetite* 52:340, 2009.

[These authors explore the psychology of food habits on both extremes of food intake: why we sometimes eat more than we should and what social factors contribute to restrained eating and self-starvation.]

Neumark-Sztainer D, Eisenberg ME, Fulkerson JA, et al: Family meals and disordered eating in adolescents. Longitudinal findings from Project EAT, *Arch Pediatr Adolesc Med* 162:17, 2008.

Vertalino M, Eisenberg ME, Story M, et al: Participation in weight-related sports is associated with higher use of unhealthful weight-control behaviors and steroid use, *J Am Diet Assoc* 107:434, 2007.

[These authors explore the role of the family, coaches, and health professionals in preventing eating disorders and combating influences on the teen culture that encourage unhealthful eating.]

Paddon-Jones D, Westman E, Mattes RD, et al: Protein, weight management, and satiety, *Am J Clin Nutr* 87(Suppl):1558S, 2008. *[Protein may have a role in weight management through its effect on satiety and overall metabolism. These authors provide some examples of its use in weight reduction diets.]*

Websites of Interest

National Heart, Lung, and Blood Institute/North American Association for the Study of Obesity: *The practical guide: identification, evaluation, and treatment of overweight and obesity in adults*, NIH Pub No 00-4084, Bethesda, Md, 2000, National Institutes of Health. This book provides a wealth of practical information on meal planning, food selection, and appropriate activity for assisting clients in developing weight control programs: www.nhlbi.nih.gov/guidelines/obesity/prctgd_c.pdf.

National Institute of Diabetes and Digestive and Kidney Diseases (NIDDK) WIN—Weight-Control Information Network. This site offers up-to-date, science-based information on weight control, obesity, physical activity, and related nutritional issues for health professionals and consumers: http://www.win.niddk.nih.gov/ (Materials are available in English and Spanish.)

National Institutes of Health and National Library of Medicine, Medline Plus: *Eating disorders.* This site offers comprehensive information on eating disorders, including causes, symptoms, treatment, and prevention: http://www.nlm.nih.gov/medlineplus/eatingdisorders.html.

National Institutes of Health and National Library of Medicine: *Weight control.* This site offers tips on food selection for weight management and links to sites that contain ideas for physical activity: http://www.nlm.nih.gov/medlineplus/weightcontrol.html.

National Institute of Mental Health: *Eating disorders.* This site provides various publications that include information about eating disorders and how to deal with this problem: http://www.nimh.nih.gov/health/publications/eating-disorders/complete-index.shtml. (Materials available in English and Spanish.)

U.S. Department of Health and Human Services, Centers for Disease Control and Prevention: *Physical activity for everyone.* This site offers physical activity programs and information for all age-groups, as well as resources for health professionals: http://www.cdc.gov/nccdphp/dnpa/physical/index.htm.

U.S. Department of Health and Human Services, U.S. Department of Agriculture: *Dietary Guidelines for Americans 2005.* The Dietary Guidelines for Americans 2005 provides information and nutrition education materials to assist with weight management: http://www.health.gov/dietaryguidelines/.

U.S. Department of Health and Human Services: *SmallStep–Adult/Teen and SmallStep–Kids.* This site offers tips on making small changes in food choices, food portions, and leisure activities that can make a difference in your body weight: http://www.smallstep.gov/(adult/teen); http://www.smallstep.gov/kids/flash/index.html (kids). (Interactive activities and printed materials are available in English and Spanish.)

Community Nutrition and the Life Cycle

9

The Food Environment and Food Safety

Eleanor D. Schlenker

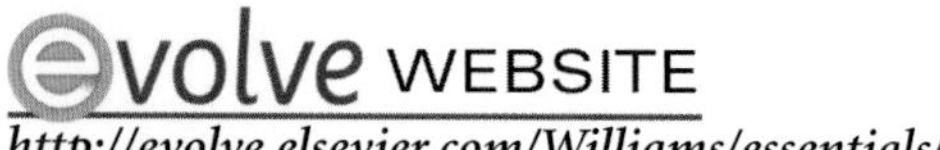

http://evolve.elsevier.com/Williams/essentials/

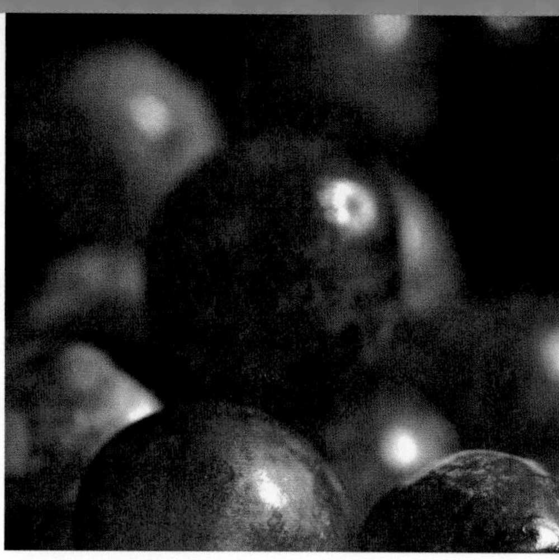

CHAPTER OUTLINE

Here we begin a two-chapter section in which we apply the principles of nutrition science to the food needs of individuals and families. Respect and concern for individual differences are as important as practical skills for applying knowledge in a useful and helpful way.

We look first at our changing food environment and the web of factors that influence personal food choices and food safety. Issues such as health and convenience have joined taste and cost as concerns of consumers in the marketplace. Although the expansion of our food supply offers a wide assortment from which to choose, this expansion has also brought the need for increased regulation of the food entering our homes. In the past, families produced most of their own food and were responsible for its wholesomeness and safety. As our sphere of food access has broadened to include our region, our country, and the world, food safety has become a responsibility of government and various enforcement agencies.

PERSONAL FOOD SELECTION

Personal food patterns, like other human behaviors, do not develop in a vacuum. Instead they grow out of our cultural, social, and psychologic environment, as well as from the unique experiences that follow each of us throughout our lives.

Cultural Influences

Cultural Identity

Culture is broadly defined as the values, beliefs, attitudes, and practices accepted by members of a group or community.[1] Often the most significant thing about a culture is what is taken for granted. Culture involves not only the obvious aspects of life—language, religion, family structure, and historical heritage—but also patterns of everyday living such as preparing and serving food and caring for children or elders. These facets of daily life are passed from generation to generation and learned as a child grows up within the community.

Food in a Culture

Foodways (food customs or traditions) are among the oldest and most deeply rooted aspects of a culture. They determine what is eaten, when and how it is eaten, and who prepares it.[1] Something considered a special treat by families in one part of the world might be an unacceptable food in another location. The geography of the land, the agriculture practiced in that locality, experiences related to health and food safety, and local history and traditions influence food choices. Within every culture certain foods are deeply infused with symbolic meaning. From early times designated foods or meals have commemorated special events of religious significance or national heritage or rites of passage. Many of these customs remain today.[2] (To learn more about food customs and culture see the *Focus on Culture* box, "Family Meals: Where Food and Culture Meet.")

FOCUS ON CULTURE

Family Meals: Where Food and Culture Meet

Over the centuries the family meal has provided a daily opportunity for children to learn about their culture. Common vocabulary, food-related customs, etiquette, food-related holidays, and intergenerational and gender relationships are learned at the family table. In most cultures, celebrations such as weddings, birthdays, religious holidays, or secular holidays involve meals more elaborate in preparation and variety than day-to-day fare; often, particular food items are served. Although Thanksgiving and Christmas mark traditional holiday meals among many cultural groups in the United States, New Year is celebrated with feasting in China. In agrarian societies, harvest dinners marked the end of the growing season and the securing of food crops for the coming winter. Sunday dinner has long been a special meal in the Appalachian culture and among African-American families, because this was the day of rest when families had time to be together.

Family meals have defined gender roles and relationships. In East Indian cultures, feeding the family is an important role of the woman of the house. Even if servants or others assist with preparation, the woman of the house delivers the food to the table. Who eats together at meal time establishes the framework of social equity among family members. In Native American, East Asian, and traditional Arab and African cultures, men and guests ate first, and then women and children ate. In comparison, African-American, Latino, and Asian families celebrated the extended family as an important social unit with grandparents, aunts, uncles, and cousins joining in communal meals. Sociologists suggest that the special cohesiveness observed among African-American families is an outgrowth of the extended family meal.

The blending of families and cultures in the United States has obscured some of these differences in traditional practice. Nevertheless, the research associating better outcomes among youth who eat regular meals with their families reinforces the importance of the learning and social interaction taking place in this environment.

BIBLIOGRAPHY

Barkoukis H: Importance of understanding food consumption patterns, *J Am Diet Assoc* 107:234, 2007.

Hooker RJ: *Food and drink in America: a history*, New York, 1981, Bobbs Merrill.

Kittler PG, Sucher KP: *Food and culture*, ed 4, Belmont, Calif, 2004, Wadsworth/Thomson.

Social Influences

Internal Factors

Food has social roles. Food is a symbol of acceptance, warmth, and friendliness. People are more likely to accept food from those they view as friends or supporters, and in many cultures the offering of food is an expected act of hospitality. Strong food patterns develop within the primary family unit, and food habits associated with family sentiments are held tenaciously throughout life (Figure 9-1). Long into adulthood, certain foods trigger a flood of childhood memories and are valued for reasons totally apart from their nutritional contribution. Nevertheless, income, local availability, and market conditions ultimately influence food choices. People eat foods that are readily available and that they have the money to buy.

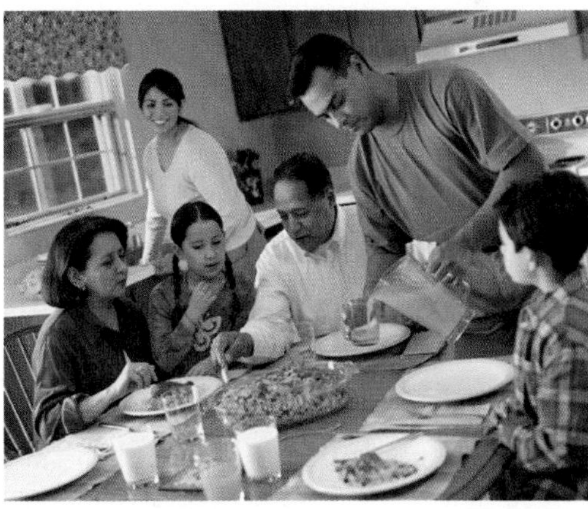

FIGURE 9-1 A family sharing food. Sharing food with visitors to your home is an established custom among many cultural and ethnic groups. (From Food and Nutrition Service, U.S. Department of Agriculture and Food and Nutrition Information Center, National Agricultural Library: Food stamp nutrition collection: photo gallery, Beltsville, Md, 2005, U.S. Department of Agriculture. Reprinted with permission. Retrieved March 20, 2009, from http://foodstamp.nal.usda.gov/foodstamp/photo_gallery.php?mode=mealtime.)

External Factors

Peer pressure influences food choices. Foods may be viewed as high-prestige foods or associated with low economic status. Those immigrating to the United States may reject their traditional foods in favor of American foods perceived to be popular among neighbors or classmates. Children plead for a particular snack item if that is what their friends eat.

Psychologic Influences

People who enjoy a bountiful food supply think less about food because it is always available,[3] whereas those with chronic hunger think, talk, and dream about food. For most of us, concern about food is associated with other needs. Maslow's classic hierarchy describes the five levels of human need, each building on the one before[4]:

1. *Basic physiologic needs:* hunger and thirst
2. *Need for safety:* physical comfort, security, and protection
3. *Need to belong:* love, giving and receiving affection
4. *Need for recognition:* self-esteem, sense of self-worth, self-confidence, and capability
5. *Need for self-actualization:* self-fulfillment and creative growth

Although these levels of need vary with time and circumstance, we can use them to help understand the needs of our

BOX 9-1 FACTORS INFLUENCING FOOD CHOICES

Environmental Factors
- Food availability
- Food technology
- Geography, agriculture, food distribution
- Personal economics, income
- Sanitation, housing
- Season, climate
- Storage and cooking facilities

Social Factors
- Advertising
- Culture
- Education, food and nutrition knowledge
- Political and economic policies
- Religion and social customs
- Social class role
- Social problems, poverty, alcoholism
- Distance from food outlets (e.g., restaurants, grocery stores)

Physiologic Factors
- Allergy, food tolerance
- Physical disability
- Health-disease status
- Personal food acceptance
- Energy or nutrient needs
- Medical nutrition therapy

clients and develop our care plan accordingly. As summarized in Box 9-1, a complex set of physical, social, and psychologic factors influence what a person eats.

TRENDS IN FOOD SELECTION

Defining a Food Pattern

All food patterns share several characteristics, although they differ in the actual foods they contain. When counseling individuals about their diet, this is one way to begin to look at their food and nutrient intake. These common dietary components are as follows[1]:

- *Core and complementary foods:* Core foods, usually complex carbohydrates, are eaten every day and provide the bulk of the energy intake. Complementary foods are those items added to improve palatability such as the vegetables or meat added to a rice meal.
- *Food flavors:* How foods are prepared and seasoned is distinctive for every group and as important as the foods themselves.
- *Meal patterns:* The number of meals or snacks eaten each day, when they are eaten, and the foods they contain, define dietary intake for individuals and cultures.

Maintaining core foods, familiar flavors, and meal sequence serves as a bridge to developing new patterns made necessary by health or other considerations.

Changing American Food Patterns

Family, ethnic, and regional patterns are strong influences in our lives, but new technology and mass media put old influences in conflict with new forces; this is true for food patterns. Traditional home cooking has given way to fast-food meals, and parents or grandparents who prided themselves on the recipes they prepared for their families are disheartened to learn that children like the "box" version better. The makeup of the typical American family is changing. Households have fewer children, and a single parent heads more families. Working parents are putting in more hours on the job and have less time for meal preparation, with the result that almost one half of the family food dollar (49%) is spent for food away from home.[5] With the busy lifestyles of parents and children, more meals are eaten on the run. One of every five restaurant meals is purchased from a car.[6] As the population ages,[7] the market for appropriate meals requiring little or no preparation will continue to expand.

BOX 9-2 CURRENT FOOD TRENDS

- Dining in—eating at home whether food is cooked at home or take-out
- The quick fix—foods easy to prepare (e.g., prewashed salad greens, frozen meal kits)
- Food talk—television food chefs and emerging cuisines
- Doing without—avoiding undesirable ingredients (e.g., trans fat, added sugar)
- Kidding around—organic baby food, refrigerated lunch kits
- Local motion—foods that are fresh, seasonal, homemade, organic
- Snacking and sharing—small packaged items and mini-meals to hold one over until mealtime

Data from Sloan AE: Top 10 food trends, *Food Technol* 61:23, 2007.

Convenience Meals

According to a food industry survey, a growing trend is "dining in" (Box 9-2), with 77% of American families eating dinner at home at least five times per week.[8] However, only 32% of dinners at home are made from scratch.[6] Consumers want foods that can be heated quickly and served in minutes after they arrive home, so frozen entrees, prepared foods from the supermarket, or fast foods are popular. Meal kits and soup and stew starters are receiving growing attention, but shoppers lament the poor selection of healthy prepared foods and frozen entrees. Frozen items are seldom available in family-sized portions, and healthy choices often cost more.[8] Many fast-food and frozen entrees are high in total fat, saturated fat, and sodium, and they are low in calcium and important vitamins. (Review Box 7-4 to compare the sodium content of processed foods and their fresh counterparts.) (See the *Perspectives in Practice* box, "Returning to Hands-On Food" for ideas on how to get started in preparing healthy meals.)

A reasonable compromise for a busy student or parent might be a combination of convenience items and fresh items that are quickly prepared. A rotisserie chicken from the supermarket or chicken from a fast-food restaurant could be combined with a frozen vegetable and a salad or fruit in place of French fries. Packaged salad greens can be washed and

PERSPECTIVES IN PRACTICE

Returning to Hands-On Food

As the pace of life quickens with the added responsibilities of work, school, and child care, preparing meals at home can appear to be a daunting task. Although a group of young adults indicated they enjoyed eating with others and thought the social aspect of meals was important, 35% of the men and 42% of the women interviewed said they lacked time to sit down and eat a meal.[1] Eating on the run led to increased intakes of soft drinks, fast-food, and saturated fat, as well as lower intakes of fruit and dark-green and orange vegetables. Not only lack of time but also poor food preparation skills adversely affect diet quality. Those who prepared a meal at home at least weekly ate more whole grains, fruits, and vegetables, and they had increased intakes of calcium.[2]

Following are ways we can develop skills for preparing meals at home:

- *Purchase a family cookbook to help you get started:* The American Dietetic Association, American Heart Association, and American Diabetes Association offer cookbooks with quick and easy recipes that can be prepared in 30 minutes and support healthy eating for all age-groups.
- *Supplement take-out foods with healthy dishes prepared at home:* Add a frozen vegetable or salad and oven-browned French fries (made with frozen potato strips) to the chicken or hamburgers purchased on the way home.
- *Try to make foods in advance to keep in your freezer for quick meals:* Instead of making a meat loaf in a loaf pan, make individual meat loaves in a muffin pan. The muffin meat loaves cook in half the time of a regular meat loaf, and leftovers can be frozen individually to thaw and heat as needed.
- *Remember that cut-up chicken cooks quickly on top of the stove or in the oven:* Look for recipes that use canned low-sodium chicken broth or low-sodium soups as ready-made sauces.
- *Look for skillet meals or casseroles that mix a protein food with pasta or vegetables:* Consider dishes such as skillet lasagna, tuna noodle casserole, macaroni and cheese, chicken and broccoli stir-fry; one-pot cooking also makes for quick cleanup.
- *Get familiar with legumes:* Lentils and dried green peas can be added directly to a recipe without soaking; make a pot of lentil soup in the evening or on a weekend afternoon to take care of dinner on a weeknight.
- *When purchasing frozen entrees, look for those lower in sodium and check the price per ounce:* For a quick dinner, supplement this purchase with a fresh or frozen vegetable or salad.
- *Get friendly with vegetables:* When fresh vegetables are out of season and costly, or when time is short, frozen vegetables that are partially processed are a good option for adding color, texture, and nutrients to your meal.

If you have not been cooking, then start by preparing just one or two meals a week. See how fast you develop both your cooking skills and some favorite recipes!

REFERENCES

1. Larson NI, Nelson MC, Neumark-Sztainer D, et al: Making time for meals: meal structure and associations with dietary intake in young adults, *J Am Diet Assoc* 109:72, 2009.
2. Larson NI, Perry CL, Story M, et al: Food preparation by young adults is associated with better diet quality, *J Am Diet Assoc* 106:2001, 2006.

served, or a frozen vegetable can be cooked in the microwave in the time it takes to set the table and get the family seated. Helping people identify nutrient-rich accompaniments to convenience items can improve the nutrition of the entire family.

Grazers

Eating frequency influences energy intake. Thirty percent of adults eat six or more times a day and consume on average about 150 kcal more than those who eat only five times and 250 kcal more than those who eat only four times.[9] Several small meals and snacks (a grazing pattern) rather than one or two very large meals represent a healthy eating pattern if the energy and nutrient content of the foods spread across the day is monitored wisely. Individuals who are physically active can benefit from eating more frequently. Older adults who had two or more snacks each day in addition to their regular meals were more likely to reach their kilocalorie (kcalorie or kcal) requirement than those who did not snack.[10] Snacking on fruits, vegetables, low-fat dairy foods, low-fat grain products, or protein foods such as peanut butter or hard cooked eggs add important nutrients with low to moderate kcalories. On the other hand, chips, baked items, and beverages high in sugar or fat escalate energy intake.

Family Meals

As families become involved in more activities outside the home, family meals with parents and children become more difficult to manage. Still, about two thirds of adolescents have dinner with their families at least three to four times each week.[11] Eating together as a family influences nutritional and emotional well-being. The more meals children eat with their parents, the greater their intakes of calcium-rich foods, fruits, and vegetables.[11] Moreover, youth who have dinner regularly with their families have an increased degree of "family connectedness," do better in school, and are less likely to use tobacco, alcohol, and drugs.[12] Meals at home also build habits that carry over into succeeding years. Young adults who ate breakfast regularly as adolescents were more likely to have breakfast as a regular meal in the years following.[13] Having a parent home in the morning increases the probability that adolescents will eat breakfast.[14] Men appear to be assuming more responsibility for meal planning and preparation,[15] providing important role models for children and youth.

Health Concerns

Americans are demonstrating greater concern about health in their shopping habits. In a survey of food shoppers, 57% indicated they were "making a lot of effort" to eat better, and

36% were trying to reduce their risk of developing a chronic health condition by choosing better foods.[16] Although taste and price still hold prominence in how Americans select their food, concern for body weight is a driving force for making dietary changes.[17] Those trying to lose weight were more likely to be reducing their portion sizes and eating fewer kcalories and less fat than following a specific diet.

Changes in food arising from new technology are receiving more attention. Mothers have reported turning to organic foods to lower their children's intakes of antibiotics, pesticides, and genetically modified (GM) foods.[6] Older adults are trying to avoid saturated fat, trans fat, and cholesterol.[6] More than 40% of shoppers in a national survey were using the nutrition label to evaluate sodium, fiber, and sugar content. Others were seeking out foods fortified with vitamins, calcium, fiber, antioxidants, and omega-3 fatty acids.[16] Healthier choices are also getting attention when dining out: main-dish salads, bottled water, milk, fruit, and diet soft drinks are among the 10 fastest-growing restaurant choices.

Although surveys indicate increasing interest in health, consumer knowledge about food is often limited. Americans know that different fats have different effects on health, yet few can name the healthy fats (e.g., monounsaturated and polyunsaturated fatty acids).[17] Shoppers who indicated an interest in lowering their fat intake were continuing to purchase high-fat foods.[18] It is often difficult to put knowledge into practice. Although 92% of a consumer group noted that breakfast is the most important meal of the day, less than half ate breakfast regularly.[17]

Ethnic and Specialty Dining

Ethnic dishes are growing in popularity, spurred by the wide variety of new cookbooks, television cooking shows, and celebrity chefs that are helping consumers learn more about international foods. Magazines are featuring recipes for traditional foods, and the growing international population in the United States has increased the availability of less common ingredients. Large supermarket sections are devoted to Asian vegetables and fruits and spices and condiments necessary for Mexican and other Latino dishes. This practice of preparing more exotic meals from fresh ingredients continues to grow, along with the general trend toward meals easy to prepare in little time.[19]

THE PROBLEM OF FOOD MISINFORMATION

Concerns for a safe and wholesome food supply have existed across the centuries. Many cultures held beliefs about the healing properties or dangers of particular foods, and certain religious food laws may reflect food safety issues. Some unsubstantiated beliefs about food or certain components of food are harmless, but others carry serious implications for health. Megadoses of vitamins or herbs that interact with a prescription drug carry financial and health costs. False information may be rooted in folklore, be built on half-truths, or stem from intentional deception and fraud.

Types of False Food Claims

Exaggerated food claims include the following:

1. Certain foods will cure specific diseases or conditions.
2. Certain food combinations have special therapeutic effects.
3. Only "natural" foods can meet body needs and prevent disease.

Why should we be concerned about food misinformation? Several reasons are outlined:

- *Danger to health:* Self-diagnosis and treatment can delay appropriate medical intervention. Patients with difficult-to-treat conditions such as cancer, diabetes, or arthritis are especially vulnerable to fraudulent claims.
- *Money spent needlessly:* As much as $18.8 billion per year is spent on dietary supplements,[20] and many are unnecessary or ineffective. If a family is low on cash, then money spent on supplements may be taken from their food budget.
- *Distrust of the food supply:* Changes in our food environment including use of chemical pesticides and newer methods of food processing have led some people to harbor suspicions about agricultural and food producers and their effects on food safety. We will discuss some of these issues later in this chapter.

Groups Vulnerable to Food Misinformation

Certain groups with particular needs and concerns are often the target for products making false claims:

- *Older adults:* Progressive physical changes and chronic disease make older individuals vulnerable to supplements promising to restore youthful vigor. Older adults with pain and disability are easy prey for exaggerated health claims and cures.
- *Teenagers:* Figure-conscious adolescent girls and muscle-minded adolescent boys often respond to crash programs in hopes of attaining the perfect body and peer acceptance.
- *Obese individuals:* Those who are desperate to lose large amounts of weight may respond to the barrage of advertisements advocating diets, pills, various devices, and special foods.
- *Athletes:* Always looking for something to give them the competitive edge, athletes can be lured by nutrition myths and false promises.

Although certain groups are especially vulnerable, no segment of the population is completely free of the appeal of unscrupulous marketers of worthless or harmful products.

Combating Food Misinformation

How do we respond to erroneous beliefs built on food misinformation or deception? Several approaches have merit, as follows:

- *Educate consumers:* Help consumers learn to evaluate advertisements about diets, food products, or dietary supplements. The U.S. Department of Health and Human Services has developed a checklist for spotting health scams and separating legitimate products and health advice from those that are harmful and waste money (Box 9-3).
- *Stay current:* Be well informed about new products—know both their content and reputed effects on the body. Search out studies by universities or government agencies that

BOX 9-3 CHECKLIST FOR SPOTTING A HEALTH SCAM

- Promises a quick or painless cure
- Claims to be made from a special, secret, or ancient formula available from only one source
- Uses testimonials or undocumented case histories from satisfied patients
- Claims to be effective for a wide range of ailments
- Claims to cure a disease such as arthritis or cancer or diabetes that is not fully understood by physicians and medical scientists
- Requires advance payment and claims limited availability of the product

Modified from National Institute on Aging, U.S. Department of Health and Human Services: Age page: *Beware of health scams*, Washington, DC, 2008, U.S. Department of Health and Human Services. Retrieved March 20, 2009, from www.nia.nih.gov/HealthInformation/Publications/quackery.htm.

evaluated advertising claims and product safety. Review publications and websites of responsible government, professional, and private organizations such as the American Dietetic Association, the American Medical Association, the U.S. Food and Drug Administration (FDA), and the International Food Information Council Foundation.

- *Think scientifically:* Use the problem-solving approach when working with children and adults. In everyday situations, look for research data to support your position and be able to answer the questions, "How do you know?" and "What is the evidence?" (Review the *Evidence-Based Practice* box in Chapter 1 for guidelines on evaluating product and practice claims.)

BIOTECHNOLOGY AND FOOD: PROMISE AND CONTROVERSY

Throughout human history, new scientific discoveries have created challenges for society. Biotechnology as related to agriculture, food processing, and protection of the environment has the potential to increase the quantity and quality of our food supply. This field of science allows us to alter the deoxyribonucleic acid (DNA) of a plant or animal species by adding or removing a particular gene, likened to cutting a circle of tape, inserting a different piece, and rejoining both ends to the new piece.[21] This was the technique used to develop a variety of rice with increased content of β-carotene. At the same time, applications of these methods to develop new plant species or enhance animal production raise questions regarding consumer safety. We examine some of these issues and the process for biosafety review in the following sections.

Bovine Growth Hormone

Growth hormone secreted by the pituitary gland has an essential role in growth, development, and health. Bovine growth hormone (BGH) extracted from the pituitary glands of cattle has long been used to boost milk production. When it became possible to synthesize bovine somatotropin (bST) using recombinant DNA methods, farmers petitioned the FDA for permission to use recombinant bovine somatotropin (rbST) in their dairy herds.[22] After intense review this use was approved. Evaluation of milk samples from retail stores in 48 states indicated that milk from rbST-treated cows does not differ in bST content from milk obtained from nontreated cows.[23] Nevertheless, this practice remains controversial.

Genetically Modified Plants

GM organisms are plants or bacteria in which the natural DNA has been changed in some way to produce a desired trait. Genetic modification can take place through plant breeding methods or through biotechnology in which a gene is transferred from one organism to another.[24] Genetic engineering was first applied in the pharmaceutical industry, and GM bacteria produce human insulin for managing diabetes.

GM food crops were introduced in the 1990s, and their use has grown dramatically. Farmers in 23 countries are planting GM species, representing 51% of the soybeans, 31% of the maize, and 5% of the rapeseed (canola oil) produced worldwide.[25] In the United States the sale and use of GM seeds are regulated by the FDA, the U.S. Environmental Protection Agency (EPA), and the U.S. Department of Agriculture (USDA).[26]

Goals for Genetic Modification

Since humans first began to cultivate plants, various practices have been used to improve the yield or desirability of particular species. Use of Mendel's principles of inheritance and the development of hybrid plants led to the green revolution and new varieties of wheat and rice with double the yields. Such advances were credited with reducing food shortages in the developing world.[27] Genetic modification of food plants has centered on the following three goals[21,27]:

1. *Resistance to disease and insects:* Plants that carry a protein acting as a built-in insecticide enable farmers to reduce their use of pesticides and herbicides.
2. *Increased tolerance to weather conditions:* Varieties able to survive more extreme environmental conditions are less likely to be destroyed by a late frost.
3. *Increased nutritional value:* Genetic modification increased the monounsaturated fatty acid content of soybean oil and scientists are working on a tomato with increased amounts of lycopene. Grains with increased protein or micronutrients will lessen the nutrient deficiencies in developing countries.

Corn, soybeans, canola (rapeseed), potatoes, and tomatoes are among the 12 genetically altered food crops approved for sale in the United States.[24]

Safety of Genetically Modified Crops

The sale and use of GM plants remain controversial. Scientists and consumer groups have voiced several concerns:

- *Risk of allergic reaction:* Transferring a known allergen into a new food (e.g., adding a peanut allergen to a corn plant) would make the modified plant unsafe for persons with the allergy.[28]
- *Potential toxicity:* All GM foods undergo toxicity testing with DNA checked against a protein database to identify any known harmful protein.[29]

- *Danger to the environment:* Plants with genes that resist insects may pass those genes along to weeds or invasive plants or may be harmful to helpful insects such as butterflies.[30] Farmers are urged to confine these plants to specific growing areas.

Current food labels are not required to identify food ingredients from GM sources *unless* the modification has increased the allergenicity or reduced the nutrient content.[24]

Biotechnology and Animal Foods

Conventional breeding methods have produced eggs with less cholesterol and beef with reduced fat. Marker-assisted breeding, combining the skills of classic breeders and molecular geneticists, offers increased potential for the development of healthy animal foods. When geneticists identify existing DNA patterns that influence traits such as fat composition, breeders can better select for these characteristics.

When assessing risk the answers are seldom clear-cut; no action by either a government agency or an individual is ever completely risk free.[31] Risk is evaluated according to potential benefits versus potential harm and usually involves numerous and often subtle variables. Available research evidence should form the basis for judgments that serve the public interest.

ENSURING A SAFE AND WHOLESOME FOOD SUPPLY

Food sources have changed dramatically over the years. No longer do families produce their own food or purchase food from their neighbors. Food from all over the world is available at local markets, and produce picked on one continent can be served at the dinner table on another continent the same day. Farmers and food processors have at their disposal a wide variety of technologies to expand and preserve our food supply and create new products in response to consumer demand. This flow of food across the nation and the world has implications for food safety and the need to monitor the overall food environment.

Government Agencies Responsible for Food Safety

A Shared Regulatory System: USDA and FDA

Regulation of the food supply began more than 100 years ago when Congress charged the USDA with ensuring the safety of the nation's food. Early on, the USDA initiated the on-site inspection of meatpacking and poultry-processing plants, an enormous job that is still continuing. Since then the FDA has been assigned responsibility for the safety of all foods except meat and poultry. These two agencies work with the EPA to ensure that pesticide residues do not exceed tolerance standards. Interagency cooperation is essential for mounting an effective response to any food-related threat to health. The USDA, FDA, and Centers for Disease Control and Prevention (CDC) work together to prevent the introduction and spread of such hazards as avian flu or to investigate and recall products associated with outbreaks of foodborne illness.

BOX 9-4 FOOD-RELATED ACTIVITIES OF THE U.S. FOOD AND DRUG ADMINISTRATION

- Ensure that processed foods are free of pathogens and contaminants
- Inspect food-processing facilities (other than meat and poultry plants)
- Approve food additives
- Monitor the content of infant formulas and medical foods
- Oversee nutrition labeling
- Check shipments of imported foods for purity
- Approve drugs and supplements added to animal feeds

Food and Drug Administration

The FDA enforces all federal regulations intended to keep our food supply safe, pure, and wholesome (Box 9-4).[32] Included in this mandate is the power to seize contaminated and unsafe food, whether grown and processed in the United States or entering from elsewhere. Because it is impossible to inspect all food products before they are sold, the FDA has put in place surveillance and risk assessment procedures in food manufacturing facilities to prevent food contamination. These procedures, referred to as *Hazard Analysis and Critical Control Points* (HACCP), identify potential sources of contamination and help plant managers set up ways to control them during production. HACCP also requires systematic testing for the presence of dangerous microbes at production points where they might enter the system. The joint efforts of the FDA and USDA to implement HACCP procedures in poultry processing are credited with reducing by 50% the number of chickens contaminated with *Salmonella.* A new responsibility of FDA is to effectively monitor the threat of food bioterrorism. (See the *Perspectives on Practice* box, "The Threat of Bioterrorism to the Food Supply: Risk Assessment and Response.")

The FDA Division of Consumer Education conducts an active program of public education through its website, electronic newsletters, and publications. Combating food and nutrition misinformation and encouraging safe food storage and preparation practices at home and in food service facilities receive special attention.

Food Safety Laws

Approval Process for Drugs

The FDA control of drugs began in 1938 with the passage of the Federal Food, Drug, and Cosmetic Act (FFDCA). When being developed, a new drug must undergo intensive testing, often extending over a period of years. The manufacturer must present convincing scientific evidence that the product meets the legal standard of "safe and effective," and formal approval is necessary before the drug can be sold.

Regulation of Food Ingredients and Food Additives

Manufacturers of all foods and food additives are legally obligated to assure the public that their products are safe. For conventional foods the FFDCA requires that the food and all ingredients not be "ordinarily injurious." Safety is assumed

PERSPECTIVES IN PRACTICE

The Threat of Bioterrorism to the Food Supply: Risk Assessment and Response

Meredith Catherine Williams

Food poisoning and foodborne illness are natural dangers that public health agencies combat continuously; however, contamination of food is usually accidental through carelessness or infection from an animal source. In recent years the threat of bioterrorism—attacks against people or agriculture using deadly biologic organisms—has become a concern for government agencies charged with food safety.

Farms and ranches are vulnerable to bioterrorism for a number of reasons:

- Many animal and crop pathogens are relatively easy to obtain and do not require sophisticated equipment or expertise for use.
- Very small amounts of a pathogen are needed to start a contamination.
- Growing crops are openly exposed, and poultry and livestock are often concentrated in large numbers on farms and feedlots.
- Animals and animal foods are shipped across wide areas in short periods of time, increasing the potential for spreading a communicable disease quickly.

The Centers for Disease Control and Prevention (CDC) have assessed the vulnerability of the U.S. food supply according to the availability of disease agents and how medically dangerous they are. Biologic agents fall into the following three categories of danger:

1. *Category A:* Includes such pathogens as *Clostridium botulinum* (botulism), neurotoxins, and anthrax that carry a high degree of morbidity and mortality and are easily spread.
2. *Category B: Salmonella, Shigella,* and *Escherichia coli* O157:H7 are easily disseminated but have significantly lower morbidity and mortality rates.
3. *Category C:* Weaker agents such as hepatitis A and *Cryptosporidium* paramecium are included in this category. Many are available in the wild or easily purchased under the guise of legitimate research.

Another component of vulnerability is the increasing centralization of food production, packaging, and distribution. The extent of damage from a bioterrorist attack would depend on the point of contamination in the supply chain and how quickly it could be contained. Increasing amounts of food entering from other countries expands the opportunities for external tampering.

Until now, detection methods for monitoring food safety were designed to protect against negligence, poor handling, and spoilage, not against direct and intentional contamination. Increased surveillance and coordination is the key to providing national and local officials with the information needed to respond quickly to contain any infection that should arise.

Food contamination incidents have shown that a deliberate attack on the food supply could lead to significant illness and death, with implications for agriculture, health care, and the economy. Tighter security in all stages of food production and distribution, improved screening and detection procedures, and increased coordination among all levels of government help to mitigate the risks of bioterrorism. Consumers also have an important role in observation and reporting of suspicious products and packaging. Although accidental and naturally occurring food-related illnesses will still take place, the chances of a successful intentional event have been greatly reduced.

BIBLIOGRAPHY

Bruemmer B: Food biosecurity, *J Am Diet Assoc* 103(6):687, 2003.

Center for Food Safety and Applied Nutrition, U.S. Food and Drug Administration: *Risk assessment for food terrorism and other food safety concerns,* Rockville, Md, 2003, U.S. Food and Drug Administration. Retrieved March 20, 2009, from www.fda.gov/OHRMS/DOCKETS/98fr/03-25850.htm.

Center for Infectious Disease Research and Policy, University of Minnesota: *Agricultural biosecurity,* Minneapolis, 2005, Regents of the University of Minnesota. Retrieved March 20, 2009, from www.cidrap.umn.edu/cidrap/content/biosecurity/ag-biosec/index.html.

Peregrin T: Bioterrorism and food safety: what nutrition professionals need to know to educate the American public, *J Am Diet Assoc* 102(1):614, 2002.

Sobel J, Khan AS, Swerdlow DL: Threat of biological terrorist attack on the U.S. food supply: the CDC perspective, *Lancet* 359:874, 2002.

U.S. Food and Drug Administration: *Consumer update: CARVER + shock: enhancing food defense,* Washington, DC, 2007, U.S. Food and Drug Administration. Retrieved August 12, 2009, from www.fda.gov/ForConsumers/ConsumerUpdates/ucm094560.htm.

for ingredients with a long history of use, and such food items may be marketed without prior FDA approval. Cookies with the ingredients of flour, brown sugar, eggs, butter, and baking soda would meet this standard.

In 1960 the FFDCA was expanded to create two legal classes of food additives:

1. *Generally recognized as safe (GRAS):* The GRAS list included all food additives and ingredients that had been marketed before 1958. Thousands of additives are on the GRAS list. One example is the yellow coloring added to margarine that has been in use since the 1930s. Under the law a food is unsafe if an additive "may render injurious" the food product. Food processors are not required to obtain FDA approval to use GRAS list additives. The presumed safety of these additives was based on their wide prior use—most have not been tested. In 1977, Congress directed the FDA to begin testing the additives on the list, and this testing is continuing.
2. *Food additives developed since 1958:* For additives in this category, the same legal standard of "may render injurious" applies, but these newer additives must undergo rigid testing and approval must be obtained before any food containing the additive may be sold. Stevia, a nonnutritive sweetener, is an example of a new additive that received FDA approval after testing.

Dietary Supplements

Dietary supplements enjoy a very favorable legal status. In 1994, Congress passed the Dietary Supplement Health and Education Act (DSHEA), which effectively deregulated the dietary supplement industry.[33] All ingredients marketed as supplements before 1994 were assumed to be safe, whether or not research evidence existed to support this claim. The dietary supplement industry markets thousands of products containing vitamins, minerals, herbs, botanical compounds, Asian medicinal herbals, and related substances. Under the law these supplements are not classified as *foods* or *drugs*. No scientific testing to demonstrate either product safety or effectiveness is required. For supplement ingredients developed after 1994, the safety standard is simply that there be no "unreasonable risk." The manufacturer must notify the FDA before marketing a product, but no prior approval is required.

The DSHEA is a controversial law. Dietary supplements are a major industry, with large advertising budgets and a wide range of products, from single vitamins to complex mixtures. Although a dietary supplement cannot claim to cure a disease, statements about how the human body will respond to the supplement, such as a claim that it will make you burn away unwanted fat, are completely unregulated and require no proof. Supplements containing growth hormone or other potentially dangerous substances said to restore youthful vitality are often marketed to older adults. Steps to ensure consumer safety along with honest claims describing appropriate use, expected effects, recommended dose, and potential drug-herb-nutrient interactions are urgently needed.

Agricultural Chemicals

American farmers have come to depend on agricultural chemicals to increase crop production. Such chemicals control destructive insects and weeds, improve seed sprouting to increase yield, prevent plant diseases, and improve market quality. However, overuse increases food pesticide residues and adds to farm workers' exposure to powerful chemicals. Universities are helping farmers reduce their use of chemical pesticides through integrated pest management, which uses the natural enemies of insect pests to decrease their population. The FDA has the difficult task of assessing health risks and establishing guidelines for the thousands of agricultural chemicals in use and development.

Organic farming—which excludes the use of chemical pesticides and herbicides—is growing in status among consumers. Retail sales of organic foods now total over $17 billion.[34] Organic farmers working with soil scientists are developing systems of sustainable agriculture for growing plant foods and raising beef and poultry. National standards have been established for producers who wish to label their food as "organic." These standards govern growing procedures and postharvest handling; the USDA must certify farmers before they can use the seal of the National Organic Program (Figure 9-2).[35]

Water Contamination

Dumping of waste has raised the concentrations of polychlorinated biphenyls (PCBs) and heavy metals such as mercury in inland and ocean waters. These pollutants are transferred to fish, shellfish, or other wildlife living in or drinking these waters, as well as to the humans who eat them. State and local health departments post advisories to fishermen regarding the safety of fish in local waters, and the FDA monitors the

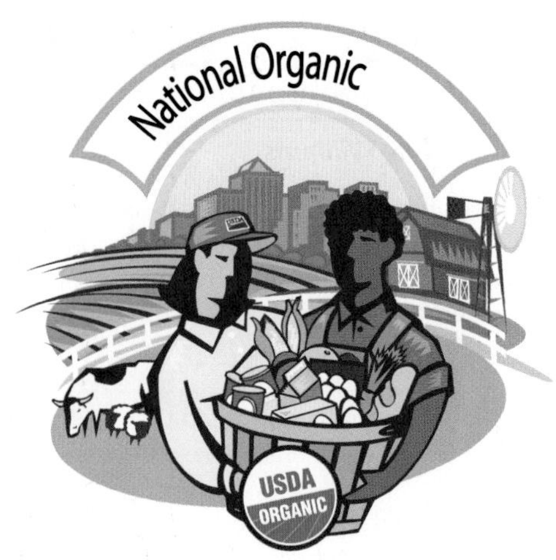

FIGURE 9-2 Seal of the National Organic Program. The U.S. Department of Agriculture (USDA) has developed a certification program to help organic farmers label their produce as *organically grown*. (From National Organic Program, Agricultural Marketing Service, U.S. Department of Agriculture: *The organic seal,* Washington, DC, 2002, U.S. Department of Agriculture. Available at www.ams.usda.gov/AMSv1.0/nop.)

BOX 9-5 MERCURY CONTENT OF FISH

Fish Lower in Mercury	Fish Higher in Mercury
• Canned light tuna*	• Shark
• Pollock	• Swordfish
• Salmon	• King mackerel
• Catfish	• Tilefish
• Shrimp	

Note: Women who are pregnant or nursing or might become pregnant should eat no more than two meals or 12 oz a week of low-mercury fish; these recommendations also apply to young children (but serve smaller portions). Fish sticks and fish sandwiches served at fast-food restaurants are generally made from fish low in mercury. Data from U.S. Department of Health and Human Services and U.S. Environmental Protection Agency: *What you need to know about mercury in fish and shellfish,* Washington, DC, 2004, U.S. Department of Health and Human Services. Retrieved March 3, 2009, from www.cfsan.fda.gov/~dms/admehg3.html.
*Albacore or white tuna is higher in mercury than light tuna.

mercury content of ocean and farm-raised fish sold in the United States. Although fish is valued for the protein and n-3 fatty acids it provides, women who are pregnant or nursing or may become pregnant should limit their intake and choose fish low in mercury to prevent harm to their unborn child or infant (Box 9-5).[36] This FDA advisory also applies to young children based on the damaging effect of mercury on the developing nervous system.

Food Labels

If people are to choose their food wisely, then they must know what nutrients they need, the amounts they need, and where to find these nutrients among the foods in the marketplace. During the past 30 years the FDA, with the advice of experts representing agriculture, foods, nutrition, and health, developed a framework of food labeling to help consumers monitor their nutrient intake.

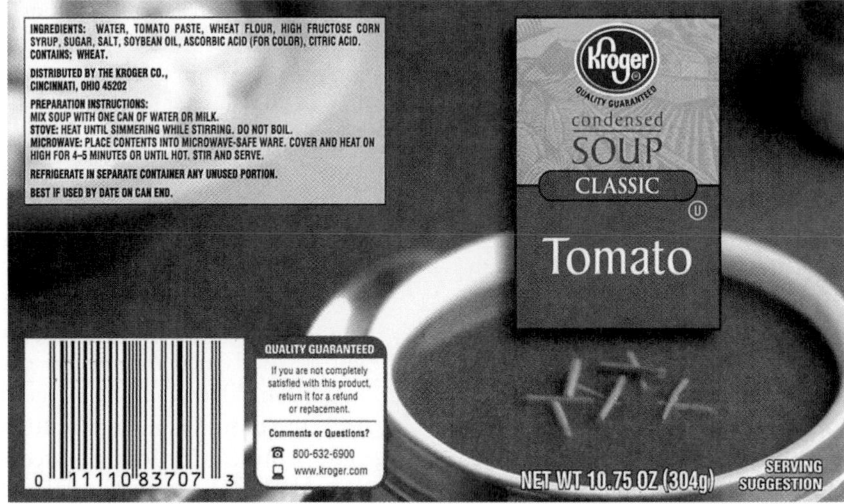

FIGURE 9-3 Example of a food label. Notice that this label also informs the consumer that the product contains wheat—one of eight food allergens that must be clearly stated on the food label to protect individuals having this allergy. (Courtesy The Kroger Company, Cincinnati, Ohio.)

Early Efforts at Food Labeling

In the middle 1970s, new requirements were set for the food label. All cans and packages had to provide content information including weight, list of ingredients, and name and address of the manufacturer (Figure 9-3). The goal at that time was to protect consumers from *economic* risk—providing true information about food weight and ingredients—not *health* risk. However, surveys indicated that consumers wanted more nutrition information, including amounts of carbohydrate, fat, and protein, total number of kcalories, and key vitamins and minerals.

Current Food Labeling Regulations

The current nutrition label became law under the Nutrition Labeling and Education Act of 1990 and has been in use since 1994 (Figure 9-4). This label is required on all prepared or processed food such as breads, cereals, canned and frozen foods, snacks, desserts, and beverages, but it is voluntary for fresh fruits, vegetables, and seafood.[37] The nutrition label describes the serving size and nutrient content as compared with recommended intakes of those nutrients. Health claims on the food label (approved by the FDA) help consumers make choices to prevent chronic disease. The USDA sets standards and controls labeling on fresh meat, poultry, and dairy products.

Nutrition Facts

Serving Size: 1/2 cup (114 g)
Servings Per Container: 4

Amount per Serving	
Calories 260	
Calories from Fat 120	
	% Daily Value*
Total Fat 13 g	20%
Saturated Fat 5 g	25%
Trans Fat 0 g	
Cholesterol 30 mg	10%
Sodium 660 mg	28%
Total Carbohydrate 31 g	11%
Dietary Fiber 0 g	0%
Sugars 5 g	
Protein 5 g	

Vitamin A 4% • Vitamin C 1%
Calcium 15% • Iron 4%

*Percents (%) of a Daily Value are based on a 2,000 calorie diet. Your Daily Values may vary higher or lower depending on your calorie needs.

Nutrient	2,000 calories	2,500 calories
Total Fat	<65 g	<80 g
Saturated Fat	<20 g	<25 g
Cholesterol	<300 mg	<300 mg
Sodium	<2,400 mg	<2,400 mg
Total Carbohydrate	300 g	375 g
Dietary Fiber	25 g	30 g

1 g Fat = 9 calories
1 g Carbohydrate = 4 calories
1 g Protein = 4 calories

FIGURE 9-4 A nutrition label. The nutrition label helps consumers evaluate the nutrient content of processed foods. (From U.S. Food and Drug Administration [FDA], Rockville, Md.)

HEALTH PROMOTION

Using the Nutrition Label

The nutrition label enables consumers to compare the nutritional value of one product with another and make informed choices about the foods they eat.[38] The major parts of the nutrition label are as follows:

- *Food amount and energy content:* Food amount is described by weight, serving size, and number of servings in the package or container. Unfortunately, the general public does not equate standard serving sizes with the amount of food they are accustomed to seeing on their plate. A food package perceived to contain two to three 1-cup portions may be labeled to contain five to six one half–cup portions, so the energy content of the portion actually consumed can be twice what was expected. Serving sizes are often presented in a way that makes the food item appear lower in kcalories. For example, a super-sized muffin that consumers might expect to represent an individual portion may be labeled as containing two servings at half the kcalories.

- *Macronutrient content:* Protein, carbohydrate, and fat are listed in grams. Individual amounts of saturated fat, trans fat, and cholesterol are required, and some processors voluntarily add monounsaturated and polyunsaturated fats. Total carbohydrate is broken down into dietary fiber and sugar (sugar total includes both naturally occurring and added sugars). For most people, grams of fat, carbohydrate, protein, or fiber hold little meaning. To help consumers compare the per-serving content to current health recommendations, suggested daily intakes are related to reference diets of 2000 or 2500 kcal.
- *Vitamin and mineral content:* Sodium and four leader nutrients—vitamin A, vitamin C, calcium, and iron—are required on the nutrition label. Sodium is listed in milligrams and as a percentage of the Tolerable Upper Intake Level (UL) (2300 mg). Vitamins and minerals appear as percentages of the Daily Reference Value (DV). The DVs were derived from the Dietary Reference Intakes (DRI) for use on food labels and represent the highest DRI value for that nutrient among the various age and gender groups. For example, the DV for iron is 18 mg, the DRI for women of childbearing age. Fortified foods such as cereals also list the vitamins and minerals added in the manufacturing process.
- *Health claims:* Health claims are label statements that imply a relationship between the consumption of a nutrient or food substance and a disease or health-related condition.[39] However, no suggestion that the substance will cure or mitigate the condition is allowed.[40] Based on the scientific evidence presented for review, the FDA has approved 12 health claims that address such relationships as calcium, vitamin D, and bone health; soluble fiber and heart health; and folate and neural tube defects (Table 9-1).[41]
- *Labels for special needs:* Additional information is included on some nutrition labels for the benefit of

TABLE 9-1 HEALTH CLAIMS APPROVED BY THE FDA FOR NUTRITION LABELS

CLAIM	FOOD REQUIREMENT	MODEL STATEMENT
Calcium and osteoporosis	High in calcium*	Regular exercise and a healthy diet with enough calcium helps teens and young adult Caucasian and Asian women maintain good bone health and may reduce their high risk of osteoporosis later in life.
Sodium and hypertension	Low in sodium	Diets low in sodium may reduce the risk of high blood pressure, a disease associated with many factors.
Dietary fat and cancer	Low fat	Development of cancer depends on many factors. A diet low in total fat may reduce the risk of some cancers.
Dietary saturated fat and cholesterol and risk of coronary heart disease	Low saturated fat Low cholesterol Low fat	Although many factors affect heart disease, diets low in saturated fat and cholesterol may reduce the risk of this disease.
Fiber-containing grain products, fruits, and vegetables and cancer	A grain product, fruit, or vegetable that contains dietary fiber Low fat Good source of dietary fiber without fortification	Low-fat diets rich in fiber-containing grain products, fruits, and vegetables may reduce the risk of some types of cancer, a disease associated with many factors.
Fruits, vegetables, and grain products that contain fiber, particularly soluble fiber, and risk of coronary heart disease	A fruit, vegetable, or grain product that contains fiber Low saturated fat Low cholesterol Low fat At least 0.6 g soluble fiber per serving (without fortification) Soluble fiber content provided on label	Diets low in saturated fat and cholesterol and rich in fruits, vegetables, and grain products that contain some types of dietary fiber, particularly soluble fiber, may reduce the risk of heart disease, a disease associated with many factors.
Fruits and vegetables and cancer	A fruit or vegetable Low fat Food source (without fortification) of at least one of the following: vitamin A, vitamin C, dietary fiber	Low-fat diets rich in fruits and vegetables (foods that are low in fat and may contain dietary fiber, vitamin A, or vitamin C) may reduce the risk of some types of cancer, a disease associated with many factors. *Example:* Broccoli is high in vitamins A and C and is a good source of dietary fiber.
Folate and neural tube defects	Good source of folate (at least 40 mcg per serving)	Healthful diets with adequate folate may reduce a woman's risk of having a child with a brain or spinal cord defect.

TABLE 9-1 **HEALTH CLAIMS APPROVED BY THE FDA FOR NUTRITION LABELS—cont'd**

CLAIM	FOOD REQUIREMENT	MODEL STATEMENT
Dietary sugar alcohols and dental caries	Sugar free Sugar alcohol must be xylitol, sorbitol, mannitol, maltitol, isomalt, lactitol, hydrogenated starch hydrolysates, hydrogenated glucose syrups, erythritol, or a combination Food must not lower plaque pH <5.7	Frequent between-meal consumption of foods high in sugars and starches promotes tooth decay. The sugar alcohols in this food do not promote tooth decay.
Soy protein and risk of coronary heart disease	At least 6.25 g soy protein per serving Low saturated fat Low cholesterol Low fat	Foods containing 25 g of soy protein a day, as part of a diet low in saturated fat and cholesterol, may reduce the risk of heart disease. The grams of soy protein that can be derived from a serving varies with the food.†
Plant sterol/stanol esters and risk of coronary heart disease	At least 0.65 g plant sterol esters per serving of spreads and salad dressings *or* At least 1.7 g plant stanol esters per serving of spreads or salad dressings Low saturated fat Low cholesterol	Foods containing at least 0.65 g per serving of vegetable oil sterol esters, eaten twice a day with meals for a daily total intake of at least 1.3 g, as part of a diet low in saturated fat and cholesterol, may reduce the risk of heart disease. The grams of vegetable oil sterol esters that can be derived from a serving varies with the food.†
Monounsaturated fat from olive oil and coronary heart disease	Must contain monounsaturated fat	Eating about 2 tbsp of olive oil daily may reduce the risk of coronary heart disease because of the monounsaturated fat in olive oil. To achieve this benefit, olive oil should replace a similar amount of saturated fat and not increase the total number of calories eaten in a day. The grams of olive oil that can be derived varies with the food.†
Omega-3 (n-3) fatty acids and coronary heart disease	Must contain both EPA and DHA omega-3 (n-3) fatty acids	Eating EPA and DHA omega-3 (n-3) fatty acids may reduce the risk of coronary heart disease. The grams of EPA and DHA fatty acids that can be derived from 1 serving varies with the food.†
Whole grain foods and risk of heart disease and certain cancers	Contains 51% or more whole grain ingredients by weight per serving Good fiber source Low fat	Diets rich in whole grain foods and other plant foods and low in total fat, saturated fat, and cholesterol may reduce the risk of heart disease and some cancers.
Potassium and the risk of high blood pressure and stroke	Good source of potassium Low sodium Low total fat Low saturated fat Low cholesterol	Diets containing foods that are a good source of potassium and low in sodium may reduce the risk of high blood pressure and stroke.

Modified from U.S. Food and Drug Administration: *Guidance for industry. A food labeling guide—Appendix C: Health claims*, Rockville, Md, 1994 (rev 1999, 2004, 2008), U.S. Food and Drug Administration. Retrieved March 9, 2009, from www.fda.gov/Food/GuidanceComplianceRegulatoryInformation/GuidanceDocuments/FoodLabelingNutrition/FoodLabelingGuide/default.htm.

DHA, Docosahexaenoic acid; *EPA,* eicosapentaenoic acid.

*Food contains without fortification at least 10% of the Daily Reference Value (DV) for the named vitamin, mineral, or fiber and less than 13 g fat, 4 g saturated fat, 60 mg cholesterol, and 480 mg sodium per serving.

†Label will list the amount found in that particular food serving.

certain groups. Animal products processed under the supervision of a rabbi that meet Jewish dietary standards are labeled as *kosher.* Foods or beverages containing aspartame must include a warning for the safety of individuals with phenylketonuria. The Food Allergen Labeling and Consumer Protection Act requires a notation regarding any major allergen known to cause **anaphylactic shock** in allergic individuals. These eight **allergens** are (1) milk (casein), (2) peanuts, (3) tree nuts, (4) fish, (5) shellfish, (6) wheat, (7) eggs, and (8) soybeans (see Figure 9-3).[40]

KEY TERMS

anaphylactic shock A serious and sometimes fatal hypersensitivity reaction to a drug, food, toxin, chemical, or other allergen; the patient experiences weakness, sweating, and shortness of breath or such life-threatening responses as loss of blood pressure and shock, respiratory congestion, or cardiac arrest.

allergens Substances that can cause a hypersensitivity reaction in the body; proteins found in milk, eggs, fish, wheat, tree nuts, peanuts, soybeans, and shellfish can produce serious and sometimes fatal reactions in allergic individuals, and the presence of these foods must be indicated on the food label.

Public attention to the energy, fat, sodium, and cholesterol content of food led to legal definitions for terms such as *low* or *reduced* to protect the public from inappropriate or misleading claims.[39] Nevertheless, confusion about serving sizes[42] and differences between the DVs used on the food label and the DRIs for vitamins and minerals create problems for users.

Food and Botanicals

New foods and beverages with added herbs or other botanicals such as ginseng are blurring the distinction between food and supplements. Manufacturers must show proof that these substances are on the GRAS list or present evidence that the intended use is safe.[43] Many products claiming to increase energy level or fitness contain excessive amounts of sugar and caffeine, which also carry dangers to health.[44]

FOOD SAFETY AND FOOD PROCESSING

Foodborne Illness

Prevalence and Causes of Foodborne Illness

Many disease-bearing microorganisms in our environment have the potential to contaminate our food and water, making foodborne illness a serious public health threat. New technologies ranging from refrigerated trucks to freeze-drying to food irradiation have brought major improvements in food handling and food safety, yet Americans are still vulnerable to foodborne pathogens. According to the CDC, 76 million persons get sick, 325,000 are hospitalized, and 5000 die of foodborne illness each year.[45]

New trends in how food is produced and consumed give foodborne pathogens new opportunities to enter the food chain. The worldwide distribution of fresh and processed food by large corporations can spread foodborne illness regionally and globally. Fruits and vegetables are often eaten raw or unpeeled, and may not have been washed thoroughly.[46] In today's fast-paced life, families eat more precooked foods, seafood salads, and deli meats. Meals are picked up at local food outlets on the way home and kept warm for extended periods, as compared with cooked meals eaten immediately after preparation. People who eat at their desks or in their cars while traveling may not take time to wash their hands or use a hand sanitizer.

Forms of Foodborne Illness

Foodborne illness caused by bacteria takes two different forms: (1) bacterial food infection and (2) bacterial food poisoning:

- Bacterial food infection occurs when individuals eat food contaminated with large colonies of bacteria.
- Toxins produced by bacteria before the food was eaten cause bacterial food poisoning.

Bacterial Food Infection. Six common bacteria cause food infection:

1. *Escherichia coli O157:H7:* Most types of *E. coli* are benign, and some even do nutritionally important work such as fermenting resistant starch. However, other strains such as *E. coli* O157:H7 produce toxins causing serious disease. Found in the intestines of animals and humans, *E. coli* O157:H7 has emerged as a major cause of individual cases and large outbreaks of inflammatory diarrhea with bloody stool and fever.[47] Serious infections can result in kidney impairment or death.

   E. coli O157:H7 is destroyed by heat, and most outbreaks arise from unpasteurized or undercooked food. Cases were reported in persons who drank unpasteurized cider made from apples that had fallen to the ground, been contaminated with animal droppings, and not thoroughly washed. A major outbreak resulted from beef that was contaminated in processing and then undercooked at a fast-food restaurant. The restaurant incident reminds us that all parties across the food chain are responsible for food safety, those who process foods and those who prepare food for immediate consumption. Ground beef must be cooked to a temperature of 165° F to ensure safety against *E. coli.*
2. *Salmonella:* Daniel Salmon (1850-1914) first isolated and identified these bacteria; they are a common cause of foodborne infections. *Salmonella* grow quickly in high-protein foods such as milk, custard, egg dishes, and sandwich filling. Seafood, especially shellfish such as oysters and clams from polluted waters, can be a source of infection. Contamination of eggs with *Salmonella enteritidis* is a worldwide problem. No one should eat raw cookie dough, drink unpasteurized beverages containing milk or egg, or eat undercooked eggs, but these rules are particularly important for older adults. According to the CDC, 40% of deaths from *Salmonella* occur in people older than age 65.[48] Symptoms develop slowly, usually 12 to 24 hours after ingestion, and range from mild to bloody diarrhea with fever.
3. *Campylobacter: Campylobacter* is a cause of acute diarrhea in America and around the world. These bacteria are found in raw and undercooked beef, poultry, and seafood; raw milk; and untreated water. They are destroyed by heating food to 160° F and appropriate water treatment. Cross-contamination of foods is a significant danger with this bacterium. One outbreak occurred when a cutting board used for raw poultry was then used to chop lettuce without appropriate cleaning.[48] *Campylobacter* infection is also associated with the development of Guillain-Barré syndrome.
4. *Shigella:* First discovered as the cause of a dysentery epidemic in Japan, *Shigella* infection is usually confined to the large intestine and varies from simple cramps and diarrhea to fatal dysentery; treatment with antibiotics may be required. Young children are at particular risk of fatal complications. *Shigella* are found in the intestinal tract of animals and in contaminated water. They are spread by insects and unsanitary food handling and grow rapidly in moist or protein foods such as milk, beans, tuna, and turkey. Apple cider or raw fruits and vegetables contaminated by animal droppings are sources of *Shigella*. Foods must be washed and cooked thoroughly and chilled quickly to prevent infection.
5. *Listeria:* This microorganism is well known as a major cause of infection after surgery, but only recently was

Listeria monocytogenes linked with foodborne illness. In older adults, pregnant women, infants, or those with suppressed immune systems, the organism produces diarrhea and flulike fever and headache. Related complications such as pneumonia, **sepsis, meningitis, endocarditis,** and miscarriage require medical intervention. Outbreaks of *Listeria*-related illness have been traced to unpasteurized dairy products, particularly soft Mexican cheeses made with unpasteurized milk. Undercooked poultry and deli foods have been implicated in *Listeria* infections.[46] Thorough cooking and careful washing of raw fruits and vegetables are preventive measures (see the *Focus on Food Safety* box, "Do I Really Need to Wash That Melon?").

6. *Vibrio:* This family of microorganisms includes *V. cholerae,* the bacterium causing cholera, which is still common in many developing countries. The species generally associated with outbreaks of foodborne illness in the United States is *V. parahaemolyticus* found in coastal waters. This is a salt-requiring organism and present in increased concentrations in warm weather. Persons eating raw or undercooked fish, oysters, clams, or other shellfish are at risk of infection. Outbreaks reported in Florida and Long Island resulted from eating raw oysters. *V. parahaemolyticus* causes a watery diarrhea with abdominal cramps, vomiting, fever, and chills that usually lasts no more than 3 days. Most cases go unreported, although it is estimated that as many as 4500 cases occur each year. Individuals with compromised immune systems or liver disease or alcoholism are at risk of serious complications and require medical attention.[49]

Bacterial Food Poisoning. Foodborne illness caused by toxins develops rapidly, with symptoms appearing within 1 to 6 hours after eating. The two most common types of bacterial food poisoning are caused by *Staphylococcus* and *Clostridia* species:

1. *Staphylococcal food poisoning: Staphylococcus aureus* is the most common cause of bacterial poisoning in the United States. Symptoms come on suddenly and include severe cramping and abdominal pain with vomiting and diarrhea, along with sweating, headache, and fever. In some cases shock and **prostration** occur. Recovery is fairly rapid but depends on the amount of toxin ingested. A common source of contamination is an infection on the hand of a food worker, often minor or unnoticed. This bacterium grows rapidly in custard- and cream-filled bakery goods, chicken and ham salads, egg products, and processed meats, cheese, and sauces—all moist foods. No change in odor, taste, or appearance of the food is seen, so the consumer has no warning.
2. *Clostridial food poisoning: Clostridium perfringens* spores are in soil, water, dust, and refuse—virtually everywhere. It multiplies in cooked meat and meat dishes and develops its toxin in foods held for extended times at warming or room temperatures. Outbreaks occur in food service facilities in which foods are held for long periods after cooking. Prevention rests with thorough cooking, prompt serving after cooking, and immediate refrigeration thereafter.

The toxins produced by another *Clostridium, C. botulinum,* cause more serious, often-fatal food poisoning. Depending on the amount of toxin consumed and the individual response, death ensues within 24 hours. Initial complaints are vomiting, weakness, and dizziness. Progressively the toxin irritates motor nerve cells and blocks transmission of neural impulses, causing gradual paralysis and ending in respiratory paralysis. *C. botulinum* spores are found in soils throughout the world and carried on harvested food to the canning process. Like all clostridia, this species is anaerobic (i.e., it develops in the absence of air). A relatively air-free environment provides ideal conditions for

FOCUS ON FOOD SAFETY

Do I Really Need to Wash That Melon?

We often associate foodborne illness with improperly cooked ground meat or poultry or deli foods left at room temperature, but 25% of reported cases of foodborne illness result from unwashed or poorly washed vegetables and fruits. Produce can become contaminated with *Escherichia coli* O157:H7, *Salmonella,* or *Cyclospora* through contact with animals, fertilizers containing animal waste, contaminated irrigation water, or poor sanitation practices of workers who pick or sort the produce.

Following are safety tips for washing fresh fruits and vegetables:

- *Rinse raw produce under running water,* even if you are not going to eat the skin or rind. Any bacteria on the outer surface will be transferred to your hands or to the knife as you peel or cut and then to the food itself. Rub firm-skinned fruits and vegetables or scrub with a small vegetable brush to remove surface dirt.
- *Remove and discard the outermost leaves* of a head of lettuce or cabbage. Wash each lettuce leaf under running water. Scrub melons thoroughly. Do not dip the entire head of lettuce or melon in a container of water. You may be rinsing in contaminated water.
- *Store fruits and vegetables in the refrigerator within 2 hours of peeling or cutting.* Be especially careful with cut melon. Melons are low in acid as compared with oranges, apples, or pineapple, and this allows more rapid growth of bacteria on cut surfaces when the melon stands at room temperature.

KEY TERMS

dysentery A general term given to a number of disorders marked by inflammation of the intestines, especially the colon, and accompanied by abdominal pain and frequent stools containing blood and mucus. Chemical irritants, bacteria, protozoa, or parasites cause it.

sepsis Presence of pathogenic microorganisms or their toxins in the blood or other tissues.

meningitis Inflammation of the meninges, the three membranes that envelop the brain and spinal cord, caused by a bacterial or viral infection and leading to high fever, severe headache, and stiff neck or back muscles.

endocarditis Inflammation of the endocardium, the serous membrane that lines the cavities of the heart.

prostration Extreme exhaustion.

toxin production if spores are not destroyed in the canning process. The commercial canning industry follows processing standards that eliminate the risk of botulism, but cases still result from foods canned at home using inappropriate methods. Boiling for 10 minutes destroys the toxin (although not the spore), so all home-canned food, no matter how well preserved, should be boiled at least 10 minutes before eating. Botulism has occurred in Alaska from native food practices involving uncooked or partially cooked meats.[50]

Table 9-2 summarizes bacterial sources of food contamination.

Viruses. Viruses from the Caliciviridae family are a common cause of gastrointestinal upset. Although these viruses can be spread by the fecal-oral route, 39% of outbreaks arise from contaminated food. Nursing homes are subject to outbreaks if health care workers disposing of vomitus, feces, or bed linens or dishes used by ill patients touch food or serving dishes without washing their hands. In food service facilities, illness can spread from worker to worker and onto the food. Vomiting and diarrhea resulting from Calicivirus contamination usually last no more than 5 days, but diarrhea can continue for as long as 28 days.[48] (Using the information you learned about the importance of family meals, using the nutrition label, and practicing food safety, complete the *Case Study* box, "Planning the Family Dinner.")

Costs of Foodborne Illness

Foodborne illness has health and economic consequences. It is estimated that medical intervention and lost productivity related to foodborne illness have an annual cost of $23 billion.[45] Microbial foodborne illness results in acute but self-limiting symptoms—diarrhea, vomiting, and abdominal pain—and most people do not seek medical attention or require only general supportive care.[51] However, for young children, older adults, and immunocompromised patients such as those with cancer, recent organ or bone marrow transplants, or autoimmune deficiency disease, foodborne pathogens result in serious illness, septicemia, acute renal failure, or death. Unfortunately, many such patients are not aware of this danger.[52] In pregnant women, foodborne illness can result in miscarriage. One in four Americans is likely to experience some form of foodborne illness each year,[48] although stomach distress is often attributed to other causes. Bottled water has been a cause of foodborne illness.[53]

TABLE 9-2 SELECTED EXAMPLES OF BACTERIAL FOODBORNE DISEASE

FOODBORNE DISEASE	CAUSATIVE ORGANISMS (GENUS AND SPECIES)	COMMON FOOD SOURCE	SYMPTOMS AND COURSE
Bacterial Food Infections			
Salmonellosis	*Salmonella* *S. typhi* *S. paratyphi*	Milk, custards, egg dishes, salad dressings, sandwich fillings, polluted shellfish	Mild to severe diarrhea, cramps, vomiting; appears 12-24 hr after eating; lasts 1-7 days
Shigellosis	*Shigella* *S. dysenteriae*	Milk and milk products, seafood, salads	Mild diarrhea to fatal dysentery (especially in young children), appears 7-36 hr after eating, lasts 3-14 days
Listeriosis	*Listeria* *L. monocytogenes*	Soft cheese, poultry, seafood, raw milk, meat products (pâté)	Severe diarrhea, fever, headache, pneumonia, meningitis, endocarditis; can cause miscarriage in pregnant women; symptoms begin after 3-21 days
Vibriosis	*Vibrio* *V. parahaemolyticus*	Raw or undercooked oysters, clams, mussels, other shellfish or finfish	Watery diarrhea, abdominal cramps, nausea, vomiting, fever, and chills; symptoms occur within 24 hours and usually continue for no more than 3 days; severe complications possible with compromised immune systems, liver disease, or alcoholism
Bacterial Food Poisoning Enterotoxins			
Staphylococcal	*Staphylococcus* *S. aureus*	Custards, cream fillings, processed meats, ham, cheese, ice cream, potato salad, sauces, casseroles	Severe abdominal pain, cramps, vomiting, diarrhea, perspiration, headache, fever, prostration; appears suddenly 1-6 hr after eating; symptoms usually subside within 24 hr
Clostridial Perfringens enteritis	*Clostridium* *C. perfringens*	Cooked meats, meat dishes held at warm or room temperature	Mild diarrhea, vomiting; appears 8-24 hr after eating; lasts ≤1 day
Botulism	*Clostridium* *C. botulinum*	Improperly home-canned foods; smoked and salted fish, ham, sausage, shellfish	Symptoms range from mild discomfort to death within 24 hr; initial nausea, vomiting, weakness, dizziness, progressing to motor and sometimes fatal breathing paralysis

Prevention of Foodborne Illness

Sanitation Procedures. Strict sanitation practices and rigid personal hygiene are essential to prevent foodborne illness. Food and everything it touches must be scrupulously clean. Attention to final cooking temperatures and holding temperatures are particularly important when supplying meals for schools or child care centers, older adults, health care facilities, or programs in which food is prepared at one location and transported to other serving centers or individual homes. Leftover food must be cooled and stored within a specific period of time (Figure 9-5) and reheated to the recommended temperature before serving.

CASE STUDY

Planning the Family Dinner

Mrs. G is a single parent with two children: a daughter in third grade and a son in ninth grade. Although they ride different buses to school, both children get home about 3:30 PM. Mrs. G is employed in a real estate office and usually does not get home until about 6:30 PM. By that time the children have already filled up on snacks and are not really hungry for a meal. Sometimes she calls ahead to tell them that she is stopping at a fast-food restaurant and they should wait to eat with her, but most of the time they get something to eat for themselves. Mrs. G's son has been gaining weight at a faster-than-expected rate and has a body mass index (BMI) of 29. At his most recent physical examination, his blood pressure was higher than normal and the physician recommended that he moderate his weight gain to improve his long-term health.

Questions for Analysis

1. Is it important that the family eat together when Mrs. G gets home? How would you approach this?
2. What are some appropriate snack foods that the children might have when they get home from school that would hold them over until dinner?
3. What are important facts on the nutrition label that Mrs. G could use in selecting after-school snacks for her children?
4. MyPyramid recommends an energy intake of 2400 kcal for a 14-year-old moderately active boy. What should be the upper level of fat and sodium included in his food for the day? If one fourth of his daily energy intake is reserved for snacks, then recommend some food combinations that would provide the appropriate amounts of kcalories, sodium, and fat.
5. What are some dinner alternatives to fast-food? What might Mrs. G bring home, or what could the children begin to prepare before she arrives home?
6. Develop five rules for food safety that the children should practice when preparing and eating their after-school snacks.

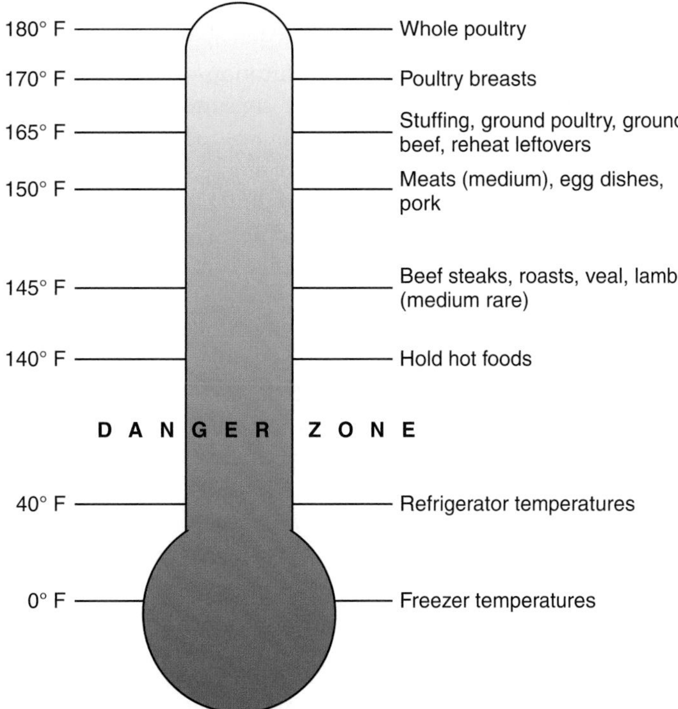

FIGURE 9-5 Chart of food temperatures. It is important to keep hot foods hot and cold foods cold. Foods should be held at temperatures less than 45° F or greater than 140° F to prevent microbial growth. Microorganisms grow rapidly between 45° F and 140° F. Meat and poultry products should be cooked to the internal temperature indicated on the chart. (From U.S. Department of Health and Human Services and U.S. Department of Agriculture: *Dietary guidelines for Americans 2005,* ed 6, Washington, DC, 2005, U.S. Government Printing Office. Retrieved August 12, 2005, from http://www.healthierus.gov/dietaryguidelines/dga2005/document/html/chapter10.htm.)

Dishwashing equipment should meet public health standards for water and drying temperatures and be used to sanitize cooking and serving utensils. Garbage or discarded food must be removed from the food preparation area immediately. Although such guidelines are well known, they are not always practiced. Frequent hand washing and use of gloves is required of all food handlers in public food service operations, food-processing and packaging plants, and public markets. Persons with any infectious disease or hand injury, however slight, must not work with food. Figure 9-6 illustrates proper hand washing.

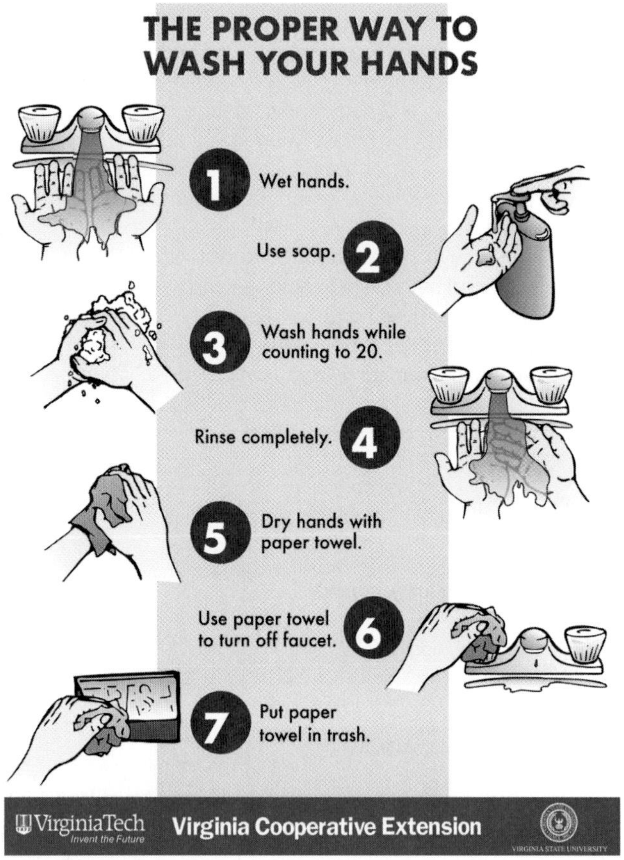

THE PROPER WAY TO WASH YOUR HANDS

1 Wet hands.

2 Use soap.

3 Wash hands while counting to 20.

4 Rinse completely.

5 Dry hands with paper towel.

6 Use paper towel to turn off faucet.

7 Put paper towel in trash.

VirginiaTech Invent the Future — Virginia Cooperative Extension

FIGURE 9-6 Seven-step process for proper hand washing. Failure to wash hands thoroughly before and after food preparation and before eating is a common cause of foodborne illness. (Courtesy Virginia Cooperative Extension, College of Agriculture and Life Sciences, Virginia Polytechnic Institute and State University, Blacksburg, Va.)

Food Irradiation. Food irradiation can extend the shelf life and increase the safety of many foods.[51] Food is irradiated using energy sources such as gamma rays, similar to microwaves, that pass through the food and safely kill harmful bacteria. Food does not become radioactive, and almost no nutrients are lost. Irradiation is used to sterilize rations for space travel and for patients requiring completely germ-free food, such as those with bone marrow transplants. Most of the cooking spices, herbs, and seasonings sold in the United States are irradiated. Irradiation destroys more than 99% of any *Escherichia coli* in ground meat and more than 99% of any *Salmonella* in fresh eggs and poultry.[54]

Although this technology is proven to be safe and effective, less than 0.1 of 1% of the fruits, vegetables, meat, and poultry sold in the United States is irradiated. Health care facilities are the primary users of irradiated foods. The sale of irradiated food has been opposed by those who erroneously believe the food becomes radioactive and by others who believe irradiation will be used to mask unsanitary processing.[51] Irradiation has been endorsed as safe by the American Medical Association, the American Dietetic Association, the World Health Organization (WHO), and the United Nations Food and Agriculture Organization.

Food Safety Education

Government agencies, food processors, and health organizations have joined forces to develop food safety education programs and certifications to meet the needs of consumers, food service professionals, and food processors. Fight BAC!—an initiative of the Partnership for Food Safety Education—offers website lessons and publicity materials for consumers and professionals (Figure 9-7). Fight BAC! contains food safety messages useful to teachers, nutritionists, nurses, or food service managers working with children or adults. The National Restaurant Association Foundation developed a 16-hour national certification program called *ServSafe* for food managers in restaurants, school food service, day care, hospitals, and nursing facilities. Many state public health departments require all food service managers to have the ServSafe certification or equivalent. Training and certification in HAACP, discussed earlier in this chapter, is available to food processors through government and university training programs. (To learn more about needs assessment for food safety education see the *Evidence-Based Practice box,* "Developing Food Safety Education Programs: Assessing Learner Needs.")

EVIDENCE-BASED PRACTICE

Developing Food Safety Education Programs: Assessing Learner Needs

We often think of evidence-based practice in terms of clinical diagnosis and intervention, but these tools can also be applied when developing nutrition education programs. As health professionals, we may believe that we know what our clients need to know and that it is up to them to pay attention. A more effective strategy is to review published studies conducted with your target group to see what they want to know. However, what if no past work exists on which you can draw? Two recent studies provide examples for assessing a target population.

Food safety behaviors of young adults: Byrd-Bredbenner and colleagues[1] surveyed over 4300 college students enrolled in introductory nutrition, biology, or psychology courses at 23 colleges and universities. Their written survey had three series of questions:

1. A list of 26 foods including safe to eat and unsafe or risky foods such as pink hamburger, runny eggs, and raw cookie dough; students were asked to indicate which they did or did not eat.

EVIDENCE-BASED PRACTICE

Developing Food Safety Education Programs: Assessing Learner Needs—cont'd

2. Were they confident in making food safety decisions, or did they need more information?
3. Were they interested in changing their food safety behavior?

In general the students indicated some risky food behaviors; 53% ate raw cookie dough and 29% consumed raw sprouts. They were reasonably confident in their ability to make food safety decisions, but many were giving some thought to changing their food safety practices and wondering how they might go about it. The authors concluded that food safety education directed toward young adults should include practical information on safe food preparation and avoiding risky foods. A short survey made up of only a few questions can provide helpful information as you plan a program for a local group.

Food safety behaviors of cancer patients: Medeiros and colleagues[2] conducted focus groups* with 31 cancer patients to learn more about (1) their food safety practices, (2) the food safety information they were given after being diagnosed, and (3) their preferences on how food safety information should be delivered to them.

Although most participants were aware that cancer patients are more vulnerable to infection, none had made major changes in their food safety behavior. They were willing to adopt several recommended practices, including avoiding raw seafood, nonpasteurized fruit juices, and products containing raw eggs, as well as heating hot dogs and deli meats to steaming before eating. However, most did not use a meat thermometer when cooking meat or poultry and were reluctant to do so. As for future food safety education, they recommended that special materials be developed for patients with cancer that are accurate, science based, and easy to read and understand. Written materials or web-based materials that they could read at home were preferred over attending classes. Determining how a group wishes to receive information is an important first step in planning a program. Although some individuals may enjoy the social setting and interacting with fellow learners, others may wish to remain at home and choose a time they find convenient for learning.

Different groups will have different educational needs and preferred formats for receiving information. Providing motivation for learning may be more difficult than developing the material to be presented. Understanding the needs and preferences of your target group must be the first step in developing a nutrition education program. (We will discuss behavioral strategies for helping individuals change their behavior in Chapter 10.)

REFERENCES

1. Byrd-Bredbenner C, Abbot JM, Wheatley V, et al: Risky eating behaviors of young adults: implications for food safety education, *J Am Diet Assoc* 108:549, 2008.
2. Medeiros LC, Chen G, Hillers VN, et al: Discovery and development of educational strategies to encourage safe food handling behaviors in cancer patients, *J Food Prot* 71:1666, 2008.

*For more information on focus groups, what they are, and how they are conducted, consider the following source: *Focus group approach to needs assessment*, Ames, Iowa, 2001, Iowa State University Extension. Retrieved March 9, 2009, from www.extension.iastate.edu/communities/tools/assess/focus.html.

FIGHT BAC!
SEPARATE
Don't cross-contaminate.
CLEAN
Wash hands and surfaces often.
CHILL
Refrigerate promptly.
COOK
Cook to proper temperatures.
BAC
Keep Food Safe From Bacteria®

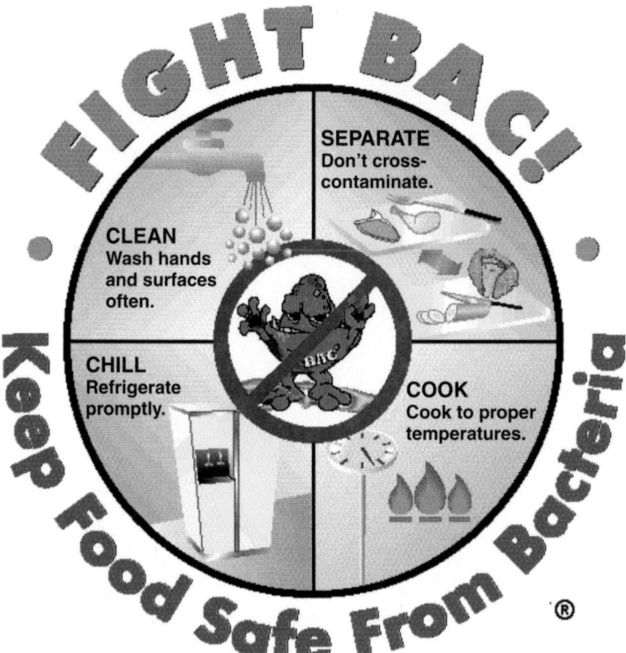

FIGURE 9-7 Fight BAC!, a program initiative of the Partnership for Food Safety Education, emphasizes four steps in food handling to prevent foodborne illness: (1) clean, (2) separate, (3) cook, and (4) chill. (Courtesy Partnership for Food Safety Education, Washington, DC. Available at www.fightbac.org/component/option,com_docman/task,cat_view/gid,24/Itemid,83/.)

Food Preservation and Processing

Preservation Methods

As consumers look for convenient foods to feed their families, food processors seek new methods of food preservation and packaging to meet the demand. Some of the methods used by commercial processors are similar to those used by consumers to keep food safe, but food scientists are always looking for new ways to control the food environment to maintain freshness and flavor and prohibit microbial growth. Following is a list of some common methods used to preserve and process food:

- *Applying heat:* Cooking procedures soften food for chewing, increase food palatability, and prepare food for digestion. Heat is also an important means of ensuring food safety in home and industrial processing. Most bacteria are killed at temperatures of 180° to 200° F.[55] Heat also inactivates enzymes that promote the deterioration of fruits and vegetables. This is why vegetables are first blanched in boiling water to prevent further enzyme activity before being frozen. Pasteurization is a means of eliminating pathogens in fluid milk and fruit juices. Canned foods are exposed to temperatures that effectively sterilize the food contents. Foods canned at home at too low a temperature carry the risk of botulism (see preceding section on foodborne illness).
- *Keeping food cold:* Microbial activity slows at temperatures less than 50° F; thus refrigeration at 45° F or lower will preserve food for a limited period of time.[55]

Freezing prevents microbial growth; however, bacteria remain alive, although dormant. Therefore it is important not to refreeze food that has been thawed for some time, allowing microorganisms to begin to multiply. Cold temperatures will decrease but not eliminate enzyme activity.

- *Removing moisture:* Drying lowers the water activity in a food, removing available water and thus preventing survival and growth of any microorganism present. Foods dried at high temperatures, such as ready-to-eat cereals, and freeze-dried foods retain more flavor and color. The removal of water from a food also slows enzyme activity and destructive oxidation reactions.
- *Adding acid, sugar, salt, or chemical additives:* Acid-containing foods lower in pH are more resistant to the growth of bacteria. Before the era of refrigeration, fermentation with the production of acid was used to turn perishable milk into yogurt or cheese that could be safely stored for a longer time. Adding salt or sugar to a food controls the growth of bacteria by limiting the available water to existing microorganisms. In this way the high sugar content of jams prevents spoilage. In earlier times, salt curing was a means of preserving meat, and pickling is still used by home and commercial food processors. Chemical additives such as sodium benzoate or calcium propionate are added to bread and grain products to retard the growth of bacteria and mold and increase shelf life.
- *Changing the atmosphere:* A new method of food preservation involves changing the atmosphere—that is, removing the oxygen necessary for bacterial growth and enzyme activity and replacing it with carbon dioxide (CO_2) or nitrogen, which slows these activities. Modified atmosphere packaging is used for highly perishable foods such as ready-to-eat chicken pieces and salad mixes.

Chemical Additives

As consumers demand new flavors, improved textures, and increased shelf life, food researchers are testing new additives and new uses for existing additives that will ensure these qualities. Additives enrich food with nutrients, provide color, standardize functional factors such as thickening, and improve flavor and mouth feel. Table 9-3 lists some examples of food additives. Vitamins acting as antioxidants are sometimes

TABLE 9-3 EXAMPLES OF FOOD ADDITIVES

TYPE	CHEMICAL COMPOUND	FUNCTION	COMMON FOOD USES
Anticaking agent	Calcium silicate, calcium stearate	Used to keep food dry and prevent caking as moisture is absorbed from the air; keep item free-flowing	Table salt, powdered sugar, baking powder
Antimicrobial agent	Calcium propionate, sodium propionate	Prevent growth of mold	Bread
Antioxidants	Butylated hydroxyanisole (BHA), butylated hydroxytoluene (BHT)	Prevents oxidation reactions and rancidity in unsaturated fatty acids	Vegetable oils, potato chips
Bleaching agent	Chlorine, benzoyl peroxide	Whiten appearance	Freshly milled wheat flour, white flour for all-purpose use or cakes
Chemical leavening systems	Sodium bicarbonate	Acts with an acid in a batter to release carbon dioxide (CO_2) for leavening	Double-acting baking powder for quick breads, cakes, and cookies
Coloring agent	Annatto (natural), FD&C red #3, FD&C yellow #5 (artificial)	Make color of food items more appealing	Margarine, candy, carbonated beverages and fruit drinks
Dough conditioners	Ammonium chloride, calcium phosphate	Improves volume	Bread
Emulsifier	Lecithin, monoglycerides and diglycerides	Keeps the water-soluble and fat-soluble ingredients evenly distributed throughout a food	Margarine, cake mixes
Humectants	Propylene glycol, sorbitol	Retain moisture, prevent food from becoming hard or stiff	Soft cookies, cake frosting, marshmallow candy
Flavoring agents	Amyl acetate, methyl salicylate, essential oils, monosodium glutamate (MSG), salt	Enhance flavor or aroma of foods	Most processed foods
Preservative	Sodium nitrate (color) Sodium nitrite (food safety)	Preserves pink color in cured meats, prevents rancidity in meats and botulism	Processed meats such as frankfurters, canned foods
Sequestrant	Citric acid	Binds with metals such as iron or copper to prevent changes in flavor, color, or appearance	Wine, juice, mayonnaise
Stabilizers and thickeners	Pectin, locust bean gum, guar gum, carrageenan	Maintain appropriate food texture and mouth feel; thickener, absorb water	Jelly, ice cream, pudding, yogurt

added to processed foods, not to increase their nutrient content but to enhance their shelf life by preventing undesirable oxidation reactions.

Nutritional Aspects of Food Processing

The effect of food processing on food nutrient content continues to concern both consumers and health advocates. In general, carbohydrates, fats, and proteins are less affected and minerals and vitamins are more affected by food processing. However, both the characteristics of a food and the methods used influence the stability or loss of nutrients. Effects on particular nutrients are summarized as follows:

- *Macronutrients:* The major change in carbohydrates and proteins is the Maillard or browning reaction that occurs between sugars and amino acids at high temperatures. This happens in normal baking and forms new sugar-amino acid compounds that cannot be digested or absorbed. The amino acid lysine enters into the browning reaction, resulting in some loss of this amino acid, although in the American diet grain foods are not major sources of lysine. Hydrogenation of liquid vegetable oils to produce solid table fats forms *trans* fatty acids that have negative effects on health. (See Chapter 4 to review fat hydrogenation.)
- *Minerals:* Major mineral losses result from the refining of cereal grains. When the germ and bran are removed from wheat or other grain to produce a finer-textured flour or cereal, iron along with zinc, chromium, and magnesium is lost. Under current food enrichment standards iron is added back to refined cereals, but the other minerals are not. Mineral content and bioavailability is retained with most other processing methods.
- *Vitamins:* No vitamin is completely stable to food processing, although losses vary from one to another. Vitamins are lost naturally during the storage of fruits and vegetables through the action of enzymes and oxidation.[56] Researchers have suggested that some synthetic vitamin forms are more stable to food processing than naturally occurring forms. However, in general, factors affecting vitamin losses influence all forms of a particular vitamin.[57]
- *Fat-soluble vitamins:* Vitamin A is relatively stable to heat. Fairly small amounts are lost in milk pasteurization, but holding milk at high temperatures for long periods increases losses. Vitamin E in oils is generally not affected by heat treatment or frying, but freezing rapidly destroys it. Naturally occurring vitamin D is not harmed by heat, but it must be protected from light and atmospheric oxygen.[57,58]
- *Water-soluble vitamins:* Thiamin is sensitive to heat, and losses occur in baking and high-temperature processing of cereals. Thiamin is also lost in foods cooked in an alkaline medium or in large amounts of water. Light is extremely destructive to riboflavin, and riboflavin-containing foods must be stored in opaque containers to avoid loss. Riboflavin does withstand the heat treatment of pasteurization, so milk remains a good food source. Niacin and pantothenic acid are generally stable in all foods. Folate is destroyed by light, and large amounts are lost in vegetables heated to high temperatures in large amounts of water. Vitamin B_6 is sensitive to light and is lost in cooking and canning of vegetables. Long exposure to heat or hot storage causes the destruction of ascorbic acid. It is best that vitamin C–containing beverages and foods be packaged with no head space, because the presence of oxygen leads to serious losses over time.[57,58]

Food processing, whether cooking at home or large-scale food manufacturing, often brings some degree of nutrient loss. When foods are refined and the bran and germ or peel is removed, nutrients and fiber are left behind. Extended cooking times, elevated temperatures, and the reduction of a natural food into smaller and smaller pieces, exert a toll on nutritional quality. Choosing whole grains and less highly processed foods more of the time and frozen entrees and dried or frozen meal starters less of the time is a positive step toward health.

TO SUM UP

Food patterns evolve from a social perspective. As our society changes, so does what we eat. More women are employed outside the home, more persons are living alone, and almost half of our food budget is spent on meals away from home. Surveys suggest the American public is becoming more conscious of nutrition and health; however, fast-food and convenience meals are the norm in many families. As more of our food comes from farmers and processors across the country and across the world, the threat of food contamination and risk of widespread outbreaks of foodborne illness increase. Two government agencies, the FDA and the USDA, carry responsibility for maintaining a safe and wholesome food supply. Although the USDA oversees meat, poultry, and dairy, the FDA regulates the processing, labeling, and formulation of all other foods, including GM foods. The nutrition label helps consumers select food to maximize their nutrient intake while limiting kcalories, sodium, and fat. Under current law, dietary supplements are largely unregulated, putting indiscriminate users at risk. The CDC monitors the incidence of foodborne illness, and various government and private agencies have joined forces to provide public and professional education to ensure safe food-handling practices. Public demand for good-tasting food, easily heated and prepared, with a long shelf life has led to increasing use of food additives and new processing methods. Consumers and health professionals must continue to monitor the nutrient content of processed food and the implications for nutrition and health.

QUESTIONS FOR REVIEW

1. What are some social and psychologic factors that influence our food habits? Give an example of a custom or special observance in your family that involves food.
2. What influences the acceptance of food misinformation? Find a print or Internet advertisement for a new dietary supplement or health cure and identify the population to whom it is directed. Using the criteria in Box 9-3, evaluate this product. Does it appear to be helpful or harmful? How would you respond to a consumer asking your advice on its use?
3. You are preparing a 15-minute lesson on use of the nutrition label as part of a nutrition education class for young families receiving food stamps. Review the educational materials found on the FDA website and develop an outline for your presentation including any visuals you would use. Develop a brochure that would be suitable for this audience.
4. A pregnant mother who has been eating more fish to obtain a good supply of n-3 fatty acids read a newspaper article indicating that all ocean fish are contaminated with mercury. She is concerned about the safety of her baby. Review the current advisory of the FDA (www.fda.gov and Box 9-5) regarding the consumption of fish by pregnant women. How would you advise her? Develop some practical menu suggestions that would help her.
5. You are helping a day care provider develop a food safety program for her facility. Compile a list of 10 guidelines for the staff that will reduce the risk of foodborne illness among their children. (Visit the Fight BAC! website at www.fightbac.org/ for some good ideas.)
6. Select a type of frozen entree and review the nutrition labels on five examples of that product. Make a table that lists the number of servings; kcalories per serving; grams of protein, fat, and fiber; milligrams of sodium; and DV for calcium, iron, vitamin A, and vitamin C. Compare the relative merits and disadvantages of each. Which is the best choice based on its contribution of protein, fiber, and vitamins and minerals? Which is the poorest choice in terms of fat, kcalories, and sodium? How do they compare in cost?
7. Name five methods of food preservation. Which methods destroy harmful bacteria and which merely retard their growth? What are the appropriate storage conditions for food preserved by each of these methods?
8. What is the difference between a bacterial infection and illness arising from a bacterial toxin? Give an example of each and the microorganism involved. Which population groups are most vulnerable to foodborne illness? What types of food are most subject to the growth of bacteria?

REFERENCES

1. Kittler PG, Sucher KP: *Food and culture*, ed 4, Belmont, Calif, 2004, Brooks/Cole, a division of Thomson Learning.
2. Counihan C, Van Esterik P: *Food and culture: a reader*, New York, 1997, Routledge.
3. Belasco W, Scranton P: *Food nations: selling taste in consumer societies*, New York, 2002, Routledge.
4. Maslow AH: *Motivation and personality*, New York, 1954, Harper & Row.
5. Economic Research Service, U.S. Department of Agriculture: *Briefing room: food CPI, prices, and expenditures*, Washington, DC, 2008, U.S. Department of Agriculture. Retrieved March 20, 2009, from www.ers.usda.gov/briefing/cpifoodandexpenditures/.
6. Sloan AE: What, when, and where America eats, *Food Technol* 60:19, 2006.
7. Federal Interagency Forum on Aging-Related Statistics: *Older Americans 2008: key indicators of well-being*, Washington, DC, 2008, U.S. Government Printing Office.
8. Sloan AE: Top 10 food trends, *Food Technol* 61(4):22, 2007.
9. Kerver JM, Yang EJ, Obayashi S, et al: Meal and snack patterns are associated with dietary intake of energy and nutrients in U.S. adults, *J Am Diet Assoc* 106:46, 2006.
10. Zizza CA, Tayie FA, Lino M: Benefits of snacking in older Americans, *J Am Diet Assoc* 107:800, 2007.
11. Neumark-Sztainer D, Hannan PJ, Story M, et al: Family meal patterns: associations with sociodemographic characteristics and improved dietary intake among adolescents, *J Am Diet Assoc* 103:317, 2003.
12. Eisenberg ME, Olsen RE, Neumark-Sztainer D, et al: Correlations between family meals and psychosocial well-being among adolescents, *Arch Pediatr Adolesc Med* 158(8):792, 2004.
13. Larson NI, Neumark-Sztainer D, Hannan PJ, et al: Family meals during adolescence are associated with higher diet quality and healthful meal patterns during young adulthood, *J Am Diet Assoc* 107:1502, 2007.
14. Merten MJ, Williams AL, Shriver LH: Breakfast consumption in adolescence and young adulthood: parental presence, community context, and obesity, *J Am Diet Assoc* 109:1384, 2009.
15. Brown D: The rise of the male cook, *J Am Diet Assoc* 107:731, 2007.
16. Sloan AE: Ten top functional food trends, *Food Technol* 62:25, 2008.
17. International Food Information Council: Consumers remain disconnected from their food: 2008 Food & Health Survey gauges consumer attitudes on nutrition and food safety, *Food Insight* July/Aug 2008. Retrieved May 17, 2010 from http://www.foodinsight.org/Newsletter.aspx.
18. Plotnikoff RC, Hotz SB, Johnson ST, et al: Readiness to shop for low-fat foods: a population study, *J Am Diet Assoc* 109:1392, 2009.
19. Heller A: Ethnic allure, *Supermarket News* 53(61):16, 2005.
20. Radimer K, Bindewald B, Hughes J, et al: Dietary supplement use by U.S. adults: data from the National Health and Nutrition Examination Survey, 1999-2000, *Am J Epidemiol* 160:339, 2004.
21. American Dietetic Association: Position of the American Dietetic Association: agricultural and food biotechnology, *J Am Diet Assoc* 106:285, 2006.
22. U.S. Food and Drug Administration: *Report on the Food and Drug Administration's review of the safety of recombinant bovine somatotropin, CFSAN*, Updated April 23, 2009, Washington, DC, U.S. Department of Health and Human Services. Retrieved August 19, 2009, from www.fda.gov/AnimalVeterinary/SafetyHealth/ProductSafetyInformation/ucm130321.htm.

23. Vicini J, Etherton T, Kris-Etherton P, et al: Survey of retail milk composition as affected by label claims regarding farm-management practices, *J Am Diet Assoc* 108:1198, 2008.
24. Wilkins J: Fact or fishberry? Answering consumer questions about genetically engineered foods, *ADA Times* 2(4):5, 2005.
25. Magana-Gomez JA: Calderon de la Barca AM: Risk assessment of genetically modified crops for nutrition and health, *Nutr Rev* 67:1, 2009.
26. Formanek R Jr: Proposed rules issued for bioengineered foods, *FDA Consum* 35(2):9, 2001.
27. Davies WP: An historical perspective from the green revolution to the gene revolution, *Nutr Rev* 61(Suppl 6):S124, 2003.
28. Lehrer SB, Bannon GA: Risks of allergic reactions to biotech proteins in foods: perception and reality, *Allergy* 60:559, 2005.
29. Dubock A: Crop conundrum, *Nutr Rev* 67:17, 2009.
30. Hampton T: Prevent genetically modified organisms from escaping into nature, report urges, *JAMA* (9):1055, 2004.
31. International Food Information Council Foundation: The myth of zero: the elusive goals of absolute safety and guaranteed benefits, *Food Insight* Nov/Dec 2008. Retrieved May 17, 2010, from http://www.foodinsight.org/Newsletter.aspx.
32. U.S. Food and Drug Administration, U.S. Department of Health and Human Services: *An overview of FDA*, Rockville, MD, 2008, U.S. Department of Health and Human Services. Retrieved February 9, 2009, from www.fda.gov/oc/opacom/fda101/sld030.html.
33. U.S. Food and Drug Administration, U.S. Department of Health and Human Services: *Dietary Supplement Health and Education Act of 1994*, Pub Law 103-417, Rockville, MD, 1994, U.S. Department of Health and Human Services. Retrieved February 9, 2009, from www.fda.gov/opacom/laws/dshea.html.
34. Organic Consumers Association: *U.S. organic food sales up 22%, hit $17 billion in 2006*, Finland, Minn, 2007, Organic Consumers Association. Retrieved March 2, 2009, from www.organicconsumers.org/articles/article_5109.cfm.
35. U.S. Department of Agriculture: *The National Organic Program*, Washington, DC, U.S. Department of Agriculture, 1990. Retrieved March 2, 2009, from http://www.ams.usda.gov/AMSv1.0/nop.
36. U.S. Department of Health and Human Services and U.S. Environmental Protection Agency: *What you need to know about mercury in fish and shellfish*, Washington, DC, 2004, U.S. Department of Health and Human Services. Retrieved March 3, 2009, from www.cfsan.fda.gov/~dms/admehg3.html.
37. U.S. Food and Drug Administration, U.S. Department of Health and Human Services: *Food labeling and nutrition overview*, Washington, DC, 2008, U.S. Department of Health and Human Services. Retrieved March 3, 2009, from www.cfsan.fda.gov/label.html.
38. Taylor CL, Wilkening VL: How the nutrition food label was developed, part 1: the Nutrition Facts Panel, *J Am Diet Assoc* 108:437, 2008.
39. Taylor CL, Wilkening VL: How the nutrition food label was developed, part 2: the purpose and promise of nutrition claims, *J Am Diet Assoc* 108:618, 2008.
40. U.S. Food and Drug Administration, U.S. Department of Health and Human Services: *A food labeling guide: guidance for industry*, Washington, DC, 2008, U.S. Department of Health and Human Services. Retrieved March 3, 2009, from www.cfsan.fda.gov/~dms/2lg-8.html#health.
41. U.S. Food and Drug Administration, U.S. Department of Health and Human Services: *Health claims meeting significant scientific agreement (SSA)*, Washington, DC, 2009, U.S. Department of Health and Human Services. Retrieved March 3, 2009, from www.fda.gov/Food/LabelingNutrition/LabelClaims/Health ClaimsMeetingSignificantScientificAgreementSSA/default.htm.
42. Seligson FH: Serving size standards: can they be harmonized, *Nutr Today* 38(6):247, 2003.
43. U.S. Food and Drug Administration, U.S. Department of Health and Human Services: *Letter to manufacturers regarding botanicals and other novel ingredients in conventional foods*, Washington, DC, 2001, U.S. Department of Health and Human Services. Retrieved August 15, 2009, from www.fda.gov/Food/DietarySupplements/GuidanceComplianceRegulatoryInformation/ucm103443.htm.
44. Clauson KA, Shields KM, McQueen CE, et al: Safety issues associated with commercially available energy drinks, *J Am Pharm Assoc* 48(3):e55–e63, 2008.
45. American Dietetic Association: Position of the American Dietetic Association: food and water safety, *J Am Diet Assoc* 109:1449, 2009.
46. Sneed J, Strohbehn CH: Trends impacting food safety in retail foodservice: implications for dietetics practice, *J Am Diet Assoc* 108:1170, 2008.
47. Foodborne Illness Primer Work Group: Foodborne illness primer for physicians and other health care professionals, *Nutr Clin Care* 7:134, 2004.
48. McCabe-Sellers BJ, Beattie SE: Food safety: emerging trends in foodborne illness surveillance and prevention, *J Am Diet Assoc* 104:1708, 2004.
49. Centers for Disease Control and Prevention: *Disease listing: Vibrio parahaemolyticus. General information/technical information, Division of Foodborne, Bacterial and Mycotic Diseases*, Atlanta, 2008, Centers for Disease Control and Prevention. Retrieved August 15, 2009, from www.cdc.gov/nczved/dfbmd/disease_listing/vibriop_gi.html.
50. Cody MM, Kunkel ME: *Food safety for professionals*, ed 2, Chicago, 2002, American Dietetic Association.
51. Walls I: Microbial foodborne diseases, *Nutr Clin Care* 7:131, 2004.
52. Medeiros LC, Chen G, Hillers VN, et al: Discovery and development of educational strategies to encourage safe food handling behaviors in cancer patients, *J Food Prot* 71:1666, 2008.
53. American Dietetic Association: Position of the American Dietetic Association: food and water safety, *J Am Diet Assoc* 103:1203, 2003.
54. Parnes RB, Lichtenstein AH: Food irradiation: a safe and useful technology, *Nutr Clin Care* 7:149, 2004.
55. Parker R: *Introduction to food science*, Delmar/Thomson Learning, 2003, Albany, NY.
56. Hotz C, Gibson RS: Traditional food-processing and preparation practices to enhance the bioavailability of micronutrients in plant-based diets, *J Nutr* 137:1097, 2007.
57. Henry CK, Chapman C, editors: *The nutrition handbook for food processors*, Boca Raton, Fla, 2002, CRC Press.
58. Finley JW, Deming DM, Smith RE: Food processing, nutrition, safety, and quality. In Shils ME, Shike M, Olson J, et al, editors: *Modern nutrition in health and disease*, ed 10, Baltimore, 2006, Lippincott Williams & Wilkins, pp. 1777–1788.

FURTHER READINGS AND RESOURCES

Further Readings

American Dietetic Association: Position of the American Dietetic Association: agricultural and food biotechnology, *J Am Diet Assoc* 106:285, 2006. *[This article describes how agricultural and health care professionals must work together to ensure a safe food supply.]*

Eisenberg ME, Olsen RE, Neumark-Sztainer D, et al: Correlations between family meals and psychosocial well-being among adolescents, *Arch Pediatr Adolesc Med* 158(8):792, 2004.

Robinson-O'Brien R, Larson N, Neumark-Sztainer D, et al: Characteristics and dietary patterns of adolescents who value eating locally grown, organic, nongenetically engineered, and nonprocessed food, *J Nutr Educ Behav* 41:11, 2009.

[These articles, from an ongoing study of food habits of children and adolescents in Minnesota, highlight the importance of family meals and family influences in the development of appropriate eating patterns. These findings can help us reinforce with parents and caregivers why their families should plan meals together.]

Foodborne Illness Primer Work Group: Foodborne illness primer for physicians and other health care professionals, *Nutr Clin Care* 7:134, 2004. *[This work group prepared an overview of foodborne illness as it relates to the health and well-being of patients. It outlines the symptoms and causes of foodborne illness that should be included in food safety education with individuals and community groups.]*

Sloan AE: What, when, and where America eats, *Food Technol* 60:19, 2006. *[Dr. Sloan provides a comprehensive review of food trends among American consumers and the implications for food scientists and nutritionists.]*

Switt J: Labeling around the globe: helping to direct food flow, *J Am Diet Assoc* 107:199, 2007.

Taylor CL, Wilkening VL: How the nutrition food label was developed, part 1: the nutrition facts panel, *J Am Diet Assoc* 108:437, 2008.

Taylor CL, Wilkening VL: How the nutrition food label was developed, part 2: the purpose and promise of nutrition claims, *J Am Diet Assoc* 108:618, 2008.

[These articles provide an overview of the nutrition label, how it was developed, and how nutrition labeling is implemented in other parts of the world.]

U.S. National Institutes of Health, National Library of Medicine: *Evaluating Internet health information: a tutorial from the National Library of Medicine*, Bethesda, Md, 2009, U.S. Department of Health and Human Services. Retrieved March 21, 2009, from http://www.nlm.nih.gov/medlineplus/webeval/webeval.html. *[This tutorial provides a framework for helping consumers evaluate claims and advertisements relating to health products and treatments.]*

Websites of Interest

American College of Allergy: *Asthma & Immunology*. This site provides medical and lifestyle resources for patients and professionals relating to the eight major food allergens: www.aaaai.org/patients/publicedmat/tips/foodallergy.stm.

American Dietetic Association: *Home Food Safety: It's in Your Hands*. This site provides comprehensive materials about food safety including heat and eat and office eating: www.homefoodsafety.org/index.jsp. (Materials available in English and Spanish.)

Center for Food Safety and Applied Nutrition, U.S. Food and Drug Administration. This site is a comprehensive source of information on food labeling, food safety, and updates on foods or drugs being recalled from the marketplace: www.cfsan.fda.gov/ (Materials available in English and Spanish.)

Fight BAC! *Partnership for Food Safety Education*. This site provides food safety materials for adults, children, and food service workers http://www.fightbac.org/. (Materials available in English and Spanish.)

Food Allergy & Anaphylaxis Network. This site provides a comprehensive resource for individuals or families with children with food allergies, including foods and recipes, working with school personnel, and anaphylaxis: www.foodallergy.org/. (Supported by a financial grant from the American College of Allergy, Asthma & Immunology.)

FoodSafety.gov—Gateway to Government Food Safety. This site provides information covering all aspects of food safety: http://www.foodsafety.gov/.

International Food Information Council. This site provides consumer information on food labeling, food additives, and food ingredients: www.ific.org/.

National Institutes of Health, U.S. Department of Health and Human Services. This site provides guidelines for evaluating sources of health information and possible treatments: www.nlm.nih.gov/medlineplus/evaluatinghealthinformation.html. (Materials available in English and Spanish.)

U.S. Department of Agriculture: *EDEN-Extension Disaster Education Network*. The EDEN website links USDA Extension educators from across the United States with resources to address natural and intentional disasters, www.eden.lsu.edu/ (Site is managed by Louisiana State University.)

U.S. National Institutes of Health, National Library of Medicine: *Medline Plus. Trusted Information for You. Food Allergy*. This site provides resource information on all food allergies and local sources of services or treatment: www.nlm.nih.gov/medlineplus/foodallergy.html.

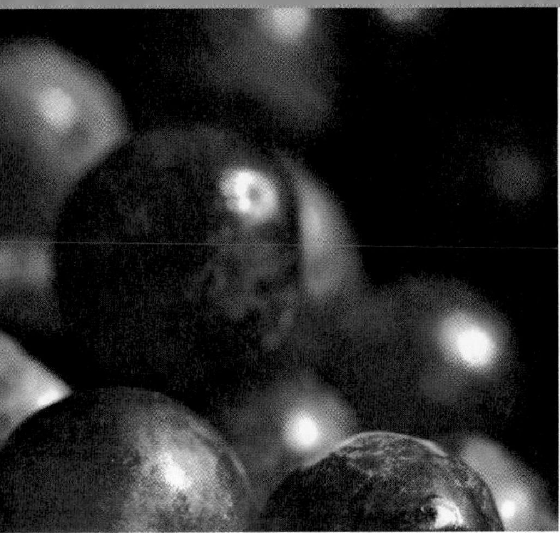

10

Community Nutrition: Promoting Healthy Eating

Eleanor D. Schlenker

evolve WEBSITE
http://evolve.elsevier.com/Williams/essentials/

CHAPTER OUTLINE

Health and nutrition professionals apply the principles of nutrition and health education in various settings. Nutrition experts in medical nutrition therapy offer instruction and support within health care facilities to individuals and their families who are learning new food patterns in response to acute or chronic illness (we will learn more about this in Part 3). Other nutrition and health educators work in community or public health programs such as schools, youth camps, weight control programs, worksite wellness programs, clinics for mothers and babies, and senior centers. They offer personal nutrition counseling or teach classes to community groups.

This chapter continues our sequence on food resources and helping individuals and families select food for optimum nutrition and best use of their food dollars. We also look at educational approaches to nutrition intervention that assist people in adopting healthy lifestyles and food patterns.

IMPLEMENTING NUTRITION EDUCATION

Framework for Wellness

In our work we promote optimum well-being through nutrition, but health and wellness are defined in various ways. The World Health Organization's (WHO's) definition of wellness includes several dimensions including physical wellness, emotional wellness, social wellness, environmental wellness, and spiritual wellness.[1] This expanded definition includes not only building a strong physical body but also developing a healthy self-concept, establishing satisfying relationships with others, and making decisions that are positive in protecting and maintaining our physical environment. The Centers for Disease Control and Prevention (CDC) has introduced the concept of "Healthy Days" to measure quality of life and health.[2] Individuals with chronic conditions such as coronary heart disease reported 10 "unhealthy days" in the previous month, as compared with those free of such conditions who reported only 5 unhealthy days.

Helping individuals and families make positive changes in their lifestyles to improve their nutrition and well-being is both an art and a science.[1] The *Dietary Reference Intakes (DRIs), MyPyramid,* and the *Dietary Guidelines for Americans* provide the science—what nutrients and foods are needed in what amounts to maintain a healthy body and postpone chronic disease—but adapting those guidelines to individuals with particular food patterns, income, living situation, and food beliefs is an art; therefore it requires patience, sensitivity, and application of behavioral theory. In the following sections we address these issues.

Framework for Nutrition Education

The terms *nutrition education* and *nutrition counseling* are sometimes used interchangeably, but they have similarities and differences. Both terms relate to helping people develop a healthy food pattern and overcome any existing barriers to good eating; however, nutrition counseling is more likely to address the prevention or treatment of a disease condition and often involves medical nutrition therapy.[3,4] Nutrition counseling can take place in a health care facility as part of patient care, with outpatients in a diabetes clinic, in a public health program serving pregnant women at risk, or with children and parents enrolled in a school obesity intervention program. Nutrition counseling is usually a one-on-one experience, with the counselor and individual (or family). *Nutrition education* is a more general term that refers to any program that assists people in making decisions about their eating practices and applies knowledge about the relationship between nutrition and health. Nutrition education often involves group education such as a school class or group weight loss program.[3,4] The qualities needed and goals for effective nutrition counseling apply equally to nutrition education.

Societies shape their own patterns of disease, and economic and **demographic** factors influence health at all ages.[5,6] Nutrition educators must recognize the food patterns of the broad ethnic and national groups that make up our cross-cultural environment. They must develop effective communication skills with people from all educational levels. Individuals new to the United States may experience difficulties in **acculturation** to a new secular and food environment.[7] Our job is to help families explore their options and make decisions based on appropriate information and personal support.

Person-Centered Goals

Family counseling must be person centered. It requires close attention to personal and family needs, nutrition and health problems, and food choices and costs. The nutrition counselor has the following goals:

1. To obtain information from the individual or family about their nutrition and health needs
2. To provide the knowledge and practical skills to meet those needs
3. To support the individual or family with encouragement, reinforcement, and referral

Model for Nutrition Counseling

Regardless of the setting, the nutrition counselor begins by carrying out a nutrition assessment, evaluating the positive aspects of the current dietary pattern and considering the need for change as appropriate. A model describing this process (Figure 10-1) emphasizes the overall goal of positive health intervention. (A protocol for nutrition assessment as applied to medical nutrition therapy and the nutrition care process is discussed in Chapter 16.)

Getting Started

The personal qualities of the counselor and the social environment he or she creates are critical to success. Early in the process the nutrition counselor must provide a foundation for future communication and trust, as follows:

- *Build a relationship:* Counseling is a dynamic and person-centered process rooted in a helping relationship. The first step in offering help is establishing a connection of trust and respect, demonstrating kindness and concern.
- *Create a positive climate:* Choose a comfortable setting with adequate space, ventilation, lighting, and low noise level. Allow sufficient time, free from interruption, and the privacy needed to ensure confidentiality. Place the desk to the side, not between you and your client (Figure 10-2).
- *Develop constructive attitudes:* This includes accepting people as they are and where they are in their personal development. You must also recognize their thoughts and ideas

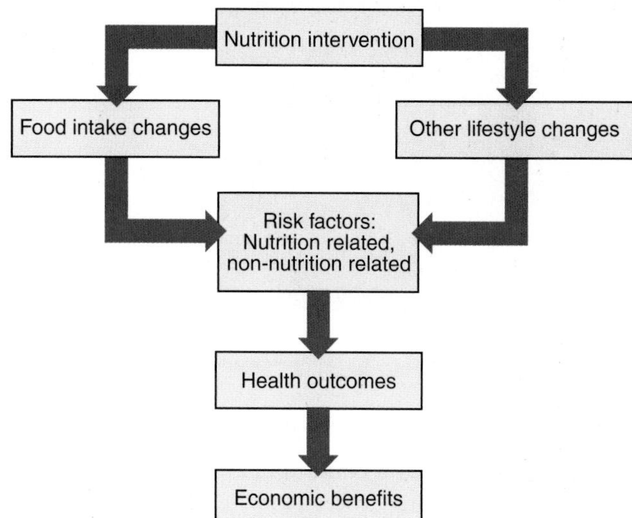

FIGURE 10-1 Model for dietary counseling. The goal of dietary counseling is to bring about a change in food and lifestyle behaviors that will lower the risk of chronic disease. (Redrawn from Olendzki MC, Tolpin HG, Buckley EL: Evaluating nutrition intervention in atherosclerosis: some theoretical and practical considerations, J Am Diet Assoc 79 (7):9, 1981. Reprinted with permission.)

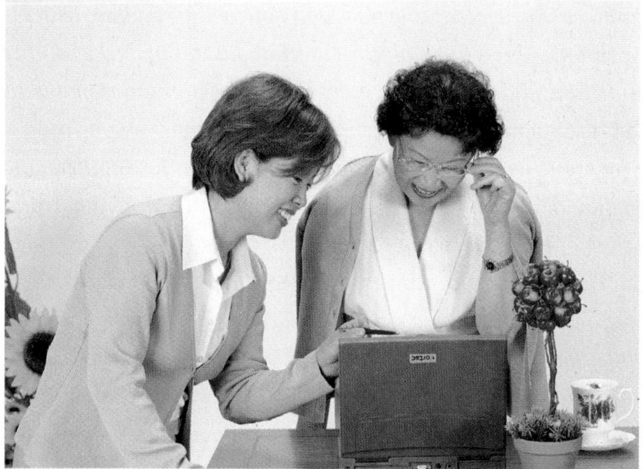

FIGURE 10-2 Sitting at a table with your client in a quiet place provides a supportive environment for communication. Online nutrition education materials can be helpful in nutrition counseling. (Copyright 2006 JupiterImages Corporation.)

KEY TERMS

demographic Statistical data describing a population according to age, income, gender, household size, ethnic or cultural group, education, or place of residence.

acculturation The process by which newcomers to a country or region begin to adopt the practices of their neighbors; this term often refers to the adoption of new foods or food patterns by individuals moving to the United States.

as important. Be aware of your own feelings and biases, and work to control them. Your evaluation of a situation must be based on facts, not opinions, assumptions, or inferences. Finally, you must hold compassion for others, accepting their emotion and absorbing its meaning.

Counseling as a Process

Nutrition counseling is a process, not something that "happens to a person" and instantly changes his or her behavior. Counseling involves small steps that over time lead to an improved nutritional status or disease condition. The goal will depend on the situation. In a clinical setting, counseling might involve helping a person newly diagnosed with diabetes to set up a meal pattern to achieve target blood glucose levels. In a school the goal for individual or group counseling might be helping children choose lower-fat snacks to support a healthy weight. In a community health center, counseling for a mother may focus on meal planning to improve the nutrient intake of her family. Regardless of the audience and goal, the steps in the process are the same, as follows:

- *Establish the need:* What is the nutritional problem or health risk of this individual? What nutrients are low in the individual or family diet? Does this person lack the resources to purchase an adequate supply of food?
- *Set the goal:* What does the individual want to do about the problem? What is his or her immediate goal? What is the long-range goal?
- *Determine the information or resources required:* What information does the client need for personal decision making? What knowledge and skills are necessary to alleviate the existing health problem or reach the goal? What referrals to other agencies or programs will be necessary? What resources do I need as a counselor to effectively intervene in this situation?
- *Plan a course of action:* What has to happen to reach the goal set by the client? What plan of action is best for solving the health problem or increasing nutrient intake? How can I best meet the client's personal needs? What steps is the client willing to take to move toward the goal?
- *Evaluate progress and readjust:* Has the action plan been effective in moving toward the goal? Is it solving the problem or meeting the need? If not, then why not? Is the client comfortable with the ongoing plan—has progress been too rapid or too slow? What changes or additions are indicated? What further information or resources are needed?

Nutrition counseling can involve one session or extended interaction over weeks or months, depending on the complexity of the problem. For an individual in good health who wishes to improve his or her nutrient intake or make better choices in the marketplace, one or two face-to-face meetings may be adequate, with a telephone follow-up to check on progress. (For further discussion of telephone counseling, see the *Evidence-Based Practice* box, "New Communication Methods: Are They Effective in Nutrition Education?")

When a patient has been diagnosed with diabetes, renal disease, or severe risk of heart disease, extended meetings over time will likely be necessary to reach short-term and long-term goals. A short-term goal may be lowering sodium

EVIDENCE-BASED PRACTICE

New Communication Methods: Are They Effective in Nutrition Education?

The complications of everyday life (i.e., work, school, and family responsibilities), along with transportation costs, make it difficult to schedule face-to-face nutrition counseling sessions. Telephone calls or text messages to monitor progress and offer advice can be a solution when long-term follow-up is needed. Evidence indicates that such methods are successful with various age- and interest groups.

Personalized Telephone Counseling

Telephone interventions used alone or in combination with other teaching methods helped participants increase their intakes of fruits, vegetables, and whole grains. Among 97 adults ranging from 21 to 84 years of age, a series of eight telephone calls over a 3-month period led to a 67% increase in vegetable servings, a 71% increase in fruit servings, and a 40% increase in servings of whole grains. Participants received calls every 3 to 4 days at the beginning of the program, which tapered off to every 10 days as the program neared completion. A 4-year intervention with breast cancer survivors used telephone calls as part of a comprehensive program that also included monthly newsletters and occasional cooking classes. Literacy- and language-appropriate materials that can supplement telephone counseling have an important role in delivering the knowledge and skills needed for chronic disease management.

The relative success of telephone counseling as compared with face-to-face counseling could depend on the age, gender, or other characteristics of participants. An activity program (offered in small groups or through biweekly telephone calls) helped people increase their physical activity. However, small group meetings were more successful with women, Hispanic and Latino participants, and those with increased body weights or multiple health conditions. The telephone intervention was more successful with participants who had a high level of social support from family or friends.

Automated Telephone Messages

An automated telephone system was used to provide ongoing encouragement and information to parents of overweight children. After an initial face-to-face meeting and distribution of written materials, parents received either no further assistance or a series of automated telephone calls asking them to report their progress and providing food or activity ideas. Children in families receiving the periodic telephone calls decreased their

Continued

EVIDENCE-BASED PRACTICE

New Communication Methods: Are They Effective in Nutrition Education?—cont'd

body mass index (BMI), whereas the other children did not. Even an automated telephone call and the expectation to report appear to provide ongoing **motivation** for change.

Short-Message Service (Text Messaging)

Short text messages may have a role in health promotion or clinical support; however, the type of information presented, the interaction between the sender and the learner, and the overall interest of the learner influences the overall success. Text messaging that supported an active interchange between the patient and the health professional was associated with reductions in blood pressure, improved glycemic control, and increased physical activity in several clinical evaluations. In contrast, programs in which the same message was sent to all participants with no opportunity for questions or report of progress resulted in little or no change in behavior. Just as in face-to-face programs, motivation has a role in the success of message programs. Random messages to individuals who have not enrolled in the message program are of little value in health promotion.

Telephone and text messages can be effective when used alone or as part of a broad-based intervention strategy; however, it is important to consider the audience and how the intended goals might best be achieved. Further research can provide a basis for decision making as to the most successful approach for a given client or group.

BIBLIOGRAPHY

Estabrooks PA, Shoup JA, Gattshall M, et al: Automated telephone counseling for parents of overweight children: a randomized controlled trial, *Am J Prev Med* 36:35, 2009.

Fjeldsoe BS, Marshall AL, Miller YD: Behavior change interventions delivered by mobile telephone short-message service, *Am J Prev Med* 36:165, 2009.

Newman VA, Flatt SW, Pierce JP: Telephone counseling promotes dietary change in healthy adults: results of a pilot trial, *J Am Diet Assoc* 108:1350, 2008.

Pierce JP, Newman VA, Natrajan L, et al: Telephone counseling helps maintain long-term adherence to a high-vegetable dietary pattern, *J Nutr* 137:2291, 2007.

Wilcox S, Dowda M, Dunn A, et al: Predictors of increased physical activity in the Active for Life program, *Prev Chronic Dis* 6(1):A25, 2009. Retrieved May 15, 2010 from http://www.cdc.gov/pcd/issues/2009/Jan/07_0244.htm.

or sugar intake, or bringing dietary intake into closer alignment with the Acceptable Macronutrient Distribution Range (AMDR). Long-term goals may involve weight loss, achieving a more favorable blood lipid profile, or decreasing blood pressure medication. Unfortunately, the cost of nutrition counseling and limited insurance reimbursement often limits the scope of intervention possible.

Effective nutrition counseling requires strong interpersonal communication skills. A simple checklist for evaluating your communication skills might include the following:

- Did you use language appropriate to the listener?
- Did you present information in a way that could be easily remembered?
- Did you provide examples that could be applied to the listener's personal situation?

Over time these methods will become an established part of your approach to nutrition education.

Communication as a Process

Successful communication involves four elements: (1) the sender, (2) the receiver, (3) the message, and (4) possible interference.[3] Each is important to the success or failure of the communication process:

1. *Sender:* Language, tone of voice, facial expression, body language, and **attitude** toward the receiver influence communication success.
2. *Receiver:* The receiver's opinion of the sender, motivation toward improving diet or health, available resources to bring about the recommended change, or feelings of hopelessness or self-efficacy will influence receptiveness to the sender and the message.
3. *Message:* Messages are verbal and nonverbal. Messages that are understood, realistic, and perceived as doable are likely to be received favorably. Directives that are condescending, impossible for the client to achieve, or include criticism of past behavior will cut short verbal communication. Nonverbal communication including dress, posture, facial expression, or evidence of listening influences the responses of both parties.
4. *Possible interference:* Environmental distractions such as a crying baby, uncomfortable conditions in the meeting room, the health condition of sender or receiver, or cultural expectations that are violated interfere with effective communication.

Effective communicators develop skills in analyzing the counseling situation and responding appropriately. When working with a client who has no interest in changing behavior, it is difficult to maintain composure or find ways to motivate that individual. Careful listening and observation, enabling you to evaluate the verbal and nonverbal communication of your client, can assist in developing a helping relationship and successful intervention. (Table 10-1 provides an example for modifying your approach according to the attitude of the client.) (To learn more about cultural influences on verbal and nonverbal communication see the *Focus on Culture* box, "Counseling and Culture: Respecting Cultural Differences.")

KEY TERMS

motivation Forces that affect individual goal-directed behavior toward satisfying needs or achieving personal goals.

attitude Aspect of personality leading to a consistent behavior toward persons, situations, or objects.

TABLE 10-1 LEVELS OF PERSONAL RESPONSIBILITY AND INTERVENTION METHODS: A DIABETES EXAMPLE

LEVEL OF PERSONAL RESPONSIBILITY	CLIENT CHARACTERISTICS	INTERVENTION METHOD
1. Having diabetes is a disaster.	Feels hopeless, helpless, defeated; self-care may be difficult	Educate family member or other caregivers
2. Having diabetes is a burden.	Blames problem on others; expects others to feel sorry for him or her; feels angry, threatened	Provide emotional support, help client accept anger to move on
3. Having diabetes is a problem.	Blames self as often as others, personal growth is possible	Reinforce attitudes that reflect sense of responsibility, examine irresponsible attitudes in a nonjudgmental way
4. Having diabetes is a challenge.	Rarely blames others for problem, recognizes responsibility but does not always act on it, good self-care expected	Point out discrepancies between stated need and actual behavior
5. Having diabetes is an opportunity.	Takes total responsibility, acts positively on decisions, optimal self-care is expected	Provide tools required for good self-care

FOCUS ON CULTURE

Counseling and Culture: Respecting Cultural Differences

Culture has sometimes been compared with an iceberg. An iceberg has a section above the water line that is clearly visible and a section below the water line that cannot be seen. This is also true of culture. All societies have underlying assumptions and values—invisible to outsiders—that guide a person's observed behavior. In working with families, we must be sensitive to not only how our clients respond but also why they respond as they do. Several differences that guide behavior across cultures are described in the following sections.

Individual or Group Orientation

In some cultures the emphasis is on the individual, or the *I*, whereas others give importance to the *we*. Those who tend to be group oriented are more likely to share whatever food or other resources they have with neighbors or their extended family. In group-oriented cultures an effort is made to save face and not make known a lack of food or inappropriate living conditions.

Locus of Control

Cultures differ in their view of a person's ability to control the forces around them and shape their own destiny. People with an internal locus of control see few limits to what they can do or become as long as they set their mind to it. Such a person with a family history of heart disease will be receptive to lifestyle changes that will lower his or her risk of a heart attack. People with an external locus of control assume that life is predetermined—what will be will be—and there is not much one can do about it. This individual could be less receptive to dietary intervention, considering such changes to be of no use in altering the health outcome.

Patterns of Communication

Messages among members of different cultures can be misunderstood. Some cultures are very direct in their communication with explicit and to-the-point words and phrases. Others have an indirect style, with understatement and nonverbal cues. In these groups what is not said may be the true message. Body language, eye contact, and tone of voice are important aspects of indirect communication. Mannerisms interpreted as rude or condescending or taken to indicate lack of interest in what is being said will quickly disrupt any rapport that had developed between counselor and client. Following are a few examples:

- *Personal space:* Americans like a lot of room. Try sitting next to the only passenger on a city bus and note the level of anxiety you create. In many other cultures, closeness is acceptable behavior. Our distance from a client may affect his or her comfort level.
- *Eye contact:* Americans show respect by looking each other straight in the eye. Asians indicate respect by looking downward. Interchanging these behaviors is often interpreted as being rude.
- *Speech inflection:* The tone of voice and its loudness and inflection can be threatening or comforting, depending on the cultural expectations of the listener.

You cannot always be aware of a client's attitudes toward body language ahead of time; however, you can take note of any signs of uneasiness and consider what might be making them uncomfortable.

BIBLIOGRAPHY

Holli BB, Calabrese RJ, O'Sullivan-Maillet J: *Communication and education skills for dietetics professionals*, ed 4, Philadelphia, 2003, Lippincott Williams & Wilkins.

Peace Corps Information Collection and Exchange: *Culture matters: the Peace Corps cross-cultural workbook*, Washington, DC, 1997, U.S. Government Printing Office.

Theories for Behavior Change

Behavioral theories are useful because they provide a framework for helping us understand why people do what they do and help us target our intervention strategies more effectively.[8] Behavior models used in nutrition education have included the health belief model, the concept of self-efficacy, and the stages of change model. We describe each of these following:

- *Health belief model:* Some individuals base their health behavior on their perceived vulnerability to a particular disease or condition. According to this model an individual would need to consider himself or herself at high risk for developing a condition, regard it as a serious threat to personal well-being, and believe that changing his or her behavior would lessen the risk.[9] This model also implies that any barriers to behavior change could be successfully overcome. A young woman planning a pregnancy might begin using a folate supplement to prevent a neural tube defect in her child or an overweight older adult might begin a walking program to lower his or her cardiovascular risk.
- *Self-efficacy model:* This theory proposes that behavior change is influenced by the demands it will make on the individual and his or her perceived ability to cope with the new situation.[3] The greater the person's confidence in his or her ability to successfully perform the new task or adapt to the new situation, the more likely it is that he or she will implement the behavior change. Successful interventions work by providing the client with the necessary tools or resources to practice the new behavior. Helping a frequent traveler develop a list of restaurant items that will fit into a lower-fat eating plan or helping a mother look at ways to add a vegetable to the evening meal increases the likelihood the goal will be achieved.
- *Stages of change:* This model was first developed to address smoking cessation[10] but has been used successfully to modify nutrition behavior.[11–13] It proposes that individuals pass through five stages of change in adopting a new behavior. How a person responds to the information presented and the type of information and resources needed differ according to stage. Table 10-2 outlines the

TABLE 10-2 STAGES OF CHANGE MODEL FOR NUTRITION BEHAVIOR

STAGE	BEHAVIORAL CHARACTERISTICS	STRATEGY	EXAMPLES
Precontemplation	Individual has no desire or intention to change, may refuse to admit a problem exists	Focus on consciousness-raising, family support may be helpful	Public service announcement about need for folate before pregnancy, poster in school cafeteria about eating fruit for quick energy, diagnosis of high blood pressure by physician
Contemplation	Individual recognizes the problem and has given some thought to what he or she might do about it—maybe in the next 6 months	Provide information that might be useful in addressing the problem	Printed materials from the health department describing food sources of folate or available supplements; leaflets available in the school cafeteria about carrying fruit in your backpack for snacks or notice of websites describing energy content of fruit; printed materials on how to reduce sodium intake or recipes for herbal mixtures to replace salt; personal evaluation of current folate, snack food, or sodium intake
Preparation	Individual is getting ready to commit to change; this stage provides the foundation for effective action	Provide resources or tools to support change	Checks availability of supplements and talks with pharmacist about options, checks out the price of fruit and availability at the school snack shop or nearby convenience store, talks with parent about putting fruit on the grocery list, looks up the kilocalorie (kcalorie or kcal) content of various fruits on the Internet, looks for low sodium recipes on several websites, talks with physician about safety of salt substitutes, joins a class at the local hospital on healthy eating
Action	Individual has implemented at least one behavior change and is trying to practice it regularly for 6 months	Encouragement and reinforcement; progress continues despite an occasional relapse	Takes a folate supplement on most days and tries to have a good folate food source at least once a day, packs an apple or banana or orange for snacking on most days rather than chips, adds no salt in cooking and less at the table, tries some new low-sodium recipes
Maintenance	Individual has successfully implemented the behavior change for more than 6 months	Continuing encouragement and reinforcement	New habits now a way of life, follows positive patterns most of the time

sequence and role of the nutrition counselor as applied to an individual or population.

Although theories are described individually, in practice they often are used in combination. Individuals passing through the stages of change are more likely to be successful if given tools that increase their feelings of self-efficacy regarding their new food behavior. As you continue to grow as a nutrition counselor, look for clues to indicate your client's current "stage" and let this guide your intervention strategy.

THE TEACHING-LEARNING PROCESS

Learning and Behavior

Despite our knowledge of behavioral theory, the myth still prevails that if health information is provided, then health practices will automatically improve. Learning is ultimately measured by a change in behavior. The need to apply new learning to self-care is especially important when working with adults. Children are accustomed to learning ideas or facts because they are expected to do so. Adults will learn only those principles for which they believe they have an immediate need.[14]

Principles of Learning

Learning follows three basic laws: (1) learning is *personal* and occurs in response to an individual need, (2) learning is *developmental* and builds on prior knowledge and experience, and (3) learning brings *change*.

Individuality

We all learn according to our own needs, in our own way and time, and for our own purpose. An initial force in learning is personal motivation. People learn only what they believe will be useful to them, and they retain only what they think they will need. The sooner a person can put new learning to use, the more likely he or she will grasp it. This highlights the importance of hands-on application and the need to provide an opportunity for the learner to practice the behavior before the counseling session or class is dismissed. As nutrition educators, we must devise new teaching strategies to meet the differing needs of learners and learning situations.

Point of Contact

Learning begins at the point of contact between prior experience and knowledge and the new concepts being presented—an overlap of the new with the familiar. Find out what the learner already knows and to what past experiences the new knowledge can be related. Search for areas of association, and relate your teaching to that point of contact.

The nutrition educator who builds on clients' needs and goals has the greatest chance for success. Encouraging learners to set personal goals promotes responsible self-care in contrast to the prescriptive approach. Personal goal setting requires more time initially but achieves far greater results over the long term.

The American Dietetic Association has developed four nutrition principles for helping individuals improve their diets[15]:

1. It is the total diet rather than one meal or one food that is important.
2. All foods can fit into a healthy diet if used in appropriate amounts and combined with physical activity.
3. Balance, variety, and moderation are key to a healthy diet.
4. Take a positive approach to food.

These principles help avoid confusion in the face of the many and often conflicting media reports about health and nutrition. Nutrition education is most effective when it builds on easy-to-understand concepts such as MyPyramid: choose a variety of fruits, vegetables, and grains; limit fats, sugars, and salt; and exercise regularly.[16]

THE ECOLOGY OF MALNUTRITION

The word *ecology* comes from the Greek word *oikos,* which means house. It refers to the relationship between individuals and their environment. Just as many forces within a family interact to influence its members, so forces in our physical and social environment interact to produce malnutrition and disease. Malnutrition occurs at all income levels but is more likely a problem for limited resource families who lack adequate funds for food. These individuals are also faced with inferior housing, limited education constraining job opportunities, and poor health care that in combination negatively influence nutrition and health. In this section, we explore the common elements of these problems and consider our role in addressing such needs.

Worldwide Prevalence of Malnutrition

Malnutrition as a worldwide public health problem continues to grow in scope. Globally, the unequal distribution of food leaves a fifth of the world's population chronically undernourished.[17] Over half of the child deaths occurring worldwide are associated with malnutrition, and about one third of children under age 5 have stunted growth.[18] Hidden hunger results in iron deficiency in women and vitamin-A deficiency in young children.[19] Problems in food and income distribution rather than a lack of available food are often the roots of malnutrition. Close to 80% of malnourished children around the world live in countries that report food surpluses.[18]

Even in the midst of plenty, millions of families have insufficient supplies of food.[20] Nearly 12% of U.S. households, representing over 38 million people and nearly 14 million children, experience food insecurity at least once within a year, meaning they have limited or uncertain availability of nutritionally safe and adequate food (Box 10-1).[20] Eight percent of these

KEY TERMS

food insecurity Limited or uncertain availability of food and the inability to obtain a sufficient supply of nutritionally safe, adequate, and acceptable food through socially acceptable means.

families are food insecure without hunger, whereas 4% are food insecure with hunger. Food insecurity is most likely in households (1) with incomes less than the federal poverty level, (2) headed by a single parent, (3) headed by an African-American or Hispanic parent or caregiver, or (4) living in cities or in the southern or western regions of the United States.

Food shortages affect emotional and physical health.[21] The worry of not having enough food brings depression, anxiety, and stress; malnutrition in pregnancy results in low birth weight, putting an infant at risk. In addition, malnutrition adds to weakness and disability among older adults. Homelessness is often associated with food insecurity. Worldwide it is estimated that hunger and malnutrition have a cost equal to 46 million years of productive life.[18]

From the biologic standpoint, malnutrition results from an inadequate supply of nutrients to support normal cell growth and function. However, the real cause of malnutrition in mothers and their children is an interconnecting set of physical, social, cultural, economic, political, and educational circumstances (Figure 10-3). Each is more or less important at a given time and place for a given individual. If the adverse conditions are only temporary, then the malnutrition is short term and quickly alleviated with no long-standing threat to life. However, chronic malnutrition carries irreparable harm and, in severe conditions, death. For the **epidemiologist,** a triad of variables influences health and disease. These three variables—(1) the agent, (2) the host, and (3) the environment—also influence malnutrition.

BOX 10-1 QUESTIONS TO IDENTIFY FOOD INSECURITY

- In the last 12 months, did you ever run out of food and have no money to purchase food?
- In the last 12 months, did you or your children ever skip a meal because you had run out of food and had no money to purchase food?
- In the last 12 months, were you or your children ever hungry but did not eat because you did not have enough food and had no money to purchase additional food?
- In the last 12 months, did you ever cut the size of your children's meals because there was not enough food in the house and you had no money to purchase additional food?

Data from Hampl JS, Hall R: Dietetic approaches to U.S. hunger and food insecurity, *J Am Diet Assoc* 102:921, 2002.

Agent

The agent in malnutrition is a lack of food. As nutrients fall in short supply, physiologic changes begin to occur. Famine, poverty, war, unequal distribution of food across a region, or unwise choices from the food available contribute to malnutrition.

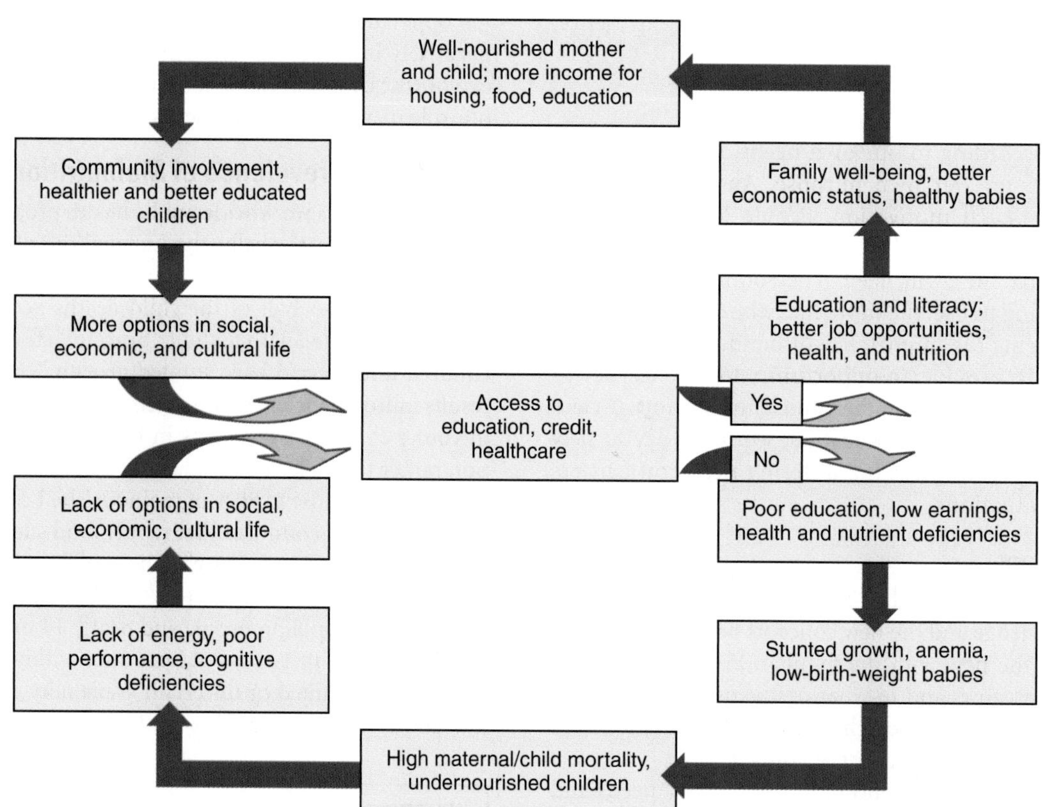

FIGURE 10-3 Breaking out of the cycle of despair. Access to education, health care, and credit enable mothers to adequately care for themselves and their children. (Redrawn from American Dietetic Association: Position of the American Dietetic Association: addressing world hunger, malnutrition, and food insecurity, *J Am Diet Assoc* 103:1046, 2003, with permission from the American Dietetic Association.)

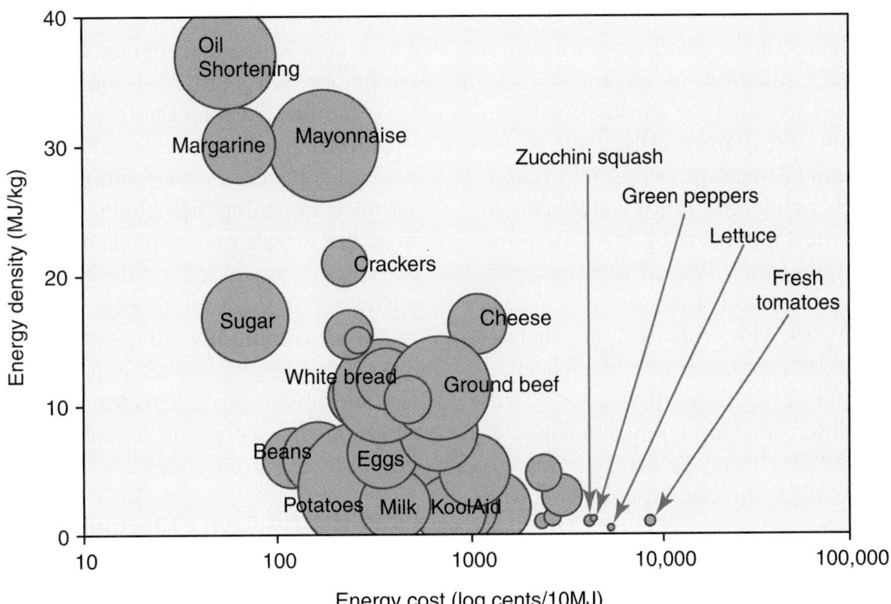

FIGURE 10-4 Relationship between energy density (megajoules/kilograms) and food costs (cents/10 MJ) for foods in the U.S. Department of Agriculture (USDA) Thrifty Food Plan. The size of the bubble indicates the amount of energy that each food contributes to the diet of a family of four during 1 week. Fresh fruits and vegetables that are expensive and contain many important vitamins and minerals make a very small contribution to energy intake. (See Chapter 8 to review measures of energy.) (Redrawn from Drewnowski A, Barratt-Fornell A: Do healthier diets cost more, *Nutr Today* 39(4):165, 2004. Used with permission.)

Host

The host is the infant, child, or adult who is malnourished. Physical characteristics such as infectious or chronic diseases; the needs of growth, pregnancy, or lactation; or heavy physical labor increase the severity of the problem. Personal factors such as emotional problems and poverty lead to malnutrition.

Environment

Lack of clean water, poor sanitation, cultural beliefs restricting appropriate food for certain groups, and poor agricultural potential are common in many places around the world. In all societies, agricultural and government policies influence food availability and distribution. Land management and erosion, government subsidies to support price structures, water distribution, or pesticide use influence food production. Food assistance programs, if available, provide nutrition support to vulnerable population groups.

The Problem of Poverty

In low-income families the constant need to obtain enough food can seem almost insurmountable. Individuals may be forced to acquire food that has been discarded by others; taking food from dumpsters despite the risk of foodborne illness.[22] They often purchase dented cans or day-old foods being sold at a reduced price. Families will fish from polluted streams or lakes despite the health risk if food is in short supply.[23] Mothers may visit more than one food pantry to obtain a sufficient amount of food for their families. When food money is limited, families purchase food that is high in kcalories and low in cost. This limits their use of fresh fruits and vegetables that supply important micronutrients.[21] Figure 10-4 compares the energy density and cost of a variety of foods. Staples such as bread, ground meat, and cereals provide more kcalories and satiety for a hungry family when food money is inadequate.[24] Low-income mothers would rather satisfy their children's hunger than provide particular fruits and vegetables that are high in nutrients but also high in cost.[25] The need to emphasize energy-dense foods plus the tendency to eat more when food is available are believed to contribute to the increased prevalence of obesity in limited resource families.[21]

Extreme pressures and difficult living conditions bring feelings of isolation, powerlessness, and insecurity—emotions that influence the use of community health services. For a family struggling day-to-day to survive, long-range preventive health practices appear to have little relevance. Health hazards inherent in poor housing and poor nutrition are often compounded by distance from sources of health care. An inadequate supply of food, with its deep psychologic and emotional influence, adds to mental and physical risk.[26]

KEY TERMS

epidemiologist A medical scientist who studies the causes, occurrence, distribution, control, and prevention of disease.

The Role of the Health Professional

If we are to be agents of constructive change, we must first understand an individual's situation in its broad social setting. The client may not see what we consider to be an overriding health problem as the most critical life factor needing his or her attention. For example, a mother who has no food in the house for her children's lunch is not likely to regard her diabetes as her most important problem. Genuine helpfulness and kindness grow from within; their basic ingredients are a concern for people and the desire to improve their situations. We must work with other team members—the physician, social worker, psychologist, nurse, pharmacist, physical therapist, and occupational therapist—to cut through the maze of conditions that hinder the implementation of health or dietary advice. It may be necessary to provide actual food resources before practical diet intervention can begin.

FAMILY ECONOMIC NEEDS: FOOD ASSISTANCE PROGRAMS

Families under economic stress often need food assistance to meet nutritional needs. Programs funded by local communities or the U.S. government supply food directly, or they increase food-buying power to provide additional nutrients. Federally funded assistance programs often target specific populations, whereas local food banks are likely to serve all age or gender groups.

United States Department of Agriculture Programs

The U.S. Department of Agriculture (USDA) oversees several food assistance programs intended to serve as a safety net for low-income Americans. Goals include (1) providing access to food, (2) promoting a healthy diet, and (3) implementing nutrition education. It is estimated that one in six Americans participates in a food assistance program.[9] Some programs are entitlement programs, in which specific income guidelines determine eligibility and guarantee participation.

Food Stamps (Supplemental Nutrition Assistance Program)

The Food Stamp program, renamed in 2008 as the *Supplemental Nutrition Assistance Program (SNAP)* with a new focus on nutrition and increased dollar benefits, increases food-buying power. SNAP is an entitlement program, reaching individuals and families having incomes within 130% of the federal poverty line. In 2006, more than 27 million people were receiving food stamps at a cost of more than $30 billion, making this the largest U.S. food assistance program.[27] Although SNAP makes a significant contribution to the food resources of low-income families, many recipients still run out of food before the end of the month and rely on local food pantries for help. The Food Stamp Act also authorizes funds for nutrition education. (Lists of items that may or may not be purchased using food stamps can be found in Appendix F.)

Meal Programs

The School Nutrition Program supervised by USDA provides all children with a nutritious lunch at moderate cost. Children from families meeting the federal poverty guidelines receive their lunch free or at reduced cost.[28] When it became apparent that many children were coming to school without breakfast, seriously impeding their ability to learn, the National School Breakfast Program was launched.[29] Children eligible for a free or reduced-cost lunch receive breakfast at the same level of payment. Local school districts, recreation departments, and nonprofit community groups sponsoring summer education or recreation programs can apply for USDA funds for breakfast and lunch meals. This food is especially important for children who depend on school meals for a significant portion of their nutrient intake.

Food Distribution Programs

The Special Supplemental Nutrition Program for Women, Infants, and Children (commonly called WIC) is administered through state health departments.[30] This program provides money for food and infant formula through food vouchers or electronic credit to low-income mothers who are pregnant, postpartum, or breast-feeding, as well as to infants and children up to the age of five who are at nutritional risk. WIC differs from entitlement programs in that income alone does not guarantee participation. Medical or nutritional risk must be certified by a health care professional for initial and continuing participation and a budgetary ceiling limits enrollment.

Programs for Older Americans

The Nutrition Program for the Elderly (NPE) enacted under the Older Americans Act is open to all adults age 60 and older, but services are targeted to those in greatest social and economic need. Particular attention is directed to low-income, minority, rural, and low-literacy seniors at risk for institutionalization.[31] Federal dollars are supplemented with state and local funds to meet the growing demand. Meals are served in congregate settings or home-delivered at noon, 5 days a week. Individuals receiving home-delivered meals must be certified as homebound by a health or social services professional. Participants are encouraged to make a donation toward the cost of the meal. Home-delivered meals programs sponsored by nonprofit community groups have a set charge, but they often offer scholarships for those who cannot afford to pay full price.

(For more information on food assistance programs and required nutrition standards, see Appendix F.)

Nutrition Education Opportunities

Food assistance programs offer unique opportunities for nutrition education. Pregnant and nursing mothers participating in WIC are helped with meal planning and use of allowable WIC foods. School food programs present examples of well-balanced meals with foods from the protein, fruit, vegetable, grain, and dairy groups, and breakfast includes milk or other high-calcium food. Teachers and school health and nutrition professionals can join together to provide educational experiences that connect the school meal with science and

TABLE 10-3 NUTRITION EDUCATION IDEAS FOR THE SCHOOL CLASSROOM

SUBJECT	ACTIVITIES FOR DIFFERENT GRADE LEVELS
Language arts	Read a story about food; keep a food diary for 3 days; write an article on nutrition for the school newspaper; write a food history of your family.
Mathematics	Using food pictures, count out the servings you need from each food group; calculate the kcalories, fat, protein, and carbohydrate in your lunch meal; look at the nutrition label on your favorite candy bar and, using the 2000-kcal diet, calculate how much fat you have left for the rest of the day.
Science	Learn about the nutrients that plants need to grow; trace the paths by which the body breaks down food to release protein, carbohydrate, and fat; do some simple microbiologic tests before and after washing your hands.
Social studies	Learn about the different breads that are eaten in various countries and how they are prepared; learn which nutrients must be listed on the nutrition label and how the U.S. Food and Drug Administration (FDA) enforces food labeling; work with the school lunch manager to have an international food day and study the culture of each country.
Art	Draw pictures of foods that we should eat every day; prepare posters advertising healthy foods offered in the school lunch; invent a healthy food and prepare a package and food label.
Health	Draw a picture of a healthy meal including all of the food groups; make a plan for obtaining 60 minutes of physical activity every day; evaluate your food diary according to the servings suggested in MyPyramid.

Ideas from Shepherd SK, Whitehead CS: *Team Nutrition's teacher handbook: tips, tools and jewels for busy educators,* Washington, DC, 1997, U.S. Department of Agriculture.

biology, social studies, and health (Table 10-3). In-school nutrition education and meals might be used to address the growing problem of child obesity.[32] For older adults the NPE offers time before or after the meal to address nutrition topics such as limiting sodium intake, low-cost meals for one or two, or good calcium sources.

EFNEP and SNAP-ED

The Expanded Food and Nutrition Education Program (EFNEP)[33] and Supplemental Nutrition Assistance Program-Nutrition Education Program (SNAP-ED)[34] funded by the USDA help limited-resource families learn about food and nutrition. EFNEP is available to all families falling below the federal poverty line, whereas SNAP-ED enrolls families on food stamps. These programs serve youth and adults and are delivered by Cooperative Extension agents, **paraprofessionals**, and volunteers. Experiential lessons offer hands-on opportunities to practice skills in food preparation, food safety, and food budgeting. Individuals are recruited through neighborhood contacts, food stamp offices, and WIC. Group classes, media methods, one-on-one instruction, and educational mailings reach different audiences. Follow-up evaluation indicated that 91% of EFNEP adults and 71% of EFNEP youth improved their food habits.[33]

Food assistance programs were intended to reduce food insecurity; however, food shortages continue to exist. Those most at risk for hunger include children, single-parent families, and older adults. It will be important for you to be aware of available food assistance programs in your community and make appropriate referrals.

Social Marketing

The concept of social marketing was first initiated about 40 years ago to describe the application of commercial marketing strategies to the development of programs that address social and health issues.[35] Just as product advertising creates a need on the part of consumers for a particular food or automobile or article of clothing, so appropriate nutrition education messages influence individuals to practice healthy behaviors. Fundamental to social marketing strategy is targeting a specific segment of society and their values, needs, and goals.[36] Programs directed at parents intended to increase fruit and vegetable servings or physical activity among young children might point to the related health benefits and reduced likelihood of early chronic disease for children observing these practices. Food safety messages often call attention to the disappointment and danger associated with poor cooking or storage of foods served at a holiday meal or family picnic. (See the Further Resources section to view some examples of social marketing campaigns.)

Social marketing also has a role in nutrition counseling. When recommending a food or lifestyle change to a patient

KEY TERMS

entitlement programs Government programs for which people are eligible or "entitled" based on income; all persons falling below a certain income level are eligible to receive food stamps.

poverty line The minimum amount of income required to provide food, clothing, shelter, and other basic necessities for a family of a given size and composition. This index is calculated by government economists and used to determine eligibility for government programs such as food stamps or free or reduced-cost school lunches.

paraprofessionals Individuals without a professional degree who work under the supervision of a health professional in providing nutrition education or other health or medical services. Paraprofessionals are often indigenous to the population or community they serve, giving them special rapport with their clients or patients.

or client, think about the intended outcome and how it might better the health or social well-being of this individual or family.

FOOD PURCHASING

Good nutrition is implemented through food; therefore helping people spend their food dollars to best advantage is integral to nutrition education.

Food Expenditures

The size and composition of a household influence the money spent for food. As household size increases, so do food costs—although the ages of the household members also make a difference in the money needed. The weekly average food cost of a preschooler is about half that of an adult, and women and girls consume less food than men and boys.[37] As household income rises, the total amount of money spent for food also rises—but not proportionately. Lower-income households are forced to spend more of their income for food as compared with higher-income households (Figure 10-5).[38] Those with increased incomes may not eat increased amounts of food, but they select more expensive food, buy more convenience items, and eat in restaurants more often.

USDA Food Plans

The USDA has developed several food plans that establish the minimum amounts of money required to purchase food for a month that will meet the DRIs and *Dietary Guidelines for Americans* for each age and gender group. They are referred to as *liberal, moderate, low, and thrifty,* with the thrifty plan used to calculate the dollar value of food stamps awarded to an individual or family.[37,39] For each food plan, a list of grocery items is provided that will meet the nutritional needs of an individual or family. (Examples of projected food costs under the various plans are found in Table 10-4.)

Developing a Family Food Plan

Each family has a specific amount of money they can spend for food and ideas as to how to divide their food dollars. When working with a family, the first step is to identify their food resources, as well as their values and preferences about food, because these will enter into their household food plan.

Food Resources and Skills

We usually consider money to be the major resource associated with a family's food, but skills that enable a person to cook a meal from scratch using simple ingredients are also a food resource. A comprehensive list of resources and skills follows:

- *Food budget in dollars:* This is the amount of money available to purchase food.

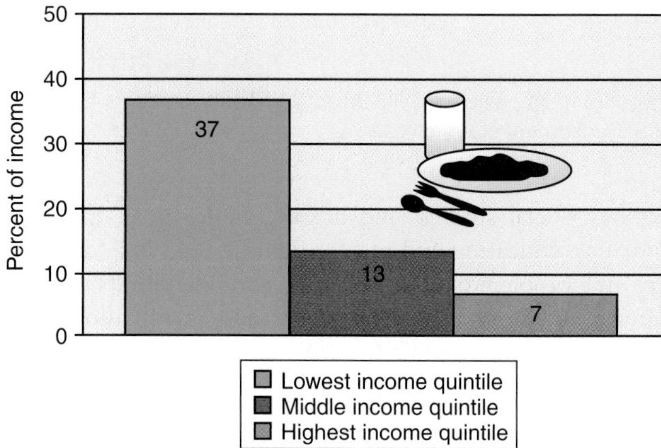

FIGURE 10-5 Lower-income families must spend a greater proportion of their income on food than higher-income families. Lower-income urban families spend 37% of their income on food compared with higher-income urban families who spend only 7%. (Data from Blisard N, Stewart H: *Food spending in American households, 2003-04,* EIB-23, Washington, DC, 2007, U.S. Department of Agriculture.)

TABLE 10-4 EXAMPLES OF USDA FOOD PLANS: AVERAGE COST OF FOOD AT HOME AT FOUR LEVELS*

	MONTHLY COST			
AGE-GENDER GROUP	**THRIFTY PLAN**	**LOW-COST PLAN**	**MODERATE-COST PLAN**	**LIBERAL PLAN**
Child, 2-3 years old	96.20	120.70	146.20	178.00
Male, 14-18 years old	162.50	226.60	282.00	323.90
Female, 19-50 years old	154.10	194.10	238.50	305.80
Couple, 51-70 years old	343.70	441.10	542.60	651.70
Couple, 19-50 years old and children—6-8 and 9-11 years old	602.50	779.40	973.80	1182.50

*The Food Plans represent a monthly food intake at four different cost levels that meets the nutrient requirements outlined in the 1997-2005 *Dietary Reference Intakes, 2005 Dietary Guidelines for Americans, and 2005 MyPyramid Food Intake Recommendations* and assumes that all meals and snacks are prepared at home. For specific foods and quantities of foods in the Food Plans, see *Thrifty Food Plan, 2006* (2007) and *The Low-Cost, Moderate-Cost, and Liberal Food Plans, 2007* (2007). Costs given are for individuals in four-person families.
This file may be accessed on the Center for Nutrition Policy and Promotion's home page: *www.cnpp.usda.gov/USDAFoodPlansCostofFood.htm.*

- *Food produced or preserved in the home:* Vegetables from a garden can be frozen or canned for later use; those in rural areas may raise animals for meat or eggs. Hunters may supplement their family food supply with fresh meat.
- *Access to food assistance programs:* Food stamps, WIC, commodity foods, free or reduced-cost meals for school-age children, meal programs for older adults, or food pantries add to family food.
- *Access to a well-stocked grocery store with competitive prices:* As supermarkets move away from the inner city to suburban areas where profit margins are increased, people living in downtown urban environments who lack transportation are forced to food shop at convenience stores with limited selection and increased prices. Older adults may have to shop at the store to which they can get a ride with a neighbor or friend. In rural areas, families may need to drive considerable distances to find a store with a good selection.
- *Time for food shopping:* Working single parents or working students may be rushed and not take time to read labels or look for the most cost-effective choice. Retired persons may see food shopping as an enjoyable way to pass the time.
- *Skills and experience in food management—planning, buying, preparation:* Adults who never learned to cook often rely on already prepared foods regardless of nutritional value or cost. Others may need help with reading food labels or understanding freshness codes. Physical limitations make it difficult to carry out food-related activities.
- *Facilities to store and cook food:* Most people have access to a cooking appliance and refrigerator, but homeless families or older persons living in single rooms lack cold storage and food preparation facilities.

Food Needs and Preferences

Food is a meaningful part of a family's relationships with each other, neighbors, and friends. Work and school patterns influence when and where family members eat. Characteristics important in developing a family food plan follow:

- *Family traditions:* Cultural, ethnic, and national groups often have specific food patterns that they wish to continue. Sometimes it is difficult to obtain certain foods or ingredients common to their meal pattern or, if available, they are high in price.
- *Special dietary needs:* Those observing a sodium-restricted diet or other meal plan related to a chronic condition may need certain foods. Severe food allergies such as gluten enteropathy require home preparation of basic foods and special ingredients.
- *Amount and kind of entertaining:* Families may enjoy sharing meals or joining potluck socials with neighbors, community organizations, or religious groups.
- *Meals away from home:* Work or school schedules can demand eating away from home, either a packed lunch or food purchased at that location. Families may enjoy eating out as part of their social framework.
- *Value placed on food and eating:* Food and mealtime may be an important part of a family's structure and interaction and hold high priority in allocation of family resources.

Extended discussion with family members about their food resources and preferences provides the framework for developing and implementing a successful food plan.

Food Shopping

Making Choices

Food marketing is a big business, and buying family food is more complex than it may seem. The typical American supermarket offers over 45,000 different food items,[40] and a single food item may be marketed in many different ways, all with different prices (Figure 10-6). Supermarket tours are effective strategies for developing decision-making skills and becoming mindful of marketing tactics that draw attention to expensive items low in nutrients. Figure 10-7 and the *Perspectives in Practice* box, "Supermarket Savvy," will help you hone your supermarket skills.

Planning Ahead

To ensure you are eating a variety of foods and the servings recommended by MyPyramid (see Chapter 1), plan meals for the week and then develop a shopping list. Review the food on hand and think about how perishable items will be used to avoid waste. Check local newspapers or store flyers for specials, and target those items that the family enjoys. Preparing a shopping list helps avoid impulse buying and extra trips to the store. To save time, grocery lists should be organized in the same order as the supermarket aisles. Avoid shopping when you are hungry or rushed because you will be more likely to buy items that you do not need or cannot afford. Limit shopping to once a week; plan to use frozen or canned items after fresh foods have been exhausted.

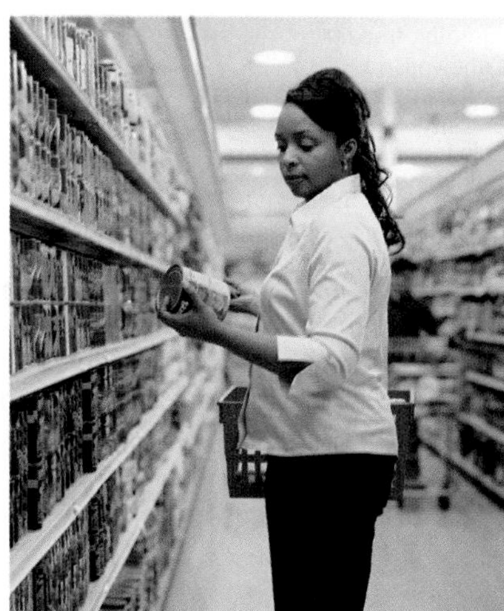

FIGURE 10-6 Shoppers are faced with a dazzling array of food choices. (From Food and Nutrition Service, U.S. Department of Agriculture and Food and Nutrition Information Center, National Agricultural Library: Food stamp nutrition collection: photo gallery, Beltsville, Md, 2005, U.S. Department of Agriculture. Retrieved August 19, 2009, from grande.nal.usda.gov/viewer.php?file=fs_recipes/imgs/shopping/shopping_vertical.jpg&file_loc=shopping_vertical.jpg. Reprinted with permission.)

Before shopping, I:	Hardly ever	Sometimes	Most of the time
Check to see what foods I have on hand	☐	☐	☐
Plan meals to include a variety of foods from each of the major food groups	☐	☐	☐
Plan food purchases to limit amounts of fat, sugars, and sodium	☐	☐	☐
Consider how much money I have to spend on food	☐	☐	☐
Make a shopping list	☐	☐	☐
While shopping, I:			
Read ingredient labels, watching for ingredients that provide fat, sugars, and sodium	☐	☐	☐
Use nutrition labels to help select food products	☐	☐	☐
Use open dating information to ensure quality and freshness	☐	☐	☐
Use unit pricing (when available) to compare prices	☐	☐	☐
After shopping, I:			
Store foods promptly and properly to maintain their nutritive value and quality	☐	☐	☐
Place newer foods in the back of refrigerator, freezer, and cabinet shelves, so older foods will be used first	☐	☐	☐
Use perishable foods promptly to avoid food waste	☐	☐	☐

FIGURE 10-7 The Super Shopper Checklist. Most people follow a general routine when they shop for food. Have your clients check the boxes that best describe what they do before, during, and after each trip to the supermarket. If "most of the time" is their answer, then they are super shoppers! (From U.S. Department of Agriculture: *Shopping for food and making meals in minutes using the dietary guidelines,* Home and Garden Bulletin No 232-10, Hyattsville, Md, U.S. Department of Agriculture.)

Buying Wisely

Food labels contain important information about food quantity, quality, and safety. Comparison shopping helps consumers get the best value for their food dollar. The following information on the food label and store shelf is helpful in comparison shopping.

- *Unit pricing:* Large packages are sometimes less expensive per unit weight than small packages, but any savings depends on how much of the product is needed and if it can be used within the appropriate time. If an item has an extended shelf life or is used regularly, then one large box rather than two smaller boxes is a wise choice. The unit pricing label on the store shelf indicates the true price per unit weight and is helpful when comparing different brands or package sizes (Box 10-2). Unit pricing tells you if the store brand is less expensive than the national brand for which you are paying the cost of advertising and any special offers.
- *Open dating:* These dates indicate the freshness of an item or how soon it must be used. Box 10-3 describes the types of dating information used on food labels. Checking the *use by* date is important when considering items reduced for quick sale.
- *Package weight or volume:* Check the food label and the nutrition label to determine the content of a package by weight or volume and the number of servings it contains. Deceptive packaging can suggest that the food content is greater than it really is.
- *List of ingredients:* Ingredients are listed by weight, from the highest to the lowest, on the food label. By reviewing this list, you can see what you are paying for. As described in Figure 10-8, fruit drinks contain sugar, water, and flavoring but little or no juice. When purchasing bread or cereal, make certain the first ingredient is a *whole grain.*
- *Convenience foods:* Use comparison shopping to evaluate the relative cost and time benefit of already prepared items, because time saved may not be worth the added cost. Fresh fruits and vegetables peeled and cut into bite-sized pieces and items packaged in single servings are handy when packing lunches or grabbing snacks, but they eat into the food budget. To save money, carrots could be peeled and packaged in lunch-size plastic bags over the weekend for use the next week. Pancake or muffin mixes or precooked meat loaves are not a prudent choice when food dollars are limited. Table 10-5 provides examples of added cost to already prepared items.

Storing Food Safely

Controlling food loss from food spoilage protects the family food dollar. Use covered containers or sealable plastic bags for dry, refrigerated, or freezer storage. Opened and partly used packages are best kept at the front of the shelf where they are visible and will be used first. Labels found on highly perishable foods such as meat, poultry, and fish give directions for preventing spoilage and contamination (Figure 10-9). Raw poultry is a source of contamination leading to foodborne illness and must be kept separate from other foods and work surfaces.

Cooking Food Well

Nutrition education for meal preparers should emphasize food preparation methods that maximize food nutrient content and control cost but also promote the joy of eating. Some ideas include the following:

- Preparation and cooking methods for fruits and vegetables that retain vitamins and minerals

PERSPECTIVES IN PRACTICE

Supermarket Savvy

As more shoppers are watching their weight and trying to choose healthy food, "supermarket savvy" is becoming a favored topic for nutrition education. Supermarket tours provide an opportunity for consumers to look at healthy alternatives across all food groups and develop more awareness of cost and nutrient quality. However, consumers also need to recognize the marketing techniques and triggers for impulse buying they will encounter when food shopping.

Topics That will Prepare Consumers for a Supermarket Visit Include the Following

When to shop: Advertised specials available at the beginning of the week are often sold out by the end of the week. In that case be sure to ask for a rain check if this is an item you will use. Weekday mornings or afternoons, or evenings, are the best times to shop because stores are less crowded, allowing more time and space for comparison shopping. On Saturdays and at dinnertime, stores are congested and checkout lines are long.

Wise use of coupons: Food manufacturers offer coupons in the newspaper, on-line, and in food packages. Most coupons do have a downside; for example, you may have to buy several packages or the largest size container to use your coupon or be enticed to buy something you do not need because it is "50 cents off." It may be that the store brand at full price is equivalent to or less than the national brand with a coupon. Make your shopping list first and then see if any of your coupons match; limit coupon use to those foods that you use regularly.

Store layout: Displays at the ends of the aisles may be set up for sale items but also are used for new or slow-moving items. Do not assume that cans or packages marked *special* are necessarily being sold at a lower price per unit weight. Stay aware of regular prices to better discern a true sale. National brands or more expensive items are usually placed at waist or neck level. Be sure to check the prices of the items on the bottom shelf as well.

The inner aisles of the supermarket usually contain less expensive staple items such as legumes, peanut butter, dry milk, canned tuna fish, bulk cereals, and canned vegetables and fruits. Fresh produce, on the other hand, is usually at the front of the store by the entrance, because it is a high-profit item and subject to impulse buying. In-store bakeries and delicatessen sections are also among the first counters passed as you begin your shopping. Be alert to these incentives to purchase foods that you do not need or cannot afford.

Unit pricing: Unit pricing is an important tool for comparison shopping, but consumers should be cautious when comparing a frozen with a canned product. Frozen vegetables contain little or no liquid as compared with canned vegetables that may contain as much as one third liquid. Even if the canned item costs less per ounce, it may not be a better buy based on the actual amount of food provided. Measure the liquid in the canned fruits and vegetables you purchase regularly to gain a perspective as to the real cost.

The USDA Cooperative Extension Service that exists in every state and county is a source of print and on-line materials to help consumers develop food shopping skills.

BIBLIOGRAPHY

Aase S: Supermarket trends: how increased demand for healthful products and services will affect food and nutritional professionals, *J Am Diet Assoc* 107:1286, 2007.

Kansas State Cooperative Extension Service: *We know.…Tips to trim food costs, MK-32,* Manhattan, Kan, 2008, Kansas State Cooperative Extension Service.

University of Kentucky Cooperative Extension Service: *Supermarket savvy,* FAM-RHF131, Lexington, Ky, 2004, University of Kentucky College of Agriculture.

- Thorough cooking and time-sensitive storage of protein foods for prevention of foodborne illness
- Use of herbs and spices rather than salt for seasoning
- Cutting down on added sugar and fat
- Using broiling, grilling, and baking as cooking methods rather than frying
- Applying principles of menu planning to provide appealing and healthful meals (Box 10-4)

People eat because they are hungry and because food looks and tastes good. Recipes that are cost-effective, nutritious, and attractive can help busy meal preparers make good use of their food dollars, especially if recipes are simple and easily remembered.[41] Many supermarket chains now provide healthy recipes on their websites or in their weekly flyers that use store specials.[40] Food demonstrations or hands-on classes with tasting are effective ways to model appropriate food safety and food preparation techniques and confirm that healthy food is good to eat.

HEALTH PROMOTION

MyPyramid Food Plan

In developing a family food plan, it is important to consider each food group and how it contributes to the overall plan. MyPyramid provides a guide for developing menus that meet the nutritional needs of all family members. Vegetables and fruits are major sources of vitamins, minerals, phytochemicals, and fiber. Aim for variety over the course of the week. A mix of fresh, frozen, and canned vegetables and fruits, depending on season and price, will help meet financial constraints. Home gardening or container gardening increases availability of vegetables. In some urban locations, community agencies sponsor gardening projects with opportunities for youth and family activities.

Grain foods are well liked, relatively inexpensive, and easily fit into meal plans. They provide complex carbohydrates and important vitamins and minerals. Whole grains are rich

BOX 10-2 UNIT PRICING

The unit price is the price per pound, ounce, quart, or other unit. Unit price labels are found on the display shelves or below canned and packaged foods. Comparing unit prices can help shoppers find the brand and size container that costs the least per unit.

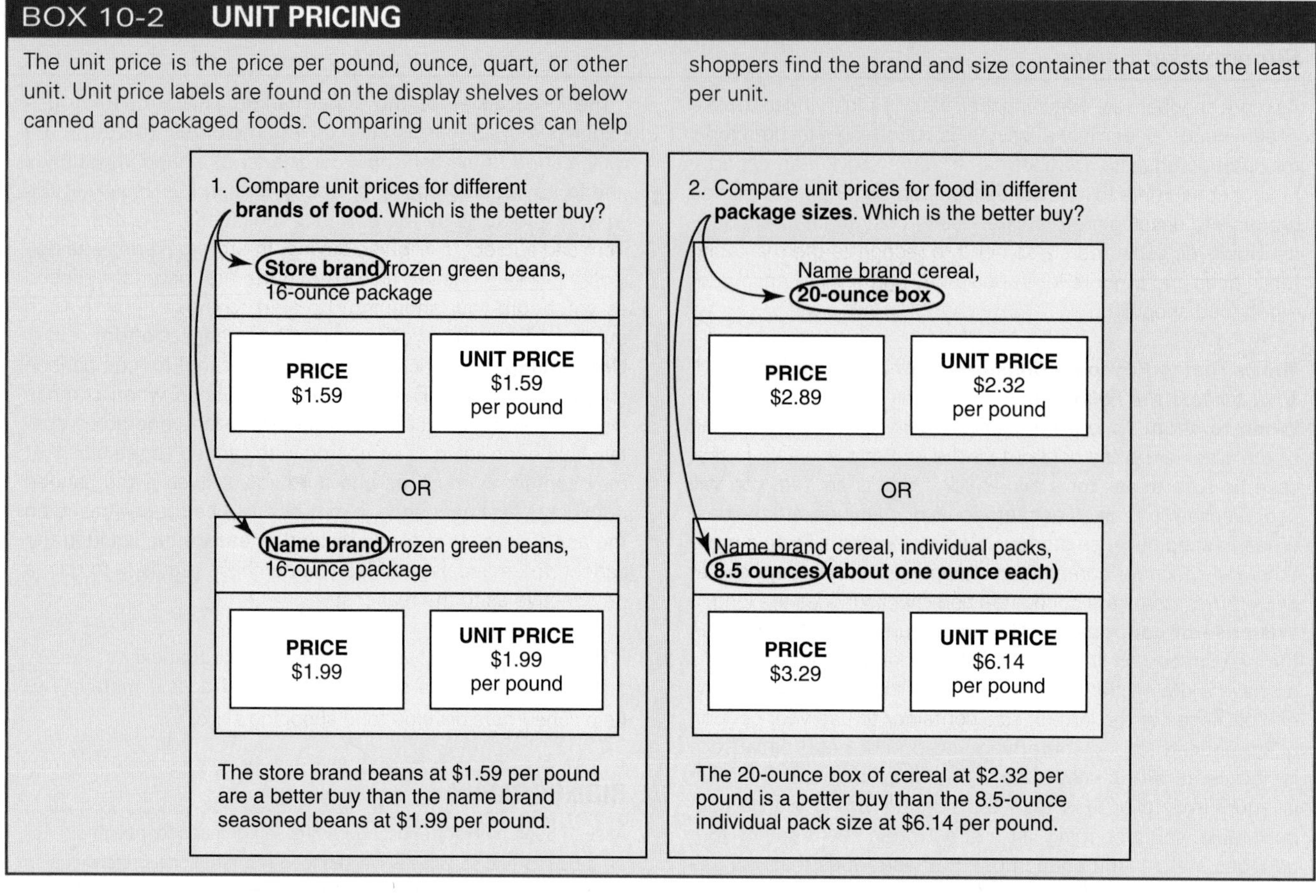

BOX 10-3 TYPES OF OPEN DATING ON FOOD LABELS

Sell by	The last date the item can be sold by the store
Best if used by	The date that indicates maximum freshness (After this date check for signs of spoilage and expect a reduced price.)
Expiration date or use by	The last date when active ingredients will be good—commonly used with yeast for baking (Do not purchase foods after their expiration date because spoilage may have occurred even if not visible.)
Pack date	The date when the food was packed (This date is commonly found on canned foods; look for a recent pack date.)

in fiber and especially high in trace minerals (Figure 10-10). At least three of our daily servings of grains should be whole grains.

Meat, fish, poultry, and eggs are complete proteins and contain B-complex vitamins and trace minerals. Eggs are relatively inexpensive sources of high-quality protein; for most people, four eggs per week is acceptable. Fish adds n-3 fatty acids to the diet (see advisory for pregnant women and children in Chapter 9). Trim visible fat and skin from meat and poultry to reduce intakes of saturated fat.

Dried beans and peas, and nuts are good sources of amino acids when combined with other plant proteins or animal foods. Legumes are low in fat, high in fiber and resistant starch, versatile in food preparation, and easy to store. Soy protein and soybeans are used to make tofu and are added to chips, pasta, trail mix, and other prepared foods.

Dairy foods provide protein and calcium, and most milk and yogurt are fortified with vitamin D. Low-fat forms of dairy foods are lower in kcalories and total and saturated fat.

Fats and oils supply the essential fatty acids and concentrated kcalories for those with high energy needs. Polyunsaturated and monounsaturated oils are the best choices and contain vitamin E. Hydrogenated fats often include *trans* fatty acids, which are harmful to health; therefore consumers should read nutrition labels carefully. Butter, high in saturated fat and a source of cholesterol, is best used in limited amounts. (Box 10-5 provides shopping hints for all major food groups; review Table 1-2 for detailed nutrient content of the major food groups.) (See the *Case Study* box, "Helping with Family Shopping" to apply principles of food shopping and planning.)

CASE STUDY

Helping with Family Shopping

The nurse at the local WIC (Supplemental Nutrition Program for Women, Infants, and Children) office has asked you to assist a family with their food selection. She is concerned about the nutrient intakes of the mother and children and their general food shopping and food preparation practices. The family consists of three adults, a woman age 26 and two men ages 27 and 69, and two children ages 5 and 2. Both children receive WIC food allocations. The mother goes food shopping almost daily and buys already prepared main dishes and any meat, dairy, and grain foods reduced for quick sale. To save money, she tries to use it all regardless of expiration or use by dates. She seldom buys fresh fruits and vegetables because they seem to be expensive, but fruit drinks are a family favorite.

Questions for Analysis

1. Based on the various food plans developed by the U.S Department of Agriculture (USDA), what is the minimum amount of money this family must spend on food to meet their nutritional requirements?
2. What questions would you ask this homemaker about her shopping practices?
3. What advice would you give her about food-buying practices to ensure food safety for her family? Which family members are most vulnerable to foodborne illness?
4. What suggestions could you give her about less expensive forms of fruits and vegetables? (See Box 10-5 and Table 10-5.) Are fruit drinks a good use of her food dollars?
5. Develop a 3-day menu for the family observing MyPyramid recommendations and using the WIC foods available to the children. Prepare a shopping list for the purchase of needed foods.

Ingredient Listing Ingredients are listed in order from the most to the least amount found in the product.

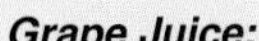

Grape Juice:

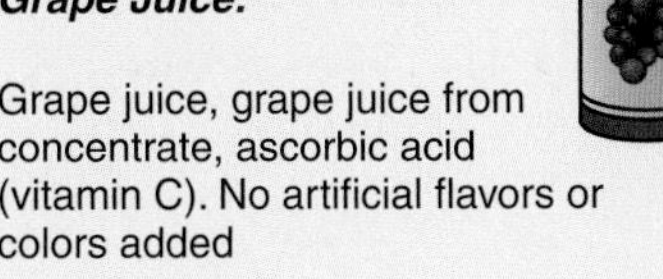

Grape juice, grape juice from concentrate, ascorbic acid (vitamin C). No artificial flavors or colors added

This label tells you:

- Mostly grape juice and juice concentrate
- Vitamin C added

Grape Juice Drink:
(10% Grape Juice)

Water; high fructose corn syrup; sugar; grape juice concentrate; fumaric, citric, and maltic acids (provide tartness); vitamin C; natural flavor; artificial color

This label tells you:

- Mostly added water, syrup, and sugar
- Some grape juice
- Vitamin C added, plus other things

Powdered Grape Drink:

Sugar, citric acid (provides tartness), natural and artificial flavor, artificial color, vitamin C

This label tells you:

- Mostly sugar
- No juice at all
- Vitamin C added, plus other things

FIGURE 10-8 Products with similar names can have very different ingredients and nutrient content. Read labels carefully to know what you are buying. (From U.S. Department of Agriculture: *Do you use unit prices to find the best buys? Make your food dollars count,* Program Aid No 1345, Washington, DC, 1984, U.S. Department of Agriculture.)

Food Shopping Locations

Supermarkets and Supercenters

Most people have access to at least one store that carries a wide variety of fresh and processed foods at reasonable prices. When several food outlets are close by, individuals can select where they want to shop or vary their location depending on the particular specials for the week. A trend in food marketing is the sale of groceries by supercenters that also sell a wide variety of nonfood merchandise. Food prices at such supercenters are 5% to 25% lower than those at more traditional supermarkets.[42] Stores serving low-income populations are generally smaller and older, have fewer checkout lines, and are open fewer hours. In urban areas, neighborhood groups are working with city governments to improve access to food supplies.[43] In rural areas often lacking public transportation, individuals may need to travel 20 miles or more to reach a supermarket.[44]

Farmers' Markets

Farmers' markets bring local produce to consumers at prices that are often lower than at supermarkets. Local fruits and vegetables are often considered to be fresher and look and taste better than similar items from a grocery store. Buying local produce also supports a local sustainable farm system.[45] The WIC program gives vouchers for use at farmers' markets.

TABLE 10-5 COST COMPARISONS OF HOME-PREPARED AND PREPREPARED FOODS

FOOD*	INGREDIENTS	SOME PREPARATION	ADDITIONAL PREPARATION
Vegetables			
Carrots	Unpeeled and uncut 3-oz serving (raw) at 18 cents	Small baby carrots peeled and washed 3-oz serving (raw) at 36 cents	Shredded carrots 3-oz serving (raw) at 81 cents
Potatoes	Fresh potatoes (from 5-lb bag, cooked/mashed) (milk and margarine added) ½ cup at 25 cents	Instant mashed potatoes (reconstituted/heated) (milk and margarine added) ½ cup at 37 cents	Refrigerated mashed potatoes (ready to heat) ½ cup at 84 cents
Protein Foods			
Chicken	Raw chicken breasts with skin and bone; 3-oz serving at 57 cents	Raw chicken breasts, skinless and boneless; 3-oz serving at 93 cents	Cooked chicken breast cut in strips for salads (no bones), 3-oz serving at $2.04
Ground beef	Ground chuck hamburger 3-oz serving (cooked) at 52 cents	Ground chuck hamburger preshaped into patties 3-oz serving (cooked) at 75 cents	Meat loaf refrigerated and ready to heat 3-oz serving (heated) at $1.32
Grains			
Oatmeal	Old-fashioned oats ¾-cup serving at 16 cents	Quick 1-minute oats ¾-cup serving at 16 cents	Instant oatmeal, unflavored ¾-cup serving (one packet) at 37 cents
Pancakes	Homemade batter One 4-inch pancake at 6 cents	Dry pancake mix, egg added One 4-inch pancake at 9 cents	Ready-to-pour batter One 4-inch pancake at 21 cents
Banana muffin	Homemade (partly whole wheat with fresh banana) 1 muffin at 14 cents	Banana muffin mix 1 muffin at 24 cents	
Sweets			
Chocolate chip cookie	Homemade cookie dough One 2-inch cookie at 7 cents	Refrigerated cookie dough (slice and bake) One 2-inch cookie at 12 cents	Packaged cookie One 2-inch cookie at 24 cents

*Costs based on market prices on the Harris Teeter Express Lane. Retrieved May 6, 2009, from www.harristeeter.com/shopping/express_lane/express_lane.aspx; ground meat calculated as cooked weight; recipes for home-prepared foods taken from Rombauer IS, Becker MR, Becker E: *Joy of cooking,* 75th anniversary ed, New York, 2006, Scribner.

Consumer Cooperatives

Consumer cooperatives offer high-quality foods at the lowest possible price. Food cooperatives usually deal in bulk sales of whole or minimally processed foods and emphasize locally grown items. Cooperatives usually require a certain number of hours of volunteer time from each member in addition to or in lieu of a membership fee.

Food Discount Stores

Food stores that stock fresh and processed foods, paper goods, and cleaning supplies at discount prices are growing in popularity. These stores offer few services, and furnishings are sparse; however, in exchange, food and other supplies are usually lower in price. Processed foods sold at food discount stores may be closeouts or excess stock that is nearing the date of expiration or best use. In addition, the units sold often include several cans or packages, so consumers must decide if the quantity being purchased can be used within the appropriate time.

Food Banks

Food banks are warehouses that collect and store donations of food from supermarkets, food processors, food distributors, growers, and the general public. These foods are made available to soup kitchens or food pantries providing meals or groceries to those in need. Food pantries offer emergency assistance when a family has no money or food stamps to purchase food. Food banks across the United States distribute more than a billion pounds of food each year.[46] USDA

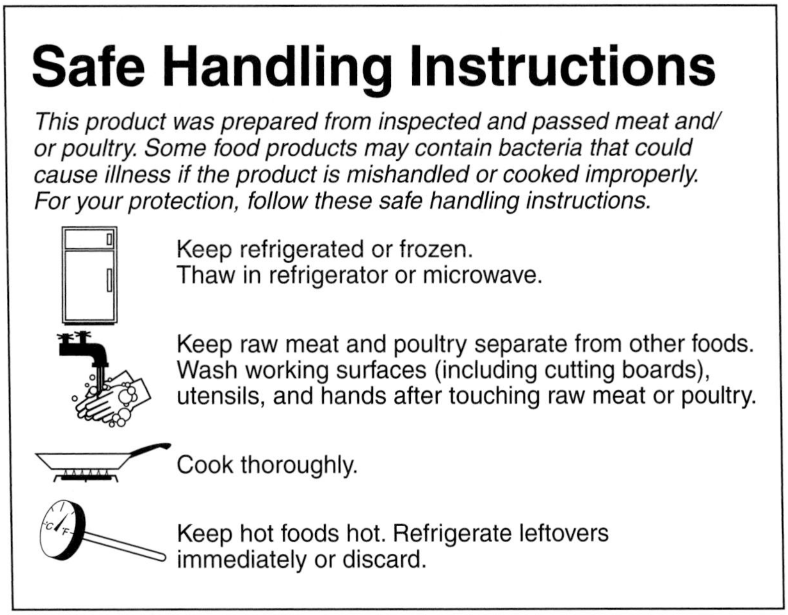

Safe Handling Instructions
This product was prepared from inspected and passed meat and/or poultry. Some food products may contain bacteria that could cause illness if the product is mishandled or cooked improperly. For your protection, follow these safe handling instructions.
Keep refrigerated or frozen. Thaw in refrigerator or microwave.
Keep raw meat and poultry separate from other foods. Wash working surfaces (including cutting boards), utensils, and hands after touching raw meat or poultry.
Cook thoroughly.
Keep hot foods hot. Refrigerate leftovers immediately or discard.

FIGURE 10-9 Food labels provide important information about safe storage and cooking of perishable foods. Labels on fresh and frozen meat, fish, and poultry advise consumers on how to store, thaw, and cook these foods to avoid foodborne illness. (From U.S. Department of Agriculture: *Safe handling label,* Washington, DC, U.S. Department of Agriculture.)

BOX 10-4 TIPS FOR MENU PLANNING

- *Strive for balance:* Try to avoid too many high-fat meals in the same week; for every high-fat meal, plan a low-fat meal on another day. If you have a high-fat item as a main dish, then serve a low-fat salad or vegetable at that meal.
- *Emphasize variety:* Try to mix raw and cooked items, for example, a casserole accompanied by raw fruit or salad greens. Do not serve the same type of food 2 days in a row, such as spaghetti with tomato sauce followed by ravioli with tomato sauce. Look to include different fruits and vegetables throughout the week to avoid monotony and obtain the various nutrients you need.
- *Add contrast:* Think about how food will look on the plate—avoid all-white or all-red meals and aim for different sizes and shapes. Mix textures with both soft and crisp foods at the same meal.
- *Consider eye appeal:* Think about color—overcooking vegetables causes loss in color. Try for the most attractive arrangement when placing food on the plate.

Adapted from U.S. Department of Agriculture: *Menu Planner for Healthy School Meals,* FNS 303, Washington, DC, Food and Nutrition Service, U.S. Department of Agriculture, 1998, Rev. 2008. Retrieved May 16, 2010, from http://teamnutrition.usda.gov/Resources/menuplanner.html.

commodity foods account for nearly 14% of the food distributed by emergency food providers, including food banks and soup kitchens.[47] (See Appendix F to learn more about commodity foods and the food items available.) Food banks tend to have more grains and meats than fruit and dairy products, limiting the vitamin A, vitamin C, and calcium available to users.[48]

Whole grain kernel
Bran
"Outer shell" protects seed
Fiber, B vitamins, trace minerals
Endosperm
Provides energy
Carbohydrates, protein
Germ
Nourishment for the seed
Antioxidants, vitamin E, B vitamins

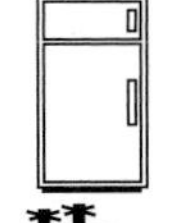

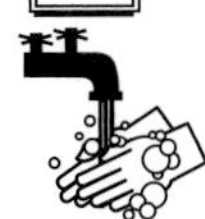

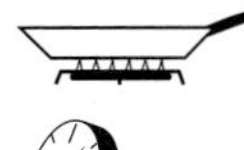

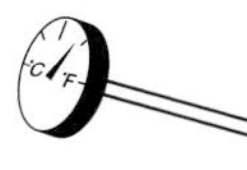

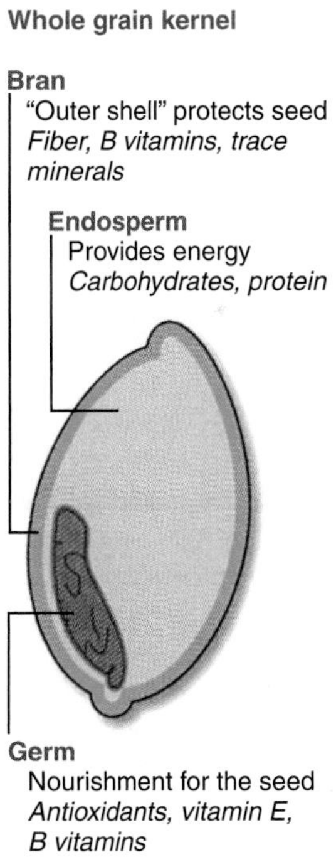

FIGURE 10-10 Nutrients in the bran and germ of whole grains are lost when grains are refined and the bran and germ are discarded. Current legislation requires that processed grains be enriched with thiamin, riboflavin, niacin, iron, and folate. (From U.S. Department of Agriculture: *Get on the grain train: putting the guidelines into practice,* Home and Garden Bulletin No 267-2, Washington, DC, 2002, U.S. Department of Agriculture.)

BOX 10-5 GETTING THE MOST FOR YOUR FOOD DOLLAR

Fruits and Vegetables

- Buy fresh fruits and vegetables in season when they cost less. Visit a farmers' market or a pick-your-own outlet to save money and enjoy a fun family activity.
- Choose produce that is firm, crisp, and free of brown or soft spots.
- Compare costs of fresh fruits and vegetables as sold by weight or count. Look for the number of items in bags sold by weight.
- Check the cost of store brands versus national brands when buying canned vegetables and fruits. Avoid fancy grades that are more expensive. Grading is based on shape, size, and perfection of pieces; lower grades are equal in food value and taste.
- Compare the cost of family-sized bags versus individual packages of frozen vegetables. It may be more cost-effective to buy the family-sized bag and pour out what you need. Return the unused portion to the freezer immediately to prevent thawing and loss of quality. Avoid frozen vegetables with special sauces that add to cost and increase fat and sodium.
- If possible, select juice- or water-packed canned fruits rather than syrup-packed canned fruits with added sugar. If using syrup-packed fruit, then rinse before serving.
- If possible, select no-sodium–added canned vegetables or rinse the higher-sodium product before using.

Breads and Cereals

- Check the weight of bread loaves when doing price comparisons, because a large loaf may not weigh more than a small loaf; higher-priced breads advertised as having fewer kcalories may be similar to other breads, just cut into thinner slices.
- Look for whole grain breads or cereals; the word *whole* should appear first on the ingredient list. Varieties include whole wheat, whole oats, oatmeal, whole rye, or whole grain corn or corn meal. (Popped corn is an easy, whole grain snack.)
- Avoid grain products with a sugar as the first or second ingredient. It is more cost-effective to add your own sugar to cereal and control the amount added; sugars commonly found on food labels include sucrose, fructose, molasses, honey, corn syrup, and high-fructose corn syrup (HFCS).
- Cereals providing 100% of the Dietary Reference Intakes (DRIs) for many vitamins and minerals cost more; if you eat a good diet, then these additional nutrients may be unnecessary. Look for those nutrients that you really need. If you eat daily multiple servings of these cereals, you may be reaching the Tolerable Upper Intake Level (UL) for certain nutrients.
- Bulgur, buckwheat, barley, and millet can be used in place of rice or potatoes or added to soup or salads; bulgur is cooked like rice and has a toastlike color and wheat flavor.
- Emphasize less-processed grains. Highly processed grains lose nutrients and fiber and have increased sodium.

Meat, Fish, Poultry, and Eggs

- Eggs are sold according to grade and size, which do not affect food value; extra-large eggs are not worth the additional cost. Shell color varies according to the breed of chicken but does not influence nutrient content.
- Check the expiration date on fresh poultry because it has a relatively short shelf life; boneless chicken pieces are more expensive because you are paying for convenience.
- Fresh fish spoils quickly, and a "fishy" odor indicates it is several days old. If fresh fish will not be used in 1 or 2 days, then it is best to freeze it. Canned fish, especially tuna, is a good buy; water-packed tuna is lower in kcalories than oil-packed tuna.
- Lower grades of beef are less expensive and lower in fat. Beef roasts keep safely in the refrigerator for several days, but ground meat with increased exposure to the air and potential pathogens should be used in 1 or 2 days or frozen.
- Trim all visible fat from beef, pork, or ham before cooking.
- When choosing meat, poultry, or fish, consider the number of portions and number of meals it will provide.

Milk, Cheese, and Other Dairy Foods

- Fluid milk can have varying levels of fat: nonfat, 1%, 2%, or 3.3% (whole milk); for persons older than 2 years of age, nonfat or low-fat milk is best. Canned evaporated milk with a long shelf life is available in fat and nonfat forms.
- Nonfat dry milk is low in cost and can be added to casseroles, mashed potatoes, or soups to increase their nutrient content; reconstituted nonfat dry milk mixed 1:1 with fluid milk is a cost-effective and palatable milk for drinking.
- Families using large amounts of milk will find it cost-effective to buy gallon containers; be sure to check the *sell by* date when buying fluid milk (see Box 10-3).
- Natural cheeses such as cheddar or Swiss contain more calcium and vitamins and are lower in fat and sodium than processed cheeses; cheeses packaged in individual slices cost more per pound than block cheeses. Shredded cheese is more expensive than a similar weight sold in wedges or blocks.
- Cottage cheese contains less calcium than an equal measure of milk or yogurt and is higher in sodium. Be sure to check the expiration date before purchase.

Fats and Oils

- Liquid oils are high in polyunsaturated fats and must be stored tightly closed in a cool dry place.
- Partially hydrogenated fats (soft-tub fats) are good table fats, but avoid those with *trans* fatty acids. Margarine with added plant sterols is more expensive.

TO SUM UP

Nutrition counselors translate food and nutrition information into ideas and action plans that help individuals and families make appropriate diet-related decisions. Health and nutrition education must focus on the needs and goals of the learner, with strategies developed jointly by the health professional and the client. Behavioral models such as the health belief model, concept of self-efficacy, and stages of change help us understand how people change their behavior and assist in developing strategies that lead to positive change. Many families are in economic stress and need help in obtaining appropriate amounts of food. Food insecurity has both nutritional and emotional consequences and occurs in the United States, as well as in developing countries. Factors relating to the individual, the environment, and the interaction between the two contribute to poverty, malnutrition, and sense of hopelessness. Food assistance programs add to a family's food resources and also serve as effective sites for nutrition education. Referral of clients with food needs to appropriate agencies is an important component of nutrition intervention. Support in developing good shopping and food-handling practices—planning ahead, buying wisely, storing safely, and cooking appropriately—help families at all income levels obtain the optimum level of nutrition possible for their food dollars.

QUESTIONS FOR REVIEW

1. Discuss the concept of wellness. How does it apply to nutrition education?
2. Nutrition counseling has been described as a process. Describe each component and give an example of its use.
3. Describe five personal qualities that you think are important for a nutrition counselor. Do you have these qualities? If not, then how might you go about developing them?
4. List the three basic principles of learning. Apply these principles to one of the following situations:
   - A low-income Hispanic mother with limited English skills whose 2-year-old son is underweight for his age
   - A 71-year-old woman with hypertension who has been told to lower her sodium intake
5. What is meant by food insecurity? How would you determine if a client was food insecure?
6. Using your local telephone directory or the Internet, compile a list of government agencies and other organizations in your community that provide food assistance. As a class project, prepare a pamphlet or booklet for distribution that lists the organization, contact information, type of assistance provided, and any requirements or qualifications for receiving assistance. Distribute the booklet to local offices or agencies serving low-income families in your community.
7. Review the different types of information provided on the food label describing package contents, freshness, and safe handling. Develop a handout to teach these concepts to a low-literacy audience.
8. Using unit pricing, compare the cost per serving of four different ready-to-eat cereals: one sugar-coated cereal, one granola cereal, one whole grain cereal, and one cereal advertised as meeting 100% of the DRIs. Which is the most expensive per serving, and which is the least expensive per serving? Which cereal provides the best nutritional value for the money? Why?
9. Obtain a global positioning satellite (GPS) navigational device or map of your city or county. Using the telephone directory or the Internet, identify supermarkets or discount food stores and input their location. Does each neighborhood or general area have access to a good source of food supplies? Visit the website of The Food Trust (www.thefoodtrust.org) to learn more about efforts to help communities and neighborhoods attract appropriate food markets.

REFERENCES

1. World Health Organization, Office of Caribbean Program Coordination: *What is health and wellness? The seven dimensions of wellness*, Geneva, Switzerland, 2007, World Health Organization. Retrieved April 19, 2009, from http://www.paho.org/English/AD/DPC/NC/7-dimensions-wellness.pdf.
2. American Dietetic Association: Position of the American Dietetic Association: the roles of registered dietitians and dietetic technicians, registered in health promotion and disease prevention, *J Am Diet Assoc* 106:1875, 2006.
3. Holli BB, Calabrese RJ, O'Sullivan-Maillet J: *Communication and education skills for dietetics professionals*, ed 4, Philadelphia, 2003, Lippincott Williams & Wilkins.
4. Curry KR, Jaffe A: *Nutrition counseling and communication skills*, Philadelphia, 1998, Saunders.
5. Hayes DK, Greenlund KJ, Denny CH, et al: Racial/ethnic and socioeconomic disparities in multiple risk factors for heart disease and stroke—United States, 2003, *MMWR Morb Mortal Wkly Rep* 54(5):113, 2005.
6. Centers for Disease Control and Prevention: *The burden of chronic diseases and their risk factors: national and state perspectives*, Atlanta, 2004, U.S. Department of Health and Human Services.
7. Kittler PG, Sucher KP: *Food and culture*, ed 4, Belmont, Calif, 2004, Brooks/Cole, a division of Thomson Learning.
8. Baranowski T: Advances in basic behavioral research will make the most important contributions to effective dietary change programs at this time, *J Am Diet Assoc* 106:808, 2006.
9. Boyle MA: *Community nutrition in action: an entrepreneurial approach*, Belmont, Calif, 2003, Wadsworth/Thomson Learning.
10. Prochaska JO, Norcross JC, Diclemente CC: *Changing for good: a revolutionary six-stage program for overcoming bad habits and moving your life positively forward*, New York, 1994, Quill, a division of HarperCollins Publisher.
11. Hildebrand DA, Betts NM: Assessment of stage of change, decisional balance, self-efficacy, and use of processes of change of low-income parents for increasing servings of fruits and vegetables to preschool-aged children, *J Nutr Educ Behav* 41:110, 2009.
12. Henry H, Reimer K, Smith C, et al: Associations of decisional balance, processes of change, and self-efficacy with stages of change for increased fruit and vegetable intake among low-income, African-American mothers, *J Am Diet Assoc* 106:841, 2006.

13. Greene GW, Fey-Yensan N, Padula C, et al: Differences in psychosocial variables by stage of change for fruits and vegetables in older adults, *J Am Diet Assoc* 104:1236, 2004.
14. Kicklighter JR: Characteristics of older adult learners: a guide for dietetics practitioners, *J Am Diet Assoc* 91(11):1418, 1991.
15. American Dietetic Association: Position of the American Dietetic Association: total diet approach to communicating food and nutrition information, *J Am Diet Assoc* 107:1224, 2007.
16. U.S. Department of Agriculture: *MyPyramid food guidance system*, Washington, DC, 2005, U.S. Department of Agriculture. Retrieved April 19, 2009, from www.mypyramid.gov.
17. Mackey M, Montgomery J: Plant biotechnology can enhance food security and nutrition in the developing world, part 1, *Nutr Today* 39:52, 2004.
18. American Dietetic Association: Position of the American Dietetic Association: addressing world hunger, malnutrition, and food insecurity, *J Am Diet Assoc* 103:1046, 2003.
19. Tanumihardjo SA, Anderson C, Kaufer-Horwitz M, et al: Poverty, obesity, and malnutrition: an international perspective recognizing the paradox, *J Am Diet Assoc* 107:1966, 2007.
20. American Dietetic Association: Position of the American Dietetic Association: food insecurity and hunger in the United States, *J Am Diet Assoc* 106:446, 2006.
21. Dinour LM, Bergen D, Yeh M-C: The food insecurity—obesity paradox: a review of the literature and the role food stamps may play, *J Am Diet Assoc* 107:1952, 2007.
22. Richards R, Smith C: The impact of homeless shelters on food access and choice among homeless families in Minnesota, *J Nutr Educ Behav* 38:96, 2006.
23. Kempson KM, Keenan DP, Sadani PS, et al: Food acquisition practices used by limited-resource individuals, *Fam Econ Nutr Rev* 14(2):44, 2002.
24. Drewnowski A, Barratt-Fornell A: Do healthier diets cost more, *Nutr Today* 39(4):161, 2004.
25. Hampl JS, Sass S: Focus groups indicate that vegetable and fruit consumption by food stamp-eligible Hispanics is affected by children and unfamiliarity with non-traditional foods, *J Am Diet Assoc* 101(6):685, 2001.
26. Chilton M, Booth S: Hunger of the body and hunger of the mind: African American women's perceptions of food insecurity, health, and violence, *J Nutr Educ Behav* 39:116, 2007.
27. Landers PS: The Food Stamp Program: history, nutrition education, and impact, *J Am Diet Assoc* 107:1945, 2007.
28. U.S. Department of Agriculture, Food and Nutrition Service: *National School Lunch Program*, Washington, DC, 2009, U.S. Department of Agriculture. Retrieved May 6, 2009, from www.fns.usda.gov/cnd/Lunch/AboutLunch/NSLPFactSheet.pdf.
29. U.S. Department of Agriculture, Food and Nutrition Service: *School Breakfast Program: program history*, Washington, DC, 2009, U.S. Department of Agriculture. Retrieved May 6, 2009 from www.fns.usda.gov/cnd/Breakfast/Default.htm.
30. U.S. Department of Agriculture, Food and Nutrition Service: *Nutrition program facts. WIC—The Special Supplemental Nutrition Program for Women, Infants and Children*, Washington, DC, 2009, U.S. Department of Agriculture. Retrieved May 6, 2009, from www.fns.usda.gov/wic/WIC-Fact-Sheet.pdf.
31. U.S. Department of Health and Human Services, Administration on Aging: *Nutrition services* (OAA Title IIIC), Washington, DC, 2009, Department of Health and Human Services, Administration on Aging. Retrieved May 6, 2009, from www.aoa.gov/AoARoot/AoA_Programs/HCLTC/Nutrition_Services/index.aspx.
32. Gleason PM, Dodd AH: School breakfast program but not school lunch program participation is associated with lower body mass index, *J Am Diet Assoc* 109:S118, 2009.
33. U.S. Department of Agriculture, Cooperative State Research, Education, and Extension Service: *EFNEP—The Expanded Food and Nutrition Education Program*, Washington, DC, 2006, U.S. Department of Agriculture. Retrieved May 6, 2009, from www.csrees.usda.gov/nea/food/efnep/pdf/2006_impact.pdf.
34. U.S. Department of Agriculture, Cooperative State Research, Education, and Extension Service: *About SNAP-ED*, Washington, DC, 2009, U.S. Department of Agriculture. Retrieved May 6, 2009, from www.csrees.usda.gov/nea/food/fsne/about.html.
35. MacFadyen L, Stead M, Hastings G: *A synopsis of social marketing, SNAP-ED connection, professional development tools: social marketing*, Washington, DC, 1999, U.S. Department of Agriculture. Retrieved August 18, 2009, from snap.nal.usda.gov/nal_display/index.php?info_center=15&tax_level=3&tax_subject=275&topic_id=1305&level3_id=5122.
36. U.S. Department of Health and Human Services, Centers for Disease Control and Prevention: *Social marketing for nutrition and physical activity*, Washington, DC, 2009, U.S. Department of Health and Human Services. Retrieved August 18, 2009, from www.cdc.gov/nccdphp/dnpa/socialmarketing/training/index.htm.
37. U.S. Department of Agriculture, Center for Nutrition Policy and Promotion: *Thrifty food plan: 2006*, CNPP-19, Washington, DC, 2007, U.S. Department of Agriculture. Retrieved May 6, 2009, from www.cnpp.usda.gov/Publications/FoodPlans/MiscPubs/TFP2006Report.pdf.
38. Blisard N, Stewart H: *Food spending in American households, 2003-04*, EIB-23, Washington, DC, 2007, U.S. Department of Agriculture.
39. U.S. Department of Agriculture, Center for Nutrition Policy and Promotion: *The low-cost, moderate-cost, and liberal food plans*, CNPP-20, *2007*, Washington, DC, 2007, U.S. Department of Agriculture. Retrieved May 6, 2009, from www.cnpp.usda.gov/Publications/FoodPlans/MiscPubs/FoodPlans2007AdminReport.pdf.
40. Aase S: Supermarket trends: how increased demand for healthful products and services will affect food and nutritional professionals, *J Am Diet Assoc* 107:1286, 2007.
41. Harper R: Easy does it, *Supermarket News* 57, Jan 17, 2005.
42. Leibtag E: Where you shop matters: store formats drive variation in retail food prices. In *Amber Waves*, vol 3 (5), Washington, DC, 2005, U.S. Department of Agriculture, p 12. Retrieved May 6, 2009, from www.ers.usda.gov/AmberWaves/November05/Features/WhereYouShop.htm.
43. The Food Trust: Philadelphia, 2009. Retrieved May 6, 2009, from www.thefoodtrust.org.
44. Sharkey JR, Horel S: Neighborhood socioeconomic deprivation and minority composition are associated with better potential spatial access to the ground-truthed food environment in a large rural area, *J Nutr* 138:620, 2008.
45. Storper B: Moving toward healthful sustainable diets, *Nutr Today* 38:57, 2003.
46. Cotugna N, Beebe PD: Food banking in the 21st century: much more than a canned handout, *J Am Diet Assoc* 102:1386, 2002.
47. Tiehen L: Stabilizing federal support for emergency food providers. In *Amber Waves*, vol 6 (5), Washington, DC, 2008, U.S. Department of Agriculture, p 4. Retrieved August 18, 2009, from www.ers.usda.gov/AmberWaves/November08/Findings/FoodProviders.htm.
48. Akobundu UO, Cohen NL, Laus MJ, et al: Vitamins A and C, calcium, fruit, and dairy products are limited in food pantries, *J Am Diet Assoc* 104:811, 2004.

FURTHER READINGS AND RESOURCES

Readings

Jonnalagadda SS: Dietary counseling is an important component of cardiac rehabilitation, *J Am Diet Assoc* 105(10):1529, 2005. *[Nutrition counseling can help individuals with chronic disease establish more healthy lifestyles. Dr. Jonnalagadda applies the principles of nutrition assessment and counseling to patients with cardiovascular disease.]*

Chilton M, Booth S: Hunger of the body and hunger of the mind: African American women's perceptions of food insecurity, health, and violence, *J Nutr Educ Behav* 39:116, 2007. *[These researchers provide an overview of the emotional, psychologic, and physical aspects of food insecurity and how we as professionals can assist clients in this situation.]*

Golan E, Stewart H, Kuchler F, et al: Can low-income Americans afford a healthy diet? In *Amber Waves*, vol 6 (5), Washington, DC, 2008, U.S. Department of Agriculture, p 25. Retrieved August 18, 2009, from www.ers.usda.gov/AmberWaves/November08/Features/AffordHealthyDiet.htm.

McCullum C, Desjardins E, Kraak VI, et al: Evidence-based strategies to build community food security, *J Am Diet Assoc* 105(2):278, 2005.

[Many low-income American families have problems obtaining sufficient amounts of healthy food, and an important source of food is the local food pantry. Dr. Golan and colleagues evaluate this situation and Dr. McCullum and colleagues provide a blueprint for how communities can work together to ensure that all families have access to the food they need.]

Popkin BM: Global nutrition dynamics: the world is shifting rapidly toward a diet linked with noncommunicable diseases, *Am J Clin Nutr* 84:289, 2006.

Dinour LM, Bergen D, Yeh MC: The food insecurity-obesity paradox: a review of the literature and the role food stamps may play, *J Am Diet Assoc* 107:1952, 2007.

[These articles address the national and international growth in obesity as a major type of malnutrition, giving insight to both causes and possible interventions.]

Liese AD, Weis KE, Pluto D, et al: Food store types, availability, and cost of foods in a rural environment, *J Am Diet Assoc* 107:1916, 2007. *[Dr. Liese and colleagues point out the problems of rural families in shopping for healthy food.]*

Websites of Interest

Center for Nutrition Policy and Promotion, U.S. Department of Agriculture. This agency produces *Nutrition Insights*, short reports that tell us about food intake and nutrition problems in the U.S. population; all can be accessed from this site: www.cnpp.usda.gov/nutritioninsights.htm.

Cooperative State Research, Education, and Extension Service, U.S. Department of Agriculture: *SNAP-ED Connection.* This site contains educational materials, recipes, and other resources useful in working with limited-resource audiences: www.snap.nal.usda.gov/nal_display/index.php?info_center=15&tax_level=1&tax_subject=245; examples of successful social marketing campaigns can be found at http://snap.nal.usda.gov/nal_display/index.php?info_center=15&tax_level=2&tax_subject=275&topic_id=1305http://snap.nal.usda.gov/nal_display/index.php?info_center=15&tax_level=2&tax_subject=275&topic_id=1305.

Food and Nutrition Service, U.S. Department of Agriculture. This site offers links to food assistance programs, including the National School Breakfast Program, the Supplemental Nutrition Assistance Program (Food Stamp Program), and the Special Supplemental Nutrition Program for Women, Infants, and Children (WIC): www.fns.usda.gov/fns/.

The Food Trust. The website of this Philadelphia-based organization describes efforts to bring nutrition education programs and appropriate food resources including supermarkets to inner-city neighborhoods: www.thefoodtrust.org/.

International Food Information Council Foundation. This site contains fact sheets and brochures for consumers and health professionals on many food-related topics including food ingredients, food processing, fats, carbohydrates, and glossary of common terms: www.ific.org/.

U.S. Agency for International Development (USAID). This agency sponsors nutrition programs in developing countries relating to vitamin-A fortification of foods, infant and child feeding, and community initiatives to ensure safe water and sanitation practices: www.usaid.gov/our_work/global_health/nut/index.html.

U.S. Department of Health and Human Services: *Healthfinder.gov. Live Well, Learn How.* This site is a gateway to health information on over 1600 topics, health news, and tools for personal assessment and intervention: www.healthfinder.gov (Materials available in English and Spanish.)

U.S. Government: *FedStats.* This site provides statistical data from all agencies of the federal government as related to population numbers and demographics, health issues, agriculture, and economic parameters; data can be accessed by topic, nation, and state: www.fedstats.gov.

11

Nutrition During Pregnancy and Lactation

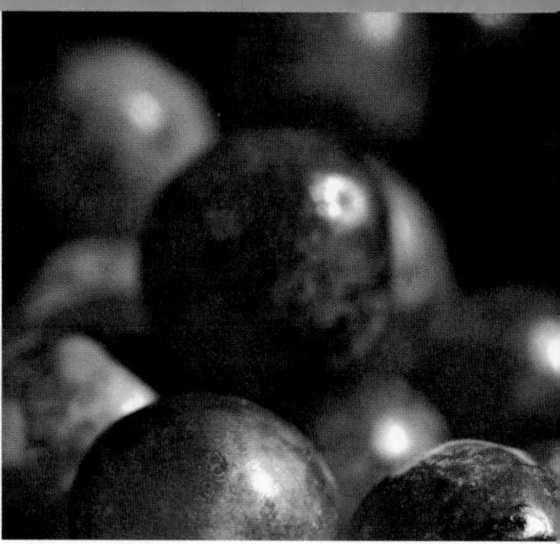

Sharon M. Nickols-Richardson

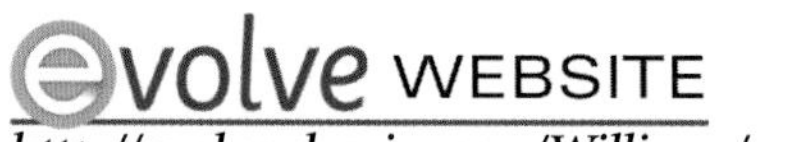

http://evolve.elsevier.com/Williams/essentials/

OUTLINE

In this chapter, we begin a three-chapter sequence on nutrition in health care throughout the life cycle. In each chapter, we will relate principles of nutrition to the remarkable process of human growth and development.

As we focus first on the beginning of new life, we examine the prenatal nutritional demands of the pregnant woman and her developing fetus, as well as maternal nutritional needs during lactation. Mother and offspring possess great adaptive abilities to meet nutritional demands during these life cycle stages.

Here, we explore the tremendous physiologic changes during pregnancy and lactation and some possible complications. You will see how vital optimal nutrition is for a successful course and outcome.

MATERNAL NUTRITION AND THE OUTCOME OF PREGNANCY

Early Medical Practice

For centuries in all cultures, a great body of folklore has surrounded pregnancy. Various traditional practices and diets have been followed, many of which have had little factual basis, and much clinical advice has been based only on supposition. For example, early obstetricians even held the notion that semistarvation of the pregnant woman was really a blessing in disguise because it produced a small baby of light weight who would be easier to deliver. To this end, they used diets restricted in kilocalories (kcalories or kcal), protein, water, and salt. Despite the lack of any scientific evidence to support such ideas, two assumptions, now known to be false, governed practice: (1) the *parasite theory* (i.e., whatever the fetus needs, it draws from maternal stores despite the maternal diet) and (2) the *maternal instinct theory* (i.e., whatever the fetus needs, the pregnant woman instinctively craves and consumes it).

Healthy Pregnancy

Until recently much of the counsel given to pregnant women during the past few decades has been based more on tradition than on scientific fact. Increasing evidence indicates that positive nutritional support of pregnancy, rather than past negative restrictions born of limited knowledge and false assumptions, promotes a successful outcome with increased health and vigor of mothers and their infants. This struggle during the past few decades, particularly to define the "healthy pregnancy," has not been easy. A healthy pregnancy has often been defined by the birth weight of the newborn, because infant mortality, or death, is low for infants with birth weights of 3500 to 4500 g.[1]

The two key factors that predict infant birth weight are (1) maternal preconception weight and (2) weight gain during pregnancy.[2] Nutrition and other lifestyle factors affect maternal weight and weight gain; many of these factors, particularly nutrition, are modifiable or may be controlled by the pregnant woman. Healthy pregnancy may also be described in broader terms of mother, infant, and family. Clinicians are beginning to understand more about what this really means, especially as they observe fetal damages from malnutrition, drug abuse, and other factors. It is clear that we must assess and support more fully the quality of life of each mother and her family if we are to achieve healthy pregnancy outcomes among women.

Directions for Current Practice

Clinical observations and developing science in nutrition and medicine have provided directions for healthier pregnancies. Previous false ideas have been refuted, and a sound base for current practice has emerged. A classic report of the National Research Council (NRC) first reflected this applied scientific base and led the way. This report, *Maternal Nutrition and the Course of Human Pregnancy,* provided an undeniable, new direction for a positive approach to the management of pregnancy.[3] Indeed, continuing research has reinforced this positive direction. On the basis of the significant NRC findings, guidelines for the nutritional care of pregnant women were then issued by the American College of Obstetrics and Gynecology and the American Dietetic Association.[4,5] These reports continue to provide useful guidelines for physicians, nutritionists, dietitians, and nurses in their prenatal care. Nutritional guidelines for pregnancy and lactation for all nutrients are also included in the Dietary Reference Intake (DRI) recommendations published by the Food and Nutrition Board of the Institute of Medicine.[6-10] These guidelines remind us that an infant is nutritionally 9 months old at birth, even older when we consider the significance of the mother's preconception status.

The *fetal origins hypothesis* supports the notion that nutrition during gestation, or the lack thereof, sets the course for chronic disease in adulthood.[11] Development of cardiovascular disease, hypertension, obesity, type 2 diabetes, metabolic syndrome, and gestational diabetes, among other chronic diseases, has been shown in the offspring of animals for which maternal dietary intakes of macronutrients and micronutrients were manipulated, as well as in human epidemiologic studies of the relationship between infant anthropometric measurements and adult disease incidence.[12,13] In these epidemiologic studies, infant body size, shape, and weight measurements served as indicators of maternal nutrition. Changes in maternal nutrition during pregnancy require that the fetus adapt. These adaptations to nutrient supplies may lead to programming, or the mechanism (or mechanisms) through which permanent changes in organ system structures and functions occur, leading to risk of chronic disease. This hypothesis presumes that nutritional insults that occur during critical stages of embryonic and fetal development are most harmful, leading to future disease risk. The merits of the fetal origins hypothesis have been debated, and much remains to be discovered.[14] Although research regarding the influence of nutrition on fetal growth and development has unique ethical and moral considerations, outcomes-based research is essential for appropriate evidence-based practice for healthy pregnancies.

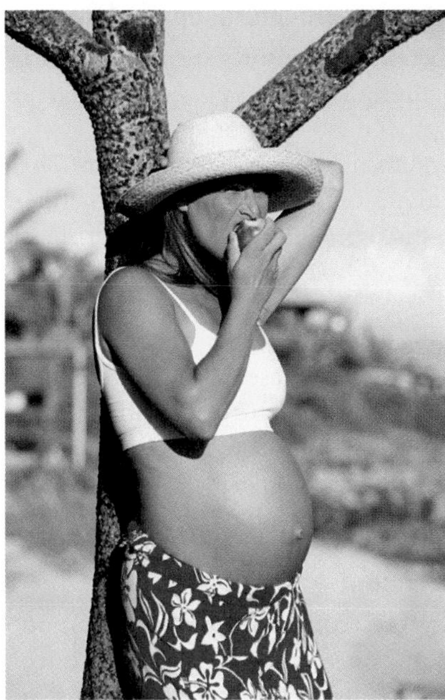

FIGURE 11-1 Adequate intake of fruits and vegetables is essential during pregnancy. (Copyright 2006 JupiterImages Corporation.)

Factors Determining Nutritional Needs

An expanding body of research and the best practices of clinicians reinforce that maternal nutrition is critically important to the mother and the newborn (Figure 11-1). It lays the fundamental foundation for the successful outcome of pregnancy—a healthy mother and infant.[15] Several vital factors that determine nutritional requirements of the woman during her pregnancy are well recognized.

Age, Gravida, and Parity

Age plays a major role in pregnancy; the teenage girl adds her own growth and maturation needs to those imposed by pregnancy. In addition, the number of pregnancies (gravida) and the number of viable offspring (parity), as well as the time intervals between them, greatly influence the woman's nutrient reserves, her increased nutritional needs, and the outcome of the pregnancy.

KEY TERMS

fetus The unborn offspring in the postembryonic period, after major structures have been outlined; in humans, the growing offspring from 7 to 8 weeks after fertilization until birth.

gestation The period of embryonic and fetal development from fertilization to birth; pregnancy.

programming The mechanism (or mechanisms) through which adaptations to nutrient supplies during gestation result in permanent changes in organ and body system structures and functions, potentially leading to chronic disease risk.

gravida A pregnant woman.

parity The condition of a woman with respect to having borne viable offspring.

Complex Physiologic Interactions of Gestation

Three distinct biologic entities are involved during gestation: the woman, the fetus, and the placenta, which nourishes fetal growth. Together they form a unique biologic whole. Constant metabolic interactions occur among them. Their functions, although unique, are at the same time interdependent. It is this unique biologic synergism that nourishes and sustains the pregnancy.

Basic Concepts Involved

As a result of our increased knowledge of pregnancy and nutrition, we can provide better nutritional guidance. Three basic concepts form a fundamental framework for assessing maternal nutritional needs and for planning supportive prenatal care for the woman.

Perinatal Concept

The prefix *peri-* comes from the Greek root meaning around, about, or surrounding. Thus the word *perinatal* refers more broadly to the scope of factors that surround a birth than merely the 9 months of the physical gestation. Certainly, as nutrition knowledge and understanding have increased, health professionals realize that all of a woman's life experiences surrounding her pregnancy must be considered. Her nutritional status and food patterns, which have developed during a number of years, and the degree to which she has established and maintained nutritional reserves are all important factors. Cultural and social influences have shaped beliefs and values of the woman about pregnancy. All of these influences come to bear on any pregnancy.

Synergism Concept

The word *synergism* is a term used to describe biologic systems in which the cooperative action of two or more factors produces a total effect greater than and different from the mere sum of the parts. In short, a new whole is created by the unified, joint effort of blending the parts in which each part makes more powerful the action of the others. Of the many biologic and physiologic examples of synergism, pregnancy is a prime case in point. Maternal organism, fetus, and placenta combine to produce a new whole, a system not existing before and producing a total effect greater than and different from the sum of the parts, all for the sole purpose of sustaining and nurturing the pregnancy and its offspring. Physiologic measures change. Blood volume and cardiac output is increased; ventilation rate and tidal volume of breathing are increased; and basal metabolic rate (BMR) is increased. The physiologic norms of the nonpregnant woman do not apply.

Thus the normal physiologic adjustments of pregnancy cannot be viewed as pathologic with application of treatment procedures for that same type of response in the nonpregnant state. For example, a normal physiologic generalized edema of pregnancy is a protective response. It reflects the normal increase in total body water necessary to support the increased metabolic work of pregnancy and is associated with enhanced reproductive performance.

Life Continuum Concept

In a real sense, throughout her life a woman is providing for the ongoing continuum of life through the food that she eats. Each offspring obviously becomes a part of this continuing process during the pregnancy, when the mother's diet directly sustains growth and development. However, in the broader sense, the mother transfers her nutritional heritage, practices, and beliefs to her growing children, who in the next generation pass on this heritage genetically and culturally. Other family members also play important roles in this generational sustenance of the life continuum.

HEALTH PROMOTION

Preconception Nutrition

A woman brings to each pregnancy all of her previous life experiences, including her diet and eating habits. Her general health and fitness and her state of nutrition at the time of conception are products of her lifelong dietary habits and her genetic heritage. The importance of preconception nutrition is increasingly recognized. The Maternal, Infant and Child Health Goal included in *Healthy People 2010: Understanding and Improving Health* (see *Further Readings and Resources* at the end of this chapter) addresses the need for improvements in preconception nutrition and health in women in the United States.[16] Preconception counseling is an avenue to such improvements. Related to nutrition, preconception counseling may include screening for medical conditions such as iron deficiency anemia, eating disorders, drug-nutrient interactions, and genetic disorders, as well as assessment of current body weight, recent and previous weight changes, body mass index (BMI), fitness and exercise status, folate status, other nutrient intakes, eating patterns, and dietary and botanical supplement use. Evaluation of existing medical conditions such as hypertension, diabetes, thyroid disease, celiac disease, phenylketonuria (PKU), and others, is important. Inquiry about the home and family environment, including income, education, safety, lead exposure, and abuse, should also be conducted during preconception counseling so that guidance, recommendations, and referrals may be thoroughly provided. Each of these nutrition and health-related factors has documented effects on pregnancy outcome, many of which are adverse. However, preconception counseling and optimal preconception nutrition may increase the odds for a healthy pregnancy and desirable infant outcome.

Excess Body Weight

Approximately 67% of adults in the United States are overweight and nearly 33% are obese. Hence many women enter their pregnancies with excess body weight. This condition increases the risks of fetal mortality and malformations, excessive weight gain during pregnancy, gestational diabetes, hypertension, and preeclampsia, as well as the likelihood of preterm delivery and infant delivery by cesarean section. Pregnancy is not a time for weight loss because of the energy and nutrient requirements of the woman and fetus. Rather, a woman with excess body weight should moderately and gradually reduce her weight before pregnancy through an individualized energy-restricted diet and exercise plan. Weight gain during pregnancy should then follow recommendations based on BMI as outlined later in this chapter.

Exercise

Women who exercise before pregnancy should continue a reasonable exercise regimen during pregnancy.[17] In fact, women who engage in prenatal exercise have been shown to have health benefits compared with nonexercising women.[18] Moderate-intensity physical activity may also be beneficial to the woman and fetus, even if the woman was sedentary before conception. Each day, a pregnant woman should strive to achieve approximately 20 to 22 minutes of aerobic activity to meet a goal of approximately 150 minutes per week.[17] As the woman's body size and shape change throughout the course of pregnancy, exercise type, duration, intensity, and frequency should be adjusted to promote safety for the woman and her fetus (Figure 11-2). Physical activities that are not recommended during pregnancy include scuba diving and those with risk of trauma to the abdominal area.[19]

The energy cost of exercise influences the kcalorie needs of the pregnant woman. Kcalories must be consumed to meet the energy cost of exercise and to promote appropriate maternal weight gain and fetal growth and development. Adequate hydration is also vital, and the woman should increase fluid intake during exercise.

NUTRITIONAL DEMANDS OF PREGNANCY

Basic Nutrient Allowances and Individual Variation

Gestation is characterized by exceedingly rapid growth and development. During this 38- to 42-week period, a single fertilized egg cell (ovum) grows into a fully developed infant weighing about 3500 g, on average. What nutrients must the woman supply to support this intense period of fetal growth and development? What must her diet provide to meet fetal nutritional demands and her own needs during this critical period?

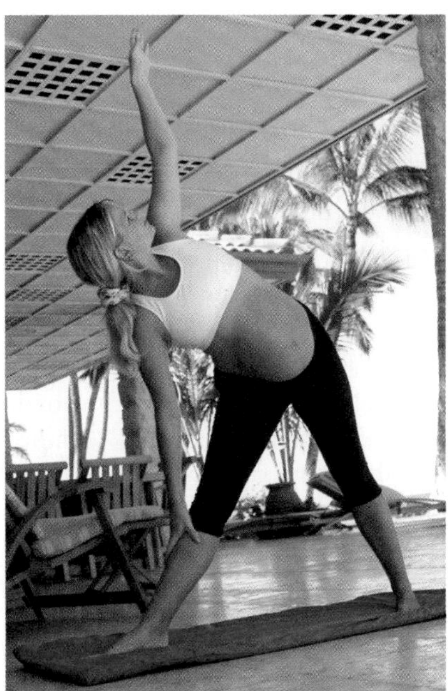

FIGURE 11-2 Physical activity during pregnancy benefits both the pregnant woman and the fetus. (Copyright 2006 JupiterImages Corporation.)

Throughout the pregnancy an increased need exists for most of the basic nutrients, as indicated by the DRI guidelines from the Food and Nutrition Board of the Institute of Medicine (Table 11-1).[6–10] However, it is important to remember that these are guidelines; individual variances in nutrient needs must be examined for each pregnancy. Individual variations such as BMR, BMI, physical activity, and health status must be considered. In addition, the quantitative need for nourishment of pregnant adolescents and multifetal pregnancies must be noted. Individual counseling and correct use of nutritional guidelines is imperative.[20] In considering the nutritional needs of the *healthy* pregnant woman, we will review here the macronutrients and selected micronutrients with increased needs, rationale for increased needs, and how such nutrients may be obtained from foods.

Energy Needs

The kcalories must be sufficient to perform the following two functions:

1. Supply the increased energy and nutrient demands created by the increased metabolic workload, including some maternal fat storage and fetal fat storage to ensure an optimal newborn size for survival.
2. Spare protein for tissue building.

The DRI standard recommends an additional amount of energy of approximately 340 kcal/day during the second trimester and 452 kcal/day during the third trimester of pregnancy to supply needs during this time of rapid growth.[10] Total daily kcalorie intake during middle and late- pregnancy should be based on the woman's nonpregnant estimated energy requirement plus the additional energy need and will typically increase about 15% to 20% beyond the woman's general prepregnancy need. This primary emphasis on sufficient kcalories is critical to ensure nutrient and energy needs to positively support the pregnancy. Appropriate weight gain during pregnancy indicates whether sufficient kcalories are being provided.

Much of our knowledge regarding the importance of sufficient energy intake during pregnancy arose from records of pregnancy and infant statistics through periods of famine during World War II. Insufficient kcalorie intake during the first trimester of pregnancy was associated with infertility and increased incidence of neural tube defects and other metabolic changes, whereas inadequate kcalorie consumption in the second and third trimesters of pregnancy was associated with

KEY TERMS

placenta Special organ developed in early pregnancy that provides nutrients to the fetus and removes metabolic waste.

synergism The joint action of separate agents in which the total effect of their combined action is greater than the sum of their separate actions.

TABLE 11-1 **DIETARY REFERENCE INTAKES PER DAY OF SOME SELECTED NUTRIENTS FOR PREGNANCY AND LACTATION**

NUTRIENTS	NONPREGNANT GIRL 9-13 YR 46 kg 101 lb	NONPREGNANT GIRL 14-18 YR 55 kg 120 lb	NONPREGNANT WOMAN 19-50 YR 63 kg 138 lb	DURING PREGNANCY 19-50 YR	LACTATION (600 mL/DAY) FIRST 6 mo	LACTATION (750 mL/DAY) SECOND 6 mo
Kilocalories	2000-2100	2300-2400	2400	No change in first trimester; + 340 kcal/day for second trimester and + 452 kcal/day for third trimester	+ 500 kcal/day (170 kcal/day from maternal stores)	+ 400 kcal/day
Protein (g)	34	46	46	71	71	71
Calcium (mg)	1300	1300	1000	1000 throughout	1000 throughout	
Iron (mg)	8	15	18	27 throughout	9 throughout	
Vitamin A (mcg RAE)*	600	700	700	770 throughout	1300 throughout	
Thiamin (mg)	0.9	1.0	1.1	1.4 throughout	1.4 throughout	
Riboflavin (mg)	0.9	1.0	1.1	1.4 throughout	1.6 throughout	
Niacin (mg NE)†	12	14	14	18 throughout	17 throughout	
Vitamin C (mg)	45	65	75	85 throughout	120 throughout	
Vitamin D (mcg)	5	5	5	5 throughout	5 throughout	
Folic acid (mcg DFE)‡	300	400	400	600 throughout	500 throughout	

Data from Food and Nutrition Board, Institute of Medicine: *Dietary Reference Intakes for calcium, phosphorus, magnesium, vitamin D, and fluoride,* Washington, DC, 1997, National Academies Press; Food and Nutrition Board, Institute of Medicine: *Dietary Reference Intakes for energy, carbohydrate, fiber, fat, fatty acids, cholesterol, protein, and amino acids (macronutrients),* Washington, DC, 2005, National Academies Press; Food and Nutrition Board, Institute of Medicine: *Dietary Reference Intakes for thiamin, riboflavin, niacin, vitamin B_6, folate, vitamin B_{12}, pantothenic acid, biotin, and choline,* Washington, DC, 1998, National Academies Press; Food and Nutrition Board, Institute of Medicine: *Dietary Reference Intakes for vitamin C, vitamin E, selenium, and carotenoids,* Washington, DC, 2000, National Academies Press; Food and Nutrition Board, Institute of Medicine: *Dietary Reference Intakes for vitamin A, vitamin K, arsenic, boron, chromium, copper, iodine, iron, manganese, molybdenum, nickel, silicon, vanadium, and zinc,* Washington, DC, 2000, National Academies Press.

*As retinol activity equivalents (RAEs): One RAE is equal to 1 mcg all-*trans* retinol or 12 mcg β-carotene.

†As niacin equivalents (NE): One NE is equal to 1 mg of niacin or 60 mg of tryptophan.

‡As dietary folate equivalents (DFEs): One DFE is equal to 1 mcg food folate or 0.6 mcg of folic acid from fortified food (or as a supplement consumed with food) or 0.5 mcg of a supplement taken on an empty stomach.

increased numbers of congenital abnormalities, infants of low birth weight, and infant mortality. Current famine and food insecurity in various locations around the world continue to support these earlier findings regarding the essential need for adequate kcalories during pregnancy to support an optimal infant outcome. Energy needs of pregnancy may be met through a balanced intake of macronutrients.

Protein, Fat, and Carbohydrate Needs

The total amount of protein recommended for a pregnant woman is 71 g/day, an increase of 25 g/day.[10] Protein, with its essential nitrogen, is the nutrient basic to tissue growth. Nitrogen balance studies suggest that a large amount of nitrogen is used by the woman and fetus during pregnancy and emphasize the importance of preconception maternal reserves to meet initial pregnancy needs. More protein is necessary for demands posed by the following:

- Rapid fetal growth.
- Enlargement of the uterus, mammary glands, and placenta.
- Increase in maternal circulating blood volume and subsequent demand for increased plasma proteins to maintain colloidal osmotic pressure and circulation of tissue fluids to nourish cells.
- Formation of **amniotic fluid.**
- Storage reserves for labor, delivery, and lactation.

Milk, egg, cheese, and meat are complete protein foods of high biologic value. Protein-rich foods also contribute other nutrients, such as calcium, iron, and B vitamins. Additional protein may be obtained from legumes and whole grains, with lesser amounts in other plant sources.

An adequate supply of essential fatty acids is also vital throughout pregnancy. Tissue growth, especially the proper development of cell membranes in nerve and brain tissue, and development of organ function, notably cognition and visual acuity, require that essential fatty acids and their converted forms reach the developing fetus in sufficient amounts. Depending on individual needs, supplementation of the mother's essential fatty acid intake may be useful to maintain adequate levels.[21] However, most pregnant women may consume adequate amounts of linoleic (13 g/day) and α-linolenic (1.4 g/day) acids through consumption of canola, soybean, and walnut oils, in addition to other dietary fat sources.[10] Docosahexaenoic acid (DHA), important for visual and cognitive development, is found in salmon, mackerel, striped bass, and other fish products. Eicosapentaenoic acid (EPA), also found in fish, fish oils, flaxseed, walnuts, and canola oil is important for blood vessel dilation, blood clotting, and attenuation of inflammation. Combined DHA and EPA intake of 500 mg/d is recommended.[22]

Carbohydrate intake of at least 175 g/day during pregnancy is important for an adequate supply of glucose and nonprotein energy.[10] Whole grain breads and cereals, as well as fruits and vegetables, should be consumed to meet maternal and fetal glucose needs and provide fiber for satiety and bowel regulation. Currently popular low-carbohydrate "diets" are not recommended during pregnancy because various phases of these diets do not provide the minimum glucose load required by the maternal and fetal bodies. In general, total daily dietary kcalorie intake should be comprised of 15% protein, 30% fat, and 55% carbohydrate, keeping in mind the individual needs of the pregnant woman and adequate macronutrient distribution ranges.

Mineral Needs

All the major and trace minerals play roles in maternal health. Four that have special functions in relation to pregnancy—(1) calcium, (2) iodine, (3) iron, and (4) zinc—deserve particular attention.

Calcium

The pregnant woman's DRI recommendation is 1000 mg of calcium per day, the same as the general recommendation for all women ages 19 to 50.[6] Calcium is the essential element for the construction and maintenance of bones and teeth. It is also an important factor in the blood-clotting mechanism and is used in normal muscle action and other essential metabolic activities. Improved absorption of calcium supplies the needs arising from the accelerated fetal mineralization of skeletal tissue during the final period of rapid growth. Dairy products are a primary source of calcium. Consumption of milk or equivalent milk foods (cheese or nonfat milk powder used in cooking) is recommended. Additional calcium is obtained in whole or fortified cereal grains and in green leafy vegetables.

Iodine

The recommendation for iodine increases by 70 mcg/day during pregnancy.[9] Iodine is vital for thyroid hormone synthesis and prevention of goiter. The need increases during gestation to support changes in maternal thyroid economy, increased maternal renal clearance, and fetal uptake of iodine. An inadequate supply of iodine to the fetus may lead to hypothyroidism in the newborn and is often associated with poor and abnormal growth, deficits in cognitive development, and poor motor function. Although infrequently encountered in the United States, infant hypothyroidism continues to be found in many developing countries. Iodine consumption is critical in the first half of pregnancy, and programs designed to provide oil- and water-based iodine supplements to women in preconception and prenatal periods in developing countries have been successful in reducing the incidence of infant hypothyroidism. Iodized salt is the primary dietary source for women in developed countries. Seafood is also a noted source of iodine.

Iron

The pregnant woman needs 27 mg of iron per day, a substantial increase beyond her general needs.[9] Some pregnant women may need supplementary iron in addition to increased dietary sources to meet the additional requirement of pregnancy. The iron cost of pregnancy is high. With increased demands for iron, often insufficient maternal stores, and inadequate provision through the usual diet, a daily supplement of 30 to 60 mg of iron per day is generally prescribed. If a woman has iron deficiency anemia at conception, then a larger therapeutic amount of 60 to 120 mg/day of iron may be necessary to reduce the risk of a preterm delivery or low-birth-weight baby (or both).

During normal pregnancy the maternal circulating blood volume expands by 40% to 50% and may increase more with multiple fetuses. This adaptation reduces the strain on the maternal heart, minimizes hemoglobin losses at delivery, and enhances nutrient flow to the fetus. Although red blood cell mass also increases during gestation, this change does not parallel blood volume expansion, resulting in hemodilution of red blood cell mass. Thus specific guidelines are used to determine iron deficiency anemia during pregnancy (see *Anemia* later in this chapter). Maternal iron is needed to supply iron to the developing placenta and fetal liver. Adequate maternal iron stores also help protect the woman against iron losses related to blood loss at delivery.

To obtain the needed amount of iron, check the percentage of elemental iron in the iron preparation being used. For example, the commonly used compound ferrous sulfate is a hydrated salt ($FeSO_4\ 7H_2O$), which contains 20% iron. It is usually dispensed in tablets containing 195, 300, or 325 mg of the ferrous sulfate compound. Each tablet, then, would contain 39, 60, or 65 mg of iron, respectively. Thus to supply a regular daily supplement of 60 mg of iron, one 300-mg tablet of ferrous sulfate is required (300 mg $FeSO_4\ 7H_2O \times 20\% =$ 60 mg iron); for a therapeutic dose of 120 mg iron, two 300-mg tablets are required.

Problems with routine iron supplementation for pregnant women include unpleasant gastrointestinal side effects (see *Effects of Iron Supplements* later in this chapter) and less motivation to maintain a good diet. Of major concern are imbalances with other trace elements, such as zinc and copper, that compete with iron for absorption. Excess iron intake, when not needed, may actually mask inadequate pregnancy-induced hemodilution. Thus some prenatal clinics follow protocols that prescribe regular prenatal vitamins with iron at the first clinic visit, adding additional iron supplementation

KEY TERMS

amniotic fluid The watery fluid within the membrane enveloping the fetus, in which the fetus is suspended.

only if hemoglobin falls to 10.5 g/dL or less at any time during the pregnancy.

A major food source of iron is liver; however, liver intake is often avoided during pregnancy. Other food sources include meat, legumes, dried fruit, green leafy vegetables, eggs, and enriched bread and cereals (see list of iron-containing foods in Chapter 7).

Zinc

During pregnancy the DRI recommendation for zinc increases from 8 to 11 mg/day.[9] Zinc is vital for enzymatic reactions and is essential to growth and development because of its role in deoxyribonucleic acid (DNA) and ribonucleic acid (RNA) synthesis and protein production. Inadequate zinc consumption during gestation has been associated with low birth weight and congenital malformations. Iron supplementation may inhibit zinc absorption; thus additional dietary sources of zinc are critical when maternal iron supplementation is prescribed. Seafood, eggs, and meat are primary sources of zinc.

Vitamin Needs

Increased amounts of vitamins A, B complex, and C are needed during pregnancy. If these needs are met, then sufficient amounts of vitamins E and K are also available. The recommended amount of vitamin D does not increase during pregnancy but is important to fetal skeletal development.

Vitamin A

The daily amount of vitamin A recommended for pregnancy is 770 mcg of retinol activity equivalents (RAE), a slight increase beyond the woman's regular need.[9] For most women in the United States, no extra amount is needed. However, malnourished, underweight women and those with multiple pregnancies need more. Vitamin A is an essential factor in cell differentiation, organ formation, maintenance of strong epithelial tissue, tooth formation, and normal bone growth. Liver, egg yolk, butter and fortified margarine, dark-green and yellow vegetables, and fruits are good food sources.

Excessive consumption of retinol and retinoic acid, two forms of vitamin A, has been associated with fetal malformations such as heart, facial, and ear defects. Overconsumption is generally related to the use of supplements or medications such as Accutane. Harmful effects are most damaging during the first few months of pregnancy, again emphasizing the need for prenatal counseling and appropriate preconception nutrition.

B Vitamins

A special need exists for various B vitamins, including thiamin, riboflavin, niacin, pyridoxine, vitamin B_{12}, pantothenic acid, and folate, during pregnancy. The B vitamins are important as coenzyme factors in a number of metabolic activities related to energy production, tissue protein synthesis, and function of muscle and nerve tissue; therefore they play key roles in the increased metabolic work of pregnancy.[23] These B vitamins are usually supplied by a well-balanced diet that is increased in quantity and quality to supply needed energy and nutrients.

A special increased metabolic need exists for the B vitamin folate during pregnancy. Folate deficiency usually occurs in conjunction with general malnutrition, making the pregnant woman in low-socioeconomic conditions especially vulnerable. A specific megaloblastic anemia caused by maternal folate deficiency sometimes occurs and warrants supplementation of the diet with folic acid. This added amount is particularly needed in situations in which such demands are increased, such as in a multiple pregnancy.

Preconception folic acid supplementation has been shown in randomized clinical trials to greatly reduce a woman's risk of bearing an infant with a neural tube defect, which is the source of the serious defects of spina bifida and anencephaly. These congenital defects in the formation of the spine develop in the first few weeks of pregnancy, when the neural tube, which forms the spinal cord, does not close completely, leaving part of one or more vertebrae of the spinal cord exposed at birth. Each year in the United States approximately 3000 infants are born with spina bifida and anencephaly, and an estimated 1500 affected fetuses are spontaneously aborted.[24] Since 1992 the U.S. Public Health Service has recommended that all women of childbearing age who are capable of becoming pregnant consume from food or supplementation 400 mcg of folic acid per day to prevent such deficiencies. This recommendation continues in the latest DRI guidelines, which recommend 400 mcg/day for nonpregnant women, rising to 600 mcg/day during pregnancy and 500 mcg/day during lactation.[7] The U.S. Food and Drug Administration (FDA), acting to increase folic acid consumption nationally, mandated in 1998 that enriched cereal grain products be fortified with folic acid.[25,26] These fortified foods are good sources of folic acid in addition to orange and pineapple juices, oranges, and dried beans.[27] (Review Chapter 6 for more discussion on neural tube defects and their prevention.)

Vitamin C

Special emphasis must be given to the pregnant woman's need for ascorbic acid. Vitamin C is essential to the formation of intercellular cement substance in developing connective tissues and vascular systems. It also increases the absorption of iron, which is needed for the increasing quantities of hemoglobin. The DRI standard recommends 85 mg/day for the pregnant woman, an increase of 10 mg/day beyond the regular female adult need of 75 mg/day.[8] Additional food sources such as citrus fruit and other vegetables and fruits should be included in the woman's diet.

Vitamin D

Women who have adequate exposure to sunlight probably need little additional vitamin D. During pregnancy, because of the need for calcium and phosphorus presented by the developing fetal skeletal tissue, vitamin D is used to promote the absorption and use of these minerals. The daily recommended amount for pregnancy is 5 mcg cholecalciferol

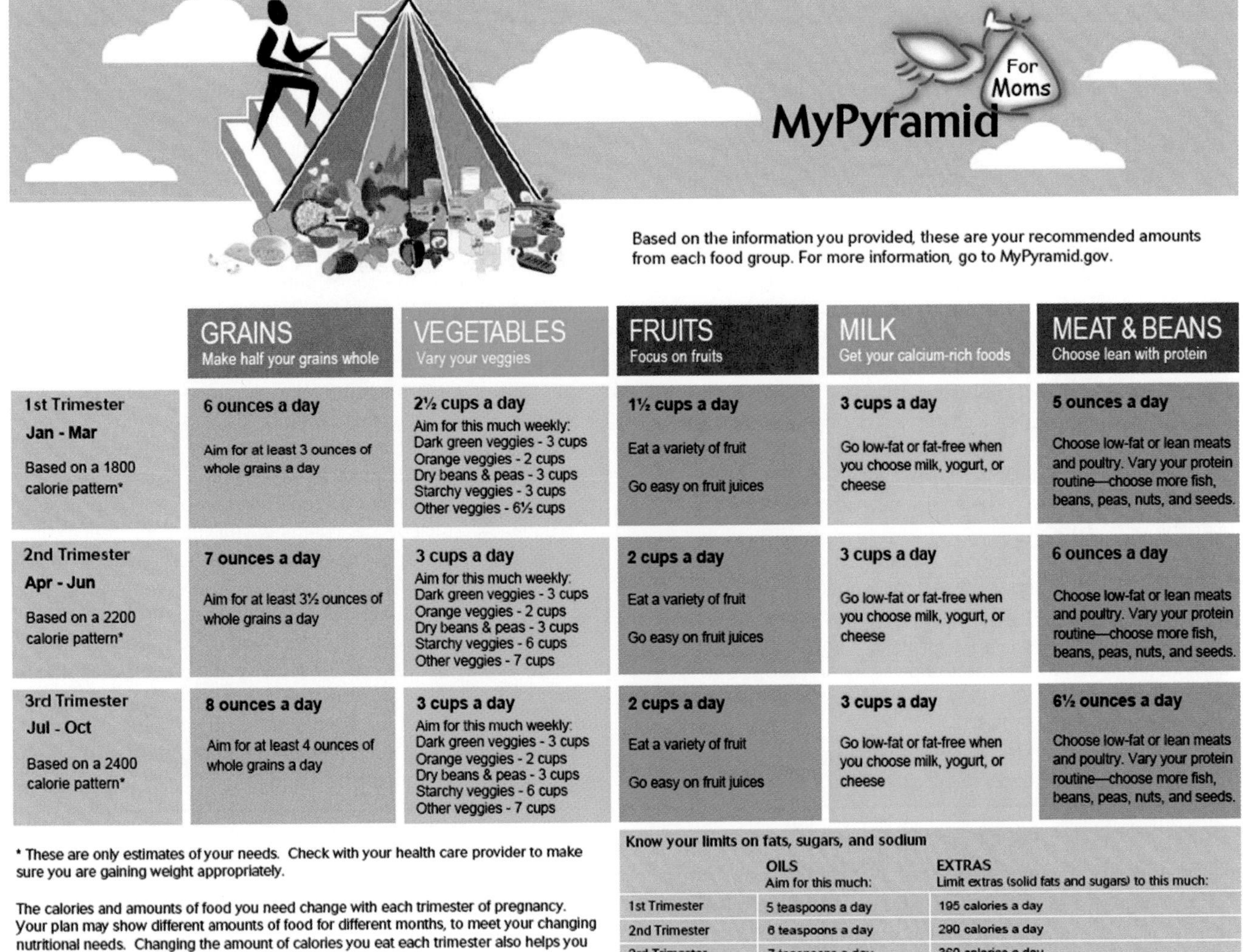
MyPyramid For Moms

Based on the information you provided, these are your recommended amounts from each food group. For more information, go to MyPyramid.gov.

	GRAINS Make half your grains whole	VEGETABLES Vary your veggies	FRUITS Focus on fruits	MILK Get your calcium-rich foods	MEAT & BEANS Choose lean with protein
1st Trimester **Jan - Mar** Based on a 1800 calorie pattern*	**6 ounces a day** Aim for at least 3 ounces of whole grains a day	**2½ cups a day** Aim for this much weekly: Dark green veggies - 3 cups Orange veggies - 2 cups Dry beans & peas - 3 cups Starchy veggies - 3 cups Other veggies - 6½ cups	**1½ cups a day** Eat a variety of fruit Go easy on fruit juices	**3 cups a day** Go low-fat or fat-free when you choose milk, yogurt, or cheese	**5 ounces a day** Choose low-fat or lean meats and poultry. Vary your protein routine—choose more fish, beans, peas, nuts, and seeds.
2nd Trimester **Apr - Jun** Based on a 2200 calorie pattern*	**7 ounces a day** Aim for at least 3½ ounces of whole grains a day	**3 cups a day** Aim for this much weekly: Dark green veggies - 3 cups Orange veggies - 2 cups Dry beans & peas - 3 cups Starchy veggies - 6 cups Other veggies - 7 cups	**2 cups a day** Eat a variety of fruit Go easy on fruit juices	**3 cups a day** Go low-fat or fat-free when you choose milk, yogurt, or cheese	**6 ounces a day** Choose low-fat or lean meats and poultry. Vary your protein routine—choose more fish, beans, peas, nuts, and seeds.
3rd Trimester **Jul - Oct** Based on a 2400 calorie pattern*	**8 ounces a day** Aim for at least 4 ounces of whole grains a day	**3 cups a day** Aim for this much weekly: Dark green veggies - 3 cups Orange veggies - 2 cups Dry beans & peas - 3 cups Starchy veggies - 6 cups Other veggies - 7 cups	**2 cups a day** Eat a variety of fruit Go easy on fruit juices	**3 cups a day** Go low-fat or fat-free when you choose milk, yogurt, or cheese	**6½ ounces a day** Choose low-fat or lean meats and poultry. Vary your protein routine—choose more fish, beans, peas, nuts, and seeds.

* These are only estimates of your needs. Check with your health care provider to make sure you are gaining weight appropriately.

The calories and amounts of food you need change with each trimester of pregnancy. Your plan may show different amounts of food for different months, to meet your changing nutritional needs. Changing the amount of calories you eat each trimester also helps you gain weight at the correct rate.

Know your limits on fats, sugars, and sodium

	OILS Aim for this much:	EXTRAS Limit extras (solid fats and sugars) to this much:
1st Trimester	5 teaspoons a day	195 calories a day
2nd Trimester	6 teaspoons a day	290 calories a day
3rd Trimester	7 teaspoons a day	360 calories a day

FIGURE 11-3 Food intake plan for a pregnant woman based on trimester of pregnancy, age, height, prepregnancy weight, and physical activity using the MyPyramid for Moms program (www.mypyramid.gov/).

(200 IU/day), which is the same as for the nonpregnant woman.[6] Food sources include fortified milk, liver, egg yolk, and fortified margarine.

Dietary Patterns: General and Alternative

General Daily Food Pattern

Two useful general principles concerning eating habits for all persons also apply during pregnancy, as follows:

1. Eat an appropriate quantity of food.
2. Eat regularly, avoiding fasting or skipping meals, especially breakfast.

During pregnancy a variety of familiar foods usually supply the woman's need for added nutrients and make eating a pleasure. The increased quantities of essential nutrients needed during pregnancy may be met in many ways by planning around a daily food pattern and using key types of suggested core foods. The MyPyramid Plan for Moms (www.mypyramid.gov/) offers a credible and easily accessible source for a woman to develop an eating plan appropriate for her trimester of pregnancy, age, height, prepregnancy weight, and physical activity level. Figure 11-3 displays one example of a dietary plan for a pregnant woman.

Lean meats and poultry, fish, dried beans, and nuts provide dietary protein, iron, zinc, and B vitamins for growth of muscles, bones, blood, and nerves; vegetable protein foods also contribute fiber. Fluid milk and dairy products provide dietary protein, calcium, and vitamin D to build strong bones, teeth, and healthy nerves and muscles and to promote normal blood clotting. Grains provide carbohydrates and B vitamins for energy and healthy nerves, as well as iron for healthy blood. At least one half of these grains should be whole grain cereal and bread products to provide fiber. Vitamin C–rich fruits and vegetables assist in preventing infection and promoting

KEY TERMS

spina bifida A congenital defect in the fetal closing of the neural tube to form a portion of the lower spine, leaving the spine unclosed and the spinal cord open in various degrees of exposure and damage.

CASE STUDY

A Baby for the Delgados

Mrs. Delgado is a 19-year-old married **primigravida,** who tested positive for urinary human chorionic gonadotropin (hCG) 2 weeks earlier. Mrs. Delgado is 160 cm (5 feet, 3 inches) tall with an average pregravid weight of 57 kg (125 lb). Her current gestational age is 6 weeks. Her history for chronic disorders and other serious health problems is negative.

During her initial nutrition interview, Mrs. Delgado indicated that the pregnancy was unplanned. She seemed especially worried about the effects of her irregular diet on the baby. As college students, she and her 21-year-old husband had erratic meals, dominated by junk food. Mrs. Delgado's 24-hour diet history revealed an inadequate intake of dark-green or red-yellow-orange vegetables and milk products, as well as meat or eggs and citrus fruits. The couple realized that these types of foods were an important part of a nutritious diet but felt inexperienced as cooks and lacked the time and money to prepare healthful meals every day.

At the end of the initial counseling session, the nutritionist told the couple about a series of prenatal group discussions conducted by members of the clinic's perinatal health team, including sessions on pregnancy, labor and delivery, and the care and feeding of the infant. These are attended primarily by a mixture of experienced parents and young, first-time parents to be and are offered as a means of introducing practical aspects of pregnancy and parenting.

The Delgados attended every prenatal group meeting and kept all consequent diet-counseling sessions. Their food choices improved in time, and Mrs. Delgado's weight gain progressed normally, to a total of 13 kg (28.5 lb) by the time of delivery. The Delgados had a healthy 4 kg (8 lb, 13 oz) baby girl.

Questions for Analysis

1. What health professionals ideally should be included on the health care team caring for Mrs. Delgado? Describe the significance of each role to the outcome of her pregnancy. What are the roles of Mr. and Mrs. Delgado?
2. What nutritional deficiencies would you expect in Mrs. Delgado's diet? What practical problems would you expect her to encounter in attempting to improve her diet?
3. Write a 1-day meal plan for Mrs. Delgado, taking into account her lifestyle and schedule, as well as the amounts of nutrients considered adequate for pregnancy.
4. Write a lesson plan for a group session on nutrition during pregnancy. Include a general description, behavioral objectives, content outline, teaching methods and materials, and evaluation tool (or tools) you would use.
5. Would you encourage Mrs. Delgado to breast-feed? If so, then why? What factors would you expect might discourage her from trying? How would you discuss these factors?
6. Write a lesson plan for an infant-feeding session, addressing breast-feeding and bottlefeeding methods. Include the components listed in questions 3 and 4.

healing; they also promote iron absorption and act as sources of fiber. Vitamin A–rich fruits and vegetables contribute β-carotene and vitamin A to prevent infection, promote night vision, and prevent constipation. Other fruits and vegetables contribute energy and fiber to the diet. Oils provide vitamin E and essential fatty acids.

Alternative Food Patterns

With the increasing ethnic diversity in the United States, it is especially important to use the woman's personal cultural food patterns in dietary counseling. We are ethnocentric if we rigidly adhere to a single dietary pattern for all pregnant women, because intake differs among women from various cultures, belief systems, and lifestyles. We must always remember that specific nutrients, not specific foods, are required for a successful pregnancy and that these nutrients are found in a wide variety of food choices. If we are wise, we will encourage our clients to use foods that serve their nutritional needs, whatever those foods might be (see the *Case Study* box, "A Baby for the Delgados"). A number of resources are available as guides for cultural, religious, and vegetarian food patterns. Suggestions for improving transcultural nutrition counseling skills are also available.[28–30]

Dietary Supplements

Often, "prenatal vitamins" are prescribed for pregnant women. These supplements include a variety of vitamins and minerals and are intended to add to nutrient intake from foods rather than replace food and nutrient consumption. Iron and folate are generally the two nutrients that require supplementation during pregnancy. Some women may need additional nutrients, however.[31] For example, pregnant women who follow vegan diets, have one or more nutritional deficiencies, smoke cigarettes, use or abuse drugs or alcohol (or both), or have multiple fetuses, need prenatal vitamin and mineral supplements that include additional nutrients.

Herbal and botanical supplement use during pregnancy is discouraged because of the potentially harmful or unknown effects on the woman and fetus. However, based on cultural and traditional medicine practices and emerging trends, pregnant women may include such products in their daily routines (see the *Case Study* box, "Nutrition Counseling in Pregnancy"). Several reference materials are available regarding the risks associated with use of specific herbals and botanicals during pregnancy (see *Further Readings and Resources* at the end of this chapter).[32–34]

WEIGHT GAIN DURING PREGNANCY

General Amount of Weight Gain

Healthy women produce healthy babies across a wide range of total weight gain. Therefore during pregnancy the nutritional focus should always be on an individualized assessment of need and the quality of the weight gain. An average weight gain during normal pregnancy is about 11 to 16 kg

CASE STUDY

Nutrition Counseling in Pregnancy

Ms. McLane is a 33-year-old Caucasian woman who is in her twenty-ninth week of pregnancy. This is her second pregnancy. During her first pregnancy (at age 29), she gained 24 lb during a normal pregnancy and had a delivery without complications. She is presently 165.1 cm (5 feet, 5 inches) tall and weighs 81.8 kg (180 lb). Her prepregnancy weight was 72.7 kg (160 lb). Ms. McLane visited her obstetrician before her second pregnancy for prepregnancy planning. She has been consuming a healthy diet and a prenatal vitamin supplement every day. After her first visit to the obstetrician during the current pregnancy (at week 10), Ms. McLane did not return for any further appointments, because of her prior positive experience with pregnancy and belief that she "didn't need anything because the first pregnancy went so well."

Ms. McLane has a positive family history for diabetes, and her mother had gestational diabetes. Ms. McLane should have been screened for gestational diabetes between the twenty-fourth and twenty-eighth weeks of her current pregnancy; however, this was not done. She experienced frequent urination and fatigue that she reported as "different" from her first pregnancy. This prompted her to return to her obstetrician. The obstetrician completed a full examination and administered an oral glucose tolerance test. One hour after consuming a 100-g solution of glucose, Ms. McLane's blood glucose concentration was 218 mg/dL. She was scheduled for follow-up testing, and gestational diabetes was confirmed. A 2200-kcal/day diabetic diet was prescribed to allow Ms. McLane to control this condition through diet.

Ms. McLane has been referred to you for nutrition counseling. This is now the thirty-first week of her pregnancy, and she shares with you that a friend suggested that she "use some natural products to help her high blood sugar." In addition to consuming her prenatal supplement on a daily basis, she takes 500 mg of burdock root and 1 tbsp of flaxseed and drinks 3 cups of hot fenugreek tea per day. Her prenatal supplement contains 400 mcg of folate, 250 mg of calcium, 40 mg of iron, 100 mg of vitamin C, 5 mcg of vitamin D, 3 mg of thiamin, 3 mg of riboflavin, 4 mg of pyridoxine, 40 mg of niacin, 10 mg of vitamin E, 5 mcg of vitamin B_{12}, 30 mg of zinc, and 10 mg of copper. Completion of a dietary intake analysis shows that Ms. McLane's kcalorie intake is 1750 per day. She reported that she has been nauseated for about 2 weeks, so she also added 300 mg of powdered ginger to each cup of the fenugreek tea. She reported some diarrhea and Braxton Hicks contractions during the last week, as well a lack of desire to be physically active.

Questions for Analysis

1. What is Ms. McLane's body mass index (BMI) based on her prepregnancy weight?
2. What is the recommended amount of weight gain for Ms. McLane based on prepregnancy weight and BMI? Has she experienced an appropriate weight gain so far?
3. Is the current level of kcalories appropriate based on her condition of gestational diabetes, BMI, and weight gain?
4. What additional information would you collect from Ms. McLane to complete a nutritional assessment?
5. How would you approach a nutritional intake plan for Ms. McLane?
6. Why would Ms. McLane's friend have recommended burdock root, flaxseed, and fenugreek? Be specific for each botanical. Are burdock root, flaxseed, fenugreek, or ginger recommended for use during pregnancy?
7. Identify at least five points that you would make during a nutrition counseling session with Ms. McLane. Discuss the priority for the first counseling session with Ms. McLane.

(25 to 35 lb).[35] Around this average, many individual variations occur. No specific rigid norm or restriction exists to which all women should be held, regardless of individual needs; therefore such a course is obviously unwise and unscientific. Current recommendations are therefore usually stated in terms of ranges to accommodate variances in needs. An initial base for evaluation, however, may be the average weight of the products of pregnancy as shown in Table 11-2. In addition to the components of growth and development usually attributed to a pregnancy, an important part is maternal stores. This laying down of extra adipose fat tissue is necessary for maternal energy reserves to sustain rapid fetal growth during the latter half of pregnancy, for labor and delivery, and for maintaining lactation after birth. Approximately 1.8 to 3.6 kg (4 to 8 lb) of adipose tissue is commonly deposited for these needs. The Institute of Medicine updated weight gain guidelines for pregnancy in May 2009, using the World Health Organization's (WHO's) classifications for prepregnancy BMI. The guidelines are as follows[35]:

- Normal-weight women with a BMI of 18.5 to 24.9 should gain from 11.5 to 16 kg (25 to 35 lb).

TABLE 11-2 APPROXIMATE WEIGHT OF PRODUCTS OF NORMAL PREGNANCY

PRODUCTS	WEIGHT
Fetus	3500 g (7.5 lb)
Placenta	450 g (1 lb)
Amniotic fluid	900 g (2 lb)
Uterus (weight increase)	1100 g (2.5 lb)
Breast tissue (weight increase)	1400 g (3 lb)
Blood volume (weight increase)	1800 g (4 lb) (1500 mL)
Maternal stores	1800-3600 g (4-8 lb)
TOTAL	10,850-12,650 g (10.9-12.7 kg, 24-28 lb)

KEY TERMS

primigravida A woman who is pregnant for the first time.

- Underweight women with a BMI of less than 18.5 should gain 12.7 to 18.1 kg (28 to 40 lb).
- Overweight women with a BMI of 25.0 to 29.9 should gain 6.8 to 11.5 kg (15 to 25 lb).
- Obese women with a BMI of 30.0 or more should gain 5.0 to 9.2 kg (11 to 20 lb).

The recommendation for adolescent girls is that they should follow the adult BMI guidelines and gain weight within the corresponding range. The recommendation for a woman carrying twins who is of normal BMI is a weight gain range of 16.8 to 24.5 kg (37 to 54 lb).[35] Overweight women carrying twins should gain 14.2 to 22.8 kg (31 to 50 lb), whereas obese women carrying twins should gain 11.5 to 19.1 kg (25 to 42 lb).[35] Compared with single-birth infants, twin-birth infants are five times more likely to be born premature (gestation of less than 37 weeks), nine and a half times more likely to be very low birth weight (<1500 g), and eight and a half times more likely to be low birth weight (<2500 g).[36]

Quality of Weight Gain

The important consideration lies in the nutritional quality of the gain. Specifically, the foods consumed should be nutrient dense, not full of empty kcalories, to meet nutrient requirements. In addition, in some cases clinicians have failed to distinguish between weight gained as a result of edema and that as a result of deposition of fat—maternal stores for energy to sustain rapid fetal growth during the latter part of pregnancy and energy for lactation to follow.[37] Analysis of the total tissue gained in an average pregnancy shows that the largest component, 62%, is water. Fat accounts for 31% and protein for 7%. Water is also the most variable component of the tissue gained, accounting for a range of 8 kg (18 lb) to as much as 11 kg (24 lb). Of the 8 kg of water usually gained, about 5.5 kg (12 lb) is associated with fetal tissue and other tissues gained in pregnancy. The remaining 2.5 kg (6 lb) accumulates in the maternal interstitial tissues.[38] Gravity causes the maternal tissue fluids to pool more in the lower extremities, leading to general swelling of the ankles, which is seen routinely in pregnant women. This fluid retention is a normal adaptive phenomenon designed to support the pregnancy and to exert a positive effect on fetal growth. Connective tissue becomes more hygroscopic as a result of the estrogen-induced changes in the ground substance and thus becomes softer and more easily distended. This facilitates delivery of the infant through the cervix and vaginal canal. In addition, the increased tissue fluid during pregnancy provides a means for handling the increased metabolic work and circulation of numerous metabolites necessary for fetal growth.

Clearly, severe kcalorie restriction is harmful to the developing fetus and the woman. It is inevitably accompanied by restriction of the vitally needed nutrients essential to the growth process.[37] Moreover, *weight reduction should never be undertaken during pregnancy.* Sufficient weight gain should be encouraged with the use of a nourishing diet.

Rate of Weight Gain

On the whole, about 0.5 to 2.0 kg (1.1 to 4.4 lb) is a target for average weight gain during the first trimester for all pregnant women.[35] Thereafter, the target for average weight gain per week is 0.5 kg (1 lb) for underweight and normal-weight women, 0.3 kg (0.6 lb) for overweight women, and 0.23 kg (0.5 lb) for obese women. No scientific justification exists for routinely limiting weight gain to lesser amounts. Moreover, an individual woman who needs to gain more should not have unrealistic patterns imposed on her. It is only unusual patterns of gain, such as a sudden sharp increase in weight after the twentieth week of pregnancy that may signal abnormal water retention, which should be monitored closely, especially if it occurs in conjunction with blood pressure elevation and proteinuria. Conversely, an insufficient or low maternal weight gain during the second or third trimester increases the risk for intrauterine growth retardation.[37,39]

Weight Gain and Sodium Intake

A moderate amount of dietary sodium is needed for two essential reasons:

1. It is the major mineral required to control the extracellular fluid compartment.
2. This vital body water is increased during pregnancy to support its successful outcome.

Current practice usually follows a regular diet with moderate sodium intake, 1.5 to 2.3 g/day, with light use of salt to taste.[40] Limiting sodium beyond this general use is contrary to physiologic need in pregnancy and is unfounded. The NRC and professional obstetric guidelines have labeled routine salt-free diets and diuretics as potentially dangerous.[3–5] Maintaining the needed increase in circulating blood volume during pregnancy requires adequate amounts of sodium and protein, as well as adequate fluid intake to prevent dehydration and possible premature contractions.

GENERAL DIETARY PROBLEMS

Functional Gastrointestinal Problems

Nausea and Vomiting

Some general dietary problems temporarily interfere with food and nutrient intake. Most are easily resolved through dietary counseling and with medical attention and have no long-term adverse effect on the quality of maternal weight gain. Symptoms of nausea and vomiting are usually mild and short term, the so-called morning sickness of early pregnancy, because it occurs more often on arising than later in the day. At least 50% of all pregnant women, most of them in their first pregnancy, experience this condition, beginning during the fifth or sixth week of the pregnancy and usually ending about the fourteenth to sixteenth week. A number of factors may contribute to the situation. Some factors are physiologic, with causal factors based on hormonal changes that occur early in pregnancy or on low blood sugar, which can be relieved by carbohydrate foods but that will return within 2 to 3 hours after a meal. Others may be psychologic, based on situational tensions or anxieties about the pregnancy itself. Still others may be dietary problems, based on poor food habits. Simple treatment generally improves food tolerance. Frequent small low-fat meals and snacks, which are fairly dry and consist chiefly of easily digested energy-yielding foods such as carbohydrates (mainly starches), are usually more readily tolerated. In addition, it may help to avoid cooking odors as much as possible. Liquids are best taken between meals instead of with meals.

Hyperemesis

In a small number of pregnant women, about 3.5:1000 pregnancies, a severe form of persistent nausea and vomiting occurs that does not respond to usual treatment. This condition, *hyperemesis*, begins early in the pregnancy and may last throughout it. It may develop into the more serious pernicious form of hyperemesis gravidarum. This persistent condition causes severe alterations in fluids and electrolytes, weight loss, and nutritional deficits, sometimes requiring hospitalization and alternative feeding by enteral or parenteral methods to sustain the pregnancy (see Chapter 19). Pyridoxine supplementation has been suggested as a preventive measure to abate nausea and vomiting, along with an increased protein and lower carbohydrate content of the diet.[41] Some prescription medications may also be useful but require physician supervision.[41] Continued personal support and reassurance are important.

Constipation

The complaint of constipation is seldom more than minor, but it contributes to discomfort and concern. Placental hormones relax the gastrointestinal muscles, and the pressure of the enlarging uterus on the lower portion of the intestine may make elimination somewhat difficult. Increased fluid intake and the use of naturally laxative foods containing dietary fiber, such as whole grains, fruits and vegetables, dried fruits (especially prunes and figs), and other fruits and juices, generally promote regularity. Laxatives should be avoided. Appropriate daily exercise is essential for overall health during pregnancy.

Hemorrhoids

A fairly common complaint during the latter part of pregnancy is that of hemorrhoids. These are enlarged veins in the anus, often protruding through the anal sphincter. This vein enlargement is usually caused by the increased weight of the fetus and its downward pressure. The hemorrhoids may cause considerable discomfort, burning, and itching. Occasionally, they may rupture and bleed under pressure of a bowel movement, causing anxiety. The problem is usually controlled by the dietary suggestions given for constipation. In addition, sufficient rest during the latter part of the day may help relieve some of the downward pressure of the uterus on the lower intestine.

Heartburn or Gastric Pressure

Pregnant women sometimes voice the related complaints of heartburn or a full feeling. These discomforts occur especially after meals and are usually caused by the pressure of the enlarging uterus crowding the stomach. Gastric reflux of some of the food mass, now a liquid chyme mixed with stomach acid, may occur in the lower esophagus, causing an irritation and a burning sensation. Obviously this common complaint has nothing to do with heart action but it receives the name because of the close proximity of the lower esophagus to the heart. The full feeling comes from general gastric pressure, lack of normal space in the area, a large meal, or gas formation. These complaints are usually remedied by dividing the day's food into a series of small meals, avoiding eating large meals at any time, and not lying down after a meal. Comfort is also improved by wearing loose-fitting clothing.

Effects of Iron Supplements

The effects of an iron supplement may include gray or black stools and sometimes nausea, constipation, or diarrhea. To help avoid food-related effects, the iron supplement should be taken 1 hour before a meal or 2 hours after it, with liquid such as water or orange juice but not with milk or tea. The absorption of iron is increased with vitamin C and decreased with milk, other dairy foods, eggs, whole grain bread and cereal, and tea. Ferrous fumarate and ferrous gluconate are alternate forms of iron supplements with good absorption properties that tend to result in less gastrointestinal distress.

HIGH-RISK PREGNANCIES

Identify Risk Factors Involved

To avoid the consequences of sustained poor nutrition during pregnancy, a first procedure is to identify women at risk. In a joint report, the American College of Obstetrics and Gynecology and the American Dietetic Association issued a set of risk factors, as shown in Box 11-1, that identify women with special nutritional needs during pregnancy.[5] These nutrition-related factors are based on clinical evidence of inadequate nutrition. However, rather than waiting for clinical symptoms of poor nutrition to appear, a better approach would be to identify poor food patterns that will induce nutritional problems and to prevent these problems from developing. On this basis, three types of dietary patterns predict failure to support optimal maternal and fetal nutrition: (1) insufficient food intake, (2) poor food selection, and (3) poor food distribution throughout the day. These patterns, added to the list of risk factors in Box 11-1, are much more sensitive for nutritional risk.

Plan Personal Care

Once early assessment identifies risk factors, practitioners can then give more careful attention to these women. By working closely with each woman and her personal food pattern

KEY TERMS

hygroscopic Taking up and retaining moisture readily.

hyperemesis gravidarum Severe vomiting during pregnancy, which is potentially fatal.

BOX 11-1 NUTRITIONAL RISK FACTORS IN PREGNANCY

Risk Factors Present at the Onset of Pregnancy

- Age: ≤15 yr or ≥35 yr
- Frequent pregnancies: three or more during a 2-year period
- Poor obstetric history or poor fetal performance
- Poverty
- Bizarre or faddist food habits
- Abuse of nicotine, alcohol, or drugs
- Therapeutic diet required for a chronic disorder
- Weight: <85% or >120% of standard weight

Risk Factors Occurring During Pregnancy

- Low hemoglobin (HGB) or hematocrit (HCT): HGB <12 g/dL, HCT <35%
- Inadequate weight gain: any weight loss *or* weight gain of <1 kg (2 lb)/month after the first trimester
- Excessive weight gain: >1 kg (2 lb)/week after the first trimester

From American College of Obstetrics and Gynecology and American Dietetic Association Task Force on Nutrition: *Assessment of maternal nutrition,* Chicago, 1978, American College of Obstetrics and Gynecology.

and living situation, a food plan can be developed with her to ensure an optimal intake of energy and nutrients to support her pregnancy and its successful outcome.

Recognize Special Counseling Needs

Several special needs require sensitive counseling. These areas of need include the age and parity of the woman; any use of harmful agents such as alcohol, cigarettes, drugs, or pica; and socioeconomic problems.

Age and Parity

Pregnancies at either age extreme of the reproductive cycle pose special problems. The National Center for Chronic Disease Prevention and Health Promotion reported that approximately 415,000 live births occurred annually to female teenagers during the years 2004 to 2006.[42] The adolescent pregnancy carries many social and nutrition-related risks associated with increased incidence of low birth weight and perinatal mortality, among other poor outcomes. The obstetric history of a woman is expressed in terms of number and order of pregnancies, or her gravida status. A **nulligravida** (no prior pregnancy) who is 15 years of age or younger is especially at risk because her own growth is incomplete; therefore sufficient weight gain and the quality of her diet are particularly important.[38] Nutrients of particular concern are those for which the adolescent female requirements are greater than the adult requirements, including calcium, magnesium, phosphorus, and zinc. These nutrients are critical for growth and development of the adolescent, as well as for her fetus. Sensitive counseling provides information and emotional support; it should involve family members or other persons significant to the adolescent. On the other hand, the older primigravida (first pregnancy), older than 35 years, also requires special attention. She may be more at risk for hypertension, either preexisting or pregnancy induced, and may need more attention to the rate of weight gain and amount of sodium used, as well as any drug therapy prescribed. In addition, several pregnancies within a limited number of years leave a mother drained of nutritional resources and entering each successive pregnancy at increased risk.

Social Habits: Alcohol, Cigarettes, and Drugs

These three personal habits may cause fetal damage and are contraindicated during pregnancy. No safe level of alcohol consumption has yet been found for pregnant women. Extensive or habitual alcohol use may lead to one of the fetal alcohol spectrum disorders known as *fetal alcohol syndrome (FAS),* which is currently a leading cause of mental retardation.[43] FAS is characterized by growth retardation, malformed facial features, joint and limb abnormalities, cardiac defects, mental retardation, and in serious cases, death. FAS signs have been seen in tests with rats as early as the human equivalent of the third week of gestation, when most women are unaware of their pregnancies. Thus moderate-to-heavy drinking among sexually active women of childbearing age may carry potential danger. Even moderate prenatal alcohol exposure has been associated with low birth weight and has effects on a child's psychomotor and cognitive development in the absence of malformations, known as *fetal alcohol effects (FAE).*[44]

Cigarette smoking during pregnancy is also contraindicated.[45] Harmful substances in tobacco and impaired oxygen transport cause fetal damage and special problems of placental abnormalities, leading to increased risk of spontaneous abortion (miscarriage), prematurity, low birth weight, impairment of mental and physical growth, and increased potential mortality.[45,46] Counseling with women and families who smoke should stress the importance of quitting for pregnancy and beyond.

Drug use, both recreational and medicinal, also poses numerous problems.[46] Self-medication with over-the-counter drugs carries potential adverse effects. The use of illicit drugs is especially hazardous, exposing the developing fetus to the risks of addiction and possibly acquired immunodeficiency syndrome (AIDS) from the woman's use of contaminated needles during drug injections. Dangers come not only from the drug itself or contaminated needles but also from impurities contained in illicit drugs. Evaluation of the effects of street drugs (marijuana, cocaine, heroin, methadone) on nutritional status is difficult because of multiple drug use, uncertain purity, unknown dose and timing, and inadequate nutritional status of many drug users. A high incidence of meconium staining (which could relate to fetal damage), poor prenatal weight gain, very short (<3 hours) or prolonged labor, operative delivery (cesarean, forceps), and other perinatal problems

KEY TERMS

nulligravida A woman who has never been pregnant.

among marijuana users has been reported. Such outcomes indicate that abstinence of marijuana use during pregnancy is prudent.

Abuse from megadosing with basic nutrients such as vitamin A or use of prescription medications such as Accutane during pregnancy may cause fetal damage as previously described (see *Further Readings and Resources* at the end of this chapter). A number of drugs are often prescribed for female patients to treat a variety of psychologic and mental health disorders. However, if taken during pregnancy, many drugs exhibit teratogenic effects. If any of these drugs are taken on a long-term basis for the treatment of serious conditions, such as clinical depression, bipolar disorder, or schizophrenia, then comprehensive medical and psychologic assessment and follow-up is needed throughout the pregnancy. Lithium has been associated with an increased risk for Epstein's anomaly (a rare cardiovascular abnormality), goiter, and diabetes insipidus, as well as neonatal toxic disturbances such as cyanosis, hypothermia, and bradycardia. A diminished suck reflex will impede attempts to nourish the infant exposed to lithium in utero. Diazepam (Valium) is associated with an abnormal fetal heart rate. The neonate risks delivery by cesarean section, with oral-facial malformations, a depressed Apgar score, and a reluctance to feed. Rats exposed to diazepam in utero have exhibited abnormal motor skills and arousal processes. *Tricyclic antidepressants* (e.g., imipramine) have led to morphologic and behavioral abnormalities in rats.

Hydantoin (Dilantin, phenytoin) is used to control seizures caused by epilepsy and other conditions. Even though this drug has caused malformations in the offspring of rats, physicians are reluctant to discontinue it for their patients with epilepsy during pregnancy. Because only 7% of children born to mothers using the drug develop malformations, and significantly more develop malformations and developmental disabilities when the mother's epilepsy is untreated, this may be one case in which prenatal drug use is more beneficial than not using it. Thus with the exception of drugs used to treat individuals with seizure disorders or natural replacement therapy (e.g., insulin for persons with type 1 diabetes), drugs should be avoided at all costs during pregnancy to ensure the health of the woman and a safe and healthy outcome of the pregnancy. The nutrition counselor is well advised to keep up with the most recent findings regarding medications (prescribed, over-the-counter, and street drugs) to evaluate the nutritional status of the woman using them and to allow the practitioner and woman to design a plan of action to safely eliminate the drug, preferably before conception. In addition, evaluation of herbal and botanical supplements, which are not regulated in the same manner as prescription and over-the-counter drugs, is necessary to inform the woman of potential safety issues and to counsel her appropriately.

Caffeine

Although milder in its effect (depending on the extent of use) than the agents just discussed, caffeine remains a widely used drug that can cross the placenta and enter fetal circulation.[47] Its use at levels of 500 mg/day or greater has been associated with an increased risk of first-trimester spontaneous abortion.[48,49] Most health agencies have recommended that pregnant women limit caffeine consumption from foods, beverages (coffee, tea, cocoa, cola), and medications to less than 300 mg/day because of the many uncertainties regarding the fetal effects of maternal caffeine consumption.[50]

Pica

Pica is the craving and consumption of unusual nonfood substances such as laundry starch, clay, dirt, or ice. This practice during pregnancy is more widespread than health care workers have believed, particularly in southern regions of the United States and among specific ethnic and cultural groups. Some pica practices have been associated with iron deficiency anemia, although the direction of causality is unknown.[51,52] Where these unusual practices exist, they must be appreciated as cultural patterns that require a respectful approach and understanding by health workers who seek to negotiate appropriate behavior changes (see the *Focus on Culture* box, "Pica During Pregnancy: Cultural Norm of Concern").[53]

FOCUS ON CULTURE

Pica During Pregnancy: Cultural Norm of Concern

Pica is the ingestion of nonfood substances or food components including but not limited to clay, dirt, chalk, cornstarch, laundry starch, baking powder, baking soda, ice, and freezer frost. These substances are often craved with subsequent consumption. Approximately 20% of pregnant women engage in pica, and the prevalence of this psychobehavioral disorder is increased in rural (compared with urban) areas and in certain cultures.

Normal Cultural Behavior or Pregnancy-Induced Disorder

In a group of women living in Kenya from a variety of ethnic and religious backgrounds, more than 80% reported consumption of approximately 1 cup of soil on a daily basis. Soil intake was more common in the latter part of pregnancy. In these cultures, pica represents a cultural norm that may increase in prevalence during pregnancy.

Nearly 45% of women born and living in western Mexico engaged in pica during pregnancy, whereas only about 30% of Mexican-born women currently residing in California practiced pica during pregnancy. Although pica may be a culturally accepted norm, changes in prevalence may be induced with acculturation into a society where this behavior is less common.

Consequences of Pica and Need for Counseling

A pregnant woman who engages in pica, regardless of cultural background, should be informed about the health consequences

Continued

FOCUS ON CULTURE

Pica During Pregnancy: Cultural Norm of Concern—cont'd

of pica. Although it is unclear if nutrient deficiencies precipitate pica behaviors or vice versa, many pica substances are capable of binding nutrients to render them unavailable for absorption. Nutritional anemias may occur, having adverse effects on both mother and baby. Exposure to toxins and teratogens from nonfood substances such as battery acid or ashes is also possible. Gastrointestinal perforation, constipation, and microbial infections are additional potential outcomes of pica.

An understanding by the health care practitioner regarding factors leading to pica is vital to affecting behavior change. For example, the pregnant woman who believes that a nonfood substance has an essential role in the body's balance or harmony with her environment may be less willing to avoid consumption of that nonfood substance. On the other hand, a pregnant woman who consumes eggshells because of the sensory cravings associated with the texture may be amenable to substituting a crunchy food substance for this nonfood product. Inquiry regarding the history of pica in the pregnant woman is important to identify sources of pica substances and to involve other family members or cultural leaders who may support such behavior and need counseling to facilitate appropriate behavior changes. Such nutrition counseling must be delivered in a culturally sensitive and appropriate manner, with emphasis on the importance of behavior changes for an optimal outcome for the infant.

BIBLIOGRAPHY

Corbett RW, Ryan C, Weinrich SP, et al: Pica in pregnancy: does it affect pregnancy outcomes? *MCN Am J Matern Child Nurs* 28(3):183, 2003.

Geissler PW, Prince RJ, Levene M, et al: Perceptions of soil-eating and anaemia among pregnant women on the Kenyan coast, *Soc Sci Med* 48(8):1069, 1999.

Mills ME: Craving more than food: the implications of pica in pregnancy, *Nurs Womens Health* 11(3):266, 2007.

Rainville AJ: Pica practices of pregnant women are associated with lower maternal hemoglobin level at delivery, *J Am Diet Assoc* 98(3):293, 1998.

Simpson E, Mull JD, Longley E, et al: Pica during pregnancy in low-income women born in Mexico, *West J Med* 173(1):20, 2000.

Socioeconomic Challenges

Special counseling is required for women and young girls facing economic challenges. Numerous studies and clinical observations indicate that lack of prenatal care, often associated with racial prejudices and fears, as well as a lack of adequate financial resources, places the expectant mother in grave difficulty. Special counseling that is sensitive to personal needs is required to help plan resources for care and financial assistance. Resources include programs such as the federally funded Special Supplemental Nutrition Program for Women, Infants, and Children (WIC), described in Appendix F, as well as numerous state and local programs. An example of a community partnership program promoting prenatal care is Stork's Nest, sponsored by the March of Dimes in affiliation with a national women's organization and local community service agencies. Another successful program targeted for low-income women is BabyCare, administered by the Virginia Department of Health (see *Further Readings and Resources* at the end of this chapter).

COMPLICATIONS OF PREGNANCY

Anemia

Anemia is common during pregnancy. It is often associated with the normal maternal blood volume increase of 40% to 50% and a disproportionate increase in red cell mass of about 20%. Of all women in large prenatal clinics in the United States, about 10% have hemoglobin concentrations of less than 10 g/dL and a hematocrit reading less than 32%. Anemia is far more prevalent among the poor, many of whom live on diets barely adequate for subsistence. However, anemia is by no means restricted to lower economic groups.

Iron Deficiency Anemia

A deficiency of iron is by far the most common cause of anemia in pregnancy. The total cost of a single normal pregnancy in iron stores is large—approximately 500 to 800 mg. Of this amount, the fetus uses nearly 300 mg. The remainder is used in the expanded maternal blood volume and its increased red blood cells and hemoglobin mass. This iron requirement typically exceeds the available reserves in the average woman. Thus in addition to including iron-rich foods in the diet, a daily supplement or increased therapeutic dose may be required as previously described.

Folate Deficiency Anemia

A less common megaloblastic anemia of pregnancy results from folate deficiency. During pregnancy, the fetus is sensitive to folate inhibitors and therefore has increased metabolic requirements for folate. To prevent this anemia the DRI standard recommends 600 mcg of folate per day during pregnancy. Women with poor diets will need supplementation to reach this intake goal.

Hemorrhagic Anemia

Anemia caused by blood loss is more likely to occur during labor and delivery than during pregnancy. Blood loss may occur earlier, as a result of abortion or ruptured tubular pregnancy. Most women undergoing these physiologic problems receive blood via transfusion, and iron therapy may be indicated for adequate replacement for hemoglobin formation.

Pregnancy-Induced Hypertension

Relation to Nutrition

A number of clinicians have presented clinical and laboratory evidence that pregnancy-induced hypertension (PIH) is a disease that principally affects young women with their first pregnancy. Although the genetic and immune-related causes of PIH are becoming clearer, diet plays a role in the risk of preeclampsia. For example, diets poor in kcalories, protein, calcium, magnesium, potassium, and dietary fiber have been associated with risk of PIH. Regardless of the underlying causes and multiorgan effects, nutritional support of the pregnancy is, as always, a primary concern. Certainly, as many practitioners have observed, PIH is classically associated with poverty, inadequate diet, and little or no prenatal care. Much of the PIH problem, which seems to develop early from the time of implantation of the fertilized ovum into the uterine lining, may be reduced by good prenatal care from the beginning of the pregnancy, which inherently includes attention to sound nutrition. It is this sound nutritional status, which a woman brings to her pregnancy and maintains throughout it, that provides her with optimal resources for adapting to the physiologic stress of gestation. Her fitness during pregnancy is a direct function of her past state of nutrition and her optimal nutrition throughout pregnancy.

Clinical Symptoms

PIH is defined according to its manifestations, which generally occur in the third trimester toward term. These symptoms are hypertension, abnormal and excessive edema, albuminuria, and, in severe cases, convulsions or coma, a state called **eclampsia**.

Treatment

Specific treatment varies according to the individual patient's symptoms and needs. Optimal nutrition is a fundamental aspect of therapy in any case. Emphasis is given to a regular diet with adequate dietary protein and calcium, as well as to a diet that is rich in fruits and vegetables, providing magnesium, potassium, and dietary fiber. Correction of plasma protein deficits stimulates the capillary fluid shift mechanism and increases circulation of tissue fluids, with subsequent correction of the **hypovolemia**. In addition, adequate salt and sources of vitamins and minerals are needed for correction and maintenance of metabolic balance.

Multiple Fetuses

The incidence of multifetal pregnancies has increased in recent decades and presents unique concerns. Infants born from a multifetal pregnancy are more likely to have lower-than-average birth weights and are at risk for preterm delivery.[36] Thus nutritional needs of these women must be given special attention. Energy intake must be increased beyond the needs of a single fetus pregnancy so that the recommended weight gain for multiple fetuses is achieved. This increase in energy intake often provides for the additional nutrient demands that exist. Attention to adequate folate intake is critical to reduce risks of low birth weights and preterm delivery. Supplemental iron may be necessary to reduce the incidence of anemia, more commonly found in women with multiple fetuses. Additional calcium and vitamin D are needed with multiple fetuses to promote adequate calcium absorption for optimal bone mineralization in utero. Zinc, copper, and pyridoxine supplementation may also be required to support multifetal growth and development.

Maternal Disease Conditions

Preexisting clinical conditions in the woman further complicate pregnancy. In each case, management of these conditions is based on general principles of care related to pregnancy and to the particular disease involved. Examples of such maternal conditions are reviewed here; they are hypertension, diabetes mellitus, PKU, AIDS, and eating disorders.

Hypertension

Preexisting hypertension in the pregnant woman can cause considerable maternal and fetal consequences. Many of these problems can be prevented by initial screening and continued monitoring by the prenatal nurse, with referral to the clinical nutritionist for a plan of care. The hypertensive disease process begins long before signs and symptoms appear, and later symptoms are inconsistent. Risk factors for hypertension before and during pregnancy are listed in Box 11-2. Nutritional therapy centers on the following three principles:

1. Prevention of weight extremes (i.e., underweight or obesity).
2. Correction of any dietary deficiencies and maintenance of optimal nutritional status during pregnancy.
3. Management of any related coexisting disease (e.g., diabetes mellitus, hyperlipidemia).

BOX 11-2 RISK FACTORS FOR PREGNANCY-INDUCED HYPERTENSION

Before Pregnancy

- Nulligravida
- Diabetes
- Preexisting condition (hypertension, renal or vascular disease)
- Family history of hypertension or vascular disease
- Diagnosis of pregnancy-induced hypertension (PIH) in a previous pregnancy
- Dietary deficiencies
- Age extremes (≤20 years old, ≥35 years old)

During Pregnancy

- Primigravida
- Large fetus
- Glomerulonephritis
- Fetal hydrops
- Hydramnios
- Multiple gestation
- Hydatidiform mole

KEY TERMS

eclampsia Advanced pregnancy-induced hypertension (PIH), manifested by convulsions.

hypovolemia Abnormally decreased volume of circulating blood in the body.

Sodium intake may be moderate but should not be unduly restricted because of its relation to fluid and electrolyte balances during pregnancy. Initial and continuing client education and a close relationship with the nurse-nutritionist care team contribute to successful management of the hypertension and prevent problems that may occur. (For a more detailed discussion of vascular disease, see Chapter 21.)

Diabetes Mellitus and Gestational Diabetes Mellitus

The management of preexisting diabetes in pregnancy presents special problems. Today, however, improved expectations for the diabetic woman's pregnancy constitute one of the success stories of modern medicine.[54] Contributing factors to this improved outlook include advances in technology for monitoring fetal development, increased knowledge of nutrition and diabetes, and management refinements in tight blood glucose control through self-monitoring.[55,56] (Chapter 22 details the care of persons with types 1 and 2 diabetes mellitus.)

During pregnancy, glycosuria is not uncommon because of the increased circulating blood volume and its load of metabolites. Routine screening protocols, typically conducted between the twenty-fourth and twenty-eighth week of gestation, are used during pregnancy to detect gestational diabetes mellitus (GDM). GDM is an intolerance of carbohydrate such that blood glucose concentration increases during pregnancy. In 95% of cases this carbohydrate or glucose intolerance resolves after delivery. Treatment during pregnancy is important because of the increased risk these women carry for fetal damage during this gestational period.[57] The most common outcome for an infant born to a mother with GDM is macrosomia, a larger than normal body size. Other infant complications include hypoglycemia, jaundice, and trauma at birth. Although GDM occurs in 2% to 13% of the pregnant population, up to 50% of women with pregnancy-induced abnormal glucose tolerance subsequently develop overt diabetes. Team management is required for adequate care of gestational and preexisting types 1 and 2 diabetes mellitus.[58,59] (See Chapter 22 for a detailed discussion of diabetes care.)

Maternal Phenylketonuria

The successful detection and management of infants with PKU through newborn screening programs in all states have ensured their normal growth and development to adulthood. PKU is a genetic metabolic disease caused by a missing enzyme for the metabolism of the essential amino acid phenylalanine. It is controlled by a special low-phenylalanine diet initiated at birth. Now a new generation of young women with PKU since birth are beginning to have children of their own. However, maternal PKU presents potential fetal hazards. Experience has shown how crucial it is for the woman to follow a strict low-phenylalanine diet before conception, whenever possible, to minimize risks of fetal damage in the early cell differentiation weeks of pregnancy.

Acquired Immunodeficiency Syndrome

Carefully monitored care throughout pregnancy and after birth is essential for pregnant women who are infected by the human immunodeficiency virus (HIV). Two goals are most important: (1) to reduce the rate of the disease progression in the woman through nutritional support and (2) to minimize the chance of HIV vertical transmission from mother to infant, either in the womb or after birth via breast-feeding. Poor weight gain and nutrient deficiencies during pregnancy are often found in HIV-positive patients. Although specific nutrient requirements for HIV-infected pregnant women have not been established, these patients may need up to 150% of normal pregnancy intakes of macronutrients and micronutrients. Continual individual monitoring and adjustment are essential. Infants can be infected by HIV during labor and delivery and through breast milk. Where safe alternatives to breast milk are available, such as commercial formula or banked human milk, a decision on breast-feeding depends on the HIV status of the newborn infant. In the United States, the Centers for Disease Control and Prevention (CDC) and the American Academy of Pediatrics recommend HIV-positive mothers do not breast-feed when the infant is not infected.[60,61]

Eating Disorders

Eating disorders, specifically anorexia nervosa (AN) and bulimia nervosa (BN), have been previously described (see Chapter 8). Diagnosis and treatment of these disorders in the nonpregnant state require multidisciplinary approaches, and even greater consideration with further specialized care is required for a pregnant woman with AN or BN. AN is uncommon during pregnancy, because amenorrhea is a diagnostic criteria for the disorder; however, ovulation and subsequent conception has been reported.[62] Compared with AN, pregnancy in a woman with BN is more likely, because of more typical menstrual patterns, weight status, and less restrictive eating. BN has been linked to spontaneous abortion, poor weight gain, low infant birth weight, premature deliveries, and congenital malformations.[63] A team approach that emphasizes nutritional needs of the growing fetus, anticipated maternal body size and shape changes, and postpartum care is critical to a successful course and outcome.[63,64]

NUTRITION DURING LACTATION

Current Breast-Feeding Trends

Data from the National Immunization Survey show that approximately 71% of mothers initiate breast-feeding.[65] Several factors contribute to this rate of breast-feeding initiation:

- More mothers are informed about the benefits of breast-feeding (Figure 11-4).[66,67]
- Practitioners recognize the ability of human milk to meet infant needs (Table 11-3) and promote immune function.[68–70]

- Maternity wards and alternative birth centers have been modified to facilitate successful lactation.
- Community support is increasingly available, even in workplaces.[71,72]
- Programs that promote breast-feeding are increasingly responsive to a wider range of maternal socioeconomic conditions and cultural backgrounds.[73–80]

Exclusive breast-feeding by well-nourished mothers can be adequate for periods ranging from 2 to 15 months.[81–84] Exclusive breast-feeding is strongly encouraged for at least 6 months. Unfortunately, exclusive breast-feeding declines to less than 43% and less than 14% of mothers by 3 months and 6 months, respectively.[65] Solid foods are usually added to the baby's diet at about 6 months of age; the American Dietetic Association's position is that breast-feeding should continue for at least the first 12 months of the infant's life.[84]

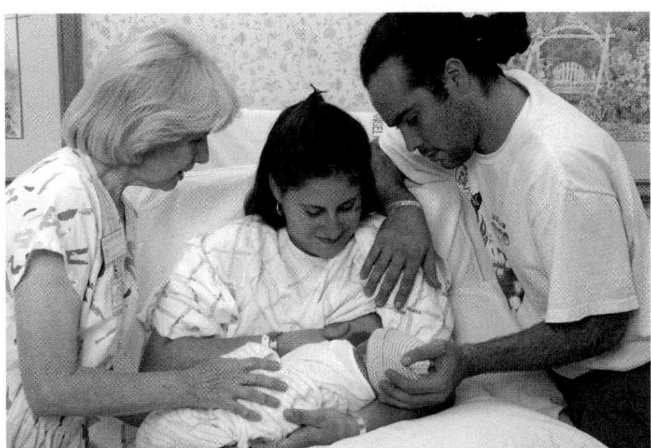

FIGURE 11-4 By teaching about the newborn and family, the nurse helps parents develop confidence in their ability to provide care for the infant. (From McKinney ES, Ashwill JW, Murray SS, et al: *Maternal-child nursing,* Philadelphia, 2000, Saunders.)

Nutritional Needs

The physiologic needs of lactation are different from those of pregnancy, and they demand adequate nutritional support (see Table 11-1). The basic nutritional needs for lactation include the following additions to the mother's prepregnancy needs.

Energy

The recommended caloric increase is 330 kcal/day (plus 170 kcal/day from maternal stores) in the first 6 months and 400 kcal/day in the second 6 months of breast-feeding (beyond the usual adult allowance). This makes a daily total of about 2700 to 2800 kcal/day for milk production and maternal energy needs.[10] This additional energy need for the overall total lactation process is based on the following four factors:

1. *Milk content:* An average daily milk production for lactating women is 780 mL (26 oz). The energy content of human milk averages 0.67 to 0.74 kcal/g. Thus 26 oz of milk has a value of about 525 kcal.
2. *Milk production:* The metabolic work involved in producing this amount of milk is about 80% efficient and requires from 400 to 450 kcal. During pregnancy the breast is developed for this purpose, stimulated by hormones from the placenta, and forms special milk-producing cells called *lobules* (Figure 11-5). After birth the mother's production of the hormone *prolactin* continues this milk-production process, which the suckling infant stimulates. Thus milk production depends on the demand of the infant. The suckling infant stimulates the brain's release of the hormone *oxytocin* from the pituitary gland to initiate the let-down reflex for the release of the milk from storage cells to travel down to the nipple. This reflex is easily inhibited by the mother's fatigue, tension, or lack of confidence, a particular source of anxiety in the new mother. She may be reassured that a comfortable and satisfying feeding routine is usually established in 2 to 3 weeks (Figure 11-6).

TABLE 11-3 SELECTED NUTRITIONAL COMPONENTS OF HUMAN MILK (per 100 mL)

MILK COMPONENT	COLOSTRUM	TRANSITIONAL	MATURE	COW'S MILK
Kilocalories	57.0	63.0	65.0	65.0
Vitamins, fat soluble				
A (mcg)	151.0	88.0	75.0	41.0
D (IU)	—	—	5.0	2.5
E (mg)	1.5	0.9	0.25	0.07
K (mcg)	—	—	1.5	6.0
Vitamins, water soluble				
Thiamin (mcg)	1.9	5.9	14.0	43.0
Riboflavin (mcg)	30.0	37.0	40.0	145.0
Niacin (mcg)	75.0	175.0	160.0	82.0
Pantothenic acid (mcg)	183.0	288.0	246.0	340.0
Biotin (mcg)	0.06	0.35	0.6	2.8
Vitamin B_{12} (mcg)	0.05	0.04	0.1	1.1
Vitamin C (mg)	5.9	7.1	5.0	1.1

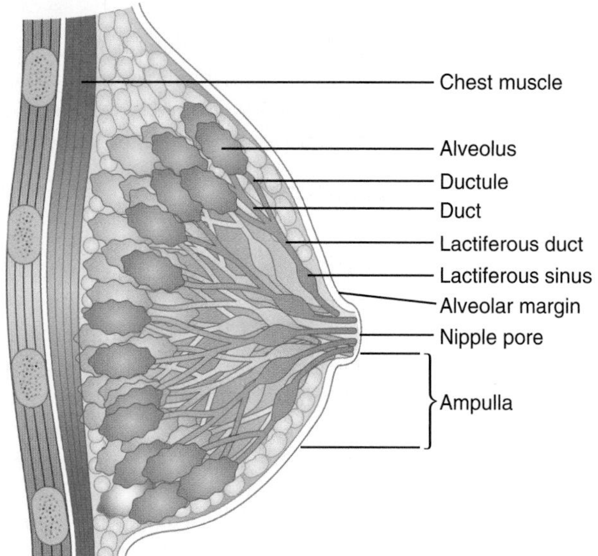

FIGURE 11-5 Structural features of the human mammary gland. (From Mahan LK, Escott-Stump S, editors: *Krause's food, nutrition, and diet therapy,* ed 11, Philadelphia, 2004, Saunders.)

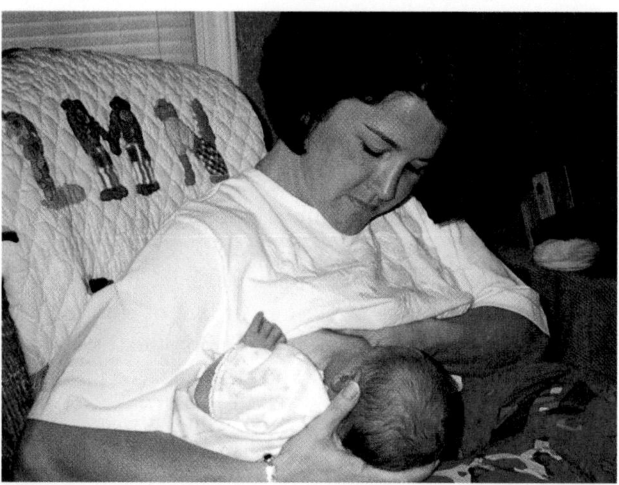

FIGURE 11-6 Breast-feeding infant and mother. (From Lowdermilk DL, Perry SE, Bobak IM: *Maternity and women's health care,* ed 7, St Louis, 2000, Mosby.)

3. *Maternal adipose tissue storage:* A component of the energy need for lactation (170 kcal/day in the first 6 months) is drawn from maternal adipose tissue stores deposited during pregnancy in normal preparation for lactation to follow in the maternal cycle. Depending on the adequacy of these stores, additional energy input may be needed in the lactating woman's daily diet.
4. *Exercise:* Lactating women generally balance energy expenditure from exercise with increased energy intake and alterations in prolactin to maintain an adequate milk supply.[85,86] In some women, the weight gained during pregnancy may be largely retained and contribute to obesity. Some overweight women who are breast-feeding have concerns whether a weight loss program might endanger the growth of their infants. Research with overweight women who were exclusively breast-feeding has shown that a diet and exercise program that led to a weight loss of around 0.5 kg/week (approximately 1 lb/week) from 4 to 14 weeks postpartum did not affect infant growth.[87] However, the mother who is involved in any specific weight loss program during lactation should be monitored closely as should her infant.[87,88]

Protein

The recommendation for protein needs during lactation is 71 g/day during both the first 6 months and the second 6 months.[10] This is an increase of about 25 g/day from the regular needs of the adult woman.

Minerals

The DRI standard for calcium during lactation is 1000 mg/day, the same as for the nonpregnant or pregnant adult woman.[6] The amount of calcium that was required during gestation for the mineralization of the fetal skeleton is now diverted into the mother's milk production. Iron, because it is not a major mineral component of milk and because of lactational amenorrhea, need not be increased during lactation.

Vitamins

The DRI standard for vitamin C during lactation is 120 mg/day.[8] This is a considerable increase from the regular 75 mg/day for adult women. Increases beyond the mother's prenatal intake are also recommended for vitamin A because it is a constituent of milk,[9] and for the B-complex vitamins because they are involved as coenzyme factors in energy metabolism.[7] Therefore the quantities of vitamins needed invariably increase as the kcalorie intake increases.

Fluids

Ample fluid intake is needed and should be based on the mother's urine color. A pale-yellow color of the urine suggests adequate fluid intake. Beverages such as juices and milk contribute fluid and kcalories.[40]

Food Intake

Figure 11-7 displays an example of a healthy food intake pattern for a breast-feeding woman. In general, 7 to 8 oz of grains, at least one half of which are whole grains; 3 cups of vegetables; 2 cups of fruits; 3 cups of fluid milk or dairy products; 6 to 6.5 oz of lean meats, poultry, fish, dried beans, and nuts; and 6 to 7 tsp of oils per day are recommended to meet nutrient needs during lactation (www.mypyramid.gov/).

Dietary Supplements

Many health practitioners recommend that women continue their prenatal nutrient supplements during lactation. Specifically, women with certain health conditions or nutrient needs may require supplements while breast-feeding.[89] For example, mothers who consume vegan diets will need vitamin-B_{12} supplementation.[90] Individual recommendations

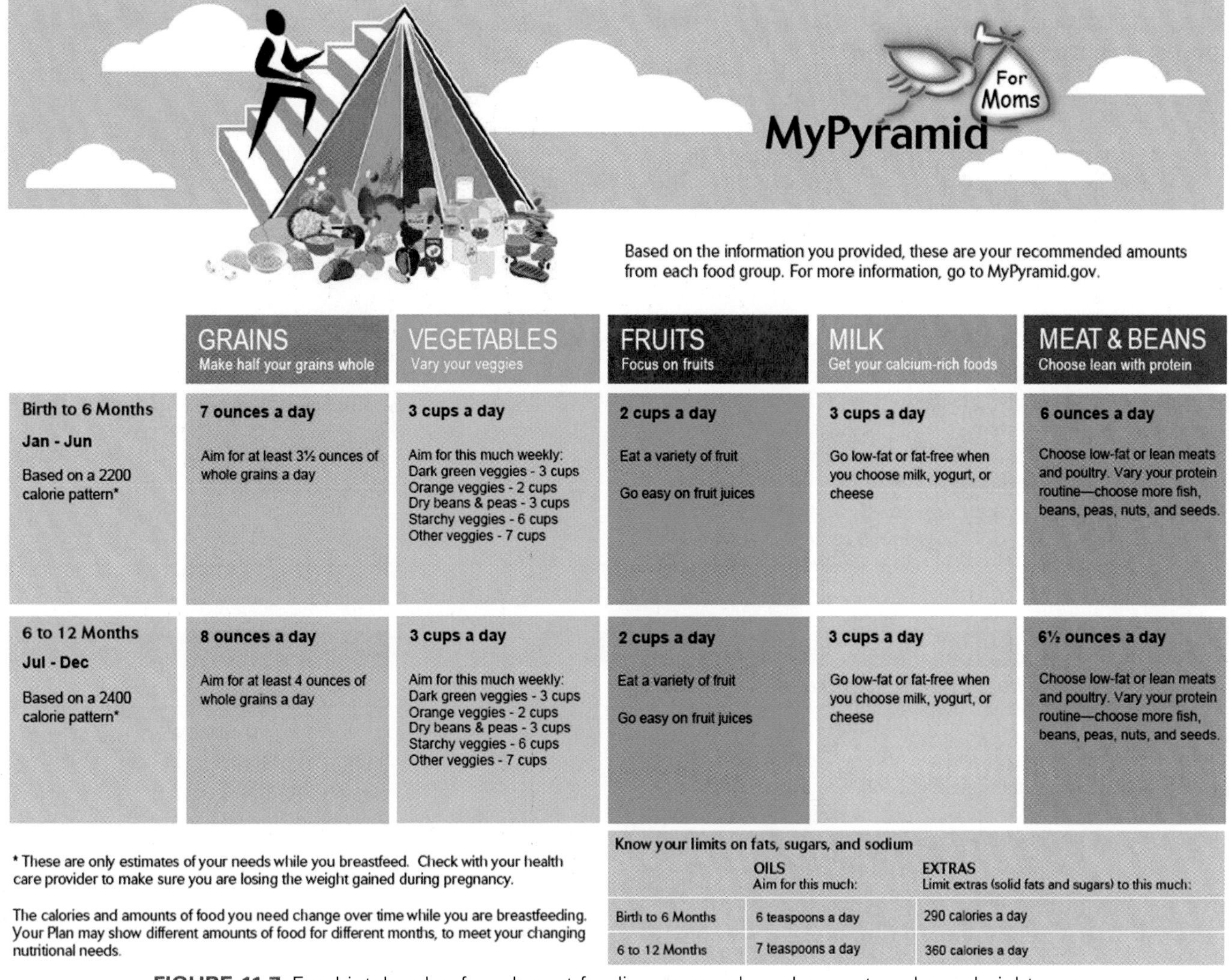

Based on the information you provided, these are your recommended amounts from each food group. For more information, go to MyPyramid.gov.

	GRAINS Make half your grains whole	VEGETABLES Vary your veggies	FRUITS Focus on fruits	MILK Get your calcium-rich foods	MEAT & BEANS Choose lean with protein
Birth to 6 Months Jan - Jun Based on a 2200 calorie pattern*	**7 ounces a day** Aim for at least 3½ ounces of whole grains a day	**3 cups a day** Aim for this much weekly: Dark green veggies - 3 cups Orange veggies - 2 cups Dry beans & peas - 3 cups Starchy veggies - 6 cups Other veggies - 7 cups	**2 cups a day** Eat a variety of fruit Go easy on fruit juices	**3 cups a day** Go low-fat or fat-free when you choose milk, yogurt, or cheese	**6 ounces a day** Choose low-fat or lean meats and poultry. Vary your protein routine—choose more fish, beans, peas, nuts, and seeds.
6 to 12 Months Jul - Dec Based on a 2400 calorie pattern*	**8 ounces a day** Aim for at least 4 ounces of whole grains a day	**3 cups a day** Aim for this much weekly: Dark green veggies - 3 cups Orange veggies - 2 cups Dry beans & peas - 3 cups Starchy veggies - 6 cups Other veggies - 7 cups	**2 cups a day** Eat a variety of fruit Go easy on fruit juices	**3 cups a day** Go low-fat or fat-free when you choose milk, yogurt, or cheese	**6½ ounces a day** Choose low-fat or lean meats and poultry. Vary your protein routine—choose more fish, beans, peas, nuts, and seeds.

* These are only estimates of your needs while you breastfeed. Check with your health care provider to make sure you are losing the weight gained during pregnancy.

The calories and amounts of food you need change over time while you are breastfeeding. Your Plan may show different amounts of food for different months, to meet your changing nutritional needs.

Know your limits on fats, sugars, and sodium

	OILS Aim for this much:	EXTRAS Limit extras (solid fats and sugars) to this much:
Birth to 6 Months	6 teaspoons a day	290 calories a day
6 to 12 Months	7 teaspoons a day	360 calories a day

FIGURE 11-7 Food intake plan for a breast-feeding woman based on maternal age, height, current weight, and physical activity, infant birth date, and exclusive breast-feeding or combination feeding using the MyPyramid for Moms program (www.mypyramid.gov/).

for nutrient supplementation during lactation should be based on a full assessment of the mother's nutritional status and other environmental factors.

Women may desire to use herbal or botanical products as *galactogogues* (agents that stimulate breast milk production), relaxants, or analgesics. The safety for mother and infant and efficacy of such products during lactation have not been adequately evaluated in randomized, placebo-controlled trials. In general, women should not use herbals and botanicals during lactation; however, some may be appropriate for use within defined quantities.[34]

Rest and Relaxation

In addition to the increased diet, the nursing mother requires rest, moderate exercise, and relaxation. Both parents may benefit from counseling focused on reducing the stresses of their new family situation, as well as meeting their own personal needs. Postpartum depression is increasingly recognized as a specific, and sometimes very serious, condition in mothers. Ranging from "baby blues" to postpartum psychosis, the relationship of this condition with nutritional status requires further investigation.[91,92] For example, iron-deficiency anemia may be a risk factor for postpartum depression (see *Evidence-Based Practice* box, "Iron and Postpartum Depression"). The connections among nutrient needs, postpartum depression, and breast-feeding duration will be of future interest.

Maternal Medical Conditions

Breast-feeding should be encouraged in most mothers (see the *Perspectives in Practice* box, "Breast-Feeding: The Dynamic Nature of Human Milk"). However, some conditions exist for which it is recommended that women in the United States not breast-feed, including HIV-positive status, active untreated tuberculosis, human T-lymphocytic virus, illicit drug use, and with specific chemotherapeutic agents. Other conditions or medications should be discussed with health practitioners.[84]

EVIDENCE-BASED PRACTICE

Iron and Postpartum Depression

Is it possible that clinical deficiencies of nutrients *cause* postpartum depression? Iron-deficiency anemia is common among women, particularly postpartum women because of iron losses with delivery and mobilization of iron stores to support fetal growth, development, and iron storage during the latter stages of pregnancy. An association between low hemoglobin concentration (≤12 g/dL) and increased self-rated symptoms of depression were reported in eight postpartum women within the first month after delivery. This was significantly different from lower self-rated symptoms of depression in 29 postpartum women with hemoglobin concentration greater than 12 g/dL. One randomized controlled trial found that self-reported depression and stress significantly decreased in 30 postpartum women with iron-deficiency anemia who were treated with 125 mg ferrous sulfate (along with folate and vitamin C), compared with 21 untreated anemic postpartum women (supplemented with only folate and vitamin C) and 30 nonanemic control women.

Questions for Analysis

1. Does this evidence suggest that postpartum women should routinely be supplemented with iron to prevent postpartum depression?
2. What additional evidence is required to establish practice guidelines regarding nutrition and prevention or treatment of postpartum depression?

BIBLIOGRAPHY

Beard JL, Hendricks MK, Perez EM, et al: Maternal iron deficiency anemia affects postpartum emotions and cognition, *J Nutr* 135:267, 2005.

Corwin EJ, Murray-Kolb LE, Beard JL: Low hemoglobin level is a risk factor for postpartum depression, *J Nutr* 133:4139, 2003.

PERSPECTIVES IN PRACTICE

Breast-Feeding: The Dynamic Nature of Human Milk

Human milk is the ideal first food for human infants. Its dynamic nature changes to match growth needs. The mother's choice to breast-feed her infant depends on a number of factors, however, especially for new mothers, who often need information and counseling from early pregnancy.

Even premature infants can thrive on human milk. Mothers and physicians have sometimes been reluctant to consider breast-feeding for infants born prematurely or delivered by cesarean section, fearing that the early birth or surgical procedure may have some negative effect on the quantity or quality of human milk. This uncertainty about the nutritional quality of mother's milk has also led physicians to encourage adding formula or solid foods (or both) to the diet to make sure the infant is well fed. These practices are usually unnecessary. They often contribute to allergies, obesity, and digestive problems because of the extra stress placed on an immature gut.

Breast Milk for the Preterm Infant

Levels of nutrients in mother's milk shift according to the gestational age of the infant at birth. The preterm infant is often denied its mother's milk by some hospital workers because they think of it as mature milk having too little protein and too much lactose to meet the child's needs. An analysis of the nutritional quality of preterm milk, however, reveals energy and fat concentrations that are 20% to 30% greater, protein levels 15% to 20% greater, and lactose levels 10% lesser than those found in mature milk. Premature milk can meet the preterm infant's needs.

Breast Milk During Weaning

Nutrient levels continue to change with time to match changing growth patterns and developing digestive abilities. Mother's milk does provide sufficient kcalories and nutrients to keep babies well fed without supplemental formula or food. Even when the infant is being weaned, the nature of human milk ensures adequate nutrients, just in case the new, solid-food diet cannot meet the child's needs. Human milk collected during gradual weaning has been found to have increased concentrations of protein, sodium, and iron. Lactose levels are lower, possibly so that increased amounts of kcalories can be supplied by fats, a more concentrated source.

Breast Milk and the Cesarean Section Infant

The quality of human milk is not influenced by the way the baby comes into the world. Many women fear that a baby born by cesarean section cannot be nursed because they think that this method of delivery delays or prevents the production of mature milk. Milk production is stimulated by the release of the placenta, which occurs whether the delivery is vaginal or not. Studies confirm that no significant difference exists in the length of time it takes for mature milk to come in after vaginal or cesarean deliveries.

Thus premature or cesarean deliveries should not discourage women from breast-feeding. Mothers should not underestimate the nutritive quality of their milk simply because it does not appear as rich and thick as cow's milk. After all, cow's milk is made for young calves, who are up and running around after birth and have a much shorter, faster growth period. For the human infant, in nutritional and immunologic terms, breast milk remains the best milk.

Mothers' Facts and Fancies About Breast-Feeding

In early counseling, mothers express a variety of concerns about breast-feeding. Following are a few such statements:

"My Breasts Aren't Big Enough."

When it comes to breast-feeding, all women are created equal. The only parts of the breast that participate in milk production are the glandular and nervous tissue and the nipple; these are basically the same in healthy women. The only difference between a size 32A and a size 42DD is the amount of fat tissue the breast contains.

PERSPECTIVES IN PRACTICE

Breast-Feeding: The Dynamic Nature of Human Milk—cont'd

"Breast-Feeding Causes Cancer."
Actually, investigators have been looking to breast-feeding as a possible means of preventing breast and ovarian cancer. Epidemiologic studies suggest a decreased risk for these cancers in women who breast-feed.

"Breast-Feeding Will Ruin My Figure."
Breast-feeding might actually help a woman regain her figure more quickly. Because the caloric demand of breast-feeding exceeds that of the nonpregnant woman by about 400 to 500 kcalories, a slightly faster rate of weight loss may be expected, although hormonal adaptations may limit the extent to which weight loss is experienced during lactation. Oxytocin, the hormone manufactured to stimulate the letdown reflex, also stimulates uterine contractions, helping reduce the uterus to its prepregnancy size more rapidly.

"Breast-Feeding Is Painful."
It may be painful in the first few days or even weeks as mother and baby establish a pattern of feeding and proper latch and release techniques. Milk should not be allowed to collect in the breast to the point of engorgement, the nipples should be kept clean and dry, and a variety of feeding positions may be used while nursing to decrease the chances of having a painful experience. *Mastitis* is a painful infection of the breast that requires medical attention and often antibiotic treatment.

"Breast Milk Is Not Nutritious."
The thin, bluish appearance of breast milk has some women convinced that it is no more nourishing than water. Let them look at Table 11-3; they will be pleasantly surprised at how well breast milk meets the nutritional needs of the infant.

"I Will Have to Change My Diet to Breast-Feed."
Foods that were eaten during pregnancy may be consumed during lactation. Some women report that after they eat onions, cauliflower, cabbage, or other foods that their infants do not like the taste of their breast milk. Other women say that eating chocolate or drinking coffee, for example, "makes their babies fussy" when breast-feeding. Scientific evidence does not discourage moderate intake of these foods or drinks. A well-balanced diet that includes a variety of colorful foods and fluids is encouraged during breast-feeding.

"I Cannot Go to Work or School if I Breast-Feed."
Breast milk can be stored for up to 5 days in the refrigerator or up to 5 months in the freezer. Many working mothers take advantage of this by expressing their milk and storing it for use by care providers. In fact, women often express milk on their breaks at school or work. (Some places of employment even have lactation rooms and provide breast pumps at the workplace.) Expressing milk not only relieves the pressure of buildup but it also allows the milk to be stored for later use at home.

Other women would like to breast-feed but are worried about special "what if" situations, such as the following:

"What if I Need a Cesarean Section?"
The method of delivery does not affect the quality or quantity of milk produced. The baby can be held in such a way (the "football hold") that he or she does not rest on the mother's abdominal stitches.

"What if the Baby Is Premature?"
Mother's milk changes to meet the infant's needs at all stages of development.

"What if the Baby Has Down Syndrome?"
Infants with Down syndrome can be nursed; however, it does require time, patience, and the use of slightly different nursing techniques. The mother should be told about the special nursing needs of infants with Down syndrome to avoid disappointment or a feeling of failure should breast-feeding become impractical for her particular living situation.

"What if I Have Twins?"
Believe it or not, it has been done. It takes time, patience, and good coordination to breast-feed twins, but it is possible. Triplets, however, are another matter altogether. Women have successfully nursed triplets, but often they did very little else until the babies were weaned. This mother will need emotional support, whether she attempts to nurse or, finding the amount of time and patience required overwhelming, prefers to bottle-feed.

"What if I Have Pierced Nipples or Have Had Breast Surgery?"
Nipple jewelry appears to interfere with breast-feeding; however, a mother who wishes to maintain her piercing while breast-feeding may use retainers. Women should be made aware that serious complications because of nipple piercing have been reported, requiring pharmaceutical or surgical treatments that have required up to 12 months for resolution. Very little is known about later breast-feeding successes or complications after earlier removal of a nipple piercing. Breast augmentation and reduction surgeries have shown mixed results related to successful breast-feeding; however, this issue has not been adequately investigated. At least one retrospective study shows that previous breast reduction did not impair the ability to breast-feed. Women should be informed about the current lack of knowledge surrounding these issues but presented with guidance for decision making.

"What if I Become Pregnant?"
Some women may purposefully choose to breast-feed to avoid pregnancy, but this is not a dependable contraception method. Well-nourished women of the world tend to be more fertile and may find themselves pregnant and breast-feeding at the same time. Women who breast-feed must understand that the lack of a menstrual period during lactation *(lactational amenorrhea)* does not mean they cannot become pregnant. Contraceptives may be required if another pregnancy is not desired at the current time. If pregnancy occurs, then the woman should discuss appropriate infant-feeding solutions with her health care team.

Advantages and Barriers to Breast-Feeding
These factors need to be reviewed with each individual mother in her particular situation. Only on this basis, can she make the informed decision that is best for the infant and for herself.

Continued

PERSPECTIVES IN PRACTICE

Breast-Feeding: The Dynamic Nature of Human Milk—cont'd

Many nutritional, physiologic, psychologic, and practical advantages to breast-feeding exist; six are identified as follows:

1. *Human milk changes* to meet changing nutrient and energy needs of the newborn and the maturing infant during the first months of life. It is always there in the correct form to meet the growing infant's needs.
2. Infants experience *fewer infections* because the mother transfers certain antibodies and immune properties in human milk to her nursing infant. In addition, no exposure of the infant to infectious organisms in the environment that can contaminate preparation and equipment for bottle-feeding, especially in poorer living situations.
3. *Fewer allergies and intolerances* occur, especially in allergy-prone infants, because cow's milk contains a number of potentially allergy-causing proteins that human milk does not have.
4. *Ease of digestion* is greater with breast milk because human milk forms a softer curd in the gastrointestinal tract that is easier for the infant to digest.
5. The *convenience and economy* of breast milk are greater because the mother is free from the time and expense involved in buying and preparing formula, and her breast milk is always ready and sterile.
6. Breast-feeding provides *psychologic bonding* because the mother and infant relate to one another during feeding, regular times of rest and enjoyment, cuddling and fulfillment.

Despite the advantages of breast-feeding, some women do have to deal with perceived barriers associated with misinformation, personal feelings of modesty, family pressures, or outside employment, among other factors. Addressing these barriers, such as the following, before delivery rather than after will increase the likelihood that the mother breast-feeds her infant:

- *Misinformation,* a major barrier, creates negative impressions and ideas. Women in today's world often lack positive role models in extended families or experienced friends with whom they can discuss their feelings and obtain much practical guidance. Experienced breast-feeding mothers or lactation consultants can fill this need, especially for young first-time mothers.
- *Personal modesty and anxiety,* or a fear of appearing immodest in breast exposure, may hinder some mothers from breast-feeding. Sensitive counseling, especially with a positive role model as described previously, can help to allay some of these personal fears. Most of women's breast-feeding is done in the privacy of the home rather than around others; therefore early support during initial experiences would be helpful.
- *Family pressures,* especially from the husband, not to breast-feed have strong influences on the mother, even though she may want to do so. Initial counseling and education about breast-feeding should include both parents whenever possible. Reasons for negative attitudes can be explored and misinformation clarified with sound education.
- *Outside employment,* with a limited maternity leave and job loss if the mother does not return to work at that time, can complicate the mother's decision, even though she may want to breast-feed her baby. However, if the mother does have the will, then it is possible to breast-feed and be employed. After breast-feeding is well established, she can regularly express milk by hand or with a breast pump into sterile disposable nursing bags to use with disposable holder, cap, and nipple ensemble. Rapid chilling and strict sanitation are required, but it can be planned, given the commitment. Some companies provide child care facilities for their employees, recognizing that helping employees with this modern need is good business. The mother can plan occasional formula feeds to fill in with the sustained breast-feeding.

All of these approaches to breast-feeding have real rewards for the infant. In addition, they can strengthen the mother's confidence in her maternal capabilities. The importance of these intangible benefits should not be underestimated.

BIBLIOGRAPHY

American Academy of Pediatrics Section on Breastfeeding: Breastfeeding and the use of human milk, *Pediatrics* 115(2):496, 2005.

Armotrading DC, Probart CK, Jackson RT: Impact of WIC utilization rate on breast-feeding among international students at a large university, *J Am Diet Assoc* 92(3):352, 1992.

Cruz-Korchin N, Korchin L: Breast-feeding after vertical mammaplasty with medial pedicle, *Plast Reconstr Surg* 114(4):890, 2004.

Ghaemi-Ahmadi S: Attitudes toward breast-feeding among Iranian, Afghan, and Southeast Asian immigrant women in the United States: implications for health and nutrition education, *J Am Diet Assoc* 92(3):354, 1992.

Jernstrom H, Lubinski J, Lynch HT, et al: Breast-feeding and the risk of breast cancer in BRCA1 and BRCA2 mutation carriers, *J Natl Cancer Inst* 96(14):1094, 2004.

Lewis CG, Wells MK, Jennings WC: *Mycobacterium fortuitum* breast infection following nipple-piercing, mimicking carcinoma, *Breast J* 10(4):363, 2004.

Martin J: Is nipple piercing compatible with breastfeeding? *J Hum Lact* 20(3):319, 2004.

Pisacane A, Toscano E, Pirri I, et al: Down syndrome and breastfeeding, *Acta Paediatr* 92(12):1479, 2003.

Position of the American Dietetic Association: Promoting and supporting breastfeeding, *J Am Diet Assoc* 105(5):810, 2005.

Siskind V, Green A, Bain C, et al: Breastfeeding, menopause, and epithelial ovarian cancer, *Epidemiology* 8(2):188, 1997.

TO SUM UP

Pregnancy involves synergistic interactions among three distinct biologic entities: (1) the fetus, (2) the placenta, and (3) the woman. Maternal needs reflect the increasing nutritional needs of the fetus and the placenta, as well as the need to meet maternal needs and to prepare for lactation. An optimal weight gain of about 11 kg (25 lb), or more or less as needed based on prepregnancy BMI, is recommended during pregnancy to accommodate rapid growth. Even more significant than the actual weight gain is the quality of the diet.

Common problems occurring during pregnancy include nausea and vomiting, heartburn, and constipation. In most cases they are easily relieved without medication by simple, often temporary, changes in the diet. Serious problems with pregnancy may be associated with preexisting chronic maternal conditions, such as diabetes mellitus, or conditions arising as a result of the physical or metabolic demands of pregnancy, such as iron deficiency anemia and PIH. Unusual or erratic eating habits, age, parity, prepartum weight status, and low income are among the many related factors that also place the woman at risk for complications.

The American Dietetic Association strongly encourages public health and clinical efforts that promote breast-feeding to optimize the indisputable nutritional, immunologic, psychologic, and economic benefits. The ultimate goal of prenatal care is a healthy infant and a mother physically capable of breast-feeding her child, should she choose to do so. Human milk provides essential nutrients in quantities required for optimal infant growth and development. It also supplies immunologic factors that offer protection against infection. Lactation requires an increase in kcalories beyond the needs of pregnancy. Adequate fluid intake is guided by the mother's natural thirst.

QUESTIONS FOR REVIEW

1. List and discuss five factors that influence the nutritional needs of the woman during pregnancy. Which factors would place a woman in a high-risk category? Why?
2. List six nutrients that are required in larger amounts during pregnancy. Describe their special role during this period. Identify four food sources of each.
3. Identify two common problems associated with pregnancy, and describe the dietary management of each.
4. List and describe the screening indicators and risk factors for hypertension and diabetes mellitus during pregnancy.
5. List and discuss five major nutritional factors of lactation.
6. Using the MyPyramid for Moms (www.mypyramid.gov) resource, determine a food intake plan for a 27-year-old woman who is 5 feet, 5 inches tall; weighs 130 pounds; exercises for less than 30 minutes per day; and is exclusively breast-feeding her 2-month-old infant.

REFERENCES

1. Mathews TJ, MacDorman MF: Infant mortality statistics from the 2005 period: linked birth/infant death data set, *Natl Vital Stat Rep* 57(2):1, 2008.
2. Nahum GG, Stanislaw H, Huffaker BJ: Accurate prediction of term birth weight from prospectively measurable maternal characteristics, *Prim Care Update Ob Gyns* 5(4):193, 1998.
3. Food and Nutrition Board Committee on Maternal Nutrition, National Research Council National Academy of Sciences: *Maternal nutrition and the course of human pregnancy*, Washington, DC, 1970, National Academies Press.
4. American College of Obstetricians and Gynecologists, Committee on Nutrition: *Nutrition in maternal health care*, Chicago, 1974, American College of Obstetricians and Gynecologists.
5. American College of Obstetrics and Gynecology and American Dietetic Association Task Force on Nutrition: *Assessment of maternal nutrition*, Chicago, 1978, American College of Obstetricians and Gynecologists.
6. Food and Nutrition Board, Institute of Medicine: *Dietary Reference Intakes for calcium, phosphorus, magnesium, vitamin D, and fluoride*, Washington, DC, 1997, National Academies Press.
7. Food and Nutrition Board, Institute of Medicine: *Dietary Reference Intakes for thiamin, riboflavin, niacin, vitamin B_6, folate, vitamin B_{12}, pantothenic acid, biotin, and choline*, Washington, DC, 1998, National Academies Press.
8. Food and Nutrition Board, Institute of Medicine: *Dietary Reference Intakes for vitamin C, vitamin E, selenium, and carotenoids*, Washington, DC, 2000, National Academies Press.
9. Food and Nutrition Board, Institute of Medicine: *Dietary Reference Intakes for vitamin A, vitamin K, arsenic, boron, chromium, copper, iodine, iron, manganese, molybdenum, nickel, silicon, vanadium, and zinc*, Washington, DC, 2000, National Academies Press.
10. Food and Nutrition Board, Institute of Medicine: *Dietary Reference Intakes for energy, carbohydrate, fiber, fat, fatty acids, cholesterol, protein, and amino acids (macronutrients)*, Washington, DC, 2005, National Academies Press.
11. Barker DJ: Fetal origins of coronary heart disease, *BMJ* 311(6998):171, 1995.
12. Barker DJ: The origins of the developmental origins theory, *J Intern Med* 261(5):412, 2007.
13. Hindmarsh PC, Geary MP, Rodeck CH, et al: Intrauterine growth and its relationship to size and shape at birth, *Pediatr Res* 52(2):263, 2002.
14. Rasmussen KM: The "fetal origins" hypothesis: challenges and opportunities for maternal and child nutrition, *Annu Rev Nutr* 21:73, 2001.

15. Nutrition-Cognition National Advisory Committee: *Statement on the link between nutrition and cognitive development in children*, Medford, Mass, 1998, Center on Hunger, Poverty, and Nutrition Policy, Tufts University.
16. U.S. Department of Health and Human Services: *Healthy people 2010: understanding and improving health*, ed 2, Washington, DC, 2000, U.S. Government Printing Office.
17. U.S. Department of Health and Human Services: *Physical activity guidelines for Americans*, ed 1, Washington, DC, 2008, U.S. Government Printing Office.
18. De Ver Dye T, Fernandez ID, Rains A, et al: Recent studies in the epidemiologic assessment of physical activity, fetal growth, and preterm delivery: a narrative review, *Clin Obstet Gynecol* 46(2):415, 2003.
19. Committee on Obstetric Practice: ACOG committee opinion: exercise during pregnancy and the postpartum period, *Int J Gynaecol Obstet* 77(1):79, 2002.
20. Food and Nutrition Board, Institute of Medicine: *Dietary Reference Intakes: applications in dietary assessment*, Washington, DC, 2000, National Academies Press.
21. Al MDM, van Houwelingen AC, Hornstra G: Long-chain polyunsaturated fatty acids, pregnancy, and pregnancy outcome, *Am J Clin Nutr* 71(Suppl 1):285S, 2000.
22. Carlson SE: Docosahexaenoic acid supplementation in pregnancy and lactation, *Am J Clin Nutr* 89(Suppl):678S, 2009.
23. Reynolds RD: Perinatal vitamin B_6 deficiency and poverty: is there a link? *Nutr Today* 35(6):222, 2000.
24. Centers for Disease Control and Prevention: Use of supplements containing folic acid among women of childbearing age: United States, 2007, *MMWR Morb Mortal Wkly Rep* 57(1):5, 2008.
25. Mills JL: Fortification of foods with folic acid: how much is enough? *N Engl J Med* 342(19):1442, 2000.
26. Mackey AD, Picciano MF: Maternal folate status during extended lactation and the effect of supplemental folic acid, *Am J Clin Nutr* 69(2):285, 1999.
27. Mosley BS, Cleves MA, Siega-Riz AM, et al: Neural tube defects and maternal folate intake among pregnancies conceived after folic acid fortification in the United States, *Am J Epidemiol* 169(1):18, 2009.
28. O'Hagan K: *Cultural competence in the caring professions*, London, 2001, Jessica Kingsley Publishers.
29. Hogan-Garcia M: *Four skills of cultural diversity competence: a process for understanding and practice*, Belmont, Calif, 1999, Brooks/Cole.
30. Bronner Y: Cultural sensitivity and nutrition counseling, *Top Clin Nutr* 9(2):13, 1994.
31. Allen LH: Multiple micronutrients in pregnancy and lactation: an overview, *Am J Clin Nutr* 81(Suppl 5):1206S, 2005.
32. Blumenthal M, Goldberg A, Brinckmann J: *Herbal medicine: expanded commission E monographs*, Boston, 2000, Integrative Medicine Communications.
33. Foster S, Tyler VE: *Tyler's honest herbal*, ed 8, Binghamton, NY, 1999, The Haworth Herbal Press.
34. *Physician's desk reference (PDR) for herbal medicine*, ed 2, Montvale, NJ, 2000, Medical Economics Co.
35. Institute of Medicine: *Weight gain during pregnancy: reexamining the guidelines*, Washington, DC, 2009, National Academies Press.
36. Luke B, Leurgans S: Maternal weight gains in ideal twin outcomes, *J Am Diet Assoc* 96(2):178, 1996.
37. Strauss RS, Dietz WH: Low maternal weight gain in the second or third trimester increases the risk for intrauterine growth retardation, *J Nutr* 129(5):988, 1999.
38. Food and Nutrition Board, Institute of Medicine: *Nutrition during pregnancy*, Washington, DC, 1990, National Academies Press.
39. Butte NF, Hopkinson JM, Mehta N, et al: Adjustments in energy expenditure and substrate utilization during late pregnancy and lactation, *Am J Clin Nutr* 69(2):299, 1999.
40. Food and Nutrition Board, Institute of Medicine: *Dietary Reference Intakes for water, potassium, sodium, chloride, and sulfate*, Washington, DC, 2004, National Academies Press.
41. Goodwin TM: Hyperemesis gravidarum, *Obstet Gynecol Clin North Am* 35:401, 2008.
42. Gavin L, MacKay AP, Brown K, et al: Sexual and reproductive health of persons aged 10-24 years—United States, 2002-2007, *MMWR Surveill Summ* 58(6):1, 2009.
43. Ikonomidou C, Bittigau P, Ishimaru MJ, et al: Ethanol-induced apoptotic neurodegeneration and fetal alcohol syndrome, *Science* 287(5455):1056, 2000.
44. Barinaga M: Neurobiology: a new clue to how alcohol damages brains, *Science* 287(5455):947, 2000.
45. Kirchengast S, Hartmann B: Nicotine consumption before and during pregnancy affects not only newborn size but also birth modus, *J Biosoc Sci* 35(2):175, 2003.
46. Ness RB, Grisso JA, Hirschinger N, et al: Cocaine and tobacco use and the risk of spontaneous abortion, *N Engl J Med* 304(5):333, 1999.
47. Eskenazi B: Caffeine: filtering the facts, *N Engl J Med* 341(22):1688, 1999.
48. Danish Epidemiology Science Centre at the Institute of Preventive Medicine: Does caffeine and alcohol intake before pregnancy predict the occurrence of spontaneous abortion? *Hum Reprod* 18(12):2704, 2003.
49. Signorello LB, McLaughlin JK: Maternal caffeine consumption and spontaneous abortion: a review of the epidemiologic evidence, *Epidemiology* 15(2):229, 2004.
50. Position of the American Dietetic Association: Nutrition and lifestyle for a healthy pregnancy outcome, *J Am Diet Assoc* 108(3):553, 2008.
51. Lopez LB, Ortega Soler CR, de Portela ML: Pica during pregnancy: a frequently underestimated problem, *Arch Latinoam Nutr* 54(1):17, 2004.
52. Rainville AJ: Pica practices of pregnant women are associated with lower maternal hemoglobin level at delivery, *J Am Diet Assoc* 98(3):293, 1998.
53. Boyle JS, Mackey MC: Pica: sorting it out, *J Transcult Nurs* 10(1):65, 1999.
54. American Diabetes Association: Diagnosis and classification of diabetes mellitus, *Diabetes Care* 29(Suppl 1):S43, 2006.
55. Langer O, Conway DL, Berkus MD, et al: A comparison of glyburide and insulin in women with gestational diabetes mellitus, *N Engl J Med* 343(16):1134, 2000.
56. Slocum J, Barcio L, Darany J, et al: Preconception to postpartum: management of pregnancy complicated by diabetes, *Diabetes Educ* 30(5):740, 2004.
57. Alberico S, Strazzanti C, De Santo D, et al: Gestational diabetes: universal or selective screening? *J Matern Fetal Neonatal Med* 16(6):331, 2004.
58. Gabbe SG, Graves CR: Management of diabetes mellitus complicating pregnancy, *Obstet Gynecol* 102(4):857, 2003.
59. Mensing C, Boucher J, Cypress M, et al: National standards for diabetes self-management education, *Diabetes Care* 28(Suppl 1):S72, 2005.
60. Wunderlich SM: Nutritional assessment and support of HIV-positive pregnant women and their children: perspective from an industrialized country, *Nutr Today* 35(3):107, 2000.

61. Taren DL: The infant feeding and HIV transmission controversy impacts public health services, *Nutr Today* 35(3):103, 2000.
62. James D: Eating disorders, fertility, and pregnancy: relationships and complications, *J Perinatal Neonatal Nurs* 15(2):36, 2001.
63. Morrill ES, Nickols-Richardson SM: Bulimia nervosa during pregnancy: a review, *J Am Diet Assoc* 101(4):448, 2001.
64. Position of the American Dietetic Association: nutrition intervention in the treatment of anorexia nervosa, bulimia nervosa, and other eating disorders, *J Am Diet Assoc* 106(12):2073, 2006.
65. Li R, Darling N, Maurice E, et al: Breastfeeding rates in the United States by characteristics of the child, mother, or family: the 2002 national immunization survey, *Pediatrics* 115(1):E31, 2005.
66. Ryan AS: The resurgence of breastfeeding in the United States, *Pediatrics* 99(4):E12, 1997.
67. World Health Organization: WHO advises: ten steps to successful breast-feeding, *World Health* 2:28, 1997.
68. Schanler RJ, O'Connor KG, Lawrence RA: Pediatricians' practices and attitudes regarding breastfeeding promotion, *Pediatrics* 103(3):E35, 1999.
69. Lawrence RA, Lawrence RM: *Breastfeeding: a guide for the medical profession*, St Louis, 1998, Mosby.
70. Emmett PM, Rogers IS: Properties of human milk and their relationship with maternal nutrition, *Early Hum Dev* 49(Suppl 1):S7, 1997.
71. Chezem J, Friesen C: Attendance at breast-feeding support meetings: relationship to demographic characteristics and duration of lactation in women planning postpartum employment, *J Am Diet Assoc* 99(1):83, 1999.
72. Wright AL, Bauer M, Naylor A, et al: Increasing breast-feeding rates to reduce infant illness at the community level, *Pediatrics* 101(5):837, 1998.
73. Carmichael SL, Prince CB, Burr R, et al: Breast-feeding practices among WIC participants in Hawaii, *J Am Diet Assoc* 101(1):57, 2001.
74. Chapman DJ, Damio G, Young S, et al: Effectiveness of breastfeeding peer counseling in a low-income, predominantly Latina population: a randomized controlled trial, *Arch Pediatr Adolesc Med* 158(9):897, 2004.
75. Philipp BL, Merewood A: The baby-friendly way: the best breastfeeding start, *Pediatr Clin North Am* 51(3):761, 2004.
76. Misra R, James DCS: Breast-feeding practices among adolescent and adult mothers in the Missouri WIC population, *J Am Diet Assoc* 100(9):1071, 2000.
77. Pobocik RS, Benavente JC, Schwab AC, et al: Effect of a breastfeeding education and support program on breastfeeding initiation and duration in a culturally diverse group of adolescents, *J Nutr Educ* 32(3):139, 2000.
78. Schmidt MM, Sigman-Grant M: Perspectives of low-income fathers' support of breastfeeding: an exploratory study, *J Nutr Educ* 32(1):31, 2000.
79. Sharma M, Petosa R: Impact of expectant fathers in breast-feeding decisions, *J Am Diet Assoc* 97(11):1311, 1997.
80. Kannan S, Carruth BR, Skinner J: Cultural influences on infant feeding beliefs of mothers, *J Am Diet Assoc* 99(1):88, 1999.
81. Kramer MS, Kakuma R: Optimal duration of exclusive breastfeeding, *Cochrane Database Syst Rev* (1):2002 CD003517.
82. Fewtrell MS, Morgan JB, Duggan C, et al: Optimal duration of exclusive breastfeeding: what is the evidence to support current recommendations? *Am J Clin Nutr* 85(Suppl):635S, 2007.
83. American Academy of Pediatrics Section on Breastfeeding: Breastfeeding and the use of human milk, *Pediatrics* 115(2):496, 2005.
84. Position of the American Dietetic Association: Promoting and supporting breastfeeding, *J Am Diet Assoc* 105(5):810, 2005.
85. Lederman SA: Influence of lactation on body weight regulation, *Nutr Rev* 62(7, part 2):S112, 2004.
86. Dewey KG: Effects of maternal caloric restriction and exercise during lactation, *J Nutr* 128(Suppl 2):386S, 1998.
87. Lovelady CA, Garner KE, Moreno KL, et al: The effect of weight loss in overweight, lactating women on the growth of their infants, *N Engl J Med* 342(7):449, 2000.
88. Butte NF: Dieting and exercise in overweight, lactating women, *N Engl J Med* 342(7):502, 2000.
89. Picciano MF: Pregnancy and lactation: physiological adjustments, nutritional requirements and the role of dietary supplements, *J Nutr* 133(Suppl 1):1997S, 2003.
90. Weiss R, Fogelman Y, Bennett M: Severe vitamin B_{12} deficiency in an infant associated with a maternal deficiency and a strict vegetarian diet, *J Pediatr Hematol Oncol* 26(4):270, 2004.
91. Brockington I: Postpartum psychiatric disorders, *Lancet* 363(9405):303, 2004.
92. Falceto OG, Giugliani ER, Fernandes CL: Influence of parental mental health on early termination of breast-feeding: a case-control study, *J Am Board Fam Pract* 17(3):173, 2004.

FURTHER READINGS AND RESOURCES

Readings

Lammi-Keefe CJ, Couch S, Phillipson E: *Handbook of nutrition and pregnancy*, ed 1, Totowa, NJ, 2008, Humana Press. *[This excellent resource provides helpful guidance for healthy pregnancies, as well as important information for identifying women at nutritional risk.]*

Picciano MF, McGuire MK: Use of dietary supplements by pregnant and lactating women in North America, *Am J Clin Nutr* 89(Suppl):633S, 2009. *[Should pregnant and lactating women consume dietary supplements? This informative article reviews the current understanding of dietary supplement use in women residing in North America who are pregnant and lactating.]*

Simmons RA: Developmental origins of adult disease, *Pediatr Clin North Am* 56:449, 2009. *[Does chronic disease begin in utero? A critical evaluation of animal and human evidence to support this hypothesis is provided. Epigenetic events and mechanisms underlying disease origins during in utero development are discussed.]*

Websites of Interest

March of Dimes Birth Defects Foundation: www.marchofdimes.com.

U.S. Department of Health and Human Services, Food and Drug Administration, Center for Food Safety and Applied Nutrition: www.cfsan.fda.gov.

U.S. Department of Health and Human Services, Office of Disease Prevention and Health Promotion: *Healthy People 2010*, www.healthypeople.gov.

U.S. Department of Health and Human Services, National Institutes of Health, National Center for Complementary and Alternative Medicine: http://nccam.nih.gov.

Virginia Department of Health, Office of Family Health Services, BabyCare: www.vahealth.org/babycare.

12

Nutrition for Normal Growth and Development

Sharon M. Nickols-Richardson

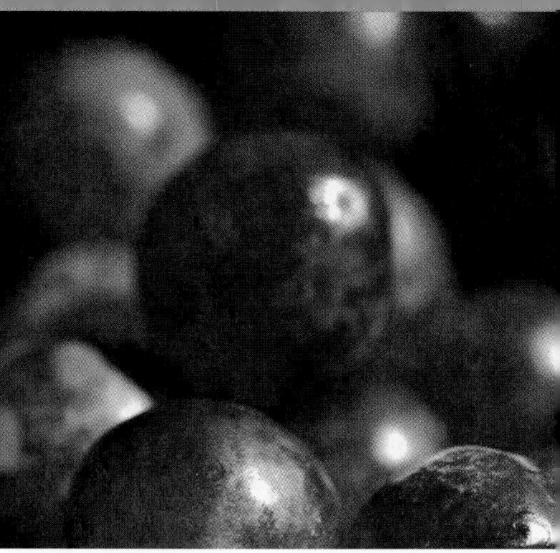

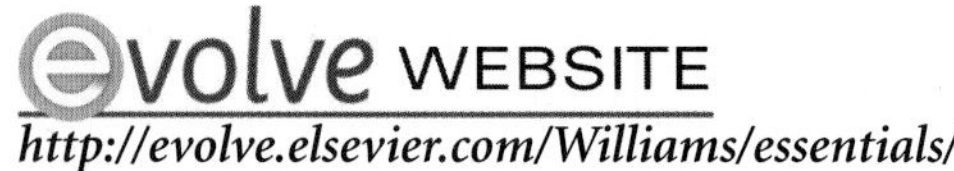

http://evolve.elsevier.com/Williams/essentials/

OUTLINE

In this second chapter in our life cycle series, we look at growing infants, children, and adolescents. We consider their physical growth and their inseparable psychosocial development at each progressive stage. This unified growth and development nurture the integrated progression of the child into the adult.

Within this dual framework of physical and psychosocial development, we consider food and feeding and their vital roles in the development of the whole child. In each age-group we relate nutritional needs and the food that supplies them to the normal physical maturation and psychosocial development achieved in that stage.

HUMAN GROWTH AND DEVELOPMENT

Individual Needs of Children

Growth may be defined as an increase in body size. Biologic growth of an organism occurs through cell multiplication (*hyperplasia*) and cell enlargement (*hypertrophy*). *Development* is the associated process by which growing tissues and organs take on a more complex function. Both of these processes are part of one whole, forming a unified and inseparable sequence of growth and development. Through these changes a small, dependent newborn is transformed into a fully functioning independent adult. However, each child is a unique entity with individual needs. This is a paramount principle in working with children. Thus we must always seek to discover these individual human needs if we are to help each child reach his or her greatest growth and development potential.[1]

Normal Life Cycle Growth Pattern

The normal human life cycle includes the following four general stages of overall growth and development: (1) infancy, (2) childhood, (3) adolescence, and (4) adulthood:

1. *Infancy:* Growth velocity is rapid during the first year of life, with the rate tapering off in the latter half of the year. At 6 months of age an infant has typically doubled its birth weight, and at 1 year he or she will likely have tripled it.
2. *Childhood:* During the latent period of childhood, after infancy and before adolescence, the growth rate slows and becomes erratic. During some periods, plateaus are reached. At other times, small spurts of growth occur. This overall growth deceleration affects appetite accordingly. At certain times, children will have little or no appetite; at other times, they will eat voraciously. Parents who know that this is a normal pattern can relax and avoid making eating a battleground with their children.
3. *Adolescence:* With the beginning of puberty, the second period of growth acceleration occurs. Because of hormonal influences involved, enormous physical changes take place, including growth and maturation of long bones, development of the sex characteristics, and gains in fat and muscle mass.
4. *Adulthood:* In the final stage of a normal life cycle, growth levels off on the adult plateau. Then it gradually declines during old age—the period of senescence.

Measuring Childhood Physical Growth

Growth Charts

Children grow at widely varying individual rates. In clinical practice a child's pattern of growth is compared with percentile growth curves derived from measurements of large numbers of children throughout the growth years. Contemporary growth chart grids, developed by the National Center for Health Statistics (NCHS), were recently revised to reflect the growth patterns of breast-fed and formula-fed infants and to provide a broad baseline for evaluating growth patterns in children today.[2] These charts are based on data from nationally representative samples of children that include various racial and ethnic groups (see *Further Readings and Resources* at the end of this chapter). Two age intervals are presented: birth to 3 years and 2 to 20 years, with separate curves for boys and girls. A variety of grids are available to monitor growth based on weight and age, length (or stature) and age, weight-for-length (or body mass index [BMI]), and head circumference and age (see Appendix I on the Evolve website for *CDC Growth Charts: United States*). Head circumference is a valuable measure in infants, but it is seldom measured routinely after 3 years of age. Directions for use of these growth charts for infants and children with special growth patterns are also available.

Nutrition Assessment

Practitioners use the nutrition care process to assess, evaluate, and monitor a child's growth and development, with growth charts and other clinical standards as points of reference. A number of methods and measures, including anthropometry, clinical signs, laboratory tests, and nutritional analysis, may be used as described in Chapter 16.

Motor, Mental, and Psychosocial Development

Motor Growth and Development

Gross motor skills, such as sitting, standing, walking, and running, develop within the first 18 months of life. Fine motor skills gradually develop over a longer period of time. Such control over and coordination of voluntary muscle develops in conjunction with mental, emotional, social, and cultural growth as the child interacts and reacts to sensory stimulants in the environment. Motor skills greatly influence feeding skills and energy needs of the child.

Mental Growth and Development

Measures of mental growth usually involve abilities in speech and other forms of communication, as well as the ability to handle abstract and symbolic material in thinking. Young children think in very literal terms. As they develop in mental capacity, they can handle more than single ideas, and they can form constructive concepts.

Emotional Growth and Development

Emotional growth is measured in the capacity for love and affection, as well as the ability to handle frustration and anxieties. It also involves the child's ability to control aggressive impulses and to channel hostility from destructive to constructive activities.

Social and Cultural Growth and Development

The social development of a child is measured as the ability to relate to others and to participate in group living and cultural activities. These social and cultural behaviors are first learned through relationships with parents and family, and these relationships greatly influence food habits and feeding patterns. As the child's horizon broadens, relationships are developed with those outside the family, with friends, and with others in the community at school or at religious or other social gatherings. For this reason, a child's play during the early years is a highly purposeful activity.

NUTRITIONAL REQUIREMENTS FOR GROWTH

Energy Needs

During childhood, the demand for kilocalories (kcalories or kcal) is relatively great. However, much variation exists in need with age and condition. For example, the total daily energy intake of a 5-year-old child is spent in the following way:

- Approximately 50% supplies basal metabolic requirements.
- Approximately 5% is used in the thermic effect of food (TEF).
- Approximately 25% goes toward daily physical activity.
- Approximately 12% is needed for tissue growth.
- Approximately 8% is lost in the feces.

Protein Needs

Protein provides amino acids, the essential building materials for tissue growth. As a child grows, the protein requirements per unit of body weight gradually decrease. For example, during the first 6 months of life an infant requires 1.52 g of protein/kg/day.[3] This amount gradually decreases throughout childhood until adulthood, when protein needs are only about 0.8 g/kg/day.[3] Usually, the healthy, active, growing child will consume the necessary amounts of kcalories and protein if a variety of food is provided. The Acceptable Macronutrient Distribution Range (AMDR) for dietary protein for children 1 year and older is 10% to 35% of total kcalories.[3]

Essential Fatty Acid Needs

Fat kcalories are important as backup energy sources but are particularly needed to supply the essential fatty acids—linoleic and α-linolenic acids. Linoleic acid is required for

KEY TERMS

growth velocity Rapidity of motion or movement; rate of childhood growth during normal periods of development compared with a population standard.

growth deceleration Period of decreased speed of growth at different points of childhood development.

growth acceleration Period of increased speed of growth at different points of childhood development.

percentile One of 100 equal parts of a measured series of values; rate or proportion per hundred.

growth chart grids Grids comparing stature (length), weight, and age of children by percentile; used for nutritional assessment to determine how their growth is progressing. The most commonly used grids are those of the National Center for Health Statistics (NCHS).

the synthesis of brain and nerve tissue and normal mental development. Infants consuming adequate amounts of breast milk or infant formula in the first 6 months of life and after complementary foods are added in the second 6 months of life are likely to meet their Adequate Intake (AI) for the essential fatty acids. Children 1 year and older may follow the AMDR of 20% to 35% of total kcalories without any adverse effect on growth and development.[3]

Carbohydrate Needs

Carbohydrates are the primary energy source and are important in sparing protein for its vital role in tissue formation. Most importantly, carbohydrates provide glucose for essential brain function.[3] The AMDR for dietary carbohydrate is 45% to 65% of total kcalories for children 1 year and older.[3]

Fiber

Many complex-carbohydrate foods also provide dietary fiber. Fiber is important to satiety and bowel regulation and affects blood lipid and glucose concentrations, as well as the vascular system. Fiber may also provide protection against some types of cancer and overweight.[3]

Water Requirements

The infant's relative need for water is greater than that of the adult. The infant's body content of water is approximately 70% to 75% of total body weight, whereas in the adult, water contributes only 60% to 65% of total body weight. In addition, a large amount of the infant's total body water is outside of cells and more easily lost. Thus prolonged water loss because of diarrhea, as occurs among infants in developing countries given formula prepared from contaminated water, is a serious threat to life and requires immediate oral hydration therapy.[4] The child's water need is related to energy intake and urine concentration. Generally, an infant drinks a daily amount of water equivalent to 10% to 15% of body weight, whereas the adult's daily water intake equals 2% to 4% of body weight. A summary of approximate daily fluid needs during the growth years is provided in Table 12-1.[5]

TABLE 12-1 APPROXIMATE DAILY FLUID NEEDS DURING GROWTH YEARS

AGE	(in mL/kg)
0-3 months	120
3-6 months	117
6-12 months	89
1-3 years	108
4-8 years	85
9-13 years	67 (boys)
	57 (girls)
14-18 years	54 (boys)
	43 (girls)

Data from Food and Nutrition Board, Institute of Medicine: *Dietary References Intakes for water, potassium, sodium, chloride, and sulfate,* Washington, DC, 2004, National Academies Press.

Mineral and Vitamin Needs

Minerals and vitamins play essential roles in tissue growth and maintenance, as well as in overall energy metabolism. Positive childhood growth and development depend on an adequate amount of these essential substances. For example, rapidly growing young bones require calcium and phosphorus. A radiograph of a newborn's body would reveal a skeleton appearing as a collection of disconnected, separate bones requiring mineralization. Calcium is also needed for tooth development, muscle contraction, nerve excitation, blood coagulation, and heart muscle action. Another mineral of concern is iron, essential for hemoglobin formation and mental and psychomotor development.[6,7] The healthy infant's fetal iron stores are depleted within 9 to 12 months after birth. Thus solid food additions around this time help supply needed iron. Such foods as iron-fortified cereals and meat assist in providing adequate dietary iron. The use of iron-fortified formulas and other foods by high-risk children enrolled in the Special Supplemental Nutrition Program for Women, Infants, and Children (WIC) assists in reducing the incidence of iron deficiency anemia among infants and young children from limited-resource families, including the homeless.[8] Generally, iron supplements are not needed during infancy.

Excess amounts of particular micronutrients are also of concern in feeding children. Excess intake is usually the result of inappropriate use of vitamin or mineral supplements and may occur because of misunderstanding, illiteracy, or carelessness. When supplements are indicated because of a specific and defined medical or nutritional condition, parents must be carefully instructed to use only the amount directed and no more. The following two nutrients pose particular hazards when consumed in excessive amounts:

1. *Vitamin A:* Symptoms of toxicity from excess vitamin A include lack of appetite, slow growth, drying and cracking of the skin, enlargement of the liver and spleen, swelling and pain in the long bones, and bone fragility.
2. *Vitamin D:* Symptoms of toxicity from excess vitamin D include nausea, diarrhea, weight loss, excess urination (especially at night), and eventual calcification of soft tissues, including the renal tubules, blood vessels, bronchi, stomach, and heart.

Summaries of the Dietary Reference Intakes (DRIs) for overall nutritional needs and growth, developed by the Food and Nutrition Board of the Institute of Medicine, are provided in Tables 12-5, 12-6, and 12-7.

STAGES OF GROWTH AND DEVELOPMENT: AGE-GROUP NEEDS

Psychosocial Development

The developmental tasks of choosing and consuming food do not develop in a vacuum. They flow as an integral part of physical, motor, and psychosocial development. In this section we discuss food and feeding practices at each of the stages of childhood and their relationship to normal physical and psychosocial maturation. Developing neuromuscular motor skills enable the child to accomplish related physical activities involved with food. Psychosocial development influences food attitudes, behavior, patterns, and habits.

Throughout the human life cycle, food and feeding not only supply nutrients for physical and motor growth but also play a role in personal and psychosocial development. The nutritional age-group needs of children cannot be understood apart from the child's overall maturation as a unique person. A leading American psychoanalyst, Erik Erikson,[9] has contributed to our understanding of human personality and growth throughout critical periods of development. His theory of human development has come to play a significant role in our view of the human life cycle.

Erikson identified eight stages in human growth and a basic psychosocial developmental problem with which the individual struggles at each stage.[9] The developmental problem at each stage has a positive ego value and a conflicting negative counterpart, as follows:

1. *Infancy:* trust versus distrust.
2. *Toddler:* autonomy versus shame and doubt.
3. *Preschooler:* initiative versus guilt.
4. *School-age child:* industry versus inferiority.
5. *Adolescent:* identity versus role confusion.
6. *Young adult:* intimacy versus isolation.
7. *Adult:* generativity versus stagnation.
8. *Older adult:* ego integrity versus despair.

Given favorable circumstances, a growing child develops positive ego strength at each life stage and builds increasing inner resources and strengths to meet the next life crisis. The struggle at any age, however, is not forever won at this point. A residue of the negative remains, and in periods of stress, such as an illness, some regression is likely to occur. However, as the child gains mastery at each stage of development, assisted by significant positive and supportive relationships, integration of self-controls takes place. Changes occurring at each stage influence food intake and the interaction of the child with family members, peers, and counselors, as follows[10]:

- *Infant:* Infants require appropriate stimulation to thrive; they enjoy seeing different colors, engaging in verbal interactions, and being physically held. Activities such as holding objects, looking at pictures, or hearing nursery rhymes support motor and cognitive development. The attention span is short, which can create problems at feeding time.
- *Toddler:* Toddlers grow rapidly and begin to demonstrate autonomy, with display of temper tantrums or other negative behaviors. They begin to develop language skills and can recall past experiences. Play is an important medium for self-expression and allows the child to express some control over his or her environment.
- *Preschooler:* The preschool years are a time for increasing social experiences, and children begin to interact more with other children. Preschoolers have an increased ability to express themselves and may try to exert control through demands for or refusal of certain foods.
- *School-age child:* The school-age child enters a formal learning environment, and attention span increases. At this age, children are more selective in choosing friends, and the influence of peers becomes more obvious. As the environment becomes more structured, physical activity may decline, despite the need for play and further coordination of motor skills.
- *Adolescent:* Adolescents become more autonomous in their actions and attempt to exert independence from parental control. Teens perceive themselves to be invulnerable to illness or injury, and risk-taking behaviors involving drugs or alcohol may begin. Obsession with body image may result in inappropriate nutrition practices.

Various related developmental tasks surround each of these stages. These learnings, when accomplished, contribute to successful resolution of the core problem.

Infant (Birth to 1 Year)

Physical Characteristics of a Full-Term Infant

The full-term infant is born after successful growth and development during a normal gestation period of about 40 weeks (280 days). During the first year of life the infant generally triples in weight, growing rapidly from an average birth weight of about 3.5 kg (7.5 lb) to a 1-year-old child ready to walk and weighing about 10 kg (22 lb). Thus energy requirements during this first year of tremendous growth are high.

Full-term infants have the ability to digest and absorb protein, a moderate amount of fat, and simple carbohydrates. They have some difficulty with starch because amylase, the starch-splitting enzyme, is not being produced at birth. However, as starch is introduced, this enzyme begins to function. The renal system functions well in infancy, but more water relative to body size is needed than in the adult to manage the renal solute load in urinary excretion. The first baby teeth do not erupt until about the fourth month; therefore food must initially be liquid and later semiliquid.

Nutrition for the Full-Term Infant

The first food for infants, breast milk or infant formula, generally provides all the nutrients required by a healthy infant for the first 6 months of life. Exclusive breast-feeding can, in fact, be adequate for the first 12 months of life; however, most mothers choose to supplement their infants' diets with complementary foods around the sixth to sev-

KEY TERMS

autonomy The state of functioning independently, without extraneous influence.

renal solute load Collective number and concentration of solute particles in a solution carried by the blood to the kidney nephrons for excretion in the urine. The particles are usually nitrogenous products from protein metabolism and the electrolyte sodium.

enth month.[11] Nearly all infants born in a hospital receive an injection of vitamin K shortly after birth to ensure an adequate level of this nutrient, and it is important that infants born at home also receive supplemental vitamin K. It may be necessary to provide vitamin D supplements to breast-fed infants, because breast milk may not supply adequate vitamin D to prevent deficiency and the development of rickets. This is especially critical in the case of African-American mothers, who are less able to initiate the synthesis of vitamin D in their skin, or for mothers who wear special clothing for religious reasons that limits their skin exposure to the sun (see the *Focus on Culture* box, "Nutritional Rickets: Role of Culture").[12] Researchers have suggested that fluoride supplements be provided for breast-fed infants or formula-fed infants older than 6 months of age in geographic regions in which the water is low in fluoride, but not all nutritionists agree on this matter.[4,13] It is important that breast-feeding mothers be well nourished to supply optimal levels of nutrients in their milk.

Infants have limited nutritional stores from gestation, and this is especially true for iron. Around the sixth to seventh month of age, semisolid foods such as iron-fortified cereals may be added to the diet to help meet increasing nutritional needs.

Psychosocial and Motor Development

The core psychosocial developmental task during infancy is the establishment of trust in others. Much of the infant's early psychosocial development is **tactile** in nature from touching and holding, especially with feeding. Feeding is the infant's primary means of establishing human relationships. The close mother-infant or caregiver-infant bonding

FOCUS ON CULTURE*

Nutritional Rickets: Role of Culture

The eradication of nutritional rickets, or the vitamin D deficiency of childhood, is one of the greatest public health success stories in the United States. Fortification of cow's milk and supplementation of infant formula with vitamin D ensured the virtual disappearance of this nutritional disease by 1970. The understanding of the importance of sunlight exposure in the initiation of the conversion of inactive to active vitamin D, in addition to adequate dietary intake, was monumental. Unfortunately, rickets is on the rise because of a variety of cultural and related behavioral factors.

Factors Linked to Rickets

Several studies describe causes of nutritional rickets. A recent study found that 46% of infants born to African-American women were vitamin D deficient at birth, whereas 10% of infants born to Caucasian women were vitamin D deficient. Vitamin D status at birth was linked to maternal vitamin D deficiency at delivery. Other common factors among such studies include exclusive and prolonged breast-feeding and inadequate sunlight exposure in infants. Although most women do not continue to breast-feed their infants beyond 6 months, certain women, primarily Caucasians of high educational and economic backgrounds, have extended periods of breast-feeding. In many cases, vitamin D supplementation is not provided to the infant; thus with an average human milk content of 68 IU/L in Caucasian women, the vitamin D source is inadequate to meet the skeletal demands for this nutrient.

Inadequate sunlight exposure of infants with darkly pigmented skin is another potential cause of rickets. For example, several case studies and larger epidemiologic investigations have shown a significant prevalence of rickets in African-American infants, even those infants residing in southern climates with an abundance of sunlight. Other reports have documented rickets in infants required to be fully covered by clothing because of religious or cultural demands.

Rickets has also been documented in infants of lactating mothers who consume vegan diets. Children who are raised on vegan diets or macrobiotic diets may also have vitamin D deficiency disorders. Often these diets are practiced to support cultural or religious beliefs.

Prevention and Treatment of Rickets

Rickets can be easily prevented, but health care practitioners must be able to recognize the clinical signs and symptoms of rickets once developed (see Chapter 6). Dietary intake assessment is often the first indicator of underlying biochemical and clinical indicators of nutritional deficiency diseases. Screening for special diets, infant-feeding method and duration, supplementation, and behaviors related to sunlight exposure of mother and child is necessary. Vitamin D supplementation of the mother, the child, or both is typically decided on a case-by-case basis. Increased sunlight exposure is another avenue to increasing vitamin D concentration in the blood. Culturally sensitive counseling is required for prevention and treatment of nutritional rickets. Targeted public health and community interventions may also help to diminish rickets once again.

BIBLIOGRAPHY

Bodnar LM: High prevalence of vitamin D insufficiency in black and white pregnant women residing in the northern United States and their neonates, *J Nutr* 137(2):447, 2007.

Greer FR: Do breastfed infants need supplemental vitamins? *Pediatr Clin North Am* 48(2):415, 2001.

Kreiter SR, Schwartz RP, Kirkman HN Jr, et al: Nutritional rickets in African American breast-fed infants, *J Pediatr* 137(2):153, 2000.

Lazol JP, Cakan N, Kamat D: 10-year case review of nutritional rickets in Children's Hospital of Michigan, *Clin Pediatr (Phila)* 47(4):379, 2008.

Lee JM, Smith JR, Philipp BL, et al: Vitamin D deficiency in a healthy group of mothers and newborn infants, *Clin Pediatr (Phila)* 46(1):42, 2007.

McCaffree J: Rickets on the rise, *J Am Diet Assoc* 101(1):16, 2001.

Tomashek KM, Nesby S, Scanlon KS, et al: Nutritional rickets in Georgia, *Pediatrics* 107(4):E45, 2001.

*The author thanks Melissa K. Zack for her assistance in creating this box.

in the feeding process fills the basic need to build trust. The need for sucking and the development of the oral organs, the lips and mouth, as sensory organs represent adaptations that ensure an adequate early food intake for survival. As a result, food becomes the infant's general means of exploring the environment and is one of the early means of communication. The infant has an additional "nonnutritive" sucking need that is satisfied, especially with the extra effort required in sucking while breast-feeding. As muscular coordination involving the tongue and the swallowing reflex develops, infants gradually learn to eat a variety of semisolid foods, beginning around 6 to 7 months of age. As physical and motor maturation proceed, infants begin to show a desire for self-feeding. When these stages of development occur, the exploration of new motor skills and autonomy should be encouraged. If their needs for food and love are fulfilled in this early relationship with the mother, father, other caregivers, and family members, then trust is developed. Infants evidence this trust by an increasing capacity to wait a few minutes for feedings until they are prepared.

Breast-Feeding

The ideal food for the human infant is human milk. It has specific characteristics that match the infant's nutritional requirements during the first year of life. The process of breast-feeding today, as in the past, is successfully initiated and maintained by most mothers who try. However, sometimes problems occur when getting started, as well as a high degree of variability among nursing mothers as to frequency of feedings, intake per feeding, and infant growth (see Chapter 11). Thus in providing support for mothers who want to breast-feed their babies, experienced nutritionists and nurses, many of whom are certified professional lactation consultants, advise flexibility rather than a rigid approach (see *Further Readings and Resources* at the end of this chapter). The World Health Organization (WHO) and the United Nations Children's Fund created the Baby Friendly Hospital Initiative (BFHI)[14,15]; this program has increased the breast-feeding initiation rate of mothers in participating hospitals.[16] Box 12-1 lists the actions that hospitals must carry out to earn BFHI status. Many hospitals use lactation consultants to oversee compliance with the actions and to promote breast-feeding practices that are optimal, yet realistic, for mother and infant.

The mother's breasts, or mammary glands, are highly specialized secretory organs, as indicated in Chapter 11 and illustrated in Figure 11-5. They are composed of glandular tissue, fat, and connective tissue. The secreting glandular tissue has 15 to 24 lobes, each containing many smaller units called *lobules.* In the lobules, secretory cells called *alveoli* form milk from the nutrient material supplied to them via a rich capillary system. During pregnancy the breasts are prepared for lactation. The alveoli enlarge and multiply, and toward the end of the prenatal period they secrete a thin, yellowish fluid called colostrum, which contains important antibodies and proteins. Hormonal components in breast milk also enhance the maturation of the gastrointestinal tract. Typically by the end of the second week, mature milk is produced; as the infant grows, the breast milk develops, adapting in composition to meet growth needs.

Breast milk is produced under the stimulating influence of the hormone *prolactin* from the anterior pituitary gland. After the milk is formed in the mammary lobules by alveoli, it is carried through converging branches of the lactiferous ducts to reservoir spaces called ampullae or the lactiferous sinus located under the areola, the pigmented area of skin surrounding the nipple. Another pituitary hormone, *oxytocin,* stimulates the ejection of the milk from the alveoli to the ducts, releasing it to the baby. This is commonly called the *let-down reflex.* It causes a tingling sensation in the breast and begins the flow of milk. The initial sucking of the baby stimulates this reflex. The newborn rooting reflex, oral need for sucking, and basic hunger drive usually induce and maintain breast-feeding by the healthy mother.

BOX 12-1 PRIORITIZING BREAST-FEEDING: THE BABY FRIENDLY HOSPITAL INITIATIVE (BFHI)

Actions to Earning BFHI Status

- Write and implement a breast-feeding policy.
- Train health care personnel to support the policy.
- Tell pregnant women how to breast-feed and about its benefits.
- Assist mothers with breast-feeding their newborns in the first 30 minutes after delivery.
- Demonstrate to mothers how to breast-feed and express breast milk.
- Provide only breast milk to infants, unless contraindicated.
- Allow infant to be with mother at all times.
- Educate mothers about on-demand feeding.
- Avoid use of pacifiers or other synthetic nipples.
- Educate mothers about breast-feeding issues and finding support after leaving the hospital.

KEY TERMS

tactile Pertaining to the touch.

colostrum Thin yellow fluid first secreted by the mammary gland a few days before and after childbirth, preceding the mature breast milk. It contains up to 20% protein, including a large amount of lactalbumin, more minerals and less lactose and fat than in mature milk, and immunoglobulins representing the antibodies found in maternal blood.

lactiferous ducts Branching channels in the mammary gland that carry breast milk to holding spaces near the nipple ready for the infant's feeding.

ampullae A general term for a flasklike wider portion of a tubular structure; spaces under the nipple of the breast for storing milk.

areola A defined space; a circular area of different color surrounding a central point, such as the darkened pigmented ring surrounding the nipple of the breast.

rooting reflex A reflex in a newborn in which stimulation of the side of the cheek or the upper or lower lip causes the infant to turn its mouth and face to the stimulus.

FOCUS ON FOOD SAFETY

Ensuring the Safety of Breast Milk and Infant Formula

Breast milk or formula can be a source of food-related illness in an infant if these fluids are not properly used and stored. All equipment used in the expression or pumping of breast milk, including pump components and containers, and in the preparation of formula, including scoops and containers, should be sterilized. Most equipment and bottle parts, including synthetic nipples, are dishwasher safe and may be sterilized in this manner. Alternatively, such components may be sterilized in boiling water for 10 to 12 minutes.

Breast milk may stand at room temperature (77° F or less) for up to 6 hours. Breast milk may be stored for no more than 8 days in a 32° to 38° F refrigerator or in a self-defrosting freezer for up to 5 months. If not used within these time frames, then breast milk should be discarded and not used to feed the infant. Some lactation consultants use the "5/5/5 rule" for breast milk handling—use breast milk that has been at room temperature within 5 hours, store breast milk in the refrigerator for no more than 5 days, and maintain breast milk in a freezer for no more than 5 months.

Mixed or reconstituted infant formula may be stored for up to 24 hours in a 32° to 38° F refrigerator. Formula should not be left to stand at room temperature and cannot be frozen. If mixed formula has been in the refrigerator for more than 24 hours or left at room temperature, then it should be thrown away and not used to feed the infant.

Whether a bottle contains breast milk or formula, any unused content should be discarded within 1 hour of when the infant began feeding from the bottle. Additional substances, such as but not limited to honey, sugar, infant cereal, soft drinks, and alcohol, should never be added to a bottle containing breast milk or infant formula.

Data from Ogundele MO: Techniques for the storage of human breast milk: implications for anti-microbial functions and safety of stored milk, *Eur J Pediatr* 159(11):793, 2000.

The mother should follow the baby's lead with an on-demand schedule. The baby's continuing rhythm of need establishes feedings, usually about every 2 to 3 hours in the first few weeks after birth.[4,13] The newborn's rooting reflex and somewhat recessed lower jaw are natural adaptations for feeding at the breast. The mother can feed the baby for about 10 to 15 minutes on each breast, burping the baby gently between each period of sucking to expel swallowed air. When the baby is satisfied, he or she can be released from the breast. The nipple should air dry to prevent irritation and soreness (see the *Focus on Food Safety* box, "Ensuring the Safety of Breast Milk and Infant Formula").

The mother's diet and rest are important factors in establishing lactation and breast-feeding. Figure 11-7 suggests a balanced diet to support ample milk production, including food choices from various food groups for meals and snacks (see Chapter 11). Natural thirst guides adequate fluid intake. Sufficient rest and relaxation for the mother are essential. An adequate energy intake is especially important in the early weeks to establish regular milk production. A gradual weight loss occurs as maternal fat stores are slowly depleted, but the mother should not expect a rapid return to her prepregnancy weight. Overweight mothers with a body mass index (BMI) between 25 and 30 kg/m^2 lost about 1 lb/week while successfully breast-feeding their infants.[17] These infants were fed on demand and grew normally; however, rigorous dieting should not be undertaken by breast-feeding mothers.

Breast-feeding may influence feeding behavior and taste preferences into childhood.[18–22] Studies suggests that breast-fed infants are less likely to become overweight as children compared with infants who are formula-fed.[23–25] Infants who develop a pattern of eating in moderation are less likely to become overweight, and breast-fed infants have more control regarding the amount of milk they consume than do formula-fed infants. Formula-fed infants may be urged to empty their bottle, even though they may turn away when they are satisfied. Force-feeding is less likely to occur in the breast-fed infant but should be avoided in all infants. Feeding should be discontinued at the first sign that the infant has had enough. Children who gain weight more rapidly during the first 4 months of life are more likely to be overweight at age 7.[26] A breast-feeding mother needs to be aware that her infant will likely gain weight more slowly than bottle-fed infants, but this should not be a concern.[27] Acceptance of a wide variety of tastes and preferences for foods may occur if the infant is breast-fed. Odorous compounds transfer into breast milk[20]; such flavor exposure during breast-feeding often affects acceptance of same-flavored foods in childhood.[21,22]

A growing public health issue in the United States and worldwide is the advisability of breast-feeding by human immunodeficiency virus (HIV)-positive mothers, because breast-feeding can be a route of HIV transmission to an infant.[28] In some countries where formula is very expensive and clean water is not readily available, the risks of bottle feeding may still outweigh the risk of HIV transmission for breast-fed infants. For the premature and low-birth-weight baby, feeding through the first year of life poses additional problems.

Bottle-Feeding

Formula feeding by bottle may be preferred by some mothers for a variety of reasons. If the mother does not choose to breast-feed or stops breast-feeding before her infant reaches the age of 1 year, then bottle-feeding of an appropriate formula is an acceptable alternative. A variety of commercial formulas that attempt to approximate the composition of human milk are available. Some of the cow's milk–based formulas are adjusted with whey protein to more nearly approximate the protein ratio in human milk.

A topic of current interest is the nutritional benefit of substantial amounts of the long-chain fatty acids *arachidonic acid* (ARA) and *docosahexaenoic acid* (DHA) provided in breast milk.[29] These fatty acids appear to play a special role in development of the brain and tissue of the retina,[30] and

TABLE 12-2 A COMPARISON OF TYPES OF FORMULAS MANUFACTURED FOR FULL-TERM INFANTS

TYPE OF FORMULA USED		PROTEIN CONTENT	FAT CONTENT	CARBOHYDRATE CONTENT
Milk-based routine	Source:	Nonfat cow's milk	Vegetable oils	Lactose
	g/100 kcal:	2.2-2.3	5.4-5.5	10.5-10.8
	% kcalories:	9	48-50	41-43
Whey-adjusted routine	Source:	Nonfat cow's milk plus demineralized whey	Vegetable and oleo oils	Lactose
	g/100 kcal:	2.2	5.4	10.8
	% kcalories:	9	48	43
Soy isolate (cow's milk sensitivity)	Source:	Soy isolate	Vegetable oils	Corn syrup solids and/or sucrose
	g/100 kcal:	2.5	5.3-5.5	10.3-10.6
	% kcalories:	10	47-50	41-42
Casein hydrolysate (protein sensitivity, galactosemia)	Source:	Casein hydrolysate	Corn oil, other vegetable oils, and MCT	Tapioca starch and glucose, sucrose, or corn syrup solids
	g/100 kcal:	2.8	5.0-5.6	10.2-11.0
	% kcalories:	11	45-50	41-44
Meat-based (cow's milk sensitivity, galactosemia)	Source:	Beef hearts	Sesame oil and beef heart fat	Tapioca starch and sucrose
	g/100 kcal:	4.0	4.8	9
	% kcalories:	16	47	37

MCT, Medium-chain triglycerides.

it has been suggested that the addition of these fatty acids to formula would be beneficial to formula-fed infants. In fact, based on the presence of ARA and DHA in human breast milk and the normal metabolic conversion of linoleic acid to ARA and α-linolenic acid to DHA (along with evidence linking ARA and DHA to visual acuity and cognitive development), the U.S. Food and Drug Administration (FDA) approved the addition of these long-chain polyunsaturated fatty acids to infant formula.[31-34]

Special formulas have been developed for infants with allergies, lactose intolerance, diarrhea, fat malabsorption, or other problems,[35] and several types of constituent proteins and carbohydrates are used. These special formulas include cow's milk protein, soy protein, casein hydrolysate, and elemental formulas (Table 12-2). Hypoallergenic formulas have been developed for infants who are allergic to cow's milk or commercial formulas based on cow's milk and have existing symptoms of that allergy.[35] Even partially hydrolyzed proteins can provoke an allergic response in infants with hypersensitivity to cow's milk. In the preparation of hypoallergenic formulas, all proteins are completely hydrolyzed to free amino acids. Although some infants allergic to cow's milk tolerate soy formulas, they are not hypoallergenic.

In recent years the use of soy protein–based infant formulas has increased. Researchers estimate that during infancy, 36% of formula-fed infants in the United States are, at some point, given this type of formula.[36] At one time, soy protein–based formula was used primarily to feed infants who could not tolerate the protein from cow's milk or the lactose found in standard formulas. However, the use of soy protein–based formulas has been increasing among parents who wish to feed their infants vegetarian diets. In addition, soy protein–based formulas have been used in the management of babies with acute diarrhea. To ensure an appropriate complement of amino acids, soy protein–based formulas are supplemented with methionine, carnitine, and taurine. Some controversy surrounds the use of soy protein–based infant formula because of the estrogen-like effects of soy, and the American Academy of Pediatrics recommends the

KEY TERMS

casein hydrolysate formulas Infant formulas composed of hydrolyzed casein, a major milk protein, produced by partially breaking down the casein into smaller peptide fragments, making a product that is more easily digested.

elemental formulas Nutrition support formulas composed of single elemental nutrient components that require no further digestive breakdown and thus are readily absorbed. Infant formula produced with elemental, ready-to-be-absorbed components of free amino acids and carbohydrate as simple sugars.

EVIDENCE-BASED PRACTICE

Soy Protein–Based Infant Formula: Effect on Reproductive Development

Soybeans, the source of protein in soy-based infant formula, contain isoflavones, which are phytochemicals that have estrogen-like properties. Concern has been raised that soy protein–based infant formula alters reproductive development in infants because of hormonal influences on reproductive tissues. Studies using animal models show contrasting results, likely because of the different sexes of the test animals, the length and quantity of exposure to soy isoflavones, and the selected endpoints. Human studies are more consistent and currently demonstrate no adverse effects of soy-based formula on reproductive development. Adults in middle life who consumed soy-based formula in infancy had no functional deficits in reproductive health in adulthood. Thus infants who have galactosemia or lactase deficiency and require a breast milk replacement can be provided with soy protein–based infant formula. Parents who prefer a vegetarian pattern of eating for their infants can offer soy protein–based infant formula to meet nutrient needs without detrimental effects on growth, development, and reproductive capacity.

Questions for Analysis

1. What future evidence might change this recommendation?
2. Are animal studies useful in forming dietary intake and nutrient recommendations in humans?

BIBLIOGRAPHY

Bhatia J, Greer F: American Academy of Pediatrics Committee on Nutrition: Use of soy protein-based formulas in infant feeding, *Pediatrics* 121:1062, 2008.

Businco L, Bruno G, Giampietro PG, et al: No oetrogens hormonal effects in long-term soy formula fed children, *J Allergy Clin Immunol* 103:S169, 1999.

Fielden MR, Samy SM, Chou KC, et al: Effect of human dietary exposure levels of genistein during gestation and lactation on long-term reproductive development and sperm quality in mice, *Food Chem Toxicol* 41:447, 2003.

Gallo D, Cantelmo F, Distefano M, et al: Reproductive effects of dietary soy in female Wistar rats, *Food Chem Toxicol* 37:493, 1999.

Lasekan JB, Ostrom KM, Jacobs JR, et al: Growth of newborn, term infants fed soy formulas for one year, *Clin Pediatr* 38:563, 1999.

Merritt RJ, Jenks BH: Safety of soy-based infant formulas containing isoflavones: the clinical evidence, *J Nutr* 134:1220S, 2004.

Newbold RR, Banks EP, Bullock B, et al: Uterine adenocarcinoma in mice treated neonatally with genistein, *Cancer Res* 61:4325, 2001.

Strom BL, Schinnar R, Ziegler EE, et al: Exposure to soy-based formula in infancy and endocrinological and reproductive outcomes in young adulthood, *JAMA* 286:807, 2001.

Wisniewski AB, Klein SL, Lakshmanan Y, et al: Exposure to genistein during gestation and lactation demasculinizes the reproductive system in rats, *J Urol* 19:1582, 2003.

use of soy protein–based infant formula only for infants with galactosemia and lactase deficiency or for infants of caregivers who prefer a vegetarian eating pattern[37] (see the *Evidence-Based Practice* box, "Soy Protein–Based Infant Formula: Effect on Reproductive Development").

Standards for the levels of nutrients required in infant formulas are based on recommendations from the American Academy of Pediatrics. Minimum levels have been established for protein, fat, and 27 micronutrients. Maximum levels have been set for 9 nutrients, including vitamins A and D and iron.[38]

When feeding formula, the baby should be cradled in the arm as in breast-feeding, keeping the baby's head upright as much as possible to avoid milk running into the ear canals and causing an ear infection. The close human touch and warmth are important. When the infant is obviously satisfied, extra milk should not be forced, regardless of the amount remaining in the bottle. Any remaining formula should be thrown away and not refrigerated for reuse (see the *Focus on Food Safety* box, "Ensuring the Safety of Breast Milk and Infant Formula" on p. 268). Infants usually take the amount of formula they need. Today most infants are fed on demand versus scheduled, which works out to be about every 2 to 3 hours. Healthy infants soon establish their individual feeding patterns according to their individual growth requirements. Only infant formula and water are appropriate for bottle-feeding; other fluids such as juice, flavored drinks, and carbonated beverages should not be provided through bottles.

Breast-Feeding and Formula-Feeding Combination

Some women may desire the flexibility of both breast-feeding and formula-feeding their infants. For example, a mother working outside of the home may choose to breast-feed her infant in the morning before work and in the evening after work and use formula during the day. This combination is possible but is recommended only after an adequate supply of breast milk and infant-feeding pattern have been established. Factors to consider include infant's acceptance of a synthetic nipple and formula's taste, mother's ability or need to express breast milk during the day, and growth of the infant.

Cow's Milk

Regular unmodified cow's milk is not suitable for infants for several reasons:

- It causes gastrointestinal bleeding.
- Its renal solute load is too concentrated for the infant's renal system to handle; this leaves too small a margin of safety for maintaining water balance, especially during illness, diarrhea, or hot weather.
- Early exposure to cow's milk increases the risk of developing allergies to milk proteins.
- It adversely affects nutrition status.[13] Cow's milk is low in iron, and iron status in the infant is lowered even further by the associated gastrointestinal bleeding and blood loss caused by this cow's milk. In addition, cow's milk is a poor source of vitamins C and E and essential fatty acids. Infants have need for fat; thus they should not be fed reduced-fat

TABLE 12-3 NUTRITIONAL VALUE OF SPECIAL FORMULAS AND HUMAN MILK FOR THE PRETERM INFANT

	ADVISABLE INTAKE FOR BIRTH WEIGHT		HUMAN MILK CONTENT		STANDARD FORMULAS		SPECIAL PREMATURE FORMULAS	
NUTRITIONAL COMPONENT	1.0 kg (2.2 lb)	1.5 kg (3.3 lb)	PRETERM	MATURE	ENFAMIL* SIMILAC† SMA‡	ENFAMIL PREMATURE LIPIL*	SIMILAC SPECIAL CARE†	"PREEMIE" SMA‡
Kcal/dL			73.0	73.0	67.0	81.0	81.0	81.0
Protein (g/200 kcal)	3.1	2.7	2.6§	1.5	2.2	6.0	2.7	2.5
Vitamins, Fat Soluble								
D (IU/120 kcal/kg/day)	600.0	600.0	—	4.0	70.0-75.0	288.0	180.0	76.0
E (IU/120 kcal/kg/day)	30.0	30.0	—	0.3	2.0-3.0	7.6	5.0	2.0
Vitamins, Water Soluble								
Folic acid (mcg/120 kcal/kg/day)	60.0	60.0	—	8.0	9.0-19.0	48.0	45.0	14.0
C (mg/120 kcal/kg/day)	60.0	60.0	—	7.0	10.0-14.0	24.0	45.0	10.0
Minerals								
Calcium (mg/100 kcal)	160.0	140.0	40.0	43.0	63.0-78.0	197.0	180.0	92.0
Phosphorus (mg/100 kcal)	108.0	95.0	18.0	20.0	42.0-53.0	99.0	100.0	49.0
Sodium (mEq/100 kcal)	2.7	2.3	1.5¶	0.8	1.0-1.8	1.8	1.9	1.7

*Mead Johnson Nutritional Division, Evansville, Ind.
†Ross Laboratories, Columbus, Ohio.
‡Wyeth Laboratories, Philadelphia.
§Range: 1.9-2.8 g/100 kcal.
¶Range: 0.9-2.3 mEq/100 kcal.

milks such as nonfat or 2% fat. Low-fat or nonfat milks do not provide (1) sufficient energy to support growth requirements, leading the infant to consume increased volumes of milk and excessive protein, and (2) sufficient linoleic acid, the essential fatty acid needed for growth and development of body tissues, found in the fat portion of milk.[13] A specific form of eczema has been observed in infants deficient in linoleic acid, and a low-fat diet in infancy may impair physical and intellectual development.

To meet the special needs of infants, the American Academy of Pediatrics recommends breast milk or formula as the major food source up to 1 year of age, with a gradual addition of appropriate foods beginning at 6 to 7 months.[4] No need exists for special formulas for older infants; such formulas also present an added expense to the family.

Premature and Small-for-Gestational-Age Infants

Infants born too early or too small have many food-related difficulties to overcome and present a special challenge in feeding. A poor sucking reflex, difficulty in swallowing, small gastric capacity, reduced intestinal motility, tiring easily from eating and being handled, and increased nutrient requirements for catch-up growth all need to be considered. The health team involved in the care of premature and small-for-gestational-age infants is faced with a myriad of decisions to overcome these feeding difficulties. Whenever possible, these infants should be fed breast milk, usually fortified with additional protein, vitamins, and minerals to the levels found in special formulas developed to meet the particular needs of premature infants. Delivery of breast milk or formula using tube feeding (enteral feeding) carries less risk of complications than the delivery of nutrients through the veins (parenteral feeding).

A comparison of the nutrient content of breast milk and special formulas for the premature infant is presented in Table 12-3. Formulas developed for the premature infant may have as much as 30% more protein per fluid volume than those developed for the normal infant, as well as increased amounts of calcium, zinc, and the B-complex vitamins. This enriched formula also supports catch-up growth in term infants who are small for gestational age.[39] Nutrition support of the high-risk infant requires a team approach that includes the pediatrician, nurse, dietitian, and a lactation consultant who can assist the mother and family in developing a routine for expressing and safely storing her breast milk to feed her infant.

Beikost: Solid Food Additions

Beikost feeding begins the transition from a predominantly liquid diet to a predominantly solid food diet.[40] Nutritional and medical authorities agree that for the first 6 to 7 months of life the optimal single food for the infant is human breast milk or an appropriate formula. No nutritional basis exists for introducing solid foods to an infant earlier than 6 to 7 months of age; before this age, it may contribute to overfeeding. Until then, the infant does not need any additional food and is not able to adequately handle other foods. In addition to nutritional reasons, developmental reasons exist for delaying the addition of solid foods until the age of 6 to 7 months. The following developmental tasks must have been mastered before the infant is prepared to receive solid foods:

- The infant can communicate desire and interest in food by opening his or her mouth and leaning forward or, conversely, leaning back or turning away, participating in the feeding process.
- The infant can sit up with support and has good control of the trunk and neck.
- The infant has developed the ability to move food to the back of the mouth for swallowing.

Developmental abilities to use the hands and fingers are required before self-feeding can be initiated. Self-feeding efforts begin first with a whole hand (palmar) grasp and then move to a more refined finger (pincer) grasp by the end of the first year. The first item for self-feeding may be a piece of Melba toast that can be grasped with the whole hand. As solid food is gradually added, the amount of breast milk or formula consumed is reduced accordingly. Box 12-2 lists the developmental milestones that correspond to feeding skills and practices.

Both cultural patterns and the age and educational level of the mother influence infant-feeding practices. Some of these practices, such as adding cereal to the infant's bottle to help the baby sleep through the night, are related more to the convenience of the mother than to the benefit of the infant.[41,42] It may not be in the infant's best interest to sleep through the night at a very early age or to adapt as early as possible to three meals a day. Smaller amounts of food, eaten on a more frequent basis, may contribute to the pattern of eating in moderation.

The traditional transition food is fortified infant cereal—specifically, infant rice cereal mixed with a little milk or formula—because rice cereal has the least potential for allergic reaction. Vegetables, fruits, potato, egg yolk, and finally meat can be added to the diet in a gradual sequence. No one sequence of food additions must be followed (a general guide is provided in Table 12-4). Single foods are given first, one at a time in small amounts, about 5 to 7 days apart; in this way, adverse reactions can be identified. These foods are usually offered before the milk feeding. Individual responses and needs can be a basis for choice, as food becomes a source of enjoyment and a new means of building warm family relationships. A basic goal during this time is to have the infant learn to enjoy many different foods. This is the perfect time to introduce a wide variety of foods, because infants appear to be more willing to taste new foods than are toddlers; in fact, the greater the variety of foods presented when the addition of solid food is begun, the greater the number of foods the infant will accept when first presented.[43] Breast-fed infants seem to be more receptive to new foods with new flavors. As stated previously, exposure to a variety of flavors in breast milk, the result of the mother's varied diet, helps prepare an infant to accept new flavors and foods.[44]

Many commercial baby foods are prepared without the formerly used ingredients of sugar, salt, or monosodium glutamate (MSG). Some mothers prefer preparing their own baby food. This can be done by cooking and straining vegetables and fruits and forming a puree using a blender, food processor, or Foley mill. These foods can be frozen in ice cube trays or in 1-tbsp amounts on a cookie sheet. The cubes or individual portions are easily stored in plastic bags in the freezer; then a single portion can be reheated conveniently for use at a feeding. When working with mothers, it is important to stress the need for a clean environment when preparing infant foods to avoid the danger of foodborne illness.

BOX 12-2 DEVELOPMENTAL MILESTONES ASSOCIATED WITH FEEDING SKILLS AND PRACTICES AT APPROXIMATE AGES IN INFANCY*

- Suckling, sucking, swallowing—breast milk or infant formula (birth to 6 to 7 months)
- Controlled head and tongue movements, independent sitting stability, tooth eruption, controlled palmer and pincer grasps, crawling, early verbalization—breast milk or infant formula; infant cereal (iron fortified); pureed fruits, vegetables, and meats (7 to 9 months)
- Controlled chewing and grasping, additional tooth eruption, use of spoon and "sippy cup"—breast milk or infant formula; infant cereal (iron fortified); well-cooked, smooth, and softly textured vegetables; mashed or sliced fruits; infant crackers (9 to 10 months)
- Standing and sitting alone, verbalization, controlled gross motor skills, early walking—breast milk or infant formula, infant cereal (iron fortified), bite-sized foods, smooth and textured foods, some "table" foods (10 to 12 months)

*Never introduce honey or cow's milk during infancy; avoid foods and food sizes that present a choking hazard; always have adult supervision of an infant during feeding.

KEY TERMS

palmar grasp Early grasp of the young infant, clasping an object in the palm and wrapping the whole hand around it.

pincer grasp Later digital grasp of the older infant; usually picking up smaller objects with a precise grip between thumb and forefinger.

TABLE 12-4 GUIDELINE FOR ADDING SOLID FOODS TO INFANT'S DIET DURING THE FIRST YEAR*

WHEN TO START	FOODS ADDED	FEEDING
Months 6-9	Infant cereal	10:00 AM and 6:00 PM
	Pureed baby foods such as cooked vegetable or fruit	2:00 PM
	Zwieback or hard toast that easily dissolves	At any feeding
Months 9-10	Potato: baked or boiled and mashed or sieved	10:00 AM and 6:00 PM
	Egg yolk (at first, hard cooked and sieved or scrambled; soft boiled or poached later)	
Suggested Meal Plan for 9 Months to 1 year or Older		
7 AM	Milk	240 mL (8 oz)
	Infant cereal	2-3 tbsp
	Strained fruit	2-3 tbsp
	Zwieback or dry toast	
Noon	Milk	240 mL (8 oz)
	Strained vegetables	2-3 tbsp
	Chopped meat or one whole egg	
	Puddings or cooked fruit	2-3 tbsp
3 PM	Milk	120 mL (4 oz)
	Toast, zwieback, or crackers	
6 PM	Milk	240 mL (8 oz)
	Whole egg or chopped meat	
	Potato: baked or mashed	2 tbsp
	Pudding or cooked fruit	2-3 tbsp
	Zwieback or toast	

*Semisolid foods should be given immediately before milk feeding. One or 2 tsp should be given first. If food is accepted and tolerated well, then the amount should be increased to 1 to 2 tbsp per feeding.

NOTE: Banana or cottage cheese may be used as substitution for any meal.

Two foods that require special attention in infant feeding are (1) honey and (2) fruit juices. Honey should never be given to an infant who is younger than 1 year, because it can lead to botulism, a fatal condition in infants. Some fruit juices, including apple, pear, and prune, contain sorbitol, which can lead to diarrhea in infants and toddlers. If given, then fruit juice should be limited to no more than 4 oz per day.

Summary Principles

The following two basic principles should guide the feeding process:

1. Nutrients are needed, not specific foods.
2. Food is a main basis of early learning.

Food not only provides for physical sustenance but also fulfills other personal development and cultural needs. Good food habits are formed early in life and continue to develop as a child grows older. By the time infants are about 9 or 10 months old, they should be able to eat many family foods that are cooked, chopped, or mashed and simply seasoned, without the need for special infant foods. Throughout the first year of life, the infant's needs for physical growth and psychosocial development will be met by breast milk or formula and a variety of solid food additions, as well as a loving and trusting relationship between parents and child (Figure 12-1).

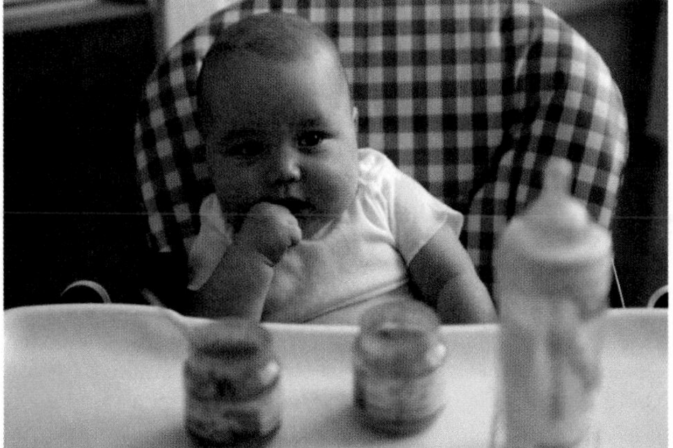

FIGURE 12-1 This child is taking a variety of solid food additions and developing wide tastes. Here, feeding serves as a source not only of physical growth but also of psychosocial development. Optimal physical development and security are evident, the result of sound nutrition and loving care. (Credit: PhotoDisc.)

Toddler (1 to 3 Years)

Physical Characteristics and Growth

After the rapid growth of the first year, the growth rate of children slows. However, although the rate of gain is less, the pattern of growth produces significant changes in body form. The legs become longer, and the child begins losing "baby fat." Less total body water exists, and more of the remaining water is inside cells. The young child begins to look and feel less like a baby and more like a child. Energy demands are lower because of the decelerated growth rate. However, important muscle development is taking place. In fact, muscle mass development accounts for about one half of the total weight gain during this period. As the child begins to walk and stand erect, more muscle is needed to strengthen the body and support these movements. For example, a special need exists for big muscles in the back, the buttocks, and the thighs. The overall rate of skeletal growth slows, with increased deposits of mineral in existing bone rather than a lengthening of bones. The increased mineralization strengthens bones to support the increasing body weight. The child has 6 to 8 teeth at the beginning of the toddler period. By 3 years of age, the remaining deciduous teeth have erupted.

Psychosocial and Motor Development

The psychosocial development of the toddler is pronounced. The core developmental problem they struggle with is the desire for autonomy. Each child has a profound increasing sense of self—of being a distinct and individual person apart from the parents, not just an extension of them. As physical mobility increases with increased gross and fine motor skill development, the sense of autonomy and independence grows. An expanding curiosity leads to much exploration of the environment, and increasingly the mouth is used as a means of exploring. Touch is important, providing the means of learning what objects are like. The constant use of the word *no* reflects the significant struggle with newly emerging ego needs in conflict with the caregiver's control efforts. The child wants to do more and more, but the attention span is fairly short and interest shifts quickly from one thing to another.

Children with neuromuscular conditions require specialized attention to meet nutrient needs that facilitate growth and development in the presence of developmental disabilities. The *Perspectives in Practice* box, "Developmental Disabilities," describes common neuromuscular conditions and related food intake problems in children.

Food and Feeding

Physical growth and psychosocial development during the toddler period influence nutrient needs (see Tables 12-5,

PERSPECTIVES IN PRACTICE

Developmental Disabilities

By Ethan Bergman and Nancy Buergel

During the developmental period of childhood, neuromuscular conditions such as cerebral palsy (CP), epilepsy, spina bifida, and Down syndrome cause eating problems that can contribute to poor growth and delayed development.

Cerebral Palsy

CP is a general term for nonprogressive disorders of muscle control of movements and posture. It affects some 500,000 children and adults in the United States at the rate of two to four children per 1000. Approximately 5000 infants are diagnosed with the condition each year. It is not a disease, and it has no "cure" per se, although training and therapy can help to improve function. CP has many causes and usually results from brain damage that occurs during fetal development or shortly after birth, probably as a result of *hypoxia*, poor oxygen supply to the brain. Other causes include premature birth, low birth weight, Rh or A-B-O blood type incompatibility between mother and infant, infection of the mother with German measles or other viral diseases in early pregnancy, and bacteria that directly or indirectly attack the infant's central nervous system (CNS).

Most affected children fall into the following three principal types: (1) spastic—muscles of one or more limbs permanently contracted, making normal movements very difficult or impossible; (2) athetoid—involuntary writhing movements; (3) ataxic—disturbed sense of balance and depth perception. An individual may possess more than one type. These continuous involuntary movements increase energy needs; research indicates increased resting metabolic rates that are approximately 15% greater than those of non-CP control subjects. Because the immune system is often compromised in persons with developmental disabilities, they are at high risk for problems related to food safety. Thus all caregivers involved should have food safety training.

Mental retardation, with an intelligence quotient (IQ) less than 70, occurs in about 75% of persons with CP, mostly in the spastic group. Important exceptions occur, mainly among those with the athetoid type; some of these individuals are highly intelligent. With patient and skillful care, features of the condition can improve throughout childhood. Improvements in methods used in obstetrics and neonatal care have led to reduced incidence of injury and death of mothers and infants. With interventions such as folate supplementation to pregnant women, immunizations, and avoidance of potentially toxic substances, it is expected that the CP rate should diminish. However, to date this has not occurred. This is partly because rates of preterm births (<37 weeks of gestation) and very preterm births (<32 weeks of gestation) have remained the same during the last 15 years.

Early nutrition therapy for CP patients focuses mainly on feeding problems. When the infant or young child cannot obtain sufficient nourishment as a result of oral motor dysfunction, a problem with body growth exists. Nutritional status, health, and body growth are most affected in children with the greatest motor dysfunction. When satisfactory oral feeding is not possible or when oral feeding is interrupted for a prolonged period because of illness or surgery, enteral nutrition support via nasoenteric or gastrostomy tube feeding

PERSPECTIVES IN PRACTICE

Developmental Disabilities—cont'd

may be necessary. For patients with severe CP, tube feeding improves quality of life for the child and the family, despite minor complications.

Oral feeding can pose numerous problems, both functional and behavioral. Feeding problems resulting from oral motor dysfunction (e.g., difficulties in sucking, swallowing, or chewing), gross motor and self-feeding impairment, lack of appetite, and food aversions can significantly reduce energy and nutrient intake, as can prolonged assisted feeding and use of pureed foods. In persons with severe physical and developmental difficulties, malnutrition and growth failure are common.

Early and ongoing nutrition assessment, intervention, and counseling are essential components of rehabilitation team care. In cases in which accurate height measures to assess growth are difficult because of joint contractures, spasticity, or inability to stand, reasonably accurate stature can be calculated from knee height measures, using the standard equations. In children with CP, growth retardation persists with age. Studies have shown that at age 2 years they are 2% shorter than their peers, and at 8 years of age they are 10% shorter. As adults, persons with spastic CP need about 500 extra kcalories per day to cover added energy needs for *athetosis*, the continuous involuntary writhing motions of the disease. Many still have feeding problems, but exercise helps promote better nutrition. Other nutritional concerns are food intolerance, food allergies, drug-nutrient interactions, constipation, and reflux.

Epilepsy

Epilepsy, literally *seizures,* is a neuromuscular disorder in which abnormal electrical activity in the brain causes recurring transient seizures. Normally the brain regulates all human activities, thoughts, perceptions, and emotions through the regular, orderly, electrical excitation of its nerve cells. During an epileptic seizure, however, an unregulated, chaotic electrical discharge occurs. Seizures often appear spontaneously, or in some cases they may be set off by some stimulus such as a flashing light. This brain dysfunction may develop for no obvious reason, or the person may have an inherited predisposition to the problem. In other cases it may result from a wide variety of diseases or injuries such as birth trauma, a metabolic imbalance in the body, head injury, brain infection (meningitis, encephalitis), stroke, brain tumor, drug intoxication, or alcohol or drug withdrawal states.

According to the American Epilepsy Society, epilepsy and seizures affect about 2.3 million Americans and result in an estimated $12.5 billion in medical costs and lost or reduced earnings and production. Approximately 10% of all Americans will experience a seizure sometime in their lives, and 3% will have had a diagnosis of epilepsy by age 80.

Usually the disorder starts in childhood or adolescence. It plateaus from ages 15 to 65 years and then rises again among older adults. About a third of these persons will outgrow the condition and will not need medication. Another third find their seizures well controlled by drug treatment and require less medication over time. The remaining third find that their condition remains the same or becomes increasingly resistant to drug therapy.

Physicians now have more drug options than ever before to treat epilepsy. Before 1990 six antiepileptic drugs (AEDs) were available for treatment of all forms of epilepsy. These are carbamazepine, phenobarbital, phenytoin, primidone, valproic acid, and ethosuximide. Since then, the FDA has approved eight new AEDs for clients with epilepsy whose care is not sufficient using only the existing drugs. The new drugs are felbamate, gabapentin (Neurontin), lamotrigine (Lamictal), topiramate (Topamax), tiagabine (Gabitril), oxcarbazepine (Trileptal), levetiracetam (Keppra), and zonisamide (Zonegran). Vigabatrin, although not currently approved in the United States, is also a possibility for future use with adults who experience partial seizures. Partial seizures begin with an electrical discharge in one limited area of the brain and may be related to head injury, brain infection, stroke, or tumor, but in most cases the cause is unknown.

These new drugs have shown some advantages in effectiveness compared with existing drugs. For example, gabapentin has been shown to be effective in treatment of newly diagnosed clients with partial epilepsy. Anticonvulsant drugs like valproic acid are often the first line of treatment for epilepsy and in most cases do lessen seizure frequency. In cases of Lennox-Gastaut syndrome, a severe form of epilepsy that usually begins in early childhood and is difficult to treat, newer AEDs such as lamotrigine and topiramate have proved to be effective and well-tolerated treatments for associated seizures. Each client needs to be evaluated for the most effective and appropriate means of controlling his or her seizures, and factors such as drug side effects must be considered. For example, phenobarbital, phenytoin, and carbamazepine have been associated with decreased bone mineral density. These drugs may not be good long-term solutions for someone who has significant risk of osteoporosis.

When medications fail to control seizure activity, other treatments are available such as vagal nerve stimulation (VNS) and a ketogenic diet. The FDA approved VNS for use in 1997 as an adjunctive therapy in adult and adolescent clients older than age 12. A flat, round battery about the size of a silver dollar is surgically implanted in the chest wall. Electrodes are threaded under the skin and wound around the vagus nerve in the neck. The therapy works by sending small regular pulses of electrical energy to the brain via the vagus nerve. The health care team initially programs electrical impulses, and the patient has the option to activate the impulses if he or she feels a seizure is about to occur. Although seizures are rarely eliminated completely, the majority of people who undergo VNS implantation experience fewer seizures and have a better sense of control. VNS has also been shown to be effective in pediatric populations younger than 12 years. Even with the effectiveness of VNS, clients still may require antiepileptic medication.

Nutrition management of epilepsy functions in several areas of care. First, it helps to ensure an appropriate diet for normal growth during childhood and adolescence and for health maintenance in adulthood. Second, it seeks to ameliorate side effects of the anticonvulsant drugs used. Third, if a ketogenic diet is used, then the clinical dietitian is responsible for its calculations and education of staff, patient, and family in its use. This special high-fat, low-carbohydrate diet was developed to control epilepsy before current anticonvulsant drugs became widely available in the 1940s. It is still successfully used with some

Continued

PERSPECTIVES IN PRACTICE

Developmental Disabilities—cont'd

children possessing intractable myoclonic epilepsy that resists drug therapy. In addition to the effectiveness of the ketogenic diet for seizure control, the diet may also help reduce costs for health care in this population. The ketogenic mechanism of seizure control is not clearly understood, although the mechanism may involve having a threshold level of ketones present, which may help control seizures by disrupting nerve transmission at the synapse. Details of the strict calculations required to achieve the necessary ratio of high fat to low carbohydrate are outlined in the American Dietetic Association's *Pediatric Manual of Clinical Dietetics.*

Clinicians have concerns about using a ketogenic diet with children because it may result in poor growth. It is recommended that adequate amounts of energy and protein be included, with an increased proportion of polyunsaturated to saturated fats. Supplementation of vitamins and minerals should also be considered.

The ketogenic diet is normally initiated in a hospital setting, with a starvation period with fluid restriction. Clinicians are concerned that this fasting period with fluid restriction may have negative effects, especially in a pediatric population. Evidence has been provided that the initial fasting period may not be necessary to provide the same beneficial effects on seizure control as long as the client reaches the ketogenic state.

Other dietary interventions are also possible and have shown some potential for effectiveness. The Atkins diet raises the levels of ketones, similarly to the ketogenic diet, but offers more protein, which would potentially be beneficial for a growing child. A calorie-restricted diet has been shown to reduce seizure activity in animal models without the presence of ketones. Use of omega-3 and omega-6 polyunsaturated fatty acids has had some success in reducing seizures.

Spina Bifida

In the United States, spina bifida is the most commonly occurring type of neural tube defect (NTD), a congenital malformation of the spine that contributes to serious developmental disabilities. It develops during early embryonic life when the neural tube, which forms the spinal cord, does not close completely, leaving part of one or more vertebrae of the spinal cord exposed at birth. Because the vertebral canal usually closes within 4 weeks of conception, this congenital defect can often be diagnosed early in the pregnancy by ultrasound scanning or by high levels of α-fetoprotein, a fetal antigen in amniotic fluid that provides an early pregnancy test for fetal malformations such as NTD, in the amniotic fluid or maternal blood. Therefore appropriate genetic counseling can be provided for the parents. Recent discovery of the cell enzyme error involved indicates that folic acid (folate) and vitamin B_{12} supplementation at time of conception through the first few months of pregnancy reduces a woman's risk that the baby will develop this devastating NTD. Mandatory fortification of cereal grain products with folate went into effect in January 1998. Between October 1998 and December 1999 the reported prevalence of spina bifida declined 31%, and the presence of anencephaly, absence of the cerebral hemispheres, was reduced by 16%. In addition, an estimated reduction in the number of NTD-affected pregnancies was noted, from 4000 in 1995 to 1996 to 3000 in 1999 to 2000.

The defect can occur anywhere along the spine but is more common in the lower back. One group study of children with myelomeningocele indicates the neurologic damage that occurs depends on the severity and level of the lesion on the spine. The incidence is about 1 per 1000 babies born, but it increases with either very young or old maternal age. A mother who has had one affected child is 10 times more likely to have another affected child.

Spina bifida has three main forms:

1. *Spina bifida occulta:* This is the least serious and most common form. The name indicates an unseen cleft in the spine. It often goes unnoticed in otherwise healthy children except for a small dimple over the area of the underlying abnormality.
2. *Myelomeningocele:* Also known as *myelocele,* this is the most severe form, and the child is usually severely disabled. Here the spinal cord *(myelo)* and its enveloping membranes *(meninges)* protrude from the spine in a sac *(cele).*
3. *Meningocele:* This form is less severe than myelomeningocele, because the nerve tissue of the spinal cord usually remains intact. Outer skin covers the bulging sac; therefore no functional problems are seen in most cases.

Ideally, necessary surgical repairs for spina bifida are performed in the first few days of life. Nutritional management of children with spina bifida focuses on growth pattern and individual degree of problems of growth retardation and short stature, low muscle mass and weakness, deformities or paralysis of lower extremities, and reduced ability to control bladder and bowels. Normal growth charts have been revised for use with nutrition assessment of these children. Nutrition care plans give attention to the main problems of short stature and poor growth, increased weight, and constipation. Obesity is a particular problem because of several factors: (1) low basal metabolic rate related to lowered amount of lean body mass, (2) little physical activity related to the disabled condition and dependency on a wheelchair, and (3) use of food and overfeeding by parents and other caregivers to reward or show love or to counteract what is seen as frailty or weakness caused by the disability. All of these factors become part of ongoing nutrition counseling. Most children born with spina bifida live well into adulthood as a result of caring professionals and the sophisticated medical techniques available today.

A growing concern is development of a latex allergy, which is a common secondary condition associated with spina bifida. A latex allergy produces symptoms of watery eyes, wheezing, hives, rash, swelling, and, in severe cases, anaphylaxis. Research has shown people with spina bifida are more susceptible because they are repeatedly exposed to latex products early in life because of medical procedures. Some common products that contain latex are catheters, elastic bandages, baby bottle nipples, pacifiers, medical gloves, and balloons.

Down Syndrome

A chromosomal abnormality accounts for the mental retardation and characteristic appearance of children with Down syndrome, a condition the English physician John L.H. Down (1828-1896) first described in the nineteenth century. Its cause remained a mystery until 1959, when modern researchers discovered persons with Down syndrome had one too many chromosomes

PERSPECTIVES IN PRACTICE

Developmental Disabilities—cont'd

in each of their cells: 47 instead of the normal 46. Because the extra chromosome is usually number 21, Down syndrome is also called *trisomy 21.* The two parent chromosomes numbered 21 fail to separate into daughter cells during the first stage of sperm or egg cell formation, and some eggs or sperm are thus formed with an extra number 21 chromosome. If one of these takes part in fertilization, then the resulting baby will have the extra chromosome and Down syndrome. This event is more likely if the mother is older than age 35, indicating that defective egg formation, rather than sperm formation, is usually the cause. Expression of the genes in a trisomy 21 condition is altered and results in modified protein production, neurobiologic development, and finally abnormal physiologic function when compared with the nontrisomy individual. However, exact dysfunction remains poorly understood.

Down syndrome occurs in about 1 in 1000 infants born. This rate has decreased from about 1 in 700 births with the number of terminated pregnancies resulting from early detection. The rate rises steeply with increased maternal age to about 1 in 40 among mothers older than 40 years. Currently more than 350,000 people living in the United States have this syndrome. Degree of mental retardation varies, with an IQ anywhere between 30 and 80, but all are capable of limited learning. Up to 50% of these individuals have congenital heart defects, which can be surgically corrected. More than 25% develop Alzheimer's disease after the age of 35, and 15% to 20% have an increased chance of developing a curable form of leukemia as a newborn and up to age 3. Despite complications associated with Down syndrome, these children are usually affectionate, cheerful, and friendly and get along well with family and friends. They thrive to their full potential in a loving family.

Early intervention in Down syndrome is important to ensure longevity and highest possible quality of life. Congenital heart defects are common in individuals with Down syndrome. Rate of congenital defects does not differ between ethnic groups. An analysis of median age of death indicates a striking improvement has occurred in longevity among Caucasian Down syndrome individuals. However, the same increase in longevity has not been seen in other ethnic groups. This difference may be caused by differential availability of access to early intervention. Prenatal diagnosis of Down syndrome is made by chromosome analysis, and screening can be conducted to help identify those who may need chromosome analysis. Currently in the United States, a blood-screening test for chromosome anomalies is given to all women in the first trimester of pregnancy. This is followed by prenatal cytogenic diagnosis, if indicated. The screening method has a 69% detection rate at present and a 5% false-positive rate. Much effort is being made to increase sensitivity of the blood test to reduce or eliminate invasive testing such as amniocentesis.

Nutrition therapy for individuals with Down syndrome focuses on delayed feeding skills; inappropriate, excessive, or inadequate intakes of food energy and nutrients; and poor eating habits. Diets need to be individualized because these children tend to gain excess weight if they are given the intakes recommended for children who do not have Down syndrome.

Early intervention often occurs in Down patients because they are commonly diagnosed before or at birth. Common problems found in Down patients include congenital heart disease, hearing loss, and ophthalmologic problems. Thyroid disease and celiac disease are common, and development of diabetes may also occur with Down patients. An awareness of these potential problems is important for the health care provider and for the family to allow prevention and early detection as the Down syndrome infant gets older. Encouraging physical activity is also important to help reduce the risk of obesity and diabetes.

BIBLIOGRAPHY

La Follette Atencio P, Ekvall SW, Oppenheimer S, et al: Effect of level of lesion and quality of ambulation on growth chart measurements in children with myelomeningocele, *J Am Diet Assoc* 92(7):858, 1992.

Brodie MJ, Dichter MA: Antiepileptic drugs, *N Engl J Med* 334(2):168, 1996.

Capone GT: Down syndrome: genetic insights and thoughts on early intervention, *Infants Young Child* 17(1):45, 2004.

Chadwick D: Vagal-nerve stimulation for epilepsy, *Lancet* 357(9270):1726, 2001.

Dustrude A, Prince A: Provision of optimal nutrition care in myelomeningocele, *Top Clin Nutr* 5(2):34, 1990.

Edelstein SF, Chisholm M: Management of intractable childhood seizures using the non-MCT oil ketogenic diet in 20 patients, *J Am Diet Assoc* 96(11):1181, 1996.

Ferrang TM, Johnson RK, Ferrara MS: Dietary and anthropometric assessment of adults with cerebral palsy, *J Am Diet Assoc* 92(9):1083, 1992.

Fung EB, Samson-Fang L, Stallings VA, et al: Feeding dysfunction is associated with poor growth and health status in children with cerebral palsy, *J Am Diet Assoc* 102(3):361, 2002.

Gonzalez L, Nazario CM, Gonzalez MJ: Nutrition related problems of pediatric patients with neuromuscular disorders, *P R Health Sci J* 19(1):35, 2000.

Gross SM, Caufield LA, Kinsman SL, et al: Inadequate folic acid intakes are prevalent among young women with neural tube defects, *J Am Diet Assoc* 101(3):342, 2001.

Harrington M, Lyman B: Special considerations for the pediatric patient. In Silkroski M, Guenter P, editors: *Tube feeding: practical guidelines and nursing protocols*, Gaithersburg, Md, 2001, Aspen.

Hogan SE: Knee height as a predictor of recumbent length for individuals with mobility-impaired cerebral palsy, *J Am Coll Nutr* 18(2):201, 1999.

Hogan SE, Evers SE: A multinational rehabilitation program for persons with severe physical and developmental disabilities, *J Am Diet Assoc* 97(2):162, 1997.

Jarra RG, Buchhalter JR: Therapeutics in pediatric epilepsy. I. The new antiepileptic drugs and the ketogenic diet, *Mayo Clinic Proc* 78(3):359, 2003.

Johnson RK, Hildreth HG, Contompasis SH, et al: Total energy expenditure in adults with cerebral palsy as assessed by doubly labeled water, *J Am Diet Assoc* 97(9):966, 1997.

Johnson RK, Ferrara MS: Estimating stature from knee height for persons with cerebral palsy: an evaluation of estimating equations, *J Am Diet Assoc* 91(10):1283, 1991.

Kim DW, Kang HC, Park JC, et al: Benefits of the nonfasting ketogenic diet compared with the initial fasting ketogenic diet, *Pediatrics* 114(6):1627, 2004.

Koman LA, Smith BP, Shilt JS: Cerebral palsy, *Lancet* 363(9421):1619, 2004.

Continued

PERSPECTIVES IN PRACTICE

Developmental Disabilities—cont'd

LaRoche SM, Helmers SL: The new antiepileptic drugs: clinical applications, *JAMA* 291(5):615, 2004.

Liu YM, Williams S, Basualdo-Hammond C, et al: A prospective study: growth and nutritional status of children treated with the ketogenic diet, *J Am Diet Assoc* 103(6):707, 2003.

Lucock M: Folic acid: nutritional biochemistry, molecular biology, and role in disease processes, *Mol Genet Metab* 71(1–2):121, 2000.

Luke A, Sutton M, Schoeller DA, et al: Nutrient intake and obesity in prepubescent children with Down syndrome, *J Am Diet Assoc* 96(12):1262, 1996.

Mandel A, Ballew M, Pina-Garza JE, et al: Medical costs are reduced when children with intractable epilepsy are successfully treated with the ketogenic diet, *J Am Diet Assoc* 102(3):396, 2002.

Centers for Disease Control and Prevention (CDC): Spina bifida and anencephaly before and after folic acid mandate—United States, 1995-1996 and 1999-2000, *Morb Mortal Wkly Rep* 53(17):362, 2004.

Mitchell LE, Adzick NS, Melchionne J, et al: Spina bifida, *Lancet* 364(9448):1885, 2004.

Morantz CA: Recommendations for prescribing new antiepileptic drugs, *Am Fam Physician* 70(6):1167, 2004.

Murphy JV, Torkelson R, Dowler I, et al: Vagal nerve stimulation in refractory epilepsy: the first 100 patients receiving vagal nerve stimulation at a pediatric epilepsy center, *Arch Pediatr Adolesc Med* 157(6):560, 2003.

Nelson KB: Can we prevent cerebral palsy? *N Engl J Med* 349(18):1765, 2003.

Nevin-Folino NL, editor: *Pediatric manual of clinical dietetics*, ed 2, Chicago, 2003, American Dietetic Association.

Yang Q, Rasmussen SA, Friedman JM: Mortality with Down's syndrome in the USA from 1983 to 1997: a population based study, *Lancet* 359(9311):1019, 2002.

Roizen NJ: The early interventionist and the medical problems of the child with Down syndrome, *Infants Young Child* 16(1):88, 2003.

Roizen NJ, Patterson D: Down's syndrome, *Lancet* 361(9365):1281, 2003.

Schmidt D, Bourgeois B: A risk-benefit assessment of therapies for Lennox-Gastaut syndrome, *Drug Saf* 22(6):467, 2000.

Smith SW, Camfield C, Camfield P: Living with cerebral palsy and tube feeding: a population-based follow up study, *J Pediatr* 135(3):307, 2000.

Stafstrom CE: Dietary approaches to epilepsy treatment: old and new options on the menu, *Epilepsy Curr* 4(6):215, 2004.

Stallings VA, Cronk CE, Zemel BS, et al: Body composition in children with spastic quadriplegic cerebral palsy, *J Pediatr* 126:1883, 1995.

Sullivan PB, Juszczak E, Lambert BR, et al: Impact of feeding problems on nutritional intake and growth: Oxford Feeding Study II, *Dev Med Child Neurol* 44(7):461, 2002.

Walter A, Cohen NL, Swicker RC: Food safety training needs exist for staff and consumers in a variety of community-based homes for people with developmental disabilities, *J Am Diet Assoc* 97(6):611, 1997.

TABLE 12-5 DIETARY REFERENCE INTAKES FOR ENERGY AND PROTEIN

	AGE	WEIGHT		HEIGHT		ENERGY*	PROTEIN
Infants	0-0.5 yr	6 kg	13 lb	62 cm	24 in	438-645 kcal	9.1 g
	0.5-1 yr	9 kg	20 lb	71cm	28 in	608-844 kcal	13.5 g
Children	1-3 yr	12 kg	27 lb	86 cm	34 in	768-1683 kcal	13 g
	4-8 yr	20 kg	44 lb	115 cm	45 in	1133-2225 kcal	19 g
Males subjects	9-13 yr	36 kg	79 lb	144 cm	57 in	1530-3038 kcal	34 g
	14-18 yr	61 kg	134 lb	174 cm	68 in	2090-3804 kcal	52 g
Female subjects	9-13 yr	37 kg	81 lb	144 cm	57 in	1415-2762 kcal	34 g
	14-18 yr	54 kg	119 lb	163 cm	64 in	1718-2858 kcal	46 g

Data from Food and Nutrition Board, Institute of Medicine: *Dietary Reference Intakes for energy, carbohydrate, fiber, fat, fatty acids, cholesterol, protein, and amino acids (macronutrients)*, Washington, DC, 2002, National Academies Press.
*Varies according to sex, body size, age, and level of physical activity.

12-6, and 12-7) and food patterns (see the *Perspectives in Practice* box, "Feeding Toddlers and Preschoolers: Eating Is a Family Affair"), as follows:

- *Energy:* The energy requirement now increases very slowly in small spurts. At about 1 year of age, children need approximately 850 kcal/day; this rises to a range of 1160 to 1680 kcal/day for boys and 1080 to 1650 kcal/day for girls by age 3.[3] The variation in energy need for toddlers is due to the wide range of physical activity. More active toddlers require more energy, whereas sedentary toddlers do not. From ages 1 to 2, some children do not eat as much as they did in the second half of infancy. Caregivers will avoid conflict with their toddler about eating if they remember this decrease in need for kcalories is normal, resulting from a slowing in the growth rate and the child's necessary struggle for autonomy and selfhood, which often involves refusal of food. Appetite varies in the toddler; therefore food intake may be irregular, with periods of good appetite and periods of disinterest in food. Encouragement is needed from caregivers, but constant conflict with the child about eating serves no useful purpose. A small plate of snacks, including finger-food pieces of raw fruit and cheese kept in the refrigerator or a few crackers on a special colorful plate, can give the child

TABLE 12-6 DIETARY REFERENCE INTAKES FOR VITAMINS

AGE	VITAMIN A (in mcg RAE)	VITAMIN D (in mcg)	VITAMIN E (in mg TE)	VITAMIN K (in mcg)	VITAMIN C (in mg)	THIAMIN (in mg)	RIBOFLAVIN (in mg)	NIACIN (in mg NE)	VITAMIN B_6 (in mg)	FOLATE (in mcg)	VITAMIN B_{12} (in mcg)
Infants 0-0.5 yr	400	5	4	2	40	0.2	0.3	2	0.1	65	0.4
Infants 0.6-1.0 yr	500	5	5	2.5	50	0.3	0.4	4	0.3	80	0.5
Children 1-3 yr	300	5	6	30	15	0.5	0.5	6	0.5	150	0.9
Children 4-8 yr	400	5	7	55	25	0.6	0.6	8	0.6	200	1.2
Boys 9-13 yr	600	5	11	60	45	0.9	0.9	12	1	300	1.8
Boys 14-18 yr	900	5	15	75	75	1.2	1.3	16	1.3	400	2.4
Girls 9-13 yr	600	5	11	60	45	0.9	0.9	12	1	300	1.8
Girls 14-18 yr	700	5	15	75	65	1.0	1.0	14	1.2	400	2.4

From Food and Nutrition Board, Institute of Medicine: *Dietary Reference Intakes for calcium, phosphorus, magnesium, vitamin D, and fluoride,* Washington, DC, 1997, National Academies Press; Food and Nutrition Board, Institute of Medicine: *Dietary Reference Intakes for thiamin, riboflavin, niacin, vitamin B_6, folate, vitamin B_{12}, pantothenic acid, biotin, and choline,* Washington, DC, 1998, National Academies Press; Food and Nutrition Board, Institute of Medicine: *Dietary Reference Intakes for vitamin C, vitamin E, selenium, and carotenoids,* Washington, DC, 2000, National Academies Press; Food and Nutrition Board, Institute of Medicine: *Dietary Reference Intakes for vitamin A, vitamin K, arsenic, boron, chromium, copper, iodine, iron, manganese, molybdenum, nickel, silicon, vanadium, and zinc,* Washington, DC, 2001, National Academies Press.
RAE, Retinol activity equivalents; *TE,* tocopherol equivalents; *NE,* niacin equivalents.

TABLE 12-7 DIETARY REFERENCE INTAKES FOR MINERALS

AGE	CALCIUM (in mg)	PHOSPHORUS (in mg)	MAGNESIUM (in mg)	IRON (in mg)	ZINC (in mg)	IODINE (in mcg)	SELENIUM (in mcg)	FLUORIDE (in mg)
Infants 0-0.5 yr	210	100	30	0.27	2	110	5	0.01
Infants 0.6-1.0 yr	270	275	75	11	3	130	20	0.5
Children 1-3 yr	500	460	80	7	3	90	20	0.7
Children 4-8 yr	800	500	130	10	5	90	30	1.0
Boys 9-13 yr	1300	1250	240	8	8	120	40	2.0
Boys 14-18 yr	1300	1250	410	11	11	150	55	3.0
Girls 9-13 yr	1300	1250	240	8	8	120	40	2.0
Girls 14-18 yr	1300	1250	360	15	9	150	55	3.0

From Food and Nutrition Board, Institute of Medicine: *Dietary Reference Intakes for calcium, phosphorus, magnesium, vitamin D, and fluoride,* Washington, DC, 1997, National Academies Press; Food and Nutrition Board, Institute of Medicine: *Dietary Reference Intakes for vitamin C, vitamin E, selenium, and carotenoids,* Washington, DC, 2000, National Academies Press; Food and Nutrition Board, Institute of Medicine: *Dietary Reference Intakes for vitamin A, vitamin K, arsenic, boron, chromium, copper, iodine, iron, manganese, molybdenum, nickel, silicon, vanadium, and zinc,* Washington, DC, 2001, National Academies Press.

a measure of positive control when hungry. Toddlers will eat when they are hungry. Positive early experiences help develop appropriate food acceptance patterns.[1]

- *Protein:* In relation to energy needs, protein needs are relatively increased during this stage of life. The toddler requires about 13 g of protein per day.[3] Muscle and other body tissues are growing rapidly. At least half of this protein should be of animal origin, because animal protein has high biologic value. However, toddlers who follow a balanced and well-planned ovolactovegetarian diet grow just as well and attain similar heights as their nonvegetarian counterparts.[4] Diets planned for vegan children will need to incorporate soy and legume protein and build on the complementarity of plant proteins (see Chapter 5).

PERSPECTIVES IN PRACTICE

Feeding Toddlers and Preschoolers: Eating Is a Family Affair

Regardless of their ages, children need the same nutrients as adults but in different amounts. The challenge for parents and caregivers is to make available appropriate and appealing foods and to set the time and place for eating. Young children must learn how to make food choices and to decide how much food they need to consume. We can help parents and caregivers develop child-feeding strategies based on the developmental needs of their young children. First, we must remind them that their children are not growing as fast as they did during the first year of life; it follows that they need less food. In addition, a child's energy needs are sporadic; therefore periods of increased food intake will vary with periods of smaller intake. Forcing food during periods of low intake may encourage overeating or food aversion, leading to food intake problems later in life.

Amount of Food

Children are not ready for adult-sized portions and may be overwhelmed by large amounts of food on their plate. It is better to serve less food than children are likely to eat and have them ask for more. In planning portion sizes, a good rule of thumb is 1 tbsp of food for every year of age. When the child begins to play with the food on the plate or seems to lose interest in eating, remove the plate and provide another activity.

Feeding Frequency

Children do best with a regular feeding schedule; try to keep meals and snacks at regular times. Young children have small stomachs, and it is difficult for them to consume enough food at one meal to last them until the next meal. They may need to eat five or six times a day. Try to allow at least 1½ or 2 hours between snacks and meals. When choosing between-meal snacks, look to foods that will provide not only additional kcalories but also protein and important vitamins and minerals. Fruit, crackers, raw vegetables (as appropriate), cheese, milk, and cereal are good snacks. It is best if children are not overtired at mealtime; if possible, then plan a short rest period immediately before a meal.

What Foods

Over time, it is important for the young child to learn to eat a variety of foods, although it may be necessary to offer a new food eight to 10 times, each including at least a taste, before it will be accepted. The child should learn to eat what other family members are eating and not be provided with special foods. However, when planning meals, be sure to have one item that the child likes and will eat. In addition, children are more willing to try a new food if it is accompanied by a favorite food; try to pair such foods at the same meal. Serve dessert, if any, with the main meal rather than later; it should not assume special importance in relation to other foods. Do allow your toddler or preschooler to make some choices about foods for meals or snacks, just as older children are able to do. This develops skills in making food choices.

Avoid Forbidding Certain Foods

All foods, including sweets, can be included in a healthy diet for young children if limited in frequency and amount. It is important that children learn how to moderate their intakes of such foods. Excluding certain foods makes them more attractive and may ultimately lead to increased intake when they do become available.

Food Safety

Two major safety considerations in feeding children are avoidance of foodborne illness and the possibility of choking. Young children are very vulnerable to foodborne illness resulting from (1) foods that are not fully cooked, such as hamburger or eggs; (2) foods that became contaminated by contact with an unwholesome food or other source of bacteria; or (3) improperly stored food with bacterial growth. Eating such foods can lead to serious illness or even death in the young child, as occurred when preschoolers ate improperly cooked hamburger at a fast-food restaurant. Children must be taught at a young age to wash their hands thoroughly after they use the bathroom and before they touch a food. Parents should ask about food-handling and other sanitary practices when evaluating the suitability of a caregiver or a care facility.

Children younger than 4 years are at greatest risk for choking and death by asphyxiation. Foods most likely to cause choking are those that are round and hard and do not dissolve in saliva. Typical items that cause choking are hot dogs, grapes, peanut butter in globs, hard pieces of raw fruits and vegetables, hard candy, or popcorn. Young children should always be supervised when eating and should eat sitting down.

Social Environment at Meal Time

Try to keep mealtime as pleasant as possible. Allow enough time for the young child to eat. Having to hurry adds stress to mealtime and takes away the pleasure of eating, especially for the child who is still learning to self-feed. Be patient about spills or accidents; it takes time to develop feeding skills. Choose appropriate utensils that are unbreakable and easy for the child to grasp. Children are less likely to accept a food that was first introduced in a negative meal situation; therefore make mealtime an enjoyable family time that reinforces positive eating behaviors. Parental modeling is an important influence in encouraging children to try new foods. Toddlers are more likely to taste a new food if they see an adult, especially a familiar adult or parent, eating it. Children model the eating behavior of parents and caregivers; be sure that others at the table are eating vegetables and drinking milk. Parental modeling is as important in the choice of snacks as it is at mealtime.

BIBLIOGRAPHY

Duyff RL: *The American Dietetic Association complete food and nutrition guide*, ed 2, Indianapolis, Ind, 2002, Wiley.

Fisher JO, Birch LL: Restricting access to palatable foods affects children's behavioral response, food selection, and intake, *Am J Clin Nutr* 69(6):1264, 1999.

Kleinman RE, editor: *Pediatric nutrition handbook,* ed 5, Elk Grove Village, Ill, 2004, American Academy of Pediatrics.

Nicklas TA, Baranowski T, Baranowski JC, et al: Family and child-care provider influences on preschool children's fruit, juice, and vegetable consumption, *Nutr Rev* 59(7):224, 2001.

Thorpe M: Parents as role models: nutrition is a family affair, *J Am Diet Assoc* 102(1):64, 2002.

Tibbs T, Haire-Joshu D, Schechtman KB, et al: The relationship between parental modeling, eating patterns, and dietary intake among African-American parents, *J Am Diet Assoc* 101(5):535, 2001.

- *Minerals:* Calcium and phosphorus are needed for bone mineralization. The bones are strengthening to keep pace with muscle development and increasing activity. Iron is needed to maintain adequate hemoglobin levels because the increase in body size requires an increasing blood volume. Adequate levels of zinc are necessary to support protein synthesis and cell division. The principle of increasing iron absorption from nonheme sources such as vegetables by including a small amount of heme iron from meat at the same meal (as discussed in Chapter 7) holds true for feeding the toddler.
- *Vitamins:* The fat-soluble and water-soluble vitamins are critical to macronutrient use and growth and development. A variety of food intake eaten in proportion to energy needs should provide adequate vitamins to the toddler.
- *Fiber:* Because solid foods make up a larger portion of the diet of toddlers than that of infants, constipation often become more prevalent. Adequate fiber of 19 g/day is recommended for children ages 1 to 3 years.[3]
- *Food choices:* About 2 to 3 cups of milk daily is sufficient for the young child's needs. Sometimes excessive milk intake, a habit carried over from infancy, excludes many solid foods from the diet. As a result, the child may lack iron and develop a so-called milk anemia. On the other hand, if a child dislikes milk as a beverage, then replacement can be made with cheese, creamed soups, puddings, or custards, or nonfat dry milk can be used in cooked cereals, mashed potatoes, meat loaf, and casseroles. Calcium-fortified foods can assist in adding calcium to the diet. Offering the child an increasing variety of foods will help to develop good food habits; food habits are learned, and little opportunity exists for learning if a child is not exposed to a wide variety of foods. Refined sweets are best avoided, reserving them for special occasions, not for habitual use or to bribe a child to eat.

Another important consideration when selecting food for the toddler is the risk of choking and death by asphyxiation. Foods that are round, hard, and not easily dissolved can cause choking. Such food items include hot dogs, grapes, peanut butter in globs, hard pieces of raw fruits and vegetables, hard candy, and popcorn. Young children should always be supervised when eating and should eat sitting down. Running when eating can lead to choking. It is best that children not eat in a moving car unless a second adult, in addition to the driver, is available to assist if needed.

Summary Principles

The following two important principles should be emphasized when working with caregivers to guide feeding practices during this period:

1. The child needs fewer kcalories but relatively more protein and minerals for physical growth; therefore a variety of foods should be offered in appropriate portion sizes to provide key nutrients. It is important that day care providers and parents work cooperatively to support the development of good food patterns.[45]

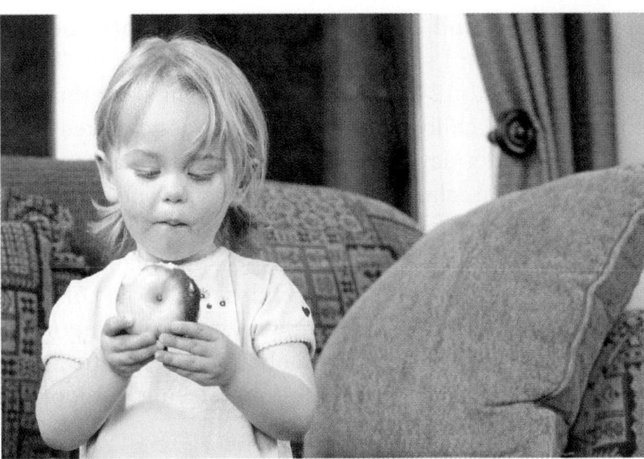

FIGURE 12-2 Fruits are an important part of the toddler's diet. (Copyright 2006 JupiterImages Corporation.)

2. The child is struggling for selfhood as part of normal psychosocial development. This struggle is expressed in refusing food and the desire to do things for self before being fully able to do them efficiently. If caregivers are patient, offer a variety of foods in small amounts, and encourage some degree of food choice and self-feeding in the child's own ceremonial manner, then eating can be a happy, positive means of development.

If we are to achieve the goal of establishing good food patterns for life, it is especially important to introduce a variety of fruits and vegetables along with grains and meats during this stage of development (Figure 12-2). A study of 72 children from 2 to 5 years of age found that they ate few fruits and vegetables and that their food choices changed very little during the 3 years.[46] Only three fruits (apples, bananas, and grapes) and four vegetables (carrots, green beans, corn, and French fries) were included among lists of 19 favorite foods given by mothers and children. Macaroni and cheese, pizza, chicken, and cereal were the four top foods, and fruit drinks, carbonated beverages, milk, and apple juice were the most commonly used beverages.[47]

Preschooler (3 to 6 Years)

Physical Characteristics and Growth

As shown in normal childhood growth charts (see the Evolve web site for *CDC Growth Charts: United States*), each child tends to settle into a regular genetic **growth channel** as physical growth continues in spurts. On occasion the child bounds with energy. Play is hard play—running, jumping, and testing new physical resources. At other times, the child will sit for increasing periods of time engrossed in passive types of activities. Mental capacities are developing, and

> **KEY TERMS**
> **growth channel** The progressive regular growth pattern of children, guided along individual genetically controlled channels, influenced by nutritional and health status.

more thinking and exploring of the environment occurs. Energy needs and specific nutrients are shown in Tables 12-5, 12-6, and 12-7. Protein requirements continue to increase as the child grows older. Preschool children need about 13 to 19 g/day of good-quality protein,[3] as found in milk, egg, meat, cheese, legumes, and soy. They continue to need calcium and iron to support growth and to build body stores. Because vitamins A and C and folate are often lacking in the diets of preschool children, a variety of fruits and vegetables should be provided. Vitamin D, important for calcium absorption, can be obtained in fortified milk or soy products or by spending time playing outdoors in the sun.

Psychosocial and Motor Development

Each stage of development builds on the previous one. The psychosocial developmental stage for preschool children involves increased socialization and initiative. They are beginning to develop their superego—the conscience. As powers of active movement increase, they have a growing imagination and curiosity. This is a period of increasing imitation. Boys and girls may imitate adults who serve as role models. Much of this becomes evident in their play by the use of grown-up clothes and role-playing in a variety of situations. Self-feeding skills increase, and eating takes on increased social aspects. The family mealtime is an important event for socialization, because children imitate their parents and others at the table.[47] Role-modeling may have longterm implications in respect to nutrient intake and health. For example, in nearly 200 girls of kindergarten age, the best predictor of their milk intakes was the milk intakes of their mothers. If the mother drank soft drinks rather than milk, then so did her daughter.[48]

Food and Feeding

The preschool child is beginning to form definite responses to various types of foods, as follows:

- *Vegetables and fruits:* Fruits are usually well liked. However, of all the food groups, vegetables usually are the least well liked by children, yet these foods contain many vitamins and minerals needed for growth. Where space or opportunity exists, involving the young child in planting and growing vegetables in a small garden or in containers is an excellent way to draw the child's interest to vegetables to be tasted. Trips to the market or learning activities in the day care setting can help a child see a variety of shapes and colors in vegetables and discover new ones that can be prepared in a variety of ways. It is important to remember that children have a keen sense of taste; therefore flavor and texture are important. Children usually dislike strong vegetables such as cabbage and onions but do like crisp raw vegetables or fruits cut in small pieces to eat as finger foods. Mixed vegetables and fruits are often less tolerated than individual ones. Children also react to consistency of vegetables, disliking them when they are overcooked. Tough strings and hard pieces are difficult to chew and swallow and should be removed.
- *Milk, cheese, egg, meat, and legumes:* It is helpful if children can set their own goals of quantities of food. Portions need to be relatively small (see the *Perspectives in Practice* box, "Feeding Toddlers and Preschoolers: Eating Is a Family Affair"). If children can pour their own milk from a small pitcher into a small glass, then they will drink more. Smaller children like their milk served closer to room temperature, not icy cold. In addition, they prefer it in small glasses that hold about 4 to 6 oz rather than in large, adult-sized glasses. Cheese is a favorite finger food or snack; however, the major source of calcium in this age-group is milk. Egg is usually well liked if hard-cooked or scrambled. Meat should be tender and easy to cut and chew; hence, ground meat is popular. Ground meat also must be well cooked to make it safe. (To avoid the risk of foodborne illness that can be fatal in the young child, ground meat should be cooked to a temperature of 160° F, the meat should have a gray-white color, and juices should be clear.)
- *Grains:* The wide variety in which grains can be eaten adds to their appeal to children who enjoy breads, cereals, and crackers. Whole grains provide important fiber. To avoid unwanted kcalories, presweetened cereals should be used infrequently if at all.
- *Temperature:* Because children prefer their foods lukewarm and not hot, some foods may remain on their plates and become dry and gummy such that the child refuses to eat them. Thus very small portions should be served at a time.
- *Single foods:* Children usually prefer single foods to combination dishes such as casseroles or stews. Preschool is also a period of language learning. Children like to learn names of foods and to be able to recognize and name them on the basis of their shape, color, texture, and taste; these identifiable characteristics need to be retained as much as possible.
- *Finger foods:* Children like to eat food they can pick up with their fingers. Often, a variety of raw fruits and vegetables cut into finger-sized pieces and offered to children for their own selection provide a source of needed nutrition.
- *Food jags:* Because of developing social and emotional needs, preschool children commonly have food jags, refusing to eat all except one particular food. This may last for several days, but it is usually short lived and of no major consequence.

Summary Principles

The preschool period is one of important growth for the young child. Lifetime food habits are forming. Food continues to play an important part in the developing personality, and group eating becomes significant as a means of socialization. The following two principles should be considered when interacting with preschoolers:

1. The social and emotional environment and companionship at mealtime with family, other caregivers, or other children greatly influence the young child's food intake and diet quality. The child learns food patterns at the family table

and follows the examples of food eaten by parents or older siblings.[49] The child may attend a day care or preschool in which group eating occurs. Food habits of preschoolers are greatly affected by peer modeling, and food preferences develop according to what the group is eating. Children in this stage of development may begin to respond to environmental cues encouraging them to consume more food than they need. In a day care setting, it was found that 5-year-old children ate more food when presented with larger portions, whereas 3½-year-old children were not affected by portion size.[50] In light of the growing numbers of overweight children, we need to encourage parents to be alert to portion size when serving their children's food.

2. Many food preferences and tolerances are established during this period. Exposure to a wide variety of foods in appropriate portion sizes may set the stage for lifetime food habits and associated patterns of health. This stage of growth is also a time for the young child to develop appropriate physical exercise habits, and games including activities such as skipping or jumping should be encouraged in a safe environment. Physical fitness established at an early age can lower the risk of overweight and obesity in childhood and adulthood, respectively.[51] Encouraging young children to participate in active games rather than sedentary pastimes such as watching videos or television may support appropriate food patterns as well (see *Further Readings and Resources* at the end of this chapter). Even a 30-second commercial for a snack food has been shown to influence the food choices of preschool-age children.[52]

School-Age Child (6 to 12 Years)

Physical Characteristics and Growth

The school-age period preceding adolescence has been called the *latent time of growth.* During this stage, the rate of growth slows and body changes occur very gradually. However, resources are being laid down for the rapid adolescent growth that lies ahead; sometimes this has been called the *lull before the storm.* By now the body type has been established, and growth rates vary widely. Girls usually outdistance boys in the latter part of this period.

Psychosocial and Motor Development

Psychosocial development during these early school years centers on the formal learning environment and its expectations. Children have widening horizons, new school experiences, and challenging learning opportunities. They develop increased cognitive capacity and the ability to problem solve. They learn to cooperate in group activities and begin to experience a sense of adequacy and accomplishment and sometimes the realities of competition. The child begins to move from a dependence on parental standards to those of peers (Figure 12-3). Pressures are generated for self-control of a growing body, and inappropriate concepts of body image that lead to chronic dieting or eating disorders likely take root during this period. Negative attitudes are sometimes expressed; these changes in temperament are evidence of the struggle for growing independence. It is a diffuse period of gangs, cliques, hero worship, pensive daydreaming, emotional stress, and learning to get along with other children. This is also a period during which nutrition and health concepts can be learned.

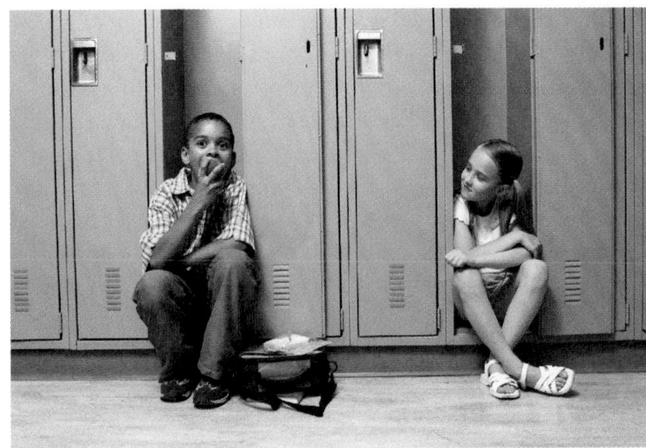

FIGURE 12-3 Peers influence the nutrition habits of school-age children. (Copyright 2006 JupiterImages Corporation.)

Food and Feeding

The slowed rate of growth during this period results in a gradual decline in the food requirement per unit of body weight. This decline continues up to the period just before approaching adolescence. Likes and dislikes are a product of earlier years. Family food attitudes are imitated; however, increasing outside activities begin to compete with family mealtimes, and family conflicts may arise.

School and the Learning Environment

Research has firmly established the close relationship between sound nutrition and childhood learning.[51] Breakfast is particularly important for the school-age child. It *breaks the fast* of the sleep hours and prepares the child for problem solving and memory in the learning hours at school.[53] The School Breakfast and Lunch Programs provide nourishing school meals that many children would not otherwise have (see Appendix F). Studies have documented the positive relationship between breakfast intake and school performance,[53,54] and innovative programs to increase school breakfast participation have been developed.[55,56] School programs implemented by the U.S. Department of Agriculture (USDA) help to maintain sound nutrition by implementing the *Dietary Guidelines for Americans* (see *Further Readings and Resources* at the end of this chapter) into child breakfast and lunch programs,[57,58] developing recipes that lower the fat in school lunch entrees and desserts,[59] and preventing the initiation of snack bars that sell soft drinks and snack foods as an alternative to the cafeteria school lunch.[60] Schools should also take a premier role in promoting lifelong physical activity patterns in children. Health professionals must take leadership roles in their communities to ensure that school meal programs provide positive examples of nutritionally appropriate meal patterns and introduce children to new foods that they may not have tasted previously.

The USDA released the *MyPyramid Food Guidance System* in September 2005. These program materials are designed to assist individuals in identifying energy needs, setting goals for food and nutrient intakes, and developing food intakes based on food groups. The *MyPyramid for Kids* (Figure 12-4) was developed for 6- to 11-year-old children to build knowledge related to food and nutrient intake along with energy intake and energy expenditure through physical activity. Classroom-based activities are available on the website of the USDA (www.teamnutrition.usda.gov/resources/mypyramidclassroom.html) for implementation in schools.

The school-age child has increasing exposure to positive and negative food habits. Television becomes a powerful source of food information. At the same time, positive learning opportunities can occur in the classroom when nutrition education is integrated with other activities and parents provide support and reinforcement at home. An important learning experience can be the preparation of simple meals; in an urban community, 35% of the children in third grade ate at least one meal a day that they prepared themselves or a brother or sister prepared.[61]

Although declines in physical activity no doubt have contributed to the growing number of overweight children, some researchers have also pointed to changes in snacking habits. A comparison of diet surveys during the past 25 years indicated that today's children do not select snacks that have more kcalories than the snacks selected by children in the past; however, they eat more snacks more often, which has added to their energy intakes.[62] An important message to children should be to snack only when they are hungry; snacking should not be a pastime, and the best snacks are those that are relatively low in kcalories but rich in protein, vitamins, and minerals.

Sound nutrition is especially critical for the child athlete. Children ages 6 to 12 years who are engaged in athletic competition need appropriate nutritional advice from parents, coaches, and trained professionals to meet their energy, protein, and fluid needs for training and competition.[63]

Summary Principles

Growth slows during the school-age years, yet development rapidly continues. Individual- and group-learning experiences greatly influence children. The following two principles should be considered when working with school-age children:

1. Energy needs decline; however, the quality of the diet is essential to provide the minerals and vitamins essential to school performance and physical demands.

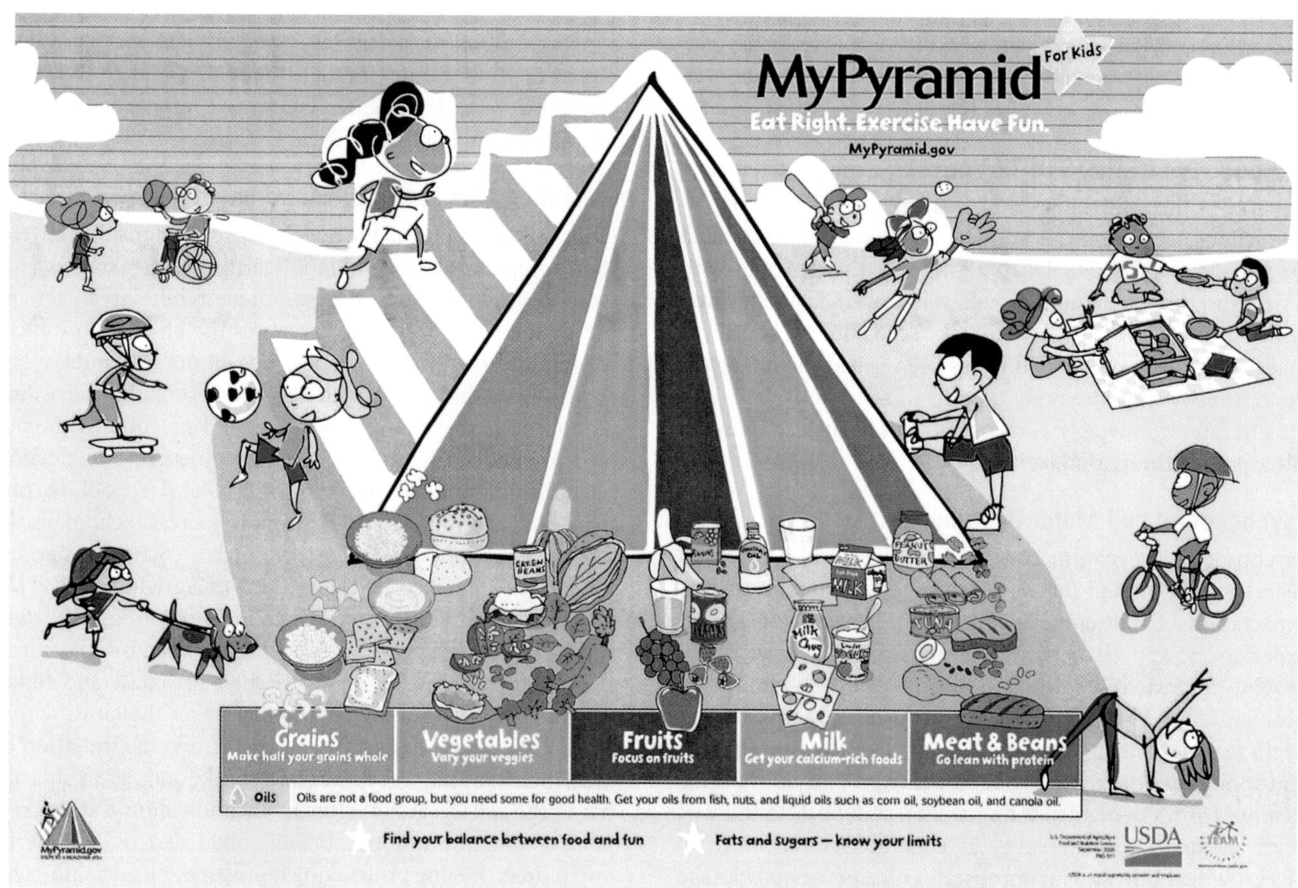

FIGURE 12-4 MyPyramid for Kids for younger children. (From U.S. Department of Agriculture, Food and Nutrition Service: *MyPyramid for Kids,* FNS381, Washington, DC, 2005, U.S. Government Printing Office.)

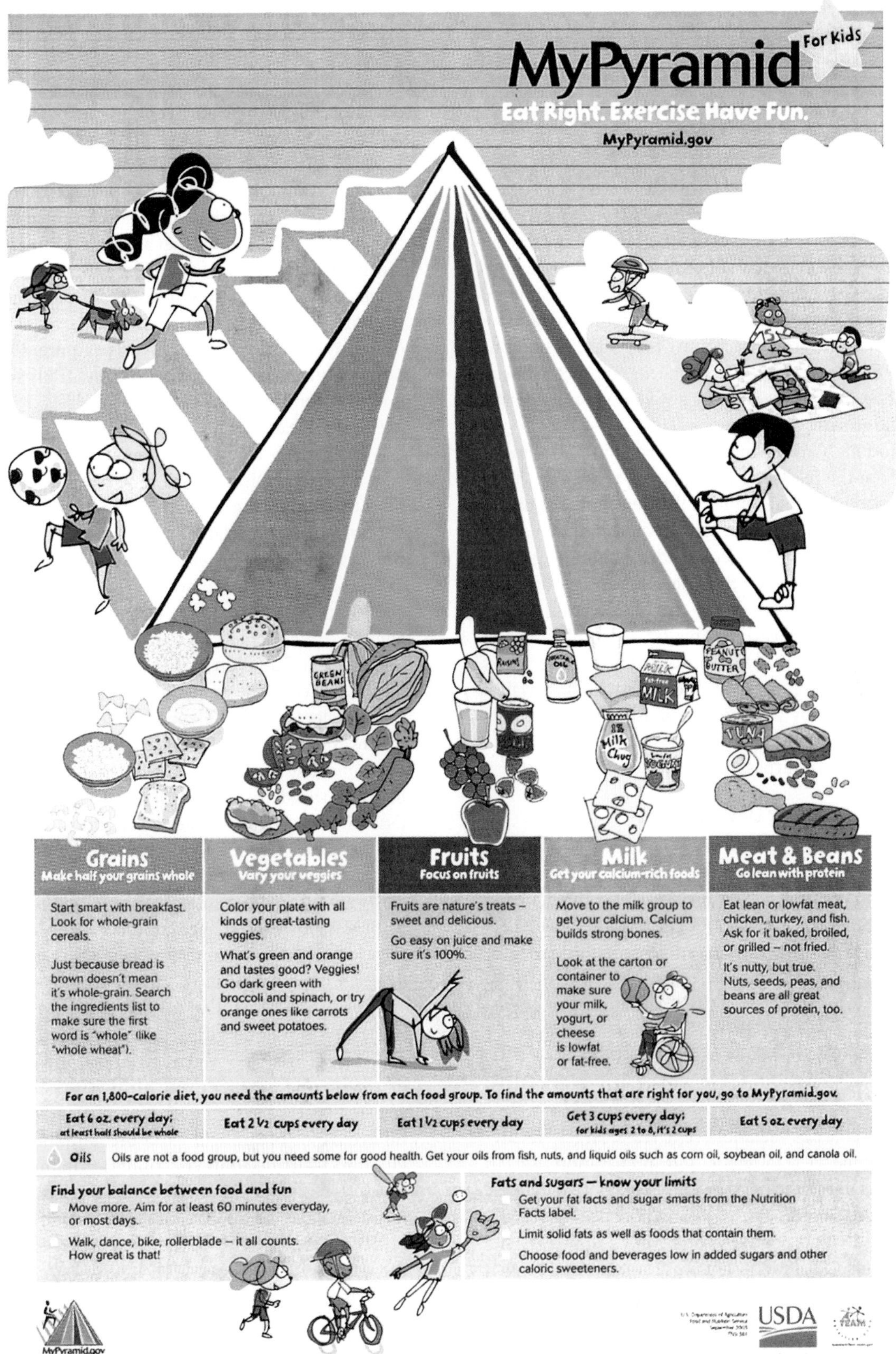

FIGURE 12-4—cont'd

2. The school and home environments must be conducive to assisting 6 to 12 year olds with making appropriate food and activity choices. These choices should be based on sound evidence related to nutritional needs of the school-age individual.

Adolescent

Physical Characteristics and Growth

During the adolescent period, with the onset of puberty, the final growth spurt of childhood occurs. Maturation during this time varies so widely that chronologic age as a reference point for discussing growth ceases to be useful. Physiologic age becomes more important in dealing with individual boys and girls. Adolescent growth accounts for wide fluctuations in physical size, metabolic rate, food needs, and even illness. These capacities can be more realistically viewed only in terms of physiologic growth.

The profound body changes occurring in the adolescent result from the release of estrogen and testosterone, the sex steroid hormones that regulate the development of the sex characteristics. The rate at which these body changes occur varies widely and is particularly distinct in the growth patterns that emerge between the sexes. In girls, the amount of subcutaneous fat increases, and the hip breadth widens in preparation for childbearing. This fat accumulation and change in body shape are often sources of anxiety to many figure-conscious young girls. In adolescent boys, physical growth is manifested by an increased muscle mass and long bone growth. Although the growth spurt in boys is slower than that of girls, boys soon surpass girls in weight and height.

Psychosocial and Motor Development

Adolescence is an ambivalent period marked by stresses and strains. On the one hand, teenagers look back to the securities of childhood; on the other hand, they reach for the maturity of adulthood. Emergence of a self-identity is the major psychosocial developmental task of the adolescent; the search for self, begun in early childhood, reaches its peak during these years. The profound body changes associated with sexual development and the capability of reproduction also result in changes in body image and resulting tensions in maturing girls and boys. Motor development and skilled coordination is complete.

The identity crisis of the adolescent years, largely revolving around sexual development and preparation for an adult role in a complex society, produces many psychologic, emotional, and social pressures. Although the period of most rapid physical growth is relatively short, only 2 or 3 years, the attendant psychosocial development continues during a much longer period. The pressure for peer group acceptance is strong, and fads in dress and food habits play out this theme. In addition, in a technologically developed society such as the United States, high values are placed on education and achievement. Social tensions and family conflicts are often created. These conflicts may have nutritional consequences as teenagers eat away from home more often and develop snacking patterns reflective of personal and peer group choices.

Food and Feeding

With the rapid growth of adolescence comes increased demands for energy, protein, vitamins, and minerals:

- *Energy:* The kcalorie needs increase with the metabolic demands of growth and energy expenditure. Although individual needs may vary, girls require fewer kcalories than boys, based on their smaller body size and body composition.[3] Sometimes the large appetite, characteristic of this rapid growth period, leads adolescents to satisfy their hunger with snack foods that are high in sugar and fat and low in essential protein, vitamins, and minerals.
- *Protein:* Adolescent growth needs for protein increase to support the pubertal changes in both sexes and the developing muscle mass in boys. Girls require 46 g/day, and boys require 52 g/day to sustain daily needs and to maintain nitrogen reserves.[3]
- *Minerals:* The calcium requirement for all adolescents rises to 1300 mg/day to meet the demands of bone growth. In fact, adolescence is a critical time for the development of bone mass under the influence of the increasing levels of the sex hormones, especially estrogen. Poor bone mineralization in adolescence increases vulnerability to bone fracture at later ages.[64] Menses and consequent iron losses in the adolescent girl predispose her to simple iron deficiency anemia. Young female athletes who begin training before menarche and develop secondary amenorrhea may in turn have reduced bone mineral density resulting from low estrogen levels.[65] For all young athletes, fluid replacement in any exercise or performance period is essential.[63]
- *Vitamins:* The B vitamins are needed in increased amounts to meet the extra demands of energy metabolism and tissue development. Intakes of vitamins C and A may be low because of erratic food intake and low intake of vegetables and fruits. A high prevalence of folate deficiency exists among adolescent girls, increasing the risk of NTDs in babies born to teenage mothers (see Chapter 6 for a review of NTDs). Vitamin D deficiency is present in up to one half of all adolescents.[66] More prevalent in the winter and spring months and in African-American and Hispanic adolescent boys and girls,[66] vitamin D deficiency is associated with rickets (overt deficiency) and increased risk of developing osteoporosis, cardiovascular disease, and certain cancers later in life.[67] Use of sunscreens, purposeful avoidance of sunlight exposure, and limited intake of vitamin D-fortified milk contribute to vitamin D deficiency in adolescents.[68] A vitamin D supplement of 10 mcg/day is recommended for adolescents who do not consume food sources of vitamin D.[68]

In the development of nutrition intervention programs for teens, it is important to consider their cultural and ethnic backgrounds, recognizing that food habits and problems may differ (see the *Case Study* box, "Nutrition Program for Adolescents"). A study of more than 2800 adolescents that included Vietnamese, Hispanic, African-American, and Caucasian students showed clearly that intakes of fruits, vegetables, and dairy products differed according to group.[69] The Vietnamese adolescents were the least likely to meet the

CASE STUDY

Nutrition Program for Adolescents

Amanda is a graduate student of clinical nutrition assigned to the "Save Our Senior High" project in a metropolitan community of 300,000 located in northwestern United States. A representative of the city's educational advisory board approached her institution for assistance in developing a program that addresses three major problems faced by the majority of high school students: (1) popularity of fad diets among athletes, (2) overweight, and (3) iron deficiency anemia.

Amanda and other members of her class met with students who were learning other health professions (medicine, dentistry, nutrition, nursing, social work), as well as several student representatives from the high school, to plan the program. After they developed goals and objectives, they decided that the nutrition topics would be addressed in a series of workshops: Nutrition and Physical Fitness, Food for the Teen Years, and Snack Facts.

The program was introduced to the students through an advance bulletin distributed at the largest high school in the city, where the project was to begin. The bulletin included an article written by Amanda: "Teenage Nutrition: A Seeming Paradox." This article responded to a common concern expressed by adolescents: the apparent preoccupation of school officials with the students' food habits when they, as a group, looked and usually felt very healthy.

Amanda's article stirred a tremendous interest in the student population. Attendance at each session was high, and the discussions were lively. The evaluation results were positive. In reviewing the evaluative data and low cost of the project, the city council asked Amanda and her classmates to repeat the program at two other high schools where these problems were also prevalent. The council approached the school board about the possibility of including the project in the citywide high school curriculum for the coming year.

Questions for Analysis

1. Outline the content of Amanda's article to reflect major points that you would have included.
2. Write a class outline for each workshop, including objectives, major topics, and questions you would expect from the students. What teaching methods and materials would you expect to be most effective in each workshop?
3. What outside influences on eating habits would you expect in this student population? How effective would you expect this educational program to be in influencing a change of behavior in eating habits?
4. Aside from in-school nutrition education programs, describe possible tactics for influencing the eating habits of teenagers.

recommended three servings of dairy products each day compared with the African-American, Hispanic, or Caucasian adolescents. Conversely, the Vietnamese students were the most likely to meet the goal of five fruits and vegetables a day. We also need to consider cost when making nutritional recommendations to students or parents. Among limited-resource mothers, fruits and some vegetables were perceived as being less filling, and one mother noted it was more important to have her son's hunger satisfied than to provide particular fruits or vegetables.[70] Nutrition counseling must be individualized, taking into consideration both cultural food preferences and other circumstances existing within the family.

Eating Habits

Physical and psychosocial pressures influence adolescent eating behavior (see the *Perspectives in Practice* box, "Food Habits of Adolescents: Where Do We Begin?"). By and large, boys fare better than girls. Their large appetites and the sheer volumes of food they consume usually ensure generally adequate nutrient intakes, but the adolescent girl may be less fortunate. The following two factors combine to increase issues surrounding nutrition and food intake in adolescent girls:

1. *Physiologic sex difference:* Because sexual maturation in girls brings about increased fat deposition during the adolescent growth period and because many teenage girls are relatively inactive, it is easy for them to gain weight.
2. *Social and personal tensions:* Social pressures dictating thinness sometimes cause adolescent girls to follow unwise and self-imposed diets for weight loss. In some cases actual self-starvation regimens lead to complex and far-reaching eating disorders such as anorexia nervosa and bulimia nervosa (see Chapter 8). These problems, which can assume severe proportions, usually involve a distorted self-image and an irrational pursuit of thinness, even when actual body weight is normal or even less than age norms. In the absence of described eating disorders, constant dieting can still result in varying degrees of poor nutrition in the teenage girl at the very time in life when her body needs to be building reserves for potential reproduction. The harmful effects that bad eating habits can have on the future course of a pregnancy are clearly indicated in many studies relating preconception nutrition status to the outcome of gestation (see Chapter 11).

Summary Principles

The following two principles should be considered when intervening with food habits during adolescence:

1. Nutrient demands are high for final growth and development; therefore the quality of the diet is vital (Figure 12-5).
2. Food choices and eating patterns may be less than optimal because of the many influential factors that affect choices during adolescence.

KEY TERMS

physiologic age Rate of biologic maturation in individual adolescents that varies widely and accounts more for wide and changing differences in their metabolic rates, nutritional needs, and food requirements than does chronologic age.

PERSPECTIVES IN PRACTICE

Food Habits of Adolescents: Where Do We Begin?

Adolescents who have entered their growth spurt seem to eat all the time. The questions for health professionals are, "What are they eating?" and "How do we help them improve their choices?" Both quantity and quality of food are important during this period of rapid growth. Lean body mass increases by about 35 kg in boys and 19 kg in girls during these years, and 45% of total bone mass is accrued. Generous supplies of iron, zinc, calcium, and essential vitamins are needed to support these changes in body size and development.

Food Intake in the Teen Years

Despite the critical nutrient needs in this life stage, national dietary surveys indicate that of all age-groups, teens have the poorest diets. Their intakes of calcium, iron, zinc, vitamin A, and folate often fall below recommended levels. Although on the average teens eat three or four servings of vegetables each day, one or two of these servings are potatoes, most likely French fries; dark-green and deep-yellow vegetables are eaten infrequently. Boys and girls between the ages of 12 and 19 years eat about one and a half servings of fruit each day, and about half comes from citrus sources. From the dairy group, boys consume only two and a half servings and girls consume only one and a half servings each day, which does not meet their need for calcium (one dairy serving = 300 mg calcium). At the same time, most adolescents are exceeding their need for protein. Foods such as hamburgers, pizza with cheese, tacos, and milkshakes, popular among teens, are good sources of protein. Foods high in sugar such as soft drinks and candy and items high in fat, including pastries, fatty meats, and fried foods, are eaten regularly by many teens. Boys and girls obtain 20% of their kcalories from added sugars, 33% from fat, and 13% from saturated fat. Twenty-one percent of adolescents use vitamin-mineral supplements, but the supplement users have better diets and obtain increased intakes of nutrients from food. Teens also indulge in risk-taking behaviors: about one third smoke, and 28% of girls and 35% of boys report at least one episode of binge drinking per month.

Lifestyle and Nutritional Behavior

Lifestyle choices in the teen years are influenced by peer pressure and teens' growing need to express their independence and make their own decisions. Teens also lead busy lives with school, sports, and jobs. Focus group interviews with teens in Minnesota indicated that (1) food taste and appeal, (2) time, and (3) convenience were the three most important factors influencing their food choices. They liked foods that looked good and chose the same foods repeatedly because they knew how they were going to taste. Foods such as pastries and other high-sugar or high-fat items were perceived as tasting better than more healthy foods such as fruits, vegetables, or dairy products. Fast-food restaurants are popular because the food is served quickly. Teens often skip breakfast. Individuals in this age-group do not want to spend time preparing food or cleaning up afterward. Food items must be easy to prepare or ready to eat, easy to eat on the go or carry in a backpack, or delivered to the house.

Unfortunately, health is often not an important personal issue at this life stage. A feeling of invulnerability and the idea that they have plenty of time in future years to worry about their health are common in teens. At the same time, body weight and appearance are major concerns for 49% of girls and 43% of boys. The need to be thin causes some adolescent girls to adopt nutritionally inadequate diets or, worse, develop anorexia or bulimia nervosa (see Chapter 8). Adolescent boys trying to increase their muscle mass or "bulk up" may resort to unproven and potentially dangerous supplements or eat high-fat foods in an effort to obtain more kcalories. When working with teens who claim to be dieting, it is necessary to talk with them individually about what kind of diet they are following. For some teens, dieting means drastically reducing their food intake or choosing foods erroneously believed to have special effects on appearance; for others, dieting refers to healthful practices like increasing their intakes of fruits and vegetables or cutting down on fats and sweets.

How Do We Help Teens Improve Their Food Choices?

Improving the food choices of this age-group will require the combined efforts of parents, health professionals, food manufacturers, restaurant personnel, and food retailers. An important message to teens is that appropriate food choices, along with regular physical activity, can help to achieve and maintain (1) a healthy weight and positive level of fitness, (2) a high energy level for school and work, and (3) an overall sense of well-being. Physical education and health teachers, nutrition educators, athletic coaches, school nurses, and parents must work together to develop programs that will reach teens at school and on the playing field.

Teens want information that they can use now, not 10 years from now. One topic of immediate use would be selecting a lower-fat or lower-kcalorie meal at a fast-food restaurant or choosing a more healthy pizza for home delivery. Snacks such as bananas, oranges, or apples; plastic containers of juice; or individual packages of ready-to-eat cereal travel well in a backpack, as do new ultrapasteurized milk drinks that do not require refrigeration. Choosing simple-to-prepare or carry-along breakfasts, such as ready-to-eat cereal or whole grain bread (or a bagel) with peanut butter, should be encouraged. Among junior high school students, ready-to-eat cereals provided a breakfast that was lower in cost, lower in fat, and higher in important nutrients including calcium, iron, vitamins A and D, and folate than fast-food breakfast meals, granola, or toaster pastries.

Because taste is the most important factor in food selection for teens, it is important that healthy foods taste good. School cafeteria managers need to produce good-tasting and satisfying food that is attractively served. This means that the school meal must be viewed as an extension of the school's educational mission and supported by teachers and parents. Salad bars have become popular among some teens, and salads "to go" might meet the need of taste and convenience. Recipes that are reduced in fat and sugar but pleasing in taste and texture need to be developed for quantity food programs.

Food manufacturers must be urged to improve the nutrient quality of ready-to-eat main dishes, as well as snack foods. Taste-testing parties with teens that compare lower-fat or reduced-sugar items with less-nutritious products may help to dispel the myth that healthy foods do not taste good. Many popular foods among teens, such as pizza or tacos, can be exceedingly healthy choices if attention is paid to reducing the levels of ingredients high in fat and saturated fat.

PERSPECTIVES IN PRACTICE

Food Habits of Adolescents: Where Do We Begin?—cont'd

Finally, food retailers who cater to the teen audience must be urged to sell and advertise healthy foods. Some fast-food restaurants include orange juice or low-fat milk as drink options in combination meals as an alternative to soft drinks. Salads are an option at many fast-food outlets, and baked potatoes may be available as an alternative to French fries. Advertisements for soft drinks or less-healthy food items often carry the endorsements of popular sports stars. Such endorsements have been applied to foods such as milk that are important to health and well-being. Community coalitions involving health professionals, educators, and parents concerned about adolescents and their future health will be necessary to bring about needed changes.

BIBLIOGRAPHY

Dixon LB, Cronin FJ, Krebs-Smith SM: Let the pyramid guide your food choices: capturing the total diet concept, *J Nutr* 131(Suppl 2): 461S, 2001.

Dwyer JT, Garcea AO, Evans M, et al: Do adolescent vitamin-mineral supplement users have better nutrient intakes than nonusers? Observations from the CATCH tracking study, *J Am Diet Assoc* 101(11):1340, 2001.

Hampl JS, Betts NM: Cigarette use during adolescence: effects on nutritional status, *Nutr Rev* 57(7):215, 1999.

Kleinman RE, editor: *Pediatric nutrition handbook*, ed 5, Elk Grove Village, Ill, 2004, American Academy of Pediatrics.

Neumark-Sztainer D, Wall M, Story M, et al: Are family meal patterns associated with disordered eating behaviors among adolescents? *J Adolesc Health* 35(5):350, 2004.

Neumark-Sztainer D, Story M, Perry C, et al: Factors influencing food choices of adolescents: findings from focus-group discussions with adolescents, *J Am Diet Assoc* 99(8):929, 1999.

Nicklas TA, McQuarrie A, Fastnaught C, et al: Efficiency of breakfast consumption patterns of ninth graders: nutrient-to-cost comparisons, *J Am Diet Assoc* 102(2):226, 2002.

O'Dea JA: Children and adolescents identify food concerns, forbidden foods, and food-related beliefs, *J Am Diet Assoc* 99(8):970, 1999.

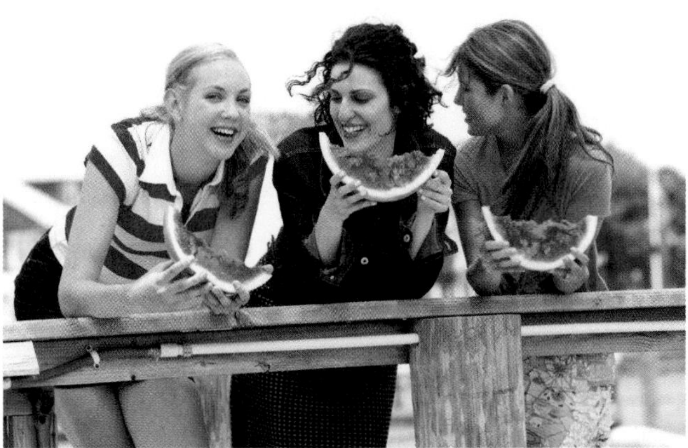

FIGURE 12-5 Fruits and vegetables help meet the high nutrient demands during adolescence. (Copyright 2006 JupiterImages Corporation.)

HEALTH PROMOTION

CHILDREN AND ADOLESCENTS: SEEKING FITNESS

The *Dietary Guidelines for Americans 2005* provides direction for the development of a healthy diet and lifestyle for all persons age 2 and older.[71] The 2005 edition set goals not only for food patterns in all age-groups but also for appropriate physical activity. Many chronic diseases that influence well-being in later life actually begin in childhood. Thus lifestyle practices that promote healthy behaviors related to diet and physical activity must be introduced at an early age, when patterns are being developed that will continue for a lifetime.

Weight Management

Body weight and physical activity are intrinsically related. A regular pattern of exercise beginning in childhood will promote lifelong heart health and prevent the accumulation of excess body fat. Large numbers of U.S. children are overweight, and the numbers continue to climb. Among 5000 children between the ages of 9 and 11, the proportion classified as overweight increased by 11% during a 2-year period.[72] Racial, ethnic, and regional differences are seen in overweight among children. Boys, African Americans, Hispanics, and those living in the Southern states are more likely to be overweight.[72] High-energy diets, coupled with inactivity patterns leading to increased body fat, are associated with the growing incidence of type 2 diabetes in children of school age.

Body fat increases rapidly during the first year of life and then slows until about age 6, when again a normal increase occurs in the size and number of body fat cells. For some children, an inappropriate accumulation of body fat begins about this time or even earlier. Figure 12-6 displays the multifaceted nature of overweight in childhood. Attention must be given to the personal or child characteristics and risk factors, parenting skills and family dynamics, and environmental factors of the community and society that contribute to this complex problem. In general, accumulation of excess body fat can be accelerated by a high energy intake in relation to energy needs or a sedentary life pattern with low energy expenditure. Although opinions about this matter differ, several experts suggest that children who are overweight do not consume more kcalories than normal-weight children; they are simply less physically active. The best insurance to prevent inappropriate accumulation of body fat in a child of any age is regular physical activity. The goal is to promote body weight gain within healthy ranges to support normal growth and development.[71] In overweight children and adolescents, the goal is to slow gains in body weight while promoting optimal growth and development.[4]

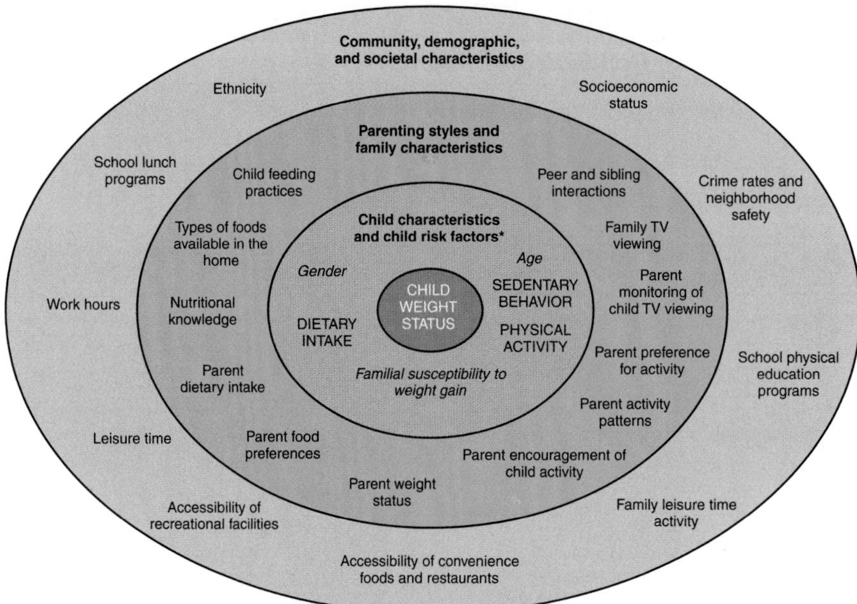

FIGURE 12-6 Ecological model of predictors of childhood overweight. (Copyright 2001 *Obesity Reviews*. From Davison KK, Birch LL: Childhood overweight: a contextual model and recommendations for future research, *Obes Rev* 2:159, 2001. Reprinted with permission.)

Inactivity
cut down

Flexibility and Strength
2-3 times a week

Active Aerobics and Recreational Activities
3-5 times a week

Everyday Activities
as often as possible

MyActivity Pyramid

Be physically active at least 60 minutes every day, or most days.
Use these suggestions to help meet your goal.

© 2006 UNIVERSITY OF MISSOURI EXTENSION

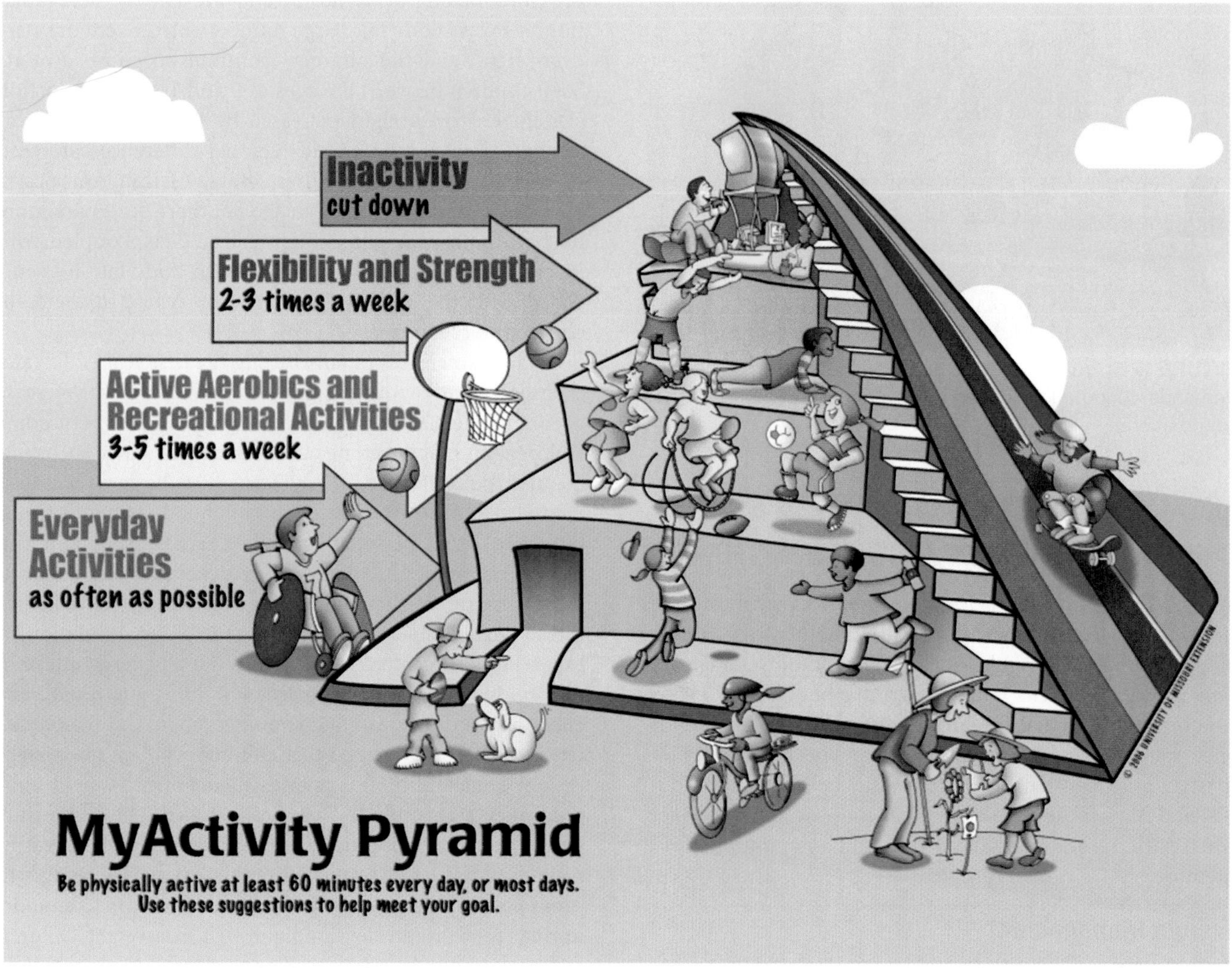

FIGURE 12-7 MyActivity Pyramid. (From University of Missouri Extension Publication N386. Reprinted with permission. Available at www.extension.missouri.edu/publications/DisplayPub.aspx?P=n386.)

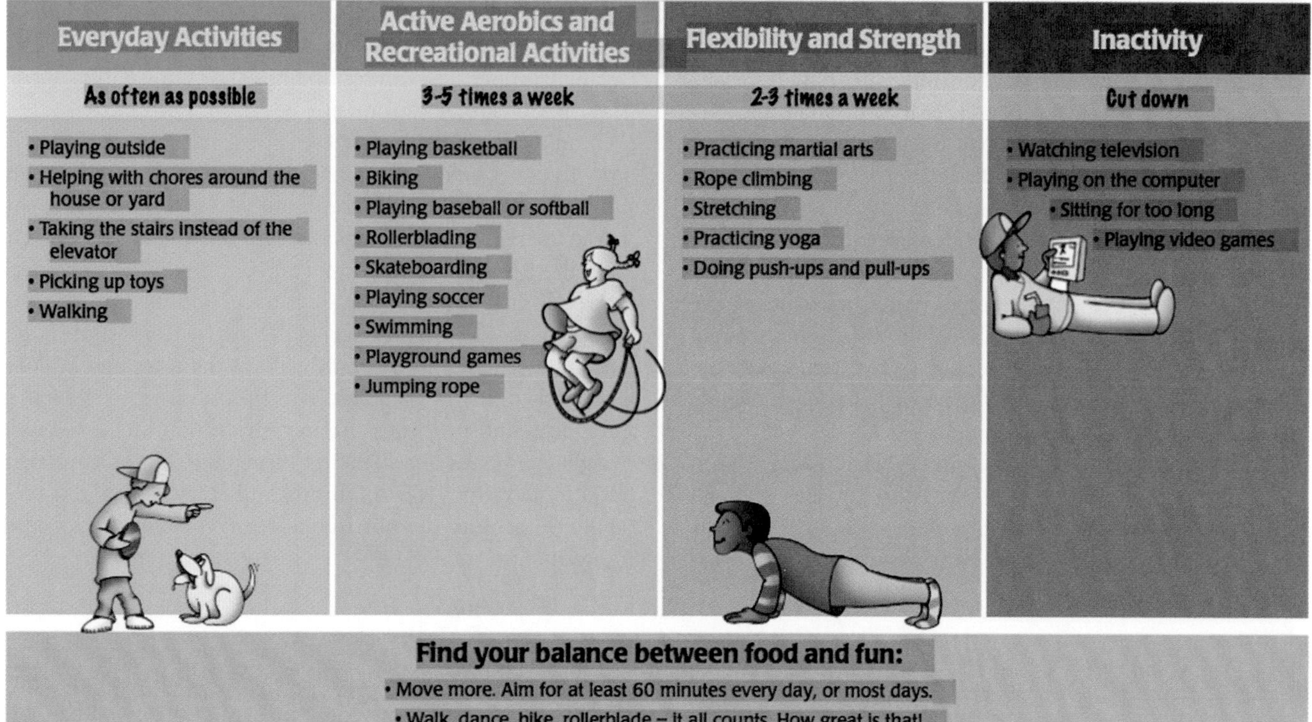

FIGURE 12-7—cont'd

Physical Activity

Although children and adolescents are typically more active than most adults, many of them appear to be settling into a sedentary lifestyle more common among adults.[73] We know that 48% of girls and 26% of boys do not exercise vigorously on a regular basis.[73] Schools now offer fewer physical education opportunities to students. During the past decade, daily participation in physical education dropped to 29%, although about half of all youth have such classes at least once each week.[73] Television, computer games, the Internet, and similar sedentary pastimes are growing in popularity. Watching television for more than 2 hours per day during childhood is related to overweight and the presence of other risk factors for chronic diseases.[74] The physical activity guideline for children and adolescents is a minimum of 1 hour of aerobic, moderate to vigorous-intensity physical activity each day.[75] Vigorous-intensity and muscle-strengthening physical activity that is weight bearing and bone health promoting should be completed at least 3 days each week.[75]

Helping Children Develop an Active Lifestyle

Parents and caregivers, schools, and communities need to work together to increase physical activity among children.[76] Children are more likely to develop an active lifestyle if parents and role models also demonstrate such behavior. Taking your teddy bear for a walk can be a meaningful activity for a preschooler who belongs to a family that walks together regularly. School games and physical education programs should focus on activities such as walking or running that allow all students to participate, rather than on games in which several students are active but the majority sit and watch. Moving away from competitive games that discourage participation by overweight or less-skilled players to such activities as kick ball, dancing, or aerobics that can be done alone to music or in groups after school are worthwhile objectives for physical education. Bike riding and jumping rope are good forms of vigorous exercise. Making school facilities such as a gymnasium or walking track available to families and students after school hours might encourage an increased level of physical activity. Figure 12-7 illustrates one example of guidelines regarding activity levels for children ages 6 to 11 years.

TO SUM UP

Normal growth and development depend on nutrition to support heightened physiologic and metabolic processes. Nutrition, in turn, depends on a multitude of social, psychosocial, cultural, and environmental influences that affect individual growth potential throughout the life cycle.

Four types of growth interact during each phase of development: (1) physical, (2) mental, (3) emotional, and (4) sociocultural. Each type of growth must be evaluated when assessing the child's nutrition status and planning an effective counseling approach. Nutritional needs change with each growth period and must be individualized according to the unique growth pattern of every child.

Infants experience rapid growth. They have immature digestive systems and limited ability to absorb and excrete metabolites efficiently. Breast-feeding is preferred during the first year of life. Solid foods are not needed or adequately tolerated until an infant is 6 to 7 months old.

Toddlers (ages 1 to 3 years), preschoolers (ages 3 to 6 years), and school-age children (ages 6 to 12 years) experience the slowed and erratic latent growth of childhood. Their energy requirements per unit of body weight are not as great as those of infants. Their nutritional needs center on protein for growth, with attendant minerals and vitamins. Social and cultural factors influence the development of food habits in these age-groups. Appropriate food behavior by parents and caregivers that can be modeled by children of these ages strongly influences the adoption of good eating habits during these periods of development.

Adolescents (ages 12 to 18 years) experience a second large growth spurt before reaching adulthood. This rapid growth involves sexual maturation and physical growth. During this period, girls increase their body proportion of fat, whereas boys increase their body proportion of muscle. Reaching peak bone mass is an important milestone for both sexes during this period of development. In general, boys (who consume larger amounts of food) more easily achieve the increased kcalorie and nutrient needs of adolescence. In contrast, girls (who may feel social and peer pressure to restrict food intake to avoid weight gain) are less likely to meet their optimal nutrient requirements for growth. This pressure may also inhibit their ability to acquire the nutritional reserves necessary for later reproduction.

QUESTIONS FOR REVIEW

1. How is physical growth measured? What are the NCHS growth charts, and how are they used? What are the limitations of these charts? What are some clinical, biochemical, and dietary measures that are helpful in assessing the nutritional status of infants and children?
2. Describe the physical and psychosocial characteristics of the newborn. What are the capabilities of the newborn's digestive and renal systems, and how do they relate to infant feeding?
3. Why is breast-feeding the preferred method for feeding infants (discuss nutritional and psychosocial factors)? Describe the anatomic and hormonal components that participate in the delivery of breast milk to the nursing infant.
4. You are planning a nutrition education class to prepare pregnant mothers for breast-feeding. Outline the material that you would present, including (a) dietary needs for the new breastfeeding mother, (b) techniques for holding and feeding the baby, and (c) nipple care.
5. You are counseling a pregnant mother who has decided not to breast-feed. Describe some types of commercial formulas that would provide an appropriate alternative feeding for her infant. Describe the feeding techniques that will be important in meeting the psychosocial needs of her infant.
6. You are working with a mother whose newborn has been found to be allergic to milk proteins. What might be an appropriate food source for this infant?
7. You are working with a low-income mother who has chosen not to breast-feed. She is concerned about the high cost of infant formula and would like to feed her infant cow's milk because it is cheaper. What would you tell her?
8. Outline a general schedule for a new mother to use as a guide for adding solid foods to her infant's diet during the first year of life; indicate both the time of addition and the items to be offered.
9. What changes in physical growth and psychosocial development influence eating habits in the (a) toddler, (b) preschool child, and (c) school-age child? How do these factors influence the nutritional needs of each age-group?
10. What factors influence the changing nutritional needs of adolescents? Who is usually at increased nutritional risk during this stage—boys or girls? Why? What nutritional deficiencies may be associated with this vulnerable age?
11. You are the director of a food service program in an elementary school and want to start a nutrition education program. You are working with a science teacher, a social studies teacher, and the school nurse to develop lessons that will connect learning in the classroom with good nutrition in the lunchroom. Visit the USDA's Food and Nutrition Information Center website for Team Nutrition (www.fns.usda.gov/tn) to find some ideas and materials that will assist you in this project. Develop a lesson plan for presentation in the science or social studies class that focuses on nutrition or food patterns, and indicate how you will connect this lesson with the lunch program.

REFERENCES

1. Chumlea WC: Physical growth and maturation. In Samour PQ, King K, editors: *Handbook of pediatric nutrition*, ed 3, Sudbury, Mass, 2005, Jones & Bartlett.
2. Kuczmarski RJ, Ogden CL, Grummer-Strawn LM, et al: *CDC growth charts: United States, advance data, vital and health statistics*, No. 314, Hyattsville, Md, 2000, Centers for Disease Control and Prevention.
3. Food and Nutrition Board, Institute of Medicine: *Dietary Reference Intakes for energy, carbohydrate, fiber, fat, fatty acids, cholesterol, protein, and amino acids (macronutrients)*, Washington, DC, 2002, National Academies Press.
4. Kleinman RE, editor: *Pediatric nutrition handbook*, ed 5, Elk Grove Village, Ill, 2004, American Academy of Pediatrics.
5. Food and Nutrition Board, Institute of Medicine: *Dietary References Intakes for water, potassium, sodium, chloride, and sulfate*, Washington, DC, 2004, National Academies Press.
6. Holst M-C: Developmental and behavioral effects of iron deficiency anemia in infants, *Nutr Today* 33(1):27, 1998.
7. Hurtado EK, Claussen AH, Scott KG: Early childhood anemia and mild or moderate mental retardation, *Am J Clin Nutr* 69(1):115, 1999.
8. Partington S, Nitzke S, Csete J: The prevalence of anemia in a WIC population: a comparison by homeless experience, *J Am Diet Assoc* 100(4):469, 2000.
9. Erikson E: *Childhood and society*, New York, 1963, WW Norton.
10. Klawitter BM: Nutrition counseling. In Samour PQ, King K, editors: *Handbook of pediatric nutrition*, ed 3, Sudbury, Mass, 2005, Jones & Bartlett.
11. Position of the American Dietetic Association: Promoting and supporting breastfeeding, *J Am Diet Assoc* 105(5):810, 2005.
12. Pettifor JM: Nutritional rickets: deficiency of vitamin D, calcium, or both? *Am J Clin Nutr* 80(Suppl 6):1725S, 2004.
13. Akers SM, Groh-Wargo SL: Normal nutrition during infancy. In Samour PQ, King K, editors: *Handbook of pediatric nutrition*, ed 3, Sudbury, Mass, 2005, Jones & Bartlett.
14. Philipp BL, Merewood A: The baby-friendly way: the best breastfeeding start, *Pediatr Clin North Am* 51(3):761, 2004.
15. Chalmers B: The Baby Friendly Hospital Initiative: where next? *BJOG* 111(3):198, 2004.
16. Philipp BL, Malone KL, Cimo S, et al: Sustained breastfeeding rates at a U.S. baby-friendly hospital, *Pediatrics* 112:234, 2003.
17. McCrory MA: Does dieting during lactation put infant growth at risk? *Nutr Rev* 59(1, part 1):18, 2001.
18. Fisher JO, Birch LL, Smiciklas-Wright H, et al: Breast-feeding through the first year predicts maternal control in feeding and subsequent toddler energy intakes, *J Am Diet Assoc* 100(6):641, 2000.
19. Hediger ML, Overpeck MD, Ruan WJ, et al: Early infant feeding and growth status of U.S.-born infants and children aged 4-71 mo: analyses from the Third National Health and Nutrition Examination Survey, 1988-1994, *Am J Clin Nutr* 72(1):159, 2000.
20. Desage M, Schaal B, Soubeyrand J, et al: Gas chromatographic-mass spectrometric method to characterize the transfer of dietary odorous compounds into plasma and milk, *J Chromatogr B Biomed Appl* 678(2):205, 1996.
21. Mennella JA, Beauchamp GK: Experience with a flavor in mother's milk modifies the infant's acceptance of flavored cereal, *Dev Psychobiol* 35(3):197, 1999.
22. Mennella JA, Griffin CE, Beauchamp GK: Flavor programming during infancy, *Pediatrics* 113(4):840, 2004.
23. Hediger ML, Overpeck MD, Kuczmarski RJ, et al: Association between infant breastfeeding and overweight in young children, *JAMA* 285(19):2453, 2001.
24. Philipsen NM, Philipsen NC: Childhood overweight: prevention strategies for parents, *J Perinat Educ* 17(7):44, 2008.
25. Stettler N: Nature and strength of epidemiological evidence for origins of childhood and adulthood obesity in the first year of life, *Int J Obes* 31(7):1035, 2007.
26. Stettler N, Zemel BS, Kumanyika S, et al: Infant weight gain and childhood overweight status in a multicenter, cohort study, *Pediatrics* 109(2):194, 2002.
27. Butte NF, Wong WW, Hopkinson JM, et al: Infant feeding mode affects early growth and body composition, *Pediatrics* 106(6):1355, 2000.
28. Humphrey J, Iliff P: Is breast not best? Feeding babies born to HIV-positive mothers: bringing balance to a complex issue, *Nutr Rev* 59(4):119, 2001.
29. Koo WW: Efficacy and safety of docosahexaenoic acid and arachidonic acid addition to infant formulas: can one buy better vision and intelligence? *J Am Coll Nutr* 22(2):101, 2003.
30. Williams C, Birch EE, Emmett PM, et al: Stereoacuity at age 3.5 y in children born full-term is associated with prenatal and postnatal dietary factors: a report from a population-based cohort study, *Am J Clin Nutr* 73(2):316, 2001.
31. Uauy R, Hoffman DR, Mena P, et al: Term infant studies of DHA and ARA supplementation on neurodevelopment: results of randomized controlled trials, *J Pediatr* 143(Suppl 4l):S17, 2003.
32. Auestad N, Scott DT, Janowsky JS, et al: Visual, cognitive, and language assessments at 39 months: a follow-up study of children fed formulas containing long-chain polyunsaturated fatty acids to 1 year of age, *Pediatrics* 112(3, part 1):E177, 2003.
33. Hoffman DR, Birch EE, Castaneda YS, et al: Visual function in breast-fed term infants weaned to formula with or without long-chain polyunsaturates at 4 to 6 months: a randomized clinical trial, *J Pediatr* 142(6):669, 2003.
34. Innis SM, Adamkin DH, Hall RT, et al: Docosahexaenoic acid and arachidonic acid enhance growth with no adverse effects in preterm infants fed formula, *J Pediatr* 140(5):547, 2002.
35. American Academy of Pediatrics, Committee on Nutrition: Hypoallergenic infant formulas, *Pediatrics* 106(2, part 1):346, 2000.
36. Merritt RJ, Jenks BH: Safety of soy-based infant formulas containing isoflavones: the clinical evidence, *J Nutr* 134:1220S, 2004.
37. Bhatia J, Greer F: American Academy of Pediatrics Committee on Nutrition: Use of soy protein-based formulas in infant feeding, *Pediatrics* 121:1062, 2008.
38. Sharpless KE, Schiller SB, Margolis SA, et al: Certification of nutrients in Standard Reference Material *1846*: infant formula, *J AOAC Int* 80(3):611, 1997.
39. Fewtrell MS, Morley R, Abbott FA, et al: Catch-up growth in small-for-gestational-age term infants: a randomized trial, *Am J Clin Nutr* 74(4):516, 2001.
40. Fomon SJ: Infant feeding in the 20th century: formula and beikost, *J Nutr* 131(2):409S, 2001.
41. Kannan S, Carruth BR, Skinner J: Cultural influences on infant feeding beliefs of mothers, *J Am Diet Assoc* 99(1):88, 1999.
42. Bronner YL, Gross SM, Caulfield L, et al: Early introduction of solid foods among urban African-American participants in WIC, *J Am Diet Assoc* 99(4):457, 1999.

43. Birch LL: Development of food preferences, *Annu Rev Nutr* 19:41, 1999.
44. Gerrish CJ, Mennella JA: Flavor variety enhances food acceptance in formula-fed infants, *Am J Clin Nutr* 73(6):1080, 2001.
45. Briley ME, Jastrow S, Vickers J, et al: Dietary intake at child-care centers and away: are parents and care providers working as partners or at cross-purposes? *J Am Diet Assoc* 99(8):950, 1999.
46. Skinner JD, Carruth BR, Houck KS, et al: Longitudinal study of nutrient and food intakes of white preschool children aged 24 to 60 months, *J Am Diet Assoc* 99(12):1514, 1999.
47. Nicklas TA, Baranowski T, Baranowski JC, et al: Family and child-care provider influences on preschool children's fruit, juice, and vegetable consumption, *Nutr Rev* 59(7):224, 2001.
48. Fisher J, Mitchell D, Smiciklas-Wright H, et al: Maternal milk consumption predicts the tradeoff between milk and soft drinks in young girls' diets, *J Nutr* 131(2):246, 2001.
49. Tibbs T, Haire-Joshu D, Schechtman KB, et al: The relationship between parental modeling, eating patterns, and dietary intake among African-American parents, *J Am Diet Assoc* 101(5):535, 2001.
50. Rolls BJ, Engell D, Birch LL: Serving portion size influences 5-year-old but not 3-year-old children's food intakes, *J Am Diet Assoc* 100(2):232, 2000.
51. Position of the American Dietetic Association: Nutrition guidance for healthy children ages 2 to 11 years, *J Am Diet Assoc* 108(6):1038, 2008.
52. Borzekowski DLG, Robinson TN: The 30-second effect: an experiment revealing the impact of television commercials on food preferences of preschoolers, *J Am Diet Assoc* 101(1):42, 2001.
53. Kleinman RE, Hall S, Green H, et al: Diet, breakfast, and academic performance in children, *Annu Nutr Metab* 46(Suppl 1):24, 2002.
54. Pollitt E, Mathews R: Breakfast and cognition: an integrative summary, *Am J Clin Nutr* 67(4):804S, 1998.
55. Gross SM, Cinelli B: Coordinated school health program and dietetics professionals: partners in promoting healthful eating, *J Am Diet Assoc* 104(5):793, 2004.
56. Kennedy E, Davis C: U.S. Department of Agriculture school breakfast program, *Am J Clin Nutr* 67(4):798S, 1998.
57. Friedman BJ, Hurd-Crixell SL, Ferris B: Texas school menu compliance with U.S. Dietary Guidelines for Americans, *J Am Diet Assoc* 98(11):1325, 1998.
58. Friedman BJ, Hurd-Crixell SL: Nutrient intake of children eating school breakfast, *J Am Diet Assoc* 99(2):219, 1999.
59. Rankin LL, Bingham M: Acceptability of oatmeal chocolate chip cookies prepared using pureed white beans as a fat ingredient substitute, *J Am Diet Assoc* 100(7):831, 2000.
60. Cullen KW, Eagan J, Baranowski T, et al: Effect of a la carte and snack bar foods at school on children's lunchtime intake of fruits and vegetables, *J Am Diet Assoc* 100(12):1482, 2000.
61. Melnick TA, Rhoades SJ, Wales KR, et al: Food consumption patterns of elementary schoolchildren in New York City, *J Am Diet Assoc* 98(2):159, 1998.
62. Jahns L, Siega-Riz AM, Popkin BM: The increasing prevalence of snacking among U.S. children from 1977 to 1996, *J Pediatr* 138(4):493, 2001.
63. Position of Dietitians of Canada, the American Dietetic Association, and the American College of Sports Medicine: Nutrition and athletic performance, *Can J Diet Pract Res* 61(4):176, 2000.
64. Wosje KS, Specker BL: Role of calcium in bone health during childhood, *Nutr Rev* 58(9):253, 2000.
65. Beals KA, Manore MM: Nutritional status of female athletes with subclinical eating disorders, *J Am Diet Assoc* 98(4):419, 1998.
66. Gordon CM, DePeter KC, Feldman HA, et al: Prevalence of vitamin D deficiency among healthy adolescents, *Arch Pediatr Adolesc Med* 158:531, 2004.
67. Huh SY, Gordon CM: Vitamin D deficiency in children and adolescents: epidemiology, impact and treatment, *Rev Endocr Metab Disord* 9:161, 2008.
68. Wagner CL, Greer FR: American Academy of Pediatrics Section on Breastfeeding; American Academy of Pediatrics Committee on Nutrition: Prevention of rickets and vitamin D deficiency in infants, children, and adolescents, *Pediatrics* 122:1142, 2008.
69. Wiecha J, Fink AK, Wiecha J, et al: Differences in dietary patterns of Vietnamese, white, African-American, and Hispanic adolescents in Worcester, Mass, *J Am Diet Assoc* 101(2):248, 2001.
70. Hampl JS, Sass S: Focus groups indicate that vegetable and fruit consumption by food stamp-eligible Hispanics is affected by children and unfamiliarity with non-traditional foods, *J Am Diet Assoc* 101(6):685, 2001.
71. U.S. Department of Health and Human Services, U.S. Department of Agriculture: *Dietary Guidelines for Americans 2005*, ed 6, Washington, DC, 2005, U.S. Government Printing Office. Available at www.healthierus.gov/dietaryguidelines/dga2005/document/default.htm. Retrieved 09 September 2009.
72. Dwyer JT, Stone EJ, Yang M, et al: Prevalence of marked overweight and obesity in a multiethnic pediatric population: findings from the Child and Adolescent Trial for Cardiovascular Health (CATCH) study, *J Am Diet Assoc* 100(10):1149, 2000.
73. Troiano RP, Macera CA, Ballard-Barbash R: Be physically active each day: how can we know? *J Nutr* 131(2, Suppl 1): 451S, 2001.
74. Hancox RJ, Milne BJ, Poulton R: Association between child and adolescent television viewing and adult health: a longitudinal birth cohort study, *Lancet* 364(9430):257, 2004.
75. U.S. Department of Health and Human Services: *Physical activity guidelines for Americans*, ed 1, Washington, DC, 2008, U.S. Government Printing Office.
76. Veugelers PJ, Fitzgerald AL: Effectiveness of school programs in preventing childhood obesity: a multilevel comparison, *Am J Public Health* 95(3):432, 2005.

FURTHER READINGS AND RESOURCES

Readings

Dwyer J: Should dietary fat recommendations for children be changed? *J Am Diet Assoc* 100(1):36, 2000.

Krebs NF, Johnson SL: Guidelines for healthy children: promoting eating, moving, and common sense, *J Am Diet Assoc* 100(1):37, 2000.

Satter E: A moderate view on fat restriction for young children, *J Am Diet Assoc* 100(1):32, 2000.

The increasing incidence of overweight in children and concern for the prevention of chronic diseases later in life have led to a discussion about the optimum level of dietary fat for children. The previous three articles discuss this controversy.

Auestad N, Scott DT, Janowsky JS, et al: Visual, cognitive, and language assessments at 39 months: a follow-up study of children fed formulas containing long-chain polyunsaturated fatty acids to 1 year of age, *Pediatrics* 112(3, part 1):E177, 2003.

Hoffman DR, Birch EE, Castaneda YS, et al: Visual function in breast-fed term infants weaned to formula with or without long-chain polyunsaturates at 4 to 6 months: a randomized clinical trial, *J Pediatr* 142(6):669, 2003.

Koo WW: Efficacy and safety of docosahexaenoic acid and arachidonic acid addition to infant formulas: can one buy better vision and intelligence? *J Am Coll Nutr* 22(2):101, 2003.

Uauy R, Hoffman DR, Mena P, et al: Term infant studies of DHA and ARA supplementation on neurodevelopment: results of randomized controlled trials, *J Pediatr* 143(Suppl 4):S17, 2003.

Is it possible that the addition of DHA and ARA to infant formula increases neurodevelopment, visual acuity, and language skills? Evidence from randomized clinical trials prompted the FDA to approve the inclusion of these long-chain polyunsaturated fatty acids into infant formula. The previous four articles discuss this subject.

Briley ME, Jastrow S, Vickers J, et al: Dietary intake at child-care centers and away: are parents and care providers working as partners or at cross-purposes? *J Am Diet Assoc* 99(8):950, 1999.

Florencio CA: Developments and variations in school-based feeding programs around the world, *Nutr Today* 36(1):29, 2001.

Gable S, Lutz S: Nutrition socialization experiences of children in the Head Start program, *J Am Diet Assoc* 101(5):572, 2001.

Position of the American Dietetic Association: Local support for nutrition integrity in schools, *J Am Diet Assoc* 100(1):108, 2000.

Children attending day care, Head Start, or schools with a breakfast and lunch program receive a major proportion of their meals for the day at that location. These articles provide some insight into the role of day care centers and schools in supporting the development of good food habits in children, as well as the role of community health professionals in supporting school food programs in the United States and developing countries.

Bronner YL, Gross SM, Caulfield L, et al: Early introduction of solid foods among urban African-American participants in WIC, *J Am Diet Assoc* 99(4):457, 1999.

Fomon SJ: Feeding normal infants: rationale for recommendations, *J Am Diet Assoc* 101(9):1002, 2001.

Mennella JA, Beauchamp GK: Early flavor expeıiences: research update, *Nutr Rev* 56(7):205, 1998.

Position of the American Dietetic Association: Promoting and supporting breastfeeding, *J Am Diet Assoc* 105(5):810, 2005.

Sills IN: Nutritional rickets: a preventable disease, *Top Clin Nutr* 17(1):36, 2001.

These articles provide some insight into early feeding experiences and nutrition issues in feeding infants.

O'Dea J: Body basics: a nutrition education program for adolescents about food, nutrition, growth, body image, and weight control, *J Am Diet Assoc* 102(Suppl 3):S68, 2002.

Reed DB, Bielamowicz MK, Frantz CL, et al: Clueless in the mall: a web site on calcium for teens, *J Am Diet Assoc* 102(Suppl 3):S73, 2002.

Sigman-Grant M: Strategies for counseling adolescents, *J Am Diet Assoc* 102(Suppl 3):S32, 2002.

Story M, Neumark-Sztainer D, French S: Individual and environmental influences on adolescent eating behaviors, *J Am Diet Assoc* 102(Suppl 3):S40, 2002.

Adolescents are an important target group for nutrition education. We need to learn more about the food-related beliefs and practices of this group and strategies to improve their nutrition and health behaviors. A supplement entitled Adolescent Nutrition: A Springboard to Health, Volume 102, March 2002, Journal of the American Dietetic Association, is devoted to issues and programs relevant to adolescent nutrition. These four articles offer practical ideas for intervention.

Websites of Interest

Centers for Disease Control and Prevention, National Center for Chronic Disease Prevention and Health Promotion, Division of Nutrition and Physical Activity: www.cdc.gov/nccdphp/dnpa.

Centers for Disease Control and Prevention, National Center for Health Statistics: *2000 CDC Growth Charts: United States*: www.cdc.gov/growthcharts.

Dietary Guidelines for Americans 2005: www.healthierus.gov/dietaryguidelines.

International Lactation Consultant Association: www.ilca.org.

La Leche League International: www.llli.org.

U.S. Department of Agriculture, Center for Nutrition Policy and Promotion: *MyPyramid Food Guidance System*: www.mypyramid.gov.

U.S. Department of Agriculture, Food and Nutrition Service, Team Nutrition: www.fns.usda.gov/tn/.

U.S. Department of Agriculture: *MyPyramid Food Guidance System for Kids*: www.mypyramid.gov/kids/.

13

Nutrition for Adults: Early, Middle, and Later Years

Eleanor D. Schlenker

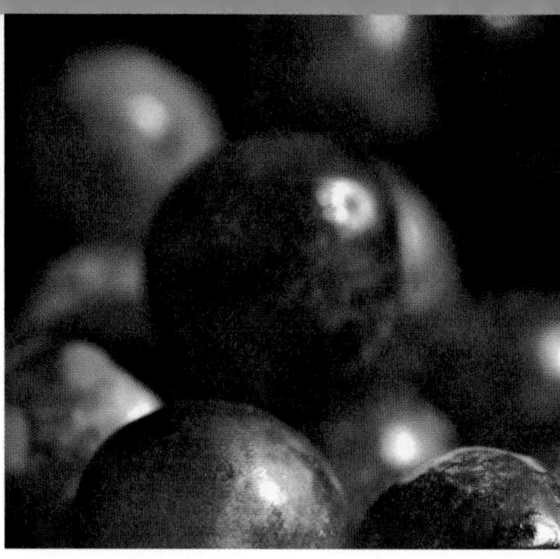

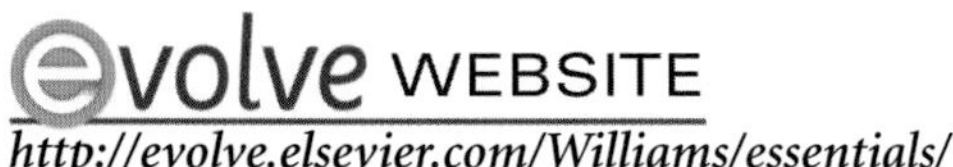

http://evolve.elsevier.com/Williams/essentials/

OUTLINE

This chapter completes our three-chapter sequence on nutrition through the life cycle. After the tumultuous adolescent years come the challenges, opportunities, and concerns of maturity and adulthood.

When adolescents come of age, they have three quarters of their potential years of life still remaining. They face a world of accelerating pace, instant communication, and broad global outlook. On the other hand, the worldwide growth in numbers of older adults has brought attention to fitness, health, and aging, and research looking at lifestyle, length of life, and prevention of chronic disease is frequently in the headlines. What you eat as a child and young adult influences your health status in middle age and beyond, but positive health habits in any stage of life reap benefits in the years ahead. It is never too late to begin choosing a healthy diet and increasing physical activity.

As we review the adult life stages—the early, middle, and later years—we will look at individual needs and the role of nutrition in optimum health.

ADULTHOOD: CONTINUING GROWTH AND DEVELOPMENT

Aging Across the Life Cycle

Although the general public holds that aging begins at a certain time in life, such as retirement or when a person starts to "look old," it actually begins at the moment of conception. Aging encompasses the whole of life as we grow and mature, not simply the end of life. All periods of life have their unique potential and fulfillment, and so do the stages of adulthood—the young, middle, and later years.

The adult years are distinguished by the attainment of optimal function in all body systems and a lifetime of experience to be used and enjoyed.[1] Two important considerations govern the development and evolution of the physiologic, psychosocial, and nutritional aspects of life across the adult years:

1. *The individual:* Gradual aging occurs across the population, but the rate of change is an individual characteristic.
2. *Life history:* Although certain changes are associated with each stage of the life span, aging is a total life process. Experiences in one stage of life hold importance for well-being in the succeeding stages.

Our genes, environment, and lifestyle influence the rate and magnitude of aging changes and development of chronic disease. As we will learn throughout this chapter, lifestyle choices enable us to exert some degree of control over our future health and aging. Even if family history puts us at risk for a chronic condition, a well-chosen diet, not smoking, maintaining a healthy weight, and regular physical activity may postpone its appearance or reduce its severity. (Our cultural and ethnic heritage also influences our health practices. See the *Focus on Culture* box, "Cultural and Ethnic Differences in Health Practices.")

Aging in America

Population shifts and new technology are affecting the lives of older adults and their families. The first of the baby boomer generation, born between 1946 and 1964, are reaching their 60s and facing a world of high-tech medical care, multiple

FOCUS ON CULTURE

Cultural and Ethnic Differences in Health Practices

Many health beliefs and practices spring from our cultural and ethnic backgrounds. The word *health* was derived from an Anglo-Saxon word meaning wholeness, or the interaction of the mind and body in reaching a state of well-being.[1] Many cultures believe that bringing our physical and spiritual beings in harmony with nature is the means to achieving health. In contrast, health care in mainstream America builds on biomedicine, applying the sciences of biology, biochemistry, and physiology to the study and treatment of human diseases. Although traditional health care focuses on the present, biomedicine focuses on the future, relating the treatment of today to physical well-being in the years to come.

The unity between physical, emotional, and psychologic health is the cornerstone of traditional health care, often referred to as *alternative* or *complementary medicine* (CAM). These healing therapies use botanical remedies and interventions such as massage or acupuncture to rectify imbalances in physical and spiritual systems. Mind-body therapies, including prayer, relaxation, or meditation are also used to prevent or cure disease by individuals favoring traditional therapies. In a national health survey, nearly 4 of 10 adults reported using CAM therapy in the past 12 months.[2] Implementation of alternative treatments to improve health or relieve problem conditions is growing in favor as individuals assert more control over their own health.

East Asian traditional medicine is based on Ayurvedic medicine developed in ancient times. *Ayur* means longevity, and *veda* means knowledge of; this system of medicine uses diet, herbal remedies, and meditation to realign the mind, body, and soul. Over time Ayurvedic botanical remedies were used to treat digestive disorders, heart problems, diabetes, and urinary tract disorders.[1] In combination with other traditional plant medicines, Ayurvedic remedies provided the foundation for many of the drugs we use today.

Various traditional home remedies making use of herbs and plants have survived the test of time. Teas made from yellow root or sassafras or ginger are used to relieve stomach distress, and many families use lemon-flavored water with honey to ease the symptoms of a cold.[1] Herbal teas prepared from peppermint, chamomile, parsley, and wormwood are used to relieve diarrhea or other illnesses. Tonics made from eggnog or malt are expected to stimulate the appetite or build strength in pale children or pregnant and postpartum women. Certain alternative medicines, however, can be hazardous. Preparations containing mercury or lead are sometimes brought into the United States from other countries, and individuals need to be warned of their danger.

It is important to know not only what health strategies your patients are observing but also the basis of their attitudes and beliefs. Those at greatest risk are often less likely to use biomedical preventive measures.[3] Low-income women who could benefit from added iron or folate are not typical supplement users. Asian and Latino Americans at risk of low bone density are not encouraged to use calcium supplements. Effective approaches must combine the strengths of biomedicine and alternative and complementary therapies.

REFERENCES

1. Kittler PG, Sucher KP: *Food and culture*, ed 4, Belmont, Calif, 2004, Brooks/Cole, a division of Thomson Learning.
2. Barnes PM, Bloom B, Nahin RL: *Complementary and alternative medicine use among adults and children: United States, 2007, Natl Health Stat Report*, Hyattsville, Md, Dec 10, 2008, National Center for Health Statistics, pp 1–23.
3. Jasti S, Siega-Riz AM, Bentley ME: Dietary supplement use in the context of health disparities: cultural, ethnic and demographic determinants of use, *J Nutr* 133:2010S, 2003.

For more information on alternative and complementary therapies visit the website of the National Center for Alternative and Complementary Medicine: *www.nccam.nih.gov/*.

medications, and spiraling costs. Medical life-support systems present difficult decisions for professionals and families caring for older patients. As the life span lengthens and the older population increases in size, their personal, social, and health care needs will be felt in all our lives.

Following are some of the characteristics of the older population and their potential impact on health and nutrition services:

- *Increase in life expectancy:* During the past 100 years, life expectancy at birth has risen from 49 years to about 78 years based on improved sanitation, the discovery of antibiotics, and increased standards of living. Life expectancy is a general measure of the overall health of a population.[2] With better prevention and treatment of heart disease, cancer, and stroke (the most common causes of death in the older population), life expectancy has also increased for persons age 65 and those age 85 (Figure 13-1). More than 5 million people in the United States are now age 85 or older,[2] and nearly 74,000 persons have reached the age of 100.

To better characterize the changing nature of the older population, the U.S. Bureau of Census developed the following three categories for those age 65 and older:

1. *The young-old:* ages 65 through 74 years
2. *The old-old:* ages 75 through 84 years
3. *The oldest-old:* ages 85 years and older

The 85 years and older group is the fastest growing age cohort in the U.S. population and is expected to double in size during the next 25 years. Given the rapid pace of biomedical research, life expectancy is likely to continue to rise, with actual numbers of older adults surpassing current projections.

As people live longer they are more likely to decline in health, develop some degree of physical disability, and require more health and community services. Individuals who are

KEY TERMS

life expectancy The number of years a person of a given age, gender, race, or ethnic group can expect to live.

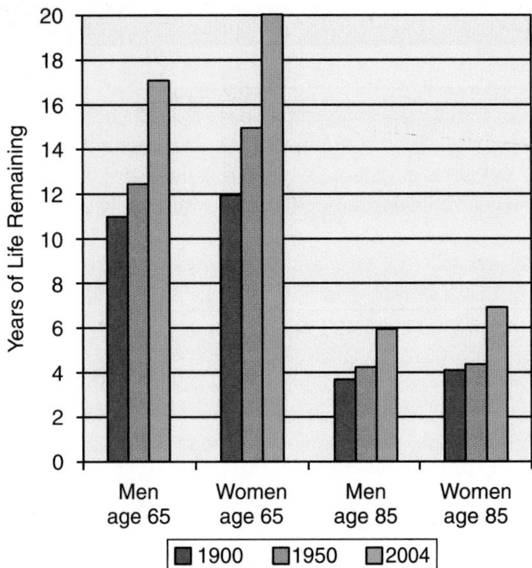

FIGURE 13-1 With increases in life expectancy, older adults are living to more advanced ages. At age 65 men can expect to live 17 more years and women can expect to live 20 more years. Even at age 85, men and women can expect to live another 6 to 7 years. (Data from Federal Interagency Forum on Aging-Related Statistics: *Older Americans 2008: key indicators of well-being,* Washington, DC, 2008, U.S. Government Printing Office.)

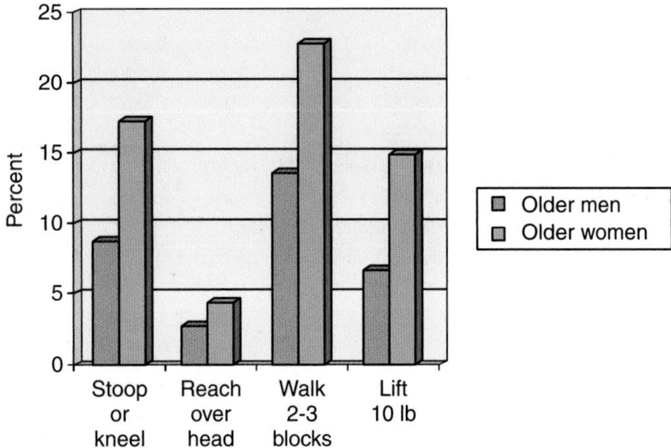

FIGURE 13-2 Percent of persons age 65 and older who are unable to perform these tasks without help. These tasks are important for an older person to remain independent. (Federal Interagency Forum on Aging-Related Statistics: *Older Americans 2008: key indicators of well-being,* Washington, DC, 2008, U.S. Government Printing Office.)

unable to stoop, reach over their heads, or lift 10 lb will have difficulty shopping for groceries and preparing meals or performing other housekeeping tasks (Figure 13-2).[2]

- *Ethnic and racial diversity:* Currently 81% of the population age 65 and older is Caucasian, but this will change. By 2050 nearly 40% of the older U.S. population will belong to another racial or ethnic group (Figure 13-3).[2] Nutrition education programs and meal services will need to adjust to different customs, food patterns, and family roles.

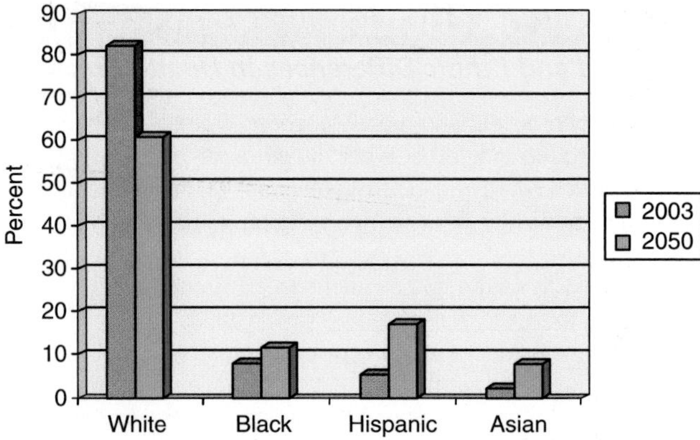

FIGURE 13-3 Percent of persons age 65 and older according to race and ethnic group. The older population will continue to become more diverse. (Federal Interagency Forum on Aging-Related Statistics: *Older Americans 2008: key indicators of well-being,* Washington, DC, 2008, U.S. Government Printing Office.)

- *Education:* In 1965 only 24% of older adults had completed high school; today 76% have high school diplomas and 19% hold bachelor's degrees.[2] However, older racial and ethnic groups differ widely in levels of education. Only 42% of Hispanic older adults and 57% of African-American older adults completed high school, compared with 75% of Caucasian older adults.[2] Those with less education who cannot read or understand labels on food or medications are disadvantaged in practicing good self-care.
- *Income:* About 9% of people age 65 and older have incomes below the poverty level; another 6% are "near poor," having incomes within 125% of the poverty level.[3] However, certain groups are more likely to be poor. Poverty rates are increased among African-American and Hispanic older adults and older persons living alone.[2,3] When food purchases are restricted, protein foods, fruits, and vegetables may be inadequate. (Review the discussion of food insecurity in Chapter 10.)
- *Living arrangements:* Because women live longer, more older women are widowed and more older men are married. About one half of all women older than age 74 live alone, whereas the majority of men this age live with a spouse.[2] Older single Asian and Hispanic women are more likely to live with other family members, whereas older single Caucasian and African-American women tend to live alone.[2] Only 4.4% of individuals age 65 and older reside in institutional settings.[4] Older men and women who are single have less food money, less help with meal preparation, and less support on sick days.

Adult Growth and Development

Adults continue to grow and develop in various ways. Physical, socioeconomic, psychosocial, and nutritional forces shape the path of adult development.

Physical Characteristics

Physical growth governed by genetic potential levels off in the late teens and early 20s. When we reach physical maturity, growth marked by increasing numbers of cells and changing body size is halted and the process of replication, forming new cells to replace old ones, begins. At older ages, physical and functional status gradually declines, as cells are lost more rapidly than they are replaced. Individual vigor reflects the lifestyle patterns of previous years. Poor food choices coupled with low physical activity accelerate normal aging and the progression of chronic disease with its toll on health.

Psychosocial Development

Three developmental tasks characterize the adult years: (1) young adults develop intimacy and expand relationships outside of their parents and siblings; (2) middle adults pursue creative expression or explore new career directions; and (3) older adults seek fulfillment and strength of purpose. Each stage affects lifestyle and health.

Socioeconomic Status

We all live our lives in a social and cultural environment. A changing world brings major social shifts—new mores and expected behaviors, fears for personal safety, and unfamiliar languages in the marketplace. Many adults experience changes in resources as they move through early, middle, and late adulthood. Financial pressures at any life stage influence food security and the availability of health care.

Nutritional Needs

Nutrient needs remain important even after physical growth and maturation are completed. Each stage of adult life provides the foundation for the one that follows. Harmful health behaviors in the teen and young adult years accelerate physiologic changes leading to hypertension, cardiovascular disease, and diabetes, as well as the risk of premature disability or death. By the same token, positive lifestyle changes in middle age—beginning a walking program that reduces waist circumference or eating more fish—slow metabolic and physical changes and reduce the severity of existing disease. Nutrient requirements remain dynamic throughout life according to age, physical activity, illness, chronic disease, or pregnancy and lactation.

ADULT STAGES: CHANGING NUTRIENT NEEDS

Young Adult (19 to 40 Years)

Physical Characteristics

After the rapid physical changes of the adolescent years, growth levels off into adult maintenance and stability. Finely regulated genes control neural and hormonal activity, maintaining a steady internal environment. Body functions are fully developed, with sexual maturation and reproductive capacity.

Psychosocial Development

The core psychosocial task of the young adult is building relationships outside of his or her core family (Figure 13-4). It is a time to become comfortable with the physical self and the demands of the adult role. If positive development is achieved, then the individual will continue to build on personal relationships leading to self-fulfillment.

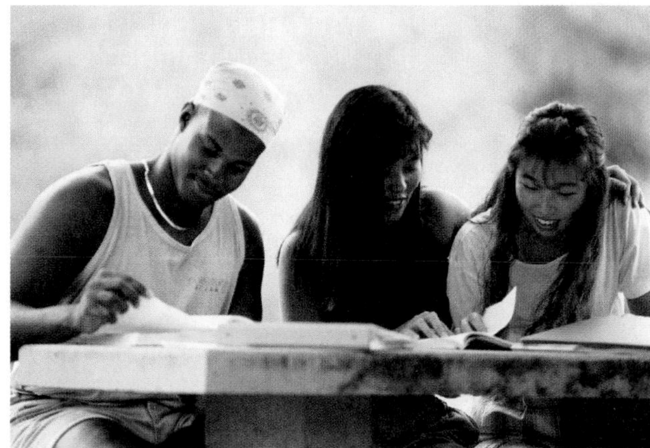

FIGURE 13-4 The early adult years center on the core problem of intimacy versus isolation. (Credit: PhotoDisc.)

Socioeconomic Status

The early adult years contain the social and economic pressures of continuing education or workforce development in preparation for adult responsibilities. Households are established and individuals may take on the parenting role. With a changing work environment, many face difficulty in meeting the life tasks of education, work, and family. Young adults ages 18 to 24 report more days of sadness or depression per month than any other adult group,[5] and life dissatisfaction is associated with risky health behaviors such as smoking, heavy drinking, and physical inactivity.[6] This is also the time when we establish lifestyle patterns that will influence our health in middle age and beyond.

Nutritional Needs

The growth patterns that emerge in adolescence are strengthened in the adult body. Young men have increased muscle mass and long bone growth. Young women develop a wider hip breadth and pelvic girdle of subcutaneous fat, genetically intended to support reproduction. Nutritional concerns for the young adult include energy, calcium, iron, and vitamins, as follows:

- *Energy:* The Recommended Dietary Allowance (RDA) for active men ages 19 to 30 is about 3000 kcal/day; for active women the RDA is about 2400 kcal/day (Table 13-1).[7] Physical activity plays an important role in maintaining

KEY TERMS

replication Making an exact copy; to repeat, duplicate, or reproduce. In genetics, replication is the process by which double-stranded deoxyribonucleic acid (DNA) makes copies of itself with each separating strand synthesizing a complementary strand. Cell replication is the process by which living cells divide to produce exact copies of themselves a programmed number of times throughout the life span of an organism.

TABLE 13-1 DIETARY REFERENCE INTAKES FOR ENERGY AND PROTEIN FOR ACTIVE ADULTS*†

AGE (in yr)	WEIGHT (in kg)	WEIGHT (in lb)	HEIGHT (in cm)	HEIGHT (in inches)	ENERGY (in kcal)	PROTEIN (in g)
Men						
19–30	70	154	177	70	3000	56
31–50	70	154	177	70	2900	56
51–70	70	154	177	70	2700	56
≥71	70	154	177	70	2500	56
Women						
19–30	57	126	163	64	2400	46
31–50	57	126	163	64	2300	46
51–70	57	126	163	64	2100	46
≥71	57	126	163	64	2000	46

Data calculated from standards found in Food and Nutrition Board, Institute of Medicine: *Dietary Reference Intakes for energy, carbohydrate, fiber, fat, fatty acids, cholesterol, protein, and amino acids (macronutrients)*, Washington, DC, 2002, National Academies Press.
*Because adults are urged to remain physically active throughout their lives, reference weights remain the same for all adult age categories.
†These energy recommendations are based on the midpoint of each age range: age 25, age 40, age 60, and age 80. Calculated values are rounded to the nearest 100. Energy needs in men decline by 10 kcal/year after the age of 19, and energy needs in women decline by 7 kcal/year.

energy balance (Figure 13-5). Additional kilocalories (kcalories or kcal) are needed to support pregnancy and lactation.

- *Protein:* The RDA is 56 g/day for men and 46 g/day for women,[7] based on a daily need of 0.8 g/kg body weight (see Table 13-1). Protein intake in young women is more than one-and-one-half times the current RDA, and young men consume about two times their RDA.[8]
- *Minerals:* The Dietary Reference Intakes (DRIs) for minerals can be met with a well-planned diet (Table 13-2); however, three minerals—calcium, iron, and potassium—warrant special attention. Young adults need to take in 1000 mg of calcium per day to ensure continued development and maintenance of peak bone mass,[9] but only 50% of men and less than 25% of women in this age-group meet the goal.[8] Median calcium intake in women ages 19 to 30 is only 75% of the Adequate Intake (AI).[8]

Iron is a problem for both young men and young women but for different reasons. Women of childbearing age must offset the iron lost through the menses, making their RDA 18 mg/day,[10] but nearly half do not reach even 67% of this amount. In contrast, young men have *mean* intakes more than twice their RDA of 8 mg,[8,10] with some exceeding four times their RDA. Such intakes over time carry risk of iron overload. Iron intake is closely related to energy intake and use of ready-to-eat cereals, bread, and beef. The iron requirement in pregnancy, 27 mg/day, is usually met with a supplement.

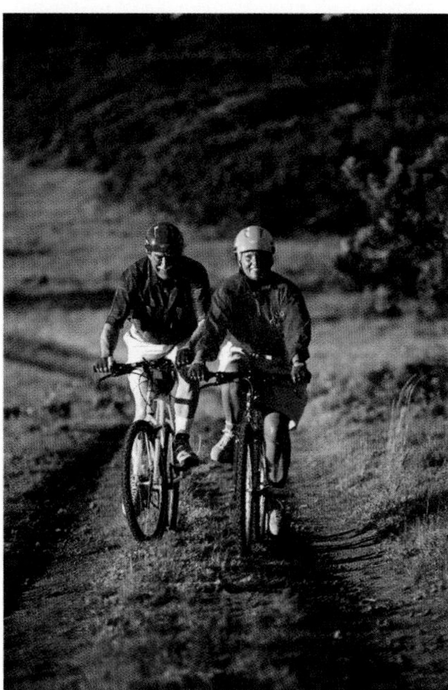

FIGURE 13-5 Energy needs vary according to level of physical activity. (Credit: PhotoDisc.)

Fruits and vegetables are major sources of potassium, and low intakes of these foods decreases the supply of this nutrient.[11] Median potassium intakes of young men are barely two thirds the AI, and median intakes of young women are less than one half the AI.[8] In light of the growing evidence associating potassium and control of blood pressure,[11] meeting this dietary recommendation could help prevent future health problems.

- *Vitamins:* Intakes of certain vitamins are less than optimal in many young adults. Folate intake including supplements is less than 400 mcg for many young women who need to build body stores before conception.[12] Young adults who spend little time in the sun and do not use vitamin D–fortified dairy products or take supplements are low in this vitamin and less able to absorb calcium. Vitamin D status is especially critical in Hispanic and African-American populations because of increased skin pigmentation and decreased ability to synthesize vitamin D.[13] Vitamin E is highly problematic, with more than 90% of adults younger than age 50 having intakes less than the RDA.[8] Nutrition education addressing the appropriate use of healthy fats along with whole grains is critical to increasing intakes of vitamin E. (Table 13-3 provides information about vitamin DRIs.)

Health Issues

Public health leaders have expressed concern about the worsening health profiles of young adults. Risk behaviors such as smoking, low physical activity, and low intakes

KEY TERMS
median In statistics, the middle number in a sequence of numbers such that half are higher and half are lower.

TABLE 13-2 **ADULT DIETARY REFERENCE INTAKES FOR MINERALS, ELECTROLYTES, AND WATER**

AGE (in yr)	CALCIUM (in mg)	PHOSPHORUS (in mg)	MAGNESIUM (in mg)	IRON (in mg)	ZINC (in mg)	IODINE (in mcg)	FLUORIDE (in mg)	POTASSIUM (in mg)	SODIUM (in mg)	WATER (in L/day)*
Men										
19–30	1000	700	400	8	11	150	4	4700	1500	3.7
31–50	1000	700	420	8	11	150	4	4700	1500	3.7
51–70	1200	700	420	8	11	150	4	4700	1300	3.7
≥71	1200	700	420	8	11	150	4	4700	1200	3.7
Women										
19–30	1000	700	310	18	8	150	3	4700	1500	2.7
31–50	1000	700	320	18	8	150	3	4700	1500	2.7
51–70	1200	700	320	8	8	150	3	4700	1300	2.7
≥71	1200	700	320	8	8	150	3	4700	1200	2.7

Data from Food and Nutrition Board, Institute of Medicine: *Dietary Reference Intakes for calcium, phosphorus, magnesium, vitamin D, and fluoride,* Washington, DC, 1997, National Academies Press; Food and Nutrition Board, Institute of Medicine: *Dietary Reference Intakes for vitamin A, vitamin K, arsenic, boron, chromium, copper, iodine, iron, manganese, molybdenum, nickel, silicon, vanadium, and zinc,* Washington, DC, 2001, National Academies Press; Food and Nutrition Board, Institute of Medicine: *Dietary Reference Intakes for water, potassium, sodium, chloride, and sulfate,* Washington, DC, 2004, National Academies Press.

*Includes water in food, beverages, and drinking water.

TABLE 13-3 **ADULT DIETARY REFERENCE INTAKES FOR VITAMINS**

AGE (in yr)	VITAMIN A (in mcg RAE)	VITAMIN D (in mcg)	VITAMIN E (in mg)	VITAMIN C (in mg)	THIAMIN (in mg)	RIBOFLAVIN (in mg)	NIACIN (in mg NE)	VITAMIN B_6 (in mg)	FOLATE (in mcg)	VITAMIN B_{12} (in mcg)
Men										
19–30	900	5	15	90	1.2	1.3	16	1.3	400	2.4
31–50	900	5	15	90	1.2	1.3	16	1.3	400	2.4
51–70	900	10	15	90	1.2	1.3	16	1.7	400	2.4
≥71	900	15	15	90	1.2	1.3	16	1.7	400	2.4
Women										
19–30	700	5	15	75	1.1	1.1	14	1.3	400	2.4
31–50	700	5	15	75	1.1	1.1	14	1.3	400	2.4
51–70	700	10	15	75	1.1	1.1	14	1.5	400	2.4
≥71	700	15	15	75	1.1	1.1	14	1.5	400	2.4

Data from Food and Nutrition Board, Institute of Medicine: *Dietary Reference Intakes for calcium, phosphorus, magnesium, vitamin D, and fluoride,* Washington, DC, 1997, National Academies Press; Food and Nutrition Board, Institute of Medicine: *Dietary Reference Intakes for thiamin, riboflavin, niacin, vitamin B_6, folate, vitamin B_{12}, pantothenic acid, biotin, and choline,* Washington, DC, 1998, National Academies Press; Food and Nutrition Board, Institute of Medicine: *Dietary Reference Intakes for vitamin A, vitamin K, arsenic, boron, chromium, copper, iodine, iron, manganese, molybdenum, nickel, silicon, vanadium, and zinc,* Washington, DC, 2001, National Academies Press; Food and Nutrition Board, Institute of Medicine: *Dietary Reference Intakes for vitamin C, vitamin E, selenium, and carotenoids,* Washington, DC, 2000, National Academies Press.
RAE, Retinol activity equivalent; *NE,* niacin equivalent.

of fruits and vegetables are most prevalent among young adults.[14] New responsibilities of home and family, along with pressures of the workplace, divert attention from healthy lifestyles. In addition, the threat of chronic disease seems remote to an individual with youthful vigor. Poor health habits such as smoking or inappropriately high computer "screen time" established in adolescence and continued into adulthood adversely affect health in succeeding years.[15,16]

Food Habits. Restaurant meals are popular among busy young adults. Many young adults eat at fast-food restaurants two or more times a week,[17,18] and follow-up studies associate frequency of fast-food meals with increases in body mass index (BMI).[17] A diverse group of young adults ages 20 to 38 consumed only one serving of fruit and two servings of vegetables (including French fries) per day but had at least two sweet snacks.[19] Less than recommended intakes of vitamins A and C and magnesium and excessive intakes of sodium are particular problems in this population group.[8] Young adults average two to four times the sodium AI of 1500 mg,[8] likely related to fast food and use of highly processed, easily prepared food items. High intakes of simple carbohydrate foods and low use of fiber foods add to the risk of obesity and elevated blood glucose levels. Excessive sodium intakes coupled with the low potassium intakes noted earlier have unfavorable effects on blood pressure in susceptible individuals. Nutrition education for this age-group might address better choices at fast-food restaurants to promote healthful eating.

Body Weight. Young adults are highly vulnerable to weight gain based on changes in living arrangements and lifestyle associated with new independence. Follow-up evaluations of young adults between the ages of 18 and 25 revealed an average increase in BMI of 2.5 kg/m^2 in men and 1.7 kg/m^2 in women.[20] Many had established households during the 7-year interval, and living with a partner increased their likelihood of weight gain. Married young adults consume more sweets and desserts, although fewer alcoholic beverages, than their unmarried counterparts.[21] About 25% of adults in their 20s are obese, and three quarters have no regular leisure physical activity.[22] Even adolescents who achieve the recommended level of daily physical activity fail to continue these patterns into adulthood.[23]

Disease Risk. A constellation of factors including BMI and waist circumference signifying overweight, elevated blood pressure, inappropriate blood lipid levels, and elevated blood glucose or insulin levels have been referred to as the *metabolic syndrome.* Although we usually associate these risk factors with middle age and beyond, they are beginning to appear in young adults with poorly chosen diets and low physical activity. In a study of young adults ages 19 to 38, more than 40% had at least one or two of these risk factors; more than 10% had three or more.[24] Young adults can lower their risk of metabolic syndrome with even modest efforts toward regular physical activity.[25] Mass media such as the Internet may be a successful route for reaching this population with nutrition and lifestyle education.

Middle Adult (40 to 65 Years)

Physical Characteristics

As individuals move into their 40s, cell replication begins to slow, with gradual loss of body cells and tissues. Men and women begin to experience age-related loss of muscle mass, with changes in muscle strength and function—a condition called *sarcopenia.*[26] Although everyone experiences some muscle loss, individuals with low physical activity

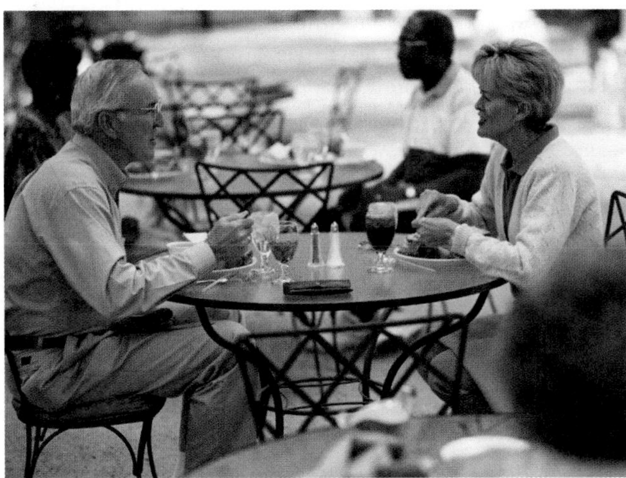

FIGURE 13-6 Middle adult years can be a time to expand personal growth. (Credit: PhotoDisc.)

levels lose significant amounts, whereas those practicing strength training lose limited amounts. (We discuss strength training in more detail in Chapter 14.) Most people increase in body fat in their middle years as a result of a sedentary lifestyle and the slow but steady decrease in basal metabolic rate (BMR) that lowers their energy needs.[27,28] Regular assessment of body weight, blood pressure, and blood lipid levels identifies health risks that respond to early intervention.

Psychosocial Development

The middle-age adult has moved beyond the period of self-analysis and early career focus to the stage of active involvement with others—family, grandchildren, and community. Some experience the "empty nest syndrome" as their children, now adults, set up their own households. Others become caregivers to grandchildren or aging family members. Individuals with fewer responsibilities have opportunities to expand their personal horizons (Figure 13-6).

Socioeconomic Status

Increasing technology in business and manufacturing, company mergers and dissolutions, and shifts in the nature of employment bring job loss for workers at all levels of responsibility. No longer can employees expect to remain with the same company all of their working lives, and reductions in salary or loss of retirement benefits wreck havoc on personal and financial well-being. Displaced workers may seek out educational opportunities or workforce training for new careers.

Nutritional Needs

Needs for particular nutrients change in the middle adult years, and intake has a critical bearing on chronic disease risk. (See Tables 13-1 to 13-3)

- *Energy:* Loss of active tissue coupled with a sedentary lifestyle lowers kcalorie requirements and, unless energy intake and activity level are adjusted, body fat will continue to accrue. This was observed in healthy middle-aged adults who, during 5 years, increased their waist circumference by 4 to 5 cm.[28]
- *Minerals:* Calcium intake assumes special importance, particularly for women. Menopause and the loss of estrogen bring about a decrease in calcium absorption and an increase in bone turnover, with a net loss of bone mass and increased risk of fracture. At age 51 the DRI for calcium increases to 1200 mg for both men and women,[9] and optimum intake helps preserve bone mass.[29,30] However, actual intakes are far less than the standard. The median intake in men ages 51 to 70 is only 813 mg; in women it is even less, at 661 mg.[8] With cessation of the menses, iron needs in women drop from 18 mg to 8 mg, becoming the same as for adult men.[10] Sodium intakes fall somewhat in middle age as compared with young adults, but they still exceed recommended levels.[8]
- *Vitamins:* The AI for vitamin D increases in people older than age 50 to ensure adequate calcium absorption[9]; yet vitamin D status is declining in this age-group. Lower milk consumption, increasing BMI, and more frequent use of sun protection lowers both dietary sources and skin production of this vitamin.[31] Vitamin E intake is less than half the recommended level despite the need for antioxidant protection as the aging process continues.[8] The requirement for vitamin B_6 increases because this vitamin is less efficiently used in the aging adult.[32]

Health Issues

The middle adult years hold the key to health in this stage of life and beyond. Those who established positive health habits as young adults enter their middle years with a minimum of chronic disease. In contrast, poor lifestyle choices prior to this time magnify the risk of overt disease, and intervention is critical to reverse the downhill slide.

Food Habits. Middle adults came to maturity during the early growth of the fast-food industry; however, about half of those living within walking distance of a fast-food restaurant reported visiting more than one or two times a week. More meals at fast-food restaurants were related to greater increases in waist circumference during the next year.[33] Use of sugar-sweetened beverages is reported by many middle-aged adults, contributing on average 160 kcal/day.[34] Although 57% of those interviewed use sugar-sweetened beverages, only 22% reported using alcohol. During the past 20 years, middle-age adults have lowered their use of red meats and luncheon meats,[35] likely in response to health messages to eat less fat. Nevertheless, fat still provides 34% to 35% of total kcalories among men and women ages 40 to 69, and saturated fat provides more than 11%.[36] The combination of salty snacks and desserts constitute almost 13% of energy intake.[35] This group's consumption of fruits and vegetables—which provide important fiber and micronutrients—fails to reach MyPyramid goals.[14] Middle-aged adults, as compared with young adults, use more dietary supplements, especially vitamins E and C, the B-complex vitamins, and calcium.[37]

BOX 13-1 MODIFIABLE RISK FACTORS FOR HEART DISEASE AND STROKE*

- High blood pressure
- High blood cholesterol
- Diabetes (type 2)
- Tobacco use
- Obesity
- Lack of exercise

From United States Department of Health and Human Services, Centers for Disease Control and Prevention: Racial/ethnic and socioeconomic disparities in multiple risk factors for heart disease and stroke—United States, 2003, *MMWR Morb Mortal Wkly Rep* 54(5):113, 2005.
*These risk factors can be modified through prevention, early recognition, and treatment.

Chronic Disease. The prevalence of cardiovascular disease, diabetes, and cancer increases during this stage of life. Nearly half in this age-group have at least two modifiable risk factors for heart disease or stroke (Box 13-1), but more than one fourth do not have their blood cholesterol level checked regularly.[38] The rise in overweight and obesity has helped fuel the rise in diabetes and younger age of diagnosis (46 versus 52 years).[39]

Food patterns influence weight gain and mortality in middle-age adults. Healthy weight individuals have more servings of fruits and vegetables than those who are overweight or obese,[40] and mortality from all causes was lower in men and women with a history of eating more fruits, vegetables, and whole grains.[41] The health implications of alcohol, however, remain controversial.[42] Additional kcalories in the form of alcohol can stimulate unwanted weight gain, and excessive intake is toxic to the liver. At the same time, limited amounts of alcohol in the form of red wine appear to offer some protection against cardiovascular disease.

Older Adult (65 to 85 Years)

Physical Characteristics

The later adult years bring a gradual waning of physical vigor, work capacity, and strength. Changes are often minimal immediately after retirement but become more pronounced as individuals move through their 70s and into their 80s. Osteoarthritis, heart disease, pulmonary disease, and diabetes can limit physical activity, adding to problems with energy balance. Advancing age brings changes in major organ systems that threaten homeostasis and response to infection or disease. Physiologic changes that influence nutritional status are summarized in the following sections.

Body Composition. Over time muscle loss affects functional capacity, with the potential loss of independence; reduction in bone mass adds to the risk of fracture. Even if body weight remains unchanged, the older adult has proportionately more fat.[43,44] Body fat also changes position, moving from the extremities to the trunk, especially the abdomen. This too has implications for health because abdominal fat releases excessive amounts of fatty acids, raising blood lipid and blood insulin levels.[45] Although some older adults experience weight gain, others undergo progressive weight loss, leading to frailty, disability, and diminished quality of life.[46]

Cardiovascular System. Changes in the heart and vascular system affect the older adult's ability to deliver nutrients and oxygen to working tissues and remove waste. The heart weakens as a pump and is less able to respond to increased demands for oxygen related to strenuous exercise, emotional stress, or acute illness. A drop in the amount of blood pumped with each beat of the heart reduces the blood supply to major organs such as the kidney and lungs. Major arteries, including those delivering nutrients to the heart muscle itself, stiffen and narrow with atherosclerotic deposition. This stiffening, limiting the ability of the arteries to stretch when blood is delivered, is responsible in part for the rise in blood pressure common to older adults.[47]

Renal System. The aging kidneys are less efficient and require more time to clear waste products from the blood. Urine cannot be concentrated to the same extent; therefore increased amounts of water are required to excrete a given amount of waste. This is why older people receiving high-protein supplements producing large amounts of nitrogen-containing waste need additional fluid. Fluid balance is poorly regulated at very high or very low intakes of water and sodium.[47]

Respiratory System. The air sacs in the aging lung become less elastic, making it more difficult to move air in and out of the lungs. Other changes in the air sacs reduce the available surface area for exchange of oxygen and carbon dioxide (CO_2). Widening areas of the lungs no longer participate in gas exchange, and this "dead space" is susceptible to the growth of pathogens. Smoking and air pollution contribute to loss of lung function and a reduced supply of oxygen for normal activity and periods of stress.[47]

Gastrointestinal System. Gastrointestinal changes influence secretions, muscles, and nerves involved in the digestion of food. Loss of gastric acid interferes with the absorption of vitamin B_{12} and reduces uptake of thiamin, folate, calcium, and iron.[9–10,32] Changes in nerve and muscle function contribute to constipation in frail older adults by increasing the time needed for food to pass through the lower digestive tract.

Psychosocial Development

Psychosocial development in the later adult years requires adaptation to new challenges as physical stamina declines and emotional supports are lost. Depending on one's resources, a sense of wholeness or a sense of despair prevails. If life's experiences have been positive, then the older individual enters this stage rich in the wisdom of the years and rewarding relationships. Nevertheless, problems with declining health, financial worries, or other circumstances over which the aging individual has no control can result in depression or failure to thrive.[48]

Socioeconomic Status

Most adults enter retirement on a fixed income, and economic uncertainty is often a constant worry. Financial resources influence nutrient intake, and lower-income older people are more likely to be food insecure than higher-income older people.[49] Social isolation can lead to depression and a lack of incentive to prepare nourishing meals.[48–50] A frail older adult living alone with no neighbors or near relatives can experience economic and social deprivation.

Nutritional Needs

The DRIs established two age categories for people older than age 50[7]:

1. Ages 51 to 70
2. Ages 71 and older

These categories recognize the physiologic changes and chronic conditions that develop as we age and influence our nutritional needs. The DRIs for persons older than age 50 are listed in Tables 13-1, 13-2, and 13-3:

- *Energy:* The energy allowance for older adults takes into consideration age-related loss of muscle and active tissue and expected levels of physical activity. A physically active 65-year-old man weighing 70 kg needs about 2700 kcal/day, and a physically active woman of this age weighing 57 kg needs about 2100 kcal/day.[7] Beyond age 70, further declines in energy expenditure are more likely the result of decreasing physical activity than the result of further changes in lean body mass.[51] Physical activity helps retain muscle mass, support cardiovascular function, and assist in weight management. Sharp declines in energy expenditure, common in older adults, are neither inevitable nor desirable.
- *Protein:* The RDA for protein is set at 0.8 g/kg body weight for younger and older adults[7]; however, this standard remains controversial. The DRI expert committee proposed that healthy older adults use protein as efficiently as healthy younger adults and therefore have no increased need for protein. However, other researchers have found that intakes of 1.0 g/kg body weight or more are needed to support nutritional well-being and prevent age-related muscle loss, especially in older individuals with chronic disease. They recommend this increased amount to ensure that needs are being met.[52–54] For older adults participating in strength training, an intake of 1.2 g/kg body weight may be optimum to support muscle building. Although intakes moderately above the RDA are believed appropriate for older adults with normal kidney function, individualized recommendations are indicated for those with any kidney impairment.[52]
- *Minerals:* The DRI for calcium increases from 1000 mg to 1200 mg for persons older than age 50 as a strategy for reducing bone loss, bone fracture, and the development of osteoporosis.[9] (Review the causes and consequences of bone mineral loss in Chapter 7.) After menopause, the iron needs of women are the same as those of men (8 mg/day), and iron supplements should be avoided unless the individual has been diagnosed with iron deficiency anemia and supplementation is supervised by a physician.[10] In general, anemia in older adults is more likely related to a vitamin B_{12} deficiency or chronic disease than to an iron deficiency. Based on the long-term consequences of any of these deficiencies, a presenting anemia must be carefully evaluated as to cause and appropriate intervention. (See Chapter 7 for more information on the anemia of chronic disease.)
- *Vitamins:* An increased DRI for vitamin B_6 continues from middle age. Vitamin B_6 is stored and metabolized mainly in muscle, so muscle loss likely changes the body's handling of this nutrient.[32] To ensure adequate vitamin D levels despite reduced sun exposure and skin synthesis, the AI increases from 10 mcg (400 IU) for those ages 51 to 70 to 15 mcg (600 IU) for persons older than age 70.[9] Vitamin D supplementation is likely to be required.

Health Issues

Socioeconomic status, physical health or disease, and mental outlook all interact to influence food intake and the subsequent health status of the older adult.

Food Intake. Energy intake continues to decline from about 1700 kcal in women ages 50 to 59 to 1500 kcal in those 70 and older. Intake falls from 2600 kcal to 2000 kcal in men in these age-groups.[36] Total fat and saturated fat lessen, although the proportion of total kcalories from fat (34% to 35%) remains the same. Older men and women exceed the Tolerable Upper Intake Level (UL) for sodium, likely complicating problems with blood pressure.[8] Although calcium intake from food decreases,[8] nonfood calcium increases, with more than one half in this age-group taking calcium supplements or using calcium-containing antiacids.[37] Nutrient intake may change as older persons are less able to prepare foods on their own and depend on heat-and-serve items that can be high in fat and sodium and low in micronutrients.

Chronic Disease. The burden of chronic disease continues to grow as the years go on, although particular risk factors are somewhat modified.[55] Elevated blood cholesterol levels and overweight diminish in importance as risk factors for cardiovascular disease in older individuals, although elevated blood pressure continues to increase vulnerability to heart attack or stroke. Cancer deaths increase in older age-groups, pointing to the continuing need for fruits, vegetables, and whole grains supplying plant-based, cancer-fighting components.

Obesity in middle age is a major contributor to morbidity and complications of cardiovascular disease and diabetes in older age. Persons with a BMI greater than 30 in middle age had annual medical costs $6500 more in their later years

KEY TERMS

failure to thrive A syndrome described in older adults characterized by loss of body weight and deterioration in physical and cognitive function and caused by inadequate food intake.

than those with a BMI between 18.5 and 29.[56] Even small differences in BMI resulted in lower medical costs. Helping the severely obese lose even modest amounts of weight at any stage of adulthood has positive dividends for long-term health.

Interest in Health Improvement. Older adults are an important target audience for nutrition and health education. Older adults who participated in a health intervention program for 10 years were most likely to make positive changes in their health behavior as compared with young and middle-aged groups.[14] These changes included stopping smoking, increasing physical activity, and increasing intakes of fruits and vegetables. Older people have a strong interest in health and must be encouraged that it is never too late to reap positive benefits from making better food choices or increasing physical activity.

Oldest-Old (85 Years and Older)

Nutritional Needs

As adults continue to age, nutrient absorption and use become less efficient, and this is especially apparent in illness or stress. Nutrient stores undergo rapid loss in acute illness or disease of long duration and are difficult to replace. At this time we know very little about the interactions between the aging process and chronic disease, as well as how these factors influence nutritional needs.

THE NATURE OF AGING

Study of Aging

To study aging the first step is to distinguish among terms. Researchers use the term *aging* to refer to all changes that occur in an individual over time—from the moment of conception until death. In the health field, we usually think of aging as those changes that occur later in life and lead to increased vulnerability, frailty, and risk of death. The term gerontology refers to the study of how and why aging happens and differs from the term geriatrics, which describes the diseases and medical conditions common to older people. The study of aging is helping us learn more about how people change as they grow older and the genetic and environmental factors that influence physical aging and the length and quality of life.

To some extent our genes control our susceptibility or resistance to particular diseases; however, environmental factors such as pollution or lifestyle choices including diet, smoking habits, alcohol use, or activity level, also have a role. Changes in organ systems and the functional decline that occurs with age are controlled by the biologic limits to cell replication, not our age in years. In fact, chronologic age is the least suitable measure of human aging. As we begin to separate the effects of chronic disease from normal aging, we can lay the groundwork for an improved end of life.

Normal Versus Successful Aging

Researchers who study the aging process have defined two types of human aging: normal aging and successful aging. In normal aging, genetic and environmental influences interact to produce degenerative changes in body systems. In successful aging, regressive changes are slowed or prevented by positive lifestyle choices and health interventions. A healthy diet, regular physical activity, a positive mental outlook, appropriate health care, and avoidance of smoking are lifestyle patterns that contribute to successful aging.

HEALTH PROMOTION

Older Americans are not only living longer but also enjoying robust and active lives. More than 80% of even the oldest-old still live in the community, and less than 5% of those ages 65 and older live in long-term care facilities.[57] Education in nutrition and self-care supports positive lifestyle interventions relating to diet and physical activity—the keys to slowing aging changes and chronic disease.

Dietary Pattern for Adult Health

Two basic tools issued by the U.S. Department of Agriculture (USDA) and the U.S. Department of Health and Human Services (USDHHS) provide a framework for planning healthy diets during the adult years. The DASH (Dietary Approaches to Stop Hypertension) Eating Plan[58] and MyPyramid[59] emphasize moderation and variety and provide an outline for food selection (see Chapters 1 and 7 to review these materials). Food guides are especially helpful as energy needs decline and people eat less food from day to day. Food guides promote the selection of foods from all major food groups and help to ensure dietary diversity. Eating a low variety of foods, even micronutrient-dense foods, can result in less than recommended intakes of kcalories, protein, vitamins, and minerals.[60] Based on the growing problem of youth and adult obesity, current nutrition and public health messages often point to reducing your fat intake, being sensitive to portion size, and selecting lower-kcalorie rather than higher-kcalorie snacks. This emphasis on reducing kcalorie intake to avoid inappropriate weight gain and the acceleration of chronic disease may be having an unwanted effect on older adults, because many older men and women are consuming less food than they should.[60]

Physical Activity for Optimal Function

Physical activity promotes fitness and helps delay age-related changes in functional capacity. There are two types of physical activity, and each has a role in maintaining optimum health in adults of all ages:

1. *Endurance exercise:* The rhythmic use of the large muscles in walking, running, or jogging promotes cardiovascular fitness. For most older individuals, walking is a safe form of endurance exercise that supports cardiovascular health, weight management, and independent living. Swimming and bicycling promote fitness and burn kcalories, and these activities are well suited to persons with joint problems. Health professionals should help older adults find an activity they enjoy and will be motivated to continue during the long term.

EVIDENCE-BASED PRACTICE

Can We Prevent Age-Related Loss of Muscle Mass?

Loss of muscle mass leads to disability and loss of independence in older adults. Decreases in muscle size and strength affect one's ability to walk with confidence, carry groceries, or perform bathing and toileting without assistance. Loss of neural connections that innervate muscle fibers, muscle fiber atrophy resulting from a sedentary lifestyle and worsened by normal aging, reduced secretion of growth hormone and testosterone, and marginal protein intake all contribute to the progressive loss of muscle mass across the adult years. By age 70, muscle mass is half what it was at age 30, and muscle strength declines at a faster rate than muscle mass, indicating that remaining muscle fibers have poorer function. At one time it was assumed that muscle loss was a result of normal aging and could not be prevented or reversed. More recently, observations of older individuals, as well as experimental intervention strategies, have helped us learn how to prevent or reverse at least a portion of this loss.

Comparisons of muscle mass and muscle strength in young (age 26), middle-age (age 51), and older (age 71) men reveal that both age and lifelong levels of physical training influence gain or loss of muscle. In each age-group those participating in regular physical training had more muscle and lean body mass than those who were sedentary. In fact, older men engaging in regular strength training had greater muscle mass and muscle strength than did untrained men who were younger. Although some muscle will be lost as part of the aging process, lifelong physical activity and strength training prevents the extreme losses that result in weakness and disability.

Clinicians at the Human Research Center on Aging at Tufts University evaluated the effect of strength training in older nursing home residents with an average age of 90. All who completed the 8-week program improved their ability to carry out activities of daily living (ADLs). Those needing assistance to get up from a chair or walk across the room before the training program were able to carry out those activities without help after the program. Radiographs of the thigh muscles of participants before and after indicated an increase in muscle area and a decrease in fat. Just 9 months of strength training increases total body fat free mass, even in frail elderly adults; however, the activity must be continued for these gains to be retained.

Strength training has been confirmed as a means of helping older adults retain or regain muscle strength and muscle mass to sustain independent living; however, it is important that such a program be approved in advance by a health care provider. Community centers often offer supervised programs for older adults beginning a strength training program, and videos are available from various reputable sources* for those wishing to implement a program at home. Adequate protein (1.0 to 1.2 g/kg body weight) and sufficient kcalories to prevent weight loss are needed to support muscle development (see Chapter 14).

BIBLIOGRAPHY

Binder EF, Yarasheski KE, Steger-May K, et al: Effects of progressive resistance training on body composition in frail older adults: results of a randomized controlled trial, *J Gerontol A Biol Sci Med Sci* 60:1425, 2005.

Campbell WW: Synergistic use of higher-protein diets or nutritional supplements with resistance training to counter sarcopenia, *Nutr Rev* 65:416, 2007.

Fiatarone MA, Marks EC, Ryan ND, et al: High intensity strength training in nonagenarians. Effects on skeletal muscle, *JAMA* 263:3029, 1990.

Goodpaster BH, Park SW, Harris TB, et al: The loss of skeletal muscle strength, mass, and quality in older adults: the health, aging and body composition study, *J Gerontol A Biol Sci Med Sci* 61:1059, 2006.

Sallinen J, Ojanen T, Karavirta L, et al: Muscle mass and strength, body composition and dietary intake in master strength athletes vs untrained men of different ages, *J Sports Med Phys Fitness* 48:190, 2008.

* *Exercise & Physical Activity: Your Everyday Guide from the National Institute on Aging,* Pub No 09-4258, Bethesda, Md, 2009, National Institute on Aging. National Institutes of Health. Copies available at no charge from the National Institute on Aging: *www.nia.nih.gov/HealthInformation/Publications/ExerciseGuide/.*

2. *Resistance exercise:* Strength training (or *resistance training,* as it is sometimes called) is a form of exercise in which the individual pushes against or lifts a set weight. This action brings about an increase in size and strength of muscle fibers, improving functional capacity and the ability to perform household tasks. Strengthening arm muscles could enable an older person to continue to carry groceries or lift cooking pots. Building strength in the lower body muscles and legs helps develop balance and prevent falls and injuries. To support strength training, a protein intake of 1.2 g/kg body weight and added kcalories sufficient to prevent unwanted weight loss are recommended.[53] (To learn more about this type of exercise, see the *Evidence-Based Practice* box, "Can We Prevent Age-Related Loss of Muscle Mass?")

NUTRITIONAL CARE OF AT-RISK OLDER ADULTS

Aging and Chronic Disease

Lifestyle choices, disease history, and environmental hazards act on each person's unique set of genes to determine the rate and severity of aging changes. As a result, older people

KEY TERMS

gerontology Study of the physiologic, biologic, psychologic, and sociologic aspects of the aging process, their effects on individuals, and potential prevention or intervention strategies.

geriatrics Branch of medicine specializing in medical problems of older adults.

chronologic age A person's age in years.

of the same age are less alike than younger people of the same age, because each has experienced a different set of genetic and environmental influences during his or her lifetime. Some individuals are physically old at age 50, whereas others maintain an active pace into their 80s or 90s. All age-groups are susceptible to sickness and disease, but in younger adults, illness is more likely an acute problem that runs its course in a few days or weeks. In comparison, conditions common to older adults are usually chronic; although managed with diet or medications, over time these conditions will impose limitations on daily activities and lifestyle. At some point, additional services provided by family members or outside agencies may be needed.

Continuing losses in physical or cognitive function may eventually require a more protective and supportive environment, such as an assisted living facility or skilled nursing home. A well-planned and appropriate diet plays a major role in slowing the downhill spiral resulting in loss of independence.

Nutrition and Preventive Care

Influences on Food Intake

Many physical, social, and environmental influences relating to the individual and the community converge to support the health and quality of life of older adults (Figure 13-7). Personal characteristics relating to health, relationships, and economic situation influence nutrient intake and physical well-being, as do community resources such as transportation services to the grocery store or physician, safe neighborhoods for walking, or meal programs for those who cannot obtain sufficient amounts of food or prepare nourishing meals. Warning signs, as described following, can alert us to developing problems before nutritional and physical health are compromised:

- *Physical changes:* The physical changes of normal aging exacerbated by chronic disease or inadequate health care adversely affect food intake. Periodontal disease and decayed teeth, or tooth loss and poorly fitting dentures (or no dentures at all) make chewing and eating painful and difficult. Those with few or no teeth consume fewer portions of fruits and vegetables and have less variety in

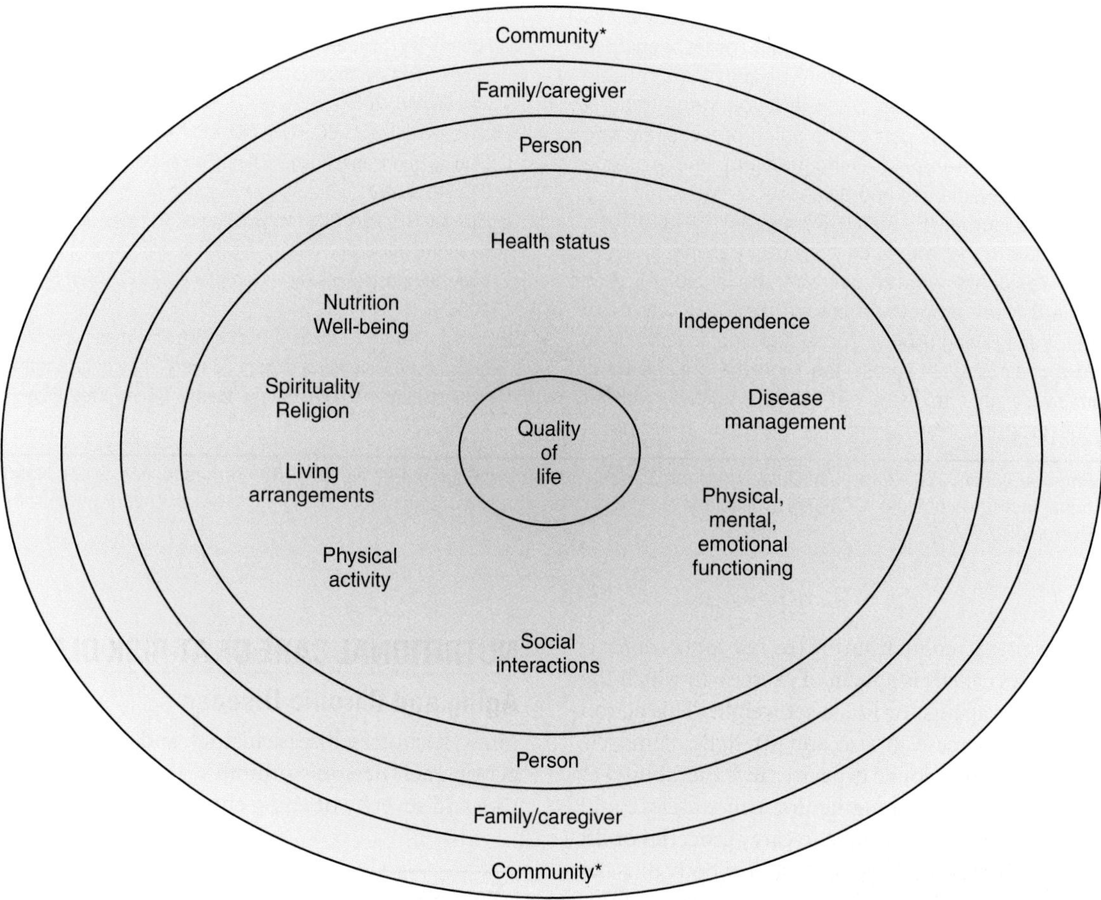

FIGURE 13-7 Many factors influence the quality of life of older adults. Personal characteristics, nearby neighbors or family caregivers, and support services available in the community help an older person remain independent. *The term *community* includes health and supportive services at local, state, and federal levels, as well as health professionals and researchers. (From American Dietetic Association: Position paper of the American Dietetic Association: nutrition across the spectrum of aging, *J Am Diet Assoc* 105:616, 2005, with permission from the American Dietetic Association.)

their diets.[61] Losses in taste, smell, or sight take away from the enjoyment of eating and lower appetite. In Chapter 2 we noted the changes in salivary secretion that lead to xerostomia (dry mouth) and make eating and swallowing troublesome. Radiation treatment or stroke that damages the nerves in the head and neck, as well as diabetes and Parkinson's disease, interfere with the swallowing reflex and cause fear of choking. Aging changes in the appetite control center of the hypothalamus reduce food intake. (See the *Case Study* box, "An Older Woman Living Alone," to see an example of these problems.)

- *Multiple medications:* Treatment regimens involving multiple drugs *(polypharmacy)* often lower food intake by producing anorexia, nausea, or unpleasant taste. Other drugs increase appetite, with higher food intake than is desirable. (We discuss nutrient-medication effects in greater detail in Chapter 18.)
- *Psychosocial distress:* Emotional loss arising from the death of a spouse, physical separation from family and friends, or fear for the future causing depression can bring disinterest in food. Older persons living alone, especially men who were unaccustomed to preparing food, may not go to the trouble of planning and cooking a meal for one person. Alcohol sometimes displaces food in the diet. A distorted body image with self-imposed food restriction (anorexia nervosa) occurs in older and younger women and men.
- *Economic problems:* Older adults living in poverty lack the resources to purchase the quantity and quality of food they should have. Even those with higher incomes but costly medications or other self-pay medical expenses may have to compromise on food. Inadequate housing with nonworking appliances or homelessness put older individuals at risk. Those living in rural areas or the inner city can be dependent on general or convenience stores with higher prices and limited selection for their food shopping.
- *Chronic illness and disability:* Food shopping and meal preparation are difficult or impossible for individuals who must use a cane or walker, can no longer drive, or have visual loss. Those who are dependent on others for transportation and shop irregularly have limited supplies of fresh fruits and vegetables and fluid milk. An inappropriately restrictive therapeutic diet that forbids favorite ethnic or comfort foods often lowers food intake. Older adults with a chronic condition such as diabetes that continues to escalate in severity requiring growing financial resources for testing supplies or medications experience worsening food insufficiency.[62] For the stroke victim who must relearn the motions necessary for self-feeding, embarrassment and frustration can severely limit food intake.

CASE STUDY

An Older Woman Living Alone

Miss E is 81 years old and lives in public housing. Her apartment kitchen has a two-unit cook top and a small refrigerator but very little storage space. She prepares and eats all her meals alone. She has always enjoyed mealtime but now has trouble with food sticking in her throat, so she cooks everything until it is very soft and seldom eats meat. She feels very tired much of the time; on days when Miss E is not well enough to fix a meal, she eats just cereal and milk. She likes fruits and vegetables but always buys them in cans because they are easier to swallow and cost less than when fresh or frozen. Miss E does her shopping at a supermarket about one half mile away. It had been her custom to walk to the market and take the bus home, but it is becoming more difficult to walk, so she rides both ways. She makes the trip twice a week so that she has fewer items to carry at one time. Because she has always liked to walk, Miss E maintained a healthy body weight, but recently she has been losing weight and now worries about her health. She wonders if she should be taking a vitamin supplement to increase her energy level.

Questions for Analysis

1. What are the physical changes influencing Miss E's food intake?
2. What are some socioeconomic or psychologic changes that may be affecting her food intake?
3. Which nutrients are likely to be low in her diet? Why?
4. What might be causing her tiredness?
5. What are your general concerns about Miss E's physical condition? What are the implications of her recent weight loss?
6. Would you recommend that Miss E begin to take a vitamin or mineral supplement? If so, then what might she take? Why would you make this recommendation?

Development of Overt Malnutrition

Protein-energy malnutrition occurs in older adults living at home, in skilled nursing facilities, or in the hospital.[49,63-65] Medical conditions accentuate the risk of undernutrition. Immune factors called *cytokines,* released in response to chronic disease or tissue injury, not only lower food intake but also interfere with the utilization of nutrients that are available so that even aggressive efforts at nutrition intervention cannot always reverse the continuing weight loss.[66] Congestive heart failure and cancer cause profound anorexia and wasting, referred to as *cardiac* and *cancer cachexia.* Undernutrition in the aging adult lowers immune function, slows production of red blood cells, and accelerates muscle loss.

Nutrition Screening

The Nutrition Screening Initiative (NSI) has promoted routine nutrition screening of older persons, drawing attention to warning signs of malnutrition that heighten the risk of chronic disease, physical disability, and loss of independence.[67] The *DETERMINE Your Nutritional Health* checklist defines seven characteristics associated with low nutrient intake (Figure 13-8) and is useful in senior centers, congregate meal

KEY TERMS

cognitive Pertaining to mental processes such as memory, judgment, and reasoning.

The Warning Signs of poor nutritional health are often overlooked. Use this checklist to find out if you or someone you know is at nutritional risk.

DETERMINE YOUR NUTRITIONAL HEALTH

Read the statements below. Circle the number in the "YES" column for those that apply to you or someone you know. For each yes answer, score the number in the box. Total your nutritional score.

	YES
I have an illness or condition that made me change the kind and/or amount of food I eat.	2
I eat fewer than 2 meals per day.	3
I eat few fruits or vegetables or milk products.	2
I have 3 or more drinks of beer, liquor, or wine almost every day.	2
I have tooth or mouth problems that make it hard for me to eat.	2
I don't always have enough money to buy the food I need.	4
I eat alone most of the time.	1
I take 3 or more different prescribed or over-the-counter drugs a day.	1
Without wanting to, I have lost or gained 10 pounds in the last 6 months.	2
I am not always physically able to shop, cook, and/or feed myself.	2
TOTAL	

Total Your Nutritional Score. If it's–

0-2 **Good!** Recheck your nutritional score in 6 months.

3-5 **You are at moderate nutritional risk.** See what can be done to improve your eating habits and lifestyle. Your office on aging, senior nutrition program, senior citizens center or health department can help. Recheck your nutritional score in 3 months.

6 or more **You are at high nutritional risk.** Bring this checklist the next time you see your doctor, dietitian, or other qualified health or social service professional. Talk with them about any problems you may have. Ask for help to improve your nutritional health.

These materials developed and distributed by the Nutrition Screening Initiative, a project of:

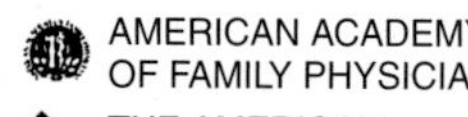
AMERICAN ACADEMY OF FAMILY PHYSICIANS

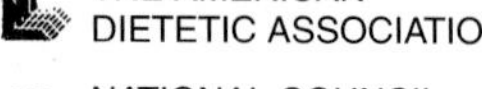
THE AMERICAN DIETETIC ASSOCIATION

NATIONAL COUNCIL ON THE AGING, INC.

Remember that warning signs suggest risk but do not represent diagnosis of any condition. Turn the page to learn more about the Warning Signs of poor nutritional health.

FIGURE 13-8 *DETERMINE Your Nutritional Health* checklist. (From Nutrition Screening Initiative: *DETERMINE Your Nutritional Health* checklist, Washington, DC, 2005, The NSI. Retrieved June 2, 2010 from http://www.mnaging.org/pdf/dynh.pdf. The Nutrition Screening Initiative [NSI] was a joint project of the American Academy of Family Physicians and the American Dietetic Association, funded in part by a grant from Ross Products Division, Abbott Laboratories Inc.)

sites, physicians' offices, or home-delivered meals programs to identify those at risk. This allows the application of intervention strategies that prevent the development of overt undernutrition. A set of warning signs for use with residents in skilled nursing facilities is found in Box 13-2.

Community Food Assistance Programs for Older Americans

Several government-supported food assistance programs help older adults meet their food needs. The Supplemental Nutrition Assistance Program (formerly referred to as *The Food Stamp Program*) extends food-buying power, making food more accessible to adults with limited resources. However, the

BOX 13-2 NUTRITION ALERTS FOR OLDER ADULTS IN LONG-TERM CARE

- Involuntary loss of 5% of body weight in 1 month or 10% in 6 months
- Leaving 25% or more of served food uneaten during the past 7 days
- BMI $\leq$21

Data from Thomas DR, Ashmen W, Morley JE, et al: Nutritional management in long-term care: development of a clinical guideline, *J Gerontol A Biol Sci Med Sci* 55A(12):M725, 2000.
BMI, Body mass index.

program having the greatest effect on the nutritional health of older Americans is the national Elderly Nutrition Program that provides congregate and home-delivered meals to adults ages 60 and older. (For more information on these programs, see Appendix F.)

Chronic Conditions and Physical Disability

Physical disability occurs in all age-groups from accident, injury, disease condition, or developmental injury, but the majority of individuals with a disability are older than age 65 and problems accelerate with age. Medical conditions resulting in functional or cognitive loss include the following:

- *Cardiovascular disease:* Congestive heart failure causing an inadequate supply of oxygen to muscles including the heart muscle limits general movement and self-care.
- *Pulmonary disease:* Chronic obstructive pulmonary disease (COPD) and emphysema bring changes in the alveoli (i.e., air sacs); less air flows in and out of the lungs and breathing becomes difficult.
- *Musculoskeletal disease:* Rheumatoid arthritis (RA) is an autoimmune disorder affecting joints in the hands, arms, and feet, with loss of movement that can restrict food shopping, meal preparation, and in severe cases, self-feeding. Osteoarthritis (degenerative joint disease) limits flexibility in hand motion and makes walking and standing difficult and painful. Osteoporosis and subsequent hip fracture often confine the individual to a wheelchair, with loss of independence and institutionalization (see Chapter 7 to review causes and interventions for osteoporosis).
- *Neuromuscular disease:* A cerebrovascular accident (stroke) can result in irreversible paralysis and loss of movement or uncontrolled movement, presenting problems with speech, walking, self-feeding, and self-care. Individuals with cerebral palsy (CP) and spinal bifida have similar problems in self-care.
- *Progressive neurologic disorders:* Individuals with advanced Parkinson's disease who have joint rigidity, body stiffness, and tremors find meal preparation and self-feeding difficult. Multiple sclerosis, myasthenia gravis, and Alzheimer's disease are other examples of neurologic disorders that affect food-related activities. (These medical conditions are discussed further in Part 3.)

One's quality of life is magnified by the opportunity to live independently in safety and comfort or perform self-care to the greatest extent possible in a supervised setting. Chronic conditions often require some adaptation of the living situation that may include assistive devices to aid in self-feeding. The ability to self-feed has implications for physical and emotional well-being. Anger, frustration, fear, and a sense of grief can accompany the loss of this fundamental skill. When a meal is dependent on the cooperation of the feeder, it is no longer driven by the inner eating pace or rhythm of the individual being fed.[68] This can lower meal satisfaction and the amount of food consumed. A variety of assistive devices can be purchased or fashioned at little or no cost to help people with limited range of motion or poor grasp self-feed (Figure 13-9).

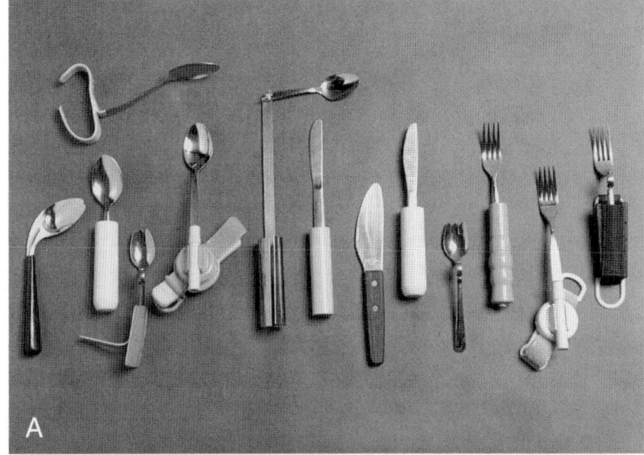

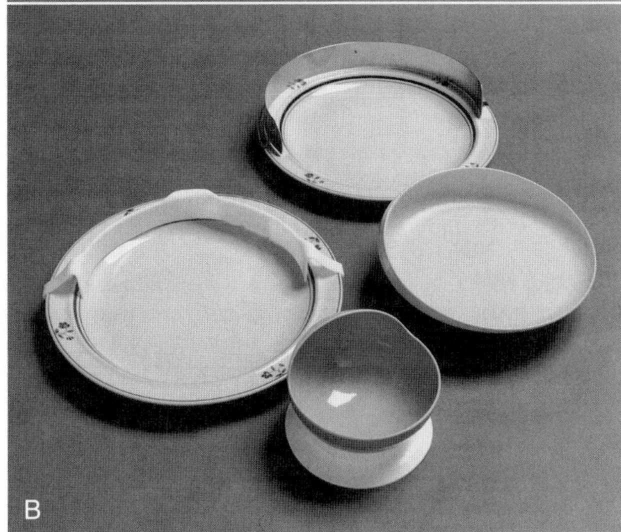

FIGURE 13-9 Various small and inexpensive aids assist individuals with disabilities to self-feed. **A,** Utensil adaptations help with length, grasp, and range of motion. **B,** Plate guards and scoop bowls provide an edge to help place food on the utensil. (From Olson DA, DeRuyter F: *Clinician's guide to assistive technology,* St Louis, 2002, Mosby.)

Efforts at rehabilitation are most successful when built on a partnership that includes the client, the client's family, and the health care professional. Together they can fashion immediate and long-term goals and provide encouragement in carrying out the nutrition care plan. Community support programs help patients and their families learn more about their condition and its management, find emotional support, and make creative decisions. Individual and group sessions providing nutrition education, physical therapy, and medical information have a positive effect on physical and psychologic well-being. Such intervention helps patients and caregivers cope with the chronic nature of the disease. (To learn about activity scales used to assess an individual's ability to remain in the community and the type of assistance or services that will be required, see the *Perspectives in Practice* box, "Community-Based Long-Term Care: How Do We Make Decisions?")

PERSPECTIVES IN PRACTICE

Community-Based Long-Term Care: How Do We Make Decisions?

At one time *long-term care* usually referred to medical, social, or personal services provided to individuals in skilled nursing homes or other resident facilities. Older adults needing help with daily tasks that could not be provided by family members moved from their homes to such a facility. Today we are placing more emphasis on community-based long-term care, developing support services that will enable older adults to remain in their own homes or in the homes of family members. The first step in planning for long-term care is evaluating the individual's functional and cognitive capabilities to determine a safe and appropriate level of care. Two evaluation scales used to assess the potential level of independence are the Activities of Daily Living (ADLs) and the Instrumental Activities of Daily Living (IADLs).

The ADLs, as listed following, focus on a person's ability to manage personal care either independently, with some level of help, or not at all:

- Bathing
- Dressing
- Feeding
- Using the toilet
- Transferring between bed and chair

An older adult requiring assistance with personal care may be able to remain in the community if family, paid caregivers, or both are available on a daily basis to provide the help needed.

The IADLs, listed as follows, evaluate an individual's ability to perform housekeeping tasks and other chores required for independent living:

- Preparing meals
- Performing housecleaning chores
- Handling money and balancing a checkbook
- Shopping without help
- Using the telephone
- Leaving home without help

A person able to perform some, if not all, of these tasks may still remain independent if food-related services such as grocery shopping or home-delivered meals can be established.

Evaluations using the ADLs or IADLs are usually performed by a health professional or trained social worker. This may occur at discharge planning after a hospitalization or convalescence or be requested by family members or health or social service professionals working with the older adult. Ongoing review is provided by a designated case manager who serves as the gatekeeper for professional and support services; he or she monitors any changes in physical or cognitive abilities requiring an adjustment in services provided or level of independence that can be sustained.

Considerations in Diet Planning: An Individual Approach

Appropriate Energy Intake

Individual needs vary with body size, metabolic needs, and physical activity. For reasonably healthy and moderately active older adults, daily energy needs range from 1600 to 2200 kcal for women and 2000 to 2800 kcal for men.[59] However, national and regional surveys tell us that many older adults take in less than these amounts, and African-American and Hispanic older adults have lower intakes than Caucasian older adults (Table 13-4).[36,69,70] In homebound elderly adults, energy intake can be less than 1000 kcal.[63] Inappropriately low kcalorie intake has serious consequences in frail older adults. For example, in a 7-year study, mortality was highest among those consuming only 65% of their recommended energy intake.[71] Chronic conditions common in older adults, including cancer, cardiac failure, and COPD, increase energy needs. In addition, older adults are less able to regulate their energy intake to compensate for day-to-day fluctuations, so temporary reductions in food intake as a result of illness or limited food availability may become the norm, with fewer kcalories consumed and progressive weight loss.[72]

Underweight is a serious situation in older adults; men and women in their 60s with a BMI less than 18.5 have a mortality risk more than twice that of their normal weight counterparts.[73] Physicians recommend that older adults maintain a BMI between 22 and 25.[74,75] Avoiding unintentional weight loss is key to continued physical and mental well-being for those in the community or long-term care.

TABLE 13-4 MEAN ENERGY INTAKES OF PERSONS AGE 60 AND OLDER

	MEN	WOMEN
Caucasian	2032 kcal	1529 kcal
African American	1704 kcal	1275 kcal
Hispanic	1748 kcal	1419 kcal

Data from Bowman SA: Socioeconomic characteristics, dietary and lifestyle patterns, and health and weight status of older adults in NHANES, 1999–2002: a comparison of Caucasians and African Americans, *J Nutr Elder* 28:30, 2009; Bermudez OI, Falcon LM, Tucker KL: Intake and food sources of macronutrients among older Hispanic adults: association with ethnicity, acculturation, and length of residence in the United States, *J Am Diet Assoc* 100:665, 2000.

Macronutrients

An appropriate diet for an older person should emphasize a variety of nutrient-dense foods in sufficient amounts to meet energy needs:

- *Carbohydrates:* Persons of all ages should obtain 45% to 65% of their total energy from carbohydrates and emphasize complex carbohydrates.[7] Diets rich in fiber reduce the need for laxatives and their potential for electrolyte disruption. Complex carbohydrates in legumes and whole grains help modulate postprandial blood glucose levels.[76]
- *Fats:* Fat intake is best contained within the range of 20% to 35% of total kcalories,[7] balancing the need for essential

fatty acids and the disease risk associated with high-fat diets. Fat is needed to absorb fat-soluble vitamins and adds to the palatability, pleasing mouth feel, and flavor of food. A diet plan with 35% of total kcalories from healthy fats can help prevent weight loss in frail older adults. Fats are generally well digested and absorbed at older ages, although the rate of fat breakdown may be slowed; dividing fat intake among all meals and snacks enhances digestion and utilization.

- *Protein:* Protein preserves muscle mass, supports optimum immune function, and maintains body tissues. The current RDA of 0.8 g/kg body weight is likely not sufficient for frail or chronically ill older adults when metabolic systems become less efficient; thus clinicians recommend an intake of 1.0 g/kg for persons older than age 70.[54] Older individuals recovering from surgery or acute illness may require as much as 1.5 g/kg for optimal recovery.[77] Overall, 10% to 35% of total kcalories should be supplied by good-quality protein.

Vitamins

Vitamins of special importance to the aging adult include the following:

- *Folate:* Optimum folate helps prevents a rise in blood homocysteine levels that damages blood vessels and accelerates atherosclerosis.[32]
- *Vitamin B_6:* As an active coenzyme in protein synthesis, vitamin B_6 is important to preserve or increase muscle mass.[32]
- *Vitamin B_{12}:* The age-related decrease in gastric acid hinders the release of vitamin B_{12} from animal protein foods. Vitamin B_{12}–fortified breads and cereals or vitamin B_{12} supplements can supply the amount needed to prevent deficiency with megaloblastic anemia and changes in cognitive function.[32]
- *Vitamin D:* Vitamin D deficiency occurs in older persons who spend most of their time indoors and do not eat vitamin D–fortified foods.[9] Aging changes in the skin reduce vitamin D synthesis regardless of sun exposure, and a supplement is likely indicated.

Minerals and Electrolytes

In planning diets for at-risk older adults, calcium, potassium, and sodium require particular attention, as follows:

- *Calcium:* The AI for calcium is 1200 mg for those ages 51 and older.[9] Fluid milk, fortified soy milk, and fortified yogurt, all good sources of calcium, also contain added vitamin D.
- *Potassium:* Various diuretics commonly prescribed for older adults bring about a loss of body potassium that must be replenished by diet. The AI for potassium (4700 mg) can be accomplished with five to nine daily servings of fruits and vegetables.[11] Potassium supplements can raise blood potassium to dangerous levels and require medical supervision.
- *Sodium:* Daily intakes should be limited to 2300 mg or less[11] to avoid unwanted fluid retention or rise in blood pressure. Meeting this sodium limitation can be difficult for frail older adults who depend on heat-and-serve food items, which are often high in sodium-containing additives.

BOX 13-3 RISK FACTORS FOR DEHYDRATION IN OLDER ADULTS

- Advanced age (85 years and older)
- Loss of thirst sensation
- Problems with mobility
- Confusion or cognitive changes
- Problems in swallowing
- Medications promoting fluid loss (diuretics, laxatives)
- Incontinence leading to self-imposed fluid restriction

Modified from Ferry M: Strategies for ensuring good hydration in the elderly, *Nutr Rev* 63(suppl 6):S22, 2005. Copyright 2005 International Life Sciences Institute.

Fluids

Dehydration is a concern for healthy and chronically ill older adults.[49,78] Physiologic changes, disease effects, medications, and environmental circumstances predispose older people to inadequate fluid intake (Box 13-3). Changes in the hypothalamus alter the thirst mechanism such that older persons do not always get thirsty and drink when or as much as they should. Age-related alterations in kidney function lessen the ability to conserve water, and changes in body water influence the dilution of medications. Dehydration affects alertness and cognitive function.[79] The general fluid recommendation of 1500 mL/day increases when temperatures outdoors or inside the home rise. In patients with fever, daily fluid needs increase by 500 mL per degree Centigrade beyond the normal temperature.[78] Older adults are also at risk of overhydration (water intoxication) when fluid intakes are inappropriately high, because excess water is less efficiently excreted.

Older persons and their caregivers should monitor their fluid intake to ensure it meets AI standards; they should also watch for signs of dehydration (see Box 13-3). In long-term care facilities, responsibility for overseeing fluid intake must be assigned and accountable.

Nutrient Supplementation

Healthy older adults who consume a variety of foods, including fortified foods, and meet the DRI for energy are unlikely to require nutrient supplements. However, those with low energy intakes and chronic health problems will benefit from prudent, individually assessed supplementation. Multiple prescription and over-the-counter medications, a limited variety of foods, isolation, and little social support put individuals at risk for nutrient deficiency.[60,63,80,81] Nutrient supplements help replenish body stores after critical or debilitating illness. However, nutritional supplements should add to—not replace—food. Using food money to purchase supplements rather than nutrient-dense food is unwise.

Surveys indicate that older adults are frequent users of dietary supplements; 37% take one supplement and 26% take four or more.[37] However, older adults should be guided in their use. Supplements can overcome existing dietary deficiencies, as is often the case with calcium. Among individuals age 60 and older, 18% used calcium supplements and another 33% used calcium-containing antacids to help meet recommended intakes.[82] At the same time, older adults may be taking in added nutrients for which their requirement is relatively low and easily met with food. Forty percent of a population age 60 and older reported using a multivitamin-multimineral supplement[37] that included iron, often in the amount required for women of child-bearing age (18 mg). In an older multi-ethnic group, 14% of the men and 11% of the women were exceeding the UL for iron, counting food and supplements.[82] On the other hand, vitamin D, often lacking in the diets of older persons, is seldom taken as a supplement unless combined with calcium. Individuals using single-nutrient supplements in addition to multivitamin-multimineral supplements are most at risk for exceeding the UL for one or more nutrients or precipitating dangerous interactions. The use of nutrient supplements should be based on an individual assessment and supervised by a health care professional. An evaluation of dietary intake, along with any available biochemical parameters assessing nutritional status, should provide the basis for any supplement recommendation.

TO SUM UP

Nutrient needs through adult life respond to the ebb and flow of continuing maturation and eventual decline. In young adults, nutrients support the physical body that has reached its full potential and build reserves for active living. Lifestyle patterns formed by young adults often continue throughout life, and sedentary living and unwanted weight gain are concerns. Middle age begins the period of physical decline, although changes occur slowly at the onset. Loss of muscle and bone mass influences functional capacity and threatens independent living in later years if allowed to continue unchecked. Attention to protein, calcium, and vitamin D, along with participation in endurance and resistance exercise, slows these processes. Patterns of healthy eating, regular physical activity, and avoidance of smoking and other addictive behaviors established in young adults support successful aging and the delay of degenerative changes.

Nutritional needs at advanced ages are influenced by changes in body composition, organ function, and worsening chronic disease. The aging process is often complicated by associated malnutrition and weight loss. Physical disability, poverty, difficulty in chewing or swallowing, isolation and depression, and multiple medications can lower food intake, adding to nutritional risk. The *DETERMINE Your Nutritional Health* checklist offers a tool to identify at-risk older adults and educate individuals and communities in preventive care.

QUESTIONS FOR REVIEW

1. Discuss the economic status, ethnic and racial composition, and living arrangements of the aging population. How might these factors influence the older person's diet or health status? What are the implications for health and support services?
2. Select one of the adult age-groups, and describe its physical characteristics, psychosocial development, socioeconomic status, and nutritional needs. What do you see as the most urgent topic for health promotion in this age-group? Why?
3. You are working with a 32-year-old man who lives alone. He has a demanding job with no time to exercise and eats fast food most of the time. He has gained 15 lb during the last 2 years and is concerned about his overall health. What questions should you ask before making any diet or lifestyle recommendations? What diet and lifestyle recommendations might be compatible with his general lifestyle?
4. You are working with a middle-age adult who is overweight, sedentary, and eats mostly meat, bread, potatoes, and desserts. Does this person represent normal aging or successful aging? What suggestions would you have for improvement?
5. What is the aging process? What are some physiologic changes that occur as we age? How do they influence food intake or nutritional status?
6. Interview a family member, neighbor, or friend who is older than age 65. What are some changes in health, living arrangements, or employment that have influenced his or her lifestyle during the past 10 years? How have these changes affected his or her eating habits?
7. You are helping a 75-year-old retired couple on a limited income with their diet. Both appear to be underweight, and you suspect that their food supplies have been limited. Using MyPyramid, plan a 3-day menu of meals and snacks that will supply each food group in the appropriate amounts. How might you increase their energy intake and still remain within the suggested ranges for the three macronutrients?
8. Distinguish between the terms *gerontology* and *geriatrics*. Go to your school library and find the *Journal of Gerontology* and the *Journal of the American Geriatrics Society*. Look for an article in each journal that discusses a nutrition problem or nutrition-related disease in older adults. Compare the articles as to the type of information presented and how they might be used.

9. Identify a food-related program for older adults in your community, and interview the director to determine (a) the target audience, (b) the types and amounts of food provided, (c) any major problems associated with the program, and (d) the major successes of the program. If possible, administer the *DETERMINE Your Nutritional Health* checklist to some of the participants. How would you characterize their nutritional risk?
10. Visit your local drugstore and review the liquid supplements being marketed to older adults. Make a table describing four different supplements listing (a) the cost and (b) the amounts of kcalories, protein, calcium, vitamin D, vitamin B_6, vitamin B_{12}, and folate per 1-cup serving. Using the nutrient analysis program on the Evolve website that accompanies your textbook, select a fortified cereal that would be eaten with 1 cup of milk. Compare the cost, kcalories, and nutrients listed previously in a 1-cup serving of the liquid supplement with the usual serving of the cereal with 1 cup of milk. Based on your findings, what would you recommend as an evening snack? Explain.

REFERENCES

1. Butler RN: *Why survive? Being old in America*, Baltimore, 2002, Johns Hopkins University Press.
2. Federal Interagency Forum on Aging-Related Statistics: *Older Americans 2008: key indicators of well-being*, Washington, DC, 2008, U.S. Government Printing Office.
3. Administration on Aging, U.S. Department of Health and Human Services: *A profile of older Americans: 2007—poverty*. Washington, DC, 2007. Retrieved October 4, 2009, from www.aoa.gov/AoAroot/Aging_Statistics/Profile/2007/10.aspx.
4. Administration on Aging, U.S. Department of Health and Human Services: *A profile of older Americans: 2007—living arrangements*. Washington, DC, 2007. Retrieved October 4, 2009, from www.aoa.gov/AoAroot/Aging_Statistics/Profile/2007/6.aspx.
5. Kobau R, Safran SA, Zack MM, et al: Sad, blue, or depressed days, health behaviors and health-related quality of life, Behavioral Risk Factor Surveillance System, 1995–2000, *Health Qual Life Outcomes* 2(1):40, 2004.
6. Strine TW, Chapman DP, Balluz LS, et al: The associations between life satisfaction and health-related quality of life, chronic illness, and health behaviors among U.S. community-dwelling adults, *J Community Health* 33:40, 2008.
7. Food and Nutrition Board, Institute of Medicine: *Dietary Reference Intakes for energy, carbohydrate, fiber, fat, fatty acids, cholesterol, protein, and amino acids (macronutrients)*, Washington, DC, 2002, National Academies Press.
8. U.S. Department of Agriculture, Agricultural Research Service: *Nutrient intakes from food: mean amounts consumed per individual, one day, 2005–2006*, Washington, DC, 2008, U.S. Government Printing Office. Retrieved October 4, 2009, from www.ars.usda.gov/SP2UserFiles/Place/12355000/pdf/0506/Table_1_NIF_05.pdf.
9. Food and Nutrition Board, Institute of Medicine: *Dietary Reference Intakes for calcium, phosphorus, magnesium, vitamin D, and fluoride*, Washington, DC, 1997, National Academies Press.
10. Food and Nutrition Board, Institute of Medicine: *Dietary Reference Intakes for vitamin A, vitamin K, arsenic, boron, chromium, copper, iodine, iron, manganese, molybdenum, nickel, silicon, vanadium, and zinc*, Washington, DC, 2001, National Academies Press.
11. Food and Nutrition Board, Institute of Medicine: *Dietary Reference Intakes for water, potassium, sodium, chloride, and sulfate*, Washington, DC, 2004, National Academies Press.
12. Cena ER, Joy AB, Heneman K, et al: Folate intake and food-related behaviors in nonpregnant, low-income women of childbearing age, *J Am Diet Assoc* 108:1364, 2008.
13. Park S, Johnson MA: Living in low-latitude regions in the United States does not prevent poor vitamin D status, *Nutr Rev* 63(6 pt 1):203, 2005.
14. Winkleby MA, Cubbin C: Changing patterns in health behaviors and risk factors related to chronic diseases, 1990–2000, *Am J Health Promot* 19(1):19, 2004.
15. Ford CA, Nonnemaker JM, Wirth KE: The influence of body mass index, physical activity, and tobacco use on blood pressure and cholesterol in young adulthood, *J Adolesc Health* 43:576, 2008.
16. Boone JE, Gordon-Larsen P, Adair LS, et al: Screen time and physical activity during adolescence: longitudinal effects on obesity in young adulthood, *Int J Behav Nutr Phys Act* 4:26, 2007.
17. Duffey KJ, Gordon-Larsen P, Jacobs DR Jr, et al: Differential associations of fast food and restaurant food consumption with 3-y change in body mass index; the Coronary Artery Risk Development in Young Adults Study, *Am J Clin Nutr* 85:201, 2007.
18. Larson NI, Nelson MC, Neumark-Sztainer D, et al: Making time for meals: meal structure and associations with dietary intake in young adults, *J Am Diet Assoc* 109:72, 2009.
19. Pletcher MJ, Varosy P, Kiefe CI, et al: Alcohol consumption, binge drinking, and early coronary calcification: findings from the Coronary Artery Risk Development in Young Adults (CARDYA) Study, *Am J Epidemiol* 161:423, 2005.
20. Burke V, Beilin LJ, Dunbar D, et al: Changes in health-related behaviours and cardiovascular risk factors in young adults: associations with living with a partner, *Prev Med* 39(4):722, 2004.
21. Deshmukh-Taskar P, Nicklas TA, Yang SJ, et al: Does food group consumption vary by differences in socioeconomic, demographic, and lifestyle factors in young adults? The Bogalusa Heart Study, *J Am Diet Assoc* 107:223, 2007.
22. National Center for Health Statistics: *Health, United States, 2008 with chartbook on the health of young adults, DHHS Pub No 2009–1232*, Hyattsville, Md, 2009, U.S. Government Printing Office.
23. Gordon-Larsen P, Nelson MC, Popkin BM: Longitudinal physical activity and sedentary behavior trends: adolescence to adulthood, *Am J Prev Med* 27(4):277, 2004.
24. Yoo S, Nicklas T, Baranowski T, et al: Comparison of dietary intakes associated with metabolic syndrome risk factors in young adults: the Bogalusa Heart Study, *Am J Clin Nutr* 80:841, 2004.
25. Yang X, Telama R, Hirvensalo M, et al: The longitudinal effects of physical activity history on metabolic syndrome, *Med Sci Sports Exerc* 40:1424, 2008.
26. Campbell WW: Synergistic use of higher-protein diets or nutritional supplements with resistance training to counter sarcopenia, *Nutr Rev* 65(9):416, 2007.

27. Hughes VA, Frontera WR, Roubenoff R, et al: Longitudinal changes in body composition in older men and women: role of body weight change and physical activity, *Am J Clin Nutr* 76:473, 2002.
28. Ekelund U, Brage S, Besson H, et al: Time spent being sedentary and weight gain in healthy adults: reverse or bidirectional causality, *Am J Clin Nutr* 88:612, 2008.
29. Macdonald HM, New SA, Golden MH, et al: Nutritional associations with bone loss during the menopausal transition: evidence for a beneficial effect of calcium, alcohol, and fruit and vegetable nutrients and of a detrimental effect of fatty acids, *Am J Clin Nutr* 79:155, 2004.
30. Dawson-Hughes B: Commentary: a revised clinician's guide to the prevention and treatment of osteoporosis, *J Clin Endocrinol Metab* 93(7):2463, 2008.
31. Looker AC, Pfeiffer CM, Lacher DA, et al: Serum 25-hydroxyvitamin D status of the U.S. population: 1988–1994 compared with 2000–2004, *Am J Clin Nutr* 88:1519, 2008.
32. Food and Nutrition Board, Institute of Medicine: *Dietary Reference Intakes for thiamin, riboflavin, niacin, vitamin B-6, folate, vitamin B-12, pantothenic acid, biotin, and choline*, Washington, DC, 1998, National Academies Press.
33. Li F, Harmer P, Cardinal BJ, et al: Build environment and 1-year change in weight and waist circumference in middle-aged and older adults, *Am J Epidemiol* 169:401, 2009.
34. Bleich SN, Wang YC, Wang Y, et al: Increasing consumption of sugar-sweetened beverages among U.S. adults: 1988–1994 to 1999–2004, *Am J Clin Nutr* 89:372, 2009.
35. Nielsen SJ, Siega-Riz AM, Popkin BM: Trends in energy intake in U.S. between 1977 and 1996: similar shifts seen across age groups, *Obes Res* 10(5):370, 2002.
36. U.S. Department of Agriculture, Agricultural Research Service: *Nutrient intakes from food: mean amounts and percentages of calories from protein, carbohydrate, fat, and alcohol, one day, 2005–2006*, Washington, DC, 2008, U.S. Government Printing Office. Retrieved September 20, 2009, from www.ars.usda.gov/SP2UserFiles/Place/12355000/pdf/0506/Table_2_NIF_05.pdf.
37. Radimer K, Bindewald B, Hughes J, et al: Dietary supplement use by U.S. adults: data from the National Health and Nutrition Examination Survey, 1999–2000, *Am J Epidemiol* 160:339, 2004.
38. U.S. Department of Health and Human Services, Centers for Disease Control and Prevention: Racial/ethnic and socioeconomic disparities in multiple risk factors for heart disease and stroke—United States, 2003, *MMWR Morb Mortal Wkly Rep* 54(5):113, 2005.
39. Koopman RJ, Mainous AG 3rd, Diaz VA, et al: Changes in age at diagnosis of type 2 diabetes mellitus in the United States, 1988 to 2000, *Ann Fam Med* 3:60, 2005.
40. Kruger J, Ham SA, Prohaska TR: Behavioral risk factors associated with overweight and obesity among older adults: the 2005 National Health Interview Survey, *Prev Chronic Dis* 6(1):A14, 2009. Retrieved September 20, 2009, from www.cdc.gov/pcd/issues/2009/jan/07_0183.htm.
41. Kant AK, Graubard BI, Schatzkin A: Dietary patterns predict mortality in a national cohort: the National Health Interview Surveys, 1987 and 1992, *J Nutr* 134:1793, 2004.
42. Suter PM: Alcohol: its role in health and nutrition. In Bowman BA, Russell RM, editors: *Present knowledge in nutrition*, ed 8, Washington, DC, 2001, International Life Sciences Institute.
43. Hughes VA, Roubenoff R, Wood M, et al: Anthropometric assessment of 10-y changes in body composition in the elderly, *Am J Clin Nutr* 80:475, 2004.
44. Kyle UG, Melzer K, Kayser B, et al: Eight-year longitudinal changes in body composition in healthy Swiss adults, *J Am Coll Nutr* 25:493, 2006.
45. Pi-Sunyer FX: The epidemiology of central fat distribution in relation to disease, *Nutr Rev* 62(7 pt 2):S120, 2004.
46. Topinkova E: Aging, disability and frailty, *Ann Nutr Metab* 52(Suppl 1):6, 2008.
47. Kane RL, Ouslander JG, Abrass IB: *Essentials of clinical geriatrics*, ed 5, New York, 2004, McGraw-Hill.
48. Rocchiccioli JT, Sanford JT: Revisiting geriatric failure to thrive: a complex and compelling clinical condition, *J Gerontol Nurs* 35:18, 2009.
49. American Dietetic Association: Position paper of the American Dietetic Association: nutrition across the spectrum of aging, *J Am Diet Assoc* 105:616, 2005.
50. Hughes G, Bennett KM, Hetherington MM: Old and alone: barriers to healthy eating in older men living on their own, *Appetite* 43:269, 2004.
51. Blanc S, Schoeller DA, Bauer D, et al: Energy requirements in the eighth decade of life, *Am J Clin Nutr* 79:303, 2004.
52. Paddon-Jones D, Short KR, Campbell WW, et al: Role of dietary protein in the sarcopenia of aging, *Am J Clin Nutr* 87(Suppl):1562S, 2008.
53. Campbell WW, Leidy HJ: Dietary protein and resistance training effects on muscle and body composition in older persons, *J Am Coll Nutr* 26:696S, 2007.
54. Chernoff R: Protein and older adults, *J Am Coll Nutr* 23(Suppl 6):627S, 2004.
55. Diehr P, O'Meara ES, Fitzpatrick A, et al: Weight, mortality, years of healthy life, and active life expectancy in older adults, *J Am Geriatr Soc* 56:76, 2008.
56. Daviglus ML, Liu K, Yan LL, et al: Relation of body mass index in young adulthood and middle age to Medicare expenditures in older age, *JAMA* 292:2743, 2004.
57. U.S. Department of Health and Human Services: *Health: United States, 1999 with chartbook on aging*, Rockville, Md, 1999, U.S. Government Printing Office.
58. U.S. Department of Health and Human Services, U.S. Department of Agriculture: *Dietary Guidelines for Americans 2005*, ed 6, Washington, DC, 2005, U.S. Government Printing Office. Retrieved September 20, 2009, from www.health.gov/dietaryguidelines/dga2005/toolkit/.
59. U.S. Department of Agriculture, Center for Nutrition Policy and Promotion: *MyPyramid food guidance system*, Washington, DC, 2005, U.S. Department of Agriculture. Retrieved September 20, 2009, from www.mypyramid.gov/.
60. Roberts SB, Hajduk CL, Howarth NC, et al: Dietary variety predicts low body mass index and inadequate macronutrient and micronutrient intakes in community-dwelling older adults, *J Gerontol A Biol Sci Med Sci* 60A:613, 2005.
61. Ervin RB: *Healthy eating index scores among adults, 60 years of age and over, by sociodemographic and health characteristics: United States, 1999–2002, advance data*, Pub No 395, Washington, DC, 2008, U.S. Department of Health and Human Services.
62. Sharkey JP: Longitudinal examination of homebound older adults who experience heightened food insufficiency: effect of diabetes status and implications for service provision, *Gerontologist* 45:773, 2005.
63. Sharkey JR: Diet and health outcomes in vulnerable populations, *Ann N Y Acad Sci* 1136:210, 2008.
64. Challa S, Sharkey JR, Chen M, et al: Association of resident, facility, and geographic characteristics with chronic undernutrition in a nationally represented sample of older residents in U.S. nursing homes, *J Nutr Health Aging* 11:179, 2007.

65. Wilson MM: Undernutrition in medical outpatients, *Clin Geriatr Med* 18:759, 2002.
66. Evans WJ, Morley JE, Argiles J, et al: Cachexia: a new definition, *Clin Nutr* 27:793, 2008.
67. American Dietetic Association, American Academy of Family Physicians: *Nutrition Screening Initiative, Washington, DC, 1989–2005*, Washington, DC, 2005, ADA-AAFP. Retrieved June 2, 2010 from http://www.mnaging.org/pdf/dynh.pdf.
68. Martinsen B, Harder I, Biering-Sorensen F: Sensitive cooperation: a basis for assisted feeding, *J Clin Nurs* 18(5):708, 2009.
69. Bowman SA: Socioeconomic characteristics, dietary and lifestyle patterns, and health and weight status of older adults in NHANES, 1999–2002: a comparison of Caucasians and African Americans, *J Nutr Elder* 28:30, 2009.
70. Bermudez OI, Falcon LM, Tucker KL: Intake and food sources of macronutrients among older Hispanic adults: association with ethnicity, acculturation, and length of residence in the United States, *J Am Diet Assoc* 100:665, 2000.
71. Leosdottir M, Nilsson P, Nilsson JA, et al: The association between total energy intake and early mortality: data from the Malmo Diet and Cancer Study, *J Intern Med* 256:499, 2004.
72. Roberts SB, Rosenberg I: Nutrition and aging: changes in the regulation of energy metabolism with aging, *Physiol Rev* 86:651, 2006.
73. Flegal KM, Graubard BI, Williamson DF, et al: Excess deaths associated with underweight, overweight, and obesity, *JAMA* 293:1861, 2005.
74. Thomas DR, Ashmen W, Morley JE, et al: Nutritional management in long-term care: development of a clinical guideline, *J Gerontol A Biol Sci Med Sci* 55A(12):M725, 2000.
75. Rivlin RS: Keeping the young-elderly healthy: is it too late to improve our health through nutrition? *Am J Clin Nutr* 86(Suppl):1572S, 2007.
76. American Dietetic Association: Position of the American Dietetic Association: health implications of dietary fiber, *J Am Diet Assoc* 108:1716, 2008.
77. Neumann M, Friedmann J, Roy MA, et al: Provision of high-protein supplement for patients recovering from hip fracture, *Nutrition* 20(5):415, 2004.
78. Ferry M: Strategies for ensuring good hydration in the elderly, *Nutr Rev* 63(6 pt 2):S22, 2005.
79. Wilson M-M, Morley JE: Impaired cognitive function and mental performance in mild dehydration, *Eur J Clin Nutr* 57(Suppl 2):S24, 2003.
80. Silver HJ, Dietrich MS, Castellanos VH: Increased energy density of the home-delivered meal improves 24-hour nutrient intakes in older adults, *J Am Diet Assoc* 108:2084, 2008.
81. Vitolins MZ, Tooze JA, Golden SL, et al: Older adults in the rural South are not meeting healthful eating guidelines, *J Am Diet Assoc* 107:265, 2007.
82. Murphy SP, White KK, Park SY, et al: Multivitamin-multimineral supplements' effect on total nutrient intake, *Am J Clin Nutr* 85(Suppl):280S, 2007.

FURTHER READINGS AND RESOURCES

Readings

Cluskey M, Grobe D: College weight gain and behavior transitions: male and female differences, *J Am Diet Assoc* 109:325, 2009.

Larson NI, Nelson MC, Neumark-Sztainer D, et al: Making time for meals: meal structure and associations with dietary intake in young adults, *J Am Diet Assoc* 109:72, 2009.

Mattes RD, Campbell WW: Effect of food form and timing of ingestion on appetite and energy intake in lean young adults and in young adults with obesity, *J Am Diet Assoc* 109:430, 2009.

National Center for Health Statistics: *Health, United States, 2008 with chartbook on the health of young adults*, DHHS Pub No 2009–1232, Hyattsville, Md, 2009, U.S. Government Printing Office. Available at www.cdc.gov/nchs/data/hus/hus08.pdf.

These articles address the growing health problems of young adults and the eating and lifestyle patterns that contribute to these problems.

James DC: Cluster analysis defines distinct dietary patterns for African-American men and women, *J Am Diet Assoc* 109:255, 2009.

Li F, Harmer P, Cardinal BJ, et al: Built environment and changes in blood pressure in middle aged and older adults, *Prev Med* 48:237, 2009.

These authors address the influence of appropriate walking environments on the health of middle-aged adults and the need to look at individual food patterns in diet planning.

American Dietetic Association: Food and nutrition programs for community-residing older adults: position of the American Dietetic Association; the American Society for Nutrition, and the Society for Nutrition Education, *J Am Diet Assoc* 110:463, 2010.

Baker EB, Wellman NS: Nutrition concerns in discharge planning for older adults: a need for multidisciplinary collaboration, *J Am Diet Assoc* 105:603, 2005.

Mattes RD: The chemical senses and nutrition in aging: challenging old assumptions, *J Am Diet Assoc* 102(2):192, 2002.

Rocchicciolі JT, Sanford JT: Revisiting geriatric failure to thrive: a complex and compelling clinical condition, *J Gerontol Nurs* 35:18, 2009.

Silver HJ, Dietrich MS, Castellanos VH: Increased energy density of the home-delivered meal improves 24-hour nutrient intakes in older adults, *J Am Diet Assoc* 108:2084, 2008.

These researchers address problems of food availability, impacts of community food programs, and general factors influencing food intake in older adults.

Websites of Interest

Administration on Aging (AoA). This site describes many activities and health-related materials available to assist older adults: www.aoa.gov/.

American Dietetic Association. This site provides food, nutrition, and lifestyle information applicable to all age-groups: www.eatright.org.

U.S. Department of Health and Human Services, National Institutes of Health: Health Information. This site assists consumers with information about healthy lifestyles and specific diseases (individual sites focus on teens, men, and women's health): http://health.nih.gov/.

U.S. National Institutes of Health, National Institute on Aging Information Center. This site lists materials and resources available to older adults and their families: www.nia.nih.gov.

USA.gov—Government Made Easy, Senior Citizens' Resources. This site covers multiple topics such as health, retirement, and grandparents raising grandchildren: www.usa.gov/Topics/Seniors.shtml.

14

Nutrition and Physical Fitness

Staci Nix

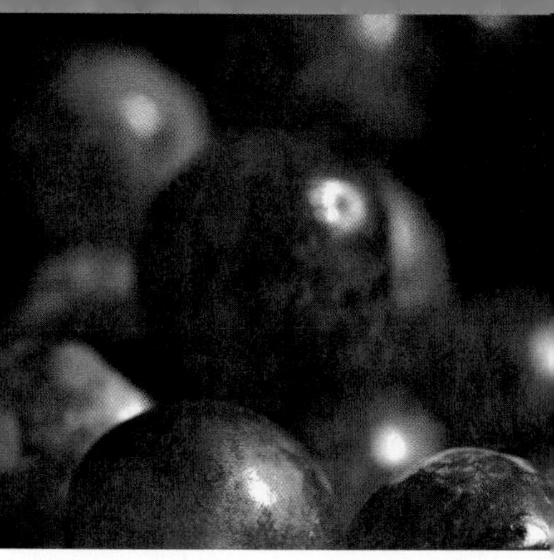

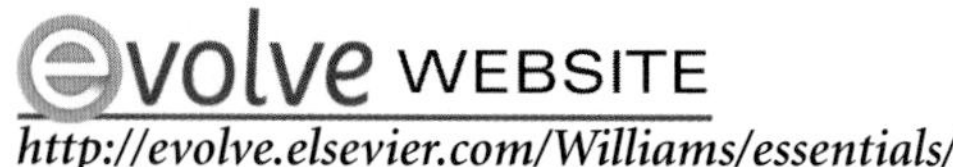

http://evolve.elsevier.com/Williams/essentials/

OUTLINE

Nutrition and physical fitness are integral to health maintenance and disease prevention. In an increasingly fast-paced and technology-dependent society, making regular physical activity part of a busy life requires commitment and effort. However, physical fitness is a vital cornerstone in the preventive approach to controlling chronic disease in modern civilization.

We examine first how nutrition provides energy for muscle action; then we apply principles to enhancing athletic performance and to building a reasonable and appropriate personal exercise program for the adult.

PHYSICAL ACTIVITY, MODERN CIVILIZATION, AND CHRONIC DISEASE

Physical Fitness and Health

The American College of Sports Medicine defines *physical activity* as "a behavior that is any bodily movement produced by the contraction of skeletal muscles that substantially increases energy expenditure."[1] Examples of physical activity would be walking or riding a bike as a form of transportation, using the stairs instead of the escalator, or manual labor such as carpentry work or farming. Physical activity differs from *exercise* based on the structure and purpose. *Exercise* generally refers to structured bouts of physical activity beyond those of normal daily activities. People engage in exercise for the purpose of training and keeping organs and bodily functions healthy. Examples of exercise include aerobic classes, jogging, swimming, cycling, weight training, and other such bouts of planned activities that are for the purpose of improving overall physical fitness.

Physical fitness is an attained set of attributes (i.e., cardiorespiratory endurance; flexibility; agility; balance; body composition; skeletal muscle endurance, strength, and power) that relates to the ability to perform physical activity.[1]

Physical *inactivity* is a global health problem and is estimated by the World Health Organization (WHO) to contribute to 1.9 million deaths annually.[2] Increased participation in regular physical activity as a part of everyday life remains a national health goal. The U.S. Department of Health and Human Services (USDHHS), in its report *Healthy People 2010: Understanding and Improving Health,* has set health-related goals for Americans in nutrition and physical fitness. The 2010 target is to reduce the percentage of individuals who do not engage in any leisure time physical activity to 20% or less in all population groups.[3] Current progress reports indicate that this goal is not likely to be met because 39% of adults still report no leisure time activity.[4] Proposed objectives for 2020 are available at www.healthypeople.gov/.

Health promotion, disease prevention, and disease management require attention to the related roles of nutrition and physical fitness. The U.S. Department of Agriculture (USDA) has published national dietary guidelines every 5 years since 1980. Starting with the *Dietary Guidelines for Americans 2000,*[5] an Aim for Fitness category was added. These guidelines encourage all people, in addition to practicing healthy eating choices, to be physically active each day and to aim for a healthy weight. The *Guidelines* encourage Americans to achieve physical fitness by including cardiovascular conditioning, stretching exercises for flexibility, and resistance exercises for muscle strength and endurance.[6] Specific recommendations include 30 to 60 minutes of moderate physical activity per day to prevent weight gain and 60 to 90 minutes per day to sustain weight loss.[6]

Modern Developed Nations and Chronic Disease

Over time and many generations, daily life in developed nations has evolved from agriculture-based societies requiring constant physical exertion to a more sedentary standard of living. Poor nutrition and inactivity contribute to a host of illnesses, the so-called *diseases of civilization,* including cardiovascular disease, type 2 diabetes, metabolic syndrome, and some forms of cancer.[7] Some researchers estimate that inactivity and poor diet will soon rank as the leading cause of death in the United States.[8]

Substantial research supports the preventive and therapeutic role of a healthy diet and physical activity on such chronic diseases as cardiovascular disease, hypertension, diabetes, metabolic syndrome, and cancer.[7]

BODY IN MOTION

Nature of Energy

The term *energy* refers to the body's ability, or power, to do work. The energy required to do work takes several different forms: mechanical, chemical, electrical, radiant, and heat. Energy, like matter, can neither be created nor destroyed. It can only be changed into another form; therefore energy is constantly cycled in the body and environment. We also speak of energy as being potential or kinetic. Potential energy is stored energy, ready to be used. Kinetic energy is active energy, being used to do work. Energy balance in physical activity requires appropriate nutrition to supply the substrate fuels, which along with oxygen and water meet widely varying levels of energy demands for body action.

Muscle Physiology

Muscle Structure

The synchronized action of millions of specialized cells that make up our skeletal muscle mass makes possible all forms of physical activity. A finely coordinated series of small bundles within the muscle fibers (Figure 14-1) produce a smooth symphony of action through simultaneous and alternating contraction and relaxation. These successively smaller muscle structures include the following:

- *Fasciculi:* This is a bundle of muscle fibers.
- *Muscle fiber:* These are muscle cells composed of bundles of still smaller strands called myofibrils.
- *Myofibril:* Each single myofibril strand of the muscle fiber is made up of the smallest of all the fiber bundles, called myofilaments. Muscular contraction occurs here.
- *Myosin and actin:* Within each myofilament are the contractile proteins, myosin and actin, which are the smallest moving parts of the muscle.

Muscle Action

Inside the muscle fiber, structures run the length of the cell that are called *myofibrils.* Myofibrils contain the contractile proteins, myosin and actin, which interact in the presence of calcium to shorten the cell (and the muscle). The muscle shortens to cause movement in different directions at the joint. When the calcium is pumped out of the surrounding fluid, the cell then "relaxes" to return the muscle elastically to its resting length. This alternating process of muscle contraction and relaxation can continue until muscle glycogen is depleted and muscle fatigue occurs.

Fuel Sources

Fuel sources at rest are a mix of carbohydrate and fat. During exercise, carbohydrate is the primary fuel, and with longer aerobic bouts, some fat is used. A fuel of last resort is protein—only used when the other fuels are exhausted. The high-energy compound driving body cells is *adenosine triphosphate* (ATP), rightly called the *energy currency* of the cell. Various forms of energy are called on for successive energy needs:

- *Immediate energy:* High-power or immediate energy demands over a short time depend on ATP being readily available within the muscle tissue. This amount is used rapidly, and a backup compound, *creatine phosphate (CP),* is made available. These high-energy compounds, however, will sustain exercise for only 5 to 8 seconds.
- *Short-term energy:* For anaerobic bursts like sprints and weight lifting, between 30 seconds and 2 minutes, *muscle glycogen* provides the only available fuel source through the lactate pathway. Although the amount of available glycogen is small, it is an important rapid source of energy for brief muscular effort.
- *Long-term energy:* Exercise continuing more than 2 minutes requires an oxygen-dependent, or *aerobic,* energy system. A constant supply of oxygen in the blood is necessary for continued exercise. Special cell organelles, the *mitochondria,* produce large amounts of ATP. The ATP is produced mainly from glucose and fatty acids and supplies the continued energy needs of the body (Figure 14-2).

KEY TERMS

potential energy Energy existing in stored fuels and ready for action but not yet released and active.

kinetic energy Energy released from body fuels by cell metabolism and now active in moving muscles and energizing all body activities.

substrate The specific organic substance on which a particular enzyme acts to produce new metabolic products.

fasciculi A general term for a small bundle or cluster of muscle, tendon, or nerve fibers.

myofibril Slender thread of muscle; runs parallel to the long axis of the muscle fiber.

myofilaments Threadlike filaments of actin or myosin, which are components of myofibrils.

myosin Myofibril protein whose synchronized meshing action in conjunction with actin causes muscles to contract and relax.

actin Myofibril protein whose synchronized meshing action in conjunction with myosin causes muscles to contract and relax.

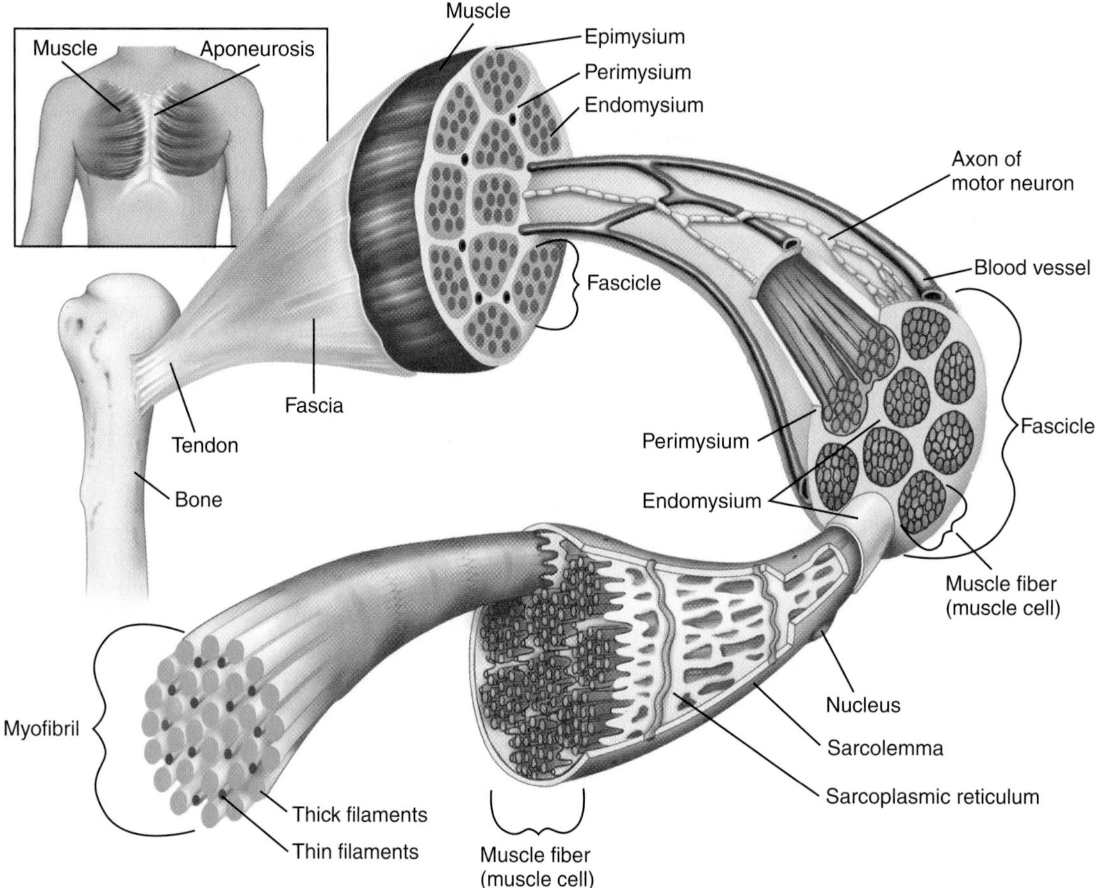

FIGURE 14-1 Skeletal muscle, showing the progressively smaller bundles within bundles. (From Thibodeau GA, Patton KT: *Anatomy & physiology,* ed 5, St Louis, 2003, Mosby.)

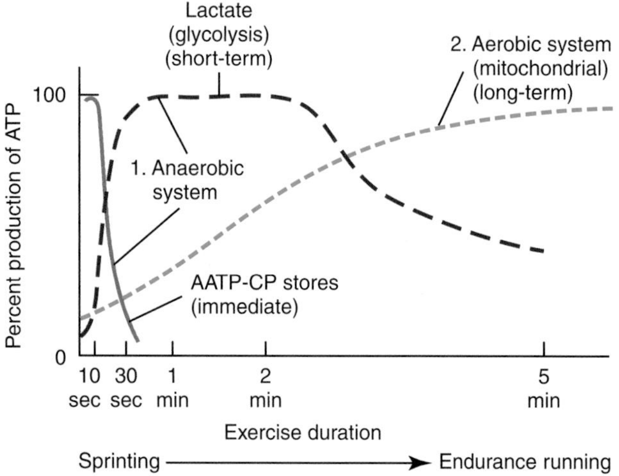

FIGURE 14-2 Contribution of the two energy systems during exercise of increasing duration. The anaerobic energy system provides adenosine triphosphate (ATP) to the working myofilaments from ATP-creatine phosphate stores and the lactate or glycolytic path. The aerobic system supplies ATP from mitochondria, which require oxygen to burn carbohydrates and fats. (Redrawn from Nieman DC: *Exercise testing and prescription,* ed 5, Boston, 2003, McGraw-Hill.)

TABLE 14-1 EFFECT OF INTENSITY ON FUEL TYPE

EXERCISE INTENSITY	FUEL USED BY MUSCLE
<30% VO_2max (easy walking)	Carbohydrates at first, then largely muscle fat stores with durations over 30 minutes
40%-60% VO_2max (jogging, brisk walking)	Fat and carbohydrate used evenly
75% VO_2max (running)	Mainly carbohydrate
≥80% VO_2max (sprinting)	Nearly 100% carbohydrate

Exercise intensity will also affect the preferred source of fuel for the active muscles. More sustained, low-intensity exercises rely primarily on muscle fat stores for energy through the aerobic pathway. As intensity increases, measured through VO_2max (discussed later in the chapter), the source of energy gradually shifts to carbohydrates and uses the lactate system more (Table 14-1).

Nutrients become depleted during continued exercise as the body draws on its stored energy. As demands for ATP increase, the body metabolizes blood glucose and muscle glycogen to provide energy via anaerobic glycolysis. With prolonged exercise of increased intensity; however, the levels of these nutrients fall too low to sustain the body's demands. Without resupply of nutrients, fatigue follows, and exercise cannot continue.

Oxygen Use and Physical Capacity

The most profound limit to exercise is the person's ability to deliver oxygen to the tissues and use it for energy production. This vital ability depends on the fitness of the pulmonary and cardiovascular systems. Because the heart is a muscle, aerobic exercise strengthens it, enabling it to pump more blood per beat, a capacity called stroke volume. The cardiac output—how much the heart pumps out in a given period—depends on the amount of blood per contraction and on the cardiac rate—the number of contractions in a given time. The following factors are influential in fitness level:

- *Cardiovascular fitness:* Cardiovascular fitness is defined in terms of aerobic capacity, which depends on the body's ability to deliver and use oxygen in sufficient quantities to meet the demands of increasing levels of exercise. Oxygen uptake increases with exercise intensity until either the demand is met or the ability to supply it is exceeded. The maximum rate the body can take in oxygen, or aerobic capacity, is called the VO_2max—the maximum uptake volume of oxygen. This capacity determines the intensity and duration of exercise that a person can perform. From the resting level, a steep rise in oxygen consumption occurs during the first 3 minutes of exercise. After approximately 6 minutes the rate levels off into a steady state, indicating equilibrium between the energy required by the exercising muscles and the aerobic energy-producing system. The aerobic capacity of an individual is measured in terms of milliliters of oxygen consumed per kilogram of body weight per minute. Thus persons of differing sizes can be compared equally.
- *Body composition:* Gender differences in aerobic capacity reflect differences in body composition. In general, men have a higher aerobic capacity because of their larger lean body mass, the active metabolic body tissue. These highly metabolic tissues of the body use more oxygen than other tissues such as fat. When oxygen consumption is expressed only in terms of lean body mass instead of body weight, however, men and women have a similar aerobic capacity. In general, women carry more body fat, a gender difference in body composition that serves critical biologic functions. Apart from stored adipose tissue fuel, essential structural and functional body fat in women is 10% to 12% of their body weight (compared with 3% to 5% in men).[1] In addition, because women must, of course, carry their entire body weight as part of their total workload, their performance will be affected accordingly.
- *Genetic influence:* A person's aerobic capacity is chiefly genetically determined. However, the genetic heritage is influenced by body composition, which is associated with gender, and by aerobic training and age. Before puberty, lean body mass is about equal in boys and girls of comparable body size, but it increases rapidly in boys at puberty under the anabolic effect of testosterone. Maximal aerobic capacity then peaks at 18 to 20 years of age and declines gradually thereafter, largely as a result of age-related losses in lean body mass.

NUTRITIONAL NEEDS DURING PHYSICAL ACTIVITY AND EXERCISE

Carbohydrates

Carbohydrates as Fuel Substrate

The major macronutrient for energy support in exercise is carbohydrate. Carbohydrates are the *only* available energy source for anaerobic fuel. Carbohydrate fuels come from two sources: (1) the circulating blood glucose and (2) glycogen stored in muscle and liver tissue. Liver glycogen contributes to blood glucose homeostasis, whereas muscle glycogen is used for the specific muscle in which it is stored.

Carbohydrates in the Diet

Carbohydrates are the preferred energy nutrient. Carbohydrate energy should contribute 45% to 65% of the kilocalories (kcalories or kcal) in the daily diet. Athletes competing in prolonged endurance events should increase their energy from carbohydrates to 60% to 70% of their daily total (6 to 10 g/kg body weight).[9,10] Complex carbohydrates (starches) are preferable to simple carbohydrates (monosaccharides and disaccharides). Starches break down gradually and help maintain blood glucose levels more evenly (avoiding low blood glucose drops), as well as maintain glycogen storage as a constant primary fuel. Simple sugars, however, can supply important immediate energy, especially for athletes in endurance events who may require as much as 5000 kcal/day.

In prolonged bouts of intense exercise, studies have found that diets low in carbohydrate have proved to be less efficient at maintaining energy homeostasis and pace.[11,12] A low-carbohydrate diet decreases the body's capacity for work, which intensifies over time. Athletes on a low-carbohydrate diet are susceptible to fatigue, ketoacidosis, and dehydration. Conversely, studies have found that a high-carbohydrate

KEY TERMS

VO_2max Maximal uptake volume of oxygen during exercise; used to measure the intensity and duration of exercise a person can perform.

stroke volume The amount of blood pumped from a ventricle (chamber of the heart releasing blood to body circulations) with each beat of the heart.

cardiac output Total volume of blood pumped by the heart in 1 minute.

aerobic capacity Milliliters of oxygen consumed per kilogram of body weight per minute; influenced by body composition and fitness level.

TABLE 14-2 MODIFIED DEPLETION-TAPER PRECOMPETITION PROGRAM FOR GLYCOGEN LOADING

DAY	EXERCISE	DIET
1	90-minute period at 70%-75% VO_2max	Mixed diet, 50% carbohydrate (350 g)
2-3	Gradual tapering of time and intensity	Day 1 diet continued
4-5	Tapering of exercise time and intensity continues	Mixed diet, 70% carbohydrate (550 g)
6	Complete rest	Days 4 and 5 diet continued
7	Day of competition	High-carbohydrate pre-event diet

From Wright ED: Carbohydrate nutrition and exercise, *Clin Nutr* 7(1):18, 1988, with permission from Elsevier.

diet enhances muscle glycogen concentrations and exercise performance.[11] In addition, carbohydrate supplementation during exercise bouts improves whole-body carbohydrate oxidation and metabolic efficiency.[13,14] Therefore athletes given carbohydrate feedings before and during exercise maintain glucose concentrations and rates of glucose oxidation necessary to exercise strenuously and delay fatigue.

Carbohydrate loading is a popular practice among endurance athletes that is intended to encourage muscles to deposit more glycogen than normal immediately before an endurance event for extra stored energy. The initial method of glycogen loading was a two-step procedure. First, athletes consumed a diet low in carbohydrates, while simultaneously exercising at high intensity; thus muscle glycogen stores were rapidly depleted. In the second step, athletes did just the opposite; they gradually decreased exercise intensity while consuming a diet high in carbohydrates (approximately 70% to 75% of total caloric intake). Table 14-2 illustrates the second phase of this procedure. Evidence indicates that glycogen storage capacity and rates are higher after glycogen depletion; however, evidence also indicates that a substantial increase in glycogen storage will still occur without the stringent first step of this plan. A recent paper by Sedlock[15] presents flexible strategies for the athlete in carbohydrate loading. Because every gram of glycogen stored requires 2.7 mL of water, potential side effects may occur. Extra water weight in muscles may result in tight or sore muscles that could ultimately hinder performance. All athletes are encouraged to experiment with carbohydrate loading before their competitive events.

Fat

Fat as Fuel Substrate

Fatty acids serve as a fuel source from stored fat tissue. In the presence of oxygen, fatty acids are oxidized to provide energy. The rate at which this can occur is determined in part by the rate of mobilization of fatty acids from storage, but not all stored fat is alike. The body stores fat in two ways: (1) *depot* fat in adipose tissue, which is destined for transport back and forth to other tissues as needed for energy, and (2) *essential* fat in metabolically active tissue, such as bone marrow, heart, lungs, liver, spleen, kidneys, intestines, muscles, and nervous system, which is reserved in these places for necessary structural and functional use only. Although storage depot fat in men and women is roughly comparable, essential fat reserves are significantly different (i.e., about three times greater in women).

Fat in the Diet

Fat, as a fuel substrate, is drawn from the body's stored adipose tissue in response to increasing levels of hormone sensitive lipase (HSL). HSL rises as blood insulin levels decrease, allowing for the mobilization of fatty acids throughout the body. It is not necessary to specifically consume extra fat in food to maintain the body's adipose tissue, because excess kcalories in the diet will be converted to fat and stored regardless of the dietary source. We do not need to eat in excess of our dietary needs to burn fat, and no danger exists of depleting our fat stores before exercise has proceeded to exhaustion. Thus no basis exists for increased levels of fat in the diet. On the other hand, a moderate level of fat is necessary in the diet for the absorption of fat-soluble vitamins and to ensure adequate intake of the essential fatty acids (linoleic and α-linolenic acids). An extremely low fat intake can be medically dangerous by creating a deficiency of the essential fatty acids. The standard recommendation that dietary fat should not exceed 20% to 35% of the total daily kcalorie intake, per the Acceptable Macronutrient Distribution Range (AMDR), is ample for most healthy individuals.

Protein

Protein as Fuel Substrate

Authorities agree that under normal circumstances protein makes a relatively insignificant and inefficient contribution to energy during exercise. Although some amino acids can feed into the basic energy cycle, the extent of this input during exercise is minimal.[16,17] In glycogen-depleted muscles, however, somewhat more protein may be used as a fuel substrate; however, exercise performance is significantly reduced in such circumstances.[18]

Protein in the Diet

A daily intake of 0.8 to 1 g of protein/kg of body weight is sufficient to meet the general needs of the *physically active* person. This amounts to the recommended daily dietary intake for adults, with 10% to 35% of the kcalories in the diet coming from protein. Misconceptions surrounding the use of and need for supplemental protein in ill-informed athletes begins as early as high school.[19] No indication exists that supplement forms of protein or amino acids are superior to food forms of protein. Excess protein in the diet cannot be stored in the body as amino acids; thus protein is converted to fat, and the amine portion (nitrogen) must be excreted. Although excess protein intake does not significantly alter hydration status, it does put a burden on the kidneys to excrete the increased urea coming from the liver.[20] High-protein diets and supplements increase intestinal calcium absorption and excretion of calcium in the urine, particularly in women.[21] Researchers do not believe that this increased calcium excretion is detrimental to bone; however, it may be problematic to individuals prone to kidney stones.

Micronutrients

Vitamins and Minerals as Catalytic Cofactors

Vitamins and minerals cannot be used as fuel substrates. They are not oxidized or expended in the process of energy production. Vitamins and minerals are, however, essential as catalytic cofactors in enzyme reactions.

Vitamins and Minerals in the Diet

Increased physical exertion during exercise or athletic training does not require a greater intake of vitamins and minerals beyond current recommendations. A well-balanced diet will supply adequate amounts of vitamins and minerals, and exercise may improve the body's efficient use of them. Because athletes, for example, have an increased dietary need for energy, their larger kcalorie intake from high-quality food sources will boost their general intake of vitamins and minerals. If, however, an athlete is restricting calories, vitamin and mineral deficiencies are a possibility. Energy-restricting behaviors often result in avoidance of animal products such as meat and dairy products, which are particularly rich sources of calcium, iron, and zinc.

On the opposite end of the spectrum, multivitamin and mineral supplementation does not improve physical performance in healthy athletes eating a well-balanced diet. In addition, the potential side effects of toxicity from megasupplements are well-known (see Chapters 6 and 7).

Hydration: Water and Electrolytes

Water and Dehydration

Dehydration limits exercise capacity in endurance- and resistance-training activities.[22,23] The extent of limitation depends on many factors, such as intensity and duration of exercise, body temperature, level of fitness, and preexercise state of hydration (see the *Case Study* box, "Fluid and Energy Needs for Endurance Athletes"). Because of dehydration, athletes may experience problems such as cramps, delirium, vomiting, hypothermia, and hyperthermia. With careful planning before athletic events, as well as providing fluid replacement during those events, many of these problems can be prevented. Regular fluid intake should be planned for all types of athletes, not just individuals participating in endurance events. Some strategies to increase fluid intake by athletes are given in Box 14-1.

Cause of Dehydration. ATP production results in significant heat release within the working muscle. During moderate-intensity physical activity, most individuals maintain a body temperature within a desirable range. However, during intense exercise, or exercise in hot or humid environments, heat production may exceed the body's acceptable temperature range for performance and the body's heat tolerance capacity.[24] Sweating is our primary mechanism for dissipating body heat. The major source of fluid loss in sweat is plasma fluid. High-intensity or long-endurance events (especially in hot climates) can cause the loss of several liters of water as sweat to regulate body temperature. Unless this fluid is replaced, consequences from dehydration and heat illness may result.

Prevention of Dehydration. The thirst mechanism may not be the most sensitive indicator of hydration needs during exercise. When someone is thirsty, he or she is already dehydrated. To prevent dehydration, athletes are advised to

---

CASE STUDY

Fluid and Energy Needs for Endurance Athletes

Jamie is a 25-year-old man training for an ultramarathon race of 50 miles. He is 5 feet, 10 inches tall and currently weighs 170 lb. On his long runs of more than 3 hours, he has been drinking water, approximately 30 oz, and consuming one GU (an energy supplement containing 100 kcal from simple sugar) at the 2-hour mark. Jamie is coming to you for advice because he is becoming increasingly weak and nauseous toward the end of his runs. He reports feeling light-headed and irritable on his long training days. Jamie states that he is eating an egg salad sandwich with two hard-boiled eggs mixed with 3 tbsp of mayonnaise on whole wheat bread about 20 minutes before his run.

Questions for Analysis

1. What sources of fuel is Jamie predominately using in this type of exercise?
2. How much fluid should he be consuming during a 3-hour run?
3. Based on his weight, how many calories and grams of carbohydrate should Jamie consume during his run?
4. On what time schedule would you recommend that he consume his fluid and carbohydrate?
5. What would you recommend regarding Jamie's preexercise meal?

BOX 14-1 STRATEGIES FOR SPORTS TEAM MEMBERS TO INCREASE FLUID INTAKE

- Establish a regular schedule; drink during warm-up exercises and between periods of play.
- Give each player a sports squeeze bottle.
- Supply players with a sports drink that tastes good while exercising.
- Make available a choice of fluids to drink.
- Offer cool fluids.
- Avoid carbonated beverages because athletes tend to drink less when the beverage is carbonated.

From Palumbo CM: Nutrition concerns related to the performance of a baseball team, *J Am Diet Assoc* 100(6):704, 2000. Copyright with permission from the American Dietetic Association.

(1) establish euhydration at least several hours before activity; (2) drink during exercise to avoid excessive water loss, defined as >2% body weight loss from water; and (3) replace fluid loss after completion of exercise (Figure 14-3).[25] The American College of Sports Medicine recommends that athletes develop a customized fluid replacement program catering to their needs and preferences (e.g., fluid temperature, taste preferences).[25] Measuring weight pre- and post-activity is an easy and appropriate method to estimate fluid loss in sweat. Hydration with fluids containing glucose and sodium reduces urinary fluid loss. Therefore during longer events (1+ hours), fluids with mild solutions of sodium and glucose are recommended to help reduce fluid loss and prevent dehydration.[26]

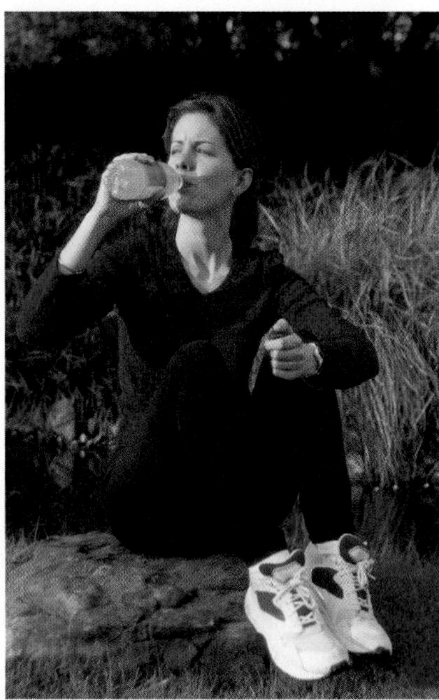

FIGURE 14-3 Frequent small drinks of cold water during extended exercise prevent dehydration. (Credit: PhotoDisc.)

Electrolytes

A number of specialty sports drinks are now available with replacement electrolytes (see the *Evidence-Based Practice* box, "Sorting Out the Sports Drinks Saga"). In the 1960s researchers believed that sodium losses exceeded water loss during vigorous activity with substantial sweat production. However, sweat is more dilute than internal fluids, and thus we lose proportionately more water than sodium. In most instances, electrolytes are replaced with the athlete's next meal. However, during longer and more demanding endurance events, especially in warm or humid environments, a mild sodium and glucose (20 to 50 mmol/L sodium and 4% to 8% glucose solution) sports drink that has rapid gastric emptying and intestinal absorption times may be beneficial.[25,26] For ultraendurance events lasting between 3 and 24 hours, fluid replacements including electrolytes are essential to adequately replace sodium losses and avoid the risk of **hyponatremia**.[26]

EVIDENCE-BASED PRACTICE

Sorting Out the Sports Drinks Saga

Problem: Sorting through the many available sports drinks and the plethora of claims that accompany each one is no easy task. Ultimately we need to answer these questions: How much and what kind of a sports drink is needed during physical activity and exercise?

The current saga of sports drinks began with a solution called *Gatorade,* a beverage its developers named for their university's football team. They reasoned that if they analyzed the sweat of their players, then they could replace the lost minerals and water in a drink containing some flavoring, coloring, and sugars to make it acceptable, and it would taste better and have more benefits than plain water. Although Gatorade is beneficial for some athletes, most do not need it during general exercise.

However, what endurance athletes do need, especially in hot weather, is water and fuel in the form of carbohydrates. For athletes losing substantial amounts of water and sodium through sweat, electrolyte replacement is also an important consideration. Hyponatremia (plasma sodium concentration <135 mEq/L), although rare, can be fatal. The most common cause of hyponatremia in endurance athletes results from excess sodium loss through sweat combined with fluid replacement of plain water. Water dilutes the plasma sodium even more, exacerbating the condition. Thus sports drinks with simple carbohydrates and electrolytes are necessary for endurance athletes.

Simply adding sugar to water holds it in the stomach longer, where it is not available for immediate needs. To meet the body's need during long events, a second category of sports drinks is available, containing glucose polymers instead of sugar, as well as less sodium. These short chains of about five glucose molecules—maltodextrins—are produced in the breakdown of starch. These drinks are less concentrated and are only slightly sweetened and flavored. In addition, they leave the stomach rapidly, thus making them ideal as a continuing fuel source for the endurance athlete.

Another category of sports drinks on the market adds large amounts of vitamins and minerals to their solutions. All of these extra vitamins do not help an athlete's performance; on a hot day a perspiring athlete could easily down a megadose in four or five bottles. However, recent studies indicate that controlled use in intermittent moderate- to high-intensity exercise improves the athlete's performance.

As a general guide, it is worth the time to sort out the costs and claims made by sports drink manufacturers. These products are not for everyone. Although special sports drinks may meet the needs of athletes competing in physically demanding endurance events, they are not required by those participating in less demanding sports activities. Water is the best solution for regular needs—and it costs far less.

BIBLIOGRAPHY

American College of Sports Medicine, American Dietetic Association, Dietitians of Canada: Joint position statement: nutrition and athletic performance, *Med Sci Sports Exerc* 32(12):2130, 2000.

NUTRITION AND ATHLETIC PERFORMANCE

Exercise and Energy

Exercise raises the body's kcalorie expenditure and has the additional benefit of helping to regulate appetite to meet these needs. Table 14-3 gives some examples of the amount of kcalories spent in various activities. The building of glycogen reserves is important for athletes such as long-distance runners who compete in endurance events and need a steady supply of energy within the muscle. Persons at moderate exercise levels have been shown to eat less than inactive persons, which may be related to an internal "set point" regulating the amount of body fat the person will carry. According to this theory, the set point is raised (i.e., more body fat is stored) when the individual becomes inactive. In any case, when exercise levels rise from mild or moderate amounts up to strenuous levels, kcaloric needs also rise to supply needed fuel.

Active people, even athletes, require no more dietary fat than their inactive counterparts. Carbohydrate is the preferred fuel and is the critical food for the active person—not only before an exercise period but also during the recovery phase. The complex carbohydrate forms (i.e., starches) sustain energy needs and supply added fiber, vitamins, and minerals. Thus the recommended composition of energy nutrients to support physical activity in highly active people is as follows[9]:

- *Carbohydrate:* 6 to 10 g/kg body weight per day
- *Protein:* 1.2 to 1.4 g/kg of body weight per day for endurance athletes and 1.6 to 1.7 g/kg body weight per day for resistance- and strength-training athletes
- *Fat:* 15% to 25% of total kcalories

TABLE 14-3 APPROXIMATE ENERGY EXPENDITURE PER HOUR DURING VARIOUS ACTIVITIES

ACTIVITY	KCALORIES PER HOUR*
Sleeping	63
Lying/sitting, awake	70
Standing, relaxed	84
Rapid typing, sitting	105
Dressing and undressing	140
Walking slowly (24 min/mile)	210
Water aerobics	280
High-impact aerobics	490
Football, flag/touch	560
Walking very fast (12 min/mile)	560
Stair, treadmill	630
Swimming, vigorous effort	700
Running (8 min/mile)	875

From Nix S: *Williams' basic nutrition & diet therapy*, ed 12, St Louis, 2005, Mosby.
*For an adult weighing 70 kg (154 lb).

Pregame and Training Meals

Protein and fat delay the emptying of the stomach, and neither contributes to the glycogen stores needed during exercise. Therefore the ideal pregame meal is approximately 200 to 300 g of carbohydrate that is eaten about 3 to 4 hours before the event, allowing adequate time for digestion and absorption.[9] An example meal is illustrated in Box 14-2. This meal should be high in complex carbohydrates, moderate in protein, and with little fat or fiber. Good food choices include pasta, bread, bagels, muffins, and cereal with nonfat milk. Throughout the period of vigorous training, a high-carbohydrate diet with 500 to 600 g/day is recommended, such as that illustrated in Table 14-4. Small amounts of carbohydrate-containing foods or drinks may be consumed briefly before the event without affecting performance for most athletes. All athletes should experiment with their own level of tolerance during training sessions.

Energy During Exercise

For activities lasting less than 1 hour, most athletes do not need exogenous sources of energy during the exercise period. However, it is well-known that performance is enhanced during longer endurance events with the interval consumption of carbohydrates. The American College of Sports Medicine, the American Dietetic Association, and the Dietitians of Canada recommend eating or drinking 0.7 g of carbohydrate per kilogram of body weight per hour (approximately 30 to 60 g/hour) during long events.[9] It is most effective to consume equal amounts of the preferred food every 15 to 20 minutes throughout the event rather than consuming the entire 30 to 60 g at once. Athletes should experiment with various forms of glucose before competition to determine what is best tolerated. A large variety of sports drinks, gels, and other forms of carbohydrates are available from which the athlete may choose. The food of choice should provide carbohydrates primarily from glucose, with little or no fat, protein, or fiber.

Energy After Exercise: Recovery

Proper nutrition is not only important to the athlete before and during exercise but also plays a major role in recovery after the event. It is well accepted that fluid and carbohydrate replacement beverages consumed immediately after

BOX 14-2 SAMPLE PREGAME MEAL

This sample pregame meal includes approximately 203 g of carbohydrates, is high in complex carbohydrates, and is low in protein, fat, and fiber:

- 1½ cups cooked spaghetti (332 kcal, 65 g carbohydrate)
- ¾ cup tomato sauce (135 kcal, 20 g carbohydrate)
- 1 slice French bread, large (281 kcal, 55 g carbohydrate)
- 1 baked potato, large (278 kcal, 63 g carbohydrate)

KEY TERMS

hyponatremia Serum sodium less than 135 mEq/L; a relative excess of body water compared with sodium.

TABLE 14-4 600-g CARBOHYDRATE DIET

MENU	CARBOHYDRATE
Breakfast	
1 orange, 2⅝ in diameter	16 g
2 cups plain oatmeal, cooked	45 g
1 cup skim milk	12 g
1 oat bran muffin, medium	55 g
1 tbsp jam	14 g
Snack	
½ cup seedless raisins	57 g
Lunch	
Lettuce salad	
1 cup romaine lettuce	2 g
½ cup garbanzo beans	27 g
½ cup tomatoes, chopped	4 g
2 tbsp French dressing	5 g
2 cups macaroni and cheese	94 g
1½ cups apple juice	43 g
Snack	
2 slices whole wheat bread	24 g
1 tbsp peanut butter	3 g
Dinner	
½ turkey breast, no skin	0 g
2 cups mashed potatoes, with whole milk	74 g
1 cup peas and onions	16 g
¾ cup fruit salad (banana, pineapple, papaya, guava)	43 g
1 cup skim milk	12 g
Snack	
1 cup cranberry juice, unsweetened	33 g
1 oz pretzels	22 g
TOTAL	601 g

Data from U.S. Department of Agriculture, Agricultural Research Service: *National nutrient database for standard reference,* Release 18, Washington, DC, 2005, U.S. Government Printing Office. Available at www.nal.usda.gov/fnic/foodcomp/search/index.html, 8/1/2009.

a glycogen-depleting endurance event will result in better glycogen synthesis and muscle recovery than if those same replacement beverages were consumed 2 hours or more after the event.[9] Beverages of 6% glucose concentration are adequate during this period, but increased concentrations may be consumed, depending on the tolerance of the athlete. For athletes taking only a short break between events (e.g., triathletes), foods and beverages ingested should be limited to primarily carbohydrate-containing substances. For athletes recovering for longer periods of time, a replacement beverage containing at least 1.2 g of carbohydrate per kilogram of body weight (over several hours) results in an increased rate of muscle glycogen recovery.[27]

Myths and Misinformation

Athletes and their coaches are particularly susceptible to myths and claims about foods and dietary supplements, relentlessly searching for the competitive edge (see the *Focus on Culture* box, "The Winning Edge—or Over the Edge?"). Knowing this, marketers unremittingly exploit this search. Manufacturers sometimes make distorted and false claims about products. For example, pangamic acid, marketed as "vitamin B_{15}" although it is not a vitamin at all, carried claims about its ability to enhance oxygen transport during exercise, to lessen muscle fatigue, and to increase endurance. Naturally, if such a compound existed, then it would be of interest to athletes and their trainers. However, scientific research has exposed these claims as unfounded.[28] Nevertheless, products and advertisements still appear for "vitamin B_{15}," although it is currently illegal to distribute pangamic acid in the United States.

Training and Precompetition Abuses Among Athletes

Weight Control Measures

The sport of wrestling has a long history of widely fluctuating weight patterns among its athletes. Wrestlers often restrict food and fluid intake to qualify for a weight classification that is less than their off-season weight, seeking to gain advantages in strength, speed, and leverage over a smaller opponent. This practice of "making weight" still seems to be an ingrained tradition that produces large, frequent, and rapid weight loss and regain cycles, with methods such as dehydration, severe

FOCUS ON CULTURE

The Winning Edge—or Over the Edge?

Athletes, their coaches, and our entire culture have become increasingly aware that the percentage of body fat versus the percentage of lean body mass is an influential factor on athletic performance. Each extra pound of body fat an athlete carries into competition is nonproductive weight. It is the muscles, the lean body mass, that provide the strength, agility, and endurance required to win.

Because of this, athletes strive to achieve as low a percentage of body fat as possible while still maintaining good health. In reaching for such a goal, however, many young athletes develop an abhorrence of body fat, resulting in food aversion and the undertaking of excessive weight loss regimens. These self-generated excesses are commonly reinforced by those surrounding the young athletes: coaches, teammates, and parents. Such an all-consuming focus may result in compulsive behaviors, driving the athlete to set unrealistic goals and abusive weight loss.

Fortunately, such excessive voluntary weight losses in young athletes are not usually the result of chronic emotional problems,

FOCUS ON CULTURE

The Winning Edge—or Over the Edge?—cont'd

as with other psychologic eating disorders. The reasons typically are more superficial, resulting from an accumulation of immediate and short-term goals and concerns. These athletes usually respond well to counseling and can reverse the excessive behavior with the support of concerned friends and teammates.

Yet for a few individuals, compulsive fixation on lean body mass and the loss of body fat becomes obsessive and enduring. For example, a compulsive runner's ideal of 5% body fat is regularly found only in ballet dancers, gymnasts, fashion models, and victims of anorexia nervosa. Unfortunately our mass media culture reinforces the view that the most desirable attributes of beauty are slimness in women and physical prowess in men. When a susceptible individual enters a time of stress in search of a firm identity, he or she may turn toward cultural and media stereotypes to provide a positive self-concept. For women this stress is usually encountered during adolescence, when some young women think being physically attractive is the key to social acceptance. For men the sense of self is more closely tied to their vocational and sexual effectiveness, both of which some men relate to their physical abilities. Thus the test of a man's abilities tends to occur more often in adulthood, which may result in his preoccupation with physical fitness as a way to deny any decline in strength or ability. This concept may explain why the majority of compulsive runners, those who believe they must run despite everything, including injury or ill health, are men. Such long-term compulsive fixation on body image in susceptible individuals may result in disordered eating requiring extensive counseling.

Our culture views compulsive dieting, as in anorexia nervosa, as a serious psychologic disorder; compulsive training, on the other hand, is seen as a positive personality trait showing dedication. In reality, both may be symptomatic of unstable self-concepts and attempts to establish a firm sense of identity. They are perceptual disorders: the anorexia nervosa victim always sees himself or herself as fat; the compulsive runner always sees himself or herself as out of shape. Such risk factors are not necessarily true for all competitive athletes. Caucasian female athletes reported the highest prevalence of disordered eating and the lowest level of self-esteem in a 2004 study examining the cultural and ethnic differences in collegiate athletes. For these individuals, no goal, once attained, is sufficiently satisfying. If 5% body fat is achieved, then the person strives for 4%. Such striving, often despite physical indications against it, has resulted in permanent disabilities and even death, sometimes from cardiac arrest caused by a linoleic acid deficiency.

The danger of athletic pressure leading to eating disorders was highlighted by the 1994 death from anorexia nervosa of 22-year-old Christy Henrich, a world-class American gymnast. At 4 feet 10 inches (147 cm) and 95 lb (43 kg), Christy won a silver medal at the 1989 U.S. National Championships. She was known as a perfectionist, who pushed herself hard, a characteristic that, when extreme, is often associated with eating disorders in athletes. She felt compelled to lose more weight and at times limited herself to only an apple a day even while continuing to train. Because of her eating disorder, she eventually lost the strength to perform and was forced to retire from competition. She weighed only 60 lb (27 kg) when she died. Although her death marked the first time an American gymnast had died from an eating disorder, such problems are widely known in competitive women's gymnastics, especially at the national and international levels.

Although physical fitness and athletic accomplishments may be admirable goals, the thrill of victory for a small percentage of participants may be a hollow one if the victory is at the expense of their health.

BIBLIOGRAPHY

Johnson C, Crosby R, Engel S, et al: Gender, ethnicity, self-esteem and disordered eating among college athletes, *Eat Behav* 5(2):147, 2004.

Obituary: Christy Henrich 1972-1994, *Int Gymnast* 36(10):1, 1994.

food restriction, and loss of food and fluid through induced vomiting and use of laxatives and diuretics. Such disordered eating affects normal growth, and progressive dehydration impairs regulation of body temperature and cardiovascular function. Other sports such as bodybuilding and gymnastics often follow similar routines, especially before competition. In gymnastics, for example, it is not uncommon for young preadolescent girls wishing to maintain a small body size in the face of advancing age to reduce food intake and body fat, sometimes developing eating disorders. As a result, a cascade of events may follow—impaired growth, delayed puberty, induced amenorrhea from low estrogen levels, disruption or delay in bone density development, and even later osteoporosis. A similar pattern has been observed among young runners.

Drug Abuse

From ancient Greek runners and discus throwers in the first Olympian contests to top competitors from around the world in current Olympic events, athletes have experimented with various ergogenic aids in their eternal search for the competitive edge or the perfect body. Modern athletes—from professional football players to their aspiring high school counterparts—are doing the same thing, trying to find the magic potion in everything from bee pollen and seaweed to freeze-dried liver flakes, gelatin, amino acid supplements, and ginseng. Such efforts have been worthless in most cases but fortunately not particularly harmful. However, in the

KEY TERMS

amenorrhea The absence of menses (menstrual cycle) entirely or no more than three periods in a year; associated with lower-than-normal estrogen levels in women.

osteoporosis Abnormal thinning of bone, producing a porous, fragile, latticelike bone tissue of enlarged spaces that is prone to fracture or deformity.

ergogenic Tendency to increase work output; various substances that increase work or exercise capacity and output.

case of *anabolic-androgenic steroids,* which are now epidemic in the sporting world, great danger and even death may lie ahead for the user. These dangers include cardiovascular health risk, impaired liver function, disturbances in normal steroid production, increased aggression and hostility, mood disturbances, and additional disturbances in psychologic and dermatologic condition.[29]

The use of legal pharmacologic agents in an illegal manner has created a black market network, which adds criminal jeopardy and street preparation impurities to the drug's inherent dangers. Abuse of anabolic steroids in the United States has moved from its early use among bodybuilders to invade almost all areas of athletics, beginning as early as adolescence.[30] In addition, other abuses amplify the dangers of steroids. For example, a large dose of a diuretic such as furosemide (Lasix, 80 to 120 mg) may be taken on the day of drug testing to dilute the urine and decrease the risk of detection. In addition, much like abused drugs, large megadoses of vitamins and minerals are used as ergogenic aids in all areas and levels of sports.

Risks for Female Athletes

Some female athletes entering highly competitive and demanding sports could face health risks related to anemia and low bone mineral density (BMD) if their diets are not meeting increased calorie needs. These risks are especially prevalent for women athletes in sports with intensive training and endurance events, such as gymnastics and running. Highly skilled dancers in the performing arts world often face similar risks.

Sports Anemia and Iron Deficiency Anemia

Normal hemoglobin (Hb) values are 12 to 15 g/dL for women and 13.8 to 17.2 g/dL for men. Iron deficiency anemia is defined as Hb levels less than these ranges. Although absolute anemia is rare among competitive athletes, low normal values are typical. As baseline plasma volume increases with aerobic training, the concentration of Hb (found within red blood cells) is reduced as a percentage of total blood. Such a situation is more appropriately referred to as *sports anemia* rather than iron deficiency anemia, because the total volume of red blood cells is normal. Additional iron intake, whether through food or supplementation, is not needed in sports anemia. However, care must be taken to appropriately distinguish sports anemia from other forms of true anemias.

True iron deficiency anemia is typically a result of inadequate iron in the diet, decreased iron absorption, or increased iron losses. Reduced Hb in an athlete's blood means reduced oxygen-carrying capacity with obvious implications for aerobic capacity and the ability to sustain an exercise workload. One of the first implications for iron deficiency anemia is exertional fatigue. Unless a woman is experiencing amenorrhea, she will have cyclic menstrual loss of iron. Some iron is lost in profuse sweating and occasionally because of *intravascular hemolysis,* which is the rupture of red blood cells caused by the stresses of heavy exercise. Neither sweat nor intravascular hemolysis is believed to be a major contributor to iron loss. Thus iron intake should be evaluated and addressed regularly.

Low Bone Mineral Density

An inadequate diet, intentionally or not, combined with an interrupted menstrual cycle can lead to low BMD (osteopenia). In some cases the bone loss may progress to a state of osteoporosis at an abnormally young age (Figure 14-4). Because of the three contributing factors—(1) energy restriction, (2) menstrual dysfunction, and (3) bone loss—it has been called the *female athlete triad* (see the *Perspectives in Practice* box, "The Female Athlete Triad: How Performance and Social Pressure Can Lead to Low Bone Mass").[31]

PERSPECTIVES IN PRACTICE

*The Female Athlete Triad: How Performance and Social Pressure Can Lead to Low Bone Mass**

The female athlete triad consists of three health afflictions: (1) disordered eating, (2) menstrual disturbances, and (3) osteopenia (low bone mass) or even osteoporosis. Low BMD is often the final result of the triad that affects women, and it is the leading cause of stress fractures and injuries throughout the body, some of which may be irreversible. Many women who are in top physical form are the most likely to develop these three linked complications, and health problems because social and performance pressure may steer women to extreme eating habits and exercise regimens. The dilemma facing women athletes today is how to maintain optimal physical performance while not provoking health risks.

Women who participate in competitive endurance sports, such as rowing or long-distance running, or who are judged partially on physical appearance, such as in ice skating, diving, gymnastics, or dancing, are more likely to be preoccupied with their weight and to have self-image issues. Social and competitive pressure for a woman to be thin can contribute to her sense of imperfection. These demands and pressures can lead to disordered eating patterns, which in combination with strenuous exercise may result in low energy levels. This drop in energy will be followed by a drop in performance as the athlete loses focus and concentration and is fatigued. Some women develop psychologic eating disorders, such as bulimia nervosa, which is characterized by binge eating followed by compensatory mechanisms, or anorexia nervosa, characterized by the refusal or inability to consume sufficient calories for daily requirements. These disorders may, in turn, progress to additional health problems including depression or low self-esteem, seizures, cardiac arrhythmia, myocardial infarction, or other health complications. The seriousness of the eating disorder is linked to the amount of stress and concern the woman feels over her body image, combined with the amount of emphasis placed on weight by the woman, her trainers, and her coaches. Athletes often believe that leanness enhances performance, and some are willing to go to great lengths to satisfy perfectionist needs.

PERSPECTIVES IN PRACTICE

The Female Athlete Triad: How Performance and Social Pressure Can Lead to Low Bone Mass—cont'd*

Poor caloric intake and disordered eating can cause menstrual irregularity. Amenorrhea is the suppression of menstrual cycles to a level of zero to three menses a year, and primary amenorrhea is the repression of all menstrual cycles until after age 16. This condition is often found in young female gymnasts who, in the most competitive circles, may actually strive to delay the onset of puberty to maintain small, childlike physiques. Some women may experience oligomenorrhea, which are sporadic cycles that occur three to nine times a year. The levels of estrogen and progesterone that regulate menses can be affected by metabolism, intensive exercise, dieting, or stress.

Several treatments are available for female athletes: hormone replacement therapy, increased caloric intake, decreased exercise, weight gain, and calcium supplements. Evidence suggests that raising estrogen and progesterone levels and increasing caloric intake are the most effective measures, yet a wide range of treatment is prescribed. Hormone therapy alone will not improve BMD. Education and further research are needed to find the optimal course.

Menstrual irregularities are related to low bone density. Before the age of 30, bone density reaches its peak, and it is vital for young women to strive for dense bones in early adulthood to maintain healthy bone density later in life. If the density of bones is compromised, then osteopenia occurs; if severe enough, it can be a signal of future osteoporosis. In active young women with inadequate diets and menstrual irregularities, cases of bone density 25% lower than normal have been reported. These thin bones increase the likelihood of stress fractures and injuries, and women are far more likely to incur such injuries than men.

Some studies, however, indicate that weight-bearing activities, such as gymnastics, seem to actually improve bone density, even perhaps in vertebrae, and they may help prevent density decreases later in life. However, the problem facing women athletes who are eating improperly is that the decline in BMD is amplified as menstrual cycles continue to be erratic. Weight-bearing sports will not overcome the tendency for participants to have low BMD if diet and exercise levels are not carefully monitored.

The best course of action is to have women athletes monitor their diets to ensure adequate caloric intake and sufficient micronutrient consumption. The prevention of osteoporosis later in life depends on habits of the individual and the modification of factors that can lead to the triad of eating disturbances, menstrual irregularity, and low bone density. Body weight is individual, depending on height and skeletal structure, and one specific weight goal should not exist for all female athletes.

The societal and competitive pressures that cause the initial step in this three-step process must be addressed. Asking female athletes to sacrifice their health for an unrealistic body image projected on them by others (as well as their coaches' and trainers' desire for vicarious victory) must not alter what constitutes acceptable eating habits. In today's weight conscious society, the emphasis must not be on a perfect image, size, or body but rather on the perfect balance of health and training. The female athlete's skeletal integrity suffers as she resorts to drastic measures in her aspiration for an overly lean physical image, but her male athlete counterpart has no such risk because his bone density is not dependent on menstrual regularity.

The need to educate trainers, athletes, and health professionals about the consequences of neglected nutrition is imperative. Young female athletes must understand that deprivation of life's essential nutrients does significant bodily harm.

BIBLIOGRAPHY

Feingold D, Hame SL: Female athlete triad and stress fractures, *Orthop Clin North Am* 37(4):575, 2006.

Fredericson M, Kent K: Normalization of bone density in a previously amenorrheic runner with osteoporosis, *Med Sci Sports Exerc* 37(9):1481, 2005.

Lloyd T, Petit MA, Lin HM, et al: Lifestyle factors and the development of bone mass and bone strength in young women, *J Pediatr* 144(6):776, 2004.

Nattiv A, Loucks AB, Manore MM, et al: American College of Sports Medicine position stand. The female athlete triad, *Med Sci Sports Exerc* 39(10):1867, 2007.

*With contribution from Meredith Catherine Williams.

An estimated 40% to 60% of a woman's normal BMD for her lifetime is created during adolescence, when her sex hormone estrogen becomes active. The diet and hormones must work together. An adequate amount of calcium must exist in the diet, as well as normal functioning of the female estrogen cycle that stimulates osteoblastic activity (bone growth). Unfortunately, many young female athletes restrict their diets in an effort to control their weight, growth, and body fat, with resulting inadequate dietary energy and calcium. Some may have more profound eating disorders, such as anorexia nervosa. At the same time, intense athletic training in women can lead to **primary** or **secondary amenorrhea.** Amenorrhea is more common in athletes than in nonathletes; it is especially prevalent among aesthetic, endurance, and weight-class sports.[32] When athletic training begins before normal menarche, the onset of puberty and its associated growth and development pattern is delayed. Such delays include the secondary sex characteristics shaping the female figure, as evidenced in the petite bodies of young gymnasts. When the menstrual cycle is delayed or interrupted, normal estrogen levels are depressed. As a result, these young women

KEY TERMS

osteopenia Below-normal level of bone mineral density, which increases the risk of stress fractures; the bone thinning is not as severe as that found in osteoporosis.

primary amenorrhea Delay of menarche past the age of 16.

secondary amenorrhea Cessation of the normal menstrual cycle after menarche.

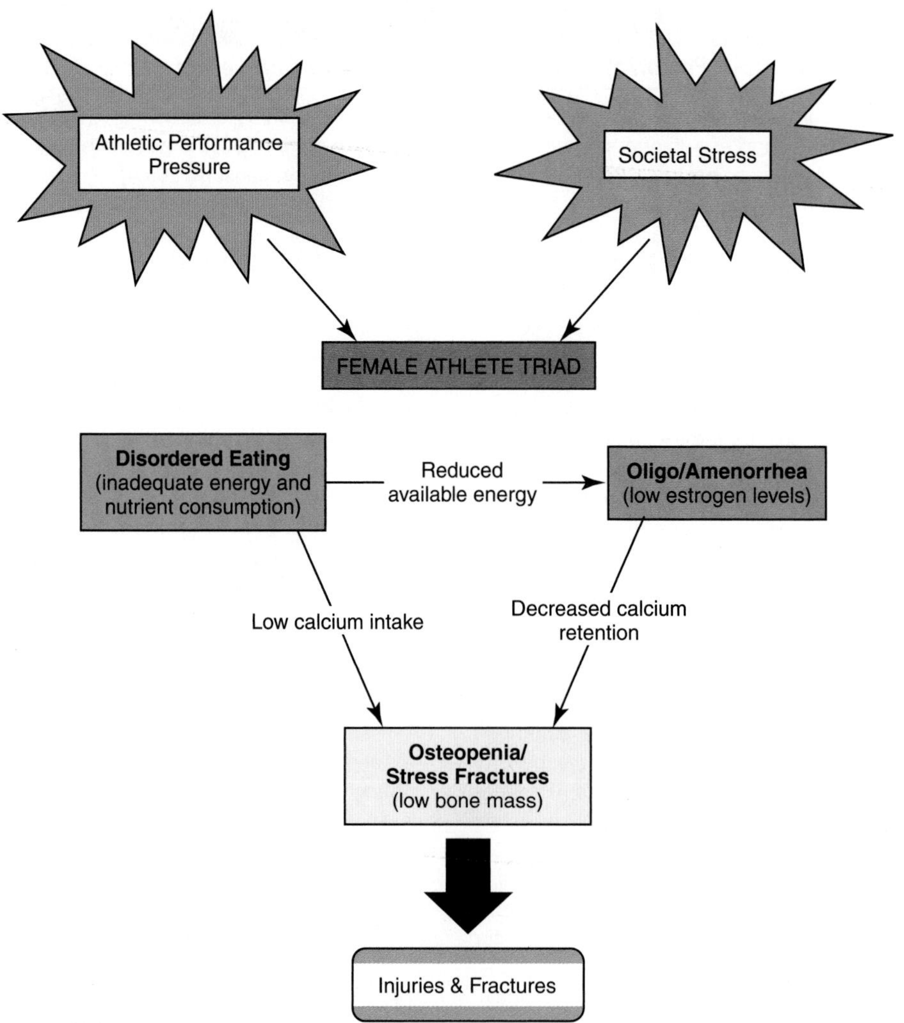

FIGURE 14-4 Female athlete triad. (From Thrash LE, Anderson JJB: The female athlete triad: nutrition, menstrual disturbances, and low bone mass, *Nutr Today* 35(5):168, 2000, with permission from Lippincott Williams & Wilkins.)

athletes are at a high risk for low BMD and stress fractures.[33] Injuries and fractures can interrupt or permanently end an athletic career, and bone mineral loss may be irreversible and become a lifelong risk.

HEALTH PROMOTION

BUILDING A PERSONAL EXERCISE PROGRAM

Exercise is a critical component in health promotion and disease prevention. The current *Dietary Guidelines for Americans* state the following[6]:

- Moderate physical activity for 30 minutes most days provides important health benefits; more than 30 minutes provides additional benefits.
- Adults need 60 minutes of moderate to vigorous physical activity most days to prevent unhealthy weight gain.
- Children and adolescents should aim for 60 minutes of moderate to vigorous physical activity most days to maintain good health and fitness and for healthy weight during growth. (See Chapter 12 for more information about children and physical activity.)
- Resistance exercise training is recommended to increase muscular strength and endurance and to maintain or increase lean body weight.

Exercise and Disease Prevention

Coronary Heart Disease

Exercise reduces risks for heart disease in several ways related to heart function, blood cholesterol levels, and oxygen transport:

- *Heart muscle function:* The heart is a four-chambered organ of muscle that is about the size of an adult fist. Exercise, especially aerobic conditioning, strengthens the heart, thereby enabling the heart to pump more blood per beat (stroke volume). A heart strengthened by exercise has an increased aerobic capacity; that is, the heart can pump more blood per minute without an undue increase in the heart rate. Therefore exercises relying primarily on the aerobic oxygen system for energy such as walking, jogging, and workouts on light cardiopulmonary exercise machines improve heart function.
- *Blood lipid levels:* A recent large-scale meta-analysis found that progressive resistance–training programs improved

blood lipid profiles by significantly lowering total cholesterol (TC), low-density lipoproteins (LDL), TC/ high-density lipoprotein (HDL) ratio, and triglycerides.[34] Improvements in HDL cholesterol in response to resistance and endurance exercise have been more modest but beneficial none the less.[35]
- *Oxygen-carrying capacity:* Exercise also enhances the circulatory system by increasing the oxygen-carrying capacity of the blood. As training continues, a person's VO_2max will improve, thus increasing the efficiency of oxygen use and uptake.

Hypertension

The risk for cardiovascular complications increases continuously with increasing levels of blood pressure. When blood pressure is measured, persons with stage 1 hypertension show a systolic blood pressure (the upper notation) of 140 to 159 mm Hg or a diastolic blood pressure (the lower notation) of 90 to 99 mm Hg (or they show both). Persons with stage 1 hypertension represent the overwhelming majority of hypertensive individuals in the general population, and exercise has become one of the most effective nondrug treatments.[36] Even for persons with elevated blood pressure, exercise has proven to be an important adjunct to drug therapy, offsetting adverse drug effects and lowering medication requirements. Normal rises in blood pressure occur during dynamic (e.g., walking, cycling) and resistance (i.e., strength training) exercise. Both forms of exercise are beneficial for individuals with hypertension. However, exercisers should avoid holding their breath during the exertion phase of heavy weight lifting to prevent severe stress on the cardiovascular system, especially those with diagnosed hypertension.

Diabetes

Regular, endurance-type exercise programs help maintain glucose homeostasis.[37] Physically active lifestyles are especially beneficial for individuals with type 2 diabetes to reduce the risk of chronic complications associated with diabetes. Exercise improves the action of a person's naturally produced insulin by increasing the sensitivity of insulin receptor sites (i.e., areas where insulin may be carried into cells). In managing type 1 diabetes mellitus, the type of exercise and when it is done must be balanced with food and insulin to prevent reactions caused by drops in blood glucose. (See Chapter 22 for a more detailed discussion of diabetes.)

Weight Management

Exercise is extremely beneficial in weight management because (1) it helps to regulate appetite, (2) it increases the basal metabolic rate (BMR), (3) it reduces the genetic fat deposit set point level, and (4) it is critical in maintenance of weight loss. Together with a well-planned diet, physical activity, planned exercise, or both correct the energy balance in favor of increased energy output (see Chapter 8). Fat is used efficiently as the fuel source for muscles during lower-intensity (30% to 60% VO_2max) aerobic exercise such as walking, jogging, swimming, and light cycling.

Stress Management

Exercise helps reduce stress-related eating. It also provides a physical outlet for working off the hormonal physiologic effects of catecholamines and corticoid hormones produced in the body by stress, thus helping to reduce a major risk factor in the development of chronic disease.[38]

Bone Disease

Weight-bearing exercises improve bone mineralization, thus reducing the risk of bone weakness and of potential osteoporosis.

Mental Health

Extended aerobic exercise stimulates the production of brain opiates, which are substances called *endorphins.* These natural substances decrease pain (this is how aspirin works, by stimulating production of endorphins) and improve the mood, including an exhilarating kind of "high."

Assessment of Personal Health and Exercise Needs

Many kinds of exercise exist. Choosing the best form depends on individual health, personal needs, the aerobic benefits involved, and personal enjoyment.

Assessing Health and Personal Needs

In planning an exercise program, it is important to assess individual health status, personal needs, present level of fitness, and resources required. Discussing an exercise program with a medical practitioner is always recommended, and getting a medical clearance before beginning an exercise program is especially important for older persons and those with chronic disease. It is wise to start slowly and build gradually rather than risk injury and discouragement. Moderation and consistency are key.

Beginning a Program

Many options exist regarding where, what, when, and how one exercises. It is important to evaluate these options before committing to any one routine. As a health care professional, you may have the responsibility of helping design exercise programs for your clients or patients. One golden rule for success is that if your clients enjoy the activity they are doing, then they are much more likely to make it part of their everyday schedule. Some individuals benefit from joining a fitness facility where they feel encouraged by others. Others, however, may shy away from fitness facilities for fear of discomfort. It is not necessary to join a fitness facility or hire a personal trainer to start an exercise program. Keeping the following questions in mind while designing an exercise program can be helpful:

1. Which is better, a fitness facility or a home program?
    - Is external encouragement helpful in maintaining a regular exercise schedule? Is company and interaction with others desirable during exercise, or is exercising alone preferable?
    - Is sticking to a schedule ideal and easy, or is it more realistic to work around other obligations and exercise when and where possible?

- Is a fitness facility located near home or work? Is it affordable?
- Is the office or home in an area that can provide uninterrupted bouts of exercise?

2. What type of exercise best fits the needs of your client?
   - It is important for everyone to determine independently what he or she *likes* to do. If the exercise chosen is not fun, then the patient or client will soon stop doing it, making it of no benefit. Encourage someone who has little exposure to various forms of physical activity to experiment with a variety of activities before committing to any one.
   - While exercising at a fitness facility, would your client or patient enjoy aerobic workouts on a bike, on a treadmill, or in a group class?
   - If your client or patient is considering exercising at home, you can ask other questions: Do you live in an area where you can run, walk, or bike? If not, then do you have access to a stationary bike, treadmill, or other aerobic machine? Try to choose an activity that he or she can stick with throughout the year, or choose a variety of activities that can be alternated during various seasons. For instance, perhaps swimming or biking can be done in the summer, whereas running or participating in aerobic classes would work in the winter.
   - For strength training, fitness facilities usually provide an assortment of free weights and resistance machines. Always encourage your client or patient to ask for help if he or she is not sure how to correctly perform any exercise. Resistance training can be done effectively at home as well, with a combination of resistance bands, small hand weights, or even cans of beans!

Determining Target Heart Rate

To build aerobic capacity, the level of exercise must raise the pulse rate to 70% of maximal heart rate (Table 14-5). Unless an exercise tolerance or stress test has been performed and the precise maximal exercising heart rate is known, an acceptable calculation to estimate maximum heart rate is 220 minus age. For aerobic benefits, 70% of maximal heart rate should then be maintained for approximately 20 minutes, three to six times per week. Resting pulse should be checked before starting the exercise period, then again during and immediately afterward, to monitor progress in developing target exercising heart rate and aerobic capacity. Heart rate monitors are a convenient way to monitor and keep track of heart rate.

Types of Exercise

Many types of exercise exist from which a participant may choose. Many of them are enjoyable and healthful but do not reach aerobic levels. For example, golf is a passion for many and gets them outdoors, but it is far too slow and sporadic to be aerobic. It is best to have a variety of exercises in any exercise plan (Figure 14-5). Even though many sports do not reach aerobic levels, if they are enjoyable they should be included.

Aerobic Exercise

Forms of exercise that can be sustained at a necessary level of intensity to provide aerobic benefits include such activities as swimming, running, jogging, bicycling, and aerobic dancing routines and workouts (Table 14-6). Perhaps the simplest and most popular form of stimulating exercise is *walking.* Figure 14-6 illustrates that aerobic walking can fit into almost anyone's lifestyle. If the pace is fast enough to elevate the pulse and maintain it for at least 20 minutes, then walking can be an excellent form of aerobic exercise. Walking is convenient, available, and appropriate for most people; in addition, it requires no equipment other than good walking shoes.

Resistance Exercise

Resistance types of exercises are designed to increase muscle strength and endurance. An ideal program would consist of

TABLE 14-5 TARGET ZONE HEART RATE ACCORDING TO AGE TO ACHIEVE AEROBIC PHYSICAL EFFECT OF EXERCISE

		TARGET ZONE	
AGE	MAXIMAL ATTAINABLE HEART RATE (PULSE: 220 MINUS AGE)	70% MAXIMAL RATE	85% MAXIMAL RATE
20 years	200	140	170
25 years	195	136	166
30 years	190	133	161
35 years	185	129	157
40 years	180	126	153
45 years	175	122	149
50 years	170	119	144
55 years	165	115	140
60 years	160	112	136
65 years	155	108	132
70 years	150	105	127
75 years	145	101	124

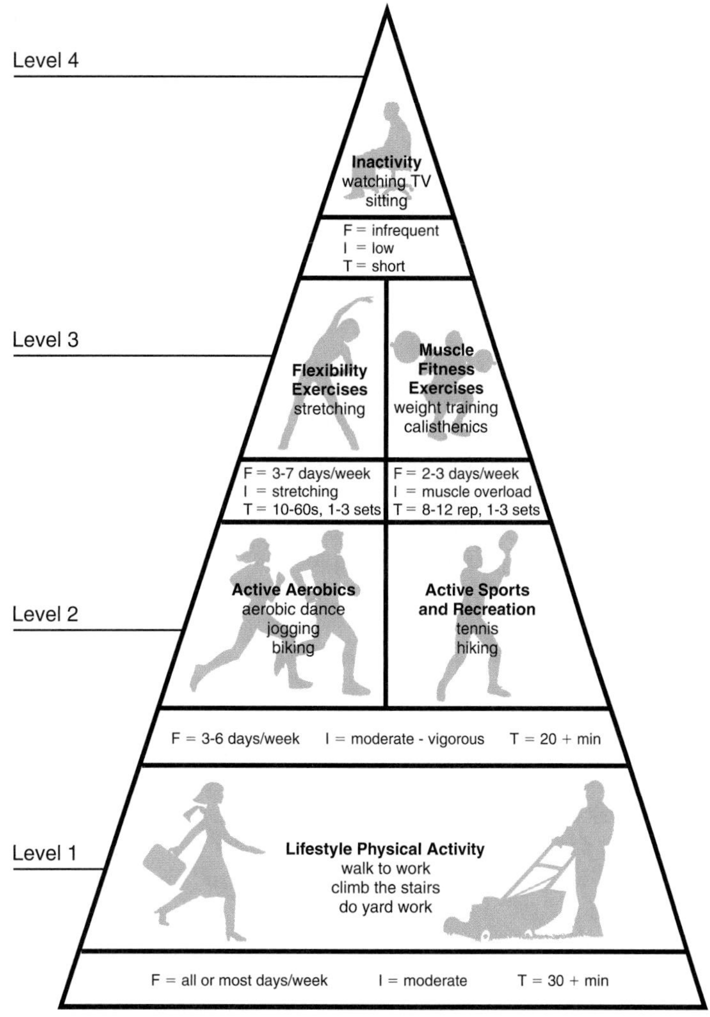

FIGURE 14-5 Physical Activity Pyramid. (Adapted with permission from Corbin CB, Lindsey R: *Fitness for life,* ed 5, Champaign, Ill, 2005, Human Kinetics, p 64.)

TABLE 14-6 **AEROBIC EXERCISES FOR PHYSICAL FITNESS***

TYPE OF EXERCISE	AEROBIC FORMS
Ball playing	Handball Racquetball Squash
Bicycling	Stationary Touring
Dancing	Aerobic routines Ballet Disco
Jumping rope	Brisk pace
Running or jogging	Brisk pace
Skating	Ice-skating Roller-skating
Skiing	Cross-country
Swimming	Steady pace
Walking	Brisk pace

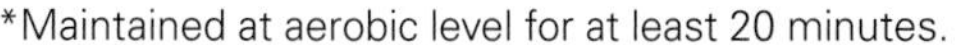
*Maintained at aerobic level for at least 20 minutes.

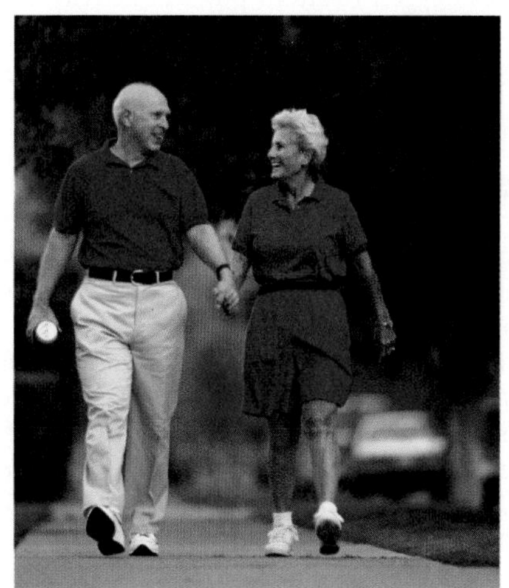

FIGURE 14-6 Aerobic walking is an enjoyable exercise that can fit into almost anyone's lifestyle. (Credit: PhotoDisc.)

8 to 10 separate exercises (with 8 to 12 repetitions of each) focusing on the major muscles of the body, performed 2 to 3 days per week. For an individual whose primary goal is to gain strength and power, the repetitions should be of high intensity with less than six repetitions to muscle fatigue. For improved endurance, a lower weight should be used that will allow at least 15 repetitions before muscle fatigue.

Weight-Bearing Exercise

Weight-bearing exercises, such as walking, jogging, aerobic dancing, or jumping rope, are important for bone structure and strength. In each of these exercises, muscles are working against gravity. Bones will adapt to the environment and load put on them during weight-bearing exercises to build more bone cells and increase bone density.

TO SUM UP

The energy molecule of the body is ATP, and the powerhouse of the cell is the mitochondrion. The cell's depot of energy is creatine phosphate. These two high-energy phosphate compounds are in limited supply. They can produce energy for only a brief initial period and need to be replenished for exercise to continue. This added supply is made available by anaerobic glycolysis, with added energy made available for continued exercise by the body's aerobic system. The process of glycolysis metabolizes only carbohydrate substrate, furnished by either blood glucose or stored glycogen. Dietary carbohydrate is necessary to replenish these fuel sources. Protein contributes little to total energy production for exercise, whereas the body's ability to burn fat as fuel depends on the level of fitness and intensity of exercise. The higher the body's efficiency in using oxygen, the more fatty acids will contribute to the energy supply. Even in the best-trained athletes, fatty acid oxidation must be accompanied by glucose metabolism.

Contrary to popular belief, exercise does not require an increased intake of protein, vitamins, or minerals. The body's increased needs are well supplied by a normal healthy diet. Exercise increases the body's need for kcalories and water. Cold water taken in small, frequent amounts is the best way to prevent dehydration in most athletic events and exercise. In most cases, electrolytes lost in sweat are replaced by a diet of adequate quality and quantity. Depending on the amount added, electrolytes or sugar in water may delay its emptying from the stomach and thus delay rehydration. A mild saline and glucose solution (4% to 8%) may supply fluid and fuel to sustain energy during longer endurance events. Some athletes use harmful practices such as food and fluid deprivation for controlling weight, as well as such ergogenic aids as illegal steroid drugs for bulking muscles.

The optimal diet for the athlete is moderate in protein and fat, with to 6 to10 g/kg body weight per day coming from carbohydrates. The pregame meal should be small, having little or no protein or fat and relying mainly on complex carbohydrates (starches).

The health benefits of general and aerobic exercise are numerous. Excellent aerobic exercises include sustained fast walking, swimming, jogging, running, and aerobic dancing or workouts. Approach any exercise sensibly, and choose those activities that are enjoyable.

QUESTIONS FOR REVIEW

1. What are the component muscle structures, and how do they produce muscular action?
2. What type of substrate fuel does the body use for immediate energy needs? For short-term needs? For long-term needs?
3. How does oxygen relate to physical activity capacity and aerobic effect?
4. Outline the nutrition and physical fitness principles to discuss with an athlete. Plan a diet for this client that would meet nutrient and energy needs.
5. Why is fluid balance vital during exercise periods? How is water and electrolyte balance achieved?
6. Describe the dangers of anabolic steroids used by some athletes for bulking muscles and gaining an edge in strength over an opponent.

REFERENCES

1. American College of Sports Medicine: *ACSM's resource manual for guidelines for exercise testing and prescription*, ed 5, Baltimore, 2006, Lippincott Williams & Wilkins.
2. World Health Organization: *Diet and physical activity: a public health priority*, Geneva, Switzerland. Retrieved February 6, 2009, from www.who.int/dietphysicalactivity/en/.
3. U.S. Department of Health and Human Services: *Healthy people 2010: understanding and improving health*, Washington, DC, 2000, U.S. Government Printing Office.
4. U.S. Department of Health and Human Services: *Progress review: physical activity and fitness*, Washington, DC, 2008, U.S. Government Printing Office.
5. U.S. Department of Agriculture: *Dietary guidelines for Americans 2000*, ed 5, Washington, DC, 2000, U.S. Government Printing Office.
6. U.S. Department of Health and Human Services, U.S. Department of Agriculture: *Dietary guidelines for Americans 2005*, ed 6, Washington, DC, 2005, U.S. Government Printing Office.
7. Roberts CK, Barnard RJ: Effects of exercise and diet on chronic disease, *J Appl Physiol* 98(1):3, 2005.
8. Mokdad AH, Marks JS, Stroup DF, et al: Actual causes of death in the United States, 2000, *JAMA* 291(10):1238, 2004.
9. Position of the American Dietetic Association, Dietitians of Canada, and the American College of Sports Medicine: Nutrition and athletic performance, *J Am Diet Assoc* 100(12):1543, 2000.

10. Rodriguez NR, DiMarco NM, Langley S: Position of the American Dietetic Association, Dietitians of Canada, and the American College of Sports Medicine: Nutrition and athletic performance, *J Am Diet Assoc* 109(3):509, 2009.
11. Green HJ, Ball-Burnett M, Jones S, et al: Mechanical and metabolic responses with exercise and dietary carbohydrate manipulation, *Med Sci Sports Exerc* 39(1):139, 2007.
12. Rauch HG, St Clair Gibson A, Lambert EV, et al: A signaling role for muscle glycogen in the regulation of pace during prolonged exercise, *Br J Sports Med* 39(1):34, 2005.
13. Harger-Domitrovich SG, McClaughry AE, Gaskill SE, et al: Exogenous carbohydrate spares muscle glycogen in men and women during 10 h of exercise, *Med Sci Sports Exerc* 39(12):2171, 2007.
14. Dumke CL, McBride JM, Nieman DC, et al: Effect of duration and exogenous carbohydrate on gross efficiency during cycling, *J Strength Cond Res* 21(4):1214, 2007.
15. Sedlock DA: The latest on carbohydrate loading: a practical approach, *Curr Sports Med Rep* 7(4):209, 2008.
16. Tarnopolsky M: Protein requirements for endurance athletes, *Nutrition* 20(7–8):662, 2004.
17. Hargreaves MH, Snow R: Amino acids and endurance exercise, *Int J Sport Nutr Exerc Metab* 11(1):133, 2001.
18. Wagenmakers AJ: Muscle amino acid metabolism at rest and during exercise: role in human physiology and metabolism, *Exerc Sport Sci Rev* 26:287, 1998.
19. Duellman MC, Lukaszuk JM, Prawitz AD, et al: Protein supplement users among high school athletes have misconceptions about effectiveness, *J Strength Cond Res* 22(4):1124, 2008.
20. Martin WF, Cerundolo LH, Pikosky MA, et al: Effects of dietary protein intake on indexes of hydration, *J Am Diet Assoc* 106(4):587, 2006.
21. Kerstetter JE, O'Brien KO, Caseria DM, et al: The impact of dietary protein on calcium absorption and kinetic measures of bone turnover in women, *J Clin Endocrinol Metab* 90(1):26, 2005.
22. Montain SJ: Hydration recommendations for sport 2008, *Curr Sports Med Rep* 7(4):187, 2008.
23. Judelson DA, Maresh CM, Farrell MJ, et al: Effect of hydration state on strength, power, and resistance exercise performance, *Med Sci Sports Exerc* 39(10):1817, 2007.
24. Armstrong LE, Casa DJ, Millard-Stafford M, et al: American College of Sports Medicine position stand. Exertional heat illness during training and competition, *Med Sci Sports Exerc* 39(3):556, 2007.
25. Sawka MN, Burke LM, Eichner ER, et al: American College of Sports Medicine position stand. Exercise and fluid replacement, *Med Sci Sports Exerc* 39(2):377, 2007.
26. Sharp RL: Role of sodium in fluid homeostasis with exercise, *J Am Coll Nutr* 25(Suppl 3):231S, 2006.
27. Millard-Stafford M, Childers WL, Conger SA, et al: Recovery nutrition: timing and composition after endurance exercise, *Curr Sports Med Rep* 7(4):193, 2008.
28. Herbert V: Pangamic acid ("vitamin B_{15}"), *Am J Clin Nutr* 32(7):1534, 1979.
29. Hartgens F, Kuipers H: Effects of androgenic-anabolic steroids in athletes, *Sports Med* 34(8):513, 2004.
30. vandenBerg P, Neumark-Sztainer D, Cafri G, et al: Steroid use among adolescents: longitudinal findings from Project EAT, *Pediatrics* 119(3):476, 2007.
31. Nattiv A, Loucks AB, Manore MM, et al: American College of Sports Medicine position stand. The female athlete triad, *Med Sci Sports Exerc* 39(10):1867, 2007.
32. Redman LM, Loucks AB: Menstrual disorders in athletes, *Sports Med* 35(9):747, 2005.
33. Joy EA, Campbell D: Stress fractures in the female athlete, *Curr Sports Med Rep* 4(6):323, 2005.
34. Kelley GA, Kelley KS: Impact of progressive resistance training on lipids and lipoproteins in adults: a meta-analysis of randomized controlled trials, *Prev Med* 48(1):9, 2009.
35. Durstine JL, Grandjean PW, Davis PG, et al: Blood lipid and lipoprotein adaptations to exercise: a quantitative analysis, *Sports Med* 31(15):1033, 2001.
36. Pescatello LS, Franklin BA, Fagard R, et al: American College of Sports Medicine position stand. Exercise and hypertension, *Med Sci Sports Exerc* 36(3):533, 2004.
37. Boule NG, Weisnagel SJ, Lakka TA, et al: Effects of exercise training on glucose homeostasis: the HERITAGE Family Study, *Diabetes Care* 28(1):108, 2005.
38. Tsatsoulis A, Fountoulakis S: The protective role of exercise on stress system dysregulation and comorbidities, *Ann N Y Acad Sci* 1083:196, 2006.

FURTHER READINGS AND RESOURCES

Readings

American College of Sports Medicine, American Dietetic Association, and Dietitians of Canada: Joint position statement: nutrition and athletic performance, *Med Sci Sports Exerc* 32(12):2130, 2000. *[This joint position statement emphasizes the importance of nutrition in physical activity, athletic performance, and recovery from exercise. The experts specifically address nutrient and fluid needs, body composition, supplements and ergogenic aids, and the roles and responsibilities of health care professionals.]*

Campbell C, Prince D, Braun M, et al: Carbohydrate-supplement form and exercise performance, *Int J Sport Nutr Exerc Metab* 18(2):179, 2008. *[The authors explore the benefits of various forms of carbohydrate, such as gels or gummy candy, and the resulting effect on performance.]*

Keim NL, Blanton CA, Kretsch MJ: America's obesity epidemic: measuring physical activity to promote an active lifestyle, *J Am Diet Assoc* 104:1398, 2004. *[The authors discuss the health benefits of physical activity, the recommendations to the public for health promotion and disease prevention, and methods of balancing the equation of energy intake versus energy output. The prevalence of overweight and inactivity are reviewed.]*

Websites of Interest

American College of Sports Medicine: www.acsm.or.

Centers for Disease Control and Prevention, National Center for Chronic Disease Prevention and Health Promotion: *Physical Activity and Health: A Report of the Surgeon General*: www.cdc.gov/nccdphp/sgr/sgr.htm.

Washington Coalition for Promoting Physical Activity: www.beactive.org.

15

The Complexity of Obesity: Beyond Energy Balance

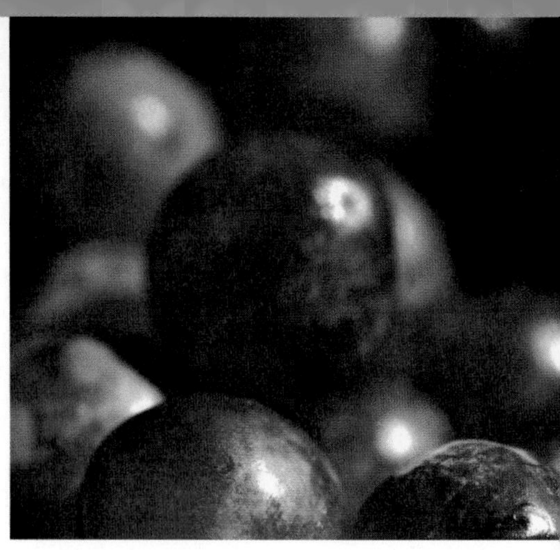

*Allan Higginbotham**

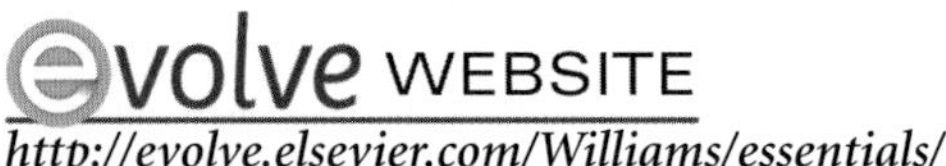

http://evolve.elsevier.com/Williams/essentials/

OUTLINE

In this chapter, we look at the complex issue of obesity. In recent years the prevalence of obesity has grown to epidemic proportions. Linked as a risk factor for many chronic disorders in the United States, the magnitude of this health care problem and its effect on the health care system is immense.

We are living in a time when the number of overweight individuals is increasing more rapidly than in earlier decades. This chapter is intended to help you understand this problem. Using an epidemiologic model of the interactions between environmental agents and the human host to explain obesity, we explore food, medications, physical inactivity, toxins, and viruses as environmental agents that interact with the genetically programmed host to disturb energy balance as causal factors in obesity. Large portion size, high fat intake, easy access to calorically sweetened beverages, and lack of any need to be physically active all play a role in the toxic environment that leads to obesity. The genetic, physiologic, and psychologic responses of the host determine whether or not this "toxic environment" will produce obesity. Reversing the current trends of obesity requires a new look at the limits of the energy balance concept and a better understanding of how environmental factors acutely and chronically change the responses of the susceptible host so that obesity becomes a chronic, relapsing disease.

*The author wishes to thank George A. Bray and Catherine M. Champagne for their contributions to this chapter in the previous edition.

REALITIES OF OBESITY

During the early part of the twentieth century, the prevalence of obesity increased slowly; however, around 1980 it began to increase more rapidly.[1-4] As illustrated in Figure 15-1, the rise in the rate of obesity has continued to the present time. In the period between 2003 and 2004, the prevalence of overweight was 66% and the prevalence of obesity was 32%.[4] This statistic means that within current definitions, nearly two thirds of American adults are defined as overweight. Prevalence of obesity and overweight increases with age. Peak age in women is between ages 60 and 70 and in men between ages 50 and 60. A higher percentage of women are overweight and obese than men. Moreover, African-American and Hispanic women have a higher prevalence of obesity than Caucasian women. This racial disparity is larger in women than in men. Overweight is also higher among people who make less money and have less education than it is among those who have a higher education and income.

Children are also affected by obesity. The prevalence was about 5% in 1960 but has increased to more than 17% in 2004.[5] For children and adults, a social stigma is associated with this weight problem. Overweight children are less liked as playmates and tend to view themselves less favorably than normal-weight children. Children are often teased at school by being labeled "fatty" and other derogatory terms. Such disparaging remarks often jeopardize feelings of self-confidence. Many overweight children and adults are traumatized by the stigma of obesity. Adults experience

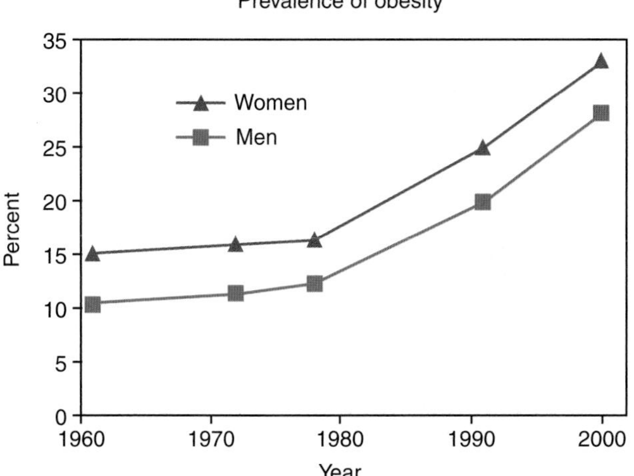

FIGURE 15-1 Graph illustrating the prevalence of obesity. The upper line shows the prevalence of obesity for women, and the lower line for men using data from several surveys of obesity done by the U.S. government beginning in the years 1960 to 1962. Obesity rose slowly from 1960 until approximately 1980, when the rate for men and women began to increase. (Data from National Center for Health Statistics: *National Health and Nutrition Examination Survey I, 1960-1962* and *National Health and Nutrition Examination Surveys 1970-1974, 1976-1980, 1988-1994, and 1999-2000,* Hyattsville, Md, 1960-2000, Centers for Disease Control and Prevention.)

prejudice in social and economic situations. Measures of quality of life show that the obese score lower on many scales and that weight loss improves their quality of life (see the *Focus on Culture* box, "Antifat Bias: The Last Acceptable Form of Cultural Discrimination").

Overweight increases the risk of developing many chronic diseases. Prominent among these is type 2 diabetes mellitus in children and adolescents.[6] This disease most often occurs in overweight or obese adolescents and adults and presages a bleak future, particularly for these children as the complications of blindness, heart disease, renal failure, and amputation disable them in the next 20 years or so. Overweight also increases the risk of gallbladder disease, heart disease, high blood pressure, and several forms of cancer. Through the development of these diseases, being overweight reduces life expectancy and shortens life span by 3 to 7 years for an individual age 40 with a body mass index (BMI) of 30 or more.

Obesity increases the cost of health care.[7] Frequency of hospital and medical office visits is increased with increasing body weight. Use of drugs to treat the complications associated with obesity also increases. The extra burden to Medicare after age 65 rises with increasing weight.

Fortunately risks associated with obesity are generally ameliorated by modest weight loss. A weight loss of 5% to 10% of initial body weight is sufficient to reduce the development of diabetes in people with prediabetes by up to 58%.[8] Weight loss that is maintained is an effective treatment for hypertension. Risks from abnormal blood lipids (dyslipidemia) are also reduced with weight loss.

To tackle the hazards of obesity for children, adolescents, and adults, we need to adopt effective strategies for prevention and, where prevention fails, for treatment of obesity.

ENERGY INTAKE, ENERGY EXPENDITURE, AND DEVELOPMENT OF OBESITY

One easy way to view the problem of obesity is with the aid of a teeter-totter—the childhood toy. On one side is the amount of food we eat expressed in calories (joules). On the other

KEY TERMS

overweight A weight beyond the upper limit of some arbitrarily set standard (see also *obesity*).

obesity An excess amount of body fat. Operationally it is usually defined by a body mass index (BMI) of 30 kg/m^2 or greater, which uses height and weight. Three subclasses of obesity are defined as follows:

- Class 1 = BMI 30-34.9 kg/m^2
- Class 2 = BMI 35-39.9 kg/m^2
- Class 3 = BMI >40 kg/m^2

prevalence This term relates the number of individuals with a particular condition at a particular time to the total number of people. If 10 people were overweight in a population of 1000, then this would indicate a prevalence of 1%.

stigma A mark or identification marking. In this context it is an increased body fat that is obvious to the viewer and that elicits emotional feelings, which are usually negative.

diabetes mellitus A disease defined by a high level of glucose in the blood, which often appears in the urine if it is high enough. Two general types of diabetes mellitus exist: type 1, which refers to the disease normally diagnosed in younger individuals (<30 years of age) in which the pancreas cannot produce enough insulin and thus not enough circulating insulin exists, and type 2, which refers to the disease normally diagnosed in older people who are often overweight or obese and in which more than enough circulating insulin exists but relatively poor response to this insulin occurs.

body mass index (BMI) Body weight in kilograms divided by the height in square meters (kg/m^2). It can be calculated from pounds and inches as 703 times body weight in pounds divided by the height in inches squared. This measurement is the common method used to define overweight and obesity.

prediabetes A condition also known as *impaired glucose tolerance* and defined as a fasting glucose between 100 and 126 mg/dL and a blood glucose between 140 and 199 mg/dL 2 hours after ingestion of 75 g of glucose.

calories The amount of heat energy needed to raise the temperature of water from 14° C to 15° C. Because this is a small unit, we usually use *kilocalories,* which are 1000 of these small calories (see also *joule*).

joules Units of energy. The International System of Units uses joules in place of calories to refer to food energy, and most nutrition journals require its use instead of calories (1 kcal = 4.184 kilojoules [kJ], often rounded to 4.2 kJ for ease in calculation). A 1000-kcal diet would be equivalent to a 4200-kJ or 4.2-MJ (megajoule) diet.

FOCUS ON CULTURE

Antifat Bias: The Last Acceptable Form of Cultural Discrimination

Our culture idealizes slimness and denigrates obesity. Discrimination based on weight bias has been recognized in many different areas of our society, including representation of obese persons in our culture. Common stereotypes of obese persons include the following:

- Warm
- Dependable
- Gluttonous
- Lazy
- Stupid
- Worthless

Popular messages in the media promote fat jokes and idealization of thin women and muscular men. Unfortunately, it appears that it is a socially acceptable in the United States to assume that obese people are fully responsible for their condition. However, do health care professionals, who are trained to understand that obesity is caused by hereditary and environmental factors and is not merely a function of personal behavior (e.g., overeating, lack of exercise), express this same bias? Regrettably, research shows that health professionals are not immune to overt or inherent antifat bias. The very people who are responsible for caring for individuals who are obese demonstrated the following attitudes toward obese patients[1-8]:

- Family practice physicians described obese patients with negative terms such as *lacking self-control.*
- Physicians reported that they would feel more negatively toward overweight patients and spend less time with them but would order more tests.
- Nurses reported the following:
  - Feeling uncomfortable caring for obese patients
  - Being "repulsed" by obese persons
  - Having a preference not to care for obese patients
- Medical students described obese patients as follows:
  - Less attractive
  - More depressed
  - Less compliant
- Registered dietitians and dietetic students reported negative attitudes toward obese individuals.
- Overweight and obese women are less likely to be screened for cervical and breast cancer.

Thus it appears the physical and psychologic consequences of obesity may stem from not only the Western culture's weight-related bias and stigma but also from the biases of health professionals. Obviously, Schwartz and colleagues[6] were right when they said, "Much more work is needed to understand and ameliorate this bias."

How about you? Are you part of the solution or part of the problem?

REFERENCES

1. Bagley CR, Conklin DN, Isherwood RT, et al: Attitudes of nurses toward obesity and obese patients, *Percept Mot Skills* 68:954, 1989.
2. Hebl MR, Xu J: Weighing the care: physicians' reaction to the size of a patient, *Int J Obes Relat Metab Disord* 25:1246, 2001.
3. Loomis GA: Attitudes and practices of military family physicians regarding obesity, *Mil Med* 166:121, 2001.
4. Maroney D, Golub S: Nurses' attitudes toward obese persons and certain ethnic groups, *Percept Mot Skills* 75:387, 1992.
5. Oberrieder H, Walker R, Monroe D, et al: Attitude of dietetics students and registered dietitians toward obesity, *J Am Diet Assoc* 95:914, 1995.
6. Schwartz M, Chambliss HO, Brownell KD, et al: Weight bias among health professionals specializing in obesity, *Obes Res* 11:1033, 2003.
7. Teachman BA, Gapinski KD, Brownell KD, et al: Demonstrations of implicit anti-fat bias: the impact of providing causal information and evoking empathy, *Health Psychol* 22:68, 2003.
8. Wigton RS, McGaghie WC: The effects of obesity on medical students' approach to patients with abdominal pain, *J Gen Intern Med* 16:262, 2001.

side is the energy we expend during the day for our various activities, which includes the energy needed to heat our bodies and keep the body temperature at 37° C (98.6° F), the energy needed to keep our hearts beating, our brains working, our kidneys excreting urine, and our intestines digesting food whether we are awake or not. Energy is also used for physical activity when we sit, stand, walk, run, or do other daily activities. When the two sides of the teeter-totter are in balance, that is, when the energy on one side is equal to the energy on the other side, we are in "energy balance." As long as we are in energy balance, we will not gain or lose weight. Overweight develops when the energy on the intake side is more than on the expenditure side, which can occur because energy intake rises, because energy expenditure falls, or both. The conservation of energy implied by the energy balance equation is often referred to as the *First Law of Thermodynamics* applied to human energy consumption and expenditure. This law was first demonstrated for human beings more than 100 years ago, and no reason exists to doubt that it provides the overall framework for understanding the way in which obesity develops. However, as we will show, it is in the details of the relation of energy intake and energy expenditure that the problem of obesity lies.

OBESITY AS A DISEASE

Obesity can be viewed as a disease. What do we mean by this? A disease has several components; it has a cause. As noted previously, this is the result of an imbalance between energy intake and energy expenditure. It has clinical signs and symptoms such as increased amount of fatness that is usually visible to the eye. No one would have difficulty distinguishing between an overweight and normal-weight individual walking down the street. Obesity also has a "pathology," by which we mean the presence of some unique features that allow one to diagnose it under a microscope, at an autopsy examination, or by defined blood tests. For obesity this is the large fat cell.

All forms of obesity have as one characteristic, an enlargement of the individual fat cells all over the body. The adult human has close to 60 billion fat cells. As people gain weight, the first change in these cells is to enlarge to accommodate the extra fat. As the cells reach their maximal size, additional cells may be recruited to store the extra fat. Fat cells are remarkable cells. They are part of the larger endocrine cellular system that secretes products into the bloodstream that have effects elsewhere. In the case of fat cells, many secreted products can affect blood clotting (plasminogen activator inhibitor-1 [PAI-1]), the removal of fats from the blood (lipoprotein lipase), inflammation (interleukin-1 [IL-1], interleukin-6 [IL-6], tumor necrosis factor-α [TNF-α]), blood pressure (angiotensinogen), and the body's recognition of the amount of its body fat (leptin). The release of this latter hormone, leptin, is an important signal from the fat cells to the brain about the amount of body fat. Circulating levels of leptin are directly related to amount of body fat. Until the amount of body fat reaches a "critical" level in women, menstruation does not occur. In many women who are ballet dancers or gymnasts, with small amounts of body fat, menstrual periods cease because leptin levels are too low. The many hormones produced and secreted from the fat cells in the body produce the pathophysiologic responses that lead to the associated diseases that we described previously. Thus obesity can be described as a chronic, relapsing, neurochemical disease.

BEYOND ENERGY BALANCE

There is no doubt that obesity results from energy imbalance and that we can predict the magnitude of the weight change over time if we know the net energy balance. However, it is what the energy balance concept *does not tell us* that is most important in dealing with obesity. The First Law of Thermodynamics does not tell us anything about the regulation of food intake or the way in which genes are involved in this process. It does not help us to understand why men and women distribute fat in different places on their bodies or to understand how fat distribution changes with age. The First Law of Thermodynamics also does not help us to understand why some drugs produce weight gain, whereas others produce weight loss, or why weight loss stops after a period of treatment with diet or medication. Understanding these mechanisms will allow us to tackle the epidemic of obesity.

One problem with the concept of energy balance is that we are never in energy balance. To study energy balance, healthy men were housed in small rooms (respiration calorimeters) in which food intake and exercise were manipulated to get as close as possible to zero energy balance—that is, when energy intake equals energy expenditure.[9] In fact, the difference was rarely closer than 50 kcal/day, or about 2.5% out of an intake of 2000 kcal/day. The values of energy imbalance for these healthy men ranged from 50 to 150 kcal/day. Had these differences been maintained for 1 year, these men would be expected to gain about 2.5 kg (5.5 lb) at the smaller error and 7.5 kg (16.5 lb) at the larger error.

To keep from gaining weight, we must make "corrective" responses in energy intake or energy expenditure to counterbalance the error that occurred on previous days. These corrective responses around a weight of relative stability make it look as though "weight regulation" exists. For some people the oscillations around this balance point can keep weight stable for many years. For others a slow upward drift occurs in this regulatory point, and weight is gradually gained. If you are fortunate enough to have robust corrective responses, then you can maintain a stable weight over many years. If it is not stable, then the following two strategies are available:

1. *Conscious control:* This method is exhibited in some people who have a pattern of eating called *restrained eating.*
2. *Regular weighing:* This second and perhaps best way to maintain weight over a long period is not to count calories but to weigh oneself regularly at the same time of day on an accurate scale and address weight increases in a timely fashion.

Consequences of energy imbalance are graphically illustrated in the movie by Morgan Spurlock entitled *Supersize Me,* in which the protagonist gained 25 lb in 1 month by eating all of his meals at McDonald's restaurants. Because we are never in energy balance, we need to view energy balance as an ideal—not a realistic goal to be obtained by counting calories.

From the perspective of energy balance, the solution to obesity should be simple: eat less and exercise more. The truth of this advice was shown by Kinsell and colleagues[10] for overweight individuals housed in a metabolic ward and provided with all of their food. During the course of several months, these patients ate diets with 1200 kcal/day. After the initial rapid weight loss because of rebalancing body fluids, subsequent weight loss was linear and was not affected by wide variations in macronutrient content of the diet. More recent studies using foods tagged with a nonradioactive isotopic carbon-13 showed that weight loss increased in relation to how well subjects adhered to a diet.[11] Thus it is adherence to diets, not diets themselves, that make the difference.

Another limitation to the concept of energy balance as the cause of obesity is the implication that if you are getting fatter, then it is your fault. You need only to control your calorie intake (food) and calorie expenditure to control the problem, which implies that we should blame our children

KEY TERMS

pathology The science of disease. Changes that reflect disease can be in organs (e.g., liver disease), tissues (e.g., skin disease), cells, or parts of cells.

leptin A peptide of 167 amino acids that is produced primarily in fat cells and released into the blood to circulate as a hormone to the brain to tell the body about long-term regulation of body fat.

pathophysiologic Term referring to the processes by which the disease develops.

for their obesity. This notion seems grossly inappropriate. If obesity were easily controlled by moderating calorie intake, then the U.S. military would not discharge up to 5000 men and women yearly for failing to meet its weight standards. If loss of livelihood is not sufficient motivation to lose weight, then the problem must be more complex.

In the very rare instance of leptin deficiency in humans, the cure of obesity involves treatment with leptin. This concept demonstrates a genetic basis for some obesity, more than simply lack of willpower.[12] Although simple in theory, applying the ideas of energy balance and calorie counting to body weight control has proven unsuccessful. More than 95% of people using dietary, behavior, and lifestyle approaches to lose weight regained it within less than 5 years.[13]

EPIDEMIOLOGIC MODEL

The current epidemic can be viewed from the perspective of an epidemiologic model, shown in Figure 15-2. Food, low physical activity, drugs, viruses, and toxins are the environmental agents that facilitate the development of obesity. One or more of these factors acting on a susceptible host can produce obesity. As the spokesperson for the Grocery Manufacturers of America said in the movie *Supersize Me*, "The food industry is part of the problem." Using this model, we can approach the problem by manipulating either the environment or the host.

Environmental Agents

Food and Its Costs as a Major Environmental Agent

Several components of our food supply may be important in determining whether or not obesity develops. The first of these is the size of food packages and restaurant portions. Convincing evidence indicates that when larger portion sizes are provided, more food is eaten. Portion sizes have dramatically increased in the past 40 years[14] and now need reduction. Calorically sweetened beverages that contain 10% high fructose corn syrup (HFCS) are available in 12-, 20-, 32-, and 44-oz containers and provide 150, 250, 400, or 550 kcal if the entire drink is consumed. Prepackaged foods list the calories per serving, but the package often contains more than one serving, encouraging larger portions.

Patterns of food consumption have changed during the past 30 years.[15] The most striking change from 1970 to 2000 was in the rising consumption of HFCS.[16] HFCS is now used as the caloric sweetener in almost all soft drinks, as well as in reconstituted juice drinks and many solid foods. The rise in HFCS consumption occurred over the same time interval as the rapid rise in the prevalence of obesity.[16] On the one hand, this relationship may be strictly coincidental. However, on the other hand, it may not be (Figure 15-3). Fructose is sweeter than either glucose or sucrose, a molecule that is a combination of fructose and glucose. In addition, HFCS is a solution of fructose and glucose as separate molecules, and thus it differs in osmotic properties from a solution with the same concentration of sucrose.

The intake of calorically sweetened beverages has been related to the epidemic of obesity.[16–18] Ludwig, Peterson, and Gortmaker[19] reported that the intake of soft drinks was a predictor of initial BMI in children in the Planet Health Study. They also showed that higher soft drink consumption also predicted an increase in BMI; during nearly 2 years of follow-up, those with the highest soft drink consumption at baseline had the highest increase in BMI. A Danish study[20] showed that individuals consuming calorically sweetened beverages during 10 weeks gained weight, whereas subjects drinking the same amount of artificially sweetened beverages lost weight. In one study, children who were focusing on reducing intake of "fizzy" drinks and replacing them with water showed slower weight gain than those not advised to reduce the intake of fizzy drinks.[21]

These studies strongly suggest that calorie-containing soft drinks could play a role in the epidemic of obesity. If so, then their consumption should be curtailed, particularly for very young children, and for schoolchildren, for whom beverages are a ready source of energy with few other nutrients.

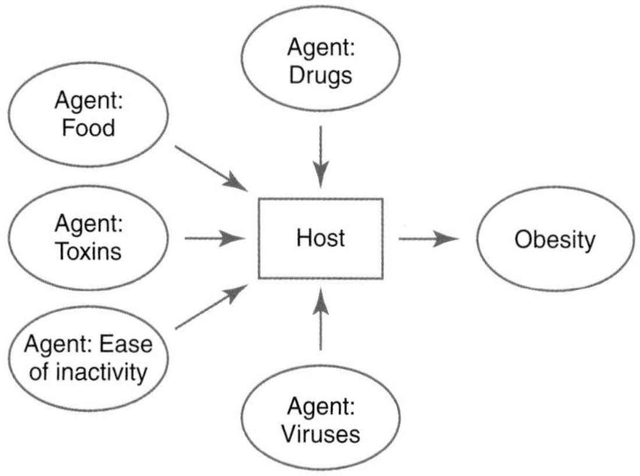

Agent: Food
Agent: Drugs
Agent: Toxins
Host
Obesity
Agent: Ease of inactivity
Agent: Viruses

FIGURE 15-2 Epidemiologic model of obesity. In this model the agent that produces obesity is "food" or food-related products. If food is in limited supply, then obesity does not develop. The food that is ingested interacts with the host. In a susceptible host the toxic effects of food produce obesity, the disease.

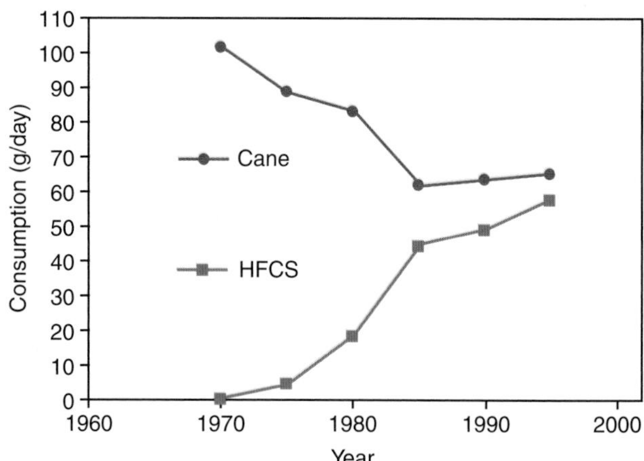

FIGURE 15-3 The consumption of high-fructose corn syrup (HFCS) and sugar (sucrose) over the years when the obesity epidemic developed. (Copyright © 2005, George A. Bray, Baton Rouge, La.)

Dietary fat is another component that may be related to the epidemic of obesity.[22] Fats contain more than twice the energy of carbohydrates (9 kcal/g). Foods combining fat and sugar may be a particular problem because they are often very palatable and usually inexpensive.[23] The Leeds Fat Study shows that people who were high-fat consumers have an increased incidence of obesity.[24] Providing palatable low-fat foods is important.

Several studies now show that when infants were given breast milk as the sole source of nutrition for more than 3 months, their risk of obesity was significantly reduced at the time of entry into school and in adolescence compared with infants who were not breast-fed or who were breast-fed for less than 3 months.[25] This may be an example of "infant imprinting." The composition of the breast milk may also be important. Over the past 50 years the proportion of n-6 fatty acids in human breast milk has increased, reflecting changes in dietary fat composition. The amount of n-3 fatty acids in breast milk has remained constant. A higher amount of n-6 fatty acids provides prostaglandin derivatives that stimulate fat cell proliferation in infants.[26] This is a concept that needs further evaluation. The rate of weight gain between ages 2 and 12 years also predicts future obesity; those children who gain the most weight have the highest risk of becoming obese.[27] Monitoring weight change early can be predictive of future obesity.

Calcium intake is another dietary factor that may be related to the development of obesity in children and adults. The level of calcium intake in population studies is inversely correlated with the risk of being overweight. In other epidemiologic studies and in feeding trials, higher dietary calcium is associated with reduced BMI or reduced incidence of insulin resistance.[28]

The cost of food is another factor in the cause of obesity. The price of items we buy influences our choices and the amount we buy. During the period from 1960 to 1980 the price of food rose more slowly than the other components in the consumer price index. Real wages also rose, providing additional money for consumption, some of which could buy a wider variety of healthy foods such as fresh fruits and vegetables, fish, and dairy products. This period was a time when the rise in the prevalence of obesity was slow. However, between 1985 and 2000 the relative cost increase in these food items was much faster than the foods with higher energy density, which contain more fat and sugar. In this period the price of fresh fruits and vegetables rose 117%, fish by 77%, and dairy products by 56%. Contrast this with sugar and sweets, which increased 47%; fats and oils, 37%; and carbonated beverages, 20%.[7] This means that your food dollar will buy relatively more food energy if the foods contain more sugar and fat or are carbonated beverages.

Low Levels of Physical Activity

Epidemiologic data show that low levels of physical activity and watching more television predict higher body weight.[29] Recent studies suggest that individuals in American cities where they had to walk more than people in other cities tended to weigh less. Low levels of physical activity also increase the risk of early mortality. Using normal-weight, physically active women as the comparison group, researchers found that the relative risk of mortality increased to 1.55 in inactive lean women, to 1.92 in active obese women, and to 2.42 in women who were obese but physically inactive.[28] It is thus better to be thin than fat and to be physically active rather than inactive.

Drugs and Chemicals That Produce Weight Gain

Several drugs can cause weight gain, including a variety of hormones and psychoactive agents.[30] The degree of weight gain is generally not sufficient to cause substantial obesity, except occasionally in patients treated with high-dose corticosteroids, as well as some psychoactive drugs such as valproate. These drugs can also increase the risk of future type 2 diabetes mellitus.

Cessation of smoking is another environmental agent that will affect body fat stores. Partially mediated by nicotine withdrawal, a weight gain of 1 to 2 kg (2.2 to 4.4 lb) is seen in the first few weeks and is often followed by an additional 2- to 3-kg weight gain over the next 4 to 6 months, resulting in an average weight gain of 4 to 5 kg or more.[31]

Viruses as Environmental Causes of Obesity

The injection of several viruses into the central nervous system (CNS) produces obesity in mice. Recent findings of antibodies to one of the adenoviruses (Ad-36) in larger amounts in obese humans raises the possibility that viruses are involved in some cases.[32] The adenoviral syndrome can be replicated in nonhuman primates and is characterized by modest obesity and a low circulating cholesterol concentration. Further studies are needed to establish that a syndrome of obesity associated with low concentrations of cholesterol clearly exists in human beings. If so, then this would enhance the value of the epidemiologic model.

Toxins

In experimental animals, exposure in the neonatal period to monosodium glutamate (MSG), a common flavoring ingredient in food, produces obesity. A similar effect of reduction in glucose can also produce obesity, suggesting that the brain of the growing animal, and possibly that of human beings, may respond with damage to the "metabolic sensors" that regulate food needs. In human beings, we know that body fat stores many "toxic" chemicals that are mobilized with weight loss. The metabolic rate can be reduced by organochlorine molecules,[33] and conceivably prolonged exposure to many

KEY TERMS

incidence The number of new cases of a particular condition that develop over time. If among 1000 people, 10 people who were not overweight initially become overweight in 1 year, then the incidence rate would be 10 cases per 1000 person-years.

energy density The amount of energy or calories in a food compared with the weight of the food.

chlorinated chemicals in our environment has affected metabolic pathways and energy metabolism. Food additives are another class of chemicals that are widely distributed and may be involved in the current epidemic of obesity.

Host

Genetic Factors

Several kinds of research indicate that genetic factors are important in regulating body weight and in whether we develop obesity. The first is family studies. For more than 75 years we have known that individuals from families with overweight parents are likely to be overweight. In contrast, individuals from families in which the parents are lean are likely to be lean. Adoption studies in which children are traced to their birth families show that the children are more like their biologic parents than like the parents who adopted them. Finally, studies in identical and nonidentical twins provide the icing on the cake, so to speak. When identical twins that have been reared in separate families from birth are identified, they are found to be more like each other than are nonidentical twins similarly reared apart. From these data we can place the role of genetic factors between 35% and 70% of the inheritance of obesity, meaning that if one individual in a given environment becomes overweight, it is highly likely that his or her identical twin would also become overweight. If one twin resists obesity, then the other identical twin would be very likely to resist obesity as well.

Further insight into the genetic causes of obesity has come from the cloning of several genes that produce obesity in human beings. Leptin, identified in 1994, was the first of these important gene products to be identified. As noted previously, it is produced in adipose tissue and secreted into the blood in relation to the amount of body fat.[34] Leptin-deficient individuals are massively obese from childhood. When they are treated with leptin, food intake falls and body fat is mobilized until body weight is nearly normalized, indicating that this is an important metabolic pathway for which the gene has been identified. This genetic defect is extremely rare, and most obese people have an appropriate level of circulation leptin for their size.

The most common single gene defect in obese children and adults is in the melanocortin-4 receptor, a key regulator of food intake.[35] When this receptor is inactive, food intake is nearly as high as when leptin is deficient. When this receptor is only partially inactivated, the food intake is only modestly beyond control levels.

Several other rare genetic defects have been identified in the regulatory process for controlling food intake that when abnormal lead to obesity. These basic biologic insights tell us that body fat has important regulation that is largely, if not completely, independent of willpower.

Intrauterine Imprinting

Several intrauterine events may lead to obesity later in life, probably because of fetal imprinting as a result of early exposure that affects brain plasticity. The Dutch winter famine of 1945 showed that starvation of infants in utero could affect long-term postnatal weight status. Another example is the infants of mothers who smoked during pregnancy, who have an increased risk of becoming overweight during their first three decades of life when compared with infants of mothers who did not smoke during pregnancy.[36] Similarly, infants of mothers who have diabetes are at higher risk of developing obesity than infants born to mothers who did not have diabetes during pregnancy.[37] Infants who are small for their birth date are at higher risk of developing central adiposity and diabetes than normal-weight infants.[38] Finally, experimental studies teach us that exposure to high levels of **insulin** during the period of brain plasticity can lead to obesity later in life.

Physiologic Control

To maintain a stable body weight over time, the body must correct daily errors in energy balance. A number of physiologic factors are known to disturb this correction. A high rate of carbohydrate oxidation, as measured by a high respiratory quotient (RQ) predicts future weight gain.[39] One explanation is that when carbohydrate oxidation is higher than carbohydrate intake, carbohydrate stores are depleted and we must eat to replace them. Obese individuals who have lost weight are less effective in increasing fat oxidation in the presence of a high-fat meal than normal-weight individuals, and this may be one reason why they are so susceptible to weight regain. Low metabolic rate may also predict future weight gain.[40]

Physical activity gradually declines with age, accounting for some increase in body fat. Recent studies suggest moderate exercise is beneficial in reducing risk of cardiovascular disease[41] and type 2 diabetes, as well as in facilitating the oxidation of fat in the diet.[9]

Fat cells in our body serve two major functions: (1) They store and release fatty acids ingested from food or from liver or fat cells, and (2) they secrete many important hormones and chemicals. The discovery of leptin catapulted the fat cell into the arena of endocrine cells.[42] In addition to leptin, the fat cell secretes a variety of other peptides (lipoprotein lipase, adipsin [complement D], complement C, adiponectin, TNF-α, IL-6, PAI-1, angiotensinogen, bradykinin, and resistin). The fat cell also releases other metabolites such as lactate, fatty acids, glycerol, and prostacyclin formed from arachidonic acid. Our understanding of fat cells as important endocrine cells continues to expand.

Production of cortisol from inactive cortisone in fat cells by the enzyme 11 β-hydroxysteroid dehydrogenase type 1 may be important in determining the quantity of visceral adipose tissue.[43] Changes in this enzyme may contribute to the risk for menopausal women to develop more visceral fat. High levels of this enzyme keep the quantity of cortisol in visceral fat high, providing a fertile environment for developing new fat cells.

Increased visceral fat seems to result in a high level of proinflamatory cytokines. The ratio of visceral fat is proportional to the risk for development of metabolic and cardiovascular problems associated with obesity. Interestingly if a substantial amount of visceral fat is surgically removed, then insulin resistance is immediately improved.[44]

Information about hunger and satiety comes from the gastrointestinal (GI) tract, where several peptides signal the body to stop or start eating. Ghrelin has received recent attention because, in contrast to other GI hormones, it stimulates food intake.[45] Levels of ghrelin are low in obesity, except for the Prader-Willi syndrome, suggesting that it may play a role.

The brain is a receiver, transducer, and transmitter of information about hunger and satiety. Several neurotransmitter systems are involved in regulation of food intake.[46] Serotonin receptors modulate the quantity of food eaten and macronutrient selection, and their loss through genetic targeting produces obesity. Peptide neurotransmitters also play a very important role in the regulation of feeding. Sleep deprivation is one way to enhance the release of peptides that produce hunger.[47] In young men allowed to sleep only 4 hours per night for 2 days, leptin decreased and ghrelin increased relative to the pattern seen with 10 hours of sleep on each of 2 nights.

OVERVIEW OF TREATING THE DISEASE OF OBESITY

Prevention of the Current Epidemic

The epidemic of obesity occurs on a genetic background that has not changed significantly in the last 100 years and certainly not since the epidemic began 20 years ago. Nonetheless, it is clear that genetic factors play a critical role in the susceptibility of becoming obese in a "toxic environment."[48] One analogy is that "genes load the gun and a permissive or toxic environment pulls the trigger." Modification of environmental factors acting on our ancient genes must be the strategy to prevent the disease. The belief that this can be done by the individual alone is to miss the argument of how environmental factors have acted on these genes to produce the current epidemic, with major emphasis on the imprinting of the plastic brain of the growing child and adolescent.

We argue that the First Law of Thermodynamics has lulled us into the uncomfortable position of believing that individuals, through willpower, increased food choices, or more places to exercise can overcome the current epidemic of obesity. Cognitive approaches relying on individual commitment and resolve have been unsuccessful in stemming the epidemic, and nothing suggests that they will be more successful in the future.

We also argue that it is what the First Law of Thermodynamics does not tell us that is important. In this context it is the unconscious host systems on which environmental factors operate that produces the disease. If the vending machines that now provide kickbacks to schools contained beverages with no added sugar or HFCS, then available calories would be reduced. We have argued that the exposure of young children to HFCS may produce detrimental imprinting of the brain, making obesity more likely and more difficult to control.

At least three preventive strategies are available to deal with the epidemic: (1) education, (2) regulation, and (3) modification of the food supply. Education in the school curriculum about good nutrition and healthy weight would be beneficial in helping all children learn how to select appropriate foods. School breakfast and lunch programs would match the educational messages.

However, it is unwise to rely on educational strategies alone, because they have not prevented the epidemic of obesity. Regulation is a second strategy. Regulating an improved food label would be one good idea. Regulations on appropriate serving sizes might be part of the information provided by restaurants when requested.

Modification in some components of the food system is a third and most important strategy. Because the energy we eat comes from food, we need to modify this system to provide smaller portions and less energy density if we are to succeed in combating the epidemic of obesity.

Treatment of Overweight People When Prevention Fails

A detailed discussion of treatment for obesity is beyond the scope of this chapter, but a few general comments about the major approaches are essential because they involve food intake and exercise. Although prevention is unlikely to be successful by relying solely on individual initiative, treatment requires individual initiative. For any change to occur, the individual must be ready for change. This idea of "stages of change" is a key component of any individual approach. The overweight person must be aware that he or she has a problem and must have moved beyond the stage of precontemplation (i.e., the stage of denial before a person is willing to do something about a problem) and into a stage of contemplation and then to action. When overweight individuals are in this state, they are ready to move forward. Their options are diet, exercise, behavioral therapy, medication, and surgery. These are the principal approaches available to those who have a weight problem that they want to address. The use of diet, exercise, and behavioral therapy are appropriate for all levels of overweight.

Dietetic professionals can play an important role in all of these approaches. First, the educated dietetic professional needs to be keenly aware of the complexity of the obesity problem. The dietitian obviously cannot alter the genetic makeup of an individual but is able to address the environmental aspects that serve to exacerbate the situation. Simply handing out diet sheets should be discouraged. Helping the obese patient requires attention to his or her overall diet history, current eating and activity patterns, and behavioral obstacles that either cause problems or prevent change. Although quick weight loss may be the patient's immediate desire, the need for permanent lifestyle changes should be the primary objective. Tips for addressing this have been outlined

KEY TERMS

insulin Hormone produced by the pancreas that lowers blood glucose by enhancing its entry into cells.

by Bray and Champagne (Box 15-1).[49] Finally, the dietitian can be an instrument of change by appealing to policymakers to modify environmental conditions such as the school vending machine situation cited previously. We can think of no better professional than the dietitian to craft this effective message to lawmakers and school officials.

BOX 15-1 PRACTICE POINTS FOR THE CLINICAL DIETITIAN

- *Focus on personal history:* More than ever, the personal history of the patient is a critical focus area for the dietitian in clinical practice who deals with patients diagnosed with the metabolic syndrome. In particular, assessment of past dietary habits using a valid food frequency questionnaire is warranted. The current dietary practices of the patient can help to highlight target areas; collecting a food record for as many days as the patient is willing to keep it will be instrumental in future counseling efforts.
- *Obtain thorough information:* Encouraging the patient to provide as much dietary information as possible will make a measurable difference in the accuracy of the dietary data for evaluation purposes. Remember to focus on the fact that no judgments will be formed; you are simply identifying areas of diet for which you will be targeting change.
- *Assess exercise habits:* Physical activity patterns are useful for designing the total lifestyle program. The dietitian may choose to collect a physical activity questionnaire from the patient and, in addition, provide the patient with an activity monitor to assess actual physical activity steps for a more accurate appraisal of daily activity levels.
- *Customize:* For increased success, dietary treatment needs to be highly individualized. It may be helpful to include a variety of weight loss strategies, such as meal replacements (for quicker initial weight loss), slightly higher protein diets, low-fat diets, and perhaps even a Mediterranean diet approach. An important point to remember: What works for one patient may not necessarily be ideal for another.
- *Consult the physician:* Working with the patient's physician to provide the ideal combination of diet, physical activity suggestions, behavior changes, and medication (if prescribed by the physician) is key to the patient's success.
- *Follow up:* Regular evaluations to monitor patient progress are key to weight management by the physician and the dietitian in clinical practice.

Data from Bray GA, Champagne CM: Obesity and the metabolic syndrome: implications for dietetics practitioners, *J Am Diet Assoc* 104:86,2004.

Diet

Popular diets have been published for more than 150 years; obviously, if any diet were significantly better than the others, it would have "won the battle" and the others would have disappeared. Popular diets can be grouped into several categories: low-energy (calorie) diets, low-fat diets, low-carbohydrate diets, and high-protein diets. A summary of data abstracted by the U.S. Department of Agriculture (USDA) is shown in Table 15-1.

Several popular diets, including the Atkins Diet (low carbohydrate), the Ornish (low fat), Weight Watchers, and the Zone diet (high protein), were recently compared and found to produce comparable weight loss, suggesting that none of these diets has an increased effect.[50] A randomized clinical trial that compared reduced-calorie diets with different macronutrient targets (low or high fat, average or high protein, low or high carbohydrate) determined that any type of reduced-calorie diet can be effective in achieving weight loss.[51]

Exercise

Increased movement, both modest and vigorous, is a way to increase energy expenditure that will burn fat deposits. Human beings expend approximately two thirds of their energy with basal activities, including maintaining body temperature, and only approximately one third in various activities. Thus to expend a significant number of calories through exercise takes time. As a rule of thumb, approximately 100 kcal are expended for each mile walked. If it takes 15 minutes to walk a mile, then you could expend up to 400 kcal in an hour of brisk walking. From a practical point of view it is often easier to eat 400 kcal less than to exercise for the extra 400 kcal. Beyond any effect on body weight, regular activity can have beneficial effects on improving cardiovascular health.

Behavioral Therapy

Since their introduction in 1967, behavioral approaches to helping overweight individuals focus on the issues that revolve around eating have been a cornerstone in the treatment of obesity. These techniques are adapted from psychologic learning theory, in which rewarding appropriate behavior tends to reinforce that behavior. The process involves familiarity with the activities associated with learning and providing consequences of eating, as well as rewards that reinforce appropriate behaviors. Among the successful techniques in this area are self-monitoring, increased physical

TABLE 15-1 FEATURES OF THE MAJOR DIETS USED BY AMERICANS

TYPE OF DIET	CALORIES	FAT, g (%)	CARBOHYDRATE, g (%)	PROTEIN, g (%)
Typical American Diet	2200	85 (35)	274 (50)	82 (15)
High-fat, low-carbohydrate diet	1400	94 (60)	35 (10)	105 (30)
Moderate-fat diet	1450	40 (25)	218 (60)	54 (15)
Low-fat and very-low-fat diet	1450	16-24 (10-15)	235-271 (65-75)	54-72 (15-20)

Modified from Freedman MR, King J, Kennedy E: Popular diets: a scientific review, *Obes Res* 9(suppl):1S, 2001, with permission from NAASO, The Obesity Society.

activity, and eating a lower-fat diet. People who are successful at maintaining a lowered body weight over time use these and other techniques.

Medication

Currently only six medications are approved by the U.S. Food and Drug Administration (FDA) for the treatment of obesity. These include four drugs that have only been approved for short-term use (benzphetamine [Didrex], diethylpropion [Tenuate], phendimetrazine [Adipost, Anorex-SR, Appecon, Bontril PDM, Bontril Slow-Release, Melfiat, Obezine, Phendiet, Plegine, Prelu-2, Statobex], and phentermine [Adipex-P, Fastin, Ionamin, Obenix, Obephen, Oby-Cap, Oby-Trim, Panshape M, Phentercot, Phentride, Pro-Fast HS, Pro-Fast SA, Pro-Fast SR, Teramine, Zantryl]) and two drugs that have been approved for longer-term use—orlistat (Xenical) and sibutramine (Meridia). Researchers believe that the four short-term drugs and sibutramine work by modifying the neurotransmitters in the CNS. Each of these drugs works in part by binding to molecules on the surface of brain cells (neurons) that transport neurotransmitters back into these neurons after they have been secreted. Because they are related to the addictive drugs amphetamine, albeit quite indirectly, the U.S. government regulated their use through the Drug Enforcement Administration (DEA). In clinical studies with these drugs, the weight loss is approximately 4 to 5 kg (8.8 to 11 lb) more than with placebo controls after 6 to 12 months of treatment. To be eligible for use of medications, an individual needs to have a BMI greater than 30 kg/m^2, unless associated problems exist, such as diabetes, heart disease, high blood pressure, or other problems that would benefit from weight loss. In that case, the lower limit for use of medications may be 27 kg/m^2 (see the *Diet-Medications Interactions* box, "Drugs Used to Treat Obesity").

Orlistat contrasts with these centrally acting drugs. It works in the intestine to block an enzyme called *lipase,* which is produced and secreted from the pancreas. At clinically used doses, it blocks digestion of approximately one third of the dietary fat. This dietary fat then passes through the intestinal tract and exits the body in the feces. When used improperly, this drug can produce significant GI tract symptoms. In clinical studies this drugs produces 2 to 4 kg (4.4 to 8.8 lb) more weight loss than placebo-treated groups and appears to be slightly less effective.[52]

The FDA is expected to approve a new class of drugs called the *cannabinoid receptor antagonists* (rimonabant [Acomplia]). These work by blocking the receptor that binds endocannabinoids (anandamide and 2-arachidonoylglycerol). Clinical studies show that rimonabant produces weight loss that is about 5 kg (11 lb) more than placebo, which is similar to other available drugs. Other new drugs are under trial and may become available fairly soon.

In addition to prescription medication, a variety of herbs and supplements are used to help individuals lose weight (see the *Complementary and Alternative Medicine [CAM]* box, "Common Herbs and Supplements Used for Weight Loss").

Surgery

Use of surgery for treatment of obesity has expanded greatly in the last decade of the twentieth century.[53] Several different types of operations are currently in use for treatment of obesity. Usually the stomach is restricted, part of the small intestine is bypassed, or both. To be eligible for surgical intervention, an overweight individual needs to have a BMI greater than 40 kg/m^2, unless the person has associated diseases such as diabetes, heart disease, sleep apnea, or osteoarthritis, in which case the BMI for considering therapy can be lowered to 35 kg/m^2. Gastric bypass is associated with the near-elimination of type 2 diabetes and improvements in cardiovascular risk factors, sleep apnea, and quality of life. Side effects include dumping syndrome, which produces nausea, flushing, bloating, and extreme diarrhea.[53,54]

HEALTH PROMOTION

Our lives are constrained by the laws of nature—gravity, momentum, and thermodynamics—with which we have been dealing in this chapter. The strategies we take to deal

KEY TERMS

benzphetamine One of the appetite-suppressant drugs that has been approved for more than 30 years for short-term use but that is regulated by the U.S. Drug Enforcement Agency (DEA) because of potential for addictive abuse (trade name, Didrex).

diethylpropion One of the appetite-suppressant drugs that has been approved for more than 30 years for short-term use but that is regulated by the DEA because of potential for addictive abuse (trade name, Tenuate).

phendimetrazine One of the appetite-suppressant drugs that has been approved for more than 30 years for short-term use but that is regulated by the DEA because of potential for addictive abuse; trade names Adipost, Anorex-SR, Appecon, Bontril PDM, Bontril Slow-Release, Melfiat, Obezine, Phendiet, Plegine, Prelu-2, and Statobex.

phentermine One of the appetite-suppressant drugs that has been approved for more than 30 years for short-term use but that is regulated by the DEA because of potential for addictive abuse; trade names Adipex-P, Fastin, Ionamin, Obenix, Obephen, Oby-Cap, Oby-Trim, Panshape M, Phentercot, Phentride, Pro-Fast HS, Pro-Fast SA, Pro-Fast SR, Teramine, and Zantryl.

orlistat Drug (trade name, Xenical) that partially blocks pancreatic lipase, thus decreasing digestion of dietary fat. It is available by prescription and over the counter.

sibutramine A newer appetite-suppressant drug that has been approved for long-term use but that is still regulated by the DEA because of potential for addictive abuse (trade name, Meridia).

pancreas Gland located near the duodenum and small intestine that has two sets of cells: (1) acinar cells, which secrete digestive enzymes into the intestine, and (2) beta-cells, which produce and secrete insulin into the blood.

DIET-MEDICATIONS INTERACTIONS

Drugs Used to Treat Obesity

GENERIC NAME	TRADE NAME	MECHANISM OF ACTION	FOOD-DRUG INTERACTIONS
Benzphetamine	Didrex	Appetite suppressant, stimulates CNS and decreases appetite (similar to amphetamine); short-term use only	Alcohol may increase the dizziness effects of this medicine.
Diethylpropion	Tenuate, Tenuate Dospan		
Phendimetrazine	Adipost, Anorex-SR, Appecon, Bontril PDM, Bontril Slow-Release, Melfiat, Obezine, Phendiet, Plegine, Preu-2, Statobex		A reduced-calorie diet must be followed while using an appetite suppressant to lose weight. In addition, to keep the lost weight from returning, changes in diet and exercise must be continued after the weight has been lost.
Phentermine	Adipex-P, Fastin, Ionamin, Obenix, Obephen, Oby-Cap, Oby-Trim, Panshape M, Phentercot, Phentride, Pro-Fast HS, Pro-Fast SA, Pro-Fast SR, Teramine, Zantryl		
Orlistat	Xenical	Blocks fat from being absorbed in intestine	This drug prevents the absorption of some dietary fat. It should be taken during the meal or within 1 hour of eating and may decrease absorption of fat-soluble vitamins from food. A multivitamin supplement should be taken once a day at least 2 hours before or after taking orlistat. The diet should contain no more than 30% of calories as fat; more fat in the diet will increase side effects. Patients who have diabetes mellitus may need to have their insulin or oral hypoglycemic agents adjusted. Patients may experience gas with leaky bowel movements, inability to hold bowel movements, increased bowel movements, oily bowel movements, and oily spotting of underclothes.
Sibutramine	Meridia	Boosts levels of serotonin, dopamine, and norepinephrine in the body	A reduced-calorie diet must be observed in conjunction with the medication to lose weight and keep it off. The patient should not drink alcohol.

with the influence of these laws on our lives include education, regulation, and product design. Deaths from the effects of the laws of momentum produced by automobile accidents provide a glimpse into the strategies we could use to minimize this effect. They also provide insights into the strategies that may be needed to deal with the epidemic of obesity. Although the laws of momentum or the laws of thermodynamics cannot be changed, their effect on producing automobile accidents and obesity can be mitigated. This goal can be achieved through better education about driving and about nutritional needs to prevent obesity. Education can be complemented in the case of cars by regulations that require seat belts, airbags, and other safety devices. In the case of obesity it can be complemented by limiting access to large portion sizes and to high energy–density foods, as well as creating an environment in which physical activity is more prevalent. Finally, product design to make cars safer partly addresses the driving problem, just as modifying the types of foods that are available helps to combat the obesity epidemic by redesigning the food environment.

COMPLEMENTARY AND ALTERNATIVE MEDICINE (CAM)

Common Herbs and Supplements Used for Weight Loss

HERB/ SUPPLEMENT	COMMON USES	DRUG/HERB INTERACTIONS	INTERACTION	SAFETY	EFFICACY
Chromium	Thought to improve insulin sensitivity, causing insulin levels to fall, thereby initiating lipolysis	Hypoglycemic agents	Possible potentiation of drug, increasing risk of hypoglycemia	Safe	Strong evidence
		Calcium carbonate and antacids	Reduce chromium absorption		
Pyruvate	Enhance fat metabolism	No known drug interactions		Formal toxicologic studies not reported	Some evidence of weight loss when used in conjunction with low-calorie diet
5-HTP (5-hydroxy-tryptophan)	Serotonin precursor	Levodopa/ carbidopa	Possible increased risk of scleroderma-like syndrome	No significant adverse effects reported in clinical trials	Some evidence it is helpful in weight loss
		SSRIs, other serotonergic drugs	Possible risk of serotonin syndrome		
Hydroxycitric acid (HCA)		No known drug interactions		No serious side effects reported, but formal safety studies not performed	Weak evidence it might be useful for weight loss
Caffeine-ephedrine	Stimulant	CNS stimulants	Potentiation of stimulant side effects Death	Use of herb ephedra instead of ephedrine may present unpredictable risks	Strong evidence it promotes short- and long-term weight loss
Conjugated linoleic acid (CLA)	Reduce body weight while retaining muscle mass	None known		Appears to be a safe nutritional substance	Contradictory evidence that CLAs might help reduce fat mass
Calcium	Weight and fat loss	Calcium channel blockers	Action may be affected by combination calcium supplements and high-dose vitamin D	Calcium supplements may increase kidney stone risk, but dietary calcium reduces risk of kidney stones	Dietary calcium facilitates more weight loss than calcium supplements (calcium carbonate)
		β-blockers	May decrease blood levels		
		Tetracycline and fluoroquinolone antibiotics	May interfere with absorption; take calcium supplements at least 2 hr before antibiotic dosing		
		Thiazide diuretics	Long-term use of thiazide diuretics tends to increase serum calcium levels by decreasing calcium excretion		
		Corticosteroids and anticonvulsants	Interfere with absorption of calcium		
Gymnema (*Gymnema sylvestre*)	Diminish ability to taste sweet substances and decrease appetite for up to 90 min	Hyperglycemic drugs or insulin	Important to monitor blood glucose levels closely	Not known	May be useful in reducing cravings for sweets

Continued

COMPLEMENTARY AND ALTERNATIVE MEDICINE (CAM)

Common Herbs and Supplements Used for Weight Loss —cont'd

HERB/ SUPPLEMENT	COMMON USES	DRUG/HERB INTERACTIONS	INTERACTION	SAFETY	EFFICACY
Yohimbe *(Pausinystalia yohimbe)*	CNS stimulant	Phenothiazines (chlorpromazine)	Increases yohimbe toxicity Side effects: priapism, hypertension or hypotension (depending on dose), irritability, migraines, dizziness, tremors, bronchospasm, insomnia, tachycardia, nausea and vomiting	Inappropriate for long-term use	Inhibits hunger
		MAOIs, tricyclic antidepressants	Hypertensive crisis		
		Antihypertensive medications (e.g., clonidine)	Antagonizes effects of drugs		

Data from Bratman S, Girman AM, for HealthGate Data Corp: *Mosby's handbook of herbs and supplements and their therapeutic uses,* St Louis, 2003, Mosby; Contributors and consultants: *Professional guide to complementary and alternative therapies,* Springhouse, Pa, 2001, Springhouse; Kuhn MA, Winston D: *Herbal therapy and supplements: a scientific and traditional approach,* Philadelphia, 2001, Lippincott Williams & Wilkins; Zemel MB, Thompson W, Milstead A, Morris K, & Campbell P: Calcium and dairy acceleration of weight and fat loss during energy restriction in obese adults, *Obes Res* 12(4):582, 2004.

TO SUM UP

Obesity is a chronic, relapsing disease characterized by an accumulation of excess body fat caused by habitual consumption of more energy than is used. Normally physiologic systems hold the body in energy balance, but environmental factors such as food, medications, physical inactivity, toxins, and viruses can interact with the host's genetic predisposition to gain weight. Obesity is a major health issue because it increases the risk for many other chronic diseases (especially type 2 diabetes), raises health care costs, and may produce psychologic stress. The increased prevalence of obesity in the last few decades has been attributed to a "toxic environment" of abundant high-energy foods with little need for physical activity. Reversing this trend requires a better understanding of how environmental factors affect the development of obesity and a redesigning of these factors.

QUESTIONS FOR REVIEW

1. Why is obesity considered to be a disease?
2. What are the psychologic, pathologic, and financial effects of obesity?
3. Why are adipose cells considered to be endocrine cells?
4. Explain how portion sizes may contribute to obesity.
5. How does high fructose corn syrup contribute to obesity?
6. What is the function of leptin?
7. What have twin studies shown about obesity?
8. What are three prevention strategies for dealing with the obesity epidemic?
9. What is the most effective popular diet?
10. What criteria must a person meet to qualify for weight loss surgery?

REFERENCES

1. Bray GA: Obesity is a chronic, relapsing neurochemical disease, *Int J Obes Relat Metab Disord* 28:34–38, 2004.
2. Flegal KM, Graubard BI: Estimates of excess deaths associated with body mass index and other anthropometric variables, *Am J Clin Nutr* 89(4):1213, 2009.
3. Hedley AA, Ogden CL, Johnson CL, et al: Prevalence of overweight and obesity among U.S. children, adolescents, and adults, 1999-2002, *JAMA* 291:2847, 2004.
4. National Center for Health Statistics: *Health, United States, 2007 with chartbook on trends in the health of Americans,* Hyattsville, Md, 2007, Centers for Disease Control and Prevention.
5. Ogden CL, Carroll MD, Flegal KM: High body mass index for age among U.S. children and adolescents, 2003-2006, *JAMA* 299:2401, 2008.
6. Klein S, Burke LE, Bray GA, et al: Clinical implications of obesity with specific focus on cardiovascular disease: a statement for professionals from the American Heart Association Council on Nutrition, Physical Activity, and Metabolism: endorsed by the American College of Cardiology Foundation, *Circulation* 110:2952, 2004.
7. Finkelstein EA, Ruhm CJ, Kosa KM: Economic causes and consequences of obesity, *Annu Rev Public Health* 26:239, 2005.
8. Knowler WC, Barrett-Connor E, Fowler SE, et al: Reduction in the incidence of type 2 diabetes with lifestyle intervention or metformin, *N Engl J Med* 346:393, 2002.
9. Smith SR, de Jong L, Zachwieja JJ, et al: Concurrent physical activity increases fat oxidation during the shift to a high-fat diet, *Am J Clin Nutr* 72(1):131, 2000.

10. Kinsell LW, Gunning B, Michaels GD, et al: Calories do count, *Metabolism* 13:195, 1964.
11. Lyon XH, Di Vetta V, Milon H, et al: Compliance to dietary advice directed towards increasing the carbohydrate to fat ratio of the everyday diet, *Int J Obes Relat Metab Disord* 19(4):260, 1995.
12. Licinio J, Caglayan S, Ozata M, et al: Phenotypic effects of leptin replacement on morbid obesity, diabetes mellitus, hypogonadism, and behavior in leptin-deficient adults, *Proc Natl Acad Sci U S A* 101:4531, 2004.
13. Institute of Medicine: *Weighing the options: criterias for evaluation weight-management programs*, Washington, DC, 1995, National Academies Press.
14. Nielsen SJ, Popkin BM: Patterns and trends in food portion sizes, 1977-1998, *JAMA* 289:450, 2003.
15. Putman JL: Absolute measurements of the activity of beta emitters, *Br J Radiol* 23:46, 1950.
16. Bray GA, Nielsen SJ, Popkin BM: Consumption of high-fructose corn syrup in beverages may play a role in the epidemic of obesity, *Am J Clin Nutr* 79:537, 2004.
17. Putman JL: Absolute measurements of the activity of beta emitters, *Br J Radiol* 23:46–63, 1950.
18. Ludwig DS, Peterson KE, Gortmaker SL: Relation between consumption of sugar-sweetened drinks and childhood obesity: a prospective, observational analysis, *Lancet* 357:505, 2001.
19. Ludwig DS, Peterson KE, Gortmaker SL: Relation between consumption of sugar-sweetened drinks and childhood obesity: a prospective, observational analysis, *Lancet* 357:505, 2001.
20. Raben A, Gerholm-Larsen L, Flint A, et al: Meals with similar energy densities but rich in protein, fat, carbohydrate, or alcohol have different effects on energy expenditure and substrate metabolism but not on appetite and energy intake, *Am J Clin Nutr* 77:91, 2003.
21. James J, Thomas P, Cavan D, et al: Preventing childhood obesity by reducing consumption of carbonated drinks: cluster randomized controlled trial, *BMJ* 328:1237, 2004.
22. Bray GA, Paeratakul S, Popkin BM: Dietary fat and obesity: a review of animal, clinical and epidemiological studies, *Physiol Behav* 83:549, 2004.
23. Drewnowski A, Specter SE: Poverty and obesity: the role of energy density and energy costs, *Am J Clin Nutr* 79:6, 2004.
24. Blundell JE, Macdiarmid JI: Fat as a risk factor for overconsumption: satiation, satiety, and patterns of eating, *J Am Diet Assoc* 97:S63, 1997.
25. Beyerlein A, Toschke AM, von Kries R: Breastfeeding and childhood obesity: shift of the entire BMI distribution or only the upper parts? *Obesity (Silver Spring)* 16:2730, 2008.
26. Ailhaud G, Guesnet P: Fatty acid composition of fats is an early determinant of childhood obesity: a short review and an opinion, *Obes Rev* 5:21, 2004.
27. Bhargava SK, Sachdev HS, Fall CH, et al: Relation of serial changes in childhood body-mass index to impaired glucose tolerance in young adulthood, *N Engl J Med* 350:865, 2004.
28. Reimer R: Milk product intake: implications for weight control and type 2 diabetes, *Can Nurse* 104:20, 2008.
29. Hancox RJ, Milne BJ, Poulton R: Association of television viewing during childhood with poor educational achievement, *Arch Pediatr Adolesc Med* 159:614, 2005.
30. Allison DB, Mentore JL, Heo M, et al: Antipsychotic-induced weight gain: a comprehensive research synthesis, *Am J Psychiatry* 156:1686, 1999.
31. O'Hara P, Connett JE, Lee WW, et al: Early and late weight gain following smoking cessation in the lung health study, *Am J Epidemiol* 148:821, 1998.
32. Dhurandhar NV, Israel BA, Kolesar JM, et al: Increased adiposity in animals due to a human virus, *Int J Obes* 24:989, 2000.
33. Tremblay A, Pelletier C, Doucet E, et al: Thermogenesis and weight loss in obese individuals: a primary association with organochlorine pollution, *Obes Res* 11:A53, 2003.
34. Zhang Y, Scarpace PJ: The role of leptin in leptin resistance and obesity, *Physiol Behav* 88:249, 2006.
35. O'Rahilly S, Farooqi IS, Yeo GSH, et al: Minireview: human obesity—lessons from monogenic disorders, *Endocrinology* 144:3757, 2003.
36. Toschke AM, Ehlin AGC, von Kries R, et al: Maternal smoking during pregnancy and appetite control in offspring, *J Perinat Med* 31:251, 2003.
37. Dabelea D, Pettitt DJ, Hanson RL, et al: Birth weight, type 2 diabetes, and insulin resistance in Pima Indian children and young adults, *Diabetes Care* 22:944, 1999.
38. Pereira MA, Jacobs DR, Van Horn L, et al: Dairy consumption, obesity, and the insulin resistance syndrome in young adults—The CARDIA study, *JAMA* 287:2081, 2002.
39. Zurlo F, Lillioja S, Esposito-Del PA, et al: Low ratio of fat to carbohydrate oxidation as predictor of weight gain: study of 24-h RQ, *Am J Physiol* 259:E650, 1990.
40. Astrup A, Gotzsche PC, van de Werken K, et al: Meta-analysis of resting metabolic rate in formerly obese subjects, *Am J Clin Nutr* 69:1117, 1999.
41. Blair SN, Lamonte MJ, Nichaman MZ: The evolution of physical activity recommendations: how much is enough? *Am J Clin Nutr* 79:913, 2004.
42. Spiegelman BM, Flier JS: Obesity and the regulation of energy balance, *Cell* 104:531, 2001.
43. Hochberg Z, Friedberg M, Yaniv L, et al: Hypothalamic regulation of adiposity: the role of 11 beta-hydroxysteroid dehydrogenase type 1, *Horm Metab Res* 36:365, 2004.
44. Esposito K, Giugliano G, Scuderi N, et al: Role of adipokines in the obesity-inflammation relationship: the effect of fat removal, *Plast Reconstr Surg* 118:1048, 2006.
45. Cummings DE, Frayo RS, Marmonier C, et al: Plasma ghrelin levels and hunger scores in humans initiating meals voluntarily without time- and food-related cues, *Am J Physiol Endicrinol Metab* 287:E297, 2004.
46. Cowley MA, Cone RD, Enriori P, et al: Electrophysiological actions of peripheral hormones on melanocortin neurons, *Ann N Y Acad Sci* 994:175, 2003.
47. Spiegel K, Tasali E, Penev P, et al: Brief communication: sleep curtailment in healthy young men is associated with decreased leptin levels, elevated ghrelin levels, and increased hunger and appetite, *Ann Intern Med* 141:846, 2004.
48. Rankinen T, Zuberi A, Chagnon YC, et al: The human obesity gene map: the 2005 update, *Obesity (Silver Spring)* 14:529, 2006.
49. Bray GA, Champagne CM: Obesity and the metabolic syndrome: implications for dietetics practitioners, *J Am Diet Assoc* 104:86, 2004.
50. Dansiger ML, Gleason JA, Griffith JL, et al: Comparison of the Atkins, Ornish, Weight Watchers, and Zone Diets for weight loss and heart disease risk reduction, *JAMA* 293(1):43, 2005.
51. Sacks FM, Bray GA, Carey VJ, et al: Comparison of weight-loss diets with different compositions of fat, protein, and carbohydrates, *N Engl J Med* 360(9):859, 2009.
52. Rucker D, Padwal R, Li SK, et al: Long term pharmacotherapy for obesity and overweight: updated meta-analysis, *BMJ* 335:1194, 2007.
53. Cummings DE, Overduin J, Foster-Schubert KE: Gastric bypass for obesity: mechanisms of weight loss and diabetes resolution, *J Clin Endocrinol Metab* 89:2608, 2004.
54. Hill JO, Catenacci VA, Wyatt HR: Obesity: etiology. In Shils ME, Shike M, Ross AC, et al, editors: *Modern nutrition in health and disease*, Baltimore, Md, 2007, Lippincott Williams & Wilkins, pp 1013–1041.

Introduction to Clinical Nutrition

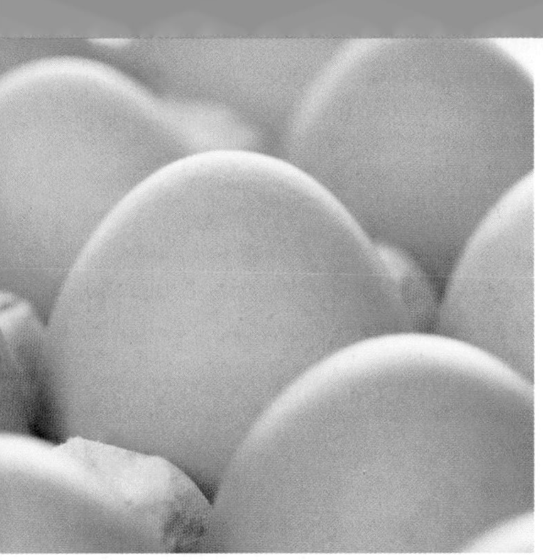

16

Nutrition Assessment and Nutrition Therapy in Patient Care

Sara Long Roth

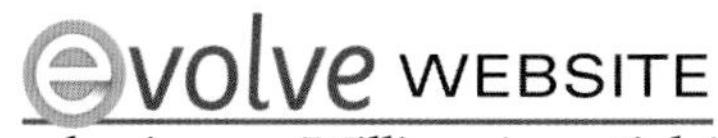

http://evolve.elsevier.com/Williams/essentials/

OUTLINE

In this chapter, we focus on the Nutrition Care Process (NCP)—the foundation of nutrition therapy. Information gathered during nutrition assessment is used to establish goals for nutrition intervention. Once interventions are initiated, monitoring and evaluation function as the point of reference from which to determine efficacy of treatment.

Nutrition assessment is defined as a "process used to evaluate nutritional status, identify disorders of nutrition, and determine which individuals need nutrition instruction and/or nutrition support."[1] Because no single test measures nutritional status, nutrition assessment draws from numerous indexes to provide a complete picture of nutritional health.[2]

ROLE OF NUTRITION IN CLINICAL CARE

Nutrition therapy plays an essential role in disease management, health care, and preventive health care and should be provided by a qualified nutrition professional.[2,3] Comprehensive nutrition assessment provides the necessary foundation for appropriate nutrition therapy based on identified needs. Nutrition assessment and nutrition therapy promote multiple goals: assisting patients in recovery from illness or injury, helping persons maintain follow-up care to promote health, and helping to control health care costs.[4] Registered dietitians (RDs) use their expertise and skills to make sound clinical judgments and to work effectively with the clinical care team. These professionals provide an essential component for successful management of the patient's plan of care.

Nutritional Status

Nutritional status can be established by measuring indicators of nutrient stores. Variations of nutrient stores result in changes in nutritional status when nutrient needs and nutrient use are increased or alterations in nutrient intake occur. Inadequacy or excess of a particular nutrient produces physiologic alteration in the body.[2]

Malnutrition

Many patients are malnourished when admitted to the hospital, whereas others may develop malnutrition during their hospital stay.[5] Hospitalized patients with hypermetabolic and physiologic stress of illness or injury can be at risk for malnutrition from increased nutritional needs. Hospital operating guidelines that provide for nutrition screening on admission combined with follow-up monitoring will identify patients at malnutrition risk and provide essential medical nutrition therapy.[2] However, potential problems arising from hospital routines may contribute to a lack of adequate nourishment in some cases, including the following:

- Highly restricted diets remaining on order and unsupplemented too long
- Unserved meals because of interference of medical procedures and clinical tests
- Unmonitored patient appetite

Each injured or ill patient is a unique person and requires special treatment and care. A formidable array of staff persons seek to determine needs and implement what each patient requires as appropriate care. When individual human needs are met with personal care, within the context of carefully developed care protocols, patients will not feel intimidated and powerless.

Undernutrition: Undernutrition subsequent to insufficient intake; altered digestion; or absorption of protein, energy, or both (calories); is called *protein-energy malnutrition (PEM)* or *protein-calorie malnutrition (PCM)*. Characteristics include weight loss, fat loss, muscle wasting and weakness, impaired immune function, poor wound healing, and reduction of protein synthesis.[1]

Overnutrition: More than two thirds of American adults are (1) overweight or (2) obese,[6] making these conditions the two most common forms of overnutrition.[1] Overweight is defined as body mass index (BMI) ≥25 and obesity as BMI ≥30 (Box 16-1). Both are associated with a number of health risks including coronary heart disease, type 2 diabetes mellitus, certain cancers (breast, endometrial, colon), hypertension, dyslipidemia, stroke, gallbladder disease, liver disease, sleep apnea, osteoarthritis, and infertility.[7]

NUTRITION SCREENING AND ASSESSMENT

Patients at nutritional risk need to be identified to allow provision of high-quality nutrition care.[8] Poor nutritional status may create complications that may lead to increased morbidity and mortality, length of stay, and cost of care.[9] Identification of nutrition risk is accomplished through the process of nutritional assessment. However, before patients can be assessed, they must first be identified. Identification takes place through the process of nutrition screening, the entry into the NCP (Box 16-2).[10]

Nutrition Screening

Nutrition screening is defined as "the process of identifying characteristics known to be associated with nutrition

BOX 16-1 BODY MASS INDEX

Calculating BMI

$$\text{BMI} = \frac{\text{Weight (kg)}}{\text{Height}^2\text{ (m)}} \text{ or BMI} = \frac{\text{Weight (lb)}}{\text{Height}^2\text{ (in)}} \times 704.5$$

Example: An individual weighs 65 kg (143 lb) and is 1.7 m (5′7″) tall. BMI = $65/(1.7)^2$ = 22.5 kg/m^2

Classification of BMI

Underweight: <18.5
Normal: 18.5-24.9
Overweight: 25.0-29.9
Obese: ≥30.0
Extreme obesity: ≥40.0

From Moore MC: *Pocket guide to nutrition assessment and care*, ed 6, St Louis, 2009, Mosby.

BOX 16-2 AMERICAN DIETETIC ASSOCIATION'S NUTRITION CARE PROCESS

Definition of the American Dietetic Association's Nutrition Care Process

Providing nutrition care using the American Dietetic Association (ADA)'s Nutrition Care Process (NCP) begins when a patient is recognized as being at nutritional risk and requiring additional support to attain or maintain positive nutritional status. The NCP is defined as "a systematic problem-solving method that dietetics professionals use to critically think and make decisions to address nutrition-related problems and provide safe and effective quality nutrition care." It is composed of the following four separate but interrelated and associated steps:

1. Nutrition assessment
2. Nutrition diagnosis
3. Nutrition intervention
4. Nutrition monitoring and evaluation

Each step builds on the preceding one, but the process is not necessarily linear. Figure 16-1 provides a visual illustration of the model.

Step 1: Nutrition Assessment

Techniques such as those outlined previously in the chapter are used to systematically obtain information necessary to determine or reassess whether or not a nutrition problem (or diagnosis) exists. If so, then the problem is diagnosed using a PES (problem, etiology, signs and symptoms) statement in step 2 of the NCP (see Figure 16-1).

Step 2: Nutrition Diagnosis

Before nutrition intervention can take place, the nutrition problem (or problems) must be identified. This is accomplished with the nutrition diagnosis. Standardized language has been developed to make the nutrition diagnosis clear to other nutrition and health care professionals. When the nutrition problem has been identified, it is labeled with a specific, standardized diagnostic term. The nutrition diagnosis statement or PES statement is organized in three distinct parts: (1) the problem (P); (2) the etiology, or cause, of the problem (E); and (3) the signs and symptoms associated with the problem (S). Typically, nutrition diagnoses fall into three categories or domains:

1. Intake
2. Clinical
3. Behavioral-environmental

Following is an example of how a nutrition diagnosis is written:

> Disordered eating pattern *related to* harmful belief about food and nutrition *as evidenced by* reported use of laxatives after meals and statements that calories are not absorbed when laxatives are used.

Step 3: Nutrition Intervention

Intervention begins once the nutritional diagnosis is identified. It is generally aimed at the etiology (E) of the nutrition diagnosis and is directed at reducing or eradicating effects of the signs and symptoms (S). Nutrition interventions are intended to modify a nutrition-related problem and are comprised of two interconnected components: (1) planning and (2) implementation. Nutrition diagnoses are prioritized in the planning component, whereby implementation is the "action phase." The plan is communicated and carried out, data are continued to be collected, and nutrition interventions are

BOX 16-2 AMERICAN DIETETIC ASSOCIATION'S NUTRITION CARE PROCESS

Definition of the American Dietetic Association's Nutrition Care Process—cont'd

revised as necessary. Four categories or domains of nutrition intervention have been identified:

1. Food and/or nutrient delivery
2. Nutrition education
3. Nutrition counseling
4. Coordination of care

Step 4: Nutrition Monitoring and Evaluation

The point of this step in the NCP is to measure improvement made by the patient in meeting nutrition care goals. Patients' progress is examined by determining if the nutrition intervention is being executed and by providing evidence that the intervention *is* or *is not* altering the patients' nutritional status. Nutrition monitoring and evaluation terms are organized into four categories or domains:

1. Food- and nutrition-related history
2. Biochemical data, medical tests, and procedures
3. Anthropometric measurements
4. Nutrition-focused physical findings

In summary, the NCP allows for continuous treatment alteration. As patients' conditions change, so do diagnoses, plans, and interventions. If patients do not respond to interventions, then new interventions can be developed for them. However, it is important to remember that any and all nutrition interventions should be planned along with patients, as well as with their caregivers or significant others. For more detailed information regarding the NCP, please refer to the references listed following.

BIBLIOGRAPHY

American Dietetic Association: *International Dietetics and Nutrition Terminology (IDNT) Reference Manual. Standardized language for the nutrition care process*, ed 2, Chicago, 2009, American Dietetic Association.

Lacey K, Pritchitt E: Nutrition Care Process and model: ADA adopts road map to quality care and outcomes management, *J Am Diet Assoc* 103(8):1061, 2003.

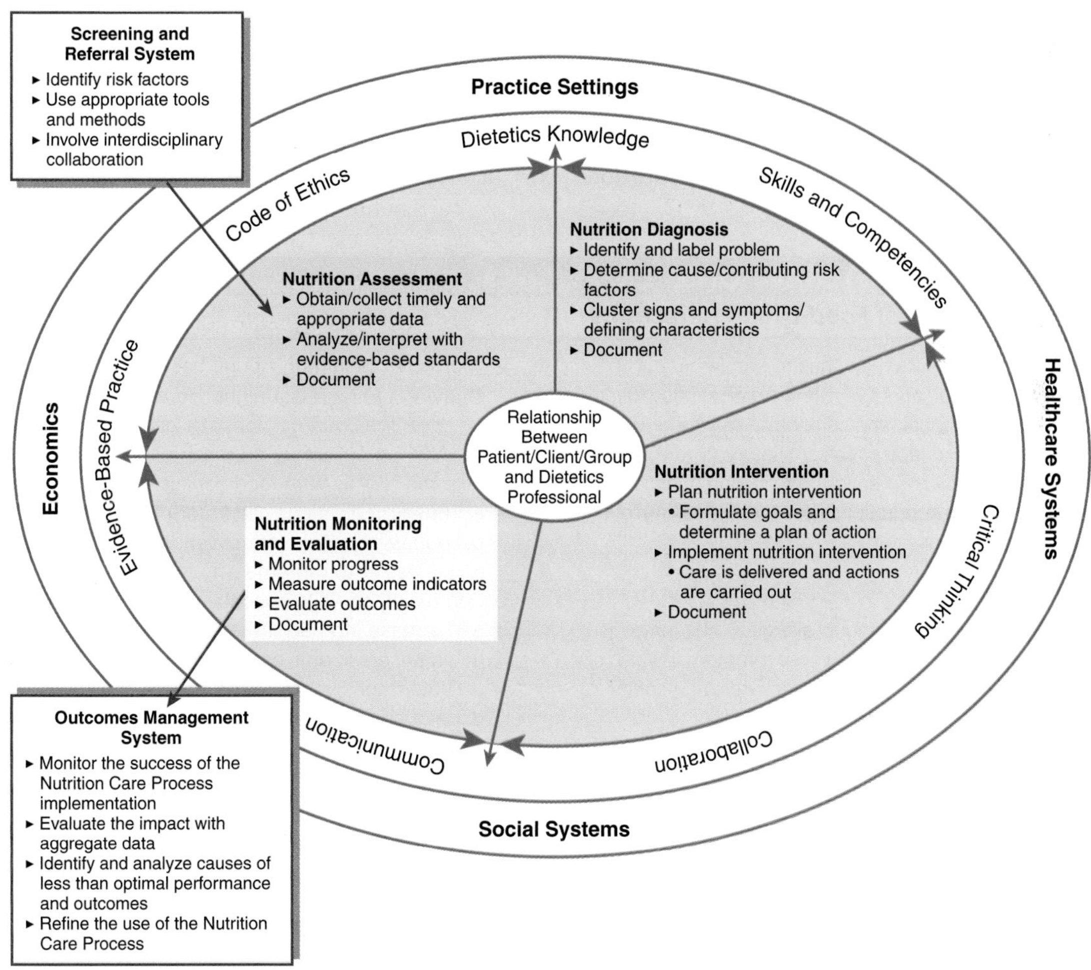

FIGURE 16-1 The Nutrition Care Process (NCP) model. (Redrawn from Lacey K, Pritchitt E: Nutrition Care Process and model: ADA adopts road map to quality care and outcomes management, *J Am Diet Assoc* 103[8]:1061, 2003, with permission from the American Dietetic Association [ADA].)

problems with the purpose of identifying individuals who are malnourished or at nutritional risk."[8,10] In long-term care, assessments must be completed on all residents within 14 days of admission. However, it is not possible or necessary to complete a full nutrition assessment on every patient hospitalized in acute care. It is necessary, however, to have a system in place to quickly identify patients at risk for nutrition problems, such as malnutrition or nutritional risk.[2] The Joint Commission requires all patients admitted to a hospital to be screened within 48 hours of admission.[11]

Nutrition screening can be executed by RDs, dietetic technicians, dietary managers, nurses, physicians, or other trained personnel.[2,8,9] Whether or not RDs are engaged in performing nutrition screening, they are responsible for providing input regarding the development of suitable screening parameters to make certain the screening process addresses the correct parameters.[8] The nutrition screening process has the following characteristics[12]:

- May be completed in any setting
- Facilitates completion of early intervention goals
- Includes collection of relevant data on risk factors and interpretation of data for intervention and treatment
- Determines need for a nutrition assessment
- Is cost-effective

Each facility or setting is responsible for determining the most appropriate mechanism for screening patients or clients. It is important to identify patients at nutritional risk.[13] Once individuals are identified, a nutrition assessment can be performed; then personalized intervention can be planned and implimented.[1] Certain criteria are used for nutrition screening[1,13]:

- Weight (i.e., BMI >25 or <18.5)
- Unintentional weight loss of ≥10% of usual body weight within 6 months or >5% of usual body weight in 1 month
- Nausea and vomiting
- Chewing and swallowing ability
- Diagnosis or presence of chronic disease
- Increased metabolic requirements (e.g., trauma, burns, systemic infection)
- Food allergies
- Diet
    - Altered intake (e.g., recent surgery, serious illness, parenteral or enteral nutrition)
    - Inadequate intake expected to continue ≥7 days
- Laboratory data (i.e., albumin, hematocrit)

If patients have been hospitalized for an extended length of time, they should be rescreened.[13] It is vital that a patient at nutritional risk is referred to an RD who will conduct the nutrition assessment, make nutrition diagnoses, and provide nutrition care.

Nutrition Assessment

The fundamental purpose of nutrition assessment in general clinical practice is to determine the following three factors:

1. Overall nutritional status of the patient
2. Current health care needs—physical, psychosocial, and personal (see *Diet-Medications Interactions* box, "Assess Your Knowledge of Food-Drug Interactions")
3. Related factors influencing these needs in the person's current life situation

DIET-MEDICATIONS INTERACTIONS

Assess Your Knowledge of Food-Drug Interactions

Medications can treat and cure many health problems, but they must be taken properly to be effective. Many medications interact with foods, beverages, alcohol, and caffeine to make them less effective or cause dangerous side effects. Assess your knowledge of food-drug interactions by answering the following questions:

1. No risk of food-drug interactions exist when taking over-the-counter medications.
   a. True
   b. False
2. Your neighbor, Greta, has serious allergies. Her physician prescribed an antihistamine to control her symptoms. Which of the following labels might appear on her prescription bottle?
   a. Take on an empty stomach.
   b. Take with food.
   c. Take only at bedtime.
   d. Take with coffee.
3. The previously mentioned label is on Greta's prescription antihistamine because:
   a. Effectiveness is increased when taken on an empty stomach.
   b. Effectiveness is increased when taken with food.
   c. The drug is metabolized more efficiently when taken at bedtime.
   d. Caffeine enhances absorption of the medication.
4. Your other neighbor, Abdul, has a horrible headache from studying too hard last night. He asks you if he should take his over-the-counter nonsteroidal antiinflammatory drug (NSAID) on an empty stomach or with a meal. He should take the NSAID with food because:
   a. These medications can irritate the stomach.
   b. Food will increase effectiveness.
   c. It is easier to remember to take them with a meal.
5. Combining NSAIDs or acetaminophen with alcohol will:
   a. Decrease stomach irritation
   b. Increase risk of liver damage
   c. Protect the liver from the effects of alcohol
   d. Have no effect whatsoever
6. Your cousin Vinny is dining on a super-sized meal at the local fast-food restaurant. Which of the following prescription medications should he avoid taking with the meal because high-fat meals may increase levels in the body?
   a. Hydrochlorothiazide (diuretic)
   b. Tetracyclines (antibiotic)
   c. NSAIDs
   d. Some forms of theophylline (bronchodilator)
7. Grandma Minnie takes a diuretic to control hypertension. Her physician told her this drug could cause hypokalemia.

DIET-MEDICATIONS INTERACTIONS

Assess Your Knowledge of Food-Drug Interactions—cont'd

Which of the following foods should she eat on a regular basis to avoid hypokalemia?
- a. Hamburgers and hot dogs
- b. Twinkies and Ding Dongs
- c. Low-fat dairy products
- d. Bananas, oranges, and potatoes

8. Uncle Joe is taking captopril (an angiotensin-converting enzyme [ACE] inhibitor) for his high blood pressure. He cannot remember if his physician told him to take the captopril with a meal or on an empty stomach. What can you tell him?
   - a. Take it with meals to increase absorption.
   - b. Take it 1 hour before or 2 hours after meals so as to not affect absorption.
   - c. Take it with breakfast but not with dinner.
9. Your roommate's cousin's uncle is taking a "statin" medication to lower serum cholesterol. Which of the following statements is true about statin medications?
   - a. Avoid drinking large amounts of alcohol because it may increase risk of liver damage.
   - b. Take with breakfast to enhance absorption.
   - c. Take with the evening meal to decrease absorption.
10. High doses of vitamin E may prolong clotting time and increase risk of bleeding. Large doses of vitamin E should be avoided when taking which of the following drugs?
    - a. Warfarin (anticoagulant)
    - b. Lovastatin (3-hydroxy-3-methylglutaryl coenzyme A [HMG-CoA] reductase inhibitor)
    - c. Furosemide (diuretic)
    - d. NSAIDs
11. Your cousin Bunny is taking oral contraceptives. Which of the following drugs may decrease effectiveness of "the pill," thereby increasing her chance of pregnancy?
    - a. Anticoagulants
    - b. NSAIDs
    - c. Antibiotics
    - d. Antidepressants
12. Bunny's pet turtle, Speedy, died. She wants to take St. John's wort because her roommate told her it would help with her depression. Are there any problems with her taking St. John's wort while she is taking oral contraceptives?
    - a. No. St. John's wort is an herb and sold at the Universal Nutrition Center at the mall. Herbal and dietary supplements cannot be sold if they are not safe.
    - b. Yes. St. John's wort will decrease effectiveness of the oral contraceptives.
13. Mr. Wilson is very excitable and nervous. Which of the following might be an explanation for this?
    - a. He took Cipro (quinolone) with his morning coffee.
    - b. He took penicillin at breakfast, which included yogurt.
    - c. He took aspirin on an empty stomach.
    - d. He just received a call from the Internal Revenue Service (IRS) to schedule an audit of last year's tax return.
14. Curt is taking tetracycline to control acne. Which of the following should he avoid?
    - a. Dairy products
    - b. Antacids
    - c. Vitamins containing iron
    - d. All of the above
15. Your favorite aunt, Constance, takes a monoamine oxidase inhibitor (MAOI). Her pharmacist cautioned her about eating foods high in tyramine (an amino acid). Why?
    - a. MAOIs combined with tyramine cause hiccups.
    - b. A rapid, potentially fatal decrease in blood pressure can occur.
    - c. A rapid, potentially fatal increase in blood pressure can occur.
    - d. None of the above will happen. Her pharmacist is mistaken.
16. Your nervous neighbor, Biff, takes alprazolam (Xanax), an antianxiety drug. He was told he should not take the Xanax with Mountain Dew. Why?
    - a. Carbonation in the soft drink will enhance effects of the Xanax.
    - b. Carbonation in the soft drink will decrease effects of the Xanax.
    - c. Caffeine in Mountain Dew may lessen the antianxiety effect of Xanax.
    - d. Caffeine in the Mountain Dew may enhance the antianxiety effect of Xanax.
17. Kevin just found out his stomach pain is being caused by excess acid production that caused an ulcer. His physician prescribed a histamine blocker and told him to avoid alcohol. Why?
    - a. Alcohol is a gastric irritant, which will make it more difficult for the stomach to heal.
    - b. Alcohol decreases the effectiveness of the histamine blocker.
    - c. Alcohol increases the effectiveness of the histamine blocker.
    - d. Kevin's physician does not want any of her patients to drink alcohol.
18. Grandpa Moe takes digoxin for his heart condition. Your cousin Sunshine brought him ginseng on her last visit. Should he take ginseng with the digoxin?
    - a. Yes. Herbal products are natural and safe.
    - b. No. Ginseng falsely elevates plasma digoxin levels.
    - c. It does not matter.
19. Trixie has a bad case of poison ivy. The physician gave her a prescription for Medrol, a corticosteroid to stop the itching. She cannot remember if the physician told her to take the Medrol on an empty stomach or with food. Can you help her?
    - a. It does not matter if Trixie takes it on an empty stomach or not.
    - b. Trixie should take the medicine on an empty stomach to decrease stomach irritation.
    - c. Trixie should take the Medrol with food or milk to decrease stomach upset.
20. Great Uncle John takes nitroglycerin (nitrate) for chest pain. Which of the following can add to the blood vessel–relaxing effect of nitrates and cause dangerously low blood pressure?
    - a. Milk and dairy products
    - b. Fruits and vegetables
    - c. Alcohol
    - d. Meats and cheeses

Answers: 1. b, 2. a, 3. a, 4. a, 5. b, 6. d, 7. d, 8. b, 9. a, 10. a, 11. c, 12. b, 13. a, 14. d, 15. c, 16. c, 17. a, 18. b, 19. c, 20. c.

The first step in nutrition assessment, as with assessing any situation to determine needs and actions, is to collect pertinent information—a database—for use in identifying needs. The clinical dietitian, assisted by other health care team members as needed, uses several basic types of activities for nutrition assessment of patients' needs, as follows:

- Anthropometric data
- Biochemical tests
- Clinical observations
- Diet evaluation and personal histories (i.e., medical, social, medications) (See the *Focus on Culture* box, "Cultural Stereotyping: Melting Pot or Salad Bowl?")

Each part of this approach is important because no single parameter directly measures individual nutritional status or determines problems or needs. Further, the overall resulting impression must be interpreted within the context of the patient's own social and health factors, because these factors have the potential to alter his or her nutritional requirements. Procedures outlined here provide a good base in general practice.

Anthropometric Measurements

Anthropometric measurements are measurements of body size, weight, and proportions. These measurements can be used to assess nutritional status, as well as growth and

FOCUS ON CULTURE

Cultural Stereotyping: Melting Pot or Salad Bowl?

Do all Southerners eat grits? Do all those who practice the Jewish religion follow orthodox food laws? Do all people of Hispanic origin eat tortillas and beans? Should you address your patient informally (by his or her first name) or more formally (e.g., Mrs. Garcia or Mr. Sato)? If your patient does not look you in the eye while talking, then is he or she being deceitful or showing respect? Why do you need to know the answer to these questions and others?

The population of the United States is growing increasingly culturally diverse. Almost 25% of the population is non–Anglo-American. By 2050, Latinos will be the largest minority group. By 2065, non-Hispanic Caucasians will most likely be a minority group. So what does this mean to you?

In terms of nutrition assessment and nutrition counseling, cultural diversity is a fact. Cultural competency is a necessity.

Cultural competency is more than recognizing and accepting cultural diversity. It is a skill critical to all dietitians and health care professionals. What good does it do to conduct a nutrition assessment or provide nutrition education if the patient's cultural background is not considered? Culture includes language, lifestyle, values, beliefs, and attitudes. These and other elements of culture influence how patients might experience illness, how they might access health care, and how they get well.

To deliver culturally competent care, dietitians and health care providers must understand beliefs, values, traditions, cultural practices. Consider the following differences in the dominant American cultural **paradigm**, the Anglo-American culture, and more traditional cultural populations:

ANGLO-AMERICAN	MORE TRADITIONAL CULTURES	WHAT THIS MAY MEAN TO YOU
Personal control of environment	Fate	Many traditional cultures believe fate, God, or other supernatural factors determine a person's destiny and directly influence health. The way they eat and exercise cannot have any influence on whether or not they develop complications of diabetes, for example.
Change	Tradition	Tradition and continuity are valued more than change. A reverence for the past takes precedence over efficiency of striving.
Time dominates	Human interaction dominates	Personal relationships determine self-worth and take priority over time schedules—promptness is not always a priority.
Human equality	Hierarchy, rank, status	In some cultures, health care professionals are more highly respected than other professionals. This may result in patients being less forthcoming if they disagree with a health care professional.
Individualism, privacy	Group or family welfare	Decision making about health issues may be a family affair.
Self-help	Birthright inheritance	Individuals may not believe they can help themselves in terms of their health.
Competition	Cooperation	Cooperation is preferred to competition.
Future orientation	Past orientation	Preventive care may not be a priority.
Action taking, goal setting, work orientated, informal approach preferred	"Being" orientation	Informality (e.g., calling people by their first names) is associated with rudeness in many traditional cultures. Clarify the patient's reference early.
Directness, openness, honesty	Formality	Individuals may not "volunteer" information.
Practicality, efficiency	Idealism, spiritualism	Idealism is stressed over practicality or expedience.

FOCUS ON CULTURE

Cultural Stereotyping: Melting Pot or Salad Bowl?—cont'd

There was a time when minorities in the United States tended to imitate the dominant middle-class culture, but this is no longer the case. Individual and cultural expression is becoming desirable. It is an expression of respect to learn about different cultures, to develop flexibility in how to approach clients and patients, and to develop cultural competency.

How Culturally Competent Are You?*

1. When the patient and dietitian come from different cultural backgrounds, the nutrition history obtained may not be accurate.
   a. True
   b. False
2. Which of the following are the correct ways to communicate with a patient through an interpreter?
   a. Making eye contact with the interpreter when you are speaking, then looking at the patient while the interpreter is telling the patient what you said
   b. Speaking slowly, pausing between words
   c. Asking the interpreter to further explain the patient's statement to get a more complete picture of the patient's condition
   d. None of the above
3. Which of the following statements is *not* true?
   a. Friendly (nonsexual) physical contact is an important part of communication for many Latin-American people.
   b. Many Asian people think it is disrespectful to ask questions of a health care professional.
   c. Most people of African heritage are either Christian or follow a traditional religion.
   d. Eastern Europeans are highly diverse in terms of customs, language, and religion.
4. Which of the following is good advice for a health care professional attempting to use and interpret nonverbal communication?
   a. The provider should recognize that a smile may express unhappiness or dissatisfaction in some cultures.
   b. To express sympathy, a health care professional can lightly touch a patient's arm or pat the patient on the back.
   c. If a patient will not make eye contact with a health care professional, then it is likely the patient is hiding the truth.
   d. When a language barrier exists, the provider can use hand gestures to bridge the gap.
5. Some symbols—a positive nod of the head, a pointing finger, a "thumbs-up" sign—are universal and can help bridge the language gap.
   a. True
   b. False
6. A female Muslim patient may avoid eye contact, physical contact, or both because:
   a. She does not want to spread germs.
   b. Muslim women are taught to be submissive.
   c. Modesty is very important in Islamic tradition.
   d. She does not like the health care professional.
7. When a patient is not compliant with prescribed nutrition therapy after several visits, which of the following approaches is *not* likely to lead to compliance?
   a. Involving family members
   b. Repeating the instructions very loudly and several times to emphasize the importance of the nutrition therapy
   c. Agreeing to a compromise in the recommended nutrition therapy
   d. Spending time listening to discussions of folk and alternative remedies
8. If a family member speaks English and the patient's native language and is willing to act as interpreter, then this is the best possible solution to the problem of interpreting.
   a. True
   b. False
9. Which of the following is *true?*
   a. People who speak the same language have the same culture.
   b. The people living in the African continent share the main features of African culture.
   c. Cultural background, diet, religious, and health practices, as well as language, can differ widely within a given country or part of the country.
   d. An alert health care professional can usually predict a patient's health behaviors by knowing what country he or she comes from.
10. Out of respect for a patient's privacy, the health care professional should always begin a relationship by seeing an adult patient alone and drawing the family in as needed.
   a. True
   b. False

Answers: 1. a, 2. d, 3. c, 4. a, 5. b, 6. c, 7. b, 8. b, 9. c, 10. b.

BIBLIOGRAPHY

Betterley C: *Increasing cultural competency of nutrition educators through travel study programs,*Unpublished paper, July 6, 2001.

Brannon C: Cultural competency—values, traditions, and effective practice, *Today's Dietitian* 6(11):14, 2004. Retrieved March 13, 2009, from www.todaysdietitian.com/newarchives/td_1104p14.shtml.

Curry KR: Multicultural competence in dietetics and nutrition, *J Am Diet Assoc* 100:1142, 2000.

U.S. Census Bureau: *Census 2000 data for the United States,* Washington, DC, 2000, U.S. Government Printing Office. Retrieved June 9, 2010, from www.census.gov.

*Quiz modified from Management Sciences for Health and the U.S. Department of Health and Human Services, Health Resources and Administration, Bureau of Primary Healthcare: *The provider's guide to quality & culture,* Boston, 2005, Management Sciences for Health. Retrieved March 13, 2009, from www.erc.msh.org/mainpage.cfm?file=1.0.htm&module=provider&language=English.

KEY TERMS

paradigm A pattern or model serving as an example; a standard or ideal for practice or behavior based on a fundamental value or theme.

development of infants and children; they are useful tools for monitoring the effects of nutritional intervention.[9]

Weight. One of the most important measurements in nutritional assessment is body weight. It is used to predict energy expenditure in prediction equations (see the *Evidence-Based Practice* box, "What is the Best Prediction Equation to Determine Energy Needs?").[9] Hospitalized patients should be weighed at consistent times—for example, before breakfast after the bladder has been emptied. Clinic patients should be weighed without shoes in light, indoor clothing or an examining gown. For accuracy, use regular clinic beam scales with nondetachable weights (Figure 16-2). Additional weight attachment is available for use with very obese persons. Metric scales with readings to the nearest 20 g provide specific data; however, the standard clinic scale is satisfactory. Scales should be checked frequently and calibrated every 3 or 4 months for continued accuracy. Nonambulatory (unable to stand or walk) persons' weight can be measured using a bed or chair scale (Figure 16-3).

After careful reading and recording of the patient's weight, ask about usual body weight. Interpret present weight in terms of percentage of usual body weight. Check for any recent weight loss: 1% to 2% in the past week, 5% during the past month, 7.5% during the previous 3 months, or 10% in the past 6 months are significant. Unintentional weight loss greater than these rates can be severe. Unexplained weight loss is a problem with persons of any age. It is particularly important in older adults, because it may be a clue to depression or a wasting disease such as cancer and needs to be on record and followed up. Values charted in the patient's record should indicate percentage of weight change.

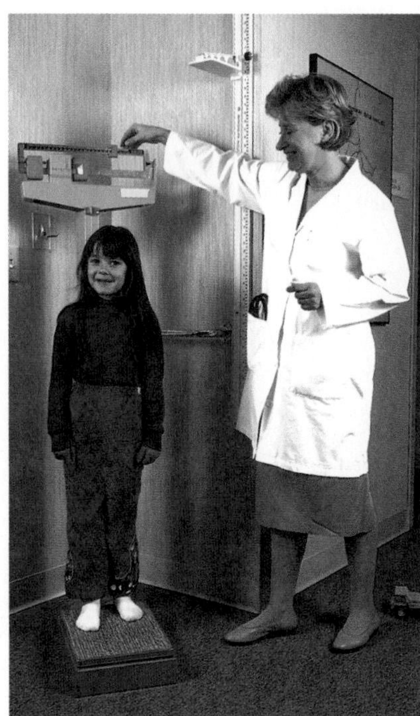

FIGURE 16-2 Balance beam scale. (From Jarvis C: *Physical examination and health assessment,* ed 3, Philadelphia, 2000, Saunders.)

Length and Stature. Measurements of length and stature (height) are easily obtained anthropometric measures. They are the most sensitive indicators of growth and development in infants and children.[9]

If possible, use a fixed measuring stick or tape on a true vertical flat surface. Have the patient stand as straight as possible, without shoes or hat, heels together, and looking straight ahead. Heels, buttocks, shoulders, and head should be touching the wall or vertical surface of the measuring rod. Read the measure carefully, and compare it with previous recordings. Children younger than 2 years should be measured using a stationary headboard and movable footboard (Figure 16-4). Note growth of children or the diminishing height of adults. Metric measures of height in centimeters provide a smaller unit of measure than inches.

Although it is always preferable to obtain standing measurements,[9] this is not always possible. Several alternative measures can provide values for estimating height and weight of persons confined to bed:

- *Knee height* (Figure 16-5) has been shown correlate well with stature.[16-18] Measurement is taken with the person lying in the supine position. The left leg is measured with

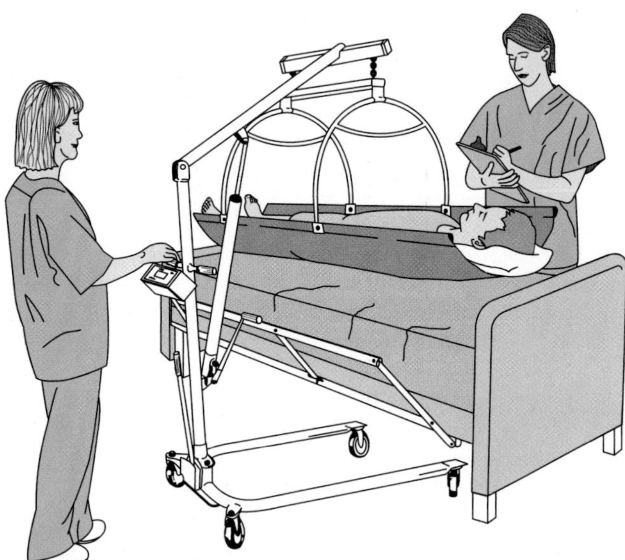

FIGURE 16-3 Bed scale. (From Grodner M, Long S, Walkingshaw BC: *Foundations and clinical applications of nutrition: a nursing approach,* ed 4, St Louis, 2007, Mosby.)

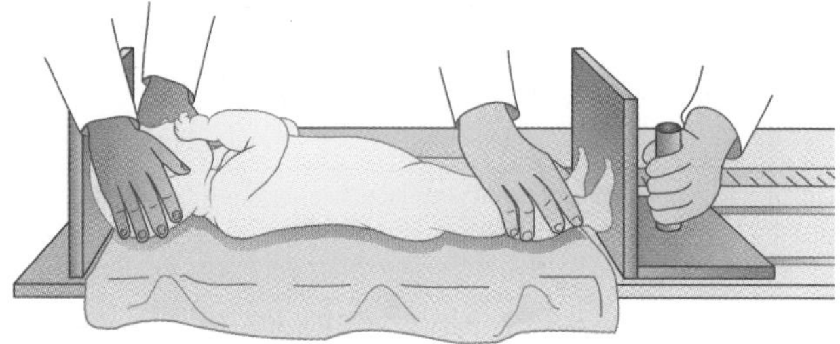

FIGURE 16-4 Measuring a baby's stature. (From Mahan LK, Escott-Stump S: *Krause's food, nutrition, & diet therapy,* ed 12, Philadelphia, 2007, Saunders.)

EVIDENCE-BASED PRACTICE

What is the Best Prediction Equation to Determine Energy Needs?

Assessment of energy needs is a necessary component in the Nutrition Care Process (NCP). Indirect calorimetry is the "gold standard" for determining resting metabolic rate (RMR) and is accurate within 5% in most cases. However, because indirect calorimetry is not always available, prediction equations are commonly used to determine RMR.

The four prediction equations most commonly used in clinical practice are as follows:

MIFFLIN-ST. JEOR

Men	RMR = (9.99 × wt in kg) + (6.25 × ht in cm) − (4.92 × age in y) + 5
Women	RMR = (9.99 × wt in kg) + (6.25 × ht in cm) − (4.92 × age in y) − 161

HARRIS-BENEDICT

Men	RMR = 66.47 + (13.75 × wt in kg) + (5.0 × ht in cm) − (6.75 × age in y)
Women	RMR = 665.09 + (9.56 × wt in kg) + (1.84 × ht in cm) − (4.67 × age in y)

OWEN

Men	RMR = 879 + (10.2 × wt in kg)
Women	RMR = 795 + (7.18 × wt in kg)

WORLD HEALTH ORGANIZATION/FOOD & AGRICULTURE ORGANIZATION/UNITED NATIONS UNIVERSITY (WHO/FAO/UNU)

Weight only (age [y])

Men	
18-30	15.3 × wt in kg + 679
31-60	11.6 × wt in kg + 879
>60	13.5 × wt in kg + 487
Women	
18-30	14.7 × wt in kg + 496
31-60	8.7 × wt in kg + 829
>60	10.5 × wt in kg + 596

Weight & height (m) (age [y])

Men	
18-30	(15.4 × wt in kg) − (27 × ht in m) + 717
31-60	(11.3 × wt in kg) + (16 × ht in m) + 901
>60	(8.8 × wt in kg) + (1128 × ht in m) − 1071
Women	
18-30	(13.3 × wt in kg) + (34 × ht in m) + 35
31-60	(8.7 × wt in kg) − (25 × ht in m) + 865
>60	(9.2 × wt in kg) + (637 × ht in m) − 302

Of the four equations listed previously, the Mifflin-St. Jeor equation was found to be the most accurate in estimating basal metabolic rate (BMR). The oldest prediction equation in clinical use, Harris-Benedict, was found to systematically overestimate basal energy expenditure (BEE) by at least 5%. The Owen equation underestimates RMR about 21% of the time and overestimates RMR 6% of the time. Accuracy of the WHO/FAO/UNU equations could not be evaluated because of how the equations have been validated. For more details about the research of these prediction equations, please refer to the Frankenfield manuscripts cited following.

BIBLIOGRAPHY

Food and Agricultural Organization/World Health Organization/United Nations University: *Energy and protein requirements. Report of a Joint FAO/WHO/UNU expert consultation,* World Health Organization Technical Report Series 724, Geneva, Switzerland, 1985, WHO.

Frankenfield DC, Muth ER, Rowe WA: The Harris-Benedict studies of human basal metabolism: history and limitations, *J Am Diet Assoc* 98(4):439, 1998.

Frankenfield D, Roth-Yousey L, Compher C: Comparison of predictive equations for resting metabolic rate in healthy nonobese and obese adults: a systematic review, *J Am Diet Assoc* 105(5):775, 2005.

Harris JA, Benedict FG: *A biometric study of basal metabolism in man,* Pub No 279, Washington, DC, 1919, Carnegie Institute of Washington.

Mifflin MD, St Jeor ST, Hill LA, et al: A new predictive equation for resting energy expenditure in healthy individuals, *Am J Clin Nutr* 51:241, 1990.

Owen OE, Kavle E, Owen RS, et al: A reappraisal of caloric requirements in healthy women, *Am J Clin Nutr* 44:1, 1986.

Owen OE, Holup JL, Dalessio DA, et al: A reappraisal of the caloric requirements of men, *Am J Clin Nutr* 46:875, 1987.

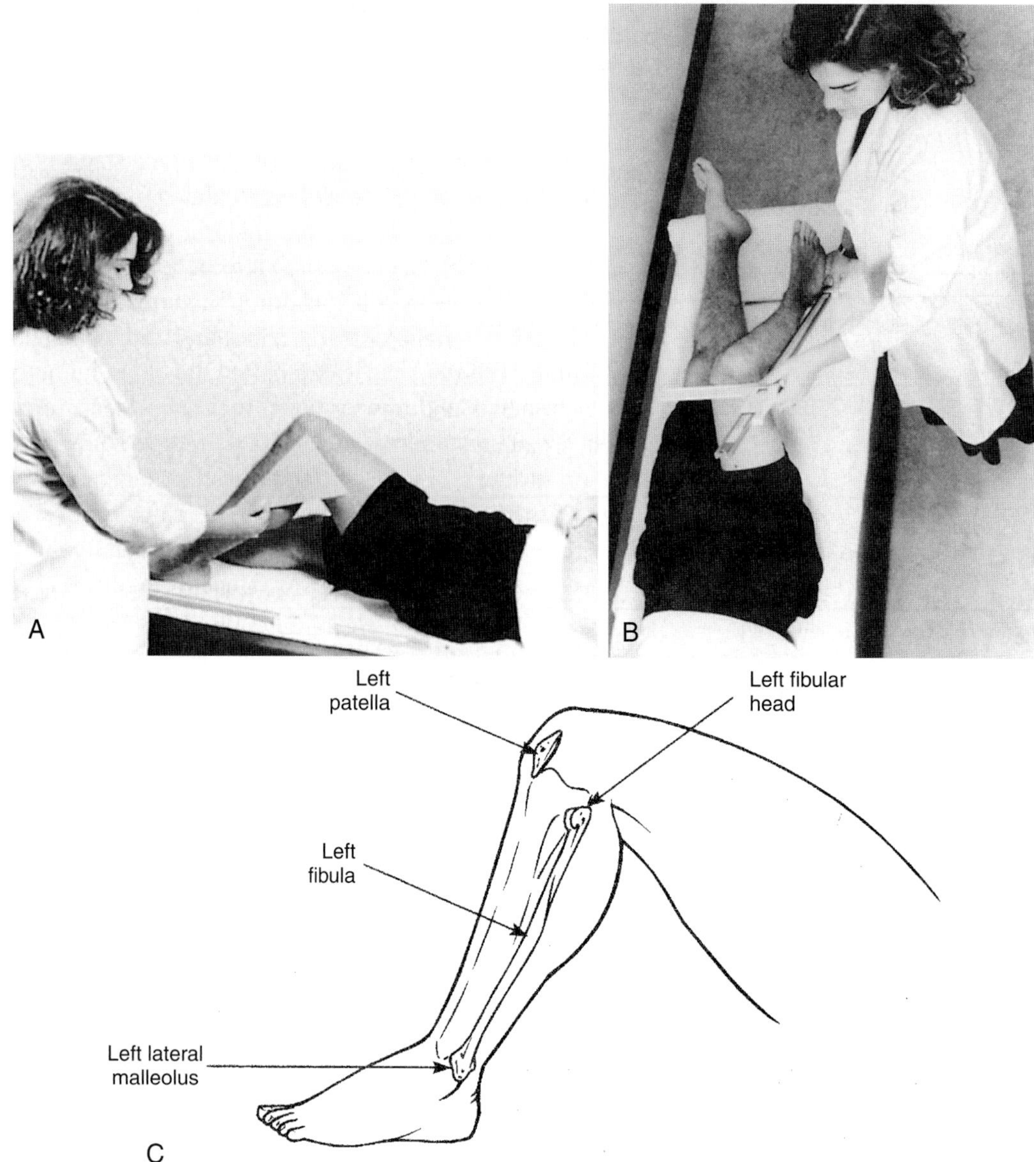

FIGURE 16-5 Knee height measurement. (From Lee RD, Nieman DC: *Nutritional assessment*, ed 4, Boston, 2007, McGraw-Hill.)

knee and ankle at a 90-degree angle using a specialized sliding caliper. Measurements are then entered into one of the following validated equations[14,16]:

Men:

$$\text{Stature (cm)} = [2.02 \times \text{knee height (cm)}] - (0.04 \times \text{age}) + 64.19$$

Women:

$$\text{Stature (cm)} = [1.83 \times \text{knee height (cm)}] - (0.24 \times \text{age}) + 84.88$$

- To estimate height of a nonambulatory person who has no skeletal abnormalities or contractures, *recumbent bed measurement* can be taken by marking the base of the heels and top of the crown on the bed sheet (Figure 16-6) on which the patient is resting in a straight line. The distance between these two lines can be measured with a tape measure.
- *Arm span* measurement taken from sternal notch to the longest finger on the dominant hand is reliable in individuals with no contractures, spinal deformities, and who can fully extend their arms. To estimate stature, multiply the number obtained by 2.[14,19]

Body Mass Index. BMI is a ratio of weight to height and has been correlated with overall mortality and nutritional risk.[2,14] It does not estimate body composition (lean body mass or adiposity); however, it is a reliable indicator of total body fat (see Box 16-1), which is related to the risk of disease.[15] Although BMI measurements are valid for men and women, they do have some limits[14,15]:

- BMI has not been validated in acutely ill patients.
- BMI may overestimate body fat in individuals who have a muscular build.
- BMI may underestimate body fat in older adults and others who have lost muscle mass.

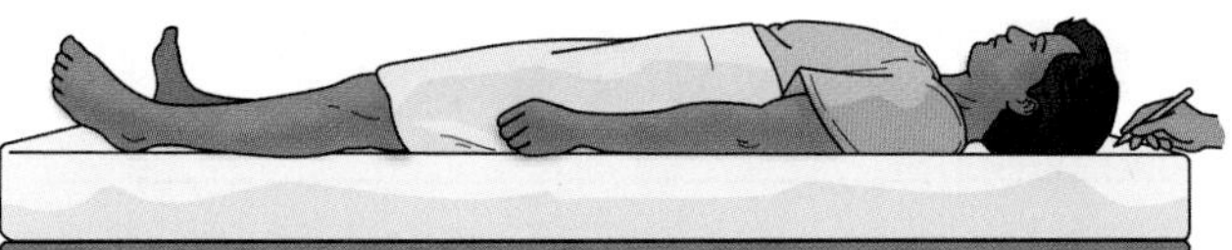

FIGURE 16-6 Recumbent bed length. (From Lee RD, Nieman DC: *Nutritional assessment,* ed 4, Boston, 2007, McGraw-Hill.)

Standardized growth charts for children can be found on the Centers for Disease Control and Prevention (CDC) website (www.cdc.gov/nchs/about/major/nhanes/growthcharts/clinical_charts.htm). These growth charts show percentile rankings of height and weight for age and weight for height, as well as BMI for age.[1]

Waist Circumference. Waist circumference is inexpensive, easy to perform, and assesses abdominal fat content. BMI and waist circumference highly correlate with obesity and risk for disease, and both should be used to classify overweight and obesity, as well as to estimate disease risk.[1,14,20] Circumference greater than 40 inches in men and greater than 35 inches in women indicates risk for disease. It should be noted that visceral adiposity may vary among racial and ethnic groups.[1]

Biochemical (Laboratory) Measurements

Biochemical (or laboratory) tests are a useful adjunct in measuring and managing nutritional status; however, their use can be problematic.[9] Precise interpretation necessitates awareness of the appropriate test, as well as nutritional and nonnutritional factors that have the potential to alter blood chemistries. Significant nonnutritional factors to be considered include disease processes, treatments, procedures, medications, and hydration status.[21] The most commonly used methods for assessing and monitoring nutritional status and planning nutrition care in clinical practice are listed here. General ranges for normal values are given in standard texts.

Protein Assessment. Usually, biochemical assessment of protein status has been undertaken from the standpoint of two protein compartments: (1) somatic and (2) visceral proteins.[9] Somatic protein is found within skeletal muscle, and visceral proteins are found in body organs, red blood cells, white blood cells, and serum proteins. Both protein pools are metabolically active, meaning the body can tap into these stores if necessary.[9] Obviously use of any proteins stored in the body means the protein is no longer available for bodily functions like synthesis of antibodies, hormones, and other vital components. Additionally, no single laboratory test or group of tests is sensitive, specific, or both for protein malnutrition. Evaluation of serum proteins necessitates simultaneous assessment of nutrient intake, physical findings, and clinical condition.[21]

Serum proteins. Serum protein concentrations can be helpful in determining protein status, risk of medical complications, and response to nutritional intervention with limitations.[9,21] A number of factors other than inadequate protein intake affect serum protein concentrations (Table 16-1).

Somatic proteins. Somatic proteins can be measured using anthropometric measures such as midarm muscle area, midarm circumference, and overall body weight.[2] A laboratory test that can be used for estimating body muscle mass is 24-hour urinary creatinine excretion.[9]

• • •

When assessing biochemical measurements, it is important to consider that a review of serial laboratory data is recommended. Direction and speed of change are more important than static value. Improvement in nutrition parameters does not always confer clinical benefit. Treat the person, not the laboratory value.[21]

Clinical Observations and Nutrition Physical Assessment

Certain information used to assess nutritional status is taken from physical examinations performed by physicians and nurses. Furthermore, RDs perform nutritional physical examinations to assess patients for signs and symptoms consistent with malnutrition or specific nutrient deficiency.[2] Techniques used in nutritional physical examinations are summarized in Table 16-2.

Clinical Signs of Malnutrition. Careful attention to physical signs of possible malnutrition provides an added dimension to the overall assessment of general nutritional status. A guide for a general examination of such signs is given in Table 16-3. A careful description of any such observations is documented in the patient's medical record.

Dietary Assessment

Collecting Information. A careful nutrition history, including nutrition information related to living situation and other personal, psychosocial, and economic problems, is a fundamental part of nutrition assessment. Obtaining accurate information about basic food patterns and actual dietary intake is not simple because some individuals misreport or underreport what they eat. Each method of diet evaluation has particular strengths and limitations.[9] However, a sensitive practitioner may obtain useful information by using one or more of the basic tools described in Table 16-4.

Evaluation of Dietary Intake. Valid patient care planning requires analysis of all nutrition data collected. On this basis, problems requiring solutions can be identified. A detailed analysis of all available nutrition information helps determine nutrition diagnosis, any primary or secondary nutritional disease, and any underlying nutrition-related conditions.

Medical tests used for nutrition assessment are generally reliable in persons of any age, but conditions in older adult patients may interfere and need to be considered in evaluating test results. For example, laboratory values are affected by hydration status, presence of chronic diseases, changes in

TABLE 16-1 LABORATORY MEASURES OF SERUM PROTEINS

SERUM PROTEIN	FUNCTION	COMMENTS
Albumin *Normal:* 3.5-5.0 g/dL *Depletion:* Mild: 3.0-3.4 g/dL Moderate: 2.4-2.9 g/dL Severe: <2.4 g/dL Half-life ~ 14-20 days	Maintains plasma oncotic pressure, carrier for small molecules	Not sensitive or specific for acute protein malnutrition or response to nutrition therapy; affected by hydration status, disease state, clinical condition Can be used as prognostic indicator of morbidity, mortality, and severity of illness
Transferrin *Normal:* 200-400 g/dL *Depletion:* Mild: 150-200 mg/dL Moderate: 100-149 mg/dL Severe: <100 mg/dL Half-life ~ 8-10 days	Binds iron in plasma and transports to bone marrow	Inversely correlated with body's iron stores; elevated concentration often indicates early iron deficiency Will decrease during acute illness Verify with laboratory whether lab is direct measurement or calculated
Prealbumin (transthyretin, thyroxin-binding prealbumin) *Normal:* 16-40 mg/dL *Depletion:* Mild: 10-15 mg/dL Moderate: 5-9 mg/dL Severe: <5 mg/dL Half-life ~ 2-3 days	Carrier protein for thyroxin Combined with retinol-binding protein, transports vitamin A	Influenced less by intravascular fluid volume Not affected as early or as significantly with liver disease (compared with albumin) More likely to be reflection of recent dietary intake than accurate indicator of nutritional status

Adapted from (compiled from components in tables and text) Moore MC: *Pocket guide to nutrition assessment and care,* ed 6, St Louis, 2009, Mosby; Lee RD, Nieman DC: *Nutritional assessment*, ed 4, Boston, 2007, McGraw-Hill; Thompson CW: Laboratory assessment. In Charney P, Malone AM: *ADA pocket guide to nutrition assessment,* ed 2, Chicago, 2009, American Dietetic Association.

TABLE 16-2 NUTRITIONAL PHYSICAL EXAMINATION

TECHNIQUE	SKILL	PURPOSE
Inspection	Systematic visual inspection	Monitor changes to normal features
Auscultation	Using a stethoscope and naked ear to identify deviations from standard sounds	Evaluate sounds produced by heart, lungs, and gastrointestinal (GI) tract such as bowel sounds
Palpation	Examination of the body using touch	Reveal conditions that have nutritional implications such as abdominal tenderness, ascites, distention, peripheral edema, nail integrity, and skin turgor
Percussion	Use of sound to distinguish deviations from standard sounds created by presence of body organs and cavities	Identify gastric air bubble, intestinal air, or fluid present in lungs

Data from Nelms MN, Sucher K, Long S: *Understanding nutrition therapy and pathophysiology,* Belmont, Calif, 2007, Wadsworth.

organ function, and drugs. Nutrition assessment is an important part of the general health care of everyone, especially of older adults. Health outreach programs for older persons, such as those in rural areas, can use brief, easily administered tools for screening and assessing nutritional status and risk of malnutrition as part of geriatric care.

NUTRITION DIAGNOSIS

Nutrition diagnosis is not to be confused with medical diagnosis. Medical diagnosis is a disease or pathologic condition that can be treated or prevented, and the diagnosis does not change as long as the condition exists.[8] Nutrition diagnosis is "identification and labeling an actual occurrence, risk of, or potential for developing a nutrition problem that dietetics professionals are responsible for treating independently."[8] Nutrition diagnoses change as patients' nutritional needs change.[8] Nutrition diagnoses provide a mechanism for dietetics practitioners to document the link between nutrition assessment and nutrition intervention and to set realistic and measurable expected outcomes for patients. Identifying diagnoses also assists dietetics practitioners in establishing priorities when planning nutrition care.[22] Nutrition diagnoses are dependent

TABLE 16-3 CLINICAL SIGNS OF NUTRITIONAL STATUS

AREA OF CONCERN	POSSIBLE DEFICIENCY	POSSIBLE EXCESS
Hair		
Dull, dry, brittle	Pro	
Easily plucked (with no pain)	Pro	
Hair loss	Pro, Zn, biotin	Vit A
Flag sign (loss of hair pigment in strips around head)	Pro, Cu	
Head and Neck		
Bulging fontanel (infants)		Vit A
Headache		Vit A, D
Epistaxis (nosebleed)	Vit K	
Thyroid enlargement	Iodine	
Eyes		
Conjunctival and corneal xerosis (dryness)	Vit A	
Pale conjunctiva	Fe	
Blue sclerae	Fe	
Corneal vascularization	Vit B_2	
Mouth		
Cheilosis or angular stomatitis (lesions at corners of mouth, Figure 16-7, *A*)	Vit B_2	
Glossitis (red, sore tongue)	Niacin, folate, vit B_{12}, and other B vit	
Gingivitis (inflamed gums)	Vit C	
Hypogeusia, dysgeusia (poor sense of taste, distorted taste)	Zn	
Dental caries	Fluoride	
Mottling of teeth		Fluoride
Atrophy of papillae on tongue	Fe, B vit	
Skin		
Dry, scaly	Vit A, Zn, EFAs	Vit A
Follicular hyperkeratosis (resembles gooseflesh)	Vit A, EFAs, B vit	
Exzematous lesions	Zn	
Petechiae, ecchymoses	Vit C, K	
Nasolabial seborrhea (greasy, scaly areas between nose and lip)	Niacin, vit B_{12}, B_6	
Darkening and peeling of skin in areas exposed to sun	Niacin	
Poor wound healing	Pro, Zn, vit C	
Nails		
Spoon-shaped nails (see Figure 16-7, *B*)	Fe	
Brittle, fragile	Pro	
Heart		
Enlargement, tachycardia, failure	Vit B_1	
Small heart	Energy	
Sudden failure, death	Se	
Arrhythmia	Mg, K, Se	
Hypertension	Ca, K	
Abdomen		
Hepatomegaly	Pro	Vit A
Ascites	Pro	

Continued

TABLE 16-3 CLINICAL SIGNS OF NUTRITIONAL STATUS—cont'd

AREA OF CONCERN	POSSIBLE DEFICIENCY	POSSIBLE EXCESS
Musculoskeletal Extremities		
Muscle wasting (especially temporal area)	Energy	
Edema	Pro, vit B_1	
Calf tenderness	Vit B_1 or C, biotin, Se	
Beading of ribs, or "rachitic rosary" (child)	Vit C, D	
Bone and joint tenderness	Vit C, D, Ca, P	
Knock-knee, bowed legs, fragile bones	Vit D, Ca, P, Cu	
Neurologic		
Paresthesias (pain and tingling or altered sensation in the extremities)	Vit B_1, B_6, B_{12}, biotin	
Weakness	Vit C, B_1, B_6, B_{12}, energy	
Ataxia, decreased position and vibratory senses	Vit B_1, B_{12}	
Tremor	Mg	
Decreased tendon reflexes	Vit B_1	
Confabulation, disorientation	Vit B_1, B_{12}	
Drowsiness, lethargy	Vit B_1	Vit A, D
Depression	Vit B_1, biotin, B_{12}	

Ca, Calcium; *Cu,* copper, *EFAs,* essential fatty acids; *Fe,* iron; *K,* potassium, *Mg,* magnesium; *Na,* sodium; *P,* phosphorus; *Pro,* protein; *Se,* selenium; *Vit,* vitamin(s); *Zn,* zinc.
Data from Moore MC: *Pocket guide to nutrition assessment and care,* ed 6, St Louis, 2009, Mosby, pp 60-63.

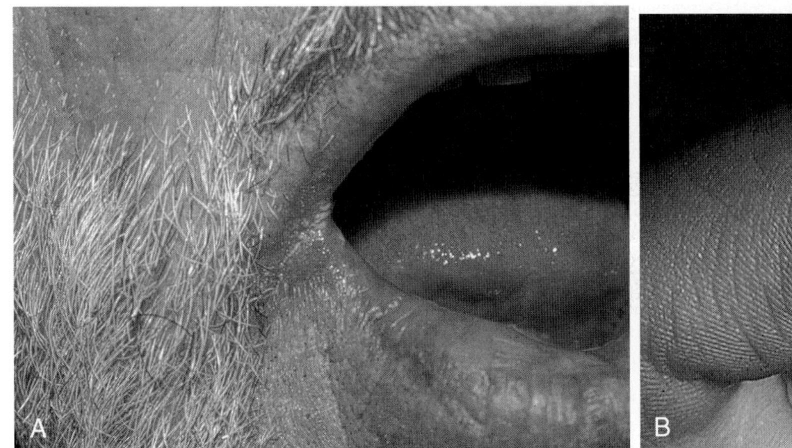

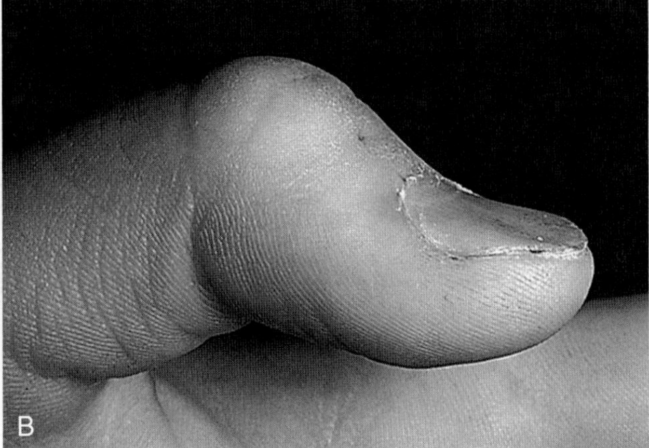

FIGURE 16-7 Examples of findings in malnourished states. (From Moore MC: *Pocket guide to nutrition assessment and care,* ed 6, St Louis, 2009, Mosby.)

on evidence-based practice and standardized language.[2,8] (More information on evidence-based practice is available for ADA members at www.adaevidencelibrary.com/default.cfm.)

Sixty nutrition diagnoses have been developed through use of standardized language and are grouped into three categories: (1) intake, (2) clinical, and (3) behavioral-environmental. Standardized language provides a means for dietetics professionals to communicate with each other, as well as with other health care professionals. It is a fundamental part of the NCP and assists dietetics professionals in better documenting nutrition care.[22] See Box 16-2 for more in-depth information and to determine how a nutrition diagnosis is written.

NUTRITION INTERVENTION: FOOD PLAN AND MANAGEMENT

Basic Concepts of Nutrition Therapy

Nutrition therapy is always based on normal nutritional requirements and personal needs for each particular patient. It is modified only as the specific disease in the specific

TABLE 16-4 STRENGTHS AND LIMITATIONS OF TECHNIQUES USED TO MEASURE DIETARY INTAKE

TECHNIQUE	BRIEF DESCRIPTION	STRENGTHS	LIMITATIONS
24-Hour food record	Trained interviewer asks respondent to recall, in detail, all food and drink consumed during a period of time in the recent past.	Requires <20 min to administer Inexpensive Easy to administer Can provide detailed information on types of foods consumed Low respondent burden More objective than dietary history Does not alter usual diet Useful in clinical settings	One recall rarely illustrative of typical intake Underreporting and overreporting problems Dependent on memory Omissions of sauces, dressings, and beverages can lead to low estimates of energy intake Data entry sometimes labor intensive
Food record or diary	Respondents record, at the time of consumption, the identity and amounts of all foods and beverages consumed for a period of time, usually ranging from 1-7 days.	Does not rely on memory Can provide detailed intake data Can provide information about eating habits Multiple-day data more representative of usual intake Reasonably valid up to 5 days	Requires high degree of cooperation Subject must be literate Takes more time to obtain data Act of recording may alter usual intake
Food frequency questionnaires	Respondents indicate how many times a day, week, month, or year they usually consume foods using a questionnaire consisting of a list of approximately >150 foods or food groups that are important contributors to the population's intake of energy and nutrients.	Can be self-administered Machine readable Modest demand on respondents Relatively inexpensive May be more representative of usual intake than a few days of diet records	May not represent usual food or portion sizes chosen by respondent Intake data can be compromised when multiple foods are grouped within single listings Depends on ability of respondent to describe diet
Diet history	Respondents are interviewed by a trained interviewer about number of meals eaten per day, their appetites, their food dislikes, the presence or absence of nausea and/or vomiting, the use of nutritional supplements and/or herbal products, cigarette smoking, as well as habits related to sleep, rest, work, and exercise.	Assesses usual nutrient intake Can detect seasonal changes Data on all nutrients can be obtained Can correlate well with biochemical measures	Lengthy interview process Requires highly trained interviewers May overestimate nutrient intake Requires cooperation of respondent with ability to recall usual diet

Modified from Lee RD, Neiman DC: *Nutrition assessment,* ed 4, Boston, 2007, McGraw-Hill.

individual necessitates. In planning and counseling for nutrition care, this is an important initial fact to grasp and impart to patients and clients. For example, it is a great source of encouragement to the parents of a child newly diagnosed with diabetes to know the food plan will be based on individual growth and development needs and will make use of regular foods.

Disease Application

Principles of a nutrition therapy will be based on modifications of nutritional components of the normal diet as a particular disease condition may require. These changes may include the following types of modifications:

- *Nutrients:* modification of one or more of the basic nutrients—protein, carbohydrate, fat, minerals, and vitamins
- *Energy:* modification in energy value as expressed in kilocalories (kcalories or kcal)
- *Texture:* modification in texture or seasoning, such as liquid or low residue

Individual Adaptation

Nutrition therapy may be theoretically correct and have well-balanced food plans, but if these plans are unacceptable to the patient, they will not be followed. A workable plan for a specific person must be based on individual food habits within

TABLE 16-5 ROUTINE HOSPITAL DIETS

FOOD	CLEAR LIQUID	SOFT	REGULAR
Soup	Clear fat-free broth, bouillon	Same, plus all cream soups	All
Cereal		Cooked cereal, cornflakes, rice, noodles, macaroni, spaghetti	All
Bread		White bread, crackers, melba toast, zwieback	All
Protein foods		Same, plus eggs (not fried), mild cheese, cottage and cream cheese, fowl, fish, sweetbreads, tender beef, veal, lamb, liver, bacon, gravy	All
Vegetables		Potatoes (baked, mashed, creamed, steamed, scalloped), tender cooked whole bland vegetables, fresh lettuce, tomatoes	All
Fruit and fruit juices	Fruit juices (as tolerated), flavored fruit drinks	Same, plus cooked fruit (peaches, pears, applesauce, peeled apricots, white cherries), ripe peaches, pears, bananas, orange and grapefruit sections without membrane	All
Desserts and gelatin	Fruit-flavored gelatin, fruit ices, and Popsicles	Same, plus plain sponge cakes, plain cookies, plain cake, puddings, pie made with allowed foods	All
Miscellaneous	Soft drinks (as tolerated), coffee and tea, decaffeinated coffee and tea, cereal beverages (e.g., Postum), sugar, honey, salt, hard candy, Polycose (Ross Laboratories), residue-free supplements	Same, plus mild salad dressings	All

the specific personal life situation. This can be achieved only through careful planning with the patient, or with the parents of a child requiring a special diet, based on an initial interview to obtain a diet history, knowledge of personal food habits, living conditions, and food security. In this way, diet principles can be understood and motivation secured. Regardless of the problems, nutrition therapy is valid only to the extent that it involves this kind of knowledge, as well as these particular skills and insights. Individual adaptations of the diet to meet individual needs are imperative for successful therapy.

Routine House Diets

A schedule of routine "house" diets, based on some type of cycle menu plan, is usually used in hospitals for patients who do not require a special diet modification. According to general patient need and tolerance, the diet order may be liquid (clear liquid), soft (in texture), and regular (a full, normal-for-age diet) (Table 16-5).

Managing the Mode of Feeding

Depending on the patient's condition, the clinical dietitian may manage nutrition therapy by using any one of the following four feeding modes.

1. **Oral diet.** As long as possible, of course, regular oral feeding is preferred. Supplements are added if needed. According to the patient's condition, he or she may need assistance in eating.
2. **Enteral nutrition and tube feeding.** If a patient is unable to eat but the gastrointestinal (GI) tract can be used, enteral delivery, or tube feeding, may provide needed nutrition support. A number of commercial formulas are available.
3. **Peripheral nutrition.** If the patient cannot take in food or formula via the GI tract, intravenous feeding is used. Solutions of dextrose, amino acids, vitamins, and minerals, with lipids as appropriate, can be fed through peripheral veins when the need is not extensive or long term.
4. **Total parenteral nutrition.** If the patient's nutritional need is great and support therapy may be required for a longer time, parenteral feeding through a large central vein is needed. Placement of this catheter is a special procedure. More concentrated special solutions can be used and monitored by a nutrition support team. Formulas are determined by the dietitian and physician, and they are prepared by trained pharmacists. This specialized nutrition support method was originally used only in hospitals, but advances in total parenteral nutrition (TPN) administration now allow its use in many health care settings and even at home with some patients.

EVALUATION: QUALITY PATIENT CARE

General Considerations

When the NCP is carried out, patient care activities need to be considered in terms of nutrition diagnosis and treatment objectives, as well as the extent to which each of the care activities helps to meet the particular goals of the patient

CASE STUDY

Nutrition Assessment and Therapy for a Patient with Cancer

Esther is a 160-cm (5 feet, 4 inches) tall, medium-frame, 43-year-old patient recovering from a *gastrectomy* performed 8 days ago to treat gastric cancer. Her weight has dropped gradually for the past 4 months, from an average of 59 kg (130 lb) before her illness began. She continues to observe a full-liquid diet, consuming 60 to 120 mL (2 to 4 oz) of milk every few hours, plus one or two soft-boiled eggs each day. Today Esther informed the nutritionist that she consumed a total of 721 mL (24 oz) of milk and two eggs.

In reviewing Esther's records, the clinical dietitian found the following nutrition assessment data: weight, 46.8 kg (103 lb); triceps skinfold, 10 mm; and midarm circumference, 17 cm. Laboratory values include serum albumin, 3 g/dL; total iron-binding capacity (TIBC), 230 mcg/dL; lymphocytes, 1200 cells/m^3 (23%); hematocrit, 35%; and hemoglobin, 10.5 g/dL. Urinalysis (24 hours) included blood urea nitrogen, 16 g; and creatinine, 1.75 g.

After reviewing the data, the clinical dietitian calculated nitrogen balance, transferrin, and creatinine-height index, which were recorded on the patient chart. Basal energy expenditure (BEE) needs, as well as the kcalories and protein needed to overcome catabolism, were also calculated, along with estimates for additional vitamin and mineral requirements.

The clinical dietitian noted the physician had ordered chemotherapy for the patient, continuing after discharge, and recommended use of total parenteral nutrition (TPN), also to be continued after discharge, as a means of meeting Esther's nutritional needs. In addition, the clinical dietitian planned ways of meeting any feeding problems that often accompany chemotherapy, such as sore mouth, nausea, and food intolerances. Observing a carefully prepared protocol developed by the hospital nutrition support team, Esther and her husband were instructed in procuring and using the home TPN treatment. The clinical dietitian also provided follow-up counseling for Esther and her husband at the office and in the group sessions for cancer patients and their families.

Questions for Analysis

1. Use a nutrition assessment data summary sheet from your hospital (or design your own) to record pertinent data given in this case study. What additional data would you collect? How would it be obtained?
2. For each test listed on your data sheet, explain what it measures and how that information contributes to an understanding of Esther's status.
3. What specific nutritional needs (nutrition diagnoses) can you identify in this case? List them in order of priority.
4. Calculate Esther's nitrogen balance and transferrin for day 8. Why are these indexes important to assessing her nutritional status?
5. What is Esther's creatinine-height Index? How does it reflect her nutritional status?
6. What nutrition problems do you expect Esther to experience after discharge? How could they be resolved? What community agencies might contribute to her sense of well-being after discharge?

and family. This evaluation is continuous and thorough, and it requires careful, objective documentation (see the *Case Study* box, "Nutrition Assessment and Therapy for a Patient with Cancer"). It seeks to validate care while it is being given, as well as to determine the effectiveness of a particular course of care. Various areas need to be investigated, as follows:

- *Estimate the achievement of nutrition therapy goals:* What is the effect of diet or mode of feeding on the illness or patient's situation? Does a need exist for any change in nutrient ratios of diet or formula as originally calculated, in meal distribution pattern, or in feeding mode?
- *Judge the accuracy of intervention actions:* Does a need exist to change any of the NCP components? For example, is it necessary to change the type of food or feeding equipment, environment for meals, procedures for counseling, or types of learning activities for nutrition education and self-care procedures?
- *Determine the patient's ability to follow the prescribed nutrition therapy:* Do any hindrances or disabilities exist that prevent the patient from observing the treatment plan? What is the effect of nutrition therapy on the patient, family, or staff? Were the necessary nutrition assessment procedures for collecting nutrition data carried out correctly? Do patient and family understand the information given for self-care? Have community resources required by the patient and family been available and convenient for use? Has any needed food assistance program been sufficient to meet needs for the patient's ongoing care?

KEY TERMS

enteral A mode of feeding that uses the gastrointestinal (GI) tract; oral or tube feeding.

parenteral A mode of feeding that does not use the GI tract; instead it provides nutrition by intravenous delivery of nutrient solutions.

TO SUM UP

The basis for an accurate assessment of the patient's nutritional needs begins with the individual patient and family. Physical, psychologic, social, economic, and cultural factors in and out of the clinical setting all play a role in evaluating the patient's health status and any possible problems with the nutrition care plan.

Nutrition assessment is based on a broad foundation of pertinent data, including food and drug uses and values. Effectiveness of an assessment based on analysis of these data depends on effective communication with the patient, family members, and significant others in the development of an appropriate care plan, as well as with other members of the health care team. The patient's medical record is a basic means of communication among health care team members.

Nutrition therapy, based on a combination of personal and physiologic needs of the patient, requires a close working relationship among nutrition, medical, and nursing staff in the health care facility. The nurse's schedule offers many opportunities to reinforce nutrition principles of the diet. Nutrition therapy does not end with the patient's discharge. Outpatient nutrition services, appropriate social services, and food resources in the community help meet the continuing needs of patients and their families.

QUESTIONS FOR REVIEW

1. Identify and discuss possible effects of various psychologic factors on the outcome of nutrition therapy.
2. Outline a general procedure for assessing the nutritional needs of a 65-year-old widower hospitalized with coronary heart disease. Include the appropriate community agencies that you would refer the patient to for follow-up care, services, and information.
3. Describe commonly used anthropometric procedures, as well as laboratory and urine tests for nutritional status information, in terms of the significance of the measure or test (i.e., what is being measured, what the results tell you).
4. Select several clinical signs used to assess nutritional status, and describe what each sign shows in a malnourished person and why.
5. Describe the nature and purpose of quality assurance plans for standards of nutrition care.

REFERENCES

1. Moore MC: *Pocket guide to nutrition assessment and care*, ed 6, St Louis, 2009, Mosby.
2. Nelms M: Assessment of nutrition status and risk. In Nelms MN, Sucher K, Long S, editors: *Understanding nutrition therapy and pathophysiology*, Belmont, Calif, 2007, Wadsworth.
3. American Dietetic Association: Position of the American Dietetic Association: integration of medical nutrition therapy and pharmacotherapy, *J Am Diet Assoc* 103:1363, 2003.
4. Wolf AM, Siadaty M, Yaeger B, et al: Effects of lifestyle intervention on health care costs: Improving Control with Activity and Nutrition (ICAN), *J Am Diet Assoc* 107:1365, 2007.
5. Fessler TA: Malnutrition: a serious concern for hospitalized patients, *Today's Dietitian* 10(7):44, 2008.
6. Weight-Control Information Network: *Statistics related to overweight and obesity*, Bethesda, Md, 2007, National Institute of Diabetes and Digestive and Kidney Diseases. Retrieved March 7, 2009, from at www.win.niddk.nih.gov/statistics/index.htm.
7. Centers for Disease Control and Prevention: *Health consequences of overweight and obesity*, Atlanta, Ga, 2009, Centers for Disease Control and Prevention. Retrieved March 7, 2009, from www.cdc.gov/nccdphp/dnpa/obesity/consequences.htm.
8. Lacey K, Pritchitt E: Nutrition Care Process and model: ADA adopts road map to quality care and outcomes management, *J Am Diet Assoc* 103(8):1061, 2003.
9. Lee RD, Nieman DC: *Nutritional assessment*, ed 4, Boston, 2007, McGraw-Hill.
10. American Dietetic Association: ADA's definitions for nutrition screening and nutrition assessment, *J Am Diet Assoc* 94:838, 1994.
11. Joint Commission on Accreditation of Healthcare Organizations: *2009 Comprehensive accreditation manual for hospitals: the official handbook (CAMH)*, Oakbrook Terrace, Ill, 2009, JCAHO.
12. Identifying patients at risk: ADA's definitions for nutrition screening and nutrition assessment, *J Am Diet Assoc* 94(8):838, 1994.
13. Charney P, Marian M: Nutrition screening and nutrition assessment. In Charney P, Malone AM, editors: *ADA pocket guide to nutrition assessment*, ed 2, Chicago, 2009, American Dietetic Association.
14. Lefton J, Malone AM: Anthropometric assessment. In Charney P, Malone AM, editors: *ADA pocket guide to nutrition assessment*, ed 2, Chicago, 2009, American Dietetic Association.
15. National Heart Lung and Blood Institute: *Obesity education initiative*, Bethesda, Md, National Heart Lung Blood Institute National Institutes of Health. Retrieved March 12, 2009, from www.nhlbi.nih.gov/health/public/heart/obesity/lose_wt/risk.htm.
16. Chumlea WC, Guo SS, Steinbaugh ML: Prediction of stature from knee height for black and white adults and children with

application to mobility-impaired or handicapped persons, *J Am Diet Assoc* 94:1385, 1994.
17. Cockram DB, Baumgartner RN: Evaluation of accuracy and reliability of calipers for measuring recumbent knee height in elderly people, *Am J Clin Nutr* 52:397, 1990.
18. Muncie HI, Sobal J, Hoopes JM, et al: A practical method of estimating stature of bedridden female nursing home patients, *J Am Geriatr Soc* 35:285, 1987.
19. Mitchell CO, Lipschitz DA: Arm length measurement as an alternative to height in the nutrition assessment of the elderly, *JPEN J Parenter Enteral Nutr* 6:226, 1982.
20. American Dietetic Association Evidence Analysis Library: *Adult weight management guidelines*, Chicago, Ill, American Dietetic Association. Retrieved March 12, 2009, from www.adaevidencelibrary.com.
21. Thompson CW: Laboratory assessment. In Charney P, Malone AM, editors: *ADA pocket guide to nutrition assessment*, ed 2, Chicago, 2009, American Dietetic Association.
22. American Dietetic Association: *International Dietetics and Nutrition Terminology (IDNT) reference manual. Standardized language for the nutrition care process*, ed 2, Chicago, 2009, American Dietetic Association.

FURTHER READINGS AND RESOURCES

Readings

American Dietetic Association: Position of the American Dietetic Association: integration of medical nutrition therapy and pharmacology, *J Am Diet Assoc* 103(10):1363, 2003.

American Dietetic Association: Position of the American Dietetic Association: ethical and legal issues in nutrition, hydration, and feeding, *J Am Diet Assoc* 108(5):873, 2008.

Websites of Interest

Nestle Nutrition, Clinical Resources and Tools. This site provides tools and resources to help identify, assess, and select appropriate products to address the nutrition challenges patients: www.nestle-nutrition.com/Clinical_Resources/Default.aspx.

U.S. Department of Agriculture, Food and Nutrition Information Center, Dietary Analysis and Intake Calculators. This site, hosted by the Food and Nutrition Information Center (FNIC) at the National Agricultural Library (NAL), provides links to numerous diet-analysis tools: http://fnic.nal.usda.gov/nal_display/index.php?info_center=4&tax_level=2&tax_subject=256&topic_id=1459.

17

Metabolic Stress

Joyce Ann Gilbert

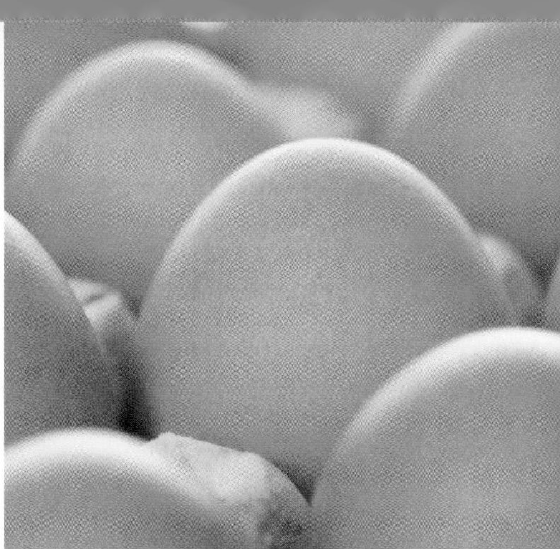

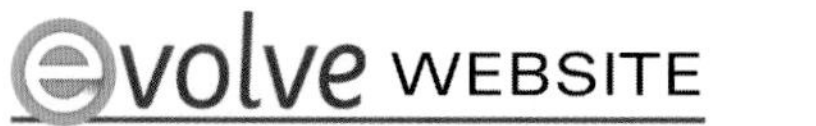

http://evolve.elsevier.com/Williams/essentials/

OUTLINE

In this chapter, various surgical procedures are discussed, with a focus on surgical procedures and situations that could bear a large nutritional consequence, particularly thermal injuries (or burns). Understanding the surgical procedure performed, with knowledge of nutritional and absorptive function and capacity of the alimentary tract, is imperative to providing optimal nutrition care of surgery patients (see the Focus on Culture box, "Physiologic Changes Related to the Aging Process That Can Affect Surgery"). An understanding of the body's response to metabolic stress is also important when determining optimal timing and type of nutrition intervention for the patient.

NUTRITIONAL NEEDS OF GENERAL SURGERY PATIENTS

Preoperative Nutrition

Nutritional needs of surgery patients vary based on several factors, including the patient's disease process, other comorbidities, and baseline nutritional status. Many general surgery patients are adequately nourished preoperatively and therefore do not have any special nutrient requirements (see the *Perspectives in Practice* box, "Energy and Protein Requirements in General Surgery Patients"). The disease itself often lends to poor nutrient intake and a hypermetabolic state that places the patient at nutritional risk. Malnutrition is associated with altered immune function, poor wound healing, and increased morbidity and mortality rates.[1] Researchers estimate that more than 50% of hospitalized patients are malnourished on hospital admission and hospital discharge.[2–5] For optimal outcome a malnourished patient should be nutritionally repleted for 7 to 10 days before surgery, if time permits.[6] Unless the gastrointestinal (GI) tract is nonfunctional, nutrient provision should be provided enterally rather than parenterally.[7] Following are some guidelines:

- *Energy:* Adequate calories should be consumed to prevent loss of endogenous stores of carbohydrate, fat, and protein. Carbohydrates should constitute the majority of calories (50% to 60%). A minimum of approximately 150 g of carbohydrates per day is needed for central nervous system (CNS) function.
- *Protein:* Most patients do not have excessive preoperative protein requirements, but body stores should be assessed. Adequate protein status is imperative to facilitate optimal wound healing.
- *Vitamins and minerals:* Any deficiency state such as anemia should be corrected. Electrolytes and fluids should be normalized and in balance with correction of dehydration, acidosis, or alkalosis.

One often-overlooked factor is the use of medicinal herbs. Many patients do not think to disclose the ingestion of herbal supplements when they are asked about medications during the preoperative interview, but some of these substances can complicate surgery. (Some common herbal supplements that can cause complications during surgery are listed in the *Diet-Medications Interactions* box, "Medicine or Poison?")

FOCUS ON CULTURE

Physiologic Changes Related to the Aging Process That Can Affect Surgery

PHYSIOLOGIC CHANGE	EFFECTS	POTENTIAL POSTOPERATIVE COMPLICATIONS
Cardiovascular		
↓ Elasticity of blood vessels ↓ Cardiac output ↓ Peripheral circulation	↓ Circulation to vital organs Slower blood flow	Shock (hypotension), thrombosis with pulmonary emboli, delayed wound healing, postoperative confusion, hypervolemia, decreased response to stress
Respiratory		
↓ Elasticity of lungs and chest wall ↓ Residual lung volume ↓ Forced expiratory volume ↓ Ciliary action Fewer alveolar capillaries	↓ Vital capacity ↓ Alveolar volume ↓ Gas exchange ↓ Cough reflex	Atelectasis, pneumonia, postoperative confusion
Urinary		
↓ Glomerular filtration rate ↓ Bladder muscle tone Weakened perineal muscles	↓ Kidney function Stasis of urine in bladder Loss of urinary control	Prolonged response to anesthesia and drugs, overhydration with intravenous fluids, hyperkalemia, urinary tract infection, urinary retention
Musculoskeletal		
↓ Muscle strength Limitation of motion	↓ Activity	Atelectasis, pneumonia, thrombophlebitis, constipation or fecal impaction
Gastrointestinal		
↓ Intestinal motility	Retention of feces	Constipation or fecal impaction
Metabolic		
↓ γ-Globulin level ↓ Plasma proteins	↓ Inflammatory response	Delayed wound healing, wound dehiscence or evisceration
Immune System		
Fewer killer T cells ↓ Response to foreign antigens	↓ Ability to protect against invasion by pathogenic microorganisms	Wound infection, wound dehiscence, pneumonia, urinary tract infection

From Keeling AW, Muro A, Long BC: Preoperative nursing. In Phipps WJ, Cassmever VL, Sands JK, editors: *Medical-surgical nursing: concepts and clinical practice,* ed 5, St Louis, 1995, Mosby.

Immediate Preoperative Period

Typical dietary preparation for surgery involves giving nothing by mouth 8 to 12 hours before surgery. The rationale is to ensure the stomach is empty of food and liquids to prevent vomiting or aspiration during surgery or anesthesia recovery. In an emergency situation, gastric suction is used to remove stomach contents. With surgery involving the GI tract, food and fecal matter may interfere with the procedure itself and cause contamination. Therefore before lower GI surgery, a low-residue diet may be prescribed to reduce fecal residue. Although restricting dietary intake may decrease the risks associated with anesthesia, it can also impair the patient's ability to respond to the metabolic stress of surgery.

Postoperative Nutrition

Nutrient provision in the postoperative period depends on several factors, including the surgical procedure performed and anticipated time to resumption of oral intake, complications of surgery and postoperative clinical status, and preoperative nutritional status. The well-nourished patient undergoing elective surgery will typically resume oral feeding by postoperative day 3 to 7, depending on return of bowel function. In this situation, supplemental nutrition in the form of enteral and parenteral nutrition is not indicated. The malnourished patient who is undergoing elective or emergency surgery and not anticipated to be able to meet his or her nutritional needs orally for a period of 7 to 10 days should receive specialized nutrition support.[6]

This nutrition support should be provided enterally rather than parenterally to minimize incidence of complications.[6] Duration of this therapy will then depend on the patient's clinical status and transition to an adequate oral dietary consumption.

Energy Requirements

In the immediate postoperative period, especially in the critically ill, the goal of nutrition support is maintenance of current lean body mass, not repletion, and should serve as an adjunct to other critical therapies. Numerous factors are present that limit effectiveness of exogenously administered nutritional substrates in preventing catabolism regardless of the level of support. It should not be expected to convert a catabolic, septic patient into an anabolic state at this time. Many undesirable metabolic complications can occur in attempting to do so, such as hypercapnia, hyperglycemia, hypertriglyceridemia, hepatic steatosis, and azotemia.[7-11] Once the hypermetabolic process is corrected, anabolism is favored and repletion can occur.

Multiple methods are available for determining energy requirements. Indirect calorimetry involves actual measurement of

EXTENT OF BODY RESERVES OF NUTRIENTS

NUTRIENT	TIME REQUIRED TO DEPLETE RESERVES IN WELL-NOURISHED INDIVIDUALS
Amino acids	Several hours
Carbohydrate	13 hours
Sodium	2-3 days
Water	4 days
Zinc	5 days
Fat	20-40 days
Thiamin	30-60 days
Vitamin C	60-120 days
Niacin	60-180 days
Riboflavin	60-180 days
Vitamin A	90-365 days
Iron	125 days (women), 750 days (men)
Iodine	1000 days
Calcium	2500 days

From Guthrie HA: *Introductory nutrition,* ed 7, St Louis, 1989, Mosby.

PERSPECTIVES IN PRACTICE

Energy and Protein Requirements in General Surgery Patients

Nutritional needs of general surgery patients vary based on several factors, including the patient's disease process, other comorbidities, surgery to be performed, and baseline nutritional status. For example, compare the following patient situations.

Adequately Nourished Preoperative Patient

For the patient with normal energy and nitrogen balance, approximately 25 kcal/kg/day and 0.8 to 1.0 g/kg/day of protein should maintain these balances.

Adequately Nourished Postoperative Patient

If no complications have occurred after surgery, then energy requirements remain about the same—25 kcal/kg/day. Protein requirements increase slightly because of increased metabolism and need for wound healing in the postoperative period to 1.0 to 1.1 g/kg/day.

Adequately Nourished Stressed Patient

This patient is assumed to have adequate nutrient stores; therefore replenishment is not the goal. Metabolic stress increases metabolic and catabolic rates, making energy and protein needs elevated. Energy needs are estimated at 25 to 30 kcal/kg/day; protein needs, 1.2 to 1.5 g/kg/day. Postoperatively the patient should be reassessed, and protein needs may increase up to 2 g/kg/day.

Nutritionally Depleted Nonstressed Patient

Upcoming Surgery: Gastrointestinal Tract Resection Resulting From Obstruction

Because of reduced dietary intake, this patient's nutrient stores (mostly glycogen and fat) may be depleted. In the nonstressed state, protein stores are spared for the most part. Energy needs are similar to those of the nourished preoperative patient at 25 kcal/kg/day. However, protein needs are slightly elevated to 1.0 to 1.2 g/kg/day. Postoperatively this patient's energy needs will remain near the same at 25 kcal/kg/day, but protein needs are increased to 1.2 to 1.5 g/kg/day.

Nutritionally Depleted Stressed Patient

This patient has elevated requirements for energy and protein because of cytokine and hormonal shifts causing a hypermetabolic and hypercatabolic state. Energy needs are 25 to 30 kcal/kg/day, with caution to avoid overfeeding. Overfeeding in a hypermetabolic state can result in hyperglycemia, hypercarbia, hepatic steatosis, and overall immune suppression. Protein needs are elevated to 1.5 to 2.0 g/kg/day. Postoperatively the nutrient needs remain about the same. At this point the goal is to minimize loss of lean body mass, not to replenish it. Once the patient is stable and anabolic, calories can be increased to 35 kcal/kg/day as needed for rehabilitation.

BIBLIOGRAPHY

A.S.P.E.N. Board of Directors: Guidelines for the use of parenteral and enteral nutrition in adult and pediatric patients, *J Parent Enteral Nutr* 26:1SA, 2002.

Frankenfield D: Energy and macrosubstrate requirements. *American Society for Enteral and Parenteral Nutrition: The science and practice of nutrition support: a case-based core,* ed 3, Dubuque, Iowa, 2001, Kendall/Hunt.

DIET-MEDICATIONS INTERACTIONS

Medicine or Poison?

"Poisons and medicines are oftentimes the same substances given with different intents."

Peter Mere Latham (1789-1875)

Medicinal herbs and pharmaceutical drugs: Both can be therapeutic at one dose and toxic at another. Patients may not think to include herbal supplements when reporting medications used during the preoperative interview. Possible surgical complications vary depending on the herbal supplement used. Following are some common herbal supplements that may cause surgical complications.

HERB	COMMON USES	POSSIBLE SURGICAL COMPLICATION
Danshen *(Salvia miltiorrhiza)*	Antibacterial, antihepatotoxin, mild sedative, antiinflammatory	May cause bleeding.
Dong quai *(Angelica sinensis)*	Menstrual disorders, menopause	May cause bleeding (interferes with warfarin).
Echinacea *(Echinacea purpurea)*	Prevent and treat common cold, treat infections, enhance wound healing	May interfere with effectiveness of immunosuppressant drugs given to prevent transplant rejection; may interfere with body's immune functioning after surgery; could impair wound healing.
Ephedra* (Ma huang, herbal ecstasy, Chinese ephedra)	Sinus congestion, weight loss (ephedrine/caffeine)	May cause cardiovascular problems (increased heart rate, arrhythmias, heart attack or stroke); interaction with anesthesia can lead to abnormal heartbeat. For patients taking maintenance doses of monoamine oxidase inhibitors (MAOIs), interaction with anesthesia and MAOIs may result in life-threatening hypertension and coma.
Feverfew *(Tanacetum parthenium)*	Migraine headaches (prophylaxis), rheumatoid arthritis (RA)	May cause bleeding.
Garlic *(Allium spp.)*	Atherosclerosis, hyperlipidemia, hypertension, antithrombotic effects, chemoprevention, insect repellant, antimicrobial	May cause bleeding or interfere with normal clotting.
Ginkgo *(Ginkgo biloba)*	Alzheimer's disease and non-Alzheimer's dementia, ordinary age-related memory loss, improving memory and mental function in the young, intermittent claudication, premenstrual syndrome, altitude sickness, tinnitus	May cause bleeding.
Ginseng *(Panax ginseng)*	Enhancing immunity, improving mental activity, diabetes, athletic performance	May cause bleeding (interferes with warfarin).
Goldenseal *(Hydrastis canadensis)*	Antimicrobial, expectorant	May cause or worsen hypertension.
Kava *(Piper methysticum)*	Anxiety	May enhance sedative effects of anesthesia.
Licorice† *(Glycyrrhiza glabra)*	Peptic ulcer disease, expectorant/antitussive	May increase blood pressure.
St. John's wort *(Hypericum perforatum)*	Major depression of mild to moderate severity, polyneuropathy	Can increase or decrease effect of some drugs used during and after surgery.
Valerian *(Valeriana officinalis)*	Insomnia, anxiety	May interfere with effects of anesthesia.

NOTE: Different herbs stay in the body for different lengths of time. An individual taking herbs may need to stop taking them 1 or 2 weeks before surgery.

BIBLIOGRAPHY

Bratman S, Girman AM: *Mosby's handbook of herbs and supplements and their therapeutic uses,* St Louis, 2003, Mosby.

Escott-Stump S: *Nutrition and diagnosis-related care,* ed 6, Philadelphia, 2007, Lippincott Williams & Wilkins.

Fugh-Berman A: Herb-drug interactions, *Lancet* 355:134, 2000.

Mayo Clinic Staff: *Herbal supplements and surgery: what you need to know,* Rochester, Minn, 2003, Mayo Foundation for Medical Education and Research. Retrieved August 14, 2005, from www.mayoclinic.com.

Winston and Kuhn's: *Herbal therapy and supplements: a scientific and traditional approach,* ed 2, Philadelphia, 2007, Lippincott Williams & Wilkins.

*Ephedra was banned by the U.S. Food and Drug Administration (FDA) in December 2003.

†Most licorice candy contains little or no herbal licorice. Consumers should consult the product ingredients. "Licorice flavoring" is safer than "licorice extract" or "natural licorice" for these purposes.

energy expenditure and remains the "gold standard."[12] However, many disadvantages to this method exist, including increased cost, the potential for improperly trained personnel, inaccurate readings in patients with an Fio_2 (fraction of inspired oxygen) of 50% or more, the possibility of malfunctioning chest tubes and endotracheal tubes, and the occurrence of bronchopleural fistulas. Because of these flaws, many institutions do not have the technology available and rely on predictive equations. Predicting energy needs can be difficult because of uncertainties regarding multiple factors of energy expenditure (Table 17-1).[13] Predictive equations (Box 17-1) may overestimate energy needs for those mechanically ventilated and sedated, and neuromuscular paralysis can decrease energy requirements by as much as 30%.[14–16] Calculated results are only as accurate as the variables used in the equation. Obesity and resuscitative water weight complicate use of these equations and lead to a tendency for overfeeding.[17] It is unclear as to whether ideal body weight (IBW) or actual body weight should be used in predictive energy equations. It has been reported that obese patients should receive 20 to 30 kilocalories (kcalories or kcal)/kg IBW per day,[18] as well as use of adjusted body weight, particularly in those weighing more than 130% IBW.[17] Predictive equations have been developed to account for obesity, using actual body weight, as well as trauma, burns, and ventilatory status.[19] Patino and colleagues[20] reported a hypocaloric-hyperproteinic nutrition regimen provided during the first days of the flow phase of the adaptive response to injury, sepsis, and critical illness. The regimen consists of a daily supply of 100 to 200 g of glucose and 1.5 to 2.0 g of protein per kilogram IBW. Overall, energy requirements for surgery patients range from 20 to 35 kcal/kg usual body weight per day.[21]

TABLE 17-1 INFLUENCES ON RESTING ENERGY EXPENDITURE

CLINICAL CONDITION	REE (%)*
Elective uncomplicated surgery	Normal
Major Abdominal, Thoracic, and Vascular Surgery	
ICU + mechanical ventilation	105-109 ± 20-28
Cardiac Surgery	
ICU + mechanical ventilation	119 ± 21
Multiple Injury	
ICU + mechanical ventilation	138 ± 23
Spontaneous ventilation	119 ± 7
Head and Multiple Injury	
ICU + mechanical ventilation	150 ± 23
Head Injury	
ICU + spontaneous ventilation	126 ± 14
ICU + mechanical ventilation	104 ± 5
Infection	
Sepsis + spontaneous ventilation	121 ± 27
ICU + septic shock + mechanical ventilation	135 ± 28
Sepsis + mechanical ventilation	155 ± 14
Septic shock + mechanical ventilation	102 ± 14
Multiple injury + sepsis + mechanical ventilation + TPN	191 ± 38

Modified from Chiolero R, Revelly JP, Tappy L: Energy metabolism in sepsis and injury, *Nutrition* 13(suppl):45S, 1997, with permission from Elsevier.

*Values are percentage of reference value (±SD).

REE, Resting energy expenditure; *ICU*, intensive care unit; *TPN*, total parenteral nutrition.

Protein Requirements

Dietary protein is required to build new and maintain existing body tissue and has many functions in the body. Protein can also be oxidized directly for adenosine triphosphate (ATP) and is critical to the body's ability to perform gluconeogenesis. Therefore protein is an important energy substrate in addition to its role in tissue building and repair.

Protein requirements in the surgical patient are typically elevated, particularly in the critically ill. Increased requirements are the result of need for tissue synthesis and wound healing, maintenance of oncotic pressure, adequate blood volume, maintenance of immune function, and energy substrate. Stressed critically ill patients require protein in the range of 1.5 to 2.0 g/kg/day.[20] Achieving positive nitrogen balance is nearly impossible immediately after metabolic insult, but after the primary insult is controlled or resolved, positive nitrogen balance is feasible. Protein requirements do not decrease with increasing age. Short-term inadequate

BOX 17-1 SELECTED METHODS FOR ESTIMATING ENERGY REQUIREMENTS

Harris-Benedict Basal Energy Expenditure (BEE) Equation

$$\text{Male}: 66.5 + 13.8(W) + 5.0(H) - 6.8(A)$$

$$\text{Female}: 655.1 + 9.6(W) + 1.9(H) - 4.7(A)$$

where *W* is weight (in kilograms); *H*, height (in centimeters); and *A*, age (in years).

Note: To predict total energy expenditure (TEE), add an injury/activity factor of 1.2 to 1.8 depending on the severity and nature of illness.

Ireton-Jones energy expenditure equations (EEEs)

Spontaneously Breathing Patients

$$EEE(s) = 629 - 11(A) + 25(W) - 609(O)$$

Ventilator-Dependent Patients

$$EEE(V) = 1784 - 11(A) + 5(W) + 244(G) + 239(T) + 804(B)$$

where *EEE* is given in kcal/day; *v*, ventilator dependent; *s*, spontaneously breathing; *A*, age (in years); *W*, body weight (in kilograms); *G*, gender (female = 0, male = 1); *V*, ventilator support (present = 1, absent = 0), *T*, diagnosis of trauma (present = 1, absent = 0); *B*, diagnosis of burn (present = 1, absent = 0); and *O*, obesity >30% more than ideal body weight (IBW) (from 1959 Metropolitan Life Insurance tables; present = 1, absent = 0).

protein intake in older adults has been shown to change skeletal muscle transcript levels that may lead to muscle wasting.[21a] Reduction in lean body mass and obligatory loss of protein during physiologic stress increase protein requirements for critically ill older patients to requirements similar to those for younger patients.[22,22a] Protein tolerance, as opposed to protein requirement, often determines amount of protein delivered. Onset of azotemia (i.e., impaired renal or hepatic function) signals the need to reduce protein delivery. Most studies that examined graded protein intakes in septic, injured, or burned patients have found no protein-sparing benefit to giving protein in excess of the previous recommendations.[23]

Fluid Requirements

Water is the medium within which all systems and subsystems function. It is necessary in digestion, absorption, transport, and use of nutrients, as well as in elimination of toxins and waste products. Total body fluid can be compartmentalized into two reservoirs: (1) intracellular and (2) extracellular. Intracellular compartment includes all water within the cell membrane and provides the environment for the metabolic reactions that take place in cells. The extracellular compartmental water includes all water external to cell membranes and allows nutrients to flow into cells and cellular waste products to return to the bloodstream. Water also provides structure to cells and is a vital component of thermoregulation. Water is the most abundant substance in the human body, accounting for approximately 60% of body weight of men and 50% of body weight of women. The majority of water intake comes from ingested fluid and food; a small amount is produced as a byproduct of metabolic processes, primarily carbohydrate metabolism. The main source of water loss is in the form of urine. However, sizeable amounts are also lost insensibly through skin and respiratory tract. Smaller amounts of water are lost in sweat and feces (Table 17-2).

TABLE 17-2 NORMAL DAILY FLUID GAINS AND LOSSES IN ADULTS

FLUID GAINS		FLUID LOSSES	
Sensible		***Sensible***	
Food	1000 mL	Urine	1500 mL
Fluid	1200 mL	Feces	100 mL
		Sweat	50 mL
Insensible		***Insensible***	
Oxidative metabolism	350 mL	Skin	500 mL
		Lungs	400 mL
TOTAL	2550 mL	**TOTAL**	2550 mL

From Whitmire SJ: Fluid and electrolytes. In Gottschlich MM, editor: *The science and practice of nutrition support: a case-based core curriculum,* Dubuque, Iowa, 2001, Kendall/Hunt, with permission from the American Society for Enteral and Parenteral Nutrition (A.S.P.E.N.). A.S.P.E.N. does not endorse the use of this material in any form other than its entirety.

Normal body water requirements can be estimated using a variety of methods. The National Research Council (NRC) recommends 1 mL/kcal energy expenditure for adults with average energy expenditure living under average environmental conditions. Fluid requirements increase with several conditions, including fever, high altitude, low humidity, profuse sweating, watery diarrhea, vomiting, hemorrhage, diuresis, surgical drains, and loss of skin integrity (e.g., burns, open wounds).

Therefore fluid balance is of vital concern after surgery. Patients often receive large volumes of fluid intraoperatively. These volumes are normally diuresed postoperatively, but occasionally the patient may require diuretics to facilitate this. Typically, surgical patients are provided with intravenous fluids until oral intake is resumed and tolerated to maintain fluid balance. Daily weight measurement of the patient provides a guideline for fluid balance.

Vitamin and Mineral Requirements

Adequate levels of vitamins and minerals are very important for optimal postoperative recovery. Vitamin C serves many functions in the body. In addition to being an antioxidant, it is required for synthesis of collagen (the structural protein found in skin, bone, tendon, and cartilage), carnitine, and neurotransmitters, as well as for immune-mediated and antibacterial functions of white blood cells. Vitamin C is also required for the scar tissue, which aids in wound healing. Iron is an essential component of hemoglobin, which is necessary for oxygen transport; of myoglobin, which is necessary for muscle iron storage; and in cytochromes, which transport electrons through the respiratory chain resulting in the oxidative production of cellular energy. Vitamin K is essential in the blood-clotting cascade by activating inactive clotting factors resulting in the formation of fibrin. Surgical patients with elevated enteric losses (e.g., ostomy, stool, fistula) are at risk for several trace element deficiencies (e.g., zinc, copper). If losses exceed 800 mL/day, then extra supplementation of micronutrients should be considered. Various GI operations may also place a surgical patient at risk for several micronutrient deficiencies, depending on the amount of remaining small intestine, the location of bowel resection, and the functional status of remaining GI tract.[1]

Diets

Oral Diet

The preferred route of nutrient delivery is for the patient to be able to consume adequate nutrients through an oral diet. Fortunately the majority of surgical patients can accomplish this by postoperative day 7 at the latest. Routine intravenous fluids are intended to provide hydration and electrolytes, not energy and protein requirements. For example, 1 L of routine intravenous fluids of a 5% dextrose solution provides 50 g of

KEY TERMS

sepsis Presence in the blood or other tissues of pathogenic microorganisms or their toxins; conditions associated with such pathogens.

dextrose, with an energy value of only 170 kcal; no protein is provided. If adequate calories and protein are not consumed, then the patient's diet may be supplemented. Often the addition of between-meal feedings consisting of soft, high-protein foods is adequate. However, sometimes commercially available oral supplements may be provided because they are a concentrated source of energy, protein, and vitamins and minerals.[24] Not all patients tolerate these supplements, because they tend to be very sweet and patients develop taste fatigue. Every effort should be made to maximize the patient's diet for his or her diet preferences to improve inadequate dietary consumption.

Routine Postoperative Diets

A diet order is typically prescribed postoperatively once the patient exhibits adequate bowel function (e.g., flatus, bowel sounds present). Historically the first diet order is a clear liquid diet (Box 17-2). This diet contains hyperosmolar fluids, calories from primarily simple sugars, very little protein, and a fair amount of sodium and chloride. Because this diet is incomplete and very unpalatable, patients should be advanced to either a full liquid or soft/regular diet as soon as the clear liquid diet is tolerated. These diets are complete diets in that calorie, protein, and vitamin and mineral requirements can be met if adequate amounts are consumed. Recently this historical diet progression after GI surgery was challenged.[25] Patients randomized to a regular diet as their first postoperative diet after abdominal surgery had equal tolerance and improved nutrient intake compared with those receiving a clear liquid diet.

BOX 17-2 TYPICAL FOODS IN POSTOPERATIVE DIETS

Clear Liquid
- Broth
- Clear juice (apple, grape, cranberry)
- Jello
- Sodas (Sprite, ginger ale)
- Tea
- Coffee

Full Liquid
- Juice (any)
- Milk
- Milkshakes
- Ice cream
- Cream soups
- Thinned oatmeal, corn grits
- Scrambled eggs (in some institutions)
- Oral liquid nutritional supplements (e.g., Ensure, Boost)

Soft/Regular
- Juice
- Canned fruits
- Cooked vegetables
- Soft meats (baked chicken, stews, roasts)
- Scrambled eggs
- Pancakes, biscuits, muffins
- Soups
- Soft sandwiches (egg, tuna, chicken salad, turkey, ham and cheese)
- Soft starches (mashed potatoes, pasta, rice)
- Milk, tea, coffee
- Ice cream
- Puddings, yogurt
- Soft desserts (cake, pies, soft cookies)

Specialized Nutrition Support

If an oral diet is not tolerated or feasible, then enteral or parenteral nutrition may be provided. Enteral nutrition is indicated for patients with an adequately functional GI tract and oral nutrient intake that is insufficient to meet estimated needs.[6] Enteral nutrition maintains nutritional, metabolic, immunologic, and barrier functions of the intestines; it is less expensive and safer than parenteral nutrition.[26] A series of studies of patients with GI cancer suggests parenteral nutrition increased the overall risk of postoperative complications by 10%. However, parenteral nutrition administered 7 to 10 days before surgery decreases postoperative complications by approximately 10%. Wound healing and surgical recovery may be impaired if parenteral nutrition is not begun within 5 to 10 days postsurgery in patients unable to eat or tolerate enteral feeding. Although enteral nutrition is the preferred route of nutrient delivery, it is not innocuous. Some situations exist in which enteral feeding is not feasible (Box 17-3), and therefore parenteral nutrition should be used. Expected length of therapy, clinical condition, risk of aspiration, and medical expertise usually determine route of administration and type of access for tube feedings. Multiple methods for obtaining enteral access exist (Box 17-4), all of which carry various levels of expertise, risk, and expense. Nasoenteric or oroenteric tubes are generally used when therapy is anticipated to be of short duration (e.g., <4 weeks) or for interim access before placement of a long-term device. Long-term access requires a percutaneous or surgically placed feeding tube. It is not always clear when enteral nutrition will be tolerated. If the needs of the individual are not met enterally, then parenteral nutrition may be implemented for either

BOX 17-3 INDICATIONS FOR PARENTERAL NUTRITION

Indications
- Bowel obstruction
- Persistent intolerance of enteral feeding (e.g., emesis, diarrhea)
- Hemodynamic instability
- Major upper gastrointestinal (GI) bleed
- Ileus
- Unable to safely access intestinal tract

Relative Indications
- Significant bowel wall edema
- Nutrient infusion proximal to recent GI anastomosis
- High-output fistula (>800 mL/day)

full nutrient provision or concurrently with enteral delivery to provide the balance of nutrients not tolerated.

The majority of postoperative surgical patients can tolerate a standard enteral formulation that provides their energy and protein requirements. Recent research studies have evaluated use of "immune-enhancing" enteral formulas in postoperative GI cancer patients, trauma patients, and patients with critical illness. These formulas are supplemented with various immune-enhancing nutrients, including L-arginine, L-glutamine, omega-3 fatty acids, nucleic acids, and various vitamins and minerals. When these diets were used in these surgical populations, decreases in infectious complications and hospital length of stay were noted.[6,27]

NUTRITIONAL CONCERNS FOR PATIENTS UNDERGOING ALIMENTARY CANAL SURGERY

The digestive tract is a metabolically active organ involved in digestion, absorption, and metabolism of many nutrients; therefore various surgical interventions involving the GI tract can result in malabsorption and maldigestion and nutritional deficiencies (Table 17-3).

Head and Neck Surgery

These patients often present for surgery malnourished because of their disease state. Many times surgical intervention is required because of a tumor that may be inhibiting the patient's ability to chew and swallow normally. Typically, loss of this ability is what makes the patient seek medical attention. Patients with head and neck cancer usually have a long history of alcohol and tobacco use, which may also affect optimal nutritional status.

Depending on the patient's treatment, optimization of nutrition preoperatively is ideal. This also depends on the individual's disease progression and ability to swallow. Many times preoperative treatment involves radiation, chemotherapy, or both to reduce the tumor size. In these situations, ability to swallow may worsen because of negative side effects of these therapies. Ideally, placement of a percutaneous endoscopic gastrostomy (PEG) feeding tube can be performed to allow for nutrition, hydration, and medication administration to maintain or improve (or both) nutritional status preoperatively. The patient may also still be able to swallow soft foods or liquids, which should be maximized for caloric and protein density. If a PEG tube is not placed preoperatively, then it can be placed intraoperatively or a nasoenteric tube may be placed. These feeding tubes are then used postoperatively until the patient is able to resume an oral diet.

Esophageal Surgery

Several medical conditions affecting the esophagus can prevent swallowing and thus nutrient intake. Common conditions include corrosive injuries and perforation, achalasia, gastroesophageal reflux disease (GERD), and partial or full obstruction caused by cancer, congenital abnormalities, or strictures. These conditions usually require surgical intervention involving removal of a segment or the entire esophagus (see the *Case Study* box, "The Patient with Esophageal Cancer"). The esophageal tract is then replaced with either the stomach

BOX 17-4 METHODS OF ENTERAL ACCESS

Short Term (<4 weeks)

Nasoenteric Feeding Tube

- Spontaneous passage
- Bedside prokinetic agent

Active Passage

- Bedside assisted
- Endoscopic
- Fluoroscopic
- Operative

Long Term (>4 weeks)

Percutaneous Feeding Tube

- Percutaneous endoscopic (percutaneous endoscopic gastrostomy [PEG])
- Gastric (PEG)
- Gastric/jejunal (PEG/jejunostomy)
- Direct jejunal (direct percutaneous endoscopic jejunostomy [DPEJ])

Laparoscopic

- Gastrostomy
- Jejunostomy

Surgical

- Gastrostomy
- Jejunostomy

KEY TERMS

malabsorption Malabsorption is a syndrome in which normal products of digestion do not traverse the intestinal mucosa and enter the lymphatic or portal venous branches.

maldigestion Maldigestion, which may be clinically similar to malabsorption, describes defects in the intraluminal phase of the digestive process caused by inadequate exposure of chyme to bile salts and pancreatic enzymes. Clinical symptoms of malabsorption include diarrhea, steatorrhea, and weight loss. Laboratory signs include depressed serum fat-soluble vitamin levels, accelerated prothrombin time, hypomagnesemia, and hypocholesterolemia. Patients with symptoms of malabsorption should have a laboratory workup to determine the presence and level of nutrient loss.

gastroesophageal reflux disease (GERD) Describes symptoms that result from reflux of gastric juices, and sometimes duodenal juices, into the esophagus. Symptoms include substernal burning (heartburn), epigastric pressure sensation, and severe epigastric pain. Prolonged and severe GERD can lead to esophageal bleeding, perforation, strictures, Barrett's epithelium, adenocarcinoma, and pulmonary fibrosis (from aspiration). Conservative dietary therapy involves weight reduction; restriction of carbonated beverages, caffeine, fatty foods, peppermint, chocolate, and ethanol; small frequent meals; and wearing of loose clothing to promote symptomatic relief.

TABLE 17-3 COMMON GASTROINTESTINAL OPERATIONS AND NUTRITIONAL CONSEQUENCES

LOCATION	POTENTIAL CONSEQUENCES
Esophagus	
Resection/replacement	Weight loss because of inadequate intake
Gastric pull-up	↑ Protein loss because of catabolism
Colonic interposition	May require enteral/parenteral nutrition until oral intake appropriate Antidumping diet; may malabsorb fat/fat-soluble vitamins, simple sugars, and various vitamins/minerals Early satiety because of reduced storage capacity (gastric pull-up)
Stomach	
Partial gastrectomy/vagotomy	Early satiety because of reduced storage capacity Delayed gastric emptying of solids because of stasis Rapid emptying of hypertonic fluids
Total gastrectomy	Weight loss because of dumping/malabsorption, early satiety, anorexia, inadequate intake, unavailability of bile acids and pancreatic enzymes because of anastomotic changes Malabsorption may lead to anemia, metabolic bone disease, protein-calorie malnutrition Bezoar formation Vitamin B_{12} deficiency because of lack of intrinsic factor
Intestine*	
Proximal	Malabsorption of vitamins/minerals (Ca^{2+}, Mg^{2+}, iron, vitamins A and D)
Gastric bypass	Protein-calorie malnutrition from malabsorption because of dumping, unavailability of bile acids and pancreatic enzymes because of anastomotic changes Bezoar formation
Distal	Malabsorption of vitamins/mineral (water soluble—folate, vitamins B_{12}, C, B_1, B_2, pyridoxine) Protein-calorie malnutrition because of dumping Fat malabsorption Bacterial overgrowth if ileocecal valve resected
Colon	Fluid and electrolyte (K^+, Na^+, Cl^-) malabsorption

*Note that consequences may occur only with extensive disease process and resection.

CASE STUDY

The Patient with Esophageal Cancer

Kevin is a 54-year-old accountant seen by his family physician for pain with swallowing and difficulty swallowing solid foods for the past 6 weeks. This has resulted in continued weight loss and fatigue. Kevin was referred to the gastrointestinal (GI) medicine service for further evaluation. After a series of tests that included endoscopy and biopsy, Kevin was found to have esophageal cancer with the tumor lying in the midesophagus. He was then referred to the GI surgery service for surgical evaluation.

A medical history revealed that Kevin smoked two packs of cigarettes per day, drank three martinis per day, and was cachectic. A referral was sent to the dietitian for nutritional evaluation and recommendations for optimizing his nutritional status for surgery. A nutrition history revealed that during the past 6 weeks, Kevin's diet had progressively decreased in consistency to the point where he could tolerate only liquids and some soft solid foods such as mashed potatoes, oatmeal, and applesauce. At a height of 178 cm (5 feet, 10 inches), Kevin's weight had dropped from 80 kg (176 lb) to 63 kg (139 lb), leaving him at 79% of his usual body weight. His blood work revealed a serum albumin level of 3.0 g/dL and prealbumin of 13.2 mg/dL. He no longer could stand long enough to make himself a meal and had to take a bath rather than shower because he became too tired. Kevin was not currently taking any medications because he could not swallow them. His current diet order was a full liquid diet.

Assessment of calorie and protein requirements estimated that Kevin required approximately 1800 kcal (basal energy expenditure + 25%) and 75 to 95 g of protein (1.2 to 1.5 g/kg) daily. Because he could eat some solid foods, the dietitian changed him to a soft diet. The dietitian modified Kevin's diet so that it contained soft, high protein–containing solids and liquids that Kevin stated he could eat and ordered a 48-hour calorie count. A liquid multivitamin was also provided. Kevin was now able to eat enough calories and protein for 14 days preoperatively that he gained 3 kg (7 lb); his albumin increased to 3.1 g/dL, and prealbumin increased to 17 mg/dL.

Kevin underwent an esophagectomy with a gastric pull-up. A feeding jejunostomy tube was placed intraoperatively. Kevin was started on low-rate enteral feedings on postoperative day 2, which were gradually advanced to his goal requirements

CASE STUDY

The Patient with Esophageal Cancer—cont'd

during the next 2 days. He was not allowed to eat until postoperative day 7 after a swallowing study for anastomotic evaluation. Once Kevin's diet was initiated and tolerated, his tube feedings were provided nocturnally because he was not able to consume 100% of his nutritional needs orally. He was discharged home with an oral postgastrectomy diet and nocturnal tube feedings to provide about 50% of his nutritional needs for 10 days, at which time his nutrition would be reevaluated.

Questions for Analysis

1. Evaluate the preoperative nutrition assessment data. Why were the particular energy and protein assessment factors chosen?
2. What dietary modifications accompany a postgastrectomy diet?
3. Why was Kevin placed on a postgastrectomy diet when his stomach was not resected?
4. At what point should his enteral tube feedings be discontinued?

(gastric pull-up) or the intestine (colonic and jejunal interposition). A gastric pull-up procedure involves drawing the stomach up to the esophageal stump, causing displacement of the stomach into the thoracic cavity. This procedure results in a reduction of stomach volume capacity, with potential delayed gastric emptying and dumping syndrome (Figure 17-1). The colonic and jejunal interposition procedure involves forming a new conduit by anastomosing the selected portion of bowel between the esophagus and stomach. Complications after this procedure include swallowing difficulties, strictures, and leakage at the anastomotic site.

Preoperative nutrition for these patients may be a tolerated oral diet (often liquids because of dysphasia and obstruction). If a patient is unable to consume his or her full nutrient needs orally, then a feeding tube may be placed if the esophagus is not obstructed. A PEG tube is not indicated if a gastric pull-up procedure is to be performed, because the stomach is used to make the esophageal conduit and a hole resulting from a gastrostomy tube would be contraindicated. These patients may require preoperative parenteral nutrition if the esophagus is obstructed. Intraoperatively, a jejunal feeding tube may be placed to allow for postoperative enteral nutrition until the anastomosis heals and oral intake is resumed. If enteral access is not obtained intraoperatively, then parenteral nutrition is indicated because these patients may not resume oral intake for 7 to 10 days.

For patients with chronic GERD, a Nissen fundoplication procedure may be performed. This is the most commonly performed antireflux procedure operation for patients with gastroesophageal reflux refractory to medical management. This procedure involves wrapping the stomach around the base of the esophagus, near the lower esophageal sphincter; this places pressure and narrows the lower esophageal opening to prevent reflux (Figure 17-2). Patients are typically placed on a pureed diet for 2 weeks after this procedure, with small frequent meals, no gulping of liquids, and crushed or liquid medications. After this time solid foods are gradually added to the diet with future avoidance of bread products, nuts, and seeds, because these can become lodged in the lower esophagus and cause an obstruction.

Gastric Surgery

A number of nutrition problems may develop after gastric surgery, depending on the type of surgical procedure and the patient's response. Several indications exist for gastric surgery, including tumor removal, ulcer disease, perforation, hemorrhage, Zollinger-Ellison syndrome, gastric polyposis, and Ménétrier's disease (giant hypertrophic gastritis). A vagotomy is often performed to eliminate gastric acid secretion. Vagotomy at certain levels can alter the normal physiologic function of the stomach, small intestine, pancreas, and biliary system. Total gastric and truncal vagotomy procedures impair proximal and distal motor function of the stomach. Digestion and emptying of solids are retarded, whereas

KEY TERMS

dumping syndrome Constellation of postprandial symptoms that result from rapid emptying of hyperosmolar gastric contents into the duodenum. The hypertonic load in the small intestine promotes reflux of vascular fluid into the bowel lumen, causing a rapid decrease in the circulating blood volume. Rapid symptoms of abdominal cramping, nausea, vomiting, palpitations, sweating, weakness, reduced blood pressure, tremors, and osmotic diarrhea occur. Symptoms of early dumping begin 10 to 30 minutes after eating; late dumping syndrome occurs 1 to 4 hours after a meal. Late dumping is a result of insulin hypersecretion in response to the carbohydrate load dumped into the small intestine. Once the carbohydrate is absorbed, the hyperinsulinemia causes hypoglycemia, which results in vasomotor symptoms such as diaphoresis, weakness, flushing, and palpitations. Individuals who have undergone gastrointestinal (GI) surgery resulting in a reduced or absent gastric pouch are more prone to dumping syndrome.

anastomosis A surgical joining of two ducts to allow flow from one to the other.

sphincter A circular band of muscle fibers that constricts a passage or closes a natural opening in the body (e.g., lower esophageal sphincter, pyloric sphincter).

Zollinger-Ellison syndrome A condition characterized by severe peptic ulceration, gastric hypersecretion, elevated serum gastrin, and gastrinoma of the pancreas or the duodenum. Total gastrectomy may be necessary.

gastric polyposis An abnormal condition characterized by the presence of numerous polyps in the stomach.

Ménétrier's disease (giant hypertrophic gastritis) Rare disease characterized by large folds of nodular gastric rugae that may cover the wall of the stomach, causing anorexia, nausea, vomiting, and abdominal distress.

vagotomy Cutting of certain branches of the vagus nerve, performed with gastric surgery, to reduce the amount of gastric acid secreted and lessen the chance of recurrence of a gastric ulcer.

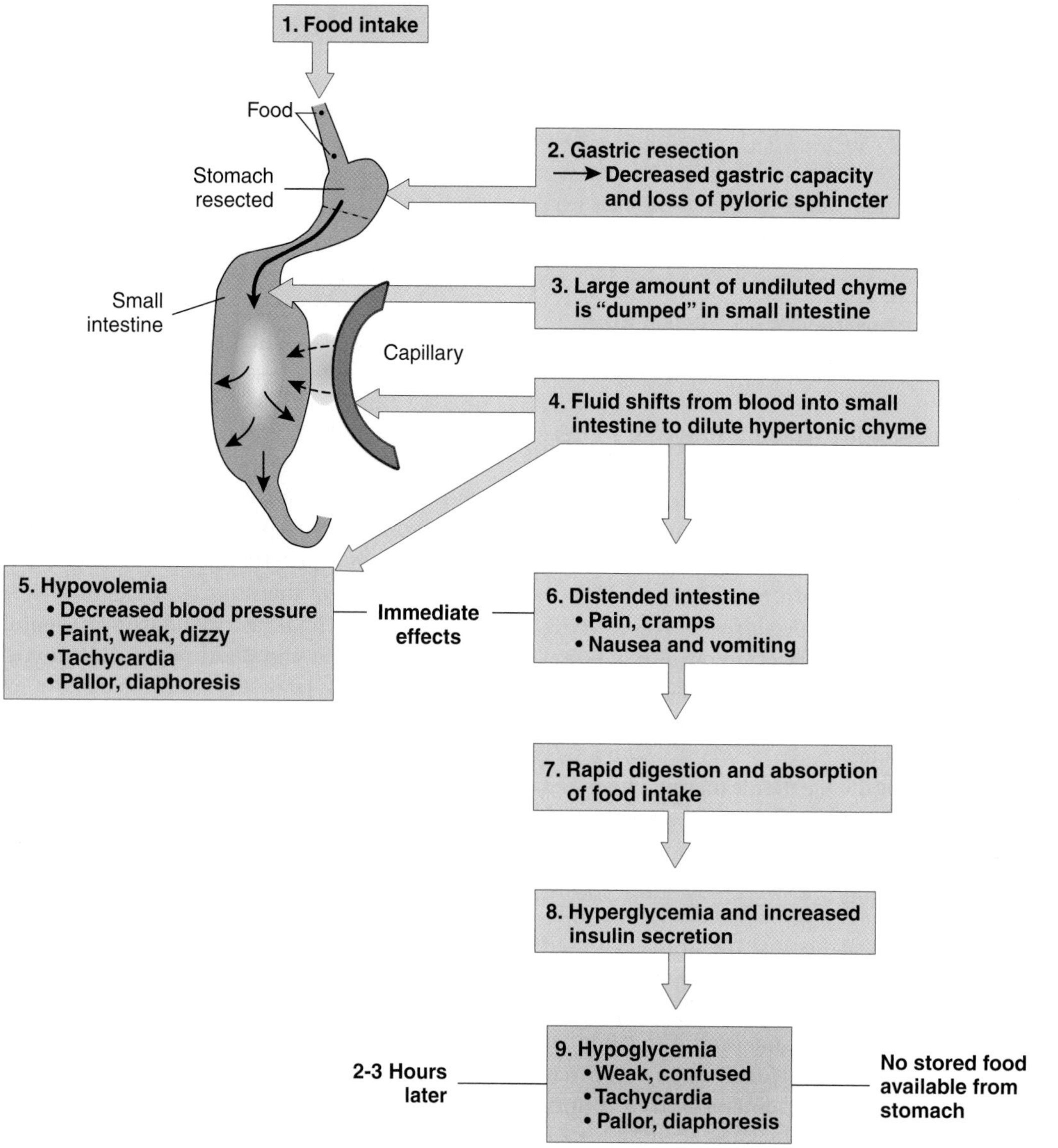

1. Food intake

Food

Stomach resected

Small intestine

Capillary

2. Gastric resection → Decreased gastric capacity and loss of pyloric sphincter

3. Large amount of undiluted chyme is "dumped" in small intestine

4. Fluid shifts from blood into small intestine to dilute hypertonic chyme

5. Hypovolemia
- Decreased blood pressure
- Faint, weak, dizzy
- Tachycardia
- Pallor, diaphoresis

Immediate effects

6. Distended intestine
- Pain, cramps
- Nausea and vomiting

7. Rapid digestion and absorption of food intake

8. Hyperglycemia and increased insulin secretion

2-3 Hours later

9. Hypoglycemia
- Weak, confused
- Tachycardia
- Pallor, diaphoresis

No stored food available from stomach

FIGURE 17-1 Dumping syndrome (postgastrectomy). (From Gould BE: *Pathophysiology for health professions,* ed 2, Philadelphia, 2002, Saunders.)

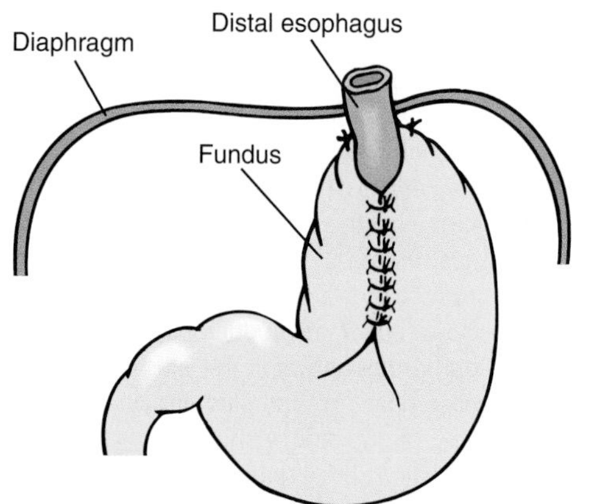

FIGURE 17-2 Nissen fundoplication. (From Lewis SM, Heitkemper MM, Dirksen SR: *Medical-surgical nursing: assessment and management of clinical problems,* ed 5, St Louis, 2000, Mosby.)

emptying of liquids is accelerated.[28] These vagotomy procedures are commonly accompanied by a drainage procedure (antrectomy or pyloroplasty) that helps the stomach to empty. Nutrition complications associated with vagotomy and pyloroplasty include dumping syndrome, steatorrhea, and bacterial overgrowth.

A total gastrectomy involves removal of the entire stomach. A storage reservoir may be created using a section of jejunum. A subtotal or partial gastrectomy involves removal of a portion of the stomach accompanied by a reconstructive procedure. A Billroth I (gastroduodenostomy) involves an anastomosis of the proximal end of the intestine (duodenum) to the distal end of the stomach (Figure 17-3). A Billroth II (gastrojejunostomy) involves an anastomosis of the stomach to the side of the jejunum, which creates a blind loop (Figure 17-4). Any gastric surgery carries some potential for development of malnutrition. Common consequences

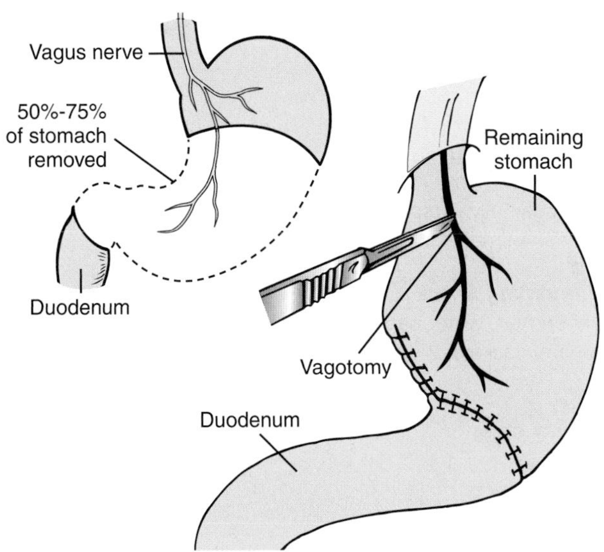

FIGURE 17-3 Billroth I (gastroduodenostomy). (From Lewis SM, Heitkemper MM, Dirksen SR: *Medical-surgical nursing: assessment and management of clinical problems,* ed 5, St Louis, 2000, Mosby.)

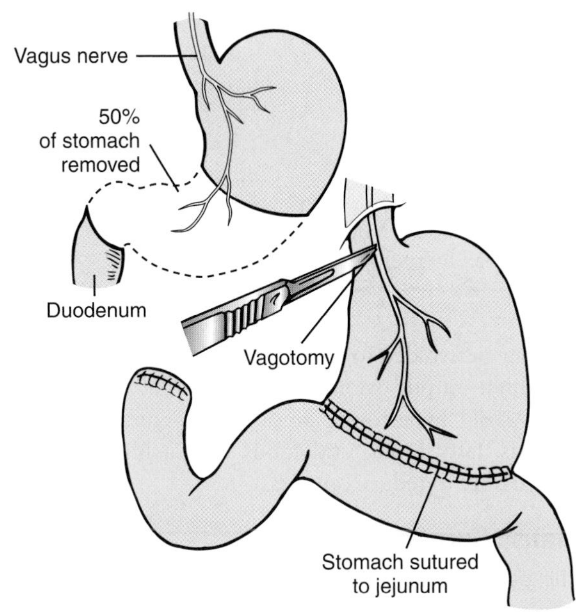

FIGURE 17-4 Billroth II (gastrojejunostomy). (From Lewis SM, Heitkemper MM, Dirksen SR: *Medical-surgical nursing: assessment and management of clinical problems,* ed 5, St Louis, 2000, Mosby.)

include weight loss, dumping syndrome, malabsorption, anemia, and metabolic bone disease. Dumping syndrome, epigastric fullness, nausea, and vomiting often occur in the early postoperative period. These symptoms are managed with dietary modifications and antiemetic medications.[28]

Generally after gastric surgery, small frequent oral feedings are resumed according to the patient's tolerance (Box 17-5). For the first 2 weeks after surgery, soft, bland foods with a low fiber content should be consumed in small portions. Simple sugars, lactose, and fried foods should be avoided; beverages should be consumed at least 30 minutes before and after meals; and foods high in complex carbohydrates and protein should be emphasized. Generally these diet modifications are necessary only for the short term because most patients can resume a regular diet. However, some individuals may need an antidumping diet indefinitely. For individuals who were malnourished preoperatively, a small bowel feeding tube may be placed intraoperatively. Low-rate enteral feedings using a standard formulation may be initiated on postoperative day 1. Tube feedings are adjusted according to the patient's clinical progress and tolerance of an oral diet. Patients may be discharged home with nocturnal tube feedings until their oral diet consumption is optimal. Oral supplements may be provided to increase nutrient intake; however, they need to be isotonic, containing no simple sugars, to avoid dumping. Unfortunately, most oral liquid supplements are hyperosmolar, containing simple sugars, and therefore are not well tolerated after gastric surgery. Parenteral nutrition is indicated only if enteral access is not available and the patient is malnourished and not able to tolerate adequate nutrients orally.

Anemia is a common consequence of gastric surgery. Anemia can be attributed to a deficiency or malabsorption of one or more nutrients, including iron, vitamin B_{12}, and folate. Assimilation of vitamin B_{12} requires liberation of the vitamin from protein and binding of the vitamin to intrinsic factor, both of which occur in the stomach. Failure of either of these reactions to occur results in vitamin B_{12} malabsorption, which with time produces anemia.[28] Total gastrectomy patients require periodic intramuscular vitamin B_{12} injections. Metabolic bone disease can be a late complication of gastric surgery. The cause of metabolic bone disease varies with the surgical procedure. The Billroth II procedure is associated with more complications than the Billroth I, because it bypasses the duodenum and upper jejunum (the site of calcium absorption). Procedures that destroy the pylorus can result in rapid gastric emptying, which may contribute to development of metabolic bone disease. Rapid gastric emptying not only reduces absorption time but also, when fats are malabsorbed, can lead to formation of insoluble calcium soaps.[28] Fat malabsorption can also lead to vitamin D malabsorption, which leads to impaired metabolism of calcium and phosphorus.

Intestinal Surgery

Surgical resections of the small and large intestine are usually well tolerated. If excessive amounts of bowel are removed, then nutritional consequences can arise, depending on the location resected. If more than 50% of the small intestine is removed, then short-bowel syndrome may occur. This syndrome is characterized by severe diarrhea or steatorrhea, malabsorption, and malnutrition, depending on the amount of remaining small intestine, the site of the resection, and the functional status of the remaining GI tract. Often the patient may require long-term parenteral nutrition to maintain his or her nutritional status and fluid and electrolyte balance (see Chapter 19).

BOX 17-5 POSTGASTRECTOMY ANTIDUMPING DIET

Principles of the Diet

After surgery some discomfort or diarrhea may occur. Therefore to reduce the likelihood of those symptoms, a healthy, nutritionally complete diet should be observed. Each person may react to food differently. Foods should be reintroduced into the diet slowly.

Steps of the Diet

1. Intake of complex carbohydrates is unlimited (e.g., bread, vegetables, rice, potatoes).
2. Intake of simple sugars (e.g., sugar, candy, cake, pies, jelly, honey) should be kept to a minimum. Artificial sweeteners may be used.
3. Fat intake should be moderate (30% of total calories).
4. Protein (e.g., meats, legumes) consumption should be unlimited because it helps with wound healing.
5. Milk contains lactose, which may be hard to digest. Introduce milk and milk products slowly several weeks after surgery.
6. Eat small, frequent meals, approximately six meals per day, to avoid loading the stomach.
7. Limit fluids to 4 oz (½ cup) during mealtimes. This prevents the rapid movement of food through the upper gastrointestinal (GI) tract.
8. Drink fluids 30 to 45 minutes before and after eating to prevent diarrhea.
9. Relatively low-roughage foods and raw foods are allowed as tolerated after postoperative day 14.
10. Eat and chew slowly.
11. Avoid extreme temperatures of foods.

Sample Menu

Breakfast

Scrambled egg, 1
Toast, 1 slice
Margarine, 1 tsp
Low-sugar jelly, 1 tsp
Banana, 1 small

Midmorning Snack

Canned fruit, water packed, ½ cup
Graham crackers, 2 squares

Lunch

Bread, 2 slices
Ham, 2 oz
Cheese, 1 oz
Mustard, 2 tsp
Canned fruit, water packed, ½ cup
Yogurt, sugar free, 4 oz

Midafternoon Snack

Saltine crackers, 3 squares
Peanut butter, 1 tbsp

Dinner

Chicken breast, 3 oz
Mashed potatoes, ½ cup
Green beans, ½ cup
Margarine, 2 tsp
Yogurt, sugar free, 4 oz

Evening Snack

Pudding, sugar free, ½ cup
Vanilla wafers, 3 pieces

Pancreaticoduodenectomy (Whipple Procedure)

In cases of ampullary, duodenal, and pancreatic malignancies, a pancreaticoduodenectomy may be performed. This procedure, one of the most difficult and technically demanding in GI surgery, involves resecting the distal stomach, distal common duct, pancreatic head, and duodenum. Three anastomoses—(1) pancreaticojejunostomy, (2) choledochojejunostomy, and (3) gastrojejunostomy (Billroth II)—must be performed. In the past few years a pyloric-sparing Whipple procedure has become more prominent, resulting in a Billroth I anastomosis. This procedure carries fewer postoperative nutritional concerns than the other, which results in a Billroth II anastomosis (Figure 17-5).

Ileostomy and Colostomy

In cases of intestinal lesions, obstruction, or inflammatory bowel disease of the entire colon or when diversion of fecal matter is required, an ileostomy or a colostomy may be the treatment of choice. These procedures involve creation of an artificial anus on the abdominal wall by incision into the colon or ileum and bringing it out to the surface, forming a stoma (Figure 17-6). A pouch is placed externally over the stoma to collect fecal matter. In general, patients with ostomies should eat regular diets. Foods that are gas forming or difficult to digest may be avoided to reduce undesired side effects. In the case of high-output ostomies (>800 mL/day), patients may need to avoid hypertonic, simple sugar–containing liquids and foods, fatty foods, and foods with a high amount of insoluble fiber to reduce outputs.

Bariatric Surgery

In the past several years, surgery for treatment of obesity has become more prevalent. Probably the most common procedure for weight loss in the world is the vertical banded gastroplasty (VBG), or gastric stapling (Figure 17-7, *A*). This technique is performed under general anesthesia and requires about 4 to 5 days in the hospital postoperatively. The VBG procedure limits food intake by creating a small pouch (½ oz) in the upper stomach, with a narrow outlet (½ inch) reinforced by a mesh band to prevent stretching. The pouch fills quickly and empties slowly with solid food, producing a feeling of fullness. Overeating results in pain or vomiting, thus restricting food intake. This procedure is preferred for those people who engage in "bulk" or "binge" eating. The disadvantage of this procedure is that weight loss is not as great as that with other procedures. It does not restrict the intake of high-caloric liquids, and the pouch can stretch with overeating. As a result, 20% of people do not lose weight, and

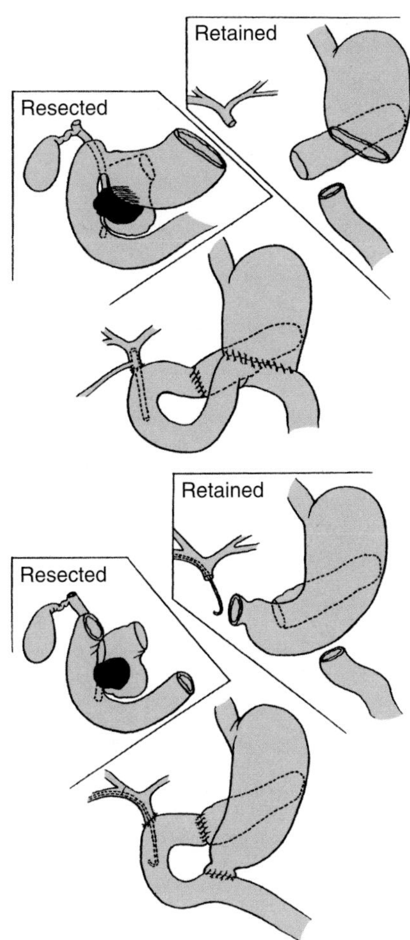

FIGURE 17-5 Whipple procedure. (From Hardy JD, editor: *Hardy's textbook of surgery,* ed 2, Philadelphia, 1988, Lippincott Williams & Wilkins.)

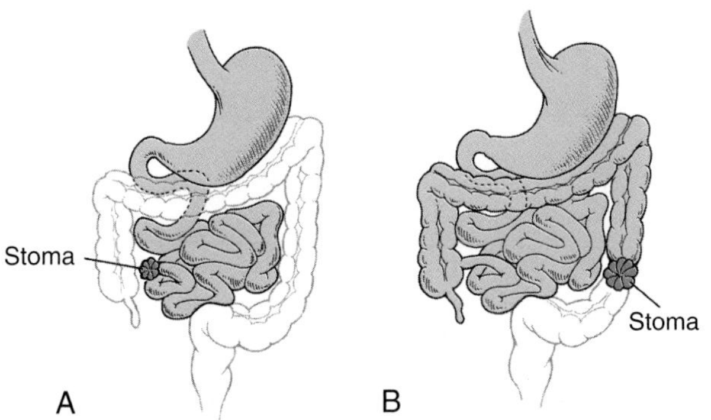

FIGURE 17-6 **A,** Ileostomy. **B,** Colostomy.

only half of people lose at least 50% of their excess weight with a VBG.

The Roux-en-Y gastric bypass (see Figure 17-7, *B*) is a combination of gastric stapling and intestinal bypass. It promotes weight loss by (1) restricting the amount of food a person can ingest by reducing the holding capacity of the stomach and (2) interfering with complete absorption of nutrients by shortening the length of small intestine through which the food travels. Unlike the VBG, this procedure discourages intake of high-calorie sweets by producing nausea, diarrhea, and other unpleasant symptoms. With this procedure a small gastric

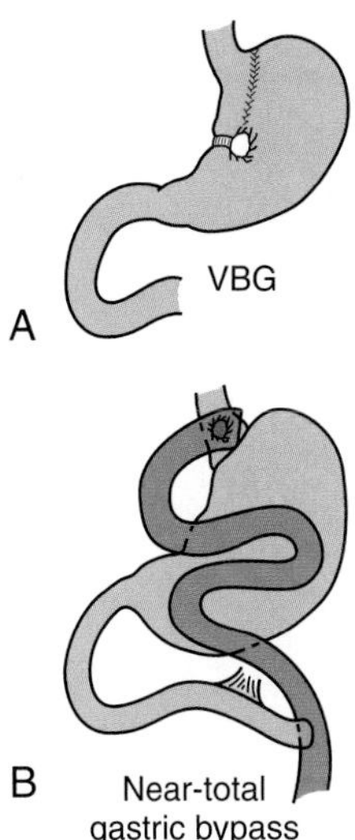

FIGURE 17-7 **A,** Vertical banded gastroplasty (VBG). **B,** Roux-en-Y gastric bypass.

pouch (15 mL) is made near where stomach and esophagus meet. The small pouch and remainder of the stomach are divided from each other with staples. An opening is made in the pouch where a portion of the small intestine is connected. This new connection between the pouch and the small intestine is called *a Roux-en-Y limb.* Food then travels down the esophagus and bypasses nearly all of the stomach and first 2 feet of small intestine. Complications related to gallstones, which tend to form during rapid weight loss, can be prevented by removal of the gallbladder. This procedure is intended for people who "graze" during the day on high-calorie and sugar-containing foods, as well as eating large amounts. Box 17-6 lists a sample meal plan after gastric bypass surgery.

Like any major abdominal operation, these bariatric surgical procedures carry risks such as bleeding, infection, bowel blockage because of scar tissue formation, hernia through the incision, and anesthesia risks. The most serious risk is leakage of fluid from the stomach or intestines resulting in abdominal infection and reoperation. Additional risks are directly related to being obese; these include blood clots in legs or lungs, pneumonia, and cardiac complications. Less immediate risks are ulcers in the stomach or intestine, dumping syndrome, bezoar formation, obstruction of stoma, and malnutrition from too rapid weight loss and loss of vitamins and minerals. Some people (10% to 15%) experience some complications from the gastric bypass; death may occur from complications in 1% to 2% of patients. Because this procedure is not risk free, strict criteria for eligibility should

KEY TERMS

bariatric A term used to describe the field of medicine that focuses on the treatment and control of obesity and diseases associated with obesity.

bezoar A hard ball of hair or vegetable fiber that may develop within the stomach and intestines; can cause an obstruction, requiring removal. Formed because of reduced gastric motility, decreased gastric mixing and churning, and reduced gastric secretions.

BOX 17-6 POSTOPERATIVE DIET FOR GASTRIC BYPASS PROCEDURE FOR MORBID OBESITY

Stage I: clear liquids—Begin once liquids allowed; continue for two to three meals

Stage II: gastric bypass—Begin after clear liquids tolerated; liquids continue for 3 to 4 weeks

Stage III: pureed—Begin after postoperative week 4; continue for 1 to 2 weeks

Stage IV: soft, solids—Begin after postoperative week 6; continue indefinitely

Gastric Bypass Liquids

- Nonfat milk
- Blenderized soups
- 100% Fruit juice (diluted ½ water and ½ juice)
- Vegetable juice (e.g., V8, tomato)
- Sugar-Free Carnation Instant Breakfast powder mixed with nonfat milk
- Grits, oatmeal, cream of wheat, mashed potatoes (thinned down enough that it could go through a straw)
- Nonfat, sugar-free milkshakes
- Thinned baby food
- Sugar-free drinks (e.g., sodas, tea)

Eating Guidelines

- Small meals: each feeding should be 4 oz total (½ cup)
- Six to eight feedings per day to consume adequate nutrients
- An hour between meals and drinking fluids
- Eat slowly/chew food well; each feeding should last at least 30 minutes
- Avoid sugars (i.e., sucrose, honey, corn syrup, fructose) and sugar-containing beverages, foods, and candy
- Low-fat foods only (avoid fried foods, gravies, excessive margarine, butter, high-fat meats, and breads)
- Eat high-protein foods (e.g., milk, yogurt, soft meats, eggs)
- Avoid soft, calorie-dense foods (e.g., ice cream, chocolate, cheese, cookies)
- Avoid obstructive foods (e.g., tough, fibrous red meat; bread made from refined flour; celery; popcorn; nuts; seeds; membranes of citrus fruits)
- Take daily complete multivitamin (liquid or chewable)
- Calcium supplements (1500 mg/day)

Sample Menu (After 8 Weeks)

Breakfast

Banana, ¼ medium
Scrambled egg, 1 egg
Toast, white, ½ slice
Margarine, ½ tsp

Morning Snack

Graham crackers, 2
Pudding, sugar free made with nonfat milk, ½ cup

Lunch

Broiled chicken breast, 2 oz
Carrots, boiled, ¼ cup
Margarine, 1 tsp
Pasta salad, ¼ cup

Afternoon Snack

Canned fruit, water packed, ½ cup

Dinner

Baked or broiled fish, 2 oz
Green beans, ¼ cup
Potato, baked, ½ small
Margarine, ½ tsp

Evening Snack

Cheese, American, 1 oz
Saltine crackers, 2 squares

NOTE: Consume nonfat milk or yogurt between meals, throughout the day. Eat and drink no more than 2 to 3 oz at a time for a daily total of 2 cups.

be made. Generally those who have at least 100 lb excess body weight (or a body mass index [BMI] of ≥40 kg/m^2) and have significant obesity-related medical problems and for whom all other serious attempts at weight reduction have failed may be candidates. A thorough medical and nutritional-behavioral evaluation is necessary to determine eligibility.

Other Related Problems

Enteric Fistulas

Enteric fistulas are abnormal communications between a portion of the intestinal tract and another organ (internal) or between the intestinal tract and the surface of the body (external or enterocutaneous).[28] The most common sites of origin are the pancreas and the large and small intestines. The majority of enteric fistulas result from surgical wound dehiscence or necrosis from bowel ischemia. Inflammatory bowel disease, cancer, trauma, and radiation to the abdomen can also lead to fistula development.

Several metabolic complications can arise as a result of an enteric fistula, including fluid and electrolyte losses, malnutrition, and sepsis. A retrospective analysis of patients with small bowel fistulas found a lower mortality rate, increased spontaneous fistula closures, and increased rate of surgical closures in those receiving parenteral nutrition.[28a] The route of nutrition intervention depends on the location of the fistula. Proximal fistulas may require that a patient be placed on parenteral nutrition if enteral access distal to the fistula cannot be achieved. This is because eating, and thus nutrients in the proximal bowel, stimulates GI secretions, thereby complicating fistula management and the likelihood of spontaneous fistula closure. Fistulas located in the distal bowel, particularly the colon, may have low output (<500 mL/day) and thus allow for oral intake of low-residue or even elemental feedings. High-output fistulas (>500 mL/day) most likely will not close spontaneously and require surgical correction.

TABLE 17-4 EBB AND FLOW PHASES

	EBB PHASE	FLOW PHASE
Hormonal and nonhormonal	↑ Glucagon ↑ Adrenocorticotropic hormone (ACTH)	↑ Counterregulatory hormones (epinephrine, norepinephrine, glucagon, cortisol) ↑ Insulin ↑ Catecholamines ↑ Cytokines (tumor necrosis factor-α [TNF-α], interleukin [IL]-1, -2, and -6)
Metabolic	Circulatory insufficiency, ↑ heart rate (vascular constriction) ↓ Digestive enzyme production ↓ Urine production	Hyperglycemia ↓ Protein synthesis/amino acid efflux ↑ Gluconeogenesis ↑ Glycogenolysis ↑↑ Urea nitrogen excretion/net (−) nitrogen balance
Clinical outcomes	Hemodynamic instability	Fluid and electrolyte imbalances Mild metabolic acidosis ↑ Resting energy expenditure (REE)

Data from Cresci G, Martindale R: Nutrition in critical illness. In Berdanier C, editor: *Handbook of nutrition and food,* Boca Raton, Fla, 2002, CRC Press; Cresci G: Metabolic stress. In Matarese L, Gottschlich M, editors: *Contemporary nutrition support practice,* ed 2, Philadelphia, 2003, Saunders.

Chylous Ascites and Chylothorax

Chylous leaks into the peritoneal and thoracic cavities can follow surgical injury or trauma to the lymphatic ducts and obstruction because of cancer or congenital anomalies. Leakage of chyle into the abdominal or thoracic cavity can cause ascites, pleural effusions, abdominal pain, anorexia, hypoalbuminemia, hyponatremia, hypocalcemia, hypocholesterolemia, and elevated alkaline phosphatase.[28] Chylous leaks may resolve with conservative management, although surgical repair can be required to ligate the duct. Conservative management involves reducing the chyle flow, which is normally 1500 to 5500 mL/day. Dietary intake (fat and fluid), blood pressure, and portal blood flow contribute to the production of chyle. Dietary manipulation is the main means of reducing chyle flow. Because dietary long-chain triglycerides (LCTs) are incorporated into chylomicrons, restriction of these fats in the diet is imperative. Depending on severity of the chyle leak and patient's response, the patient may be allowed oral dietary intake with no LCTs, enteral feeding with no LCTs, or parenteral nutrition. Medium-chain triglycerides (MCTs) are allowed enterally because these are absorbed directly via the portal vein, not the lymphatic system. A diet without or limited to less than 4% of calories as LCTs is not advised for more than 10 to 14 days because it lacks essential fatty acids (linoleic and linolenic acid), causing the patient to develop a deficiency. Resolution of lymphatic leaks conservatively can take up to 6 weeks; therefore adequate nutrition during this period is important to maintain nutritional status.

NUTRITIONAL NEEDS IN THERMAL INJURIES

Patients with trauma and burns exhibit similar metabolic alterations as previously described, but metabolic alterations often occur to a much greater extent. Few traumatic injuries result in a hypermetabolic state comparable to that of a major burn. An understanding of the cause of metabolic response and implications for nutritional requirements is necessary with traumatic and burn injuries for a nutrition care plan to be designed to minimize the effects of hypermetabolism and hypercatabolism, as well as for support immunocompetence to be developed.

Metabolic Response to Injury

Stressed patients undergo several metabolic phases as a series of ebb and flow states reflecting a patient's response to the severity of the stress. The initial ebb phase occurs immediately after injury and is associated with shock. If the injured patient survives, then the ebb phase evolves into the flow phase. Table 17-4 lists hormonal, metabolic, and clinical outcome comparisons between the two phases.

Clinical efforts in the ebb phase are focused on maintaining heart action and blood circulation. The flow state is a hyperdynamic phase in which substrates are mobilized for energy production while increased cellular activity and hormonal stimulation are noted. An energy expenditure distinction exists for each phase, making the goals of nutrition therapy variable depending on the stage in question. During ebb phase a decrease in metabolic needs occurs. Typically, because of hemodynamic instability and need for resuscitation, nutrition intervention is not pursued during this phase. Flow phase brings hypermetabolism, yielding increased proteolysis and nitrogen loss, accelerated gluconeogenesis, hyperglycemia and increased glucose use, and retention of salt and water. Mobilization of protein, fat, and glycogen is believed to be mediated through release of cytokines such as tumor necrosis factor-α (TNF-α); interleukin (IL)-1, -2, and -6; and

KEY TERMS

chyle The fat-containing, creamy white fluid that is formed in the lacteals of the intestine during digestion, is transported through the lymphatics, and enters the venous circulation via the thoracic duct.

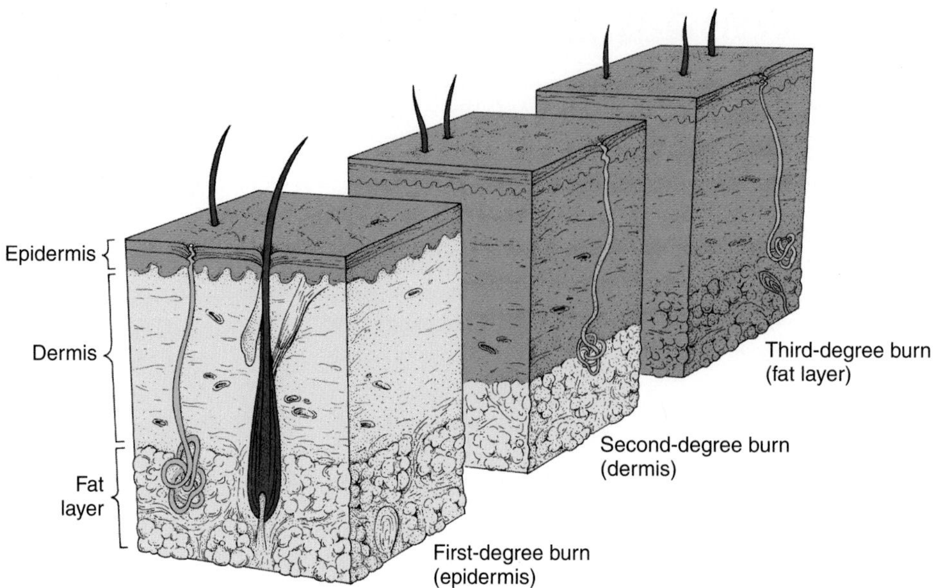

FIGURE 17-8 Depth of skin area involved in burns.

counterregulatory hormones such as epinephrine, norepinephrine, glucagon, and cortisol. Circulating levels of insulin are also elevated in most metabolically stressed patients, but responsiveness of tissues to insulin, especially skeletal muscle, is severely blunted. Researchers believe this relative insulin resistance to be caused by the effects of the counterregulatory hormones. The hormonal milieu normalizes only after the injury or metabolic stress has resolved. As long as the patient is in a hyperdynamic catabolic state, optimal nutrition support is needed but can only at best approach zero nitrogen balance in attempts to minimize further protein wasting.

Burn Wounds

Size and depth of the burn wound affect its healing process and overall prognosis (Figure 17-8). Burns are usually classified by degree using the **rule of nines,** as follows:

1. *First-degree burns:* **erythema** involving cell necrosis above the basal layer of the epidermis
2. *Second-degree burns:* erythema and blistering, and necrosis within the dermis
3. *Third-degree burns:* full-thickness skin loss, including fat layer
4. *Fourth-degree burns:* exposed bone and tendon

Burns of first- and second-degree depths generally reepithelialize without surgical intervention. Third-degree burns will not heal independent of excision and grafting. Fourth-degree burns typically involve the use of muscle flaps because skin grafting onto bone is not a viable therapy option.

Extent of the burn directly affects fluid resuscitation, surgical needs, immunocompetence, metabolic sequelae, and nutrition intervention. Second- and third-degree burns covering 15% to 20% or more of the total body surface area (TBSA), or 10% in children and older adults, usually cause extensive fluid loss and require intravenous fluid and electrolyte replacement therapy. Burns of severe depth covering more than 50% of the TBSA are often fatal, especially in infants and older adults. Thermal injury permits the loss of heat, water, nitrogen, whole proteins, and micronutrients through the open wound. Loss of the protective skin barrier allows microorganisms to access subcutaneous tissue and potentiates systemic infectious processes, contributing to the postburn hypermetabolic state. Loss of plasma volume and electrolytes through the open wound predispose the burned patient to acid-base imbalance and cardiovascular, pulmonary, and renal instability. Adequate fluid and electrolyte resuscitation during the first 24 to 48 hours of postburn hypovolemia is essential for hemodynamic stability. Extensive fluid shifts, unique to burn injury, drive the characteristic edema process of resuscitation by increasing intracellular and interstitial fluid volumes. Fluids given during the resuscitative period should be titrated in accordance with urine output to prevent overresuscitation and underresuscitation. The replacement of extracellular sodium chloride, most commonly in the form of **lactated Ringer's solution,** is obligatory for successful resuscitation.[29]

In addition, certain herbs and botanicals have been suggested for use in patients with thermal injuries. (For an

KEY TERMS

rule of nines Describes the percentage of the body surface represented by various anatomic areas. For example, each upper limb, 9%; each lower limb, 18%; anterior and posterior trunk, each 18%; head and neck, 9%; and perineum and genitalia, 1%.

erythema Redness of the skin produced by coagulation of the capillaries.

lactated Ringer's solution Sterile solution of calcium chloride, potassium chloride, sodium chloride, and sodium lactate in water administered to replenish fluid and electrolytes.

COMPLEMENTARY AND ALTERNATIVE MEDICINE (CAM)

Feel the Burn?

The following herbs and botanical supplements have been suggested for use with thermal injury.

HERB/BOTANICAL AND USE IN BURNS	EFFICACY	SAFETY ISSUES	DRUG INTERACTIONS
Aloe *(Aloe vera)* Aloe is a topical gel used to heal burns and reduce burn pain.	It may help heal abrasions and burns; research indicates aloe significantly delays healing of deep surgical wounds.	It produces an occasional allergic reaction and may lower blood glucose levels. Aloe is considered safe, but comprehensive safety studies are lacking.	None are known. Aloe gel may be a useful adjuvant therapy when combined with hydrocortisone acetate cream. If gel is taken internally, then it can reduce absorption of many medications.
Echinacea *(E. purpurea, E. pallida, E. angustifolia)* Echinacea is used topically to enhance wound healing.	Several research studies have provided evidence that various *Echinacea* species can significantly reduce the duration and severity of illness, but little demonstration of efficacy in wound healing is reported.	Oral echinacea causes few side effects; most common reports include bad taste and minor GI symptoms.	*E. angustifolia* (the most popular species in North America) root might inhibit cytochrome P_{450} 3A4 (CYP3A4).
Garlic (*Allium* spp.) Garlic is used orally and topically to fight infections.	Little research, if any, is available to substantiate this claim.	Garlic is on the FDA's GRAS list. Raw garlic taken in excessive doses can cause numerous symptoms such as stomach upset, heartburn, nausea, vomiting, diarrhea, flatulence, facial flushing, rapid pulse, and insomnia. Topical garlic can cause skin irritation, blistering, even third-degree burns.	When taken with anticoagulants, NSAIDs, antiplatelet agents, or other herbs that exert anticoagulation effects (feverfew, ginkgo), garlic may increase bleeding time. Blood glucose level may be decreased with hypoglycemic agents.
Gotu kola *(Centella asiatica)* Gotu kola is used in Europe as treatment for scarring.	No substantial evidence exists to support this claim.	Rare allergic reactions occur to topical gotu kola.	None are known.
Plantain *(Plantago ovata, P. psyllium, P. lanceolata, P. major)* Plantain is used topically for skin inflammation.	Efficacy has not been validated scientifically.	Plantain is safe; long-term use shows no toxicity.	None are known.
St. John's wort *(Hypericum perforatum)* Hypericum tincture or oil is used topically for inflammation and burns.	It speeds healing of burns.	Noted side effects are related to ingestion of the herb.	Interactions are related to ingestion of the herb.

BIBLIOGRAPHY

Bascom A, Breiner MA, Brigs M, et al: *Professional guide to complementary and alternative therapies*, Springhouse, Pa, 2001, Springhouse.

Bratman S, Girman AM: *Mosby's handbook of herbs and supplements and their therapeutic uses*, St Louis, 2003, Mosby.

Escott-Stump S: *Nutrition and diagnosis-related care*, ed 6, Philadelphia, 2007, Lippincott Williams & Wilkins.

Kuhn MA, Winston D: *Winston and Kuhn's: Herbal therapy and supplements: a scientific and traditional approach*, ed 2, Philadelphia, 2007, Lippincott Williams & Wilkins.

FDA, U.S Food and Drug Administration; *GI,* Gastrointestinal; *GRAS,* generally recognized as safe; *NSAIDs,* nonsteroidal antiinflammatory drug.

outline of these herbs and additional information on their efficacy, safety, and possible interaction with other drugs, see the *Complementary and Alternative Medicine [CAM]* box, "Feel the Burn?")

Nutrition Therapy After Burn Injury

Thermal injury induces hypermetabolism of varying intensity and duration depending on extent and depth of the body surface affected, presence of infection, and efficacy of early treatment. Energy requirements peak at approximately postburn day 12 and typically slowly normalize as the percentage of open wound decreases with reepithelialization or skin grafting.

Energy

Burn patients require individualized nutrition plans to provide optimal energy and protein to accelerate muscle and protein synthesis and minimize proteolysis. Numerous predictive equations are used to estimate energy needs. Several studies have reviewed the accuracy of predictive equations in determining energy requirements in burn patients. Consensus indicates that predictive equations tend to overestimate energy expenditure; therefore the preferred method of determining energy requirements is by using indirect calorimetry. If indirect calorimetry is not available in the clinical situation, then resting energy expenditure (REE) can be estimated at 50% to 60% more than the Harris-Benedict equation for burns of more than 20% of TBSA.[30]

Carbohydrate

During the flow phase of metabolic stress, hyperglycemia is present because of the increased glucagon-to-insulin ratio that activates gluconeogenesis. Tissue insulin resistance further exacerbates glucose intolerance. Despite these metabolic aberrations, carbohydrate should be the primary energy source provided for the burned patient. For burns exceeding 25% TBSA, carbohydrate should compose 60% to 65% of the calories.[29] Patients should be monitored closely for hyperglycemia and glucosuria with exogenous insulin provided to maintain blood glucose levels at less than 180 mg/dL.[6] Complications of hyperglycemia include osmotic diuresis with resulting dehydration and hypovolemia, lipogenesis, fatty liver, and carbon dioxide (CO_2) retention inhibiting ventilatory weaning.

Protein

Trauma, burns, and sepsis initiate a cascade of events that leads to accelerated protein degradation, decreased rates of synthesis of selected proteins, and increased amino acid catabolism and nitrogen loss. Clinical consequences of these metabolic alterations can increase morbidity and mortality rates of patients, causing serious organ dysfunction and impaired host defenses. Therefore trauma and burn patients require increased amounts of protein in attempts to minimize endogenous proteolysis, as well as to support the large losses from wound exudate. Providing 20% to 25% of calories as protein to those with burns of greater than 25% TBSA promotes improved nutrition laboratory values, immunity, nitrogen balance, and survival.[31] Overall recommendations are to provide protein in the amount of 1.5 to 2.0, rarely up to 3.0 g/kg body weight per day in an attempt to minimize protein losses. Providing these increased levels of protein requires continuous monitoring of fluid status, blood urea nitrogen, and serum creatinine because of high renal solute load. In addition to quantity of protein provided, protein quality is also significant. Use of protein of high biologic value is preferred for burn patients. Consumption of whey protein has been recommended more than use of casein because of its beneficial effects on burned children, improvement in tube-feeding tolerance, enhanced solubility at low gastric pH, increased digestibility, and improved nitrogen retention. Pharmacologic doses of the single amino acids arginine and glutamine have also been explored regarding their benefit in critical illness and burns.

Fat

Lipid is an important component of a trauma or burn patient's diet for many reasons; at 9 kcal/g it is an isosmotic concentrated energy source for these patients. Dietary lipid is also a carrier for fat-soluble vitamins, as well as a provider of the essential fatty acids linoleic and linolenic acid. Even though lipids are required in critical illness, excess lipid can be detrimental. Excessive lipid administration has been associated with hyperlipidemia, fatty liver immunosuppression, and impaired clotting ability. For burn and multiple trauma patients, the recommended amount of total fat delivery is 12% to 15% of total calories. A minimum of 4% of calories in the diet should consist of essential fatty acids to prevent deficiencies, which often equates to about 10% of total calories as fat because most sources do not solely contain essential fatty acid. Formulations supplemented with fish oil, a rich source of n-3 fatty acids (eicosapentaenoic acid [EPA] and docosahexaenoic acid [DHA]) and canola oil (α-linolenic acid) are of particular interest for their potential antiinflammatory and immune-enhancing benefits.[30]

Vitamins and Minerals

Micronutrients function as coenzymes and cofactors in metabolic pathways at the cellular level. With increased energy and protein demands associated with traumatic and burn injury, one would also expect an increased need for vitamins and minerals. In addition, increased nutrient losses from open wounds and altered metabolism, absorption, and excretion would also be suspect for requirements beyond that of the Recommended Dietary Allowance (RDA). Various vitamins and minerals have also been found to aid with wound healing, immune function, and other biologic functions. Unfortunately, little concrete data are available to support exact requirements during these hypermetabolic states. However, in addition to a daily multivitamin, burn patients may benefit from additional vitamin A (5000 IU/1000 kcal of enteral nutrition), vitamin C (500 mg twice daily), and zinc (45 mg elemental zinc per day).

Nutrient Delivery

Oral intake is generally adequate in children and adults with burns of less than 25% TBSA and in young children and infants with less than 15% TBSA. Adequate oral intake can be achieved by providing patient food preferences; high-calorie, high-protein supplements; and modular calorie and protein enhancement of foods.[29] However, patients with burns of greater than 25% TBSA often require enteral tube feeding. Gastric feedings are frequently interrupted in burn patients for multiple reasons such as the presence of gastric ileus, dressing changes, physical therapy, prone positioning, respiratory treatments, and surgery. Enteral feeding is well tolerated in burn patients when delivered in the small intestine because the small bowel maintains its absorptive capacity. Therefore a nasoenteric feeding tube is preferred. Small bowel feeding may also reduce incidence of aspiration. Enteral nutrient delivery should be initiated as soon as postinjury allows (during the resuscitative period). Early enteral feedings, within the first 6 hours after the burn, have been shown to decrease the level of catabolic hormones, improve nitrogen balance, maintain gut mucosal integrity, lower the incidence of diarrhea, and decrease hospital stay.[32] A full-strength, intact protein formula at low rate (20 to 30 mL/hr) advanced by 5 to 20 mL/hr to the desired volume is typically tolerated.[29] Parenteral nutrition is indicated only if enteral nutrition is not tolerated or grossly inadequate, because it has been associated with metabolic and immunologic complications.[32] Whenever possible, low-rate enteral feedings should accompany parenteral nutrition to prevent villous atrophy.

HEALTH PROMOTION

IMMUNONUTRITION

It is known that malnutrition leads to suppressed immune responses. Providing nutrition support using standard enteral formulations has shown improvements in various clinical indexes of nutritional status when adequate calories and protein are given; however, a lack of demonstrated effect is seen on morbidity and mortality. During the past 20 years the field of immunology has exploded and expanded into nearly every area of medicine, including nutrition. Certain dietary components have been classified as *immune-enhancing nutrients.* Compared with standard nutrients, an immune-enhancing nutrient is a substance that provides positive effects on the immune system when provided in certain quantities. Of the many immune-enhancing nutrients identified in human clinical trials, the ones that appear to be most beneficial are L-arginine, L-glutamine, nucleotides, omega-3 fatty acids (EPA and DHA), and various vitamins and minerals (zinc and vitamins A, E, and C). Several special enteral nutrient formulations have been categorized as immune-enhancing formulations (IEFs). Each of these formulas contains various combinations or levels (or both) of these immune-enhancing nutrients.[33]

Immune-Enhancing Formulations

Glutamine is known to be a major fuel source for rapidly dividing cells such as enterocytes, reticulocytes, and lymphocytes. In normal metabolic states, glutamine is a nonessential amino acid. However, during times of metabolic stress, glutamine is implicated as being conditionally essential because it is needed for maintenance of gut metabolism, structure, and function. Despite the accelerated skeletal muscle release of amino acids, blood glutamine levels are not increased after burns. In fact, decreased plasma glutamine levels have been reported after severe burn, multiple trauma, or multiple organ failure.[34]

A number of studies have shown beneficial effects with supplemental glutamine, its precursors (ornithine α-ketoglutarate, α-ketoglutarate), or glutamine dipeptides (alanine-glutamine, glycine-glutamine). These studies deliver glutamine in pharmacologic doses of 25% to 35% of the dietary protein. Supplemental glutamine has been shown to have multiple benefits that include increased nitrogen retention and muscle mass, maintenance of the GI mucosa and its permeability, preserved immune function and reduced infections, and preserved organ glutathione levels. These protective effects of glutamine supplementation could have significant effects on morbidity and mortality rates in trauma and burn patients. Safety and cost-effectiveness of glutamine supplementation in trauma and burns continue to be researched.

Arginine, like glutamine, is considered a conditionally essential amino acid. Arginine is the specific precursor for nitric oxide production, as well as a potent secretagogue for anabolic hormones such as insulin, prolactin, and growth hormone. Under normal circumstances, arginine is considered a nonessential amino acid because it is adequately synthesized endogenously via the urea cycle. However, research suggests that during times of metabolic stress, optimal amounts of arginine are not synthesized to promote tissue regeneration or positive nitrogen balance.

Studies in animals and humans have investigated the effects of supplemental arginine in various injury models. Positive outcomes from supplementation include improved nitrogen balance, wound healing, and immune function, as well as increased anabolic hormones (insulin and growth hormone). The outcomes are of special interest in the post-trauma and postburn patient during the flow phase, when enhancement of these processes would yield the greatest advantage. However, despite these positive effects, caution with excessive arginine supplementation is warranted in burn patients because of its potential adverse effects on nitric oxide production.

Even though *lipids* are required, excess lipid can be detrimental. Excessive lipid administration has been associated with hyperlipidemia, fatty liver immunosuppression, and impaired clotting ability. All long-chain fatty acids share the same enzyme systems because they are elongated and desaturated with each pathway competitive in nature based on substrate availability. Dietary fatty acids modulate the phospholipid cell membrane composition and the type and quantities of eicosanoids produced. Prostaglandins of the 3 series (PGE_3) and series 5 leukotrienes have proved to be antiinflammatory and immune-enhancing agents. In addition, PGE_3 is a potent vasodilator. These concepts have received considerable attention for the potential of n-3 fatty acids to enhance immune function and reduce acute and chronic inflammation.

In most standard enteral formulations, the fat source is predominantly n-6 fatty acids, with a portion coming from MCTs. Formulations supplemented with fish oil, a rich source of n-3 fatty acids (EPA and DHA) and canola oil (α-linolenic acid), are available. Clinical trials using these formulations have shown positive benefits in patients with psoriasis, rheumatoid arthritis (RA), burns, sepsis, and trauma. Researchers believe these results are caused by alterations in eicosanoid and leukotriene production, with decreased arachidonic acid metabolites (e.g., PGE_2), as well as increased production of the less biologically active trienoic prostaglandins and pentaenoic leukotrienes.

Clinical Outcomes with Immune-Enhancing Formulas

Trauma Outcomes

IEFs have been used in trauma patients and are associated with decreased incidence of intraabdominal abscess, multiple organ failure, infections, and systemic inflammatory response syndrome (SIRS), as well as decreased hospital length of stay and days of therapeutic antibiotic use.

Intensive Care Unit and Sepsis Outcomes

The intensive care unit population involves a very heterogeneous group, making data interpretation difficult. This population involves differing severity and pathologic processes of various disease states. Studies conducted with this population contain differences in study design and methods of reporting data, adding to the complexity of comparing results between investigations. A few studies have been conducted with various diagnoses, such as cardiac failure, pulmonary failure, transplantation, trauma, and GI surgery. Positive outcomes in the form of decreased incidence of infections, requirement for mechanical ventilation, incidence of bacteremia, and length of stay were reported when using IEFs.

Surgery Outcomes

Research in surgical populations using IEFs has been performed with preoperative, postoperative, or combined nutrition therapies. The majority of procedures performed in these studies involved upper GI cancer or head and neck cancer surgery. Significantly improved outcomes in the IEF groups include fewer infections and wound complications, decreased severity of complications, and shorter postoperative and hospital length of stay.[35]

Other Populations (Burns, Head Injury, Human Immunodeficiency Virus and Acquired Immunodeficiency Syndrome)

Study of the use of IEFs in these patient populations is limited. Currently only two studies investigating the effect of IEFs on immune function and nutritional status of patients with acquired immunodeficiency syndrome (AIDS) have been published. Improved weight gain was found in one of the studies when IEF was provided (but not in the other study).[36] Burn patients appear to benefit when provided with IEFs, exhibiting decreased infections and length of hospital stay. Head injury patients theoretically should benefit from IEFs because of severe hypermetabolism and the likelihood of infectious complications. However, no clinical data are available to support this theory. More research using IEFs in these populations is needed.

TO SUM UP

Nutritional status of the patient should be addressed before the patient is even considered for surgery. If the patient has any nutrient deficiencies, then these should be corrected before surgery if time allows. Postoperatively the patient should be provided with nutrition as soon as feasible to improve surgical outcomes.

Postoperative nutrition may be supplied in a number of ways. The oral route is preferred; however, often it is not feasible or adequate to support metabolic needs. Enteral or parenteral nutrition may be provided for those unable to achieve adequate nutrient intake and absorption orally. Enteral feeding is preferred to parenteral feeding. Because alimentary tract surgery often alters the flow of nutrients, resulting in several potential metabolic and nutrition complications, postoperative diets are described to help minimize these effects.

QUESTIONS FOR REVIEW

1. Discuss requirements for energy, protein, vitamins, and minerals and means of providing them during the various stages of surgery (preoperative, immediately preoperative, postoperative).
2. Describe potential nutritional consequences that may result after surgery of the head and neck, esophagus, stomach, and intestine.
3. Develop a menu plan for a patient undergoing gastric bypass surgery for morbid obesity; include all phases of the diet progression.
4. Describe metabolic alterations that occur during metabolic stress.
5. Develop a nutrition care plan for a patient sustaining third-degree burns covering 40% TBSA.

REFERENCES

1. Klein S, Kinney J, Jeejeebhoy K, et al: Nutrition support in clinical practice: review of published data and recommendations for future research directions, *JPEN J Parenter Enteral Nutr* 21:133, 1997.
2. Vitello J: Prevalence of malnutrition in hospitalized patients remains high, *J Am Coll Nutr* 12:589, 1993.
3. Naber T, Schermer T, De Bree A: Prevalence of malnutrition in nonsurgical hospitalized patients and its association with disease complication, *Am J Clin Nutr* 66:1232, 1997.
4. Coats K, Morgan SL, Bartolucci AA, et al: Hospital-associated malnutrition: a reevaluation 12 years later, *J Am Diet Assoc* 93:27, 1993.

5. Kelly I, Tessier S, Cahill A, et al: Still hungry in hospital: identifying malnutrition in acute hospital admissions, *Q J Med* 93:93, 2000.
6. A.S.P.E.N. Board of Directors: Guidelines for the use of parenteral and enteral nutrition in adult and pediatric patients, *JPEN J Parenter Enteral Nutr* 26:1SA, 2002.
7. VA TPN Cooperative Study: Perioperative total parenteral nutrition in surgical patients, *N Engl J Med* 325:525, 1991.
8. Cerra B, Benitez MR, Blackburn GL, et al: Applied nutrition in ICU patients: a consensus statement of the American College of Chest Physicians, *Chest* 111:769, 1997.
9. Klein C, Stanek G, Willes C: Overfeeding macronutrients to critically ill adults: metabolic complications, *J Am Diet Assoc* 98:795, 1998.
10. Pomposelli JJ, Baxter JK, Babineau TJ, et al: Early postoperative glucose control predicts nosocomial infection rate in diabetic patients, *JPEN J Parenter Enteral Nutr* 22:77, 1998.
11. Pomposelli JJ, Bistrian BR: Is total parenteral nutrition immunosuppressive? *New Horiz* 2:224, 1994.
12. Flancbaum L, Choban PS, Sambucco S, et al: Comparison of indirect calorimetry, the Fick method, and prediction equations in estimating the energy requirements of critically ill patients, *Am J Clin Nutr* 69:461, 1999.
13. Chiolero R, Revelly JP, Tappy L: Energy metabolism in sepsis and injury, *Nutrition* 13(Suppl):45S, 1997.
14. Frankenfield DC, Rowe WA, Smith JS, et al: Validation of several established equations for resting metabolic rate in obese and nonobese people, *J Am Diet Assoc* 103:1152, 2003.
15. Frankenfield DC, Roth-Yousey L, Compher C: Comparison of predictive equations for resting metabolic rate in healthy nonobese and obese adults: a systematic review, *J Am Diet Assoc* 105:775, 2005.
16. Barton RG: Nutrition support in critical illness, *Nutr Clin Pract* 10:129, 1994.
17. Cutts M, Dowdy RP, Ellersieck MR, et al: Predicting energy needs in ventilator-dependent critically ill patients: effect of adjusting weight for edema or adiposity, *Am J Clin Nutr* 66:1250, 1997.
18. Marik P, Varon J: The obese patient in the ICU, *Chest* 113:492, 1998.
19. Ireton-Jones CS, Turner WW Jr, Liepa GU, et al: Equations for estimation of energy expenditures in patients with burns with special reference to ventilatory status, *J Burn Care Rehabil* 13:330, 1992.
20. Patino J, de Pimiento SE, Vergara A, et al: Hypocaloric support in the critically ill, *World J Surg* 23:553, 1999.
21. Cresci GA, Martindale RG: Nutrition support in trauma. In *American Society for Enteral and Parenteral Nutrition: The science and practice of nutrition support: a case-based core*, ed 3, Dubuque, Iowa, 2001, Kendall/Hunt.
21a. Thalacker-Mercer A, Fleet JC, Craig BA, et al: Inadequate protein intake affects skeletal muscle transcript profiles in older humans, *Am J Clin Nutr* 85:1344, 2007.
22. Campbell WW, Crim MC, Dallal GE, et al: Increased protein requirements in elderly people: new data and retrospective reassessments, *Am J Clin Nutr* 60:501, 1994.
22a. Campbell WW, Johnson CA, McCabe GP, et al: Dietary protein requirements of younger and older adults, *Am J Clin Nutr* 88:1322, 2008.
23. Dabrowski G, Rombeau J: Practical nutritional management in the trauma intensive care unit, *Surg Clin North Am* 80:92, 2000.
24. Keele AM, Bray MJ, Emery PW, et al: Two-phase randomized controlled clinical trial of prospective oral dietary supplements in surgical patients, *Gut* 40:343, 1997.
25. Jeffery KM, Harkins JB, Cresci GA, et al: The clear liquid diet is no longer a necessity in the routine postoperative management of surgical patients, *Am Surg* 62:167, 1996.
26. Lipman T: Grains or veins: is enteral nutrition really better than parenteral nutrition? A look at the evidence, *JPEN J Parenter Enteral Nutr* 22:167, 1998.
27. Heyland DK, Novak F, Drover JW, et al: Should immunonutrition become routine in critically ill patients? A systematic review of the evidence, *JAMA* 286:944, 2001.
28. Sullivan M, Alonso E: Gastrointestinal and pancreatic disease. In Matarese L, Gottschlich M, editors: *Contemporary nutrition support practice*, Philadelphia, 1998, Saunders.
28a. Himal HS, Allard JR, Nadeau JE, et al: The importance of adequate nutrition in closure of small intestinal fistulas, *Br J Surg* 61:724, 1974.
29. Mayes T, Gottschlich M: Burns and wound healing. In *American Society for Enteral and Parenteral Nutrition: The science and practice of nutrition support: a case-based core*, ed 3, Dubuque, Iowa, 2001, Kendall/Hunt.
30. Khorram-Sefat R, Behrendt W, Heiden A, et al: Long-term measurements of energy expenditure in severe burn injury, *West J Med Surg* 23:115, 1999.
31. Alexander JW, MacMillan BG, Stinnett JD, et al: Beneficial effects of aggressive protein feeding in severely burned children, *Ann Surg* 192:505, 1980.
32. Rose J, et al: Advances in burn care. In Cameron J, editor: *Advances in surgery*, vol 30, Chicago, 1996, Mosby-Year Book.
33. Hillhouse J: Immune-enhancing enteral formulas: effect on patient outcome, *Support Line* 23:16, 2001.
34. Martindale R, Cresci G: The use of immune enhancing diets in burns, *JPEN J Parenter Enteral Nutr* 25(Suppl):S24, 2001.
35. Sax H: Effect of immune enhancing formulas in general surgery patients, *JPEN J Parenter Enteral Nutr* 25(Suppl): S19, 2001.
36. Schloerb P: Immune-enhancing diets: products, components, and their rationales, *JPEN J Parenter Enteral Nutr* 25(Suppl):S3, 2001.

FURTHER READINGS AND RESOURCES

Readings

Cerra FB: How nutrition intervention changes what getting sick means, *JPEN J Parenter Enteral Nutr* 14(Suppl 5):164, 1990. *[This article provides a good review of three basic factors that influence what is observed at an ill patient's bedside when considering the effects of nutrition intervention: (1) the disease process inherent in the metabolic response to injury, (2) the presence of starvation, and (3) the presence of the nutrition intervention.]*

Hustler DA: Nutritional monitoring of a pediatric burn patient, *Nutr Clin Pract* 6:11, 1991. *[This experienced dietitian-specialist on a burn center team provides a case report of a young boy who sustained mostly full-thickness burns on 56% of his total body surface area (TBSA). She describes in detail the challenge of initial evaluation and therapy, constant close monitoring, and appropriate responses to changing needs.]*

Tynes JJ, Austhof SI, Chima CS, et al: Diet tolerance and stool frequency in patients with ileoanal reservoirs, *J Am Diet Assoc* 92(7):861, 1992. *[This brief report of a survey of patients with ileoanal reservoirs provides helpful background information about this recently developed alternative surgical procedure to the ileostomy, with practical guidance for nutritional management and patient counseling.]*

Websites of Interest

American Academy of Physical Medicine and Rehabilitation. Website of the only organization exclusively serving the specialty of physicians who specialize in physical medicine and rehabilitation: www.aapmr.org.

American Botanical Council. An independent, not-for-profit research and education organization dedicated to providing accurate and reliable information for consumers, healthcare practitioners, researchers, educators, industry, and the media: www.herbalgram.org.

National for Complementary and Alternative Medicine. Lead agency of the U.S. Government for scientific research on diverse medial and health care systems, practices, and products not generally considered part of conventional medicine: www.nccam.nih.gov/.

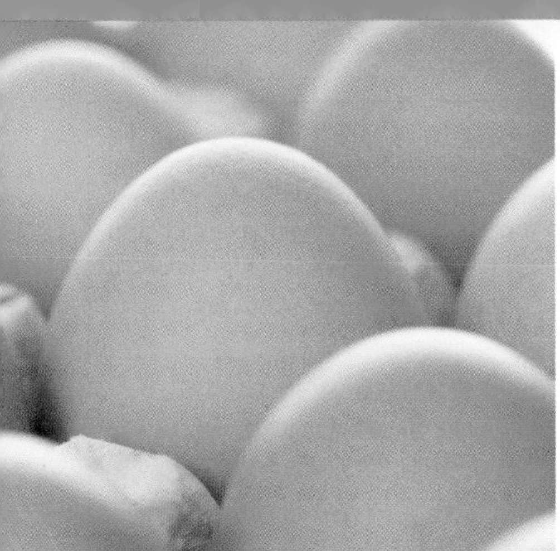

18

Drug-Nutrient Interactions

Sara Long Roth

evolve WEBSITE

http://evolve.elsevier.com/Williams/essentials/

OUTLINE

In this chapter, continuing our clinical nutrition sequence, we look briefly at some main effects of combining food and nutrients with drugs. We will see how these interactions affect nutrition therapy.

Today consumers are generally better informed about drug misuse. However, many are dangerously uninformed or misinformed about the specific drugs they may be taking, especially in relation to the food they eat.

All members of the health care team must have knowledge of drug actions and nutrition to make the wisest and most effective use of drugs and nutrition therapy. Here we examine some of these drug-nutrient effects and how these interactions affect nutrition therapy and education.

DRUG-NUTRIENT PROBLEMS IN MODERN MEDICINE

Problem Significance: Causes, Extent, and Effects

Medications and food can work together in various manners. Various nutrients interfere with the medication's absorption and efficacy. In addition, medications can disturb ingestion, digestion, and absorption of nutrients. During this century, unprecedented medical progress has resulted in decreased childhood mortality rates and increased life expectancy. As we live longer, incidence of chronic diseases such as cardiovascular disease, type 2 diabetes mellitus, hypertension, and arthritis will continue to increase, often in comorbid manner. Furthermore, treatment of these and other chronic diseases often involves long-term use of medications, often resulting in polypharmacy, in addition to alternative and herbal therapies (see the *Focus on Culture* box, "Are We Speaking the Same Language?").[1] To this we can then add the large volume of nonprescription drugs that Americans purchase without a physician's guidance (Figure 18-1).

Drug Use and Nutritional Status

Drug Administration

Drugs are administered several different ways. Administration route depends on chemical properties of the drug, desired effect, and patient characteristics that affect administration of the drug. Drug administration routes are described in Table 18-1.

Older Adults at Risk

All of us, at any age, risk harmful drug-drug or drug-nutrient interactions. However, older adults are particularly vulnerable, and this will only become more serious. Today, adults older than age 65 represent approximately 14% of the U.S. population. It is projected this number will increase to 20% to 22% by 2050.[2] Older adults take a much larger percentage of prescription and nonprescription medications than their younger counterparts (Figure 18-2). Several factors contribute to an increased risk among older adults, including the following[3]:

- They are likely to be taking more drugs for longer periods to control chronic diseases.
- Their drugs are likely to be more toxic.
- They respond to drugs with increased variability.
- They have less capability of handling drugs efficiently.
- Their nutritional status is more likely to be deficient.

FOCUS ON CULTURE

Are We Speaking the Same Language?

Consider the following prescription label directions written half in English and half in Spanish:

Aplicarse once cada dia til rash is clear.

What does it mean to you? If you do not read Spanish, then it probably does not mean much (although you can pick out the words *once* and *til rash is clear*). In addition, if you study this phrase hard enough, then you might figure out it says something about using the medication once a day until the rash is gone.

If you read Spanish, then the meaning may be entirely different. *Once* means eleven in Spanish. If this is a mild topical medication, then perhaps no permanent harm would result if you used it 11 times a day. However, if this is an oral medication, then the results could be fatal.

Many people using prescription or over-the-counter (OTC) medications, herbal products, or vitamin and mineral supplements use a language other than English as their primary language. Foreign-born individuals make up 11% of the U.S. population. The majority of immigrants are of Hispanic origin. Although many members of these groups have good reading and writing skills in their native languages, they do not possess the same skills in English. How then are they supposed to read and understand directions regarding how to take medications or supplements? How can they adhere to a prescribed medical regimen if they are unable to read the label? This language barrier may make the individuals more susceptible to food-drug interactions.

Another barrier to health is literacy. More than 40% of patients with chronic illnesses are functionally illiterate. Almost 25% of all adult Americans read at or below a fifth-grade level, whereas medical information is typically written at a tenth-grade level or greater. The National Adult Literacy Survey (NALS) found almost 25% of patients with inadequate functional health literacy did not know how to take medications.

Limited health literacy and language barriers have many consequences. Patients who do not understand prescription directions and instructions for preventative care and self-care may make the following mistakes:

- Incorrect doses (e.g., improper infant formula preparation and feeding)
- Incorrect schedules of administration (e.g., four times a day versus four pills at one time)
- Incorrect routes of administration (e.g., teens who have misunderstood directions for contraceptive jelly and have eaten it on toast every morning to prevent pregnancy)

Low health literacy risk groups include pediatric patients, older adult patients, and patients with language barriers. Pediatric patients are at increased risk of incorrect doses. Older adult patients take multiple medications, which increases risk for errors. In addition, patients older than age 60 may have hearing loss, memory loss, short attention span, and low energy levels, thus exacerbating the problems. Patients who speak English as their second language are vulnerable to misinterpretation of information.

Following are some solutions to this problem:

- Provide written materials in several languages and at a fifth-grade reading level or lower.
- Offer small amounts of information at a time.
- Avoid using "medical speak" (medical terms that are used every day in the clinical setting but are unfamiliar to patients).
- Employ a multilingual staff.
- Have patients repeat instruction to ensure the message was received and understood.
- Use identifiers such as time-of-day references (e.g., "Take one tablet in the morning when you wake up and the second tablet at bedtime.").
- Use visual images when possible.

BIBLIOGRAPHY

Hardin LR: Frontline pharmacist: counseling patients with low health literacy, *Am J Health Syst Pharm* 62:364, 2005.

Institute for Safe Medication Practices: *Hospitals need to take action now to reduce threat of medication errors with magnesium sulfate, ISMP Medication Safety Alert!*, March 12, Horsham, PA, 1997, Retrieved April 11, 2009, from www.ismp.org/MSAarticles/calendar/Mar97.html.

Institute for Safe Medication Practices: *To promote understanding, assume every patient has a health literacy problem, ISMP Medication Safety Alert!* October 31, 2001. Retrieved April 11, 2009, from www.ismp.org/MSAarticles/calendar/Oct01.html#Oct31, 2001.

Literacy Partners of Manitoba: *Literacy and health resources*, Manitoba, Canada, 2005, Literacy Partners of Manitoba. Retrieved April 11, 2009, from www.health.mb.literacy.ca/health.htm.

National Institute for Literacy: *Literacy fact sheets: scope of the literacy need*, Washington, DC, 2001, National Institute for Literacy. Retrieved July 1, 2010, from http://factfinder.census.gov/servlet/DatasetMainPageServlet?_program=ACS&_submenuid=&_lang=en&_ts=%29Available at www.nifl.gov.

Census Bureau US: *Profile of selected social characteristics: 2000, Census 2000 supplementary survey summary tables*, Washington, DC, 2001, U.S. Government Printing Office.

Wallendorf M: Literally literacy, *J Consum Res* 27:505, 2001.

- They are more likely to make increased errors in self-care because of illness, mental confusion, or lack of drug information.

As a result of these problems, concerned physicians, nutritionists, pharmacists, and nurses are increasingly working together as a team to provide drug and nutrition education and therapy on a more sound basis. A number of drug-nutrient interactions demand this type of teamwork in patient care.[1]

Nutritional Status

Poor nutritional status can have a major effect on risk for complications of drug-nutrient reactions. Nutrient-drug mechanisms that influence nutritional status include those affecting the following:

- Stimulated or suppressed appetite
- Decreased intestinal absorption
- Increased renal excretion

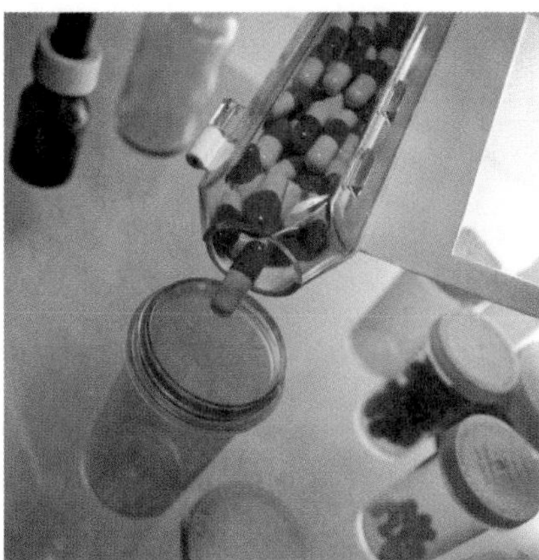

FIGURE 18-1 Prescription and nonprescription drugs have become part of American life. (Copyright 2006 JupiterImages Corporation.)

TABLE 18-1 DRUG ADMINISTRATION ROUTES

ADMINISTRATION ROUTE	CHARACTERISTICS
Oral	Requires ability to swallow and absorb the medication
Sublingual	Medication placed under tongue to dissolve; absorbed quickly across mucous membrane
Buccal	Medication placed in cheek to dissolve; absorbed quickly across mucous membrane
Parenteral	Injection in circulatory system
Subcutaneous (SC)	Injection under the skin
Intradermal (ID)	Injection under outermost layer of skin
Intramuscular (IM)	Injection into muscle
Intraperitoneal (IP)	Injection into peritoneal cavity
Intravenous (IV)	Injection into a vein
Topical	Applied to skin
Inhalation	Medication breathed into respiratory system
Ophthalmic	Placement of medication into eye
Otic	Placement of medication into ear
Epidural	Placement of medication into spinal fluid
Intrathecal	Placement of medication into membrane surrounding central nervous system (CNS)

Adapted from Nelms M: Pharmacology. In Nelms MN, Sucher K, Long S: *Understanding nutrition therapy and pathophysiology,* Belmont, Calif, 2007, Wadsworth.

- Competition or displacement of nutrients for carrier protein sites
- Interference with synthesis of necessary enzyme, coenzyme, or carrier
- Hormonal effects on genetic systems

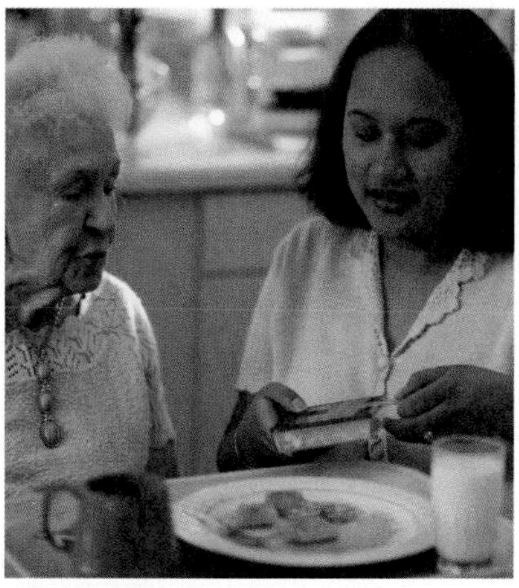

FIGURE 18-2 Older adults make up a large percentage of those taking prescription and nonprescription medications in the United States.

- Drug delivery system
- Components in drug formulation

In general, drugs are grouped according to primary action. Following we review the various effects of drugs on food and nutrients and the effects of food and nutrients on drugs. In each case we give some examples for your reference in patient care.

DRUG EFFECTS ON FOOD AND NUTRIENTS

Drug Effects on Food Intake

Appetite Changes

The following drugs may stimulate appetite, weight gain, or both[4]:

- *Antihistamines:* These drugs can lead to marked increase in appetite and subsequent weight gain. Cyproheptadine hydrochloride (Periactin) is an antihistamine also used as an appetite stimulant.
- *Antianxiety drugs:* Some drugs in this classification may lead to hyperphagia, or excessive eating. Some of these drugs include chlordiazepoxide hydrochloride (Librium), diazepam (Valium), and alprazolam (Xanax).
- *Tricyclic antidepressants:* Tricyclic antidepressants and most antipsychotic drugs such as amitriptyline hydrochloride (Elavil), olanzapine (Zyprexa), chlorpromazine hydrochloride (Thorazine), and clozapine (Clozaril) may promote appetite and lead to significant weight gain.
- *Insulin:* Hypoglycemia can occur in persons with type 1 diabetes if food is not taken immediately after their insulin injection (see Chapter 22). If some food is not readily available to counteract the rapid progression of the unrelieved severe hypoglycemia, then coma and death occur. If excess food is consumed to avoid or treat hypoglycemia, then weight gain may occur.
- *Steroids:* Anabolic steroids, including testosterone, promote nitrogen retention, increased lean body mass, and subsequent weight gain.

CASE STUDY

Drug-Herb Interaction

Ivanna is a 20-year-old exchange student from Germany. She lives with three roommates and is in her junior year at the local university. Ivanna is seeking medical attention at the urging of her roommates, who report her mood has become increasingly depressed during the past two semesters. She has become withdrawn and moody but is otherwise a healthy young woman. She is 5 feet, 11 inches tall and weighs 160 lb on admission.

Ivanna reports a 5-lb weight loss in the past 3 months. She takes oral contraceptives, smokes ½ pack of cigarettes per day, and drinks four to five beers on the weekends. Her mother has been treated for depression with St. John's wort by the family physician in Germany for the past 10 years. Her admitting diagnosis is depression. Physician's orders are as follows: Zoloft, 50 mg every day, referral to house psychologist for counseling, and nutrition consult for her poor eating habits.

Questions for Analysis

1. Ivanna's physician ordered Zoloft to treat her depression. Zoloft is a selective serotonin reuptake inhibitor (SSRI). Are there any pertinent nutritional considerations when using this medicine?
2. How do SSRIs work?
3. During the diet history, you ask Ivanna if she uses any over-the-counter (OTC) vitamins, minerals, or herbal supplements. She tells you her mother suggested she try *Hypericum perforatum* (St. John's wort) because in Germany it is prescribed to treat depression. Ivanna did as her mother suggested, because it is available without prescription in the United States. What is St. John's wort?
4. How is St. John's wort used in the United States?
5. How does St. John's wort work as an antidepressant?
6. Does St. John's wort have any side effects?
7. How is St. John's wort regulated in the United States? How is it used in Europe?
8. What is your immediate concern regarding Ivanna's use of St. John's wort?

Modified from Nelms MN, Long S, Lacey K: *Medical nutrition therapy: a case study approach*, ed 3, Belmont, Calif, 2008, Wadsworth.

The following drugs may depress appetite[4]:

- *Selective serotonin reuptake inhibitor (SSRI):* This class of antidepressants may cause anorexia and weight loss; an example is fluoxetine (Prozac). (See the *Case Study* box, "Drug-Herb Interaction," for an application of the use of SSRIs.)
- *Amphetamines:* These drugs act as stimulants to the central nervous system (CNS) and have the effect of depressing the desire for food, thus leading to marked loss of weight. For this reason, they have been used in the past as appetite-depressant drugs in the treatment of obesity. However, long-term use of these drugs for such treatment has caused problems, such as addiction. For this reason, amphetamines are rarely used now for this purpose. Children taking amphetamines show dose-dependent growth retardation.
- *Alcohol:* Abuse of alcohol can lead to loss of appetite, reduced food intake, and malnutrition. The anorexia, or loss of appetite, can stem from various effects of alcoholism such as gastritis, hepatitis, cirrhosis, ketosis, pancreatitis, alcoholic brain syndrome, drunkenness, and withdrawal symptoms. The resulting reduced food intake can then lead to malnutrition, which further complicates the anorexia.

PERSPECTIVES IN PRACTICE

Counseling Patients About Potential Food-Medication Interactions

- Provision of relevant medication information: drug name, drug indications, duration of therapy
- Information detailing how to take the medication
- Probable side effects and dietary suggestions to lessen symptoms
- Nutritional difficulties that may develop, particularly if dietary intake is poor
- Dietary alteration that may change drug action
- Food and beverages to avoid or consume in moderation while taking the medication
- Implications of alcohol ingestion
- Potential for interactions involving medications and vitamin and mineral supplements (or other food supplements)
- Significance of staying on a special diet prescription for treatment of medical condition
- Individualization of dietary prescription to that person only
- Consultation with prescribing physician before modifying drug or diet prescription
- Consultation with a registered dietitian (RD) for in-depth nutrition information
- Consultation with a registered pharmacist (RPh) for questions regarding drug action or possible side effects

Adapted from Pronsky ZM: *Food medication interactions,* ed 15, Birchrunville, Penn, 2008, Food Medication Interactions.

Taste and Smell Changes

Drugs such as the tricyclic antidepressant amitriptyline (Elavil) may impair salivary flow, causing dry mouth along with a sour or metallic taste.[4] The antibiotic clarithromycin (Biaxin) is secreted into saliva, causing a bitter taste.[4] Antibiotics such as tetracycline may suppress natural oral bacteria, resulting in oral yeast overgrowth or candidiasis. Metronidazole (Flagyl), an antibiotic, may cause *dysgeusia* (abnormal or impaired sense of taste) by causing a metallic taste in the mouth.[4] Antineoplastic medications (cisplatin or methotrexate) may damage rapidly growing cells, causing stomatitis, glossitis, or esophagitis (or a combination of these problems)[4] (see the *Perspectives in Practice* box, "Counseling Patients About Potential Food-Medication Interactions").

Gastrointestinal Effects

Many drugs can affect the stomach and cause nausea, vomiting, bleeding, or ulceration; intestinal peristalsis; or changes in intestinal flora. Nonsteroidal antiinflammatory drugs (NSAIDs) such as aspirin (acetylsalicylic acid [ASA]), ibuprofen (Advil, Motrin), and naproxen (Aleve, Anaprox) cause stomach irritation.[4] Sometimes the irritation is so severe as to cause sudden and serious gastric bleeding.[4] Anticholinergic medications (antipsychotics, antidepressants, antihistamines) slow peristalsis, resulting in constipation. Ciprofloxacin (Cipro) is an antibiotic that can allow for the overgrowth of *Clostridium difficile,* resulting in pseudomembranous colitis.[4]

Drug Effects on Nutrient Absorption and Metabolism

Nutrient Absorption

A number of drugs can increase nutrient absorption and thus benefit nutritional status. For example, cimetidine (Tagamet), a gastric antisecretory agent, helps patients with bowel resection in several ways.[4] The drug reduces gastric acid and volume output; it also lowers duodenal acid load and volume and reduces jejunal flow.[4] It maintains pH of secretions and decreases fecal fat, nitrogen, and volume, thus improving absorption of macronutrients.[4] This drug is therefore helpful in the treatment of various gastrointestinal (GI) disorders, including peptic ulcer disease (see Chapter 20).[4] On the other hand, prolonged use of cimetidine may cause decreased absorption of vitamin B_{12}, thiamin, and iron.[4]

A number of drugs can contribute to primary malabsorption. Questran (antihyperlipidemic, bile acid sequestrant [cholestyramine]) binds vitamins A, D, E, and K in the GI tract, preventing absorption of these nutrients.[4] Colchicine, a drug used in the treatment of gout, leads to vitamin B_{12} deficiency, causing megaloblastic anemia.[4] Alcohol abuse can provoke malabsorption of thiamin and folic acid, causing peripheral neuritis and anemia.[4] Laxatives can produce severe malabsorption, leading to conditions such as osteomalacia.[4]

Secondary malabsorption may also be drug induced. For example, the antibiotic neomycin causes tissue changes in the intestinal villi, precipitates bile salts, prevents fat breakdown by inhibiting pancreatic lipase, and decreases bile acid absorption.[4] These effects can lead to steatorrhea and failure to absorb the fat-soluble vitamins A, D, E, and K.[4] Malabsorption of vitamin D in turn leads to a calcium deficiency. Other drugs cause malabsorption of folic acid or impair its use. Methotrexate, for example, used in cancer chemotherapy, is a folic acid antagonist that impairs the intestinal absorption of calcium.[4] Summaries of medications affecting food and nutrients can be found in Table 18-2.

Mineral Depletion

Certain drugs can lead to mineral depletion through induced GI losses or renal excretion[5]:

- *Diuretics:* Diuretic drugs are intentionally used to reduce levels of excess tissue water and sodium, but they may also result in loss of other minerals, such as potassium, magnesium, and zinc. Potassium deficiency brings weakness, anorexia, nausea, vomiting, listlessness, apprehension, and sometimes diffuse pain, drowsiness, stupor, and irrational behavior. On the contrary, potassium-retaining diuretics such as spironolactone, as well as overuse of potassium supplementation, may cause the opposite effect of hyperkalemia.
- *Chelating agents:* Penicillamine attaches to metals and can lead to the deficiency of such key trace elements as zinc and copper.
- *Alcohol:* Abuse of alcohol can lead to diminished levels of potassium, magnesium, and zinc.
- *Antacids:* These commonly used OTC medications are of concern because they can produce phosphate deficiency, with symptoms of anorexia, malaise, paresthesia, profound muscle weakness, and convulsions, as well as calcification of soft tissues from the prolonged hypercalcemia.
- *Aspirin:* Salicylates such as ASA (aspirin) can induce iron deficiency by causing low-level blood loss from erosions in the stomach or intestinal tissue when taken incorrectly (see Health Promotion section for discussion).

Vitamin Depletion

Certain drugs act as metabolic antagonists and can cause deficiencies of the vitamins involved:

- *Vitamin antagonists:* Various drugs have been used successfully to treat disease because they are antagonists of certain vitamins and thus can control key metabolic reactions in which that vitamin is involved. For example, warfarin (Coumadin) anticoagulants inhibit regeneration of vitamin K, which is necessary for blood clotting. In addition, some cancer chemotherapy drugs such as methotrexate have multiple antagonist effects on folate metabolism, thus inhibiting the synthesis of cell reproduction substances—deoxyribonucleic acid (DNA) and ribonucleic acid (RNA)—and protein. In a similar manner, the antimalaria drug pyrimethamine inhibits the action of folate in protein synthesis.

Special Adverse Reactions

Several reactions are related to specific drug interactions with particular nutrients, as follows:

- *Monoamine oxidase inhibitors (MAOIs):* These antidepressant drugs can increase the vascular effect of simple vasoactive amines, such as tyramine and dopamine, from food.[5] The resulting tyramine syndrome is marked by headache, pallor, nausea, and restlessness. With increased absorption, symptoms may escalate to apprehension, sweating, palpitations, chest pain, fever, and increased blood pressure, at times, although rarely, to the extent of hypertensive crisis and stroke.

KEY TERMS

paresthesia Abnormal sensations such as prickling, burning, and crawling of skin.

vasoactive Having an effect on the diameter of blood vessels.

TABLE 18-2 MEDICATIONS AFFECTING FOOD AND NUTRIENTS

DRUG CLASS	EXAMPLES	ACTION	NUTRIENTS AFFECTED	HOW TO AVOID
Alcohol, particularly excessive use	Beer, wine, spirits	Increases turnover of some vitamins; substitution of alcohol for food	Vitamin B_{12}, folate, and magnesium	Limit alcohol consumption to <2 drinks per day for men, <1 drink per day for women
Analgesic, NSAID, and antiinflammatory agents	Salicylates (aspirin), ibuprofen (Motrin, Advil), naproxen (Anaprox, Aleve, Naprosyn), acetaminophen (Tylenol)	Increases loss of vitamin C and competes with folate and vitamin K	Vitamin C, folate, vitamin K	Increase intake of foods high in vitamin C, folate, and vitamin K; take with 8 oz water
Antacid agents	Aluminum antacids, H_2 blockers	Inactivates thiamin; decreases absorption of some nutrients	Thiamin B_1	Foods containing thiamin (B_1) should be consumed at a different time; depends on antacid; possibly magnesium, phosphorus, iron, vitamin A, and folate Take antacid after meals; take iron, magnesium, or folate supplements separately by 2 hours; take separately from citrus fruit or juices or calcium citrate by 3 hours
Antiulcer agents (histamine blockers)	Ranitidine (Zantac), Cimetidine (Tagamet), famotidine (Pepcid)	Decreases vitamin absorption	Vitamin B_{12}	Consult physician or RD regarding vitamin B_{12} supplementation
Antibiotic agents	Tetracycline, Ciprofloxacin (Cipro)	Chelation of minerals; ingestion with caffeine may increase excitability and nervousness	Calcium, magnesium, iron, and zinc; caffeine	Take tetracycline at least 1 hr before or 2 hr after a meal; do not take with caffeine-containing products
Antineoplastic agents	Methotrexate	Causes mucosal damage, which may cause decreased nutrient absorption	Folate and vitamin B_{12}, (also see *Antibiotics*)	Consult physician or RD regarding supplementation
Anticholinergic agents	Amitriptyline (Elavil), chlorpromazine (Thorazine)	Saliva thickens and loses ability to prevent tooth decay	Fluids	Increase intake of fluids
Anticonvulsant agents	Phenobarbital, phenytoin (Dilantin)	Increases metabolism of folate (possibly leading to megaloblastic anemia), vitamin D (especially in children), and vitamin K	Folate, vitamin D, and vitamin K	Increase folate, vitamins D and K intake

Antidepressant agents	Lithium carbonate, Lithane, Lithobid, Lithonate, Lithotabs, Eskalith	May cause metallic taste, nausea, vomiting, dry mouth, anorexia, weight gain, and increased thirst	Fluids	Drink 2-3 L of water per day and take with food, consistent sodium intake
Antihyperlipidemic agents	Cholestyramine (Questran), colestipol (Colestid)	Binds bile salts and nutrients	Fat-soluble vitamins (A, D, E, K), folate, vitamin B_{12}, and iron	Include rich sources of these vitamins and minerals in diet
Antituberculosis agents	Isoniazid (INH)	Inhibits conversion of vitamin B_6 to active form	Vitamin B_6	Vitamin B_6 supplementation is necessary to prevent deficiency and peripheral neuropathy
Corticosteroid agents	Prednisone, Solu-Medrol, hydrocortisone	Increases excretion	Protein, potassium, calcium, magnesium, zinc, vitamin C, and vitamin B_6	Increase intake of foods high in protein, potassium, calcium, magnesium, zinc, vitamin C, and vitamin B_6
Loop diuretic agents	Furosemide (Lasix)	Increases mineral excretion in urine	Potassium, calcium, magnesium, zinc, sodium, and chloride	Include fresh fruits and vegetables in diet
Thiazide diuretic agents	Hydrochlorothiazide (HCTZ)	Increases excretion of most electrolytes, but enhances reabsorption of calcium	Potassium, calcium, magnesium, zinc, sodium, chloride, and calcium	Increase intake of foods high in potassium, calcium, magnesium, zinc, sodium, chloride, and calcium
Potassium-sparing diuretic agents	Triamterene (Dyrenium)	Hyperkalemia	Potassium	Avoid potassium-based salt substitutes
Laxative agents	Fibercon, Mitrolan	Decreases nutrient absorption	Vitamins and minerals	Consult physician or RD regarding supplementation
Sedative agents	Barbiturates	Increases metabolism of vitamins	Folate, vitamin D, vitamin B_{12}, thiamin, and vitamin C	Increase intake of foods high in folate, vitamin D, vitamin B_{12}, thiamin, and vitamin C
Mineral oil	Agoral Plain	Decreases absorption	Fat-soluble vitamins (A, D, E, K), β-carotene, calcium, phosphorus, and potassium	Take 2 hr apart from food and fat-soluble vitamins
Oral contraceptive agents	Estrogen/progestin	May cause selective malabsorption or increased metabolism and turnover	Vitamin B_6 and folate	Increase foods high in B_6 and folate

Data from Anderson J, Bland SE: Drug-food interactions, *J Pharm Soc Wisc*, p 28, Nov/Dec 1998; Bobroff LB, Lentz A, Turner RE: Food/drug and drug/nutrient interactions: what you should know about your medications, Gainesville, 1994, University of Florida Cooperative Extension Service, Institute of Food and Agricultural Science. Available at www.edis.ifas.ufl.edu; Food and Drug Administration/National Consumers League: Food & drug interactions, Washington, DC, U.S. Government Printing Office. Retrieved April 11, 2009, from www.nclnet.org/Food%20&%20Drug.pdf.

NSAID, Nonsteroidal antiinflammatory drug; *RD,* registered dietitian.

- *Flushing reaction:* A number of drugs react with alcohol to produce a flushing reaction along with dyspnea and headache. CNS depressants, including hypnotic sedatives, antihistamines, phenothiazines, and narcotic analgesics, may cause a loss of consciousness if taken in combination with alcohol. Extreme caution must be exercised with these medications, and patients should be alerted to the dangers of mixing them with alcohol.
- *Hypoglycemia:* Drugs such as chlorpropamide (Diabinese) and similar oral medications used to control type 2 diabetes mellitus are hypoglycemic agents. They precipitate a rapid release of insulin, which may provoke a hypoglycemic reaction. This response of a rapidly reduced blood glucose level is especially strong when the drugs are used with alcohol. Symptoms of hypoglycemia include weakness, mental confusion, and irrational behavior. If not treated, then loss of consciousness can follow.
- *Disulfiram reaction:* The drug disulfiram, commonly called *Antabuse,* is used in the treatment of alcoholism. It combats alcohol consumption by producing extremely unpleasant side effects when taken with alcohol. Within 15 minutes, flushing ensues, followed by headache, nausea, vomiting, and chest or abdominal pain. Other drugs, including aldehyde dehydrogenase inhibitors, may have a similar effect.

FOOD AND NUTRIENT EFFECTS ON DRUGS

Physiologic Factors in Drug Absorption

Absorption of drugs is a complex matter. Physiologic events are important in a number of ways.

Solution

Before an orally administered tablet or capsule can dissolve, it must first disintegrate. The absorption of the drug, either from solution in acid gastric secretions or in the more alkaline medium of the intestine, may be more or less complete, depending on its degree of solubility (see the *Evidence-Based Practice* box, "Grapefruit 'Juices' Certain Medications"). Food may affect eventual drug absorption at any of these points. Table 18-3 provides some examples of drugs that are better used when taken without food and those that should be taken with food. The drug then passes through the intestinal mucosa and liver circulation before entering systemic circulation. In the systemic blood circulation system, it may be subject to metabolism, deactivation, and elimination through the so-called first-pass mechanism.

Stomach-Emptying Rate

Composition of the diet affects the rate at which food enters the small intestine from the stomach. Slow emptying of food from the stomach has the effect of doling out small portions of a drug, creating more optimal saturation rates on the absorptive sites in the small intestine. Fats, high temperatures, and solid meals prolong the time the food stays in the stomach. Food usually increases secretion of bile, acid, and gut enzymes. It also enhances intestinal motility and splanchnic blood flow. Certain food particles may adsorb drugs.

Clinical Significance

Whether these physiologic events have clinical significance depends on the extent of the effect and nature of the drug. A small change in absorption is critical for a drug with a steep dose response curve but perhaps unnoticeable for a drug with a wide range of effective concentrations. In general, the amount of absorption is clinically more important than the rate of absorption, because it has increased effect on the steady-state plasma concentration of the drug after multiple doses.

Effects of Food on Drug Absorption

Increased Drug Absorption

In summary, the following five basic circumstances contribute to increased absorption of a drug:

1. *Dissolving characteristics:* When a drug does not dissolve rapidly after it has been taken, the time it remains in the stomach with food is prolonged. This increased time in the stomach may increase its effective dissolution and consequent absorption. In some instances, the drug may not dissolve properly because of either the drug or gastric pH and is excreted, thus decreasing absorption of the drug.
2. *Gastric-emptying time:* Delayed emptying of food from the stomach can have the effect of doling out small portions of a drug, creating more optimal saturation rates on the absorption sites in the small intestine.
3. *Nutrients:* Some nutrients can promote absorption of certain drugs. For example, high-fat diets increase absorption of the antifungal drug griseofulvin. This drug is fat soluble, and high-fat diets stimulate the secretion of bile acids, which aid in absorption of the drug. Vitamin C, as well as gastric acid, enhances iron absorption. Recent studies indicate that citrus fruit reduced lipoprotein oxidation in persons consuming a high-saturated fat diet.[6] Anticoagulant drugs interact with dietary factors, and a consistent dietary intake of vitamin K is important.[7,8] Folic acid supplementation is needed when phenytoin is used for seizure control in epileptic patients.[9]
4. *Blood flow:* Food intake increases splanchnic blood flow carrying any ingested drugs. This direct circulation to abdominal visceral organs stimulates absorption and results in an increased availability of the accompanying drugs.

KEY TERMS

flushing reaction Short-term reaction resulting in redness of neck and face.

dyspnea Labored, difficult breathing.

disulfiram White to off-white crystalline antioxidant; inhibits oxidation of the acetaldehyde metabolized from alcohol. It is used in the treatment of alcoholism, producing extremely uncomfortable symptoms when alcohol is ingested after oral administration of the drug.

TABLE 18-3 **FOODS AND NUTRIENTS AFFECTING MEDICATIONS**

DRUG CLASS	EXAMPLES	USE	ACTION	FOOD/NUTRIENTS	HOW TO AVOID
Alcohol, particularly excessive use	Beer, wine, spirits	Lower inhibitions, CNS depressant	Slows absorption	Food	Consume alcohol with food or meals
Analgesic and NSAID agents	Salicylates (aspirin), ibuprofen (Motrin, Advil), naproxen (Anaprox, Aleve, Naprosyn), acetaminophen (Tylenol)	Pain and fever	Alcohol ingestion increases hepatotoxicity, liver damage, or stomach bleeding	Alcohol	Limit alcohol intake to <2 drinks per day for men, <1 drink per day for women
Antiulcer agents (histamine blockers)	Cimetidine (Tagamet)	Ulcers	Increased blood alcohol levels, reduced caffeine clearance	Alcohol, caffeine-containing foods and beverages	Limit caffeine intake; limit alcohol intake to <2 drinks per day for men, <1 drink per day for women
Antibiotic agents	Ciprofloxacin (Cipro)	Infection	Decreases absorption	Dairy products	Avoid dairy products
Anticoagulant agents	Warfarin (Coumadin)	Blood clots	Reduced efficacy, increased anticoagulation	Vitamins K and E (supplements) may reduce efficacy, alcohol and garlic may increase anticoagulation	Limit foods high in vitamin K: broccoli, spinach, kale, turnip greens, cauliflower, brussels sprouts; avoid high dose of vitamin E (400 IU or more)
Antineoplastic agents	Methotrexate	Cancer	Increased hepatotoxicity with chronic alcohol use	Alcohol	Avoid alcohol
Antiemetic agents	Amitriptyline HCl (Elavil), chlorpromazine HCl (Thorazine)	Antidepressant; antipsychotic/antiemetic	Increased sedation	Alcohol	Avoid alcohol
Anticonvulsant agents	Phenobarbital	Seizures, epilepsy	Increased sedation	Alcohol	Avoid alcohol
Antidepressant agents: MAOIs	Phenelzine (Nardil), tranylcypromine (Parnate)	Depression, anxiety	Rapid, potentially fatal increase in blood pressure	Foods or alcoholic beverages containing tyramine	Avoid beer; red wine; American processed, cheddar, bleu, Brie, mozzarella, and Parmesan cheeses; yogurt; sour cream; beef or chicken liver; cured meats such as sausage and salami; game meats; caviar; dried fish; avocados; bananas; yeast extracts; raisins; sauerkraut; soy sauce; miso soup; broad (fava) beans; ginseng; caffeine-containing products (colas, chocolate, coffee, tea)
Antihistamine agents	Fexofenadine (Allegra), loratadine (Claritin), cetirizine (Zyrtec), astemizole (Hismanal)	Allergies	Increases drowsiness and slows mental and motor performance	Alcohol	Use caution when operating machinery/driving

Continued

TABLE 18-3 FOODS AND NUTRIENTS AFFECTING MEDICATIONS—cont'd

DRUG CLASS	EXAMPLES	USE	ACTION	FOOD/NUTRIENTS	HOW TO AVOID
Antihypertensive agents	ACE-inhibitors, angiotensin II receptor antagonists, β-blockers, verapamil HCl	Hypertension	Reduced effectiveness	Natural licorice *(Glycyrrhiza glabra)* and tyramine-rich foods	Avoid these foods
Antihyperlipidemic agents (HMG-CoA reductase inhibitors) or statin agents	Atorvastatin (Lipitor), lovastatin (Mevacor), pravastatin (Pravachol), simvastatin (Zocor)	High serum LDL cholesterol	Enhances absorption, increases risk of liver damage	Food/meals, alcohol	Lovastatin should be taken with evening meal to enhance absorption; avoid large amounts of alcohol
Antiparkinsonian agents	Levodopa (Dopar, Larodopa)	Parkinson's disease	Decreased absorption	High-protein foods (eggs, meat, protein supplements), vitamin B_6	Spread protein intake equally in 3-6 meals per day to minimize reaction; avoid vitamin B_6 supplements or multivitamin supplement in doses <10 mg
Antituberculosis agents	Isoniazid (INH)	Tuberculosis	Reduced absorption with foods, increased hepatotoxicity and reduced INH levels with alcohol	Alcohol	Take on empty stomach, avoid alcohol
Bronchodilator agents	Theophylline (Slo-Bid, Theo-Dur)	Asthma, chronic bronchitis, emphysema	Increased stimulation of CNS; alcohol can increase nausea, vomiting, headache, and irritability	Caffeine, alcohol	Avoid caffeine-containing foods/ beverages (chocolate, colas, teas, coffee); avoid alcohol if taking theophylline medications
Corticosteroid agents	Prednisolone (Pediapred, Prelone), methylprednisolone (Solu-Medrol), hydrocortisone	Inflammation/ itching	Stomach irritation	Food	Take with food or milk to decrease stomach upset
Hypoglycemic agents	Chlorpropamide (Diabinese), metformin (Glucophage)	Diabetes	Severe nausea and vomiting	Alcohol	Avoid alcohol

Data from Bland SE: Drug-food interactions, *J Pharm Soc Wisc* p 28, Nov/Dec 1998; Bobroff LB, Lentz A, Turner RE: *Food/drug and drug/nutrient interactions: what you should know about your medications,* Gainesville, 1994, University of Florida Cooperative Extension Service, Institute of Food and Agricultural Science. Available at www.edis.ifas.ufl.edu; Brown CH: Overview of drug interactions, *US Pharm* 25(5), 2000. Retrieved April 11, 2009, from www.uspharmacist.com; Food and Drug Administration/National Consumers League: Food & drug interactions, Washington, DC, U.S. Government Printing Office. Retrieved April 11, 2009, from www.nclnet.org/Food%20&%20Drug.pdf.

CNS, Central nervous system; *NSAID,* nonsteroidal antiinflammatory drug; *MAOIs,* monoamine oxidase inhibitors; *ACE,* angiotensin-converting enzyme; *HMG-CoA,* 3-hydroxy-3-methylglutaryl coenzyme A; *LDL,* low-density lipoprotein.

EVIDENCE-BASED PRACTICE

Grapefruit "Juices" Certain Medications

Almost all oral drugs are subject to first-pass metabolism. That is, any substance the body views as a toxin (e.g., drugs, alcohol) goes through the liver via hepatic portal circulation, thus removing some of the active substance from blood before it enters general circulation. This means a fraction of the original dose of the drug will not be "available" to systemic circulation because it has undergone biotransformation. In other words, bioavailability of the drug has been altered, or lowered. One mechanism responsible for this is an enzyme system found in the intestinal wall and liver. Cytochrome P_{450} 3A4 (CYP3A4) system, specifically CYP3A4-mediated drug metabolism, is responsible for first-pass metabolism of many medications. Most medications are lipid soluble and readily absorbed. To eliminate toxins (i.e., drugs) from the body, however, the CYP3A4 system either breaks them down in the gut or changes the drug into a more water-soluble version in the liver, allowing it to be eliminated via urine.

Where does grapefruit juice come into play? Grapefruit juice blocks CYP3A4 enzyme in the wall of the small intestine, thus increasing bioavailability of the drug. This means an increased serum drug level, which may cause unpleasant consequences, including side effects, toxicity, or both.

What is it in grapefruit juice that does this? The precise chemical nature of the substance responsible for inhibiting gut wall CYP3A4 enzyme is unknown, but it is believed that more than one component present in grapefruit juice may contribute to the inhibitory effect on CYP3A4.

A single glass (8 oz) of grapefruit juice has the potential to increase bioavailability and enhance beneficial or adverse effects of a broad range of medications. These effects can persist up to 72 hours after grapefruit consumption, until more CYP3A4 has been metabolized. Interactions have been found between grapefruit juice and drugs, as outlined in the following table.

Interactions Between Grapefruit Juice and Medications

CATEGORY	GENERIC NAME	BRAND NAME	EFFECT
Antihypertensive (calcium channel blockers) agents	Felodipine	Plendil	Flushing, headache, tachycardia, decreased blood pressure
	Nifedipine	Procardia, Adalat	
	Nimodipine	Nimotop	
	Nisoldipine	Sular	
	Nicardipine	Cardene	
	Isradipine	DynaCirc	
	Verapamil	Calan, Isoptin	Same as previously stated plus bradycardia and block
Nonsedating antihistamine agents	Astemizole	Hismanal	No studies available; recommended to avoid taking grapefruit juice with astemizole
Immunosuppressant agents	Cyclosporine	Neoral, Sandimmune, SangCya	Kidney toxicity, increased susceptibility to infections
	Tacrolimus	Prograf	
Statin (HMG-CoA reductase inhibitors) agents	Atorvastatin Lovastatin	Lipitor Mevacor	Headache, GI complaints, muscle pain, increased risk of myopathy
Caffeine	Simvastatin	Zocor	Nervousness, overstimulation
Antianxiety, insomnia, or antidepressant agents	Buspirone	BuSpar	Increased sedation
	Diazepam	Valium	
	Alprazolam	Xanax	
	Midazolam	Versed	
	Triazolam	Halcion	
	Zaleplon	Sonata	
	Carbamazepine	Tegretol	
	Clomipramine	Anafranil	
	Trazodone	Desyrel	
Protease inhibitor agents	Saquinavir	Fortovase, Invirase	Doubles bioavailability, resulting in increased efficacy or toxicity depending on dose and patient variability
Sexual dysfunction agents	Sildenafil	Viagra	Delayed absorption (takes longer to become effective)

Continued

EVIDENCE-BASED PRACTICE

Grapefruit "Juices" Certain Medications—cont'd

Interactions Between Grapefruit Juice and Medications—cont'd

CATEGORY	GENERIC NAME	BRAND NAME	EFFECT
Medications Considered Safe for Use With Grapefruit			
	Cetirizine	Zyrtec, Reactine	
	Fexofenadine	Allegra	
	Fluvastatin	Lescol	
	Loratadine	Claritin	
	Pravastatin	Pravachol	

BIBLIOGRAPHY

Bailey DG, Malcolm J, Arnold O, et al: Grapefruit juice-drug interactions, *Br J Clin Pharmacol* 46(2):101, 1998.

Guo L, Fukuda K, Ohta T, et al: Role of furanocoumarin derivatives on grapefruit juice–mediated inhibition of human CYP3A activity, *Drug Metab Dispos* 28:766, 2000.

Ho PC, Saville DJ: Inhibition of human CYP3A4 activity by grapefruit flavonoids, furanocoumarins and related compounds, *J Pharm Pharm Sci* 4(3):217, 2001.

Hyland R, Roe EGH, Jones BC, et al: Identification of the cytochrome P450 enzymes involved in the N-demethylation of sildenafil, *Clin Pharmacol* 51:239, 2000.

Jetter A, Kinzig-Schippers M, Walchner-Bonjean M: Effects of grapefruit juice on the pharmacokinetics of sildenafil, *Clin Pharmacol Ther* 71(1):21, 2002.

Kane GC, Lipsky JJ: Drug-grapefruit juice interactions, *Mayo Clin Proc* 75:933, 2000.

Pronsky ZM: *Food medication interactions*, ed 15, Birchrunville, Penn, 2008, Food Medication Interactions.

Schmiedlin-Ren P, Edwards DJ, Fitzsimmons ME, et al: Mechanisms of enhanced oral availability of CYP3A4 substrates by grapefruit constituents, *Drug Metab Dispos* 25(1):1228, 1997.

University of Illinois Chicago College of Pharmacy Drug Information Center: *Grapefruit juice interactions*, Chicago, 2005, University of Illinois. Retrieved July 1, 2010, from https://www.uic.edu/pharmacy/services/di/grapefru.htmwww.uic.edu/pharmacy/services/di/grapefru.htm.

AV, Atrioventricular; *HMG-CoA*, 3-hydroxy-3-methylglutaryl coenzyme A; *GI*, gastrointestinal.

5. *Nutritional status:* In addition to the presence of specific nutrients, nutritional status may also affect the bioavailability of certain drugs in different ways. For example, the antibiotic chloramphenicol is absorbed more slowly in children with protein-energy malnutrition, but elimination of the drug is slower in well-nourished children. In both cases the effect is a net increased bioavailability of the drug.

Decreased Drug Absorption

Absorption of some drugs is delayed or reduced by the presence of food:

- *Aspirin:* Absorption of aspirin is reduced or delayed by food. It should be taken on an empty stomach with ample water, preferably cold (see Health Promotion section for discussion).
- *Tetracycline:* Nutritional status may also have an effect on drug absorption. For example, tetracycline absorption is impaired in malnourished individuals. Absorption of this commonly used antibiotic is also hindered when it is taken with milk, as well as with antacids or iron supplements. The drug combines with these materials to form new insoluble compounds that the body cannot absorb, causing loss of the minerals involved, that is, calcium or iron.[6]
- *Phenytoin:* The presence of protein inhibits absorption of phenytoin. Carbohydrate increases its absorption, but fat has no effect.

Effects of Food on Drug Distribution and Metabolism

Carbohydrates and Fat

Dietary carbohydrates and fat, especially their relative quantities, influence liver enzymes that metabolize drugs. For example, presence of fat increases the activity of diazepam (Valium). Fat increases the concentration of the unbound active drug by displacing it from binding sites in plasma and tissue protein.

Licorice

Licorice, a sweet-tasting plant extract used in making chewing tobacco, candy, and certain drugs, causes sodium retention and increased hypertension.[10] A person being treated for hypertension needs to avoid any natural licorice-containing product. The active ingredient in licorice is glycyrrhizic acid, which is named for its natural plant source, *Glycyrrhiza glabra*, meaning sweet root, a member of the legume family. An analogue of this active part of licorice is marketed under the trade names Biogastrone and Duogastrone, which are widely used, especially in Europe, for healing gastric ulcers, but hypertension is a side effect.

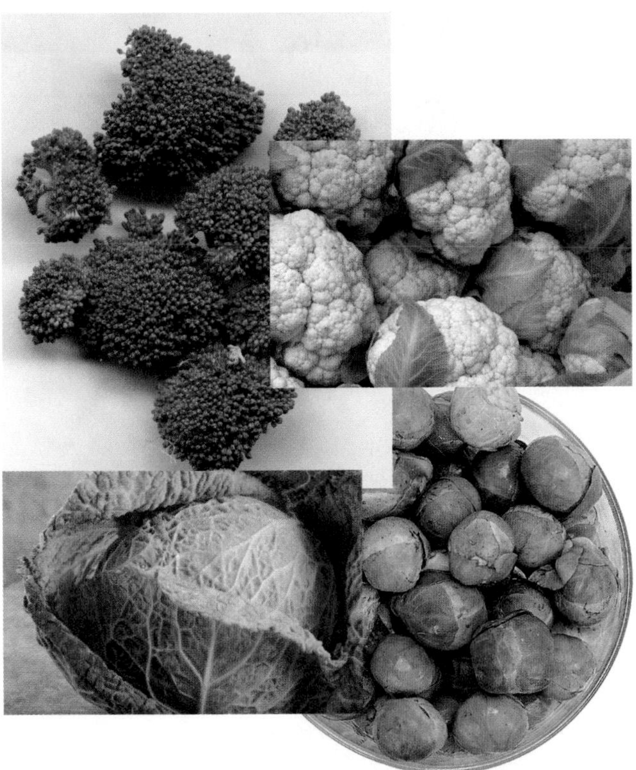

FIGURE 18-3 Examples of cruciferous vegetables. (Copyright 2006 JupiterImages Corporation.)

Indoles

Indoles in cruciferous vegetables (e.g., cabbage, brussels sprouts, broccoli, cauliflower) (Figure 18-3) can speed up the rate of drug metabolism. They apparently induce mixed-function oxidase enzyme systems in the liver.

Cooking Methods

The method of cooking foods may alter rate of drug metabolism. Charcoal broiling, for example, increases hepatic drug metabolism through enzyme induction.

Vitamin Effects on Drug Action

Vitamin Effects on Drug Effectiveness

Pharmacologic doses or large megadoses beyond nutritional need of vitamins decrease blood levels of drugs when vitamins interact with the drugs. For example, large doses of folate or pyridoxine can reduce the blood level and effectiveness of anticonvulsive drugs such as phenytoin (Dilantin) or phenobarbital that are used for seizure control. Unwise self-medication with large drug-level doses of vitamins can cause severe toxic complications (see the *Complementary and Alternative Medicine (CAM)* box, "At Least It's Natural!"). On the other hand, vitamins themselves may become important medications when used as part of the medical treatment for a secondary deficiency induced by a childhood genetic or metabolic disease. Such is the case with biotin in treating certain organic acidemias or with riboflavin in treating certain defects in fatty acid metabolism.

Control of Drug Intoxication

Riboflavin is useful in treating boric acid poisoning. Boric acid combines with the ribitol side chain of riboflavin and is excreted in the urine. In addition, vitamin E combats pulmonary oxygen toxicity. Premature human infants at risk for development of bronchopulmonary dysplasia by oxygen treatment have been protected by vitamin E administration during the acute phase of respiratory distress requiring oxygen treatment.

NUTRITION-PHARMACY TEAM

A decade or so ago, hospitalized patients as a whole were less severely ill than they are today. Now, however, as a reflection of our more complex medical system and economic reform efforts, patients who are hospitalized are more acutely ill. They are more at risk for nutritional deficits and more likely to develop malnutrition, which leads to increased lengths of stay and increased costs. The task of monitoring food and drug interactions is complex and requires team responsibilities. Coordinating the pharmacy, food service, and clinical nutrition minimizes adverse drug-nutrient interactions (Table 18-4).

Hospitals and other health care facilities concentrate on key processes and functions, such as drug-nutrient interactions in this case, rather than traditional strictly compartmentalized tasks of departments. Current standards continue to focus on departmental or service roles, but this is changing because of economic necessity, as well as philosophy of care. This changing focus is being shaped, for example, in the work of The Joint Commission.[11]

The Joint Commission's accreditation manual reflects the philosophy that key functions often involve different disciplines coming together as partners with clearly defined responsibilities. The team of clinical nutritionist and clinical pharmacologist is clearly one of these partnerships. Current guidelines mandate monitoring of drug therapy and counseling with patients about adverse drug-nutrient interactions.[11]

HEALTH PROMOTION

"THE PAIN RELIEVER DOCTORS RECOMMEND MOST"

Aspirin (Figure 18-4) has a venerable history. Being a buffered form of salicylic acid, it is a modified version of an ancient folk remedy of willow bark that had been used for

KEY TERMS

indoles Compounds produced in the intestines by the decomposition of tryptophan; also found in the oil of jasmine and clove.

cruciferous Bearing a cross; botanical term for plants belonging to the botanical family Cruciferae or Brassicaceae, the mustard family, so-called because of crosslike four-petaled flowers; name given to certain vegetables of this family, such as broccoli, cabbage, brussels sprouts, and cauliflower.

COMPLEMENTARY AND ALTERNATIVE MEDICINE (CAM)

At Least It's Natural!

The U.S. Food and Drug Administration (FDA) does not regulate herbal remedies and dietary supplements, so the purity, potency, and safety of these products can and do vary. Manufacturers' claims of efficacy and safety are not subject to the same rigorous testing mandatory for medications. It is likely for herbs and dietary supplements to be contaminated with other herbs, pesticides, herbicides, and other products during growth, harvesting, preparation, and storage. Moreover, active chemical components in the herb may not be standardized. This leads to dissimilar potencies from lot to lot or even from capsule to capsule within the same lot. Safety, toxicity, and the likelihood of adverse interactions with other medications or treatments frequently have not been tested, particularly in children. Patients contemplating use of herbs and dietary supplements should proceed with caution and seek out products only from reliable manufacturers.

The reason many people give for using herbal remedies and food supplements is based in tradition (e.g., The Chinese have been using it for thousands of years!), as well as in their belief in the extensive and aggressive marketing claims that tout certain herbal remedies as "miracle cures," regardless of the lack of scientific data available to support such statements. Many turn to herbal remedies because they are considered natural and therefore seen as harmless. However, it is important to remember that hemlock, nightshade, mistletoe berries, belladonna, and poison ivy are all "natural" plants. What many do not realize is that the term *natural* is not synonymous with *safe*—especially when they combine herbs with medications.

HERB	TRADITIONAL USE*	DRUG(S) THAT INTERACT WITH THE HERB	ADVERSE EFFECTS/DRUG INTERACTIONS
Chamomile (English) *(Chamaemelum nobile, Matricaria recutita)*	Indigestion, reduce tension, and induce sleep; eczema, irritation of mucous membranes after chemotherapy or radiation (for cancer)	Anticoagulants: heparin, warfarin (Coumadin)	May increase bleeding time
		Benzodiazepines: alprazolam (Xanax), chlordiazepoxide (Librium), diazepam (Valium), flurazepam (Dalmane), lorazepam (Ativan), temazepam (Restoril), triazolam (Halcion)	Binds to benzodiazepine receptors, which may alter effect of drug
		Central nervous system (CNS) depressants: alcohol, anticonvulsants, antiemetics, antihistamines, antipsychotics, antivertigo drugs, barbiturates, hypnotics, opioids, tricyclic antidepressants, paraldehyde (Paral)	May add to sedative effect
Chasteberry *(Vitex agnus-castus)*	Premenstrual syndrome (PMS), menopausal symptoms, amenorrhea, and other menstrual irregularities; fibrocystic breasts	Hormone replacement therapy, oral contraceptives	Herb binds to estrogen receptor, may counteract oral contraceptives
Dong quai *(Angelica sinensis)*	Menstrual irregularities, menopausal complaints	Anticoagulants	May increase bleeding time; if using concurrently, then obtain prothrombin time and International Normalized Ratio (INR) to rule out interactions
Echinacea *(Echinacea angustifolia, E. pallida, E. purpurea)*	Decrease duration of colds	Immunosuppressants: azathioprine, basiliximab, cyclosporine, daclizumab, interferon, muromonab CD3, mycophenolate, sirolimus, tacrolimus, corticosteroids	May decrease immunosuppressant effect
Ma Huang, ephedra *(Ephedra sinica, E. equisetina, E. intermedia)*	Bronchodilator, decongestant, CNS stimulant, diuretic	Amitriptyline (Elavil)	Drug may decrease hypertensive effect of ephedrine
		Anticonvulsants	Sympathomimetic effects, which may interfere with drug
		General anesthetics	Concurrent use may result in arrhythmias
		Caffeine and other xanthine alkaloids	Increased effects and potential toxicity
		Monoamine oxidase inhibitors (MAOIs)	Increased sympathomimetic effects
		Antihypertensives: angiotensin-converting enzyme (ACE) inhibitors, α-blockers, angiotensin II receptor blockers, β-blockers, calcium channel blockers, diuretics	May decrease effectiveness of drug caused by stimulant effect
		Insulin/oral hypoglycemic agents	Possible hyperglycemia with concurrent use
		Methylphenidate (Ritalin)	May displace drug from adrenergic neurons, which may decrease effectiveness of drug

COMPLEMENTARY AND ALTERNATIVE MEDICINE (CAM)

At Least It's Natural!—cont'd

HERB	TRADITIONAL USE*	DRUG(S) THAT INTERACT WITH THE HERB	ADVERSE EFFECTS/DRUG INTERACTIONS
Ma Huang, ephedra—cont'd		Morphine	Increases analgesic effect
		Oxytocin (Pitocin)	Possible hypertension
Evening primrose oil *(Oenothera biennis L)*	PMS, eczema, diabetic neuropathy, fibrocystic breasts, rheumatoid arthritis (RA)	Phenothiazines: chlorpromazine (Thorazine), fluphenazine (Prolixin), prochlorperazine (Compazine), promethazine hydrochloride (Phenergan)	May increase risk of seizures
		Anticoagulants	May increase risk of bleeding
Ginkgo *(Ginkgo biloba)*	Improved blood flow, protection against free-radical damage, attention–deficit hyperactivity disorder (ADHD), dementia, macular degeneration, mental performance	Aspirin or Coumadin	May increase risk of bleeding
Ginseng American *(Panax quinquefolius)* Panax or Asian *(Panax ginseng)*	ADHD, stress reduction, chronic fatigue syndrome, fibromyalgia, age-related memory loss, menopausal cloudy thinking	Insulin/oral hypoglycemic agents	May enhance hypoglycemic effect
		Oral contraceptives/hormone replacement therapy	May alter effectiveness of exogenous hormones
		General anesthetics	Should be discontinued 7 days before surgery; herb increases risk of hypoglycemia and bleeding
		Caffeine and other stimulants	Red ginseng (steamed) may be additive to stimulant effect
		Immunosuppressants	Ginseng has immunostimulant activity and should not be used concurrently
		MAOIs	Potentiates phenelzine, causing manic symptoms
Kava (or kava kava) *(Piper methysticum)*	Sleep disorders, antianxiety, tension headaches, menopausal anxiety, fibromyalgia	Alprazolam (Xanax)	Synergistic CNS activity of alprazolam
		Alcohol, tranquilizers (barbiturates), and antidepressants	May potentiate action
		Antiparkinsonian drugs	May increase tremors and make medications less effective
			May reduce intestinal absorption
Senna *(Cassia senna)*	Laxative, weight loss	Any drug	May reduce intestinal absorption
		Antiarrhythmics	May potentiate drug
		Corticosteroids	May cause hypokalemia
		Digoxin/cardiac glycosides	May increase effects
		Diuretics	May interfere with potassium-sparing effect
St. John's wort	Depression, seasonal affective disorder	Theophylline and β_2-agonists	Possibility of increased anxiety
		Selective serotonin reuptake inhibitors (SSRIs)	Serotonin syndrome (sweating, agitation, tremor)
Valerian *(Valeriana officinalis)*	Sleep disorders, ADHD, menstrual cramps	Sedatives, barbiturates, CNS depressants, general anesthetics, thiopental	May intensify effects

Data from Kemper K, Gardiner P, Chan E: "At least it's natural." Herbs and dietary supplements in ADHD, *Contemp Pediatr* 9:116, 2000. Retrieved April 11, 2009, from www.contemporarypediatrics.com; Kemper K, Gardiner P, Conboy LA: Herbs and adolescent girls: avoiding the hazards of self-treatment, *Contemp Pediatr* 3:133, 2000. Retrieved April 11, 2009, from www.contemporarypediatrics.com; Kuhn MA, Winston D: *Herbal therapy and supplements. a scientific and traditional approach,* ed 2, Philadelphia, 2007, Lippincott Williams & Wilkins.

*Not an exhaustive listing.

TABLE 18-4 ADVERSE DRUG REACTIONS CAUSED BY ALCOHOL AND SPECIFIC FOODS

TYPE OF REACTION	DRUGS	ALCOHOL/FOODS	EFFECTS
Flushing	Chlorpropamide (diabetes), griseofulvin, tetrachloroethylene	Alcohol	Dyspnea, headache, flushing
Disulfiram reaction	Aldehyde dehydrogenase inhibitors: disulfiram (Antabuse), calcium carbamide, metronidazole, nitrofurantoin, sulfonylureas	Alcohol, foods containing alcohol	Abdominal and chest pain, flushing, headache, nausea and vomiting
Hypoglycemia	Insulin-releasing agents: oral hypoglycemic drugs	Alcohol, sugar, sweets	Mental confusion, weakness, irrational behavior, unconsciousness
Tyramine reaction	Monoamine oxidase inhibitors (MAOIs): antidepressants such as phenelzine, procarbazine, isoniazid (isonicotinic acid hydrazide)	Foods containing large amounts of tyramine: cheese, red wines, chicken liver, broad beans, yeast	Cerebrovascular accident, flushing, hypertension

Modified from Roe DA: Interactions between drugs and nutrients, *Med Clin North Am* 63:985, 1979; Roe DA: *Diet and drug interactions,* ed 2, New York, 1979, AVI Books.

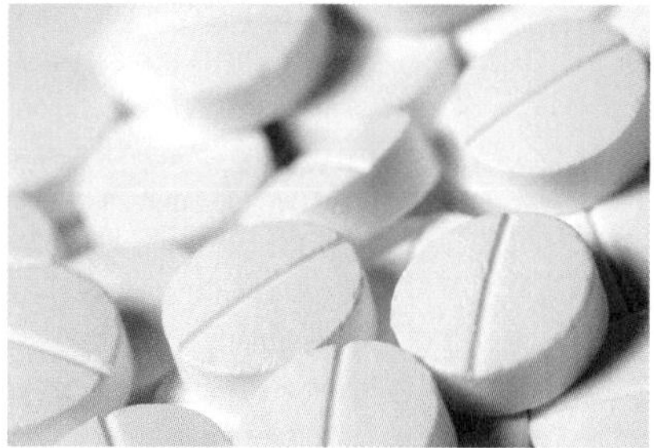

FIGURE 18-4 Aspirin remains one of the most popular pain relievers in the United States. (Copyright 2006 JupiterImages Corporation.)

many hundreds of years for fever, aches, and pain. However, the acetyl group in ASA makes aspirin easier on the stomach than willow bark.

Aspirin is an analgesic agent, an effect enhanced in combination with caffeine[12] that is used for the relief of minor aches and pains. Its mechanism of action is through inhibition of certain prostaglandins (see Chapter 4), which have a profound influence on a spectrum of physiologic functions, including blood clotting, blood pressure, inflammatory process, contraction of voluntary muscles, and transmission of nerve impulses (Table 18-5).

Studies implicate aspirin in alleviating many disorders, dangers, and discomforts, including the following:

- Risk of repeated transient ischemic attacks (TIAs), or little strokes, is reduced by 50% in men (but not in women) who have already had one.
- Many studies indicate aspirin is effective in reducing risk for myocardial infarction.
- Aspirin is one of the most effective antiinflammatory drugs and is effective in long-term treatment of arthritis.
- Aspirin may play a role in inhibiting spread of some cancers through its action of inhibiting production of prostaglandin E_2.
- Aspirin's effect as an anticoagulant is important in treatment of phlebitis and other clot-related disorders.
- Aspirin may be effective in promoting sleep. Many scientists now believe aspirin is as effective as most prescription sedatives, and it has far fewer and less serious side effects.

It is important to remember aspirin is a drug. Many of the benefits of aspirin stem from its systemic, wide-reaching effects on metabolism, which may have unforeseen, short- and long-term detrimental results. We do know that aspirin is to be strictly avoided by persons with hemophilia. In addition, allergic reactions to aspirin can be severe. Aspirin seems to be implicated in asthma. Children are especially vulnerable to side effects and should not be given aspirin without a physician's instructions.

Aspirin is an irritant to the stomach and intestine. Its continuous use is associated with low-level chronic loss of iron caused by mucosal erosion. This can lead to iron deficiency anemia. Aspirin has been linked to birth defects, especially when it is taken later in the course of pregnancy. It increases risk of infant and neonatal mortality, low birth weight, and intracranial hemorrhage.

The best way to take aspirin is on an empty stomach with a full glass of water. This is important: absorption of aspirin is facilitated by a large volume of liquid and inhibited by the presence of food. In addition, taking aspirin—especially on an empty stomach—without a large fluid intake invites erosion of the stomach lining.[13] However, aspirin should never be taken when using alcohol because it increases the bioavailability of alcohol, raising the blood concentration and thus the effect of alcohol on brain centers.[14]

TABLE 18-5 IS THERE A DIFFERENCE IN PAIN RELIEVERS?

	EFFECTS			
ANALGESIC	**PAIN RELIEF**	**FEVER REDUCTION**	**OTHER EFFECTS**	**TRADE NAMES**
Aspirin (acetylsalicylic acid [ASA])	✓	✓	Antiinflammatory Reduces blood clotting Gastric irritation May cause Reye's syndrome in children with viral infection Allergic reaction	Ascriptin, Bayer, Bufferin, Ecotrin
Acetaminophen	✓	✓	Large doses can injure the liver or kidneys Use by persons who have three or more alcoholic drinks per day may cause liver damage	Tylenol
Ibuprofen	✓	✓	Antiinflammatory Gastric irritation Reduces blood clotting Worsens existing kidney problems	Advil, Motrin IB
Naproxen sodium	✓	✓	Antiinflammatory Reduces blood clotting Worsens existing kidney problems	Aleve
Ketoprofen	✓	✓	Antiinflammatory Gastric irritation Use by persons who have three or more alcoholic drinks per day may cause gastric bleeding	Orudis, Orudis KT

Data from Mayo Clinic Staff: *Over-the-counter pain reliever guide: compare before choosing,* Rochester, Minn, 2005, Mayo Foundation for Medical Education and Research. MayoClinic.com (www.mayoclinic.com).

TO SUM UP

Drugs can have multiple effects on the body's absorption, metabolism, retention, and nutrient status. They can provoke adverse reactions in combination with certain foods and can influence appetite, either repressing it or artificially stimulating it. Drugs can either increase an individual's absorption of nutrients or, more commonly, decrease absorption, sometimes leading to clinical deficiencies. Drugs can also induce mineral and vitamin deficiencies by their mode of action.

Just as drugs affect our use of food, food affects our use of drugs. Food can affect the absorption of drugs in a variety of ways. Foods also have an effect on subsequent distribution and metabolism of drugs. Vitamins may interfere with drug effectiveness, especially if they are taken in large doses. On the other hand, large doses of specific vitamins can be effective in countering certain toxicity conditions or a specific secondary deficiency induced by a genetic disease.

QUESTIONS FOR REVIEW

1. Name four ways food may affect drug use, and give examples of each.
2. If your patient were using a prescribed MAOI such as tranylcypromine sulfate (Parnate), then what foods would you instruct the patient to avoid?
3. What is the most effective way to take aspirin? With what type of liquid should it be taken? Should it be taken with or without food? Why?
4. What foods would you suggest to a hypertensive patient on the diuretic drug hydrochlorothiazide (HCTZ) as good sources of potassium replacement?
5. Outline suggestions you would discuss with a patient experiencing a drug-induced taste loss. How would you explain the cause of the taste loss?

REFERENCES

1. Cresci G: Patient history. In Charney P, Malone AM, editors: *ADA pocket guide to nutrition assessment*, ed 2, Chicago, 2009, American Dietetic Association.
2. U.S. Census Bureau: *Profiles of general demographic characteristics 2006*, Washington, DC, U.S. Government Printing Office. Retrieved April 11, 2009, from www.census.gov/.
3. Nelms M: Pharmacology. In Nelms MN, Sucher K, Long S, editors: *Understanding nutrition therapy and pathophysiology*, Belmont, Calif, 2007, Wadsworth.
4. Pronsky ZM: *Food medication interactions*, ed 15, Birchrunville, Penn, 2008, Food Medication Interactions.
5. Merriman SH: Monoamine oxidase drugs and diet, *J Hum Nutr Diet* 12:21, 1999.
6. Harats D, Chevion S, Nahir M, et al: Citrus fruit supplementation reduces lipoprotein oxidation in young men ingesting a diet high in saturated fat: vitamin E presumptive evidence for an interaction between vitamins C and E in vivo, *Am J Clin Nutr* 67(2):240, 1998.
7. Harris JE: Interaction of dietary factors with oral anticoagulants: review and applications, *J Am Diet Assoc* 95(5):580, 1995.
8. Booth SL, Charnley JM, Sadowski JA, et al: Dietary vitamin K and stability of oral anticoagulation: proposal of a diet with constant vitamin K content, *Thromb Haemost* 77(3):408, 1997.
9. Lewis DP, Van Dyke DC, Willhite LA, et al: Phenytoin-folic acid interaction, *Ann Pharmacother* 29(7/8):726, 1995.
10. Morris DJ, Davis E, Latif SA, et al: Licorice, chewing tobacco, and hypertension, *N Engl J Med* 322:849, 1990.
11. The Joint Commission: *2009 Comprehensive accreditation manual for hospitals: the official handbook (CAMH)*, Oakbrook Terrace, Ill, 2009, The Joint Commission.
12. Schachtel BP, Fillingim MD, Lane AC, et al: Caffeine as an analgesic adjuvant, *Arch Intern Med* 151:733, 1991.
13. Koch PA, Schultz CA, Wills RJ, et al: Influence of food and fluid ingestion on aspirin bioavailability, *J Pharm Sci* 67(11):1533, 1978.
14. Roine R, Genry RT, Munõz RH, et al: Aspirin increases blood alcohol concentration in humans after ingestion of ethanol, *JAMA* 264(18):2406, 1990.

FURTHER READINGS AND RESOURCES

Websites of Interest

American Academy of Family Physicians. This consumer-focused site provides links to the Family Doctor website: www.familydoctor.org/121.xml.

Center for Food-Drug Interaction Research and Education. This site, co-sponsored by the University of Florida and Tufts University, provides education about risk and potential significance of food-drug interactions based on scientifically-founded evidence: http://www.druginteractioncenter.org/.

Grapefruit-Drug Interactions. Created for pharmacists and other allied health professionals, this page is designed to provide up-to-date information in the large body of research on grapefruit-drug interactions: www.powernetdesign.com/grapefruit/.

Medline Plus. This site has gathered facts from the National Library of Medicine, National Institutes of Health, and other government agencies and health-related organizations to provide information on thousands of prescription and over-the-counter medicines: www.nlm.nih.gov/medlineplus/druginformation.html.

Rx List: The Internet Drug List, sponsored by WebMD. This site provides food drug interaction information for consumers and health professionals: www.rxlist.com/.

U.S. Pharmacist. *U.S. Pharmacist* is a monthly journal dedicated to providing up-to-date, authoritative, peer-reviewed clinical articles relevant to contemporary pharmacy practice in a variety of settings: www.uspharmacist.com/.

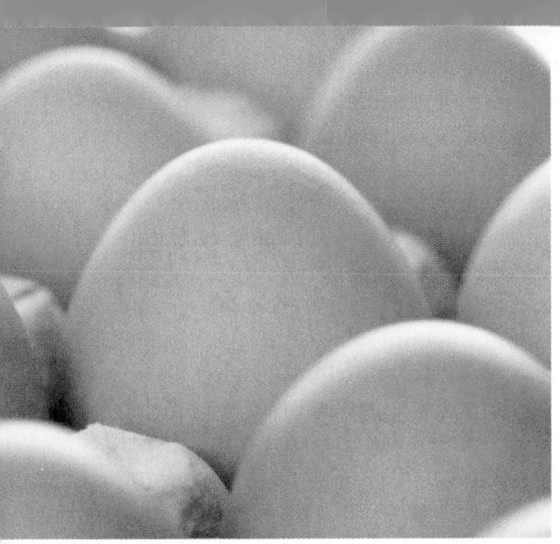

19

Nutrition Support: Enteral and Parenteral Nutrition

Kenneth Byrne

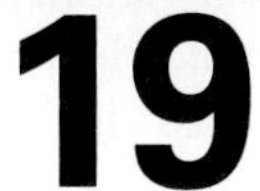

http://evolve.elsevier.com/Williams/essentials/

OUTLINE

In this chapter, we look at alternate modes of feeding to provide nutrition support for patients with special needs. We examine ways of feeding when the gastrointestinal (GI) tract can be used—enteral nutrition (EN) given orally or through a feeding tube. Then we review nutrient feeding directly into a vein when the GI tract cannot be used—parenteral nutrition (PN).

Malnutrition, preexisting and hospital-induced, is a serious concern in hospitalized patients, especially those with critical illness or injury. Nutrition care provided by a skilled nutrition support team or clinician can have a positive effect on patient survival and recovery. This chapter will examine enteral and PN support formulas, solutions, and delivery systems for use in hospital and home.

NUTRITION ASSESSMENT

Nutrition Support and Degree of Malnutrition

It is an easier task to maintain nutrition than to replenish body stores from malnutrition. The effect of starvation on the body, even during relatively brief periods, is well documented.[1] The small amount of glycogen stored in the liver is a crucial immediate energy source. Glycogen breakdown for fuel begins 2 to 3 hours after a meal, and glycogen stores are depleted after 30 hours of fasting in the absence of metabolic stress. Release of amino acids from body tissue proteins begins after 4 to 6 hours of fasting to provide a source of blood glucose. In addition, fatty acids are mobilized from the body's adipose tissues to provide keto acids as a principal fuel for heart, brain, and other vital organs. As adaptation to starvation occurs, the body relies less on amino acids from protein for fuel and uses more ketones from fat to meet metabolic needs. This reduces nitrogen losses and preserves lean body mass. During critical illness this adaptation to insufficient energy to meet needs does not occur. Severely ill patients rely heavily on large amounts of glucose and protein for fuel. They often have elevated insulin levels, which inhibit the mobilization of fat for energy production and thus increase reliance on amino acids from protein with a urinary nitrogen loss of 10 to 15 g/day or more that continues unchecked. Critical illness can lead to severe depletion of lean body mass. Nutrition provided during critical illness reduces but does not reverse the process.

For example, two healthy people are hiking in the mountains and get lost. They have a limited supply of food but adequate water available from mountain streams. Hiker #1 is severely injured in a fall while the two are searching for the way back to civilization. Both have inadequate food supply to meet their energy needs. Hiker #2 will initially use glycogen stores followed by breakdown of lean body mass and fat for energy needs. However, after several days the body will decrease its use of protein for energy and start relying on fat so that lean body mass is preserved as long as possible. This is the adaptation to starvation. Hiker #1 will not adapt to starvation. He will continue to use protein for energy and rely much less on fat for fuel and thus will lose more lean body mass during the period of inadequate energy supply than Hiker #2.

Any medical treatment has less chance of success if the patient is malnourished. The patient who becomes malnourished during hospitalization (iatrogenic malnutrition) has been referred to as *the skeleton in the hospital closet,* with several reports of general malnutrition among hospitalized patients.[2–6] Lack of adequate nutrition to meet metabolic demands is increasingly recognized as a serious concern in medical and surgical patients. Malnutrition can be defined as any disorder of nutrition status including disorders resulting from a deficiency of nutrient intake, impaired nutrient metabolism, or overnutrition.[7] Braunschweig and colleagues[6] reported that as many as 54% of patients admitted to the hospital were malnourished, and 31% of these patients declined nutritionally during hospitalization.

In addition, the disease process itself imposes a nutritional risk and affects nutrient requirements. Deterioration of a patient's nutritional status during hospitalization contributes to increased length of hospital stay, development of comorbidities, and increased cost.[6] Persons with underlying chronic disease, traumatic injury, and older adults are particularly at risk. Thus assessment, monitoring, and reassessment of nutritional status become an important part of overall care, especially for hospitalized patients (see Chapter 16). For the severely malnourished patient, especially those facing problems such as organ failure or extensive surgery, adequate and consistent provision of nutrition support is indicated. The guiding principle for provision of nutrition support is, "If the gut works, then use it." Studies have shown patients experience fewer infectious complications and shorter length of stay and recover more rapidly when fed enterally rather than parenterally.[8,9]

A general screening and assessment program used at hospital admission should be a routine procedure to identify those already in states of malnutrition, as well as those at risk of potential malnutrition because of their underlying disease or injury.[6] In the hospital the attending nurse or another health care professional may discover eating problems or disorders in a patient and confer with the registered dietitian (RD), who can evaluate any malnutrition risks associated with the current hospitalization and perform a full nutrition assessment.

The RD conducts the initial nutrition assessment and performs ongoing monitoring of nutritional status. Initial assessment data supply the necessary basis for (1) identifying patients requiring nutrition intervention, (2) determining appropriate nutrition support route (i.e., **enteral** or **parenteral**), (3) calculating the patient's nutrient requirements, (4) determining specific formulations to meet requirements, and (5) identifying measurable nutrition-related outcomes for determining if the nutrition care plan is appropriate and effective. Once therapy begins, careful monitoring maintains optimal therapy and discourages metabolic, septic, and GI complications.

Guidelines for Nutrition Assessment

Nutrition assessment is done through a standard approach and includes six key parameters: (1) evaluation of nutrient intake and adequacy, (2) nutrition-focused physical assessment, (3) biochemical laboratory data, (4) anthropometrics, (5) comprehensive review of medical and surgical histories, and (6) nutrition diagnosis.[10,11] Nutrition assessment techniques and parameters are described in detail in Chapter 16. However, standard nutrition assessment parameters are adversely affected by critical illness and inflammatory response. Weight is often affected by fluid status and may no longer reflect usual or current body weight. Laboratory values are often not reflective of nutrition, particularly if the patient has inadequate liver or renal function, acid-base imbalance, or abnormal hydration status. Constitutive hepatic proteins such as serum albumin, transferrin, and prealbumin are decreased as a result of inflammation and do not reflect nutritional status; therefore the clinician must rely primarily on subjective global assessment (Box 19-1) and astute clinical judgment to perform and interpret assessment of nutritional status.[5,12] Subjective global assessment focuses on two features: (1) history and (2) physical examination.[5] This technique eliminates the ambiguity and nonspecific, nonsensitive nature of laboratory values during critical illness and inflammation.

History

History includes all aspects of the patient's health: weight change, nutrient intake, GI function and symptoms, functional capacity, and diagnosis, and its nutritional effect. The clinician should identify whether the patient has experienced an intentional or nonintentional weight change from normal or usual weight and time frame during which the weight change occurred. Quantifying weight loss is not always easy, particularly if the patient has lost lean body mass but weight is unchanged because the patient is retaining fluid as occurs with end-stage liver, heart, and kidney diseases. Current or actual body weight (ABW) and height are interpreted according to

BOX 19-1 SUBJECTIVE GLOBAL ASSESSMENT COMPONENTS

History
- Change in weight
- Change in dietary intake
- Gastrointestinal (GI) symptoms
- Functional capacity
- Nutritional requirements of disease

Physical Assessment
- Loss of subcutaneous fat
- Muscle loss
- Fluid retention
  - Ankle and sacral edema
  - Ascites

From Detsky AS, McLaughlin JR, Baker JP, et al: What is subjective global assessment of nutritional status? *JPEN J Parenter Enteral Nutr* 11(1):8, 1987. Reprinted with permission of SAGE Publications.

changes from usual body weight (UBW) and the percent of recent weight change:

$$\text{Percent UBW} = \text{ABW} \div \text{UBW} \times 100$$

$$\text{Percent weight change} = [(\text{UBW} - \text{ABW}) \div \text{UBW}] \times 100$$

The amount of recent weight change is compared with values associated with malnutrition (Table 19-1).

Changes in appetite and dietary intake must be assessed to identify overall nutrient adequacy of the diet and potential contributing factors for reported weight loss. It is important to identify diet modifications observed and nutritional supplements consumed by the patient. The clinician must verify whether nutritional supplements are being taken in addition to meals or used as a meal replacement. GI function determines the ability to assimilate nutrients. Presence of nausea, vomiting, diarrhea, and anorexia inhibits nutrient intake and availability. Assessment of functional capacity of the patient determines whether the patient can perform activities of daily living (ADLs), completely or in part, or if the patient is bedridden and totally dependent on others for care. Medical and surgical history entails examination of the past and current medical problems and enables the clinician to identify potential risks for nutrient inadequacies, deficiencies, excesses, and toxicities.

Physical Examination

During the physical assessment the clinician looks for signs of muscle and fat wasting. Inspection of the upper body can identify temporal, clavicular, and torso wasting of skeletal muscle mass and subcutaneous fat. Signs of edema and ascites indicate inability to keep fluid in the vascular space with subsequent interstitial fluid accumulation. Physical signs and symptoms are then correlated to the patient's disease process and current medical condition.

Basal Energy Expenditure

An estimate of an adult patient's energy or kilocalorie (kcalorie or kcal) needs can be performed using more than 200 different calculations. However, one formula will suffice, and the Mifflin-St. Jeor regression equation has been validated in a number of studies. Daily energy requirements are estimated by combining basal energy expenditures (BEEs), disease and injury energy needs, and physical activity (see Chapter 8). A healthy person's energy requirements will not include a factor for disease and injury. The hospitalized patient's increased disease and injury energy requirement is often offset by decreased physical activity.

Another equation, the Harris-Benedict equation, has been found to overestimate energy needs by 5% to 15%. The Mifflin-St. Jeor equations were published in 1990 and are more accurate than Harris-Benedict equation in normal weight and obese patients.[14,15] In addition, the Mifflin-St. Jeor equation development included obese patients. The Mifflin-St. Jeor equation uses measures of weight in kilograms, height in centimeters, and age in years to calculate resting energy expenditure (REE):

$$\text{Women: REE} = (10 \times \text{wt}) + (6.25 \times \text{ht}) - (5 \times \text{age}) - 161$$

$$\text{Men: REE} = (10 \times \text{wt}) + (6.25 \times \text{ht}) - (5 \times \text{age}) + 5$$

For example, for a 35-year-old woman, 60 kg (132 lb), 165 cm (5 feet, 5 inches):

$$(10 \times 60) + (6.25 \times 165) - (5 \times 35) - 161$$
$$= 600 + 1031 - 175 - 161 = 1295 \text{ kcal/day}$$

The term *REE* is often used interchangeably with BEE in discussing basal energy needs. In general, energy provision to critically ill patients should not exceed 20% beyond BEE/REE. However, metabolic conditions such as severe burns or head injury create energy needs up to 50% to 100% beyond BEE.

Energy requirements for hospitalized patients on nutrition support vary with amount of metabolic stress but generally range from 20 to 35 kcal/kg. Regardless of the calculation used to estimate energy expenditure, it is important to monitor the effect of nutrients provided to determine changes needed to maintain or replete the patient. Energy and nutrients are adjusted based on patient tolerance and desire versus actual response to nutrient provision.

The more malnourished a patient is, the more carefully resumption of nutrition should be done. Refeeding syndrome is a life-threatening response to overaggressive provision of energy to a patient who has been chronically starved. Hallmark symptoms of refeeding are a shift of electrolytes from blood into the cell, resulting in decreased blood levels of potassium, phosphorus, and magnesium, along with increased blood glucose levels and fluid retention.[16] The end result can be cardiac collapse and death.

Critically ill patients with major trauma, sepsis, and inflammation demonstrate catabolism (i.e., breakdown of

TABLE 19-1 CATEGORIZATION OF SEVERITY OF WEIGHT LOSS BY PERCENTAGE OF WEIGHT LOST OVER TIME

TIME PERIOD	SIGNIFICANT WEIGHT LOSS (%)	SEVERE WEIGHT LOSS (%)
1 week	1-2	>2
1 month	5	>5
3 months	7.5	>7.5
6 months	10	>10

Modified from the American Society for Parenteral and Enteral Nutrition (A.S.P.E.N.): Nutritional and metabolic assessment of the hospitalized patient, *JPEN J Parenter Enteral Nutr* 1(1):11, 1977. Reprinted with permission of SAGE Publications.

KEY TERMS

enteral A feeding modality that provides nutrients, either orally or by tube feeding through the gastrointestinal (GI) tract.

parenteral A feeding modality that provides nutrient solutions intravenously rather than through the gastrointestinal (GI) tract.

body tissue) resulting in a net loss of body mass. When protein is broken down, the nitrogen component of amino acids is released and excreted in urine. Nitrogen lost in urine can be as high as 15 to 30 g over 24 hours. This can result in a negative nitrogen balance if the patient is losing more nitrogen in urine than is provided from protein in the diet. Catabolic periods with losses of lean body mass are inevitable after trauma and extensive surgery. The catabolic process increases nutrient demand and requirements. Initiating nutrition support in these patients reduces, but does not eliminate, negative nitrogen balance that occurs after traumatic injury or critical illness.

Nitrogen Balance

Nitrogen balance studies are calculations that estimate the amount of catabolism. The patient's intake of protein (nitrogen) is subtracted from nitrogen output through urinary and insensible losses:

$$\text{Nitrogen balance} = \text{Nitrogen intake} - \text{Nitrogen loss}$$

$$\text{Nitrogen intake} = \text{Protein intake} \div 6.25^*$$

$$\text{Nitrogen loss} = \text{Urinary urea nitrogen} + 4^\dagger$$

For example, a patient receiving 50 g of protein per day in an enteral tube feeding is getting 8 g of nitrogen per day (50 g ÷ 6.25 = 8 g). If that individual's nitrogen losses are 10 g per 24 hours (6 g in urine per nitrogen balance study + 4 g of insensible losses), then the patient's nitrogen balance is −2 g/24 hours. Increasing protein in the enteral tube feeding to more than 62.5 g protein per day will result in a positive nitrogen balance.

However, nitrogen balance calculation is not accurate with renal failure or retained nitrogen such as elevated blood urea nitrogen (BUN). Other sources of nitrogen such as blood products, as well as losses of nitrogen from wounds, stool, nasogastric suction, and bleeding, must also be taken into account when calculating nitrogen balance. The 4 g of insensible nitrogen loss may not be an accurate estimate and could affect accuracy of the results. Measurement of urinary urea nitrogen requires an accurate 24-hour urine collection. Nitrogen balance should be performed serially (e.g., weekly) to monitor changes in status because the patient's condition does not remain constant.

Hepatic Proteins as Nutrition Indicators

Hepatic proteins, albumin, transferrin, and prealbumin are often used to determine the patient's nutritional status. During critical illness, hepatic production of **constitutive proteins**—albumin, transferrin, and prealbumin—is decreased in favor of increased production of acute phase reactants required for survival.[12,17] A decreased serum value of albumin, prealbumin, or transferrin therefore signifies an inflammatory process (or how sick the patient is) and does not provide information about the patient's nutritional status or response to nutrition therapy. These proteins are better used as prognostic indicators of the patient's risk of complications (morbidity) and death (mortality).

Management of Nutrition Support Patients

Management of nutrition support is ideally performed by an official interdisciplinary nutrition support committee or team composed of designated members from the departments of medicine, surgery, nutrition, nursing, and pharmacy.[18] Each team member should be certified in nutrition support by an accrediting body such as the National Board of Nutrition Support Certification and the Board of Pharmaceutical Specialties. The American Society for Parenteral and Enteral Nutrition (A.S.P.E.N.) has developed standards of practice for nutrition support professionals and interdisciplinary nutrition support competencies.[19–23] However, in many facilities, nutrition support management is overseen by an informal collection of interested clinicians, a sole nutrition support practitioner, or no one person in particular. Standards of The Joint Commission and the Accreditation Manual for Hospitals (AMH) have focused on key multidisciplinary processes that ensure performance of nutrition screening and assessment to promote quality patient outcomes.[24] (For additional considerations surrounding nutrition support, see the *Focus on Culture* box, "What's Religion Got to Do with It?")

Baseline nutrition data obtained before starting nutrition support provide a means of measuring effectiveness of treatment. At designated periods during therapy, certain tests are repeated to monitor the patient's course and reduce metabolic complications. Specific protocols vary in different medical centers. However, a general guide for standard monitoring data is summarized in Box 19-2.[25]

Generally, clinicians give primary importance to the following three major monitoring parameters: (1) serial weights to determine adequacy of total energy provision and to monitor fluid status, (2) physical examination for micronutrient adequacy and changes in body fat and muscle mass, and, ultimately (3) improvement in functional status.

All baseline and monitoring data are recorded in the patient's chart, along with all enteral and parenteral solution orders.

No evidence-based "rules" exist for the time to start nutrition support with either EN or PN. Determination of when to initiate nutrition support depends on the patient's nutritional status and the anticipated time period before oral diet can be resumed and tolerated. American Society for Parenteral and Enteral Nutrition (A.S.P.E.N.) Guidelines[7] recommend that nutrition support should be considered when the patient has had an inadequate oral intake for 7 to 14 days or the patient's oral intake is anticipated to remain inadequate for 7 to 14 days. A 5- to 10-day timeline is recommended for critically ill patients. Other guidelines available to identify when to feed are the "rule of five" and amount of weight loss. The rule of five states that if a patient has had no food for 5 days and is unable to tolerate an oral diet for an additional 5 days, nutrition support should be considered to reduce the risk of developing malnutrition. The weight loss rule stratifies patients according to percentage of weight loss of their usual body weight over a designated period (see

*6.25 g of protein yields 1 g nitrogen.

†Estimated insensible losses of nitrogen.

FOCUS ON CULTURE

What's Religion Got To Do with It?

"That was not a natural death. It was an imposed death," said Cardinal Renato Martino, a top Vatican official. "When you deprive somebody of food and water, what else is it? Nothing else but murder." In this impassioned statement, the Cardinal was referring to the landmark battle over the life of Terri Schiavo after her death after nearly 2 weeks without any nutrition support. Over 15 years had passed since Terri Schiavo had suffered severe brain damage stemming from heart failure and had relied on EN for survival ever since. The legal decision to stop her tube feeding created a national uproar and sparked many debates over end-of-life issues, including nutrition support. The Catholic Church fervently opposed the legal action taken and was especially vocal in the events surrounding Terri Schiavo's death because she was Catholic.

What role does religion have in issues such as nutrition support? In this section we will encapsulate beliefs of three religions, focusing on end-of-life issues, particularly nutrition support.

Catholicism

Because Catholics believe they are stewards of their bodies and life is to be respected, the act of withholding nutrition support is not something to be taken lightly. However, bodily life is not to be maintained at all costs. The late John Paul II wrote: "Certainly there is a moral obligation to care for oneself and allow oneself to be cared for, but this duty must take account for concrete circumstances. It needs to be determined whether the means of treatment available are objectively proportionate to the prospects for improvement."

In short, withdrawal of nutrition support is not condemned, but rather only recommended when quality of life is so low nutrition is of absolutely no benefit. Although it is hard to know where the point of "no benefit" is, it is the duty of a Catholic to promote a social order in which a certain level of responsibility exists for those who are marginalized or in a vegetative state. Each case merits special consideration, and in most cases nutrition is considered a basic form of care likened to warmth and cleanliness.

Judaism

According to Judaism, life possesses an intrinsic value as a divine gift of creation. As in Catholicism, humans are thought to be only a temporary steward of the body and therefore must treat the body with utmost respect and sensitivity. Jewish law mandates humans must do everything in their power to heal themselves when ill and must also strive to save the lives of others. This obligation, however, applies only to those therapies that have a reasonable chance of success, and although some believe tube feeding is equivalent to medical treatments, Jewish tradition disagrees with this opinion. According to Jewish authorities, nutrition in any form is a basic human need and should be provided to all patients unless feeding itself causes suffering. Consequently, Jewish law further accentuates feeding must be done in a kind and compassionate manner, emphasizing the importance this religion places on nourishment.

Islam

Not unlike the other religions mentioned in this section, in Islam humans are thought of as stewards of their bodies, which are viewed as a gift from God. Sanctity of life is a monumental principle, and every moment of life is deemed precious and must be preserved. Even so, death is believed to be a natural part of life, and treatment does not have to be provided if it merely prolongs the final stages of a terminal illness. Nutrition support—especially EN—is considered part of basic care rather than a treatment; therefore it is a religious obligation to provide nourishment unless such an act shortens life.

Religion and end-of-life issues like nutrition support are complicated and sensitive matters that must be approached with understanding and tolerance. People from different religious backgrounds can have varying views on this subject that can drastically affect the choice of care provided. The Terri Schiavo case brought to life a plethora of issues that will not likely be resolved any time soon; however, when dealing with nutrition support cases, it is important to consider the implications that the patient's religion can have for your decisions and actions.

BIBLIOGRAPHY

Associated Press: Vatican: Schiavo's death "cruel", *Fox News* March 31, 2005 (news broadcast).

Clarfield AM, Gordon M, Markwell H, et al: Ethical issues in end-of-life geriatric care: the approach of three monotheistic religions—Judaism, Catholicism, and Islam, *J Am Geriatr Soc* 51:1149, 2003.

Cooley M: Faith, ethics help many in agonizing dilemma, *The Spokesman-Review,* p A1, March 27, 2005.

Huggins C: *Survey finds physicians willing to allow patients' religion to trump medical advice.* New York, August 9, 2005, Reuters Health (news release).

Jotkowitz A, Clarfield A, Slick S: The care of patients with dementia: a modern Jewish ethical perspective, *J Am Geriatr Soc* 53:881, 2005.

Sunshine E: Truncating Catholic tradition: Florida bishops avoid full consideration of ethical issues in Schiavo case, *Natl Cathol Report* 41:23, April 8, 2005. Retrieved December 22, 2005, from http://www.natcath.com/NCR_Online/archives2/2005b/040805/040805k.php.

Table 19-1). Patients who have undergone severe weight loss and are unable to tolerate oral nutrition for 5 to 7 days or longer are candidates for nutrition support.

ENTERAL NUTRITION VERSUS PARENTERAL NUTRITION

Debate continues concerning evidence-based effectiveness of PN and EN support. Questions focus on what constitutes early EN, how to select the most appropriate enteral tube feeding formula according to each patient's specific disease state, what is the preferred method of formula delivery, and which factors contribute to enteral tube feeding–related complications, such as diarrhea or respiratory problems.[26,27] In all cases when the GI tract is functioning, EN support should be used to restore or maintain an optimal

KEY TERMS

constitutive proteins Albumin, prealbumin, transferrin. Plasma proteins often used to assess the response to nutrition support. Serum levels are nonspecific and nonsensitive to nutritional status or requirements.

state of nutrition. PN should be reserved for patients with a nonfunctional GI tract or an inadequately functional GI tract that prevents the patient from meeting nutrient needs enterally. In some cases the patient can take some enteral feeding, but impairment in either digestive or absorptive capacity requires supplementation with parenteral therapy. The Veterans Affairs Cooperative Study showed perioperative nutrition support was beneficial for severely malnourished patients but contributed to increased complications in mild to moderately malnourished patients.[28] The GI tract should always be the first choice for nutrition support. Figure 19-1 provides an algorithm for determining the route of nutrition support.[7]

PN is associated with serious complications, as shown in Box 19-3. Reliance on PN when the GI tract is functional can contribute to disuse of the GI tract with subsequent bacterial overgrowth, hepatic abnormalities, deterioration of GI integrity with subsequent migration of intestinal bacteria into the

KEY TERMS

osmolarity The number of millimoles of liquid or solid in a liter of solution; parenteral nutrition (PN) solutions given by central vein have an osmolarity around 1800 mOsm/L; peripheral parenteral solutions are limited to 600 to 900 mOsm/L (dextrose and amino acids have the greatest effect on a solution's osmolarity).

BOX 19-2 CLINICAL PARAMETERS TO MONITOR DURING NUTRITION SUPPORT

Daily intake and output (I/O)
Daily weights
Physical examination
Temperature, pulse, respirations
Laboratory parameters:
- Acid-base status
- Blood urea nitrogen (BUN)
- Complete blood cell count (CBC)
- Creatinine
- Electrolytes
- Glucose
- International Normalized Ratio (INR)
- Liver function tests
- **Osmolarity,** serum and urine
- Platelet count
- Prothrombin time (PT)
- Triglyceride level
- Urinary urea nitrogen
- Urine specific gravity
- Vitamins and minerals

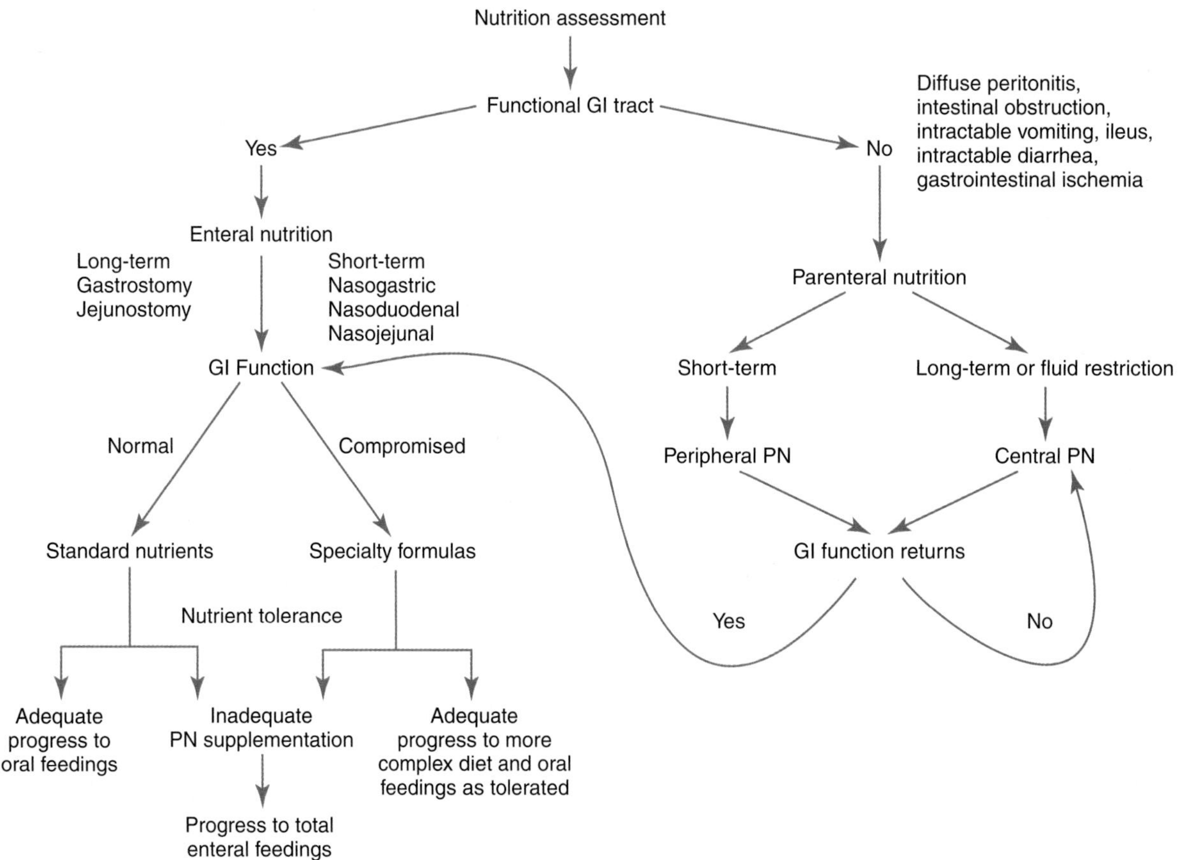

FIGURE 19-1 Route of administration of specialized nutrition support. (Redrawn from A.S.P.E.N. Board of Directors: *Clinical pathways and algorithms for delivery of parenteral and enteral nutrition support in adults,* Silver Spring, Md, 1998, A.S.P.E.N. A.S.P.E.N. does not endorse the use of this material in any form other than its entirety.)

BOX 19-3 COMPLICATIONS ASSOCIATED WITH PARENTERAL NUTRITION

Catheter-Related Complications
- Air embolism
- Catheter embolization
- Catheter occlusion
- Improper tip location
- Phlebitis
- Pneumothorax
- Sepsis
- Venous thrombosis

Gastrointestinal (GI) Complications
- Fatty liver
- Gastric hyperacidity
- GI atrophy
- Hepatic cholestasis

Metabolic Complications
- Acid-base imbalance
- Electrolyte abnormalities
- Essential fatty acid deficiency
- Fluid imbalance
- Glucose intolerance
- Metabolic bone disease
- Mineral abnormalities
- Overfeeding
- Refeeding syndrome
- Triglyceride elevation

systemic circulation, and sepsis. Patients reliant solely on PN are at risk for septic and hepatic complications that can contribute to morbidity and mortality. The GI tract is the body's largest immunal organ. Continued research on the immunal contributions of the GI tract have resulted in numerous publications on the subject. (To learn more about probiotics and how they contribute to enteral and PN, read the *Evidence-Based Practice* box, "Probiotics.") GI disease that prevents or reduces use of the GI tract may itself contribute to adverse effects often associated with PN. Therefore it may not be the route of feeding, but rather the inability to use the gut that increases infectious and metabolic complications.[29] Some adverse effects of PN may be related to inability to provide all necessary nutrients parenterally. Parenteral solutions are not as "complete" (i.e., do not contain the wide variety of nutrients) as enteral formulas or oral diet because of the complexity of adding all nutrients found in nature to an intravenous solution.

ENTERAL TUBE FEEDING IN CLINICAL NUTRITION

Modes of Enteral Nutrition Support

Many patients with a functioning GI tract do not or cannot eat a sufficient amount of nutrients by mouth to restore, repair, or maintain physiologic systems or body tissues. The first option for providing adequate nutrition should be to deliver nutrients orally. The patient can be given small, frequent, nutrient-dense meals with an oral liquid

EVIDENCE-BASED PRACTICE

Probiotics

The popularity of probiotics has increased greatly in recent years, but the truth is that probiotics have been the subject of research for some time now. In fact, probiotics have been researched so often that a joint effort by the Food and Agriculture Organization of the United Nations (FAO) and World Health Organization (WHO) established guidelines for the evaluation of probiotics in food back in October of 2001.[1]

Probiotics have been defined as "live microorganisms that, when administered in adequate amounts, confer a health benefit on the host."[1] Some of the confirmed positive consequences of ingested probiotics include enhanced lactose digestion for individuals with lactose intolerance, reduced incidence of sepsis, and enhanced hepatic function for patients with alcohol-related or hepatitis C–related cirrhosis to name just a few.[1,3] The negative side effects of probiotic ingestion are at best, rare, and limited to individuals with underlying medical conditions.[1]

Intestinal microflora survive by consuming very small amounts of indigestible food that people eat. The waste products of the microflora can be beneficial, including the production of vitamin K and medium-chain fatty acids, which the host can use.[4] During periods of fasting, or when the diet does not supply sufficient nutrition for the microflora, they decrease in number.

Periods of fasting and decreased gastric motility are often found hand in hand with patients on PN or EN. Decreased gastric motility is a common and serious problem in critically ill patients as well. The decreased motility can affect EN efforts, atrophy of intestinal mucosa, sepsis, and multiple organ failure. Although probiotics have not been found to effectively reverse the effects of inhibited gastric motility, they have been proven effective in managing all forms of diarrhea. To understand the importance of effectively managing diarrhea, see the *Case Study* box at the end of this chapter.

Because of the nature of many procedures performed in hospitals, many patients are, at least in the short term, left in a fasting state for the purpose of surgical preparation, as well as for other reasons. Probiotics have been shown to have beneficial effects on patients during fasting periods, and administering probiotics can help maintain nutritional status, including enhanced recovery from malnutrition and reduced mucosal atrophy, at least in animal models.[2]

However, probiotics may have little clinical significance in critically ill patients. In one study the probiotic *Lactobacillus plantarum* 299v was enterally fed to critically ill patients.[4] A significantly delayed attenuation of systemic inflammatory response (SIRS) was found in the treatment group versus the probiotic group, although the design of the study could not confirm this delayed attenuation was affected by the probiotics. The end result of the study concluded that probiotics may play a hand in delaying SIRS but could not reduce morbidity or mortality in critically ill patients.

Continued

EVIDENCE-BASED PRACTICE

Probiotics—cont'd

In the end, consumer acceptance and researcher curiosity is spurring the demand for more research into the beneficial effects of probiotics. Probiotics are being studied at an increasing rate, and research is showing promising results; however, not enough consistent information is available to make a professional recommendation to use probiotics in the treatment of patients on EN or PN. Perhaps with more time, probiotics may find a place in assisting those on EN or PN, but for now, we will simply have to accept that probiotics only have a place in the intestines of the healthy.

REFERENCES

1. *FAO/WHO guidelines for the evaluation of probiotics in food. Joint FAO/WHO Working Group report on drafting guidelines for the evaluation of probiotics in food*, London, Ontario, 2002, pp 1–11.
2. Dock DB, Latorraca MQ, Aguilar-Nacimento JE, et al: Probiotics enhance recovery from malnutrition and lessen colonic mucosal atrophy after short-term fasting in rats, *Nutrition* 20:473, 2004.
3. O'Brien A, Williams R: Nutrition in end-stage liver disease: principles and practice, *Gastroenterology* 134:1729, 2008.
4. McNaught CE, Woodcock NP, Anderson AD, et al: A prospective randomized trial of probiotics in critically ill patients, *Am J Clin Nutr* 24:211, 2005.

nutritional supplement. If oral intake remains suboptimal despite attempts to increase nutrient intake with nutritional supplements and diet changes, then enteral tube feeding can be initiated to meet nutrient and energy requirements. If it is not feasible to use the GI tract for feeding or if the GI tract cannot effectively provide consistent and adequate nutrition, then PN may be an appropriate feeding modality. Therefore the following questions must be answered:

- Does the patient require nutrition support?
- What is the optimal route of feeding: oral, tube feeding, parenteral?
- Will the enteral route alone be sufficient to meet nutrient and energy requirements?
- What type of formula is needed, and how should it be provided?
- Does the patient require long-term nutrition support?

Oral Diet

When a patient does not consume a nutritionally complete diet, the energy value of foods in the oral diet can be increased according to patient tolerance and preference with added sauces, seasonings, and dressings. Frequent, less bulky, concentrated small meals may be helpful so that the patient is not overwhelmed or discouraged by a tray full of food. If a patient is on a modified diet (e.g., a low-fat, low-sodium, or diabetic diet), then liberalization of the diet as much as is medically feasible can help improve oral intake. For example, changing from a regimented 1800-kcal diabetic diet to a carbohydrate-counting diet allows the patient more flexibility in food selection. In some cases it may be necessary to liberalize to an unrestricted or regular diet to increase oral intake. Depending on the patient's condition and food preferences, an oral liquid nutritional supplement, commercially available or made in-house, can be provided with or between meals. However, taste fatigue can happen fairly rapidly when patients are receiving two to six cans of an oral nutritional supplement per day. Patients may use their nutritional supplements as meal replacements, therefore not increasing overall energy and nutrient intake. It is important to offer nutritional supplements in a variety of flavors and textures to maintain adequate consumption. Some facilities, particularly those specializing in long-term care, have found that dispensing oral nutritional supplements in small amounts of 30 to 60 mL during times when medications are administered improved oral nutritional supplement intake and nutrient delivery.[30,31]

Enteral Tube Feeding

If a sufficient oral intake of nutrients and energy is not possible, then the next option is EN by tube feeding, either as a supplement to oral dietary intake or as the sole source of nutrition.

Indications for Enteral Tube Feeding

A.S.P.E.N. has published guidelines for indications for nutrition support.[7] Enteral tube feeding is indicated for patients who are (or who are likely to become) malnourished and unable or unwilling to consume adequate nutrition by mouth. Factors that affect the decision to provide enteral tube feeding include the patient's preadmission nutritional status, risk for malnutrition based on current disease or condition, ability to consume a nutritionally complete oral diet, and functional status of the GI tract. Research found no benefit to aggressive early enteral tube feeding for patients who were not malnourished versus those who waited 6 days to begin an oral diet.[32]

ENTERAL TUBE FEEDING FORMULAS

Complete Enteral Tube Feeding Formulas

Blenderized Formulas

Our current age of advanced nutrition science and technology has brought a variety of commercial enteral formulas and

COMPLEMENTARY AND ALTERNATIVE MEDICINE (CAM)

Homemade Enteral Formulas: A Recipe for Trouble?

Home-based enteral nutrition (EN) support is a common and safe practice that has been in existence for decades. Many people have benefited from the freedom and medical support it provides, and they can maintain a healthy nutritional status in spite of the fact they cannot consume an oral diet. Advancements in pumps, tubes, and placement of tubes are all contributing factors to the success rate of home tube feeding, but another major improvement of note is the development of enteral feeding solutions. Over the years, commercial enteral feeding solutions have grown to encompass many brands and formulas specialized for nutrient needs or even a particular disease state. Most formulas can supply total nutrition to the recipient of EN support and cause few side effects if administered and calculated correctly. Therefore with all of the options commercially available, why would someone want to make "homemade" enteral solutions? More importantly, is it safe to do so?

In the past, homemade enteral solutions were a widely used and accepted entity for EN support at home and even in hospitals. Many people, particularly home caretakers, considered homemade solutions a more economical and personally fulfilling feeding method. Home caretakers such as mothers, fathers, or spouses believed making the solutions was a more affectionate and devoted method as opposed to simply opening a can. Even so, current consensus directs the consumer away from these homemade solutions, not only because of the advancements in commercial formulas but also because of potential problems with homemade solutions.

As mentioned previously, commercial formulas are nutritionally complete and specialized for a wide array of nutritional and disease states. These commercial feedings are also consistent in their formulation and, as such, are easily quantifiable to readily meet the recipient's needs. Conversely, homemade solutions of varying composition have no exact method of quantification or verification of nutritional content. Furthermore, these solutions are not tested for digestive and absorptive properties like commercial solutions, which can lead to a host of problems such as dehydration, constipation, vitamin deficiency, and even severe malnourishment.

Sanitation is a critical variable to consider when dealing with nutrition support and choosing an enteral feeding solution. Its importance cannot be overstated. Although no way exists to totally avoid contamination of enteral feeding, use of commercially prepared solutions can considerably limit the chance of a health risk. Points of potential contamination such as preparation, cooking, and blenderizing are all omitted, leaving the caretaker with less of a chance of exposing the recipient to a potentially serious bacterial or viral infection; this can be especially important for those who have an altered immune system. In addition, commercially available formulas lessen the workload of the administer and guard the recipient from clogs associated with underblenderized feedings.

For the vast majority of those receiving EN support, commercially available enteral tube feeding solutions are the appropriate choice. The advantages of being easily quantifiable and safe from foodborne illness and providing complete nutritional content far outweigh any advantages of a homemade solution. Guiding those who might otherwise use homemade tube feedings can simplify nutrition support and protect them from potential complications.

BIBLIOGRAPHY

Duperret E, Trautlein J: *Homemade tube feeding formula … two dietitians' perspective*, Tucson, Ariz, November 20, 2003, Mealtime Notions, LLC. Retrieved December 22, 2005, from http://www.mealtimenotions.com/GuestOpinions/GuestOpinion1HomemadeTubeFeedingFormula.htm.

Malone A: Enteral formula selection: a review of selected categories, *Pract Gastroenterol* (series 28):44 June 2005.

Mokhalalati JK, Druyan ME, Shott SB, et al: Microbial, nutritional and physical quality of commercial and hospital prepared tube feedings in Saudi Arabia, *Saudi Med J* 25(3):331, 2004.

Stanley D: Forward, *JPEN J Parenter Enter Nutr* 25(Suppl 5):S2, 2002.

Sullivan MM, Sorreda-Esguerra P, Platon MB, et al: Nutritional analysis of blenderized enteral diets in the Philippines, *Asia Pac J Clin Nutr* 13(4):385, 2004.

smaller, safer, more comfortable feeding tubes. The majority of enteral tube feedings in health care facilities are given with a defined, commercially prepared enteral tube feeding formula. However, financial or personal reasons may motivate a patient or family to use blenderized formulas for home enteral tube feeding. Although emotional comfort may be achieved by using home-prepared food, its use does create problems (see the *Complementary and Alternative Medicine [CAM]* box, "Homemade Enteral Formulas: A Recipe for Trouble?"). These problems involve its physical form, which could cause tube clogging, an increased risk of bacterial contamination, and inconsistent nutrient adequacy based on the foods chosen and preparation techniques used. The blenderized formula must be given into the stomach and requires a normal GI tract to digest and absorb the nutrients contained in the formula. Use of blenderized formulas has decreased over the past 20 years, with the proliferation of commercially available enteral tube feeding formulas.

Commercial Enteral Tube Feeding Formulas

In contrast, commercial enteral tube feeding formulas provide sterile, nutritionally complete, homogenized solutions suitable for small-bore enteral feeding tubes. Enteral tube feeding formulas are available as polymeric, semielemental or oligomeric, and elemental or monomeric formulas (Table 19-2).[33] It is important to keep abreast of products currently available because new formulations and enteral tube feeding products are constantly being developed. Polymeric enteral tube feeding formulas require digestion and are available with and without fiber. Macronutrients and micronutrients of a polymeric tube feeding formula can be modified for specific needs of patients with various disease states. Semielemental or oligomeric tube feeding formulas are partially digested or hydrolyzed. Smaller molecules increase the osmolality of the formula. Elemental or monomeric tube feeding formulas are completely predigested and require only absorption for assimilation into the body. These formulas have the highest osmolality, lowest viscosity, and worst taste of all enteral

KEY TERMS

osmolality The ability of a solution to create osmotic pressure and determine the movement of water between fluid compartments; determined by the number of osmotically active particles per kilogram of solvent; serum osmolality is 280 to 300 mOsm/kg.

TABLE 19-2 CATEGORIES AND MACRONUTRIENT SOURCES FOR VARIOUS TYPES OF ENTERNAL FORMULAS

TYPE OF FORMULA	PROTEIN SOURCES	CARBOHYDRATE SOURCES	FAT SOURCES	Kcal/mL	PROTEIN CONTENT	NONPROTEIN CALORIE-TO-NITROGEN RATIO	EXAMPLES
Intact (Polymeric)							
	Calcium and magnesium caseinates Sodium and calcium caseinates Soy protein isolate Calcium-potassium caseinate Delactosed lactalbumin Egg white solids Beef Nonfat milk	Maltodextrin Corn syrup solids Sucrose Cornstarch Glucose polymers Sugar Vegtables Fruits Nonfat milk	Medium-chain triglycerides Canola oil Corn oil Lecithin Soybean oil Partially hydrogenated soybean oil High-oleic safflower oil Beef fat	1-2	30-84 g/L	75-177:1	Boost (No) Compleat (No) Fibersource (No) Isocal (No) Isosource (No) Jevity (R) Nutren (Ne) Osmolite (R) Resource (No) TwoCal HN (R) Ultracal (No)
Hydrolyzed (Oligomeric or Monomeric)							
	Enzymatically hydrolyzed whey or casein Soybean or lactalbumin hydrolysate Whey protein Soy protein hydrolysate	Hydrolyzed cornstarch Sucrose Fructose Maltodextrin Tapioca starch Glucose oligosaccharides	Medium-chain triglycerides Sunflower oil Lecithin Soybean oil Safflower oil Corn oil Coconut oil Canola oil Sardine oil	1-1.33	21-52.5 g/L	67-282:1	Advera (R) AlitraQ (R) Criticare HN (No) Crucial (Ne) Peptamen (Ne) Perative (R) Tolerex (No) Vital HN (R) Vivonex Plus (No)

Modular							
Protein	Low-lacotose whey and casein Calcium caseinate Free amino acids	—	—	**Per 100 g** 370-424	**Per 100 g** 75 -88.5	—	Casec (No) ProMod (R) Resource Protein Powder (No)
Carbohydrate	—	Maltodextrin Hydrolyzed cornstarch	—	**Per 100 g** 380-386	—	—	Modular (No) Polycose (R)
Fat	—	—	Safflower oil Polyglycerol esters of fatty acids Soybean oil Lecithin Medium-chain triglycerides Fish oil	**Per 1 tbsp** 67.5-115	—	—	MCT Oil (No) Microlipid (No)

Modified from Gottschlich MM, Shronts EP, Hutchins AM: Defined formula diets. In Rombeau JL, Rolandelli RH, editors: *Clinical nutrition: enteral and tube feeding,* ed 3, Philadelphia, 1997, Saunders.

No, Novartis; *R*, Ross; *Ne,* Nestle.

tube feeding formulas. Enteral tube feeding formulas will also vary according to nutrient density from 1 to 2 kcal/mL. More concentrated formulas are designed for patients with fluid intolerance, such as those with renal, hepatic, or cardiac failure, as well as for patients who desire less volume or fewer feedings per day. However, it is imperative to provide adequate water for patients without a fluid restriction receiving a concentrated enteral tube feeding formula so that they do not become dehydrated.

Nutrient Components

Carbohydrates

Approximately 50% to 60% of the energy in the American diet comes from carbohydrates, starches, and sugars. Carbohydrates are the body's primary energy source (see Chapter 3). Although large starch molecules are well tolerated and easily digested by most patients, their relative insolubility creates problems in enteral tube feeding formulas. Thus smaller sugars formed by partial or complete breakdown of cornstarch and other glucose polymers are common tube feeding formula components (see Table 19-2).[33] Very few enteral tube feeding formulas contain lactose, because lactose intolerance is common among hospitalized patients. Tube feeding formulas can also contain soluble and insoluble fiber. Considerable controversy exists as to the benefit of providing fiber in enteral tube feeding formulations.[26,33] Insoluble fiber increases stool volume and thus is used to treat problems with gastric motility: constipation and diarrhea. Soluble fiber has been promoted to improve blood sugar control, reduce serum cholesterol levels, and maintain colon health. The focus on maintaining normal intestinal bacteria has resulted in increased research and availability of prebiotics and probiotics given with or in enteral tube feeding formulas. Prebiotics, nondigestible food components, provide fuels to enhance repletion of normal bacterial found in the GI tract, whereas probiotics, live nonpathogenic microbes, are designed to repopulate by providing "good" bacteria directly to the GI tract.[34] The strain of probiotic and combination of strains most effective depends on the therapeutic intent (see *Evidence-Based Practice* box, "Probiotics" for more information).

Protein

Protein content of standard enteral tube feeding formulas is designed to maintain body cell mass and promote tissue synthesis and repair (see Chapter 5). Biologic quality of dietary protein depends on its amino acid profile, especially its relative proportions of essential amino acids. To supply these needs, the following three major forms of protein are used in nutrition support enteral tube feeding formulas: (1) intact proteins, (2) hydrolyzed proteins, and (3) crystalline amino acids (see Table 19-2).[33]

1. *Intact proteins:* Intact proteins are the complete and original forms as found in foods, although protein isolates such as lactalbumin and casein from milk are intact proteins that have been separated from their original food source. These larger polypeptides and proteins must be broken down further (digested) before they can be absorbed.
2. *Hydrolyzed proteins:* Hydrolyzed proteins are protein sources that have been broken down by enzymes into smaller protein fragments and amino acids. These smaller products—tripeptides, dipeptides, and free amino acids—are absorbed more readily into the blood circulation.
3. *Crystalline amino acids:* Pure crystalline amino acids are easily absorbed. Small size of the amino acid results in an increase in osmolality of the formula. Amino acids result in a bitter-tasting formula. If an elemental tube feeding formula is used as an oral supplement, then it requires flavoring aids or special preparation methods to improve taste (e.g., pudding, frozen slush, Popsicle). However, despite flavorings, the taste can still be unacceptable to a sick patient or can quickly lead to taste fatigue and refusal by the patient.

Fat

Major roles of fat in an enteral tube feeding formula are to supply a concentrated energy source, essential fatty acids, and a transport mechanism for fat-soluble vitamins. Major forms of fat used in standard formulas are butterfat in milk-based mixtures; vegetable oils from corn, soy, safflowers, or sunflowers; medium-chain triglycerides (MCT); and lecithin (see Table 19-2).[33] Vegetable oils supply a rich source of the essential fatty acids—linoleic and linolenic acids. Researchers continue to examine outcomes related to enteral tube feeding formulas containing various combinations of short-chain fatty acids, medium-chain fatty acids, and omega-3 fatty acids (see Chapter 4).[35,36]

Vitamins and Minerals

Standard whole diet commercial tube feeding formulas provide 100% of the Recommended Dietary Allowance (RDA) and Dietary Reference Intake (DRI) for vitamins and minerals when the formula is provided at a specific volume per day. The volume required to provide the RDA-DRI varies with each tube feeding formula and the nutrient requirements of the patient. Delivery of a reduced volume and use of diluted formulas may require supplementation with vitamin and mineral preparations. Patients with nutrient deficiencies may require supplementation of specific vitamins and minerals in addition to the standard vitamin and mineral composition of the enteral tube feeding formula. Several enteral tube feeding formulas are designed for specific patient populations and contain micronutrients designed to meet the requirements of the particular disease state or condition.

Physical Properties

After selecting a tube feeding formula according to the patient's nutritional requirements and GI function, the clinician must consider physical properties of the formula that can affect tolerance. Individual intolerance is reflected in delayed gastric emptying, abdominal distention, cramping and pain, diarrhea, or constipation. A factor often evaluated when a patient demonstrates intolerance is osmolality of the enteral tube feeding formula. Osmolality is based on concentration of the formula and defined as number of osmotic particles per kilogram of solvent (water), energy-nutrient density, and residue content. However, no evidence indicates that enteral tube feeding formula osmolality is the primary contributor to formula intolerance. Enteral tube feeding formulas can approximate 700 mOsm, whereas some medications are 4000 mOsm or more. Signs and symptoms of enteral tube feeding intolerance, of which diarrhea is the most common, are more often related to inappropriate tube feeding techniques or drug interactions.

Medical Foods for Special Needs

Certain tube feeding formulas designed for special nutrition therapy are called medical foods. The U.S. Food and Drug Administration (FDA) first recognized the concept of medical foods as distinct from drugs in 1972, when the first special formula was developed for treatment of the genetic disease phenylketonuria (PKU) in newborns (see Chapter 12). The definition of medical foods remained rather murky as medical research developed an increasing number of special formulas. The Orphan Drug Act has defined medical foods as a food that is formulated to be consumed or administered enterally under the supervision of a physician and that is intended for the specific dietary management of a disease or condition for which distinctive nutritional requirements, based on recognized scientific principles, are established by medical evaluation.[37] The Orphan Drug Act was subsequently incorporated into the reformed Nutrition Labeling and Education Act of 1990.

An explosion of specialty enteral tube feeding formulas has occurred over the past 10 years. Several products are available in each category of disease- or condition-specific formulation: (1) end-stage renal disease, (2) hepatic disease, (3) pulmonary disease, (4) diabetes mellitus, (5) malabsorption syndromes, (6) immunoincompetence, (7) oncology, and (8) metabolic stress. Every patient with one of the previous diagnoses does not need a specialty tube feeding formula. Indications for specialty tube feeding formulas are limited to a small subset of patients within each disease state classification for which a specialty formula is designed. Considerable debate exists regarding the treatment value and cost-effectiveness of specialty tube feeding formulas; therefore scientific evidence to support their use is continually needed.[26]

Modular Enteral Tube Feeding Formulas

Commercially available nutritionally complete enteral formula products for tube feeding are designed with a fixed ratio of nutrients to meet general standards for nutritional needs. However, some patients' particular needs are not met by these standard fixed-ratio tube feeding formulas, and they require an individualized modular formula. An individual formula, composed completely of modular components, is planned, calculated, prepared, and administered with the expertise of the RD. Modular enteral components are listed in Table 19-2. However, the more common use of modular components is the addition of carbohydrate, fat, or protein to a commercial formula to individualize the calorie and protein content of the formula for the patient. For example, additional protein powder can be added to increase the amount of protein per liter, or more carbohydrate or fat can be added to increase energy concentration. Other modular nutrients such as fiber and probiotics or prebiotics can also be added to the feeding regimen but should be given separately through the feeding tube and not added directly to the commercial tube feeding formulation. Every component added to an enteral tube feeding formula can increase the osmolality and viscosity of the formula and contribute to feeding intolerance, bacterial contamination, or clogging of the feeding tube.

Blue food dye is often added to tube feeding formulas to detect aspiration of formula into the trachea and lungs. Concern exists as to safety, specificity, and sensitivity of blue dye in identifying aspiration in tube-fed patients.[38-40] Addition of blue food dye increases risk of bacterial contamination, false-positive occult stool test, discoloration of the skin and body fluids, and death. In addition, no standardization exists for how much food dye to add per liter of tube feeding formula, with formula hues ranging from pale to cobalt blue. Methylene blue should not be added to tube feeding formulas because it can adversely affect cellular function.[41] Colored dyes are not diagnostic for aspiration, are potentially harmful, and should not be added to tube feedings.[40] Nonrecumbent positioning (elevating the head of the bed 30 to 40 degrees) is an evidence-based method for aspiration prevention and should be emphasized in all tube-fed patients.[40]

ENTERAL TUBE FEEDING DELIVERY SYSTEMS

Tube Feeding Equipment

Nasoenteric Feeding Tubes

Small-bore nasoenteric feeding tubes, generally from 8 to 12 French, made of softer, more flexible polyurethane and silicone materials have replaced former large-bore stiff tubing. Small-bore feeding tubes are more comfortable for patients and permit the infusion of commercially available enteral tube feeding formulas. Nasoenteric tubes can be inserted into either the stomach or beyond the pyloric valve into the small intestine: duodenum or jejunum (Figure 19-2).[42] Distal placement of a feeding tube beyond the ligament of Treitz into the jejunum is often preferred for patients with a history or risk of aspiration, impaired gastric emptying, depressed gag reflex, neurologic impairment, and critical illness.[27] Feeding tube insertion can be done blindly at the bedside or using radiographic visualization. Placement of a feeding tube should be performed by experienced, trained personnel. Feeding tube placement is an invasive procedure and carries the risk of misplacement into the lungs or brain, as well as perforation of

> **KEY TERMS**
>
> **medical foods** Specially formulated nutrient mixtures for use under medical supervision to treat various metabolic diseases.

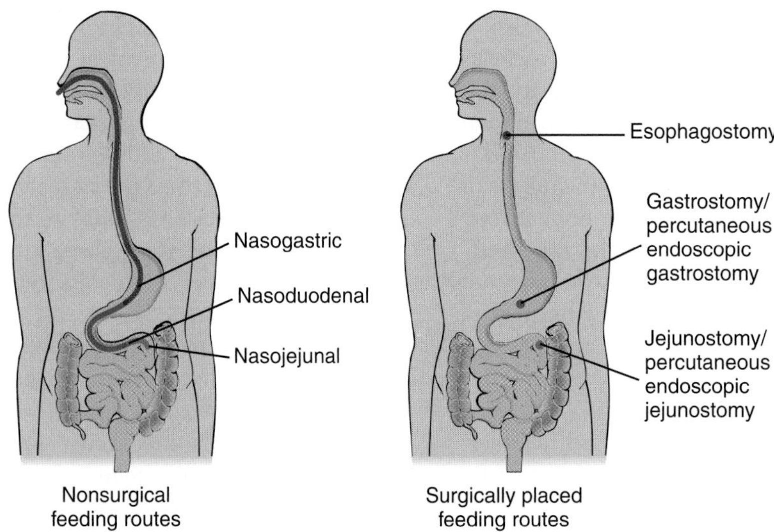

FIGURE 19-2 Types of enteral feeding routes. (From Rolin Graphics in Grodner M, Anderson SL, DeYoung S: *Foundations and clinical applications of nutrition: a nursing approach,* ed 2, St Louis, 2000, Mosby.)

the GI tract. During placement, aspirates of GI contents can be checked for pH and enzyme concentration, as well as visually inspected to reduce the number of radiographs required to determine when the desired location has been reached.[43] However, no tube feeding should be infused until feeding tube placement is confirmed by radiography.

Tube Feeding Enterostomies

Nasoenteric tube placement is usually indicated for short-term therapy. However, for enteral feeding anticipated to last more than 3 to 4 weeks, surgically or endoscopically placed enterostomies are preferred[42] (see Figure 19-2), as follows:

- *Esophagostomy:* A cervical esophagostomy can be placed at the level of the cervical spine to the side of the neck after head and neck surgeries for cancer or traumatic injury. This removes the discomfort of a nasoenteric tube, and the entry point can be concealed under clothing.
- *Gastrostomy:* A gastrostomy tube is surgically or endoscopically placed in the stomach if the patient is not at risk for aspiration and has normal gastric motility.
- *Jejunostomy:* A jejunostomy tube is surgically or endoscopically placed past the ligament of Treitz in the jejunum, the middle section of the small intestine. This procedure is indicated for patients with neurologic impairment, a risk or history of aspiration, an incompetent gag reflex, or gastric dysfunction. Gastric dysfunction can be related to gastric atony, gastroparesis, gastric cancer, gastric outlet obstruction, or gastric ulcerative disease.

Care and Maintenance of Enteral Feeding Tubes

Enteral feeding tubes should be flushed routinely with water to maintain patency and prevent clogging. Tap water is generally sufficient. If concern exists regarding safety of the water source or if the patient is immunosuppressed, then sterile water should be used to flush the feeding tube. Standard flushing volumes are 30 mL of water every 4 hours during continuous feedings. Water flushes for intermittent and bolus enteral feedings are a minimum of 30 mL immediately after each feeding. The amount of water flushed through the tube is adjusted according to the patient's fluid requirements and tolerance. Larger fluid volumes will be needed for patients who cannot drink water for hydration; smaller fluid volumes are needed for patients on fluid restrictions.

General Comfort Tips for Patients with Nasoenteric Tube Feedings

- *Thirst, oral dryness:* Lubricate lips, chew sugarless gum, brush teeth, rinse mouth frequently with water, and suck lemon drops occasionally. If a small amount of water by mouth is permitted, then let ice cubes melt in the mouth to soothe mouth and esophagus.
- *Tube discomfort:* Gargle with a mixture of warm water and mouthwash, gently blow the nose, and clean the tube regularly with water-soluble lubricant. If discomfort persists, then pull the tube out gently, clean it, and reinsert a new tube. (Many long-term users of tube feeding have learned to pass their own nasogastric tubes.)
- *Tension, fullness:* Relax and breathe deeply after each tube feeding infusion.
- *Loud stomach noises:* Take feedings in private.
- *Limited mobility:* Change positions in bed or chair, and walk around the house or hospital corridor. Perform range-of-motion exercises while confined to bed.
- *General gustatory distress with feeding:* Warm or chill the tube feeding formula, but avoid making the formula too cold because that increases risk of diarrhea.
- *Persistent hunger:* Chew a favorite food, then spit it out; chew gum; or suck lemon drops.
- *Inability to drink:* Rinse the mouth frequently with water or other liquids.

DIET-MEDICATIONS INTERACTIONS

Drug-Nutrient 'Enteralactions'

Even though enteral nutrition (EN) support is becoming rather ordinary, relatively few clinical studies are available documenting drug-nutrient interactions associated with enteral feeding solutions. This relates to the fact that administration of drugs through a feeding tube should be considered a last resort, but it can also be linked to the theory that interactions are so common and varied they are simply not reported. However, potential consequences of interactions should not be taken lightly. Use of EN support poses many pharmaceutic and dietary complications that can physically interfere with administration of nutrition, alter bioavailability of a given drug, or cause long-term vitamin and mineral deficiencies.

Physical interferences with nutrition support are problems related to manipulation of the delivery system of nutrition support or the drug before it enters the body. Physical interferences are the most commonly reported problems and include but are not limited to occlusion of the feeding tube related to medication administration, manipulation of solid-dose forms of drugs, and exposure of photosensitive drugs to light for extended periods of time. No medication is formulated to be administered in combination with EN support; therefore the composition can sometimes alter viscosity of enteral feeding solutions and cause occlusion of the feeding tube. Furthermore, when crushing a solid-dose pill for administration through a feeding tube, occlusion is not only risked but also bioavailability of the medication and its time release properties will be altered considerably. Any type of drug added to a feeding solution will have longer exposure to ultraviolet light than if taken orally, which in some cases can compromise therapeutic effects.

The recipient of EN support is able to obtain total nutrition from his or her enteral feeding solutions; however, composition of these enteral feeds differ considerably from orally fed diets. Enteral feeds contain increased concentrations of proteins, vitamins, and minerals, which can bind drugs or alter the mechanism by which they are metabolized. Closely related, but resulting in a more long-term effect are vitamin and mineral binding. Chronic problems such as osteoporosis can develop over time as a result of an interaction that goes unnoticed. The following is a brief list of some classically noted drug-nutrient interactions related to EN support.

DRUG	INTERACTION	POSSIBLE REMEDY
Phenytoin	Probable cause of interaction is the binding of phenytoin to caseinate proteins found in enteral feeds, preventing its absorption from the gastrointestinal (GI) tract.	Withhold feedings for 2 hours after administration of phenytoin. Increased dose might be in order.
Quinolones	Concurrent administration of a quinolone and enteral feed could compromise antimicrobial efficiency. This is related to the divalent cations found in enteral nutrition (EN) formulas.	Withhold feedings 1 hour before and 1 hour after administration of quinolones. Increase dose when converting from intravenous to oral form.
Warfarin	Decreased bioavailability of this drug results from high binding of warfarin to proteins found in EN. In addition, vitamin K was formerly found to reverse anticoagulant effects of warfarin, but most current enteral feeds contain little or no vitamin K.	Avoid concurrent administration of warfarin and EN solutions. Choose EN supplements that contain limited vitamin K content.

Working as a team with physicians, nurses, speech pathologists, and pharmacists can substantially reduce interactions stemming from EN support. By educating those who administer and prescribe medications, risks involved can be controlled and monitored correctly.

BIBLIOGRAPHY

A.S.P.E.N. Board of Directors: Section IX: drug nutrient interactions, *JPEN J Parenter Enter Nutr* 26:1, 2002.

British Association for Parenteral and Enteral Nutrition, The British Pharmaceutical Nutrition Group: *Drug administration via enteral feeding tubes: a guide for general practitioners and community pharmacists*, Redditch, UK, 2001, BAPEM.

Finch C, Self T: Medication and enteral tube feedings: clinically significant interactions, *J Crit Illn* 16:20–21, 2001.

Fitzgerald M: What do I need to know about drug interactions with enteral feeding? *Medscape Nurses* 7:1, 2005. Retrieved July 1, 2010, from http://www.medscape.com/viewarticle/498270.

Ideally no medications should be put down small-bore feeding tubes because medications are a primary contributor to feeding tube clogs. However, the reality of life often requires administration of medications via feeding tubes. Flush with 30 mL of water before and after medication administration. Each medication should be administered separately with 5 mL of water flushed through the tube between each medication. Check with a pharmacist when determining which medications are compatible with administration through a feeding tube (see the *Diet-Medications Interactions* box, "Drug-Nutrient 'Enteralactions'"). Medications should never be added directly to the tube feeding formula because of the risk of drug-nutrient interactions. Warm water, a 30- to 60-mL syringe, and a pumping action can be used to dislodge a clog within the feeding tube. No evidence supports the use of other liquids such as soft drinks or juices to declog feeding tubes.[44] A pancreatic enzyme and bicarbonate mixture may be effective against formula clogs but will not dissolve medication clogs.[45]

Tube Feeding Containers and Pumps

The enteric tube feeding system includes the formula container, connection tubing, and often an infusion pump. A variety of tube feeding containers and feeding sets are available. Tube feeding formulas can be administered by syringe, gravity drip, or a volumetric pump. A pump may be needed for more accurate control, which is essential for tube feedings given directly into the small intestine, tube feedings infused at slow rates, and tube feedings using more viscous formulas. Critically ill patients should also be tube fed by volumetric pump to increase tolerance to EN support.

Tube feeding delivery systems are categorized as either *open* or *closed.* An open delivery system involves pouring a volume of formula from a can or mixing bowl (or container) into an empty tube feeding bag, syringe, or infusion container. The infusion bag or container is reopened and refilled periodically with more formula. Clean technique is required when decanting the tube feeding formula into the bag and when handling the tubing connections. Formula hang time is limited to 8 hours or less.[24,46] Hang time is further reduced if additives such as protein powder are placed into the formula. The tube feeding infusion bag should be rinsed with sterile water before initial filling and subsequent refilling with formula.[24] The tube feeding administration set, tubing and infusion bag, should be changed every 24 hours. The primary benefit of the open system is the ability to modulate the tube feeding formula.

The closed system is composed of a sterile vessel that is purchased prefilled with tube feeding formula. The container is spiked and connected to an infusion pump. Hang time is expanded to 24 to 48 hours (refer to manufacturer's guidelines for hang time of product being used). Benefits of the closed system are a reduction of time, labor, and contamination risk.[47,48] Caveats of the closed system are its increased cost and inability to modulate the formula. Regardless of the system used, good hand washing is essential for reduction in bacterial contamination. Clinicians working with patients on tube feedings need to be familiar with different delivery systems, types of enteral feeding tubes, and features of enteral feeding pumps to determine which products are preferable for their facility and patient population.

Infusion of Enteral Tube Feeding

Tube feedings can be provided via bolus, intermittent, or continuous infusion through a feeding tube. Patients can progress from one infusion modality to another as their medical condition changes. All enteral tube feedings should be initiated at full strength. Tolerance to tube feeding has not been shown to be improved with dilution of the formula.[49] Enteral tube feedings should be introduced gradually and progressed per patient tolerance. Gastric tube feedings can be given as bolus, intermittent, or continuous feedings. Small bowel tube feedings are given as continuous feedings.

Bolus tube feeding is generally initiated with 120 to 240 mL of formula every 3 to 4 hours and increased by 60 to 240 mL every 8 to 12 hours, depending on the level of illness and tolerance. The infusion period is relatively short, 10 to 20 minutes, and is infused through a syringe or from a bag by the flow of gravity.[50] The infusion should not exceed 40 to 60 mL/min. Gravity infusion is controlled by a roller clamp, raising or lowering the formula container, or advancing the plunger into the syringe.

Intermittent tube feedings are similar to bolus feedings but are given over a longer time period of 30 to 60 minutes every 3 to 6 hours. The enteral tube feeding formula is placed in a bag with rate controlled by a roller clamp. This method is used to provide periodic gastric feedings to patients who do not tolerate the more rapid infusion of a bolus feeding. Maximum amount of formula given by bolus or intermittent feedings varies from 240 to 500 mL per feeding and is based on patient tolerance and requirements.

Continuous tube feedings are provided over a defined period, with the formula infused by gravity or pump. Continuous feedings can be given over 24 hours or cycled over a shorter period, such as 8 to 20 hours per day. Enteral tube feeding tolerance is generally better in critically ill patients who are fed continuously regardless of whether fed into the stomach or small bowel.

All patients fed through a feeding tube should have the head of the bed elevated 30 to 45 degrees to reduce the risk of aspiration.[51] Patients fed with a tube into the small bowel can still aspirate gastric contents and may require concomitant gastric decompression during small bowel feeding.[52] Patients who must lie flat or in Trendelenburg's position should have enteral feedings stopped.

MONITORING THE TUBE-FED PATIENT

Monitoring of the tube-fed patient should focus on transitioning to an oral diet and reducing or eliminating dependency on tube feeding. All patients being nourished by tube feeding should be carefully monitored for signs and symptoms of enteral tube feeding intolerance. Tolerance to enteral tube feeding is determined by GI signs of vomiting, abdominal distention or bloating, and frequency and consistency of bowel movements. If problems occur, then the tube feeding formula may need to be replaced, the infusion rate adjusted, or the method of administration changed until tolerance improves and symptoms subside. In most instances the tube feeding formula itself is not the causative agent for the intolerance. Two parameters—(1) residual volume and (2) diarrhea—are often used to determine tolerance to tube feeding. Both are terms that have no standardized definition within each institution, much less nationwide standard definitions.

Diarrhea is generally defined by the person cleaning it up and can be based on volume, frequency, or consistency of the stools (or a combination of these factors). Fourteen definitions of diarrhea are found in the literature.[53] Commonly used definitions are more than three stools per day or more than 500 mL of stool per day for 2 consecutive days.[54] Each health care facility should define diarrhea and then create an algorithm or protocol for treatment to reduce unnecessary interruptions of enteral feeding.[54] The most common cause of diarrhea in the tube-fed patient is medications, primarily antibiotics and medications containing sorbitol (see Health Promotion later in this chapter for a discussion).

Residual volume interpretation is also often determined by caregiver experience and not evidence-based guidelines. Enteral feeds are interrupted for gastric residual volumes ranging from 50 to 200 mL.[55] A research study defined acceptable residual volume as less than 200 mL with a nasogastric tube and less than 100 mL with a gastrostomy tube.[56] The authors suggested high residual volumes be correlated with the presence of physical signs of intolerance before stopping enteral feeding. Another study found that if patients were given a prophylactic prokinetic agent, then a residual volume of 250 mL was tolerated.[57] The A.S.P.E.N. Guidelines[7] and the Canadian Clinical Practice Guidelines[58] state a high residual volume is more than 200 mL for two consecutive checks and more than 250 mL, respectively. In contrast, according to a survey of intensive care unit (ICU) nurses, the nurses believed a residual volume greater than 100 mL was excessive.[59] A patient with a history of aspiration or reflux is at risk of aspiration even with low gastric residuals; therefore residual volumes do not always correlate with risk of aspiration.

GI aspirates containing gastric enzymes and hydrochloric acid (HCl) required for digestion, electrolytes, enteral formula, and fluid should be returned to the patient after determining the volume. However, if doing so would make the patient uncomfortable or if the volume removed exceeds 300 mL, then the residuals should be discarded and rechecked in 1 to 2 hours. The feeding tube should be flushed with 30 mL water after checking and returning residuals to be sure gastric contents with digestive enzymes are no longer within the lumen of the feeding tube. Patient tolerance of tube feeding formula, state of hydration, and nutritional response to tube feeding should be monitored using data collected from a variety of sources, including laboratory, anthropometric, physical and clinical assessment, and nursing records. Protocols for enteral tube feeding can provide guidelines for troubleshooting problems and improve nutrient delivery.[60,61]

Clinical and Laboratory Parameters to Monitor

Daily blood and urine tests for glucose during the first week or so, according to protocol, reflect carbohydrate tolerance. Patients who have diabetes or those who are severely stressed or septic may have difficulty metabolizing carbohydrate and are monitored closely. It is important not to overfeed patients on nutrition support. Historically insulin has been provided as needed to maintain serum glucose level at less than 200 mg/dL. However, a growing body of evidence indicates that glycemic control less than 110 mg/dL[62] and less than 140 mg/dL[63] can significantly reduce mortality and morbidity in ICU patients.

Daily weights, compared with a baseline weight before start of the tube feeding, along with daily input and output measures are essential for an accurate assessment of patient tolerance and nutrient adequacy. Routine monitoring also includes serum tests for potassium, sodium, chloride, carbon dioxide (CO_2), creatinine, as well as BUN and CBC, along with periodic tests for urine specific gravity. Sudden weight changes can indicate fluid imbalance and need to be investigated. (See Box 19-2 for a list of nutrition support monitoring parameters.)

Hydration Status

Signs of volume deficit or dehydration include weight loss, poor skin turgor, dry mucous membranes, and low blood pressure from decreased blood volume. Patients also demonstrate increased serum levels of sodium, albumin, hematocrit, and BUN, as well as elevated urine specific gravity levels. Severe dehydration is critical and life threatening. Fluid requirements can be estimated by several available formulas, such as 1 mL of water per kcalorie or 30 to 35 mL/kg. Water content of the enteral tube feeding formula and the amount of water given with medications and routine flushing of the feeding tube, as well as the patient's medical condition, are taken into consideration when determining the patient's fluid requirements. Fluids must be monitored for adequacy and adjusted as necessary to attain and maintain adequate hydration. Patients with large fluid losses from fistulas, ostomies, and drains may require intravenous hydration in conjunction with enteral tube feeding nutrition.

Signs of volume excess or overhydration include weight gain, edema, jugular vein distention, elevated blood pressure, and decreased serum levels of sodium, albumin, BUN, and hematocrit. Patients with renal, cardiac, and hepatic impairment may require less fluid than do other patients.

Documentation of the Enteral Nutrition Tube Feeding

The patient's medical record is an essential means of communication among members of the health care team. The health care team is involved in actions and documentation related to (1) all ongoing nutritional analyses of actual tube feeding formula intake; (2) tolerance of the formula and any complications; (3) desired versus actual outcomes; (4) recommendations for adjustments in tube feeding formula, routine tube flushing, and method and rate of delivery; and (5) education of patient and family.

PARENTERAL FEEDING IN CLINICAL NUTRITION

PN should be reserved for patients unable to receive adequate nutrition via the enteral route. A.S.P.E.N. has published general guidelines to determine when PN support is appropriate.[7] Indications and contraindications for PN are listed in Box 19-4.

KEY TERMS

viscous Physical property of a substance dependent on the friction of its component molecules as they slide by one another; viscosity.

BOX 19-4 INDICATIONS AND CONTRAINDICATIONS FOR PARENTERAL NUTRITION

Indications

1. Nonfunctional gastrointestinal (GI) tract
   a. Obstruction
   b. Intractable vomiting or diarrhea
   c. Short-bowel syndrome
   d. Paralytic ileus
2. Inability to adequately use GI tract
   a. Slow progression of enteral nutrition (EN)
   b. Limited tolerance of EN
3. Perioperative condition
   a. Severely malnourished
   b. Nothing by mouth (NPO) for at least 1 week before surgery

Contraindications

1. No central venous access
2. Grim prognosis when parenteral nutrition (PN) will be of no benefit
3. EN is an alternative means of support

Conditions Previously Treated with PN That Benefit from Enteral Feeding

1. Inflammatory bowel disease
2. Pancreatitis

Modified from Fuhrman MP: Parenteral nutrition, *Dietitian's Edge* 2(1):53, 2001.

BOX 19-6 EXAMPLE OF A BASIC PARENTERAL NUTRITION FORMULA FOR A 65-kg PATIENT PROVIDING APPROXIMATELY 25 kcal/kg AND 1.2 g PROTEIN PER KILOGRAM

Base Solution

70% Dextrose	350 mL	245 g	833 kcal
10% Amino acids	800 mL	80 g	320 kcal
20% Lipid	250 mL	50 g	500 kcal
TOTAL	1400 mL		1653 kcal

Additives

Standard Electrolytes	Amount per day
Sodium chloride	20 mEq
Sodium acetate	50 mEq
Potassium chloride	30 mEq
Potassium phosphate	30 mEq (20 mmol phosphorus)
Calcium gluconate	10 mEq
Magnesium sulfate	10 mEq
Multivitamin preparation	10 mL
Trace element preparation	1 mL

Medications

Regular insulin	Only with hyperglycemia
H_2-antagonists Famotidine 40 mg	Dose depends on H_2-antagonist and renal functions

BOX 19-5 GUIDELINES FOR ORDERING PARENTERAL NUTRITION

1. Determine that the patient has central intravenous access.
2. Identify amount of energy, protein, and fluid desired.
3. Determine desired distribution of dextrose and lipids.
4. Indicate additives desired.
   a. Vitamins
   b. Minerals
   c. Electrolytes
   d. Medsications
   e. Sterile water
5. Determine infusion rate based on compounded volume and time of infusion.

Basic Technique

Guidelines for ordering PN are given in Box 19-5, and an example of a basic PN solution is given in Box 19-6. PN refers to any intravenous feeding method. Nutrients are infused directly into the blood when the GI tract cannot or should not be used. The following two parenteral routes are available (Figure 19-3)[64]:

1. *Central parenteral nutrition (CPN):* A large central vein is used to deliver concentrated solutions for nutrition support. Osmolarity of central vein parenteral formulas can be as high as 1700 to 1900 mOsm/L. High formula osmolarity requires infusion of the formula into a large vessel with rapid blood flow. A central line generally originates from the subclavian, internal jugular, or femoral vein, with the tip in the superior vena cava, right atrium of the heart, or inferior vena cava. Central line access can also be achieved with a peripherally inserted central catheter (PICC) that is inserted in the basilic vein, with the tip in the superior vena cava or right atrium.
2. *Peripheral parenteral nutrition (PPN):* A smaller peripheral vein, usually in the distal arm or hand, is used to deliver less-concentrated solutions for periods less than 14 days. Osmolarity of PPN is limited to 900 mOsm/L or less to reduce risk of thrombophlebitis in smaller vessels of the upper distal extremities.[65]

Parenteral Nutrition Development

The pioneering work of American surgeons such as Jonathan Rhodes and Stanley Dudrick in the late 1960s propelled PN from theory into reality.[66] In the proceeding years, development of the surgical technique, equipment, and solutions to meet nutritional requirements of catabolic illness and injury, as well as development of certain antibiotics and diuretics, led to its widespread use and continuing development.[26,67] PN was preferentially used to treat critically ill patients until a resurgence in EN in the 1990s when more was learned about the importance of maintaining GI integrity. PN is associated with potentially serious mechanical, metabolic, and GI complications (see Box 19-3). PN should be used judiciously

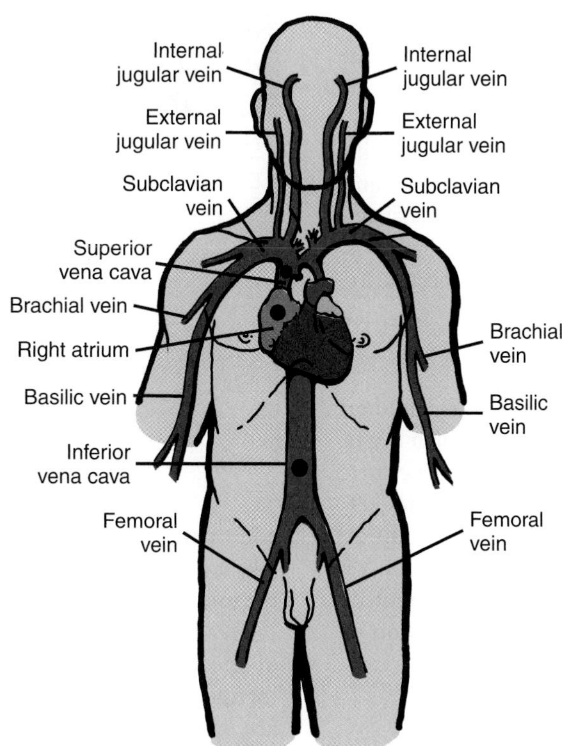

FIGURE 19-3 Sites of central venous access for parenteral nutrition (PN). (From Fuhrman MP: Management of complications of parenteral nutrition. In Matarese LE, Gottschlich MM, editors: *Contemporary nutrition support practice: a clinical guide,* Philadelphia, 1998, Saunders.)

to minimize the risks involved. PPN can be used in many cases as a viable alternative for brief periods for patients without central vein access.[68]

Basic factors govern decisions about use of PN: availability and functional capacity of the GI tract, prognosis, and availability of central intravenous access.[7] The cost of PN is generally more than that of enteral feeding, and institutions have demonstrated cost savings when inappropriate use of PN have been decreased.[69,70] Patients must have central intravenous access to receive PN with one port designated exclusively for PN. Thus careful assessment of each situation should weigh benefits and burdens of providing PN for nutrition support.

Indications for PN include inability to access or malfunction of the GI tract. Patients may have inadequate absorption of nutrients in the GI tract because of reduced bowel length or inflammation. Examples of indications for PN are obstruction, fistula, severe inflammation, intractable vomiting or diarrhea, or GI bleeding (see Box 19-4). If the GI tract is functional but the patient cannot or will not consume sufficient nutrients orally, then enteral tube feeding should be considered. Many conditions that had been previously thought to be an indication for PN are treated with enteral tube feeding, such as pancreatitis, severe malnutrition, ileus, and coma.

Candidates for Parenteral Nutrition

PN should be reserved for patients unable to receive or tolerate adequate nutrients via the enteral route. On the basis of these general considerations, a number of clinical situations suggest a need for aggressive PN support:

- *Preoperative nutrition intervention:* This measure may benefit moderately to severely malnourished patients who can receive nutrition support for a minimum of 7 to 14 days preoperatively.[7] PN should be given only if EN support is not feasible or tolerated. The Veterans Affairs Cooperative Study[28] demonstrated the greatest benefit of perioperative PN was experienced by severely malnourished patients.
- *Postoperative surgical complications:* Complications that often result in initiation of PN are prolonged paralytic ileus and obstruction; stomal dysfunction; short-bowel syndrome; enterocutaneous, biliary, or pancreatic fistula; chylothorax; chylous ascites; and peritonitis. However, reports exist of successful enteral feeding with short-bowel syndrome, fistula, and chylous leaks when patients are given an elemental or semielemental, low-fat enteral formula.[71–73] PN is not indicated in patients who can resume EN within 7 to 10 days postoperatively.[7]
- *Bowel inflammation:* Intractable gastroenteritis, regional enteritis, ulcerative colitis, extensive diverticulitis, and

KEY TERMS

fistula Abnormal connection between two internal organs, an internal organ and the skin, or an internal organ and a body cavity.

radiation enteritis may require PN if the GI inflammation is severe and prolonged.[7] Studies have shown that in some cases enteral feeding can be feasible and beneficial in diseases with bowel inflammation.[74]

- *Malabsorption:* Nutrient losses and interference with nutrient absorption occur with chemotherapy and radiation therapy. The malabsorption that is associated with severe GI inflammation, acute severe pancreatitis, and massive burns can exceed the ability to meet nutrient requirements enterally.

Peripheral Parenteral Nutrition

Generally, decisions to use PPN instead of CPN are based on energy demands, anticipated time of use, and availability of intravenous access. Characteristics of PPN include caloric value generally less than 2000 kcal/day, of which 50% to 60% is provided by lipids; infusion volume of 2 to 3 L (dilution of the formula is required for peripheral vein tolerance); and use of infusion for less than 14 days.[68] PPN cannot be used when the patient has problems with fluid retention or hyperlipidemia.

PARENTERAL SOLUTIONS

Parenteral Nutrition Prescription

The PN prescription and plan of care are based on the calculation of basic nutritional requirements plus additional needs resulting from the patient's level of illness or injury, malnutrition, and physical activity. An example of a basic PN formula is shown in Box 19-6. The same principles of nutrition therapy are applied whether the patient is fed enterally or parenterally. Nutritional needs are fundamental—energy, protein, electrolytes, minerals, and vitamins. Guidelines are available that address PN labeling, compounding, formulations, stability, and filtering.[75] The guidelines are designed to reduce errors and complications in prescribing, preparing, labeling, and infusing parenteral solutions.

Preparation of the Parenteral Nutrition Solution

A variety of PN component solutions exist, with varying concentrations and nutrient compositions. Standard components of PN can include dextrose, lipids, amino acids, electrolytes, vitamins, minerals, and medications. Although PN is compounded with modular components and hence an ability to adjust dextrose, lipid, and protein independent of each other, the energy provided to meet estimated or measured energy needs should include total energy (kcalories) from carbohydrate, fat, and protein (Table 19-3). Estimated and measured energy equations are based on total energy (kcalories) requirements.

Protein-Nitrogen Source

Nitrogen is supplied by essential and nonessential crystalline amino acids in the PN solution. Standard commercial amino acid solutions range in concentration from 3% to 20%. Standard amino acid solutions are appropriate for almost all adult patients receiving PN. Protein has an energy value of 4 kcal/g (see Table 19-3) and usually provides 10% to 20% of the total energy provided in PN.

TABLE 19-3 CALORIC VALUE PER MILLILITER OF PARENTERAL COMPONENTS

NUTRIENT	CONCENTRATION (%)	kcal/mL
Dextrose	70.0	2.38
	50.0	1.85
Lipids	30.0	3.0
	20.0	2.0
	10.0	1.1
Amino acids	15.0	0.6
	10.0	0.4
	8.5	0.34

In addition to standard amino acid solutions, three types of specialized amino acid solutions have been formulated for specific disease states. The two disease-specific formulas are more expensive than standard solutions, and their effectiveness has not been demonstrated. One type is enriched with the branched-chain amino acids (BCAAs) isoleucine, leucine, and valine and is designed for patients with liver failure. A renal failure formula contains only essential amino acids to prevent the development of hyperuremia. Neither disease-specific formula has been found to improve outcomes in these patient populations.[7] Infusion of BCAA may be beneficial in a very small population of patients with chronic hepatic encephalopathy that is unresponsive to drug therapy.[7] The third type of specialized amino acid formula is designed specifically for the needs of pediatric patients and is selected based on the age and nutrient requirements of the child.

Carbohydrate-Dextrose

Dextrose is the most common and least expensive source of energy used for PN support. Dextrose is available in concentrations ranging from 2.5% to 70%. Hypertonic solutions of 50% to 70% dextrose are often used in PN formulations and provide 50 or 70 g of dextrose per 100 mL, respectively. Glucose used in PN support is commercially available as dextrose monohydrate ($C_6H_{12}O_6H_2O$), which has an energy value of 3.4 kcal/g versus the energy value of 4 kcal/g of dietary glucose ($C_6H_{12}O_6$). The caloric values of dextrose solutions are given in Table 19-3. Initial dextrose content of PN should not exceed 200 g. Gradual introduction of dextrose enables the clinician to evaluate blood sugar response and, if necessary, then institute insulin therapy. The amount of dextrose provided is increased to goal according to patient tolerance and should not exceed 5 mg/kg/min.

Glycerol is another form of carbohydrate used in parenteral solutions. It provides 4.3 kcal/g and is available as a component along with amino acids in a commercially available PPN solution.

Fat-Lipids

Lipid emulsions provide a concentrated energy source, 9 kcal/g, as well as the essential fatty acids linoleic and linolenic acid. A minimum of 4% to 10% of the daily energy intake should consist of fat to prevent essential fatty acid deficiency. Lipids are available in 10% (1.1 kcal/mL), 20% (2 kcal/mL), and 30% (3 kcal/mL) products (see Table 19-3). A 500-mL bottle of 10%, 20%, or 30% fat emulsion provides 550, 1000, and 1500 kcal, respectively. Commercial lipid emulsion products consist of soybean and safflower oils combined or soybean oil alone. Content of lipid in a parenteral solution is usually limited to 20% to 30% of total energy because lipids have been reported to adversely affect the immune system.[76] However, infusion of lipids over 24 hours may limit this adverse effect. Research on alternative lipid sources includes forms such as short-chain fatty acids, medium-chain fatty acids, omega-3 fatty acids, and blended or structured lipids. However, these alternatives are not available for commercial use in the United States. Lipid emulsions can be infused separately through the Y-port of the intravenous catheter (piggybacked) or combined with the dextrose and amino acid base in what is called a *total nutrient admixture* (TNA) or *3-in-1*.[75]

Electrolytes

The body maintains a balance of fluid and electrolytes in intracellular and extracellular spaces of all tissues to maintain homeostasis (see Chapter 7). Electrolyte status is affected by disease state and metabolic condition of the patient. Electrolytes in PN formulas are based on normal electrolyte balance with adjustments according to individual patient requirements. Electrolytes should be routinely monitored to determine electrolyte requirements in PN.

In general, basic electrolyte recommendations are as shown in Table 19-4, with chloride and acetate balanced among the salts. Commercial amino acid formulations are available with or without added electrolytes. Amounts of electrolytes present in the amino acid solution must be taken into account when calculating additions of electrolytes for a specific patient. Guidelines for electrolyte management include the following:

1. Identify and correct any preexisting deficits before initiating PN.
2. Determine the cause of electrolyte abnormalities.
3. Replace excessive fluid and electrolyte losses.
4. Monitor and assess electrolyte status daily.

Depending on requirements for electrolyte replacement, it may be necessary to give additional electrolytes outside the PN, because limitations exist regarding what can be added to a parenteral solution based on solution stability and compatibility.[72] Selected electrolytes can be omitted from the parenteral solution when serum levels exceed normal values, such as potassium and phosphorus with renal failure. Electrolyte levels should be checked in all patients before starting PN and routinely throughout PN therapy.

Vitamins

Vitamin requirements are based on normal standards (see Chapter 6), with adjustments made according to metabolic states that require either more or less of a specific vitamin. All patients on PN should receive vitamins daily. Serum levels of vitamins should be monitored in patients requiring long-term PN or when deficiencies or excesses are suspected.

The Nutrition Advisory Group of the American Medical Association has established guidelines for parenteral administration of 12 vitamins: A, D, E, thiamin, riboflavin, niacin, pantothenic acid, pyridoxine, folic acid, biotin, cyanocobalamin, and ascorbic acid (see Table 19-4).[77] Multivitamin infusion preparations based on these guidelines are commercially available. Vitamin K has not historically been a component of any injectable vitamin formulation for adults. The FDA mandated changes in parenteral vitamin formulations that included addition of 150 mcg of vitamin K to injectable multivitamin preparations.[78] It will be important to monitor International Normalized Ratio (INR) levels, particularly for patients on anticoagulation therapy started or stopped on PN containing vitamin K. An injectable multivitamin preparation without vitamin K is also available.

Trace Elements

The American Medical Association has set guidelines for addition of four trace elements in PN solutions: zinc, copper, manganese, and chromium (see Table 19-4).[79] Trace element preparations are available with combinations of the aforementioned four trace elements only, the standard four plus selenium, or the standard four plus selenium, molybdenum, and iodine. Each trace element is also available as a single injectable mineral product. A growing amount of literature demonstrates the importance of providing selenium to PN patients who are critically ill[80,81] and those who require long-term PN.[82] Iron is not routinely added to PN because of incompatibility with intravenous lipids, as well as the potential adverse effects of iron dextran. Other forms of intravenous iron have less adverse effects but are not approved for addition to the PN solution. Intravenous iron should only be given to patients with iron deficiency anemia and administered apart from the PN admixture or added to a 2-in-1 PN solution.[75] A dose of 25 to 50 mg of iron dextran once a month should be sufficient to meet iron needs in a patient without blood loss.[75]

Patients on long-term PN without trace element supplementation are at risk for micronutrient deficiencies.[82,83] In addition, reports exist of excess trace element levels with infusion of standard trace element preparations.[84] Patients requiring long-term PN should be routinely monitored for potential trace element deficiencies and toxicities.

KEY TERMS

admixture A mixture of ingredients that each retain their own physical properties; a combination of two or more substances that are not chemically united or that exist in no fixed proportion to each other.

TABLE 19-4 MICRONUTRIENTS AND PARENTERAL NUTRITION FOR ADULTS

MICRONUTRIENTS	STANDARD DAILY AMOUNTS
Electrolytes	
Potassium (K)	1-2 mEq/kg
Sodium (Na)	1-2 mEq/kg
Phosphate (HPO_4)	20-40 mmol
Magnesium (Mg)	8-20 mEq
Calcium (Ca)	10-15 mEq
Acetate	Balance with chloride to maintain acid-base balance
Chloride	Balance with acetate to maintain acid-base balance
Vitamins	
Vitamin A	3300 IU
Vitamin D	200 IU
Vitamin E	10 IU
Vitamin K	150 mcg
Thiamin (B_1)	6 mg
Riboflavin (B_2)	3.6 mg
Niacin (B_3)	40 mg
Folic acid	600 mcg
Pantothenic acid	15 mg
Pyridoxine (B_6)	6 mg
Cyanocobalamin (B_{12})	5 mcg
Biotin	60 mcg
Ascorbic acid (vitamin C)	200 mcg
Trace Elements	
Chromium	10-15 mcg
Copper	0.3-0.5 mcg
Iodine	Not routinely provided
	50 mcg for pregnant women
Iron	Not routinely provided
	25-50 mg per month without blood loss
Manganese	60-100 mcg
Selenium	20-60 mcg
Zinc	2.5-5.0 mg
Molybdenum	Not routinely provided

Data from Fuhrman MP: Complication management in parenteral nutrition. In Matarese LE, Gottschlich MM, editors: *Contemporary nutrition support practice: a clinical guide,* ed 2, Philadelphia, 2003, Saunders; Task force for the revision of safe practices for parenteral nutrition: Safe practices for parenteral nutrition, *JPEN J Parenter Enteral Nutr* 28(suppl):S39, 2004; American Medical Association, AMA Department of Foods and Nutrition: Multivitamin preparations for parenteral use: a statement by the Nutrition Advisory Group, *JPEN J Parenter Enteral Nutr* 3:258, 1979; Parenteral multivitamin products; drugs for human use; drug efficacy study implementation; amendment (21 CFR 5.70), *Fed Register* 65:21200, 2000; Expert Panel for Nutrition Advisory Group, AMA Department of Foods and Nutrition: Guidelines for essential trace element preparations for parenteral use, *JAMA* 241:2051, 1979.

Medications

Medications often added to PN include insulin, H_2-antagonists, heparin, metoclopramide, and octreotide. Inclusion of these medications and others will depend on each institution's guidelines and protocols for addition of medications to PN solutions. Many issues exist concerning compatibility, bioavailability, efficacy, interactions, and safety when including medications in PN solutions. Consult a pharmacist whenever considering the addition of a medication to PN solutions.

PARENTERAL NUTRITION DELIVERY SYSTEM

Equipment

Strict aseptic technique throughout PN administration by all health care personnel is absolutely essential. This includes (1) solution preparation by the pharmacist, (2) surgical placement of the venous catheter by the physician, (3) care of the catheter site and all external equipment, and (4) administration of the solution by the nurse. At every step of the PN process, strict infection control is a primary responsibility of all health care professionals.

Venous Access

Surgical placement of the venous catheter is done by the physician at the bedside or in a surgical suite, using local or general anesthesia. Intravenous catheters are available with single, double, triple, or quadruple lumens. Inconsistent data exist as to whether the number of lumens contributes to the risk of catheter-related infection.[85-87] Catheters are also categorized as either *temporary* or *permanent.* Temporary catheters involve a direct percutaneous puncture into a major vessel and are used short-term during hospitalization. Permanent catheters are designed for long-term use and are available as implanted ports, tunneled catheters, and PICCs. The tip of a central venous catheter is located in the inferior or superior vena cava, which leads directly into the heart (see Figure 19-3).[64] Placement of the catheter tip in the vena cava allows infusion of concentrated solutions, five times the concentration of blood plasma, to be infused at a rate of 2 to 3 mL/min. Hypertonic solutions are immediately diluted by the large blood flow of 2 to 5 L/min in the vena cava.

Catheter-related sepsis is a serious complication, particularly with the increase in colonization of resistant strains of microorganisms that limit available treatment options. Antibiotic-impregnated catheters and dressings are available and are associated with reduced catheter-related septic complications.[88-90] Filters (0.22 μm) on intravenous catheter tubing prevent infusion of not only particulate matter but also certain microorganisms.[75] However, a larger filter (2.1 μm) that is less effective against microorganisms must be used with PN containing lipids. Clinicians must use aseptic technique when inserting and caring for intravenous catheters.

PERSPECTIVES IN PRACTICE

Parenteral Nutrition Administration

Of all the various ways of nourishing the human body—normal eating, liquid diets, enteral nutrition (EN), and parenteral nutrition (PN)—PN requires the highest level of skilled and precise administration. A risk of potentially life-threatening complication and infection exists. Trained nutrition support clinicians are central to the success of PN. The nutrition support nurse administers the PN solution according to the nutrition support team protocol, monitoring the entire PN system frequently to see that it is operating accurately.

Specific clinical protocols will vary somewhat, but they usually include the following points:

- *Start slowly:* Give the patient time to adapt to the glucose and electrolyte concentration of the solution.
- *Schedule carefully:* PN volume can vary from 1 to 3 L and should be infused with an infusion pump. The infusion rate is based on the total volume of the compounded solution.
- *Monitor closely:* Note metabolic effects of glucose and electrolytes. Blood glucose levels should not exceed 200 mg/dL during initiation of PN and should not exceed 110 to 150 mg/dL when the patient is stable on the formula. First-day formulas generally contain no more than 200 g dextrose. Monitor glycemic tolerance closely, particularly the first couple of days, as the feeding is advanced. Electrolyte status and glucose levels should be determined before and throughout PN administration. Increase energy provision only as patient tolerates macronutrient content.
- *Make changes cautiously:* Monitor and report the effect of all changes, and proceed slowly.
- *Maintain a constant rate:* Keep to the correct hourly infusion rate, with no "catch-up" or "slow-down" effort to meet the original volume order.
- *Discontinue PN:* Reduce the rate by one half for 1 hour before discontinuing. If patient has had insulin added to PN and is not receiving enteral tube feeding, then monitor for rebound hypoglycemia (check serum glucose 2 hours after stopping PN infusion).

Solution Infusion and Administration

Volumetric infusion pumps should be used to deliver the parenteral solution at a constant rate to prevent metabolic complications. Protocols for external delivery system tubing changes are provided by infection control guidelines. Routine flushing of intravenous catheters is recommended to maintain catheter patency. Needleless intravenous access devices reduce risk of needlestick injuries but can increase risk of catheter-related infections. According to the Intravenous Nurses Society standards of practice, needleless devices should be changed every 24 hours, the injection port should be disinfected with alcohol before accessing, and all junctions should be secured with Luer-Lok, clasps, or threaded devices.[91]

Infusion of PN is generally over 24 hours, particularly in the critically ill. PN is usually cycled for patients at home or who need "time off" during hospitalization for physical therapy or other routine activities. PN can be cycled over 10 to 12 hours if desired and if the patient can tolerate the larger volume over a shorter period. Rate of infusion is based on the final compounded volume and length of time the infusion is to be given. Administration of PN should be adjusted based on the patient's response and tolerance to the regimen (see the *Perspectives in Practice* box, "Parenteral Nutrition Administration"). When PN is being discontinued, the infusion rate should be cut by one half for 1 hour and then stopped. Abrupt interruption of PN infusion may require hanging 10% dextrose to prevent possible rebound hypoglycemia.[75]

Monitoring

Complications of PN include catheter, GI, and metabolic problems (see Box 19-3). In the hands of well-trained PN clinicians, risks can be minimized and complications controlled.[92] Specific evidence-based protocols, updated periodically, guide continuing assessment and monitoring.[93] Every patient on PN should undergo a routine nutrition reassessment with adjustments made in the feeding regimen according to the patient's metabolic and nutritional needs. Every effort should be made to transition the patient from PN to enteral tube feeding or oral diet whenever feasible or appropriate. Providing at least a portion of energy via the GI tract may help reduce the adverse effects associated with PN.[64]

HOME NUTRITION SUPPORT

Patients being discharged with home nutrition support and those started on nutrition support while in the home require special consideration. Several factors must be evaluated to ensure that the home environment is safe and the patient and family are able and willing to accept the responsibility of home infusion therapy. The home should have refrigeration, running water, electricity, and adequate storage for supplies. The patient and family must be capable of and willing to learn techniques required to administer and manage the feeding access. It is also important that the patient and family accept responsibility to comply with the infusion regimen so that the patient receives nutrients as prescribed. Ongoing communication occurs among the patient, physician, and home infusion provider, but ultimately the patient must self-manage the therapy and work closely with the home nutrition support team. The Oley Foundation (www.oley.org) provides a network of support for patients on chronic, long-term home enteral and parenteral therapies. Reimbursement for services must be confirmed before sending a patient home on nutrition support. The process can require additional diagnostic testing and documentation in order for the patient to qualify, particularly when Medicare is the source of reimbursement.

Home Enteral Tube Feeding

Patient Selection

Developments in enteral tube feeding formulas and portable, lightweight infusion equipment have simplified home tube feeding and made it easier to manage. As a result, the number of patients receiving home tube feeding continues to grow as a means of cutting hospital costs and allowing earlier family support at home. Success of home infusion of enteral tube feeding relies on the education and training of patient and family.[94]

Teaching Plan

Educating the patient and family for home infusion of enteral tube feeding is a team responsibility. This team may be hospital based or affiliated with the home infusion company that will manage the patient's care after discharge. The RD, nurse, and pharmacist develop and carry out a teaching plan, which includes topics and related tasks in preparing patients and families for discharge on home enteral feeding (Box 19-7).[89] The goal is to promote self-care and monitoring.

The hospital or home infusion company should provide a teaching manual with illustrations to guide the teaching-learning process and to be used as a reference at home. The teaching plan should start as soon as the decision for home tube feeding is made. A social worker identifies and, if possible, resolves any personal, psychosocial, safety, or economic issues with home infusion.

Finally, the teaching plan should allow sufficient time before discharge for the patient and family to demonstrate competency in (1) administering the tube feeding formula and (2) recording all necessary information about formula and fluid intake, formula tolerance, and complications. Directions for recording information are included in the home infusion manual. Records are reviewed regularly by the home nutrition support team and the patient's physician.

Follow-Up Monitoring

The plan for follow-up monitoring should be guided by specific protocols developed by the home infusion provider for laboratory, clinical, and home nutrition assessments. The home nutrition support team checks the patient's progress and works with the patient and family to troubleshoot any problems that arise and make required adjustments in the formula or tube feeding plan. Whenever feasible and appropriate, the RD works closely with the patient and family to transition from tube feeding to oral intake. A study by Silver and colleagues[95] reported older adults receiving home enteral tube feeding with no consistent clinical follow-up experienced complications associated with unscheduled health care visits and readmissions to the hospital. This study demonstrated the potential for improving outcomes with more frequent monitoring, reassessment, and intervention by a home nutrition support team that includes an RD.

BOX 19-7 HOME ENTERAL TUBE FEEDING EDUCATION TOPICS AND TASKS

- Which enteral formulation is used and why
- How to prepare the tube feeding formula for infusion
- How to infuse the formula through the feeding tube
- How to correctly use and troubleshoot problems with the equipment
- How much water and how often to flush the feeding tube
- How to care for the tube site
- How to recognize tube feeding formula intolerance
- How to avoid and treat complications
- How to give medications and other separate nutrients through the feeding tube
- When to call the physician or home infusion provider

Home Parenteral Nutrition

The patient sent home with PN requires education and training on the provision of PN in the outpatient setting. In the hands of knowledgeable and capable patients and their families, home PN allows mobility and independence. Equipment used in the home is small and portable—fitting in a backpack to allow patients to resume normal activities. The patient and family must be trained to use aseptic technique for adding micronutrients and medications to the solution and for accessing the intravenous catheter or port. Special equipment, solutions, and guidelines for training and supervising patients and families have been developed and are successfully used by hundreds of patients. Ongoing assessment of GI function must be performed to determine if the patient is ready to transition to enteral feedings (either oral or via feeding tube). Patients are also monitored closely for the development of complications associated with long-term PN infusion.

A study in complex inflammatory bowel disease patients demonstrated home PN could be successfully used to delay or avoid surgery.[96] The study also found anxiety about managing PN at home decreased for most of the patients after 1 week at home.

HEALTH PROMOTION

TROUBLESHOOTING DIARRHEA IN TUBE-FED PATIENTS

Diarrhea is one of the most common complications associated with tube feeding, yet the reported incidence ranges widely, from as little as 2% to as much as 70% in general patient populations to as high as 80% in ICU patients. Questions that relate to this wide variance and that plague investigators apparently center on definition and cause. However, the ultimate bottom line for patients, their families, and health insurers is the cost of the clinical search for the cause of diarrhea in these patients and the appropriate method of treatment. Although clinicians search for an effective treatment, diarrhea results in reduced energy intake, dehydration, electrolyte abnormalities, and skin breakdown. Diarrhea also causes the patient discomfort, embarrassment, and frustration.

Problem of Definition

If we are ever going to determine an accurate occurrence rate, cause, and treatment of diarrhea, we need a precise operational definition on which to establish a research design and evaluate results. As stated previously, at least 14 definitions exist for diarrhea in the literature. However, little agreement exists concerning which definition most accurately reflects diarrhea that requires intervention. Common definitions include output of more than 500 mL on 2 consecutive days or more than three stools per day. From a nursing standpoint, collection and measurement of stool outputs are much less desirable than tracking number of occurrences. However, the true definition of diarrhea may need to reflect consistency and volume and not just number of stools per 24 hours. Most institutions do not have a standard definition for diarrhea; therefore in most cases, diarrhea is defined by the person cleaning it up. Diagnosis of the cause of diarrhea and subsequent treatment consume time and health care resources. Meanwhile the patient is losing fluid, electrolytes, and nutrients through uncontrolled stool output. This can further exacerbate impaired nutritional status. Diarrhea not only takes a physical and nutritional toll on the patient but also has a psychologic effect of embarrassment and humiliation from an inability to control bodily functions and the loss of privacy.

A recently reported case of unexplained diarrhea in a tube-fed patient illustrates the difficult—and often expensive—search for the cause (see the *Case Study* box, "Case of the Costly Chase").

Factors Contributing to Diarrhea

Reported causes of diarrhea in tube-fed patients also vary. The finger of blame for diarrhea usually is aimed at the tube feeding formula. This results in manipulation of the formula—selection and concentration and infusion methods—usually to no avail because feeding intolerance is generally a manifestation, not the cause, of diarrhea. A variety of causes for diarrhea have been reported. The most common contributors to diarrhea in tube-fed patients are medications or some aspect of the patient's condition. However, many times a combination of events or therapies (not a single contributor) results in diarrhea.[53,54,87–100]

CASE STUDY

Case of the Costly Chase

A reported case of unexplained diarrhea in a tube-fed patient illustrates the difficult, and often costly, search for the cause. Max was a 55-year-old man who had had an aortic aneurysm and underwent emergency surgery to repair it. In the intensive care unit (ICU), the postoperative course was complicated by respiratory problems requiring ventilator assistance. He was administered a bronchodilator drug, theophylline, in tablet form, crushed and administered by nasogastric tube with water. When Max was started on an enteral tube feeding with an isotonic formula, crushed theophylline tablets were changed to a sugar-free theophylline solution. Within a day Max began to have progressive abdominal distention and continuous liquid diarrhea. To rule out an abdominal catastrophe related to the aneurysm or surgery, a computed abdominal tomography scan, an aortogram, and colonoscopy were performed, but all of these studies produced normal results.

Despite stopping the enteral tube feeding, the distention and diarrhea continued. Stool specimens were tested for fecal leukocytes, parasites, and *Clostridium difficile* toxin, and an enteric pathogen culture was prepared. All were nondiagnostic. Extensive additional serum and urine tests, as well as a sigmoidoscopy with rectal biopsy, gave no clue. Then stool electrolytes and osmolality measures suggested an osmotic diarrhea. Because Max was not receiving enteral tube feedings, his physicians thought a secretory bacterial toxin was probably causing continuing diarrhea, so the previous studies were repeated to confirm the osmotic nature of the diarrhea. In addition, all medications were reviewed, but none appeared to be the cause.

Because the continued diarrhea prohibited enteral tube feeding and Max needed to be fed, parenteral nutrition (PN) was ordered. This move immediately brought an automatic nutrition support service consultation, which included assessment of medications. This evaluation revealed that the sugar-free theophylline solution was 65% sorbitol.

Sorbitol is a polyhydric alcohol used as a sweetener in many sugar-free products such as dietetic foods and chewing gum. Because sorbitol is considered an "inactive" ingredient, the package label and insert contained no information about it. Sorbitol content was obtained by contacting the manufacturer.

Fortunately for Max, however, the nutrition support team did know the components of the medication and found the hidden culprit. The registered dietitian (RD) knew sorbitol in larger doses is a laxative! Calculations of the regular daily amount of theophylline Max was taking showed he was receiving nearly 300 g of sorbitol daily when the usual laxative dose was only 20 to 50 g. The nutrition support team immediately recommended that this sorbitol-sweetened solution of theophylline be discontinued and a sorbitol-free form of the medication be used instead. Almost immediately the diarrhea began to decrease, and in 3 days it was gone.

The extent of this costly chase was revealed in Max's hospital bill. He had continued to receive the faulty drug for almost half of his 3-month hospital stay, during which time the diarrhea prevented enteral tube feeding and he had to have the more expensive PN. The PN cost $5000 more than enteral feedings would have cost for the same period. In addition, all the extensive investigations to find the cause of the diarrhea cost $5300, which together with the indirect costs for extra days of care and supplies made a total hospital bill of about $200,000.

Causes of diarrhea in tube-fed patients are many, but in the hands of a skilled nutrition support team, the formula is seldom one of them. It is often found in the medications. Just remember what this medication's hidden ingredient—sorbitol—cost Max.

Data from Wong K: The role of fiber in diarrhea management, *Support Line* 20:16, 1998.

Formula

Tube feeding formula osmolality or concentration and rate of delivery are often blamed for instigating diarrhea. However, reports have shown no increase in incidence of diarrhea when the formula concentration varied widely from 145 to 430 mOsm/L, and no significant association has been made between malabsorption and formula osmolality or rate of delivery. Formulas providing more than 30% of total kcalories as fat have been associated with an increased incidence of diarrhea, whereas those providing 20% fat rarely were involved. Further study of fat composition is needed, specifically comparing medium-chain triglycerides (MCT) versus long chain triglycerides (LCT) and omega-3 versus omega-6 fatty acids. Studies of the role of fiber in tube feedings have had conflicting results. No consistency is seen in the types and amount of fiber in enteral tube feeding formulas. Soluble fiber can increase colonic absorption of water. However, when the fiber given to a patient is increased rapidly, the patient will experience flatulence, abdominal distention, and constipation. Reviewers have found the studies thus far have been few, models used variable, limitations substantial, and conclusions of investigators mixed. In general, amount and type of fiber in enteral formulas are not significant enough to prevent or contribute to diarrhea.[53,54,97–100]

Bacterial Contamination

Studies have shown the more manipulation and additives, such as modular components, that are added to an enteral formula, the more likely the formula will become contaminated. Tube feeding formula hang time, open versus closed delivery systems, and preparation technique can affect the risk of bacterial contamination of the enteral tube feeding formula. Formula added to open delivery systems should hang no longer than 8 hours (even shorter periods of time if additives are combined with the formula). Closed systems that use containers prefilled with formula can hang 24 to 48 hours. The fewer times any system is handled and opened, the less chance exists for contamination. Commercial formula manufacturers are making formulas now that contain microbial inhibitors to reduce the risk of bacterial contamination of the enteral formula itself.[53,54,97–100]

Infusion Method

Intragastric feedings are associated with an increased incidence of diarrhea. Infusion of a large amount of energy into the stomach stimulates the colon to secret water, sodium, and chloride with resulting inability of the colon to absorb nutrients.[53,54,97–100]

Patient's Condition

Malnourished or critically ill patients are more susceptible to mucosal tissue breakdown and malabsorption leading to diarrhea. Hypoalbuminemia has also been reported to be a potential cause of diarrhea because of its effect on reducing colloidal osmotic pressure within blood vessels, which could lead to edema of the intestinal mucosa, malabsorption, and diarrhea. However, no correlation has been found between patients with hypoalbuminemia and incidence of diarrhea. Patients with pancreatic insufficiency, celiac disease, short-bowel syndrome, fecal impaction, diabetes mellitus, or GI inflammation are at increased risk for diarrhea.[53,54,97–100]

Medications

Multiple medications routinely given to hospitalized patients have been related to diarrhea. Antibiotics are most often associated with GI side effects. However, patients more susceptible to developing diarrhea are those who are critically ill and on multiple medications. Extensive treatment with antibiotics and disuse of the GI tract contribute to a change in the bacterial milieu of the intestine, with proliferation of the enteric pathogen *Clostridium difficile.* Other medications associated with development of diarrhea are H_2-blockers, lactulose or laxatives, magnesium-containing antacids, potassium and phosphorus supplements, antineoplastic agents, and quinidine. Medications are often hyperosmolar and require dilution before infusion through a feeding tube. In general, drug reactions may relate to the metabolically active agent or to another ingredient added for its physical properties in the form of the drug, such as tablet or liquid (as the case in the *Case Study* box illustrates). Probiotics, nonpathogenic lactic acid bacteria, are receiving more attention as a potential treatment of diarrhea and as a means of preventing bacterial overgrowth and *C. difficile* infections.[53,54,97–100]

TO SUM UP

For patients with functioning GI tracts, EN support has proved to be a potent tool against present or potential malnutrition. EN support is achieved by an oral diet with nutrient-dense supplementation or alternately by tube feeding when the patient cannot, will not, or should not eat. Commercial tube feeding formulas with or without modular enhancement provide complete nutrition when provided in adequate amounts. Enteral tube feeding can be provided through nasoenteric or enterostomy feeding tubes with an open or closed delivery system. Tubing and container adaptations and development of small, mobile infusion pumps, together with a comprehensive teaching plan for patient and family and follow-up monitoring by a clinical team, allow many patients the option of home tube feeding.

For patients with a dysfunctional GI tract, PN is a life-sustaining therapy. This feeding method depends heavily on biomedical technology for the development of tubes, bags, pumps, and other equipment for feeding nutrients directly into the vein. Route of entry may be a large central vein for intravenous feeding over a long period or a smaller peripheral vein for feeding less-concentrated solutions for a shorter period. Home PN is successfully used by many patients with the support of family, friends, and a home nutrition support team.

QUESTIONS FOR REVIEW

1. Describe several types of patient situations in which enteral tube feeding may be indicated. What nutrition assessment procedures may help to identify these individuals?
2. Describe nutrient components of a typical complete polymeric enteral formula. How does it differ from a modular formula? How does it differ from a semielemental and an elemental formula?
3. Define PN, and identify examples of conditions in which it would be used.

The following questions apply to the case of a man referred to nutrition support services. Imagine you are caring for this patient.

> A previously healthy 45-year-old man, while on a long transport haul as a truck driver, was in an accident in which he sustained a severe abdominal injury requiring extensive surgical repair and leaving the GI tract unavailable for use for an undetermined period. He is referred to the nutrition support team for PN. Early in this care he asks you how this feeding works.

4. How would you describe and explain the PN feeding process?
5. What nutrition assessment parameters would be beneficial in identifying his risk of developing malnutrition and his tolerance of parenteral therapy?
6. List typical components of a basic PN formula he may require, and describe the purpose of each to help reassure him of its adequacy and importance.
7. Sufficient energy (kcalorie) intake is essential to immediately meet his metabolic needs after surgery. Assume a normal preinjury weight (175 lb) and height (70 inches) and an added stress factor of 1.2 times his BEE. Calculate his total energy requirement, using the Harris-Benedict equation and the Mifflin-St. Jeor equation. Compare the results.
8. Define hepatic proteins, and describe why they are not appropriate indicators of nutritional status. How can you monitor the effectiveness of the PN formula in meeting his nutrition support needs for recovery?

REFERENCES

1. Borum PR: Nutrient metabolism. In Gottschlich MM, Fuhrman T, Hammond K, et al, editors: *The science and practice of nutrition support: a case-based core curriculum*, Dubuque, Iowa, 2001, Kendall/Hunt Publishing.
2. Butterworth CE: The skeleton in the hospital closet, *Nutr Today* 9:4, 1974.
3. Bistrian BR, Blackburn GL, Hallowell E, et al: Protein status of general surgical patients, *JAMA* 230:858, 1974.
4. Naber T, Schermer T, de Bree A, et al: Prevalence of malnutrition in nonsurgical hospitalized patients and its association with disease complications, *Am J Clin Nutr* 66:1232, 1997.
5. Detsky AS, McLaughlin JR, Baker JP, et al: What is subjective global assessment of nutritional status? *JPEN J Parenter Enteral Nutr* 11(1):8, 1987.
6. Braunschweig C, Gomez S, Sheean PM, et al: Impact of declines in nutritional status on outcomes in adult patients hospitalized for more than seven days, *J Am Diet Assoc* 100:1316, 2000.
7. A.S.P.E.N. Board of Directors and the Clinical Guidelines Task Force: Guidelines for the use of parenteral and enteral nutrition in adult and pediatric patients, *JPEN J Parenter Enteral Nutr* 26:1SA, 2002.
8. Moore FA, Feliciano DV, Andrassy RJ, et al: Early enteral feeding, compared with parenteral, reduces postoperative septic complications: the results of a meta-analysis, *Ann Surg* 216:172, 1992.
9. Lipman TO: Grains or veins: is enteral nutrition really better than parenteral nutrition? A look at the evidence, *JPEN J Parenter Enteral Nutr* 22:167, 1998.
10. Shopbell JM, Hopkins JB, Shronts EP, et al: Nutrition screening and assessment. In Gottschlich MM, Fuhrman T, Hammond K, et al, editors: *The science and practice of nutrition support: a case-based core curriculum*, Dubuque, Iowa, 2001, Kendall/Hunt Publishing.
11. Lacey K, Pritchett E: Nutrition care process and model: ADA adopts road map to quality care and outcomes management, *J Am Diet Assoc* 103:1061, 2003.
12. Fuhrman MP, Charney P, Mueller CM, et al: Hepatic proteins and nutrition assessment, *J Am Diet Assoc* 104:1258, 2004.
13. Reference deleted in proofs.
14. Mifflin MD, St. Jeor ST. Hill LA, et al: A new predictive equation for resting energy expenditure in healthy individuals, *Am J Clin Nutr* 51(2):241, 1990.
15. Frankenfield DC, Rowe WA, Smith JS, et al: Validation of several established equations for resting metabolic rate in obese and nonobese people, *J Am Diet Assoc* 103:1152, 2003.
16. Crook MA, Hally V, Panteli JV, et al: The importance of the refeeding syndrome, *Nutrition* 17:632, 2001.
17. Vanek VW: The use of serum albumin as a prognostic or nutritional marker and the pros and cons of IV albumin therapy, *Nutr Clin Pract* 13:110, 1998.
18. Meyer J, Lund D, Smith J, et al: Benefits of a nutrition support service in an HMO setting, *Nutr Clin Pract* 16:25, 2001.
19. American Society for Parenteral and Enteral Nutrition Board of Directors: Standards of practice for nutrition support nurses, *Nutr Clin Pract* 16:56, 2001.
20. American Society for Parenteral and Enteral Nutrition Board of Directors: Standards of practice for nutrition support pharmacists, *Nutr Clin Pract* 14:275, 1999.
21. American Society for Parenteral and Enteral Nutrition Board of Directors: Standards of practice for nutrition support physicians, *Nutr Clin Pract* 18:270, 2003.
22. American Society for Parenteral and Enteral Nutrition Board of Directors: Standards of practice for nutrition support dietitians, *Nutr Clin Pract* 15:53, 2000.
23. Board of Directors, American Society for Parenteral and Enteral Nutrition: Interdisciplinary nutrition support core competencies, *Nutr Clin Pract* 14:331, 1999.

24. JCAHO Board of Directors: *Comprehensive accreditation manual for hospitals*, Oakbrook Terrace, Ill, 2000, Joint Commission on Accreditation of Healthcare Organizations.
25. Fuhrman MP: Parenteral nutrition: a clinician's perspective, *Dietitians Edge* 2(1):53, 2001.
26. Charney P: Enteral nutrition: indications, options and formulations. In Gottschlich MM, Fuhrman T, Hammond K, et al, editors: *The science and practice of nutrition support: a case-based core curriculum*, Dubuque, Iowa, 2001, Kendall/Hunt Publishing.
27. Roth JL, Clohessy S: Administration of enteral nutrition: initiation, progression, and transition. In Rolandelli RH, editor: *Clinical nutrition: enteral and tube feeding*, ed 4, Philadelphia, 2005, Saunders.
28. Veterans Affairs Total Parenteral Nutrition Cooperative Study Group: Perioperative total parenteral nutrition in surgical patients, *N Engl J Med* 325:525, 1992.
29. Jeejeebhoy KN: Total parenteral nutrition: potion or poison? *Am J Clin Nutr* 74:160, 2001.
30. Lewis DA, Boyle K: Nutritional supplement use during medication administration: selected case studies, *J Nutr Elder* 17(4):53, 1998.
31. Turic A, Gordon KL, Craig LD, et al: Nutrition supplementation enables elderly residents in long-term care facilities to meet or exceed RDAs without displacing energy or nutrient intakes from meals, *J Am Diet Assoc* 98:1457, 1998.
32. Watters JM, Kirkpatrick SM, Norris SB, et al: Immediate postoperative enteral feeding results in impaired respiratory mechanics and decreased mobility, *Ann Surg* 266:369, 1997.
33. Charney P, Russell M: Enteral formulations: standard. In Rolandelli RH, editor: *Clinical nutrition: enteral and tube feeding*, ed 4, Philadelphia, 2005, Saunders.
34. Matarese LE, Seidner DL, Steiger E, et al: The role of probiotics in gastrointestinal disease, *Nutr Clin Pract* 18:507, 2003.
35. Gadek JE, DeMichele SJ, Karlstad MD, et al: Effect of enteral feeding with eicosapentaenoic acid, α-linolenic acid, and antioxidants in patients with acute respiratory distress syndrome, *Crit Care Med* 27:1409, 1999.
36. Consensus recommendations from the U.S. Summit on Immune-Enhancing Enteral Therapy, *JPEN J Parenter Enteral Nutr* 25:S61, 2001.
37. Reference deleted in proofs.
38. Metheny NA, Clouse RE: Bedside methods for detecting aspiration in tube-fed patients, *Chest* 111:724, 1997.
39. Maloney JP, Halbower AC, Fouty BF, et al: Systemic absorption of food dye in patients with sepsis, *N Engl J Med* 343:1047, 2000.
40. Maloney JP, Ryan TA: Detection of aspiration in enterally fed patients: a requiem for bedside monitors of aspiration, *JPEN J Parenter Enteral Nutr* 26:S34, 2002.
41. Cannon R, et al: *Methods and tubes for establishing enteral access: discussion. Enteral nutrition support for the 1990s: innovations in nutrition, technology, and techniques*, Columbus, Ohio, 1992, Ross Products Division, Abbott Laboratories.
42. Moore MC, editor: Enteral nutrition. *Mosby's pocket guide series: nutritional care*, ed 4, St Louis, 2001, Mosby.
43. Metheny NA, Stewart BJ, Smith L, et al: pH and concentration of bilirubin in feeding tube aspirates as predictors of tube placement, *Nurs Res* 48(4):189, 1999.
44. Metheny N, Eisenberg P, McSweeney M, et al: Effect of feeding tube properties and three irrigants on clogging rates, *Nurs Res* 37:165, 1988.
45. Sriram K, Jayanthi V, Lakshmi RG, et al: Prophylactic locking of enteral feeding tubes with pancreatic enzymes, *JPEN J Parenter Enteral Nutr* 21(6):353, 1997.
46. Marian M, Carlson SJ: Enteral formulations. In A.S.P.E.N, Merritt R, DeLegge MH, Holcombe B, et al, editors: *A.S.P.E.N. nutrition support practice manual*, Silver Spring, Md, 2005, American Society for Parenteral and Enteral Nutrition.
47. Vanek VW: Closed versus open enteral delivery systems: a quality improvement study, *Nutr Clin Pract* 15:234, 2000.
48. Herlick SJ, Vogt C, Pangman V, et al: Comparison of open versus closed systems of intermittent enteral feeding in two long-term care facilities, *Nutr Clin Pract* 15:287, 2000.
49. Keohane PP, Attrill H, Love M, et al: Relation between osmolarity of the diet and gastrointestinal side effects in enteral nutrition, *BJM* 288:678, 1984.
50. Lysen LK: Enteral equipment. In Matarese LE, Gottschlich MM, editors: *Contemporary nutrition support practice: a clinical guide*, ed 2, Philadelphia, 2003, Saunders.
51. Ibáñaez J, Peñafiel A, Raurich JM, et al: Gastroesophageal reflux in intubated patients receiving enteral nutrition: effect of supine and semirecumbent positions, *JPEN J Parenter Enteral Nutr* 16:419, 1992.
52. Cogen R, Weinryb J, Pomerantz C, et al: Complications of jejunostomy tube feeding in nursing facility patients, *Am J Gastroenterol* 86:1610, 1991.
53. Mobarhan S, Demeo M: Diarrhea induced by enteral feeding, *Nutr Rev* 53:67, 1995.
54. Fuhrman MP: Diarrhea and tube feeding, *Nutr Clin Pract* 14:83, 1999.
55. Kirby DF, Delegge MH, Fleming CR, et al: American Gastroenterological Association technical review on tube feeding for enteral nutrition, *Gastroenterology* 108:1282, 1995.
56. McClave SA, Snider HL, Lowen CC, et al: Use of residual volume as a marker for enteral feeding tolerance: prospective, blinded comparison with physical examination and radiographic findings, *JPEN J Parenter Enteral Nutr* 16(2):99, 1992.
57. Pinilla JC, Samphire J, Arnold C, et al: Comparison of gastrointestinal tolerance to two enteral feeding protocols in critically ill patients: a prospective, randomized trial, *JPEN J Parenter Enteral Nutr* 25:81, 2001.
58. Heyland DK, Dhaliwal R, Drover JW, et al: Canadian clinical practice guidelines for nutrition support in mechanically ventilated, critically ill adult patients, *JPEN J Parenter Enteral Nutr* 27:355, 2003.
59. Mateo MA: Nursing management of enteral tube feeding, *Heart Lung* 25:318, 1996.
60. Spain DA, McClave SA, Sexton LK, et al: Infusion protocol improves delivery of enteral tube feeding in the critical care unit, *JPEN J Parenter Enteral Nutr* 23:288, 1999.
61. Heyland DK, Dhaliwal R, Day A, et al: Validation of the Canadian clinical practice guidelines for nutrition support in mechanically ventilated, critically ill adult patients: results of a prospective observational study, *Crit Care Med* 32:2260, 2004.
62. van den Berghe G, Wouters P, Weekers F, et al: Intensive insulin therapy in critically ill patients, *N Engl J Med* 345:1359, 2001.
63. Krinsley JS: Effect of an intensive glucose management protocol on the mortality of critically ill adult patients, *Mayo Clin Proc* 79:992, 2004.
64. Fuhrman MP: Complication management in parenteral nutrition. In Matarese LE, Gottschlich MM, editors: *Contemporary nutrition support practice: a clinical guide*, ed 2 Philadelphia, 2003, Saunders.

65. Mirtallo JM: Introduction to parenteral nutrition. In Gottschlich MM, Fuhrman T, Hammond K, et al, editors: *The science and practice of nutrition support: a case-based core curriculum*, Dubuque, Iowa, 2001, Kendall/Hunt Publishing.
66. Dudrick SJ, Wilmore DW, Vars HM, et al: Can intravenous feeding as the sole means of nutrition support growth in the child and restore weight loss in an adult? *Ann Surg* 169:974, 1969.
67. Klein S, Kinney J, Jeejeebhoy K, et al: Nutrition support in clinical practice: review of published data on recommendations for future directions, *JPEN J Parenter Enter Nutr* 21(3):133, 1997.
68. Stokes MA, Hill GL: Peripheral parenteral nutrition: a preliminary report on its efficacy and safety, *JPEN J Parenter Enteral Nutr* 17(2):145, 1993.
69. Trujillo ED, Young LS, Chertow GM, et al: Metabolic and monetary costs of avoidable parenteral nutrition use, *JPEN J Parenter Enteral Nutr* 23:109, 1999.
70. Speerhas RA: Five year follow-up of a program to minimize inappropriate use of parenteral nutrition, *JPEN J Parenter Enteral Nutr* 25:S4, 2001.
71. Tulsyan N, Abkin AD, Storch KJ, et al: Enterocutaneous fistulas, *Nutr Clin Pract* 16:74, 2001.
72. Byrne TA, Veglia L, Celio M, et al: Beyond the prescription: optimizing the diet of patients with short bowel syndrome, *Nutr Clin Pract* 15:306, 2000.
73. Spain DA, McClave SA: Chylothorax and chylous ascites. In Gottschlich MM, Fuhrman T, Hammond K, et al, editors: *The science and practice of nutrition support: a case-based core curriculum*, Dubuque, Iowa, 2001, Kendall/Hunt Publishing.
74. Kelly DG, Nehra V: Gastrointestinal disease. In Gottschlich MM, Fuhrman T, Hammond K, et al, editors: *The science and practice of nutrition support: a case-based core curriculum*, Dubuque, Iowa, 2001, Kendall/ Hunt Publishing.
75. Task force for the revision of safe practices for parenteral nutrition, et al: Safe practices for parenteral nutrition, *JPEN J Parenter Enteral Nutr* 28(Suppl):S39, 2004.
76. Seidner DL, Mascioli EA, Istfan NW, et al: Effect of long-chain triglyceride emulsions on reticuloendothelial system function in humans, *JPEN J Parenter Enteral Nutr* 13:614, 1989.
77. American Medical Association, AMA Department of Foods and Nutrition: Multivitamin preparations for parenteral use: a statement by the Nutrition Advisory Group, *JPEN J Parenter Enteral Nutr* 3:258, 1979.
78. Parenteral multivitamin products; drugs for human use; drug efficacy study implementation; amendment (21 CFR 5.70), *Fed Regist* 65:21200, 2000.
79. Expert Panel for Nutrition Advisory Group, AMA Department of Foods and Nutrition: Guidelines for essential trace element preparations for parenteral use, *JAMA* 241:2051, 1979.
80. Forceville X, Vitoux D, Gauzit R, et al: Selenium, systemic immune response syndrome, sepsis, and outcome in critically ill patients, *Crit Care Med* 26:1536, 1998.
81. Angstwurm MAW, Schottdorf J, Schopohl J, et al: Selenium replacement in patients with severe systemic inflammatory response syndrome improves clinical outcome, *Crit Care Med* 27:1807, 1999.
82. Cohen HJ, Brown MR, Hamilton D, et al: Glutathione peroxidase and selenium deficiency in patients receiving home parenteral nutrition: time course for development of deficiency and repletion of the enzyme activity in plasma and blood cells, *Am J Clin Nutr* 49:132, 1989.
83. Fuhrman MP, Herrmann V, Masidonski P, et al: Pancytopenia following removal of copper from TPN, *JPEN J Parenter Enteral Nutr* 24:361, 2000.
84. Masumoto K, Suita S, Taguchi T, et al: Manganese intoxication during intermittent parenteral nutrition: report of two cases, *JPEN J Parenter Enteral Nutr* 25:95, 2001.
85. Pemberton L, Lyman B, Lander V, et al: Sepsis from triple- vs single-lumen catheters during total parenteral nutrition in surgical or critically ill patients, *Arch Surg* 121:591, 1986.
86. Farkas J, Liu N, Bier P, et al: Single-versus-triple-lumen central–catheter-related sepsis: a prospective randomized study in a critically ill population, *Am J Med* 93:277, 1992.
87. Savage AP, Picard M, Hopkins CC, et al: Complications and survival of multilumen central venous catheters used for total parenteral nutrition, *Br J Surg* 80:1287, 1993.
88. Maki DG, Stolz SM, Wheler S, et al: Prevention of central venous catheter-related bloodstream infection by use of an antiseptic-impregnated catheter: a randomized, controlled trial, *Ann Intern Med* 127:257, 1997.
89. Veenstra DL, Saint S, Sullivan SD, et al: Cost-effectiveness of antiseptic-impregnated central venous catheters for the prevention of catheter-related bloodstream infection, *J Am Med Assoc* 282:554, 1999.
90. Centers for Disease Control and Prevention: Guidelines for the prevention of intravascular catheter-related infections, *MMWR Morb Mortal Wkly Rep* 51(RR-10):1, 2002.
91. Intravenous Nurses Society: Infusion nursing standards of practice, *J Intraven Nurs* 23(Suppl 6):S1, 2000.
92. Dodds ES, Murray JD, Texler KM, et al: Metabolic occurrences in total parenteral nutrition patients managed by a nutrition support team, *Nutr Clin Pract* 16:78, 2001.
93. Klein CJ, Stanek GS, Wiles CE, et al: Nutrition support care map targets monitoring and reassessment to improve outcomes in trauma patients, *Nutr Clin Pract* 16:85, 2001.
94. American Society for Parenteral and Enteral Nutrition Board of Directors: Standards for home nutrition support, *Nutr Clin Pract* 14:151, 1998.
95. Silver HJ, Wellman NS, Arnold DJ, et al: Older adults receiving home enteral nutrition: enteral regimen, provider involvement, and health care outcomes, *JPEN J Parenter Enteral Nutr* 28:92, 2004.
96. Evans JP, Steinhart AH, Cohen Z, et al: Home total parenteral nutrition: an alternative to early surgery for complicated inflammatory bowel disease, *J Gastrointest Surg* 7:562, 2003.
97. Bowling TE: Enteral-feeding-related diarrhea: proposed causes and possible solutions, *Proc Nutr Soc* 54:579, 1995.
98. Ringel AF, Jameson GL, Foster ES: Diarrhea in the intensive care patient, *Crit Care Clin North Am* 11:465, 1995.
99. Wong K: The role of fiber in diarrhea management, *Support Line* 20:16, 1998.
100. Williams MS, Harpter R, Magnuson B, et al: Diarrhea management in enterally fed patient, *Nutr Clin Pract* 13:225, 1998.
101. A.S.P.E.N.: Definition of terms, style and conventions used in A.S.P.E.N. guidelines and standards, *Nutr Clin Pract* 20:281, 2005.
102. 21 U.S.C. 360ee: Grants and contracts for development of drugs for rare diseases and conditions, 2007.

FURTHER READINGS AND RESOURCES

Readings

American Society for Parenteral and Enteral Nutrition Board of Directors and Task Force on Standards for Specialized Nutrition Support of Hospitalized Adult Patients, Standards for Specialized Nutrition Support: Adult hospitalized patients, *Nutr Clin Pract* 17:384, 2002.

A.S.P.E.N. Board of Directors and the Clinical Guidelines Task Force: Guidelines for the use of parenteral and enteral nutrition in adult and pediatric patients, *JPEN J Parenter Enteral Nutr* 26(Suppl):1SA, 2002.

Heyland DK, Dhaliwal R, Drover JW, et al: Canadian clinical practice guidelines for nutrition support in mechanically ventilated, critically ill adult patients, *JPEN J Parenter Enteral Nutr* 27:355, 2003.

Task Force for the Revision of Safe Practices for Parenteral Nutrition and the A.S.P.E.N. Board of Directors: Safe practices for parenteral nutrition, *JPEN J Parenter Enteral Nutr* 28(Suppl):S30, 2004.

Websites of Interest

The American Society for Parenteral and Enteral Nutrition (A.S.P.E.N.). An interdisciplinary organization involved in provision of clinical nutrition therapies including parenteral and enteral nutrition: www.nutritioncare.org.

American Dietetic Association. The world's largest organization of food and nutrition professionals committed to improving the nation's health and advancing the profession of dietetics through research, education, and advocacy: www.eatright.org.

CIGNA Medicare. This site offers free Medicare training for clinicians regarding Medicare qualifications for home enteral and parenteral nutrition: www.cignamedicare.com/webtraining.

Dietitians in Nutrition Support. Dietetic practitioners integrating the science of enteral and parenteral nutrition to provide appropriate nutrition support to individuals in inpatient and outpatient settings: www.dnsdpg.org.

The Oley Foundation. This non-profit organization provides information and psychosocial support of consumers of home parenteral and enteral nutrition: www.oley.org.

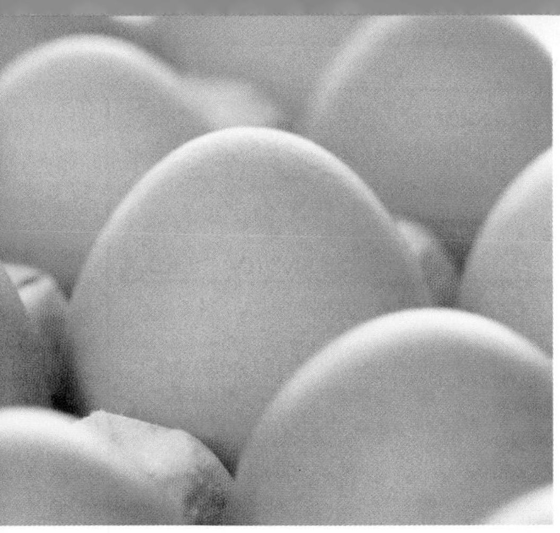

20

Gastrointestinal Diseases

Sara Long Roth

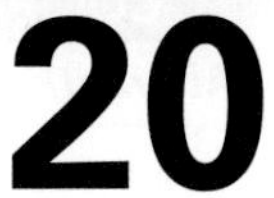

http://evolve.elsevier.com/Williams/essentials/

OUTLINE

In this chapter, we consider diseases of the gastrointestinal (GI) tract and surrounding accessory organs—liver, gallbladder, and pancreas. In health, digestion and absorption of food are accomplished through a series of intimately interrelated actions among and within these organ systems. To the extent disease or malfunction at any point interferes with this finely interwoven process, adequate nutrition is provided either through quantitative or qualitative modifications to food.

The GI tract is a sensitive mirror of the individual human condition. Its physiologic function often reflects physical and psychologic conditioning. In this chapter, these basic functions, healing process, nutrition therapy indicated, and individuals' personal needs will be discussed. The Complementary and Alternative Medicine box, "Alternative Treatments for Diseases of the Gastrointestinal Tract," outlines the effectiveness of alternative treatments for diseases of the GI tract.

DIGESTIVE PROCESS

When food is taken into the mouth, the act of eating stimulates the GI tract into accelerated action. Throughout the digestive process, highly coordinated systems and interactive functions respond (Figure 20-1). Secretory functions provide the necessary environment and agents for chemical digestion. *Peristalsis* and gravity move the food mass along. Nutrients are absorbed into circulation and carried to cells that take up what is needed to nourish the body. Emotional factors influence overall individual response pattern. This highly individual and interrelated functional network forms the basis for nutrition therapy in disease.

After food is taken into the mouth and masticated (forming a bolus), swallowing occurs, allowing the bolus to pass from the laryngopharynx into the esophagus entrance at the upper esophageal sphincter (UES) (Figure 20-2). Food is pushed through the esophagus by gravity and involuntary muscular movements, called *peristalsis,* controlled by the medulla oblongata. Circular muscle fibers contract, constricting the esophageal wall and squeezing the bolus toward the stomach. The lower esophageal sphincter (LES) muscle at the entry to the stomach forms a controlling valve, relaxing to receive the bolus and then closing to hold each bolus for some initial digestive action of enzymes. Stomach cells produce enzymes to partially break down food particles and other secretions to protect themselves from being broken down. Passage of food from mouth to stomach takes about 4 to 8 seconds.

Chyme (semiliquid mass) is released by the stomach through the pyloric sphincter into the duodenum, the first section of the small intestine, where most digestion occurs. A number of small intestine and accessory organ conditions may interfere with normal food passage and digestive processes and create malabsorption problems. These overall conditions vary widely from brief periods of functional discomfort to serious disease and complete obstruction. In making nutrition therapy recommendations for food choices and feeding mode, the dietetics practitioner will take into account the degree of dysfunction.

COMPLEMENTARY AND ALTERNATIVE MEDICINE (CAM)

Alternative Treatments for Diseases of the Gastrointestinal Tract

What Is Known from the Scientific Evidence about CAM Modalities for Gastrointestinal Disorders?

No well-documented herbal treatments exist for gastrointestinal (GI) disorders, although use of probiotics to treat Crohn's disease shows some promise.

What CAM Therapies Might Be Used to Treat Gastrointestinal Disorders?

GASTROINTESTINAL DISORDER	HERB	SCIENTIFIC NAME	ACTIVE INGREDIENT	EFFICACY	SIDE EFFECTS AND/OR RISKS
Cirrhosis	Milk thistle (plant)	*Silybum marianum*	Silymarin (found in the fruit)	Results are inconsistent.	It is generally well tolerated but can cause laxative effects and allergic reactions in people allergic to ragweed, chrysanthemum, marigold, and daisy.
Crohn's disease	Fish oil	Docosahexaenoic acid (DHA), eicosapentaenoic acid (EPA), omega-3 fatty acids, omega-3 oils		Results are mixed as to whether or not fish oil helped keep the disease controlled in patients who were in remission.	Possible risk of bleeding complications.
Dyspepsia	Curcumin	*Curcuma longa*	Polyphenol	It stimulates contraction of the gallbladder; it provides full or partial relief of symptoms.	It could present risks in individuals with gallbladder disease. Maximum safe doses in individuals with severe hepatic or renal disease are not known.
Hepatitis C virus (HCV)	Milk thistle (plant)	*Silybum marianum*	Silymarin (found in the fruit)	Although some benefits might be seen, none are definitively beneficial in treating HCV.	See above.
	Licorice root (plant)	*Glycyrrhiza glabra*	Glycyrrhizin	It might have antiviral properties in vitro and has the potential for reducing long-term complications of chronic HCV in patients who do not respond to interferon. It does not reduce the amount of HCV in patients' blood.	Licorice intake over a long period of time can lead to hypertension, salt and water retention, swelling, depletion of potassium, headache, and/or sluggishness. In addition, it can worsen ascites and can interact with certain drugs (diuretics, digitalis, antiarrhythmic agents, and corticosteroids) (see Chapter 18).
	Thymus extract (gland)	(Should not be confused with the prescription drug thymosin α_1)	Peptides from thymus glands of cows or calves sold as dietary supplements	Very little research exists, but no studies found the product beneficial for patients with HCV.	Thrombocytopenia (a drop in number of platelet cells in blood) is possible. Concern exists regarding possible contamination from diseased animal parts (people on immunosuppressive drugs should use caution).
	Schisandra (plant)	*Schisandra chinensis, S. sphenanthera*	Extracts from its fruits	Some antioxidant effects are possible. No reports exist regarding the safety and effectiveness of using schisandra alone to treat HCV in humans.	It is found as an ingredient in herbal formulas and considered generally safe. In some patients it may cause heartburn, acid indigestion, decreased appetite, stomach pain, or allergic skin rashes.
	Colloidal silver	Silver	Metallic element	Silver has no known function in the human body and is not an essential mineral supplement. Claims of silver "deficiency" in the body are unfounded.	Silver builds up in body tissues: argyria—a bluish gray discoloration of the body, especially skin, other organs, deep tissues, nails, and gums. Argyria is not treatable or reversible. Other possible complications include neurologic problems (e.g., seizures), kidney damage, stomach distress, headaches, fatigue, and skin irritation. It might interfere with absorption of the following drugs: penicillamine, quinolones, tetracyclines, and thyroxine.

COMPLEMENTARY AND ALTERNATIVE MEDICINE (CAM)

Alternative Treatments for Diseases of the Gastrointestinal Tract—cont'd

GASTROINTESTINAL DISORDER	HERB	SCIENTIFIC NAME	ACTIVE INGREDIENT	EFFICACY	SIDE EFFECTS AND/OR RISKS
Irritable bowel syndrome (IBS)	Peppermint oil	*Menthe piperita*	Menthol	It provides antispasmodic properties and might provide some relief from crampy abdominal pain.	Enteric-coated peppermint is believed to be reasonably safe in healthy adults; nonenteric-coated peppermint oil can cause heartburn. Maximum doses in individuals with severe hepatic or renal disease is not known.
	Probiotics	*Lactobacillus plantarum*	Acidophilus	Evidence of efficacy is mixed; it might reduce intestinal gas and pain.	No known safety issues exist.
	Flaxseed	*Linum usitatissimum*	Lignans, α-linolenic acid	It helps relieve constipation, abdominal pain, and bloating.	It is not associated with any significant adverse effects.
Nausea	Ginger	*Zingiber officinale*		It is as effective for motion sickness as standard pharmaceutical agents. In addition, it is effective in reducing nausea in pregnancy.	No drug interactions are known. Ginger should be used with care in patients using anticoagulant or antiplatelet agents.
Peptic ulcer disease (PUD)	Licorice, deglycyrrhizinated (DGL)	*Glycyrrhiza glabra*	DGL is a specially processed form of licorice that does not produce pseudohyperaldosteronemia.	No evidence indicates that DGL eradicates *Helicobacter pylori*; it may protect gastric lining from NSAID-induced gastritis. It is no more effective than antacids in providing relief.	It may reduce testosterone levels in men. The maximum safe doses in those with severe hepatic or renal disease is not known. Licorice appears to potentiate topical and oral corticosteroids. It should be used with caution in patients taking thiazide or loop diuretics and/or digitalis.
	Probiotics	*Lactobacillus plantarum*	Acidophilus	It exerts inhibitory action on *H. pylori* but not enough to eradicate the bacterium. It may be a useful adjunct to standard antibiotic therapy.	See above.
Ulcerative colitis (UC)	Probiotics	*Escherichia coli* spp.	Nonpathogenic strain of *E. coli*	It can prevent acute attacks of UC as effectively as mesalazine.	See above.
	Essential fatty acids	DHA, EPA, omega-3 fatty acids, omega-3 oils	Fish oils	It might be helpful for reducing symptoms of UC; regular use does not appear to help prevent disease flare-ups.	See above.
	Essential fatty acids	Omega-6 fatty acid GLA	Evening primrose oil	Somewhat beneficial in preventing flare-ups.	See above.

Data from National Center for Complementary and Alternative Medicine: *CAM and hepatitis C: a focus on herbal supplements,* NCCAM Pub No D422, Bethesda, Md, 2008, NCCAM. Retrieved May 14, 2009, from www.nccam.nih.gov/health/hepatitisc/; Bratman S, Girman AM: *Mosby's handbook of herbs and supplements and their therapeutic use,* St Louis, 2003, Mosby.
NSAID, Nonsteroidal antiinflammatory drug; *GLA,* γ-linolenic acid.

PROBLEMS OF THE MOUTH AND ESOPHAGUS

Mouth Problems

Teeth and jaw muscles in the mouth work together to break down food into a form that can be easily swallowed. Conditions that interfere with this process interfere with nutritional intake.

Tissue Inflammation

Tissues of the mouth often reflect a person's basic nutritional status. In malnutrition, tissues of the mouth deteriorate and become inflamed and are more vulnerable to local infection or injury, causing pain and difficulty with eating. These conditions (Figure 20-3) in the oral cavity include (1) *gingivitis,* inflammation of the gums, involving the mucous membrane with its supporting fibrous tissue circling the base of the teeth (see Figure 20-3, *A*); (2) *stomatitis,* inflammation of the oral mucosa lining the mouth (see Figure 20-3, *B*); (3) *glossitis,* inflammation of the tongue (see Figure 20-3, *C*); and (4) *cheilosis,* a cracking and dry scaling process at the corners of the mouth affecting the lips and corner angles, making opening the mouth to receive food difficult (see Figure 20-3, *D*).

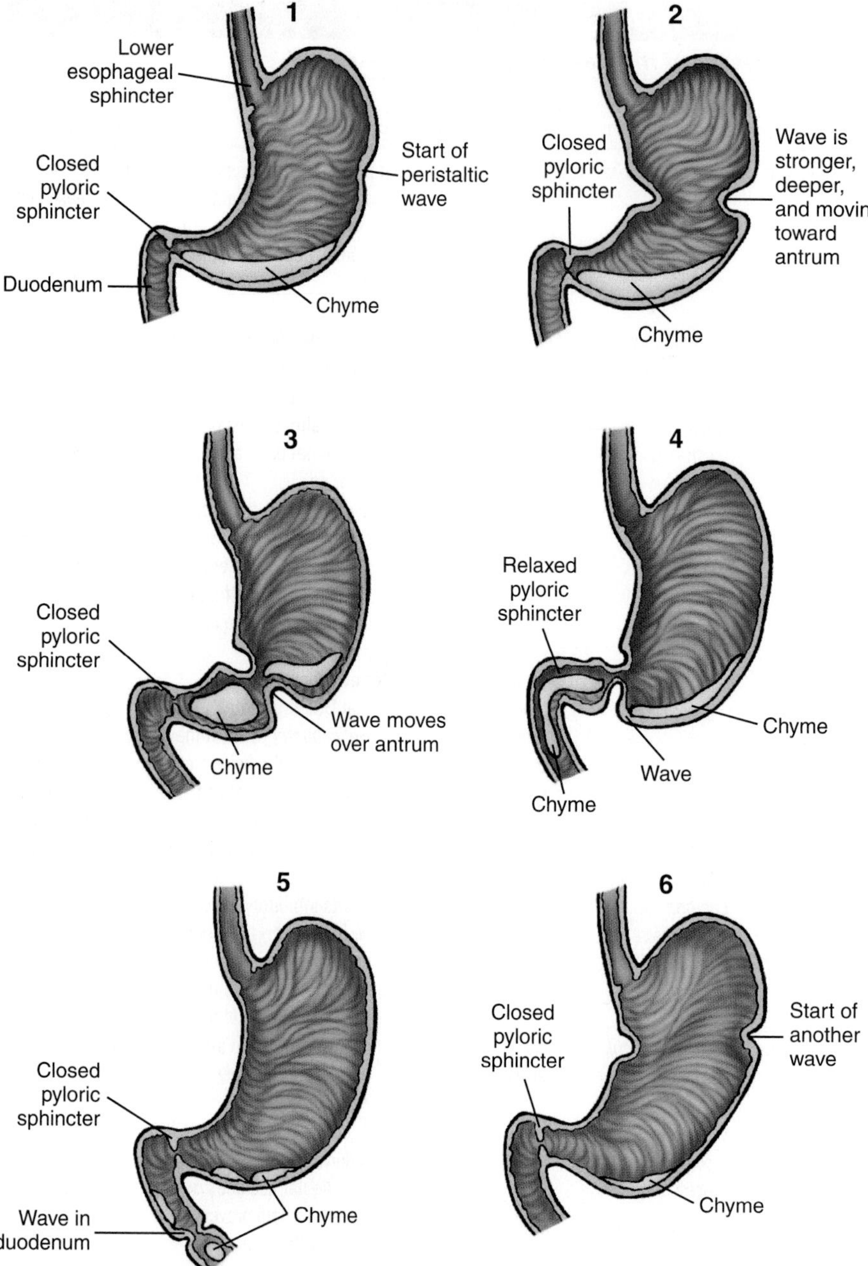

FIGURE 20-1 Peristaltic waves force chyme toward the pyloric sphincter. Meanwhile, a small amount of chyme is squirted into the duodenum, and the remainder is forced back into the stomach, where further mixing occurs. (From Monahan FD, Neighbors M: *Medical-surgical nursing: foundations for clinical practice,* ed 2, Philadelphia, 1998, Saunders.)

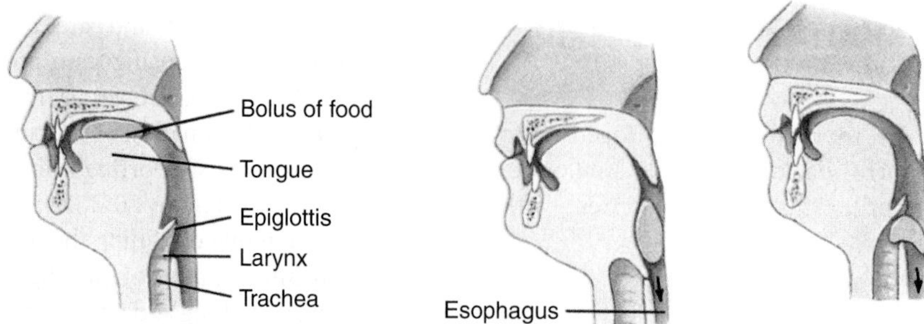

FIGURE 20-2 Parts of the mouth, pharynx, and esophagus involved in the swallowing process. (From Wardlaw GM, Insel PM: *Perspectives in nutrition,* ed 2, New York, 1993, McGraw-Hill.)

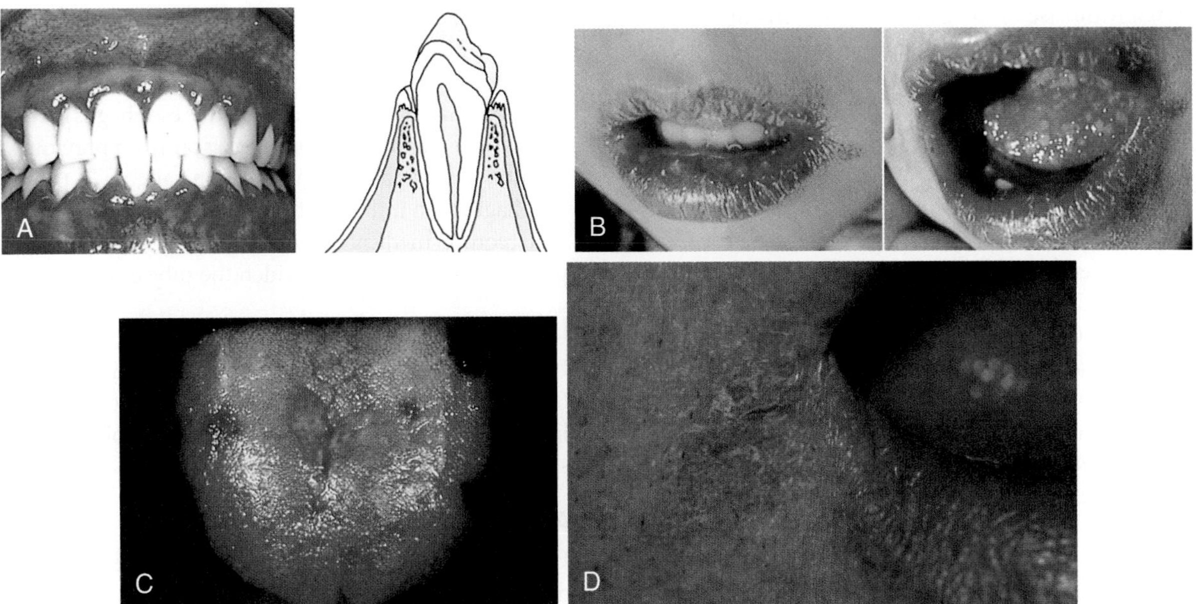

FIGURE 20-3 Tissue inflammation of the mouth. **A,** Gingivitis. **B,** Stomatitis. **C,** Glossitis. **D,** Cheilosis. (**A** from Murray PR, Rosenthal KS, Pfaller MD: *Medical microbiology,* ed 2, St Louis, 1994, Mosby; **B** from Doughty DB, Broadwell-Jackson D: *Gastrointestinal disorders,* St Louis, 1993, Mosby; **C** courtesy Hoffbrand AV, Pettit JE, Vyas P: *Color atlas of clinical hematology,* ed 4, Philadelphia, 2010, Saunders; **D** from Lemmi FO, Lemmi CAE: *Physical assessment findings,* Philadelphia, 2000, Saunders.)

These oral tissue problems may also be nonspecific and unrelated to nutritional factors. In some cases, gingivitis and stomatitis occur in mild form in relation to another disease or stress. Occasionally a severe form of acute necrotizing ulcerative gingivitis occurs. It is caused by a specific infectious bacterium, *Fusobacterium nucleatum,* often in conjunction with the spirochete *Treponema vincentii*; it is also known as *Vincent's disease,* from the Paris physician Henri Vincent (1862-1950), who first identified the disease process. Gums around the bases of teeth become puffy, shiny, and tender, overlapping the teeth margins. Affected gums often bleed, especially during tooth brushing. This serious condition destroys gum tissue and supporting tissues of the teeth and requires a course of antibiotic treatment.

Mouth pain in these conditions often causes decreased food intake. Maintaining adequate nutritional intake then becomes a major problem. Generally patients are given high-protein, high-kilocalorie (kcalorie or kcal) liquids and then soft foods, usually nonacidic and without strong spices to avoid irritation. Temperature extremes may also be avoided if they cause pain. Gradually foods are increased according to toleration, and foods are often supplemented with vitamins and minerals. In severe disease, use of a mouthwash containing a mild topical local anesthetic before meals helps relieve the pain of eating.

Dental Problems

Incidence of dental caries has recently been reduced in children and young adults. However, it is still present in many children and older adults, especially those unable to afford regular dental care, and causes tooth loss and chewing problems. In older adults, periodontal disease is a major cause of tooth loss. Especially if dental caries is untreated or if dental hygiene is poor, then gum tissue at the base of the teeth becomes damaged and pockets form between the gums and the teeth. Dental plaque forms from a sticky deposit of mucus, food particles, and bacteria. Plaque hardens into *calculus,* a mineralized coating developed from plaque and saliva. These hardened particles then collect in pocket openings at the base of the teeth where bacteria attack periodontal tissue. The result is bacterial erosion of bone tissue surrounding affected teeth and subsequent tooth loss. Preventive care through daily dental care with fluoridated toothpaste, careful flossing, and periodic plaque removal by the dental hygienist forms the best approach. Extensive tooth loss leads to the need for tooth replacement with dentures. In many older adults these dentures become ill fitting, especially when weight loss occurs, and hinder adequate chewing. All of these dental problems need to be reviewed as part of the physical assessment in any patient's nutrition history so that food textures and forms can be adjusted to individual needs.

Salivary Glands and Salivation

Disorders of the salivary glands affect eating because saliva carries an *amylase* that begins starch breakdown and is vital in moistening food to facilitate chewing. Problems may arise from infection, such as infection with the mumps virus that attacks the parotid gland. Other problems come from excessive salivation, which occurs in numerous disorders affecting the nervous system, such as Parkinson's disease, and from local disorders such as mouth infections or injury. Problems may arise from any disease or drug that causes overactivity of the parasympathetic division of the autonomic nervous system, which controls the salivary glands.

Conversely, lack of salivation, which causes *xerostomia* (dry mouth), may be a temporary condition caused by fear, salivary gland infection, or action of anticholinergic drugs that hinder the normal action of neurotransmitters. Clients with dry mouth best tolerate moist, soft foods with added gravies and sauces. Permanent xerostomia is rare but does occur in Sjögren's syndrome, a symptom complex of unknown cause thought to be an abnormal immune response. It occurs in middle-aged or older women and is marked by dry mouth and enlargement of parotid glands; it is often associated with rheumatoid arthritis (RA) or radiation therapy. Difficulty occurs in swallowing and speaking; problems also include tooth decay and interference with taste. Salty foods dry the mouth and should be avoided. Chewing gum or sucking on sugarless candy can increase salivary secretions. Extreme mouth dryness may be partially relieved by spraying the inside of the mouth with an artificial saliva solution.

Swallowing Disorders

Most people take swallowing for granted. Each day we eat, chew, and swallow without giving it a second thought. However, the process of swallowing involves highly integrated actions of mouth, pharynx, and esophagus (see Figure 20-2). Swallowing difficulty, known medically as *dysphagia,* is a fairly common problem arising from many causes, including stroke, aging, developmental disabilities, and nervous system diseases. It may be only temporary, such as a piece of food lodged in the back of the throat, for which the Heimlich maneuver is appropriate first aid, or it may be involved with insufficient production of saliva and xerostomia. Such dysfunctional swallowing often causes individuals to aspirate food particles, in turn causing coughing and choking episodes. Dysphagia is of concern for many reasons. Foods may enter the trachea and aspirate into the lungs, allowing bacteria to multiply, leading to pneumonia. Clients with dysphagia are usually referred to a special interdisciplinary team that includes a physician, speech pathologist, nurse, clinical dietitian, physical therapist, and an occupational therapist, with special training in swallowing problems. Thin liquids are the most difficult food form to swallow. Depending on the level of dysphagia, liquids may need to be thickened. Thickening agents include baby rice, commercially prepared thickeners, potato flakes, or mashed potatoes. Levels of thickness include thick (yogurt or pudding consistency) and medium thick (nectar consistency).

Esophageal Problems

Central Problems

The esophagus is a long, muscular tube lined with mucous membranes that extends from the pharynx, or throat, to the stomach (see Figure 20-2). It is bounded on both ends by circular muscles, or sphincters, that act as valves to control food passage. The upper sphincter remains closed except during swallowing, thus preventing airflow into the esophagus and stomach. Disorders along the tube that may disrupt normal swallowing and food passage include esophageal spasm (uncoordinated contractions of the esophagus), esophageal stricture (a narrowing caused by a scar from previous inflammation, ingestion of caustic chemicals, or a tumor), and esophagitis (an inflammation). These problems hinder eating and require medical attention through dilation, stretching procedures, or surgery to widen the tube or drug therapy.

Lower Esophageal Sphincter Problems

Defects in the operation of the LES muscles may come from changes in smooth muscle itself or from nerve-muscle hormonal control. In general, these LES problems arise from spasm, stricture, or incompetence.

Achalasia

If the LES does not relax normally when presented with food during swallowing, the uncommon condition of achalasia (*a* meaning without and *chalasia* meaning relaxation) occurs. A primary esophageal motility ailment, achalasia is characterized by absence of esophageal peristalsis and failure of the LES to relax on swallowing. These aberrations bring about a functional obstruction at the gastroesophageal junction. Signs and symptoms characterizing achalasia are dysphagia (most common), regurgitation, chest pain, heartburn, and weight loss.[1]

The exact cause of achalasia is unknown, but it is thought to be an autoimmune disorder, infectious agent, or both.[1] Medical intervention and treatments are outlined in Table 20-1. Nutritional requirements of patients with achalasia vary with severity of the disease and approach to treatment. Generally, nutrient-dense liquids and semisolid foods, taken at moderate temperatures, in small quantities, and at frequent intervals are usually tolerated by patients with achalasia.[2]

Gastroesophageal Reflux Disease

Gastroesophageal reflux disease (GERD), backflow or regurgitation of gastric contents from the stomach into the esophagus, is a very common disease. Regurgitation of acid gastric contents into the lower part of the esophagus creates constant tissue irritation because the wall of the esophagus is not protected from the acid of the stomach. During reflux, many patients feel a burning sensation behind the sternum that radiates toward the mouth, producing the most common symptom of GERD: heartburn (pyrosis), which is unrelated to disease of the heart (see the *Diet-Medications Interactions* box, "Potential Food Interactions with Drugs Used to Treat Heartburn"). Additional symptoms of GERD include acid indigestion and regurgitation, which often have a negative effect on quality of life.[2]

Other less common symptoms include iron deficiency anemia with chronic bleeding and aspiration, which may cause cough, dyspnea, or pneumonitis. Sometimes substernal pain radiates into the neck and jaw or down the arms. Acid reflux may be worsened by a hiatal hernia, pregnancy (estrogen and progesterone have been shown to reduce LES pressure),

TABLE 20-1 MEDICAL INTERVENTIONS AND TREATMENT OF ACHALASIA

TYPE	DESCRIPTION AND EFFICACY
Pharmacologic: calcium channel blockers, nitrates, phosophodiesterase inhibitors	This intervention is used to reduce LES pressure and is of limited value.
Mechanical: dilation by pneumatic balloons	This intervention involves esophageal dilation to decrease LES pressure. It is successful in decreasing LES pressure in 42% to 85% of patients.
Botulism toxin: Botox	This intervention decreases LES pressure by blocking the release of neurotransmitters at presynaptic cholinergic nerve endings.
	The best results have been seen in patients with vigorous achalasia. Effective duration of treatment varies but takes 6 to 12 months in most patients.
Surgical: esophageal myotomy	This intervention, surgery, is considered to be the primary treatment. The procedure involves controlled division of muscle fibers of the lower esophagus and proximal stomach, followed by a partial fundoplication to prevent reflux. It relieves symptoms in 80% to 100% of patients.

Data from Pohl D, Tutuian R: Achalasia: an overview of diagnosis and treatment, *J Gastrointestin Liver Dis* 16(3):297, 2007.
LES, Lower esophageal sphincter.

DIET-MEDICATIONS INTERACTIONS

Potential Food Interactions with Drugs Used to Treat Heartburn

Drugs and nutrients share related characteristics in the body. They are most often absorbed from the same sites in the intestine. Both can alter physiologic processes, and both can be toxic in high doses. Drugs used to treat heartburn, gastroesophageal reflux disease (GERD), and peptic ulcer disease (PUD) are commonly used. Many are available without prescription. Following is a discussion of common drug-nutrient and herb-drug interactions.

Antacids and Alginates

Antacids may have an effect on absorption of vitamins and iron. Antacids should be taken at least 2 hours before or after iron preparations. The effect of aluminum-containing antacids may be decreased by high-protein meals. Prolonged antacid use, along with excessive consumption of calcium, may cause high calcium levels and result in serious metabolic disease. Antacids may impair folate absorption, which may increase risk of neural tube defects and congenital anomalies of heart, palate, and urinary tract. Folate supplementation may offset this increased risk. Concurrent ingestion of antacids and manganese may reduce manganese absorption.

H_2-Receptor Antagonists

The H_2-blocker cimetidine reacts with many drugs, including caffeine and alcohol. Cimetidine may also increase the likelihood of alcohol intoxication. H_2-blockers decrease the body's ability to excrete caffeine; consequently, large quantities of caffeine may cause tremors, insomnia, or heart palpitations. Folate absorption or use may be impaired by H_2-blockers, which may increase risk of neural tube defects and congenital anomalies of heart, palate, and urinary tract. Folate supplementation may offset this increased risk.

H_2-blockers may impair iron absorption through effects on the pH of the digestive tract. H_2-blockers may also impair absorption of selenium. Vitamin B_{12} from food is impaired by H_2-blockers, but absorption of B_{12} supplements is not affected. Magnesium supplements can interfere with absorption of H_2-blockers. Magnesium supplements should be taken at least 2 hours before or after this medication.

Proton Pump Inhibitors

Proton pump inhibitors (PPIs) may hinder absorption of iron products, thus lessening their effectiveness. PPIs may also impair absorption of selenium. Vitamin B_{12} from food is impaired by PPIs, but absorption of B_{12} supplements is not affected. PPIs may potentiate phototoxic effects of *Hypericum* (St. John's wort).

Data from Bratman S, Girman AM: *Mosby's handbook of herbs and supplements and their therapeutic use,* St Louis, 2003, Mosby.

KEY TERMS

Heimlich maneuver A first-aid maneuver to relieve a person who is choking from blockage of the breathing passageway by a swallowed foreign object or food particle. Standing behind the person, clasp the victim around the waist, placing one fist under the sternum (breastbone) and grasping the fist with the other hand. Then make a quick, hard, thrusting movement inward and upward.

achalasia Failure to relax the smooth muscle fibers of the gastrointestinal (GI) tract at any point of juncture of its parts; especially failure of the esophagogastric sphincter to relax when swallowing, as a result of degeneration of ganglion cells in the wall of the organ. The lower esophagus also loses its normal peristaltic activity. Also called *cardiospasm.*

pyrosis Heartburn.

obesity, pernicious vomiting, or nasogastric tubes. A number of drugs also lower LES pressure, causing GERD and heartburn to be a side effect of drugs used in the treatment of other conditions.

Acid and pepsin cause tissue erosion with symptoms of substernal burning, cramping, pressure sensation, or severe pain.[2] Symptoms are aggravated by lying down or any increase of abdominal pressure, such as that caused by tight clothing. The condition is related to (1) a nonfunctioning gastroesophageal sphincter, (2) frequency and duration of the acid reflux, and (3) inability of the esophagus to produce normal secondary peristaltic waves to prevent prolonged contact of the mucosa with the acid pepsin. A hiatal hernia (Figure 20-4) may or may not be present. The most common complications of GERD are stenosis and esophageal ulcer.

Treatment of GERD is aimed at one or more aspects that cause or continue symptoms (Table 20-2). Nutrition therapy plays only a minor role in the management (Box 20-1) of GERD, and none of the dietary measures can be classified as *evidence-based treatment.*

Hiatal Hernia

The esophagus normally enters the chest cavity at the *hiatus,* an opening in the diaphragm membrane, and immediately joins the upper portion of the stomach. A hiatal hernia occurs when a portion of the upper part of the stomach at this entry

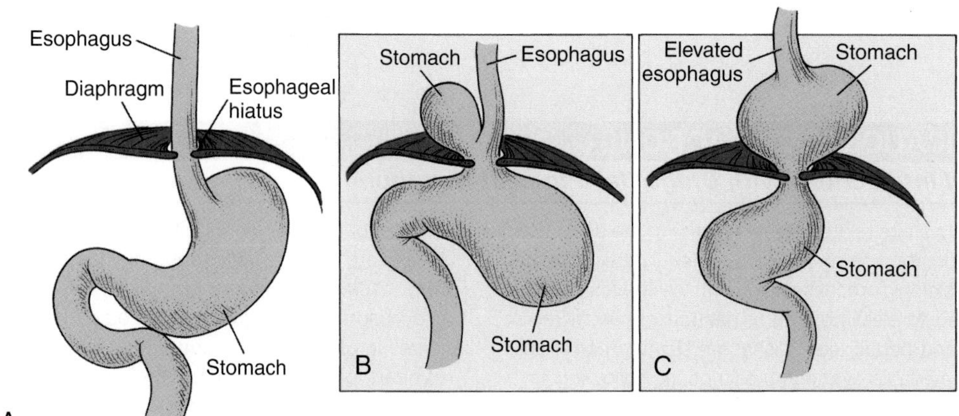

FIGURE 20-4 Hiatal hernia compared with normal stomach placement. **A,** Normal stomach. **B,** Paraesophageal hernia (esophagus in normal position). **C,** Esophageal hiatal hernia (elevated esophagus).

TABLE 20-2 TREATMENT OF GASTROESOPHAGEAL REFLUX DISEASE STAGES

CATEGORY	RECOMMENDED TREATMENTS
Mild heartburn only (occasional bouts for >1 week)	Early low-fat dinners Elevation of head of bed H_2-antagonist >6 weeks and alkali antacids prn
Moderately severe heartburn (months of daily symptoms of heartburn/chest pressure) or poor response to H_2-receptor antagonist	PPIs single dose >6 weeks
Recurrence and persistence of moderately severe GERD symptoms (rapid recurrence of symptoms after course of PPI therapy; occasional odynophagia/dysphagia)	Gastroenterology consultation; endoscopy and biopsy of esophageal-gastric junction for Barrett's metaplasia Recurrent courses of PPI therapy
Severe, persistent GERD symptoms (daily symptoms, often with odynophagia; dysphagia)	Continuous PPI therapy (often two capsules per day) Add cisapride Consider referral for laparoscopic fundoplication
Recalcitrant GERD symptoms (persistent daily/nightly symptoms with regurgitation; odynophagia, dysphagia, poor response to full drug therapy)	Maximal PPI therapy and cisapride Laparoscopic fundoplication

Data from Gray GM: *Gastro-esophageal reflux disease (GERD): the spectrum of esophagitis, Barrett's, dysphagia, and cancer,* New York, 1996-2010, interMDnet Corporation. Retrieved May 14, 2009, from www.cyberounds.com.

PPIs, Proton pump inhibitors; *prn,* as needed; *GERD,* gastroesophageal reflux disease.

point of the esophagus protrudes through the hiatus alongside the lower portion of the esophagus (see Figure 20-4). Food is easily held in this herniated area of the stomach and mixed with acid and pepsin; then it is regurgitated back up into the lower part of the esophagus. Gastritis can occur in this herniated portion of the stomach and cause bleeding and anemia. Reflux of gastric acid contents causes symptoms similar to those described earlier.

A regular diet of choice using frequent small feedings for comfort is usually tolerated. In addition, because obesity is often associated with hiatal hernia, weight reduction is a primary goal. Avoiding tight clothing helps relieve discomfort. Patients will need to avoid leaning over or lying down immediately after meals and should sleep with the head of the bed elevated. Antacids help relieve the burning sensation. Large hiatal hernias or smaller sliding hernias may require surgical repair.

PROBLEMS OF THE STOMACH AND DUODENUM

Peptic Ulcer Disease

One in 10 Americans will be affected by peptic ulcer disease (PUD) during their lives, and approximately 10% of patients seen in emergency departments with abdominal pain are diagnosed with PUD.[2]

An *ulcer* is the loss of tissue on the surface of the mucosa. In the GI tract, an ulcer extends through mucosa, submucosa, and often into the muscle layer. *Peptic ulcer* is the general term for an eroded mucosal lesion in the central portion of the GI tract. A peptic ulcer can occur in any area of the stomach exposed to pepsin. Areas affected include the lower portion of the esophagus, stomach, and first portion of the duodenum, called the *duodenal bulb.* Esophageal and gastric ulcers are less common. Most ulcers occur in the duodenal bulb, where gastric contents emptying into the duodenum through the pyloric valve are most concentrated. Gastric ulcers occur usually along the lesser curvature of the stomach. PUD itself is a benign disease, but ulcers do tend to recur. Gastric ulcers are more prone to develop into malignant disease. Weight loss is common in patients with gastric ulcers. Patients with duodenal ulcers may gain weight from frequent eating to counteract pain.

Peptic ulcer is caused by *Helicobacter pylori* in the stomach or intake of nonsteroidal antiinflammatory drugs (NSAIDs).[3] Nutrition or diet is not thought to play a significant role in the cause. *H. pylori* is a short, spiral-shaped, microaerophilic gram-negative bacillus (Figure 20-5) that attaches itself to gastric mucosa.[3] It is able to survive the acidic environment of the stomach by secreting enzymes to neutralize the acid. This allows *H. pylori* to find its way to the protective mucous lining of the stomach, and its spiral shape facilitates burrowing through the lining.[4]

Intake of aspirin or other NSAIDs such as ibuprofen (Motrin), naproxen (Naprosyn), and etodolac (Lodine) induce ulcer formation by interfering with formation of prostaglandins, the chemicals that help the mucosal lining resist caustic acid damage.[5] They irritate gastric mucosa and cause bleeding, erosion, and ulceration, especially with prolonged or excessive use. The NSAID group of drugs is so

BOX 20-1 MANAGEMENT OF GASTROESOPHAGEAL REFLUX DISEASE

Self-Care
- Over-the-counter (OTC) therapy
  - Antacids
  - Alginate/antacids
  - H_2-receptor antagonists

Lifestyle
- Stop smoking
- Avoid alcohol, chocolate, fatty foods, large meals at night
- Refrain from lying down after meal
- Elevate head of bed or use pillows

Primary Care (Primary Care Physicians)
- Proton pump inhibitors (PPIs) or combination of alginate/antacid and acid suppressive therapy

Secondary Care (Specialists)
- Endoscopic examination
- PPIs

Modified from Tytgat GN, McColl K, Tack J, et al: New algorithm for the treatment of gastro-oesophageal reflux disease, *Aliment Pharmacol Ther* 27(3):249, 2008.

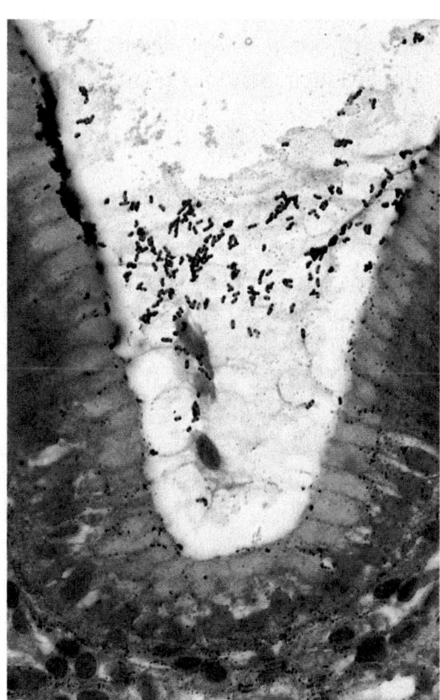

FIGURE 20-5 *Helicobacter pylori.* (From Kumar V, Abbas AK, Fausto N: *Robbins and Cotran pathologic basis of disease,* ed 7, Philadelphia, 2005, Saunders.)

KEY TERMS

gastritis Inflammation of the stomach.

named to distinguish them from the corticosteroids, synthetic variants of the natural adrenal hormones. The NSAIDs include a dozen antiinflammatory drugs.

Clinical Symptoms

Basic symptoms of peptic ulcer are increased gastric tone and painful hunger contractions when the stomach is empty. In duodenal ulcer, amount and concentration of hydrochloric acid (HCl) are increased. In gastric ulcer, amount and concentration of HCl may be normal. Nutritional deficiencies are evident in low plasma protein levels, anemia, and loss of weight. Hemorrhage may be the first sign in some patients. Diagnosis is based on clinical findings, radiographs, or visualization by fiber-optic gastroscopy.

The primary goal of medical management for PUD is control of *H. pylori.* Additional supportive goals are to (1) alleviate symptoms, (2) promote healing, (3) prevent recurrences, and (4) prevent complications. In addition to general traditional measures, the rapidly expanding knowledge base and development of a number of new drugs have increased the physician's available management tools.

General Therapeutic Measures

Adequate rest, relaxation, and sleep have long been a foundation for general care of PUD to enhance the body's natural healing process. Positive stress-coping and relaxation skills, which help patients deal with personal psychosocial stressors, can be learned and practiced. Simple encouragement to talk about anxieties, anger, and frustrations helps to make patients feel better, and as soon as they are able, appropriate physical activity helps work out tensions. Habits that contribute to ulcer development, such as smoking and alcohol use, should be eliminated. Common drugs such as aspirin and NSAIDs should be avoided.

Pharmacologic Management

Current pharmacologic management of PUD includes a wider choice of drugs to control underlying physiologic cause and clinical symptoms, as well as to support healing. In various ways the following five types of drugs suppress gastric acid and pepsin secretion, protect mucosal tissue, buffer acid, and eliminate infection:

1. *H_2-receptor antagonists:* These agents, commonly called *H_2-blockers,* are popular drugs for controlling gastric acid secretion. They decrease HCl production by competing with histamine for receptor sites on parietal cells. Normally histamine attaches to its specific cellular receptors (type H_2) on acid-producing parietal cells of gastric mucosa and mediates secretion of HCl. Thus the blocking action of these agents effectively controls acid and pepsin because inactive pepsinogen requires acid for activation. The four drugs in this classification have now been reclassified for OTC purchase: (1) cimetidine (Tagamet), (2) ranitidine (Zantac), (3) famotidine (Pepcid), and (4) nizatidine (Axid).
2. *PPIs:* This newer class of drugs, more potent than H_2-blockers, also suppresses gastric acid but by a different action. Without competition, in parietal cells they irreversibly prevent action of a key enzyme that actively secretes hydrogen ions needed for HCl production. Without available H_2 ions, HCl cannot be made. Then without acid, ulcers heal rapidly. The U.S. Food and Drug Administration (FDA) has approved five drugs in this category: (1) lansoprazole (Prevacid), (2) omeprazole (Prilosec), (3) esomeprazole (Nexium), (4) rabeprazole (Aciphex), and (5) pantoprazole (Protonix). PPIs may interfere with liver metabolism of anticoagulants, diazepam (Valium), or phenytoin (Dilantin). Serum levels of these drugs should be monitored during concurrent therapy.
3. *Mucosal protectors:* Drugs of this type act as cytoprotective agents by helping the stomach heal itself. They produce a gel-like suspension that binds to the ulcer base and covers it and surrounding normal mucosal tissue to protect involved tissue from harm while it heals. This drug also forms complexes with pepsin that inactivates pepsin. An example of this type of drug is sucralfate (Carafate). These drugs are not as effective as the other options.
4. *Antacids:* These well-known substances counteract or neutralize acidity. They are safe and inexpensive to use. Two main types are (1) magnesium-aluminum compounds (Maalox, Mylanta) and (2) aluminum hydroxide (Basaljel, Amphojel). Aluminum-based preparations may cause constipation; magnesium-based preparations may cause diarrhea.
5. *Antibiotics:* Drugs of this type are used to control the *Helicobacter pylori* infection associated with PUD. Treatment using one or two antibiotics such as amoxicillin, tetracycline (not to be used for children younger than age 12), metronidazole, or clarithromycin is recommended for 10 days to 2 weeks, in conjunction with either ranitidine bismuth citrate, bismuth subsalicylate, or a PPI. The combination of acid suppression by the H_2-blocker or PPI with antibiotics helps alleviate ulcer-related symptoms (e.g., abdominal pain, nausea), heal inflammation, and may enhance efficacy of the antibiotics.[5] Currently the FDA has approved eight *H. pylori* treatment regimens (Box 20-2), although other combinations have been used effectively. Better eradication rates have been demonstrated using triple-therapy regimens rather than dual therapy, longer length of treatment (14 days instead of 10 days), or both. Major reasons for treatment failure are antibiotic resistance and patient noncompliance.[5]

Nutritional Management

Pharmacologic therapy is the treatment of choice for PUD. No evidence indicates that diet plays a significant role in treatment when compared with pharmacologic regimens.[6] Dietary recommendations are formed from individual tolerance and should be considered supplemental to pharmacologic therapy. No conclusive evidence supports use of a traditional "bland" diet to decrease gastric acid secretion or increase the time it takes to heal ulcers.[2] In short, individuals with PUD should be encouraged to eat a healthy diet from foods they enjoy.

BOX 20-2 U.S. FOOD AND DRUG ADMINISTRATION–APPROVED TREATMENT OPTIONS FOR PEPTIC ULCER DISEASE

Proton Pump Inhibitor (PPI)–Based Triple Therapies
- PPI (lansoprazole or omeprazole), amoxicillin, and clarithromycin
- The above three packaged together: Prevpac (using the PPI lansoprazole)
- PPI (lansoprazole or omeprazole), metronidazole, and clarithromycin or amoxicillin

"Conventional Triple Therapy" for *Helicobacter pylori*
- Bismuth (Pepto-Bismol), metronidazole, and tetracycline or amoxicillin, combined with an H_2-blocker (cimetidine, famotidine, nizatidine or ranitidine) or a PPI (lansoprazole or omeprazole)
- The three packaged together: Helidac combined with an H_2-blocker (cimetidine, famotidine, nizatidine, or ranitidine) or a PPI (lansoprazole or omeprazole)

Note: Dual therapy of single PPI and a single antibiotic is not recommended.
Modified from Stratemeier MW, Vignogna L, Hale KL. Peptic ulcers. eMedicine. Retrieved July 2, 2010 from http://www.emedicinehealth.com/peptic_ulcers/article_em.htm.

General nutritional therapeutic recommendations include the following[7]:

- Emphasize a balanced, nutritious diet.
- Limit the following foods and seasonings, and encourage avoidance of lifestyle habits known to increase acid secretion, inhibit healing, or both:
  - Caffeine (including coffee, tea, or decaffeinated coffee)
  - Black pepper
  - Chocolate
  - Foods that are irritating or not well tolerated
  - Alcohol
  - Eating less than 2 hours before bedtime

Personal Focus

Sound nutritional management plays an important supportive role in total medical care of persons with PUD. The individual must be the focus of treatment. The patient is not *an ulcer;* he or she is a person *with an ulcer.* Course of the disease is conditioned by the individuality of the patient and his or her life situation. Presence of the ulcer affects the patient's life and quality of life. In the long run a wide range of foods, attractive to the eye and the taste, and regular, unhurried eating habits provide the best course of action (see the *Case Study* box, "The Patient with Peptic Ulcer Disease").

CASE STUDY

The Patient with Peptic Ulcer Disease

Lowell is a 40-year-old businessman who was admitted to the city hospital 3 weeks ago after vomiting bright-red blood. A medical history revealed that a dull, gnawing pain in the upper abdomen began several months ago and has increased in severity during that time. It became more severe after his most recent out-of-state trip to one of his stores. Because the pain was usually accompanied by headaches, he took aspirin to help relieve it.

Initial hospital treatment consisted of blood transfusions, intravenous fluids and electrolytes, and vitamin C. Lowell continued to feel nauseated and weak, but he stopped vomiting. However, he passed several large, tarry stools during the first 24 hours. His initial nutrition assessment results included weight 68 kg (150 lb), height 175 cm (5 feet, 9 inches), albumin 2.8 g/dL, prealbumin 14 mg/dL, transferrin 18% saturation value, hemoglobin (Hb) 11 g/dL, and hematocrit 35%. His medications included cimetidine, sucralfate, magnesium-aluminum hydroxide, and triple antibiotic therapy.

The patient began slowly to tolerate sips of clear liquids and then advanced to a regular diet as tolerated, showing continued improvement. Before he was discharged at the end of the second week, the registered dietitian (RD) discussed general nutritional needs with Lowell and his wife. He was advised to eat meals regularly in as relaxed a setting and manner as possible, eliminate his frequent between-meal snacks, and take his multivitamin supplement daily with his meals. In addition, general guidelines and a list of a few food-related items or habits to avoid were reviewed. He was also advised to stop smoking and to rest as much as possible before returning to work. His physician had also advised him to reduce his workload and scheduled a follow-up appointment in 1 week.

Lowell's wife accompanied him to the next appointment and reported she was pleased with his ability to put aside business duties and take more time to enjoy his family. Lowell stated his two teenage sons had been surprisingly supportive in assisting him in following the prescribed regimen, and he plans to make it his general habit.

Questions for Analysis

1. The radiographic diagnosis of Lowell's illness was a gastric ulcer in the antrum lesser curvature. What does this mean? Where do most ulcers occur? Why?
2. What factors contributed to Lowell's ulcer? What effect did each of them have?
3. Evaluate the results of Lowell's initial nutrition assessment data. How would you use this information in nutrition counseling?
4. Identify Lowell's basic nutritional needs. Outline a teaching plan based on these needs that you would use to help him with his new diet plan. How would you include his wife in formulating and implementing his nutrition care plan?
5. What role does vitamin C play in Lowell's therapy?
6. Why should Lowell give up coffee, cigarettes, and alcohol? What problems do you think he may encounter in trying to change these habits?

DISORDERS OF THE SMALL INTESTINE

Diarrhea and Malabsorption

Diarrhea

Diarrhea is not a disease; it is a symptom that can be attributed to many medical conditions (see the *Perspectives in Practice* box, "Nutritional Aspects of Diarrhea"). *Diarrhea* is defined as an increase in frequency of bowel moments compared with the usual pattern, an excess water content of stools affecting consistency or volume, or both. Diarrhea most directly involves the large intestine but may be caused by disease of the small intestine, pancreas, or gallbladder. General diarrhea may result from basic dietary excesses. Fermentation of sugars or excess fiber stimulation of intestinal muscle function may be involved.

PERSPECTIVES IN PRACTICE

Nutritional Aspects of Diarrhea

Gastrointestinal (GI) disease so often presents barriers to efficient nutrient absorption that nutritional deficiencies are planned for automatically. Unfortunately, many of these conditions also frequently lead to diarrhea, which results in further loss of fluids and electrolytes. As expected, replacement of these fluids is the initial and primary concern of therapy. However, different types of diarrhea also present other differences; control of type-specific problems requires different modes of treatment coordinated with treatment of the disease it accompanies. Before looking into possible treatment modes, three of the most common types of diarrhea should be examined: (1) watery, (2) fatty, and (3) small volume.

Watery diarrhea occurs when the amount of water and electrolytes moving into intestinal mucosa exceeds that amount absorbed into the bloodstream. This movement of water and electrolytes into the mucosa may be secretive or osmotic. If this movement of water and electrolytes into the mucosa is secretive, then it may be active or passive. Active movement occurs with excessive gastric hydrochloric acid (HCl) secretion or enterotoxin-induced infections such as cholera. Passive movement occurs with a rise in hydrostatic pressure that accompanies such infectious diseases as salmonellosis or tuberculosis, nonbacterial infections, fungal infections, renal failure, irradiation enteritis, and inflammatory bowel disease (IBD). Other conditions associated with watery diarrhea include hyperthyroidism, thyroid carcinoma, and hypermotility of the GI tract.

If this movement of water and electrolytes into the mucosa is osmotic, it will occur when nutrients are not absorbed because of intolerable levels of nonabsorbable particles present in intestinal chyme. Such particles include lactose (milk sugar) in individuals with lactase deficiency or gluten (a cereal protein found in wheat and rye and to a lesser degree in barley and oats) in persons with a reduced GI transit time caused by the removal of part of the intestinal tract.

Fatty diarrhea, or *steatorrhea,* occurs with maldigestion or malabsorption. Maldigestion involves a lack of enzymatic activity required to completely digest food, such as reduced pancreatic exocrine activity (release of intestinal enzymes from the pancreas) caused by pancreatic insufficiency. Malabsorption means digested materials do not make it across the intestinal mucosa to enter the bloodstream. This failure occurs in conditions in which the intestinal villi are destroyed, such as celiac disease (CD).

Small-volume diarrhea occurs mainly when the rectosigmoid area of the colon is irritated, such as in IBD (Crohn's disease or ulcerative colitis [UC]). It also occurs when inflammatory conditions affect areas adjacent to the colon, as in pelvic inflammatory disease, diverticulitis, appendicitis, or hemorrhagic ovarian cysts.

Metabolic consequences of each type of diarrhea are similar. Uncontrolled, they result in syncope, hypokalemia, acid-base imbalances, and hypovolemia, with resulting renal failure. They may also be accompanied by low levels of fat-soluble vitamins, vitamin B_{12}, or folic acid or eventually lead to protein-energy malnutrition (PEM). In addition to these conditions, each type also manifests problems associated with the disorder they accompany. Workers with the Memorial Sloan-Kettering Cancer Center in New York and the Department of Medicine at Brooke Army Medical Center in Texas have developed recommendations for treating GI diseases associated with each type of diarrhea. These are summarized as follows, with the focus on the diarrheal aspects of disease:

- Watery diarrhea often accompanies inflammatory bowel conditions, such as Crohn's disease, for which nutrition therapy involves (1) increased protein and kcalories, (2) low fats and lactose, and (3) avoidance of foods that stimulate peristalsis. Thus secretive diarrhea is reduced by eliminating foods that may stimulate gastric acid secretion, and all types of watery diarrhea are avoided by reducing the motility of the GI tract. In other conditions in which osmotic diarrhea occurs, such as dumping syndrome, this problem is prevented by giving fluids between meals to avoid any extreme difference in osmotic pressures on either side of the intestinal wall. Small, frequent meals also help prevent this problem, as well as painful distention.
- Steatorrhea frequently accompanies conditions associated with maldigestion such as chronic pancreatitis. Nutritional management of this disease involves (1) frequent meals high in protein and carbohydrates and low in fat; (2) use of medium-chain triglycerides (MCTs), which are more easily absorbed under adverse conditions; and (3) avoiding gastric stimulants, especially caffeine and alcohol. Steatorrhea also accompanies conditions of malabsorption, such as gluten-sensitive enteropathy. In addition to nutritional management strategies listed, treating this type of diarrhea requires removal of products that damage the mucosal villi, including lactose and gluten, which is found in wheat, rye, barley, and oats, and food products and fillers such as hydrolyzed vegetable protein products. It sometimes requires restricting fat as well. In both cases, the primary concern is to monitor fats that would otherwise appear in the feces. As therapy progresses, fat content of the meal can be increased as tolerated to normal levels to improve palatability.
- Small-volume diarrhea may accompany diverticulosis of the colon. A high-residue diet is recommended to increase fecal bulk, thereby preventing diarrhea. To prevent flatulence and distention, fiber should be added to the diet gradually.

All types of diarrhea can result in malnutrition, primarily because of electrolyte and fluid losses. It is important to identify the type of diarrhea occurring with each patient; only then can an effective nutritional management strategy be designed to replace those losses, as well as to eliminate or prevent other nutrition-related problems that are possible for each case.

Chronic diarrhea may occur as a result of GI tract motility dysfunction such as irritable bowel syndrome (IBS), malabsorption, metabolic disorders, food intolerances (e.g., lactose intolerance), food poisoning, infections, and human immunodeficiency virus (HIV) infection. In the case of lactose intolerance, accumulated concentration of undigested lactose in the intestine, resulting from the lack of the enzyme lactase, creates increased osmotic pressure. This pressure effectively draws water into the gut and stimulates hypermotility, abdominal cramping, and diarrhea. Milk treated with lactase enzyme is tolerated by these persons without the difficulty encountered with regular milk. Secretory, osmotic, and inflammatory processes in the intestine result in increased losses of fluid and electrolytes from diarrhea.[8]

Malabsorption

In a normally functioning body, foods are digested and then nutrients are absorbed into the bloodstream, mostly from the small intestine. Malabsorption occurs either because a disorder interferes with how food is digested or because a disorder interferes with how nutrients are absorbed. Multiple causes of a malabsorption condition exist.[8] Symptoms of malabsorption include a change in bowel habits, apathy, fatigue, and a smooth surface on the lateral tongue. Some of these causes include the following:

- *Maldigestion problems:* pancreatic disorders, biliary disease, bacterial overgrowth, ileal disease (inflammatory bowel disease [IBD])
- *Intestinal mucosal changes:* mucosal surface alterations, intestinal surgery such as resections that shorten the bowel, lymphatic obstruction, intestinal stasis
- *Genetic disease:* cystic fibrosis (CF), with its complications of pancreatic insufficiency and lack of the pancreatic enzymes lipase, trypsin, and amylase
- *Intestinal enzyme deficiency:* lactose intolerance caused by lactase deficiency
- *Cancer and its treatment:* absorbing surface effect of radiation and chemotherapy
- *Metabolic biochemical defects:* absorbing surface effects of pernicious anemia or gluten-induced enteropathy (celiac sprue)

Here we briefly review four of these malabsorptive conditions: (1) celiac sprue, (2) CF, (3) IBD, and (4) short-bowel syndrome (SBS).

Celiac Disease

Metabolic Defect

In 1889 a London physician named Gee observed a number of malnourished children having steatorrhea and distended abdomens. He gave the name *celiac* to the general clinical condition from the Greek word *kolia,* meaning belly or abdomen. It was not until the mid-1950s that the Dutch pediatrician Willem-Karel Dicke and his associates discovered the causative agent. Their tissue studies confirmed that the gliadin fraction of the protein gluten in wheat produced the fat malabsorption; further, what had been called *celiac disease (CD)* in children and *nontropical sprue* in adults was a single disease, which came to be called *celiac sprue.*[9] As currently used, the alternative terms *CD* and *gluten-sensitive enteropathy* are synonymous with celiac sprue. In all cases, such diseased tissues consistently show an eroded mucosal surface lacking the number and form of normal villi and having few microvilli, resulting in malabsorption of most nutrients (Figure 20-6). (For more information regarding genetic malabsorption diseases, see the *Evidence Based Practice* box, "Food Intolerances from Genetic-Metabolic Disease," and the *Focus on Culture* box, "Did Your Ancestors Herd Dairy Cattle?")

Gluten molecules trigger an autoimmune and inflammatory response in the small intestine, causing the usually brush-like lining of the intestine to flatten, thereby being much less able to digest and absorb foods. Damage is reversed when gluten is removed from the diet. It is unclear why an immunologic response occurs when gluten is ingested by genetically predisposed persons.[10] Resulting malabsorption promotes malnutrition and severe debilitation.[8] Gluten is a protein present in some grains such as wheat, rye, and barley but not oats, rice, or corn.

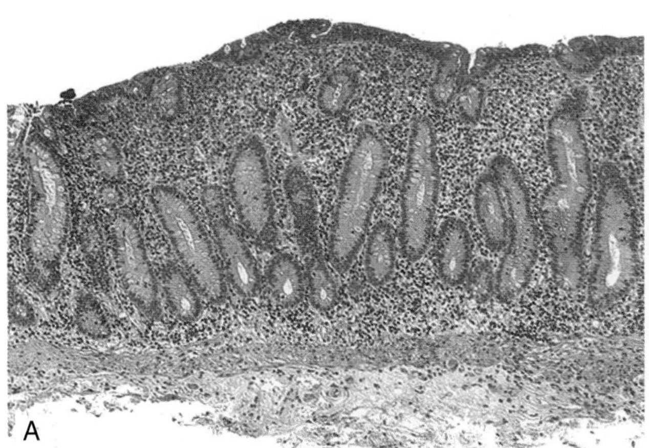

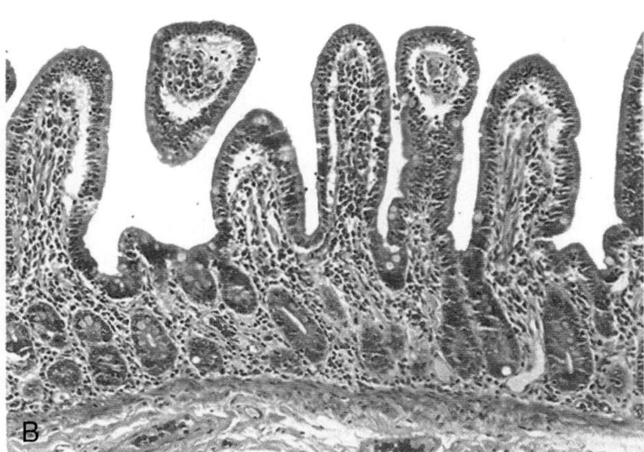

FIGURE 20-6 Comparison of normal intestinal villi and those in an individual with celiac disease (CD). **A,** A biopsy specimen of diseased mucosa shows diffuse severe atrophy and blunting of villi. **B,** A normal mucosal biopsy specimen. (From Kumar V, Abbas AK, Fausto N: *Robbins and Cotran pathologic basis of disease,* ed 7, Philadelphia, 2005, Saunders.)

EVIDENCE-BASED PRACTICE

Food Intolerances from Genetic-Metabolic Disease

Certain food intolerances may stem from underlying genetic disease that affects metabolism of one or more specific nutrients. Genetic disease results from the individual's specific gene inheritance. Genes in each cell control the metabolic functions of the cell. They regulate synthesis of some 1000 or more specific cell enzymes that control metabolism within the cell. When a specific gene is abnormal *(mutant)*, the enzyme for which that gene controls its synthesis cannot be made. In turn, specific metabolic reaction controlled by that specific missing enzyme cannot take place. Specific genetic disease caused by this metabolic block then manifests clinical symptoms connected with resulting abnormal metabolic products. As primary examples here, we look briefly at two such genetic diseases affecting food-nutrient intolerances: (1) phenylketonuria (PKU), which affects amino acid metabolism and hence protein foods, and (2) galactosemia, which affects carbohydrate metabolism, specifically food sources of lactose. Both are detected by newborn screening procedures that are mandatory by law.

Phenylketonuria

PKU results from the missing cell enzyme phenylalanine hydroxylase, which metabolizes one of the essential amino acids, phenylalanine, to tyrosine, another nonessential amino acid. Phenylalanine then accumulates in the blood, and its alternate metabolites, the phenyl acids, are excreted in the urine. One of these urinary acids, phenylpyruvic acid, is a phenylketone; hence the name of the disease. Untreated, PKU can produce devastating effects, but present nutrition therapy can avoid these results. In past years, before current newborn screening laws and dietary treatment practices from birth, the most profound effect observed in persons with untreated PKU was severe mental retardation. The intelligence quotient (IQ) of affected persons was usually less than 50 and often less than 20. Central nervous system (CNS) damage caused irritability, hyperactivity, convulsive seizures, and bizarre behavior.

PKU can now be well controlled by special nutrition therapy. After screening at birth, a special low-phenylalanine diet effectively controls serum phenylalanine levels so that they are maintained at appropriate amounts to prevent clinical symptoms and promote normal growth and development. Because phenylalanine is an essential amino acid necessary for growth, it cannot be totally removed from the diet. Blood levels of phenylalanine are constantly monitored, and the metabolic team nutritionist calculates the special diet for each infant and child to allow only limited amount of phenylalanine tolerated. Based on extensive studies, guidelines for nutritional management of PKU are currently being used effectively to build lifetime habits; research now indicates that no safe age exists at which a child may discontinue the diet. This dietary management is built on two basic components: (1) a substitute for milk (a special medical food continued past infancy and childhood into adolescence and adulthood) and (2) guidelines for adding solid foods (both regular and special low-protein products) and then building continuing food habits.

Initial education and continuing support of parents is essential, because dietary management of PKU is the only known effective method of treatment and maintaining the diet becomes more difficult as the child grows older. Parents must understand and accept the necessity of the diet, and this requires patience, understanding, and continued reinforcement. The PKU team, together with parents, provides initial and continuing care so that the child with PKU will grow and develop normally. When PKU is diagnosed at birth, as a result of widespread screening programs, a child can have a healthy and happy life, instead of the profound disease consequences experienced in the past. Current practice of long-term nutritional management is especially critical for young women with PKU who are considering pregnancy. At least 6 months before becoming pregnant, women with PKU should meet with a metabolic team to discuss treatment and follow-up. It is possible for women with PKU to have normal children. However, maternal PKU presents the possibility of a potentially high-risk pregnancy if a low-phenylalanine diet is not strictly followed.

Galactosemia

This genetic disease affects carbohydrate metabolism so that the body cannot use the monosaccharide galactose. Three enzymes are responsibly for conversion of galactose to glucose, and in galactosemia at least one of the enzymes is defective or missing. Milk, infants' first food, contains a large amount of the precursor lactose (milk sugar). When infants with galactosemia are given breast milk or regular infant formula, they vomit and have diarrhea. After galactose is initially combined with phosphate to begin metabolic conversion to glucose, it cannot proceed further in the infant with galactosemia. Galactose rapidly accumulates in the blood and in various body tissues. In the past, excess tissue accumulations of galactose caused rapid damage in the untreated infant. Clinical symptoms appeared soon after birth, and the child failed to thrive. Continued liver damage brought **jaundice,** an enlarged liver with **cirrhosis,** enlarged spleen, and ascites. Without treatment, death usually resulted from liver failure. If the infant survived, then continuing tissue damage and hypoglycemia in the optic lens and the brain caused cataracts and mental retardation. Now, however, with newborn screening programs, infants with galactosemia are diagnosed at birth and started on special dietary management. With this vital nutrition therapy, children can grow and develop normally.

The main indirect source of dietary galactose is the lactose in milk. A galactose-free diet (free of all forms of milk and lactose) is observed, and the infant is fed a soy-based formula. Breastfeeding is not an option when this genetic condition is present. The body synthesizes the amount of galactose needed for body structures. As solid foods are added to the infant's diet at about 6 months of age, careful attention must be given to avoiding lactose from other food sources. Parents quickly learn to check labels carefully on all commercial products to detect any lactose or lactose-containing substances.

WEBSITES OF INTEREST

Galactosemia

National Organization for Rare Disorders: www.rarediseases.org.

Parents of Galactosemic Children, Inc.: www.galactosemia.org.

Phenylketonuria (PKU)

Children's PKU Network: www.pkunetwork.org.

National Coalition for PKU and Allied Disorders: www.pku-allieddisorders.org.

National PKU News: www.pkunews.org.

The Arc: *Q & A on PKU*: http://www.thearc.org/NetCommunity/Page.aspx?pid=183.

Data from Nelms MN, Sucher K, Long S: *Understanding nutrition therapy and pathophysiology,* Belmont, Calif, 2007, Wadsworth/Thomson Learning.

FOCUS ON CULTURE

Did Your Ancestors Herd Dairy Cattle?

Do you or any one you know experience these symptoms—cramps, bloating, gas, diarrhea, nausea—anywhere from 30 minutes to 2 hours after consuming a food or beverage containing lactose? As you learned in Chapter 3, lactose is found in milk and some dairy products, and the enzyme lactase is necessary for us to digest lactose. Lack of this enzyme, lactase, results in a condition called *lactose intolerance*.

Humans are the only mammals that continue to drink milk past weaning. Most mammals produce lactase until they are weaned and stop drinking milk. Cessation of milk drinking and lactase production characterizes most of the world's population, especially those of Asian and African ancestry. For children older than 5 years, 90% to 95% of people of color (African Americans, Asians, Hispanics) are lactose intolerant, whereas only 20% to 25% of those of northern European descent do not tolerate dairy products. Lactose intolerance is usually referred to as a *disease* or *disorder*. Does this seem logical? Why is a trait found in 90% to 95% of the world's population abnormal? Perhaps lactose intolerance should be considered a normal adult condition.

Researchers from Cornell University believe lactose tolerance is the outcome of a genetic mutation that sustains the functionality of lactase production into adulthood, allowing consumption of milk throughout life. This mutation occurs commonly among populations from Northern Europe, where raising cattle and other ruminant animals has been practiced for centuries because the environment made it safe and economical to do so.

It appears that the ability to produce lactase and absorb lactose is nutritionally beneficial for adults only if milk is consistently available. To test this theory, data were collected on adult lactose absorption and malabsorption from 270 indigenous African and Eurasian populations. Adult lactose malabsorption was found to be associated with extreme hot or cold climates (high and low latitudes). In addition to the geographic and climatic features of these regions that preclude the raising of dairy herds, historical evidence (pre-1900) indicates that nine deadly communicable cattle diseases occurred in them. The researchers conclude that areas of the world in which adult lactose malabsorption predominates are the same areas in which it is dangerous or impossible to sustain dairy herds. Thus the ability to digest lactose appears for the most part to be a genetic mutation.

Data from Bloom G, Sherman PW: Dairying barriers affect the distribution of lactose malabsorption, *Evol Hum Behav* 26(4):301, 2005.

CD occurs in roughly 1 in 133 persons in the United States, but only a small percentage of people with it have been diagnosed. CD, as a rule, commonly occurs in women, Caucasians and others of European ancestry, and first-degree relatives. It can occur at any age from infancy to late adulthood.[11]

Clinical Symptoms

Symptoms vary significantly from person to person. They may be intestinal or nonintestinal in nature, which makes diagnosis difficult. One person may present with diarrhea, another with constipation, and yet another with no stool elimination problems.[11] Children with CD most often display failure to thrive, with or without malabsorption. Adults most frequently present with anemia caused by iron or folate deficiency (or both).[11] A partial listing of GI symptoms is summarized in Table 20-3.

TABLE 20-3 GASTROINTESTINAL SYMPTOMS ASSOCIATED WITH CELIAC DISEASE

SYMPTOM	COMMENTS
Abdominal pain	
Abdominal distention	Bloating, gas, indigestion
Constipation	
Decreased appetite	May also be increased or unchanged
Diarrhea	Chronic or occasional
Lactose intolerance	Common on diagnosis; usually resolves after treatment
Nausea and vomiting	
Steatorrhea	Stools that float, are foul smelling, bloody, or "fatty"
Weight loss	Unexplained (people can be overweight or normal weight on diagnosis)

Data from U.S. National Library of Medicine, National Institutes of Health: *Medline Plus A.D.A.M. medical encyclopedia: celiac disease-sprue,* Atlanta, 2005, A.D.A.M. Inc. Retrieved May 14, 2009, from www.nlm.nih.gov/medlineplus/ency/article/000233.htm.

Diagnosis

Individuals in the general population may not be identified by clinical symptoms, therefore remaining underdiagnosed, yet screening still remains controversial. Antitransglutaminase (tissue TGA) has been found to be a sensitive marker for CD.[11] Intestinal biopsy is then used to confirm diagnosis in patients with positive serologic tests. Depending on the degree of intestinal involvement, a complete blood count (CBC); levels of serum iron or ferritin, red cell folate, vitamin B_{12}, serum calcium, alkaline phosphatase, albumin, and β-carotene; and prothrombin time (PT) should be obtained in patients suspected of malabsorption problems.

Nutritional Management

The goal of nutritional management is to control intake of dietary gluten and prevent malnutrition. The diet is better

KEY TERMS

jaundice A syndrome characterized by hyperbilirubinemia and deposits of bile pigment in the skin, mucous membranes, and sclera, giving a yellow appearance to the patient.

cirrhosis Chronic liver disease, characterized by loss of functional cells, with fibrous and nodular regeneration.

defined as *low gluten* rather than *gluten free* because it is impossible to remove all gluten. Newer products labeled *gluten free* can contain wheat starch as a thickening agent, which cannot be recommended.[12] Wheat and rye are the main sources of gluten-like proteins; it is also present in oats and barley. Thus these four grains have always been eliminated from the diet. However, a growing body of evidence suggests that moderate amounts of oats may be safely used in diets of most adults with CD.[13] Corn and rice are usually the substitute grains used. Parents of children with CD need special instructions about food products to avoid, what constitutes a basic meal pattern, and recipes for food preparation. Careful label reading must be discussed, because many commercial products use the offending grains as thickeners or fillers, and parents' knowledge of gluten-containing food products is highly variable and influences the child's attitudes toward dietary compliance. Good dietary management varies according to the child's age, pathologic conditions, and clinical status. Generally, a dietary program based on the low-gluten diet should be followed (Box 20-3). In a small subgroup of patients, symptoms persist despite strict adherence to the diet. In rare instances, persons with such a refractory form of the disease respond only to parenteral nutrition (PN) support.

Cystic Fibrosis

Genetic-Metabolic Defect

CF is inherited as an autosomal recessive trait in about 3% of the Caucasian population. It is the most common fatal genetic disease among Caucasians, occurring in about 1 in 3300 live Caucasian births, 1 in 15,300 African-American births, and 1 in 32,000 Asian-American births.[14] Approximately one third of CF cases in the United States involve adults. The leading characteristic of CF is hypersecretion of abnormal, thick mucus that obstructs exocrine glands and ducts.[14] Therefore it can be classified as a *respiratory disease* or *GI disorder.*

BOX 20-3 SAMPLE GLUTEN-FREE MENU

Breakfast

Denver omelet made with low-fat natural cheddar or Monterey Jack cheese and fresh vegetables

Rice cake (ingredient list should be checked to ascertain it is gluten free) topped with fruit jelly

Orange juice

Lunch

Burrito made with corn tortilla, black beans, fresh vegetables, low-fat natural cheese

Fresh green salad with oil and vinegar dressing

Homemade lemon/limeade

Evening Meal

Shrimp and fresh vegetable stir-fry in oil and spices

Brown rice or enriched white rice, plain

Sorbet

Cranberry juice/seltzer water spritzer

Snack

All-natural yogurt mixed with fresh peaches (or other fruit in season)

The CF gene (found on chromosome 7q) is very large, and over 600 mutations causing CF have been described.[14] The gene product is the cystic fibrosis transmembrane regulator (CFTR) protein, which regulates chloride transport and water flux across epithelial cells.[14] This results in an abnormally high concentration of sodium in perspiration and low water content in mucus.[14] CF primarily affects the pancreas, intestinal tract, sweat glands, and lungs; it causes infertility in male patients (Figure 20-7).[14]

Clinical Symptoms

Classic clinical symptoms of CF include the following effects in body organ systems[14]:

- Thick mucus in the lungs that accumulates and clogs air passages, damages epithelial tissue of these airways, and leads to chronic obstructive pulmonary disease (COPD) and frequent respiratory infections, both contributing to increased metabolism and increased energy-nutrient needs
- Pancreatic insufficiency caused by progressive clogging of pancreatic ducts and functional tissue degeneration, resulting in lack of normal pancreatic enzymes leading to bulky, foul-smelling, oily stools (steatorrhea); progressive loss of functional insulin-producing beta cells in the islets of Langerhans', resulting in type 1 diabetes mellitus.
- Malabsorption of undigested food nutrients and extensive malnutrition and stunted growth

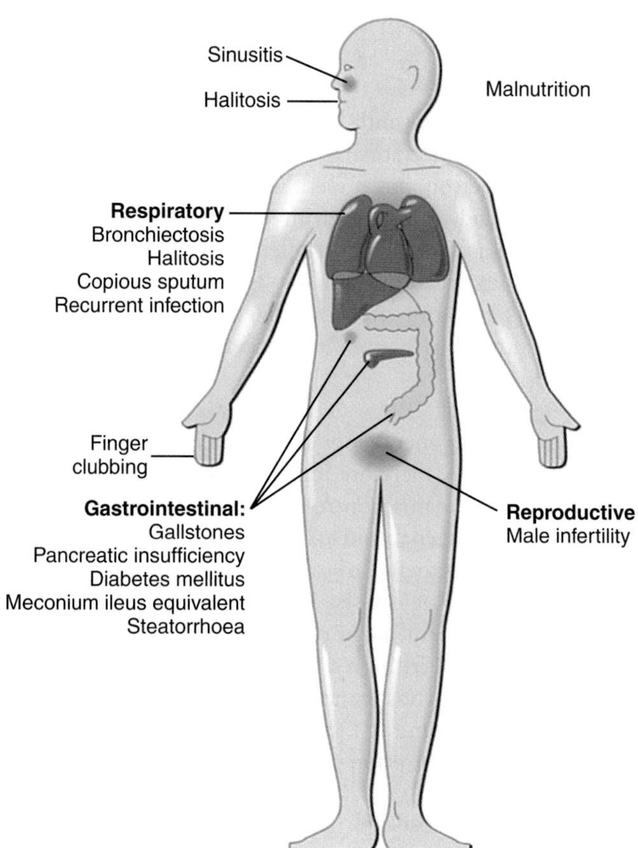

FIGURE 20-7 Cystic fibrosis (CF). (From Axford JS, O'Callaghan CA: *Medicine,* ed 2, Malden, Mass, 2004, Blackwell Science.)

- Excessive sweating in hot weather that may lead to dehydration and circulatory failure
- Biliary cirrhosis caused by progressive clogging of bile ducts producing biliary obstruction and functional liver tissue degeneration
- Inflammatory complications that may include arthritis, finger clubbing (Figure 20-8), or vasculitis
- Gallbladder disease, PUD, GERD, or episodes of partial intestinal obstruction
- Delayed puberty and maturity, probably the result of chronic malnutrition (Men are typically infertile because the vas deferens fails to develop.)

Nutritional Management

The overall nutritional goal is to support normal nutrition and growth for all ages[15]:

- Unrestricted diet, including high-fat foods and additives
- Three meals and two to three snacks each day
- Vitamin supplementation
- Pancreatic enzymes
- Supplements and nutrient-dense nourishments may help
- Encouragement to consume whole grains, nuts, fruits, and vegetables for adequate vitamin and mineral intake
- Extra salt to replace that lost in sweat
- Adequate calcium, vitamin D, and vitamin K

Nutrition intervention is based on an initial and ongoing schedule for assessment, including anthropometrics, laboratory studies, and nutrition evaluation (Table 20-4). Related therapy is then outlined in five levels according to individual assessment results and nutrition care needs and actions (Table 20-5).

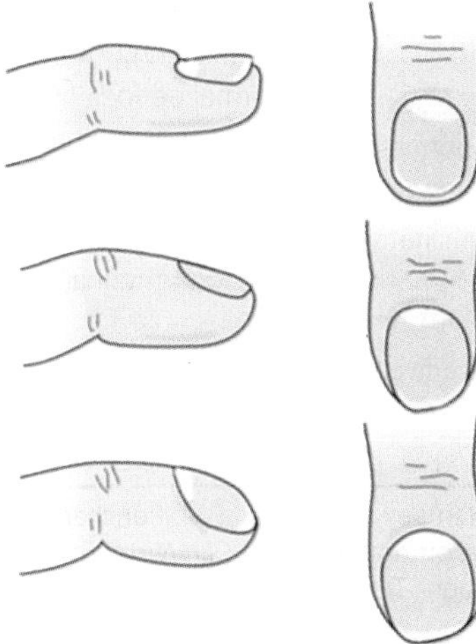

FIGURE 20-8 Clubbing of the fingers. (From Axford JS, O'Callaghan CA: *Medicine,* ed 2, Malden, Mass, 2004, Blackwell Science.)

TABLE 20-4 BASIC NUTRITION ASSESSMENT FOR NUTRITIONAL MANAGEMENT OF CYSTIC FIBROSIS

KEY ASSESSMENTS	MONITORING SCHEDULE AND INDICATIONS
Anthropometry	
Weight	Every 3 months or as needed for growth evaluation
Height (length)	
BMI (adults)	
Head circumference (until child is age 2)	
Midarm circumference	
Triceps skinfold	
Midarm muscle circumference (derived)*	
Biochemical Data	
CBC TIBC, serum iron, ferritin	Yearly routine care, interim as needed to detect deficiencies, iron status
Plasma/serum retinol, α-tocopherol Albumin, prealbumin	As indicated, weight loss, growth failure, clinical deterioration
Electrolytes, acid-base balance	Summer heat, prolonged fever
Random glucose	Annually to detect CFDM
Dietary Evaluation	
Dietary intake	As indicated, history and food records, full energy-nutrient analysis
Three-day fat balance study†	As indicated, weight loss, growth failure, clinical deterioration
Anticipatory guidance	Yearly, interim as needed according to growth or situational needs

Data from Hollander FM, De Roos NM, De Vries JH, et al: Assessment of nutritional status in adult patients with cystic fibrosis: whole-body bioimpedance vs body mass index, skinfolds, and leg-to-leg bioimpedance, *J Am Diet Assoc* 105(4):549, 2005; Ramsey BW, Farrell PM, Pencharz P: Nutritional assessment and management in cystic fibrosis: a consensus report—The Consensus Committee, *Am J Clin Nutr* 55:108, 1992; Yankaskas JR: Cystic fibrosis adult care: consensus conference report, *Chest* 125:1S, 2004.

CBC, Complete blood count; *TIBC,* total iron-binding capacity; *BMI,* body mass index; *CFDM,* cystic fibrosis–related diabetes mellitus.

*See Chapter 16 for equations.

†Three-day food records for analysis of fat intake; stool collections for analysis of fat content and degree of malabsorption.

TABLE 20-5 LEVELS OF NUTRITION CARE FOR MANAGEMENT OF CYSTIC FIBROSIS

LEVELS OF CARE	PATIENT GROUPS	NUTRITION ACTIONS
Level I—routine care	All	Diet counseling, food plans, enzyme replacement, vitamin supplements, nutrition education, exploration of problems
Level II—anticipatory guidance	Greater than 90% ideal weight-height index but at risk of energy imbalance; severe pancreatic insufficiency, frequent pulmonary infections, normal periods of rapid growth	Increased monitoring of dietary intake, complete energy-nutrient analysis, increased kcaloric density as needed; assess behavioral needs; provide counseling, nutrition education
Level III—supportive intervention	85%-90% ideal weight-height index, decreased weight-growth velocity	Reinforce all previously mentioned actions, add oral supplements (energy-nutrient dense)
Level IV—rehabilitative care	Consistently less than 85% ideal weight-height index, nutritional and growth failure	All of the previously mentioned plus EN support by nasoenteric or enterostomy tube feeding (see Chapter 19)
Level V—resuscitative or palliative care	Less than 75% ideal weight-height index, progressive nutritional failure	All of the previously mentioned plus continuous enteral tube feedings or TPN (see Chapter 19)

Modified from Ramsey BW, Farrell PM, Pencharz P: Nutritional assessment and management in cystic fibrosis: a consensus report—The Consensus Committee, *Am J Clin Nutr* 55:108, 1992.
EN, Enteral nutrition; *TPN,* total parenteral nutrition.

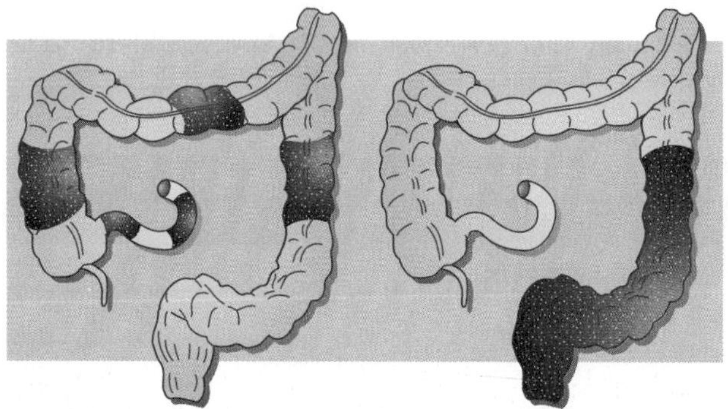

FIGURE 20-9 Crohn's disease *(left)* and ulcerative colitis (UC) *(right)*. Crohn's disease typically involves the small and large intestine in a segmental manner; UC generally starts in the rectum and progresses to involvement of varying lengths of the colon. (Modified from Cotran CS, Kumar V, Robbins SJ: *Robbins' pathologic basis of disease,* ed 4, Philadelphia, 1989, Saunders.)

Inflammatory Bowel Diseases

Nature and Incidence

The two most common forms of IBD are Crohn's disease and ulcerative colitis (UC).[16] Both conditions produce extended mucosal tissue lesions, although these lesions differ in extent and nature (Figure 20-9). However, they have been classified medically in a *single group,* because they are similar in their clinical symptoms and management. Their causes remain unknown, although heredity, environment, and immune functions are thought to be contributing factors.[16] Incidence of these diseases, especially Crohn's disease, has increased worldwide. Crohn's disease is particularly prevalent in industrialized areas of the world. It also appears among otherwise low-risk persons who move from rural to urban centers, with incidence being highest in people from 20 to 40 years of age and those of Jewish heritage.

Clinical Manifestations

Also called *regional enteritis* and *granulomatous colitis,* inflammation produced by Crohn's disease extends through all layers of the intestinal wall, most commonly in the proximal portion of the colon and less often the terminal ileum.[17] UC is an inflammatory disease of mucosal layers of the rectum and colon.[18] Similarities and differences between the two diseases are summarized in Table 20-6.

Medical Management

Because the cause of IBD is unknown, treatment is focused on alleviating and reducing inflammation. Similar drug therapies are used for Crohn's disease and UC: antibiotics, immunosuppressants, immunomodulators, and biologic therapies.[2,18] A small percentage of patients with UC require surgery.[18] Most common surgical procedures include total colectomy or ileostomy (Figure 20-10). Approximately 80% of patients with Crohn's disease will eventually require surgery. Fifty percent of these patients will require a second surgery within 10 years as a result of disease recurrence. Strictures often require minimal resection; colitis may require colectomy with ileorectal anastomosis or ileostomy. Abscesses are drained, and enteric fistulae are resected.[17,18]

Nutrition Therapy

Nutrition therapy centers on supporting the healing process and avoiding nutritional deficiency states and will be contingent on functional condition of the GI tract. Nutrition intervention depends on the functional status of the GI tract: extent of exacerbation, extent of diarrheal output, obstruction, surgery, and bleeding. When an oral diet cannot meet nutritional needs, enteral nutrition (EN) or PN is used:[19]

TABLE 20-6 **SIMILARITIES AND DIFFERENCES BETWEEN CROHN'S DISEASE AND ULCERATIVE COLITIS**

MANIFESTATION	CROHN'S DISEASE	ULCERATIVE COLITIS
CAUSE	**UNKNOWN**	**UNKNOWN**
Genetics	Increased prevalence in first-degree relatives; NOD2 gene mutation on chromosome 16	Increased prevalence in first-degree relatives; susceptibility loci on chromosomes 2 and 6
Site of inflammation	Any part of the gastrointestinal (GI) tract	Rectum (and spreads proximally)
Mucosal layers affected		Epithelial
Abdominal pain	Common	Common
Diarrhea	Common	Common
Rectal bleeding	Sometimes	Common
Perforations	Common	Yes
Fibrosis, stricture, and fistulas	Common	No
Toxic megacolon	Rare	Common
Weight loss	Common	Common
Steatorrhea	Sometimes	No
Perianal disease	Common	No
Fever	Yes	No
Epidemiology	Developed countries, major age peak at ages 20-40, more common in women	Developed countries, major age peak at ages 20-40, more common in women
Relapses and remissions	Chronic	Usually no symptoms between attacks
Complications	Abscess, obstruction, fistulas, perianal disease, increased risk of colon cancer, malabsorption, kidney stones (oxalate and uric acid), gallstones	Many and varied including joint disorders, fatty liver, disorders of the eyes and skin
Prophylactic therapy	Not well established	Colonoscopy with multiple biopsies every 1-3 years
Prognosis	Recurrent morbidity throughout lives; risk of death approximately twice the general population	Mortality rate similar to general population

Data from Sartin JS: Gastrointestinal disorders. In Copstead LC, Banasik JL: *Pathophysiology,* ed 4, St Louis, 2009, Saunders.

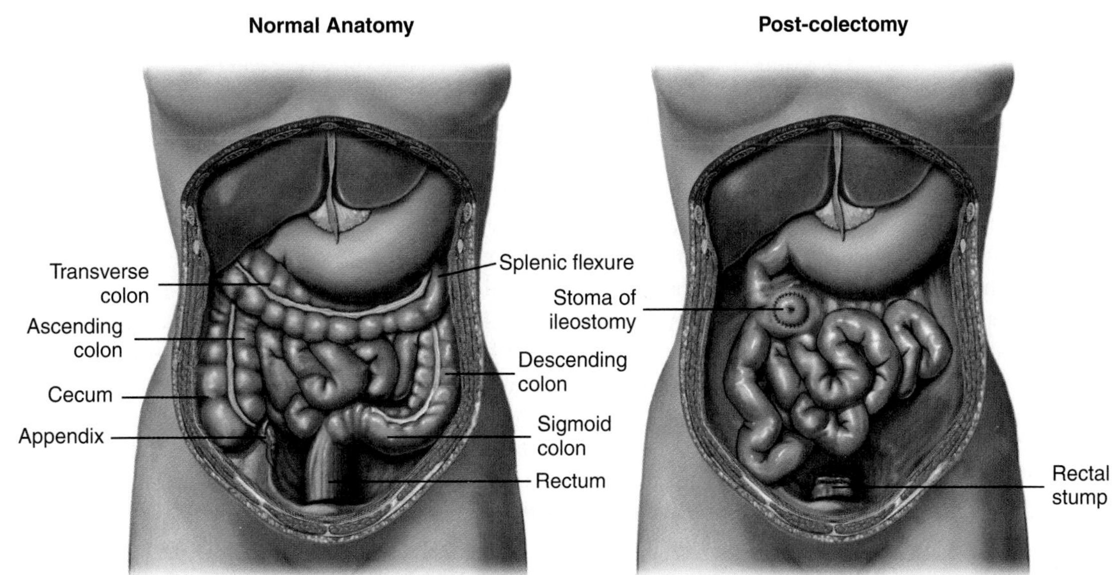

FIGURE 20-10 Colectomy (colon removal) with ileostomy. (Medical Illustration Copyright © 2006 Nucleus Medical Art, All rights reserved. www.nucleusinc.com.)

- Enteral feedings or total parenteral nutrition (TPN)
- Progression to low-fat, low-residue, high-protein, high-calorie, small, frequent meals
- Vitamin and mineral supplements: vitamin D, zinc, calcium, magnesium, folate, vitamin B_{12}, iron

Nutrition Therapy During Remission

Nutrition therapy in remission includes the following[19]:

- Tailor for patient's current GI function
- Energy and protein at levels to maintain weight and replenish nutrient stores
- Avoid foods high in oxalate (Appendix C)
- Increase antioxidant intake (see Chapter 6)
- Consider supplementation with omega-3-fatty acids and glutamine
- Use probiotics and prebiotics
- Diet as complete as possible

Short-Bowel Syndrome

Cause

SBS is a malabsorptive condition secondary to surgical removal of parts of the small intestine with extensive dysfunction of the remaining portion of the organ. Severity of malabsorption is contingent on amount and location of bowel resection. Removal of the distal two thirds of ileum and ileocecal valve often results in severe malnutrition because the ileocecal valve controls transit time of intestinal contents. Removal often promotes a transit time too rapid for sufficient absorption of nutrients. Absorption of water, electrolytes, protein, fat, carbohydrates, vitamins, and minerals is significantly reduced when large portions of the small intestine are lost.[8,20]

Typically, in an adult the small intestine is 20 feet long and the large intestine is 7 feet long. A general definition for SBS is a resection of more than 50% of the small intestine. Resections result from inherent conditions such as Crohn's disease or radiation enteritis, surgical bypass, or massive abdominal injury and trauma. They may also be required for vascular problems such as blood clots causing death of involved tissue or for extensive fistula formation, radiation injury, congenital abnormalities, or cancer. After resection, the remaining small intestine has remarkable ability to adapt.[2] Remaining villi may enlarge and lengthen, consequently increasing absorptive surface area of the remaining intestine. Nutrients must be ingested orally for this adaptive sequence to take place, and gradual increase in oral intake after resection could promote gradual recovery in absorptive capability. PN support may be necessary for the short term or indefinitely after surgical shortening of the gut.

Nutritional Management

Degrees of surgical resection create different problems, and nutrition therapy must be tailored to individual functional capacity remaining. Initial nutritional needs are usually supplied by early EN or PN support (see Chapter 19). Frequent monitoring of responses to nutrition support, especially fluid and electrolyte balances and malnutrition signs, is essential. The patient is weaned from nutrition support to an oral diet as tolerated, accompanied by vitamin and mineral supplementation. Nutritional status should continue to be monitored. As adaptation progresses, early restriction of fat may be liberalized somewhat with moderate use of the more easily absorbed MCT oil to obtain needed kcalories.

Bowel Transplantation

Patients with complications from or failure of TPN such as recurrent sepsis, thrombosis of access sites, metabolic disorders, cholestasis, and hepatic dysfunction may be considered candidates for intestine transplant, which may involve the entire small intestine or just a segment of it. Most intestine transplants are whole organ transplants and are often performed in combination with a liver transplant.

Patients undergoing small-bowel transplantation can have problems transitioning to oral nutrition. Furthermore, special feeding considerations should be taken into consideration during the initial posttransplant phase when the graft begins to function (Table 20-7). Large amounts of fluids lost after surgery must be replaced to prevent dehydration. Oral rehydration solutions may be used, although intravenous fluids may be required to replace not only lost fluids but also magnesium, zinc, bicarbonate, potassium, and sodium. Fiber, pectin, paregoric, and loperamide may enhance intestinal absorption by slowing transit time.

DISORDERS OF THE LARGE INTESTINE

Flatulence

Everyone has it. Most believe they have too much, and everyone is embarrassed if they pass gas in the wrong place at the wrong time. History views flatulence with mixed reviews. Hippocrates professed, "Passing gas is necessary to well-being." The Roman Emperor Claudius decreed, "All Roman citizens shall be allowed to pass gas whenever necessary." Regrettably for flatulent Romans, Emperor Constantine later overturned this pronouncement.

Cause

Flatulence is the condition of having excessive stomach or intestinal gas. Gas in the gut is the result of swallowed air or production in the intestines. Air swallowing (aerophagia) is a common cause of gas in the stomach. Small amounts of air are swallowed when eating and drinking. Some people swallow additional air while they eat or drink rapidly, chew gum, smoke, or wear dentures that are too loose. Most swallowed air is expelled from the stomach by burping or belching. Residual gas moves into the small intestine and is partially absorbed. A small quantity of gas travels to the large intestine and is expelled through the rectum.

Gas is produced in the intestines when normal, harmless bacteria in the large intestine break down undigested foods humans cannot because of a lack of specific digestive enzymes. Gas in the intestines is made of primarily odorless vapors—carbon dioxide (CO_2), oxygen, nitrogen, hydrogen,

TABLE 20-7 GUIDELINES FOR INITIATING ENTERAL NUTRITION IN INTESTINE TRANSPLANT RECIPIENTS

NUTRIENT	GUIDELINE	COMMENT
Carbohydrates	Concentrated sweets and hyperosmolar fruit juice may cause osmotic diarrhea.	Carbohydrate malabsorption and secondary lactase deficiency may increase luminal osmolarity and increase stomal output.
Fat	MCT or intravenous lipids short term.	Lacteals and lymphatics of small intestine are severed during organ retrieval causing fat malabsorption initially.
Glutamine	Long-chain fatty acid absorption may improve within 2-6 weeks as lacteals and lymphatics are regenerated.	Glutamine is a conditionally essential amino acid and fuel for enterocytes.
Bicarbonate	An enteral formula enriched with glutamine may theoretically improve absorptive function and mucosal structure after transplantation.	Bicarbonate losses from the ostomy are often increased.
Fluid	Supplement. Rehydration solutions may be helpful.	High intestinal losses are common.

Modified from Hasse JM: Nutrition assessment and support of organ transplant recipients, *JPEN J Parenter Enteral Nutr* 25:120, 2001. Reprinted with permission of SAGE Publications.
MCT, Medium-chain triglycerides.

and sometimes methane. The unpleasant odor of flatulence is produced by bacteria in the large intestine that release small amounts of gases that contain sulfur. These gases eventually exit the body through the rectum. Hydrogen and CO_2 are produced after ingestion of certain fruits and vegetables containing indigestible carbohydrates and in those with malabsorption syndromes (CF, CD, pancreatic insufficiency). Large amounts of disaccharides pass into the colon and are fermented to hydrogen in those with lactose deficiency. Methane is produced in approximately one third of the population and is influenced minimally by food ingestion. Tendency to produce methane appears to be a familial trait.[21] Foods that produce gas in one person may not produce gas in another. Most foods that produce gas contain carbohydrates (Table 20-8); fats and proteins cause little gas.

Medical Management

The most common ways to reduce production of gas are changing diet, taking medications, and reducing amount of air swallowed. The difficulty in suggesting dietary modification is individual tolerances. The quantity of gas produced by particular foods varies from person to person. Effective dietary change is typically the result of learning by way of trial and error.

Few well-controlled studies have demonstrated clear-cut benefit from any drug.[22] Some OTC medicines are available to help reduce symptoms (Table 20-9). Although gas may be unpleasant and embarrassing, it is not life threatening. Education concerning causes, ways to reduce symptoms, and treatment help most people find relief.[22]

Irritable Bowel Syndrome

Cause

Sometimes called *spastic colon,* IBS is a recurring functional disorder typified by abdominal pain or discomfort with alternating diarrhea and constipation for which no

TABLE 20-8 FOODS THAT MAY CAUSE GAS

CATEGORY		FOOD SOURCES
Sugars	Raffinose	Beans, cabbage, brussels sprouts, broccoli, asparagus, other vegetables, whole grains
	Lactose	Milk, milk products (cheese, ice cream, processed foods)
	Fructose	Onions, artichokes, peas, wheat (fructose also used as a sweetener in some soft drinks and fruit drinks)
	Sorbitol	Fruits: apples, pears, peaches, prunes (sorbitol also used as an artificial sweetener in many dietetic foods and sugar-free candies and gums)
Starches		Potatoes, corn, noodles, wheat products (only starch that does not produce gas is rice)
Fiber	Soluble	Oat bran, beans, peas, most fruits
	Insoluble	Wheat bran, some vegetables

Modified from National Digestive Disease Information Clearinghouse (NDDIC), National Institute of Diabetes and Digestive and Kidney Diseases (NIDDK), National Institutes of Health (NIH): *Gas in the digestive tract,* NIH Pub No 08-883, Bethesda, Md, 2008, National Digestive Diseases Information Clearinghouse. Retrieved May 14, 2009, from www.digestive.niddk.nih.gov/ddiseases/pubs/gas/.

KEY TERMS

probiotics Microbial foods or supplements that can be used to modify or reestablish intestinal flora and improve health of the host.

prebiotics Nondigestible food products that promote growth of symbiotic bacterial species already present in the colon.

TABLE 20-9 NONPRESCRIPTION MEDICATIONS USED TO TREAT FLATULENCE

MEDICATION	CLASSIFICATION	ACTION
Simethicone Mylanta II Maalox II Di-Gel	Antacid	Foaming agent that joins gas bubbles in the stomach, making gas more easily belched away; no effect on intestinal gas
Lactase Lactaid Lactrase	Enzyme	Aids lactose digestion
Beano	Enzyme supplement	Contains sugar-digesting enzyme the body lacks to digest sugar in beans and many vegetables; has no effect on gas caused by lactose or fiber
Charcocaps	Activated charcoal	May produce relief from gas produced in colon

Data from National Digestive Disease Information Clearinghouse (NDDIC), National Institute of Diabetes and Digestive and Kidney Diseases (NIDDK), National Institutes of Health (NIH): *Gas in the digestive tract,* NIH Pub No 08-883, Bethesda, Md, 2008, NIH. Retrieved May 14, 2009, from www.digestive.niddk.nih.gov/ddiseases/pubs/gas/; Maslar J, Kreplick LW: *Flatulence (gas),* Omaha, Neb, 2005, eMedicine Consumer Health. Retrieved May 14, 2009, from www.emedicinehealth.com/Articles/5940-1.asp.

organic explanation is available.[8] For those with IBS, quantity of symptoms is not as important as quality of life. Work, social life, and even sexual intercourse can be disrupted by IBS.[8] IBS is an extremely common disorder, affecting up to 20% of the U.S. population, but most never seek medical attention.[2]

Clinical Symptoms

Manifestation of IBS may differ to a great extent from person to person. Some experience only diarrhea or constipation, whereas others experience an alternating pattern of both problems.[8] Some symptoms may be more marked than others. No physical findings or diagnostic tests confirm the diagnosis of IBS.[23] Diagnosis is determined in the presence of congruent symptoms and after ruling out organic diseases.[23] More than half of those diagnosed with IBS are female patients.

The symptom-based Rome III diagnostic criteria for IBS emphasize a clear-cut diagnosis instead of excluding other medical conditions.[23] These criteria are based on a detailed history, physical examination, and limited diagnostic tests, as well as presentation of a particular set of symptoms (for the last 3 months, with symptom onset at least 6 months before diagnosis) as follows[24]:

- Recurrent abdominal pain or discomfort* at least 3 days per month in the last 3 months associated with two or more of the following:
  1. Improvement with defecation
  2. Onset associated with a change in frequency of stool
  3. Onset associated with a change in form (appearance) of stool
- The following other symptoms support, but are not essential, to the diagnosis of IBS:
  - More than three bowel movements per day or fewer than three bowel movements per week
  - Lumpy-hard or loose-watery stool form
  - Abnormal stool passage (straining, urgency, or feeling of incomplete evacuation)
  - Passage of mucus
  - Bloating or feeling of abdominal distention

Medical Management

Possibly the most helpful treatment intervention is to proffer assurance and a straightforward explanation of the functional nature of symptoms. Patients should be assured that their symptoms are real (i.e., not caused by stress or a psychologic or psychiatric disorder), although in some individuals stress can trigger or exacerbate symptoms of IBS.[24,25]

A chronic disorder, IBS can be treated but not cured. Therapy is directed at specific symptoms.[25] Antidiarrheal agents can decrease motility and increase consistency of stools for patients with diarrhea-predominant IBS. An α-adrenergic stimulating agent is sometimes used to treat diarrhea and abdominal pain by inhibiting norepinephrine activity. Other medications often used to treat IBS and assist in pain control are tricyclic antidepressants and selective serotonin reuptake inhibitors (SSRIs). Constipation-predominant IBS is often treated with bulking agents and osmotic laxatives. The newest medications for IBS are medications that work as 5-HT_4 receptor agonists and are effective in treating constipation-predominant IBS.[2]

Nutritional Management

Dietary triggers of IBS have not been established; however, dietary modification may provide symptomatic benefit. For some, a food diary in which food intake, symptoms, and activities are recorded may uncover dietary or psychosocial aspects that predispose symptoms. Malabsorption of lactose, fructose, and sorbitol can cause bloating, distention, flatulence, and diarrhea. An assortment of foods can trigger flatulence (see Table 20-8), which may cause pain and distention in some patients.

For patients presenting primarily with constipation, a high-fiber diet (20 to 30 g/day) may ease symptoms. Bran powder (1 tbsp two to three times daily with food or in 8 oz or more of liquid) provides the recommended amount.

**Discomfort* means an uncomfortable sensation not described as pain.

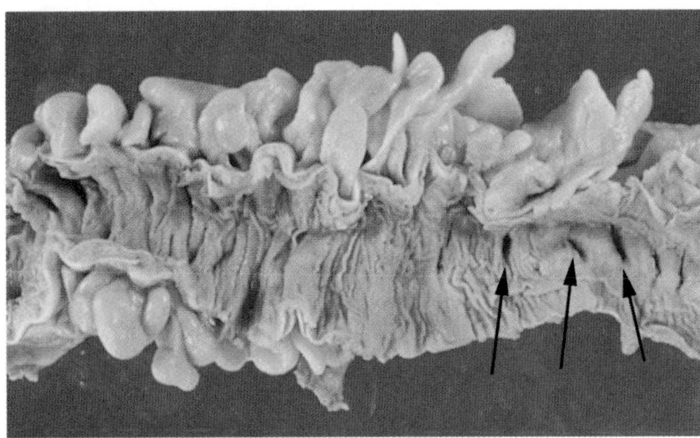

FIGURE 20-11 Diverticula. (From Lewis SM, Heitkemper M, Dirksen S: *Medical-surgical nursing: assessment and management of clinical problems,* ed 6, St Louis, 2004, Mosby.)

Some patients may describe increased gas and distention from fiber supplementation with bran; therefore psyllium, methylcellulose, or polycarbophil are often better tolerated.

Diverticular Disease

Nature and Cause

A *diverticulum* is a small tubular sac that protrudes from a main canal or cavity in the body (Figure 20-11). Formation and presence of small diverticula protruding from the intestinal lumen, usually the colon, produce the condition diverticulosis. More often diverticulosis occurs in older adults. It develops at points of weakened musculature in the bowel wall, along the track of blood vessels entering the bowel from within. Direct cause is a progressive increase in pressure within the bowel from segmental circular muscle contractions that normally move the remaining food mass along and form the feces for elimination. When pressures become sufficiently high in one of these segments and dietary fiber is insufficient to maintain the necessary bulk for preventing high internal pressures within the colon, diverticula, small protrusions of the muscle layer, develop at that point. The condition causes no problem unless small diverticula become infected and inflamed from fecal irritation and colon bacteria. This diseased state is called *diverticulitis.* The commonly used collective term covering diverticulosis and diverticulitis is *diverticular disease.*

Clinical Symptoms

As the inflammatory process grows, increased hypermotility and pressures from luminal segmentation cause pain. Pain and tenderness are usually localized in the lower left side of the abdomen and are accompanied by nausea, vomiting, distention, diarrhea, intestinal spasm, and fever. If the process continues, then intestinal obstruction or perforation may necessitate surgical intervention.

Nutritional Management

Diverticular disease is a common GI disorder among middle-aged persons and older adults. Aggressive nutrition therapy hastens recovery from an attack, shortens hospital stay, and reduces costs. Numerous studies and extensive clinical practice have demonstrated better management of chronic diverticular disease with an increased amount of dietary fiber than with old practices of restricting fiber. In acute episodes of active disease, however, the amount of dietary fiber should be reduced. The relationship of dietary fiber and diverticular disease has been further reinforced by studies of populations, such as those in Japan, that have recently experienced the westernization of their culture. Chapter 3 provides an extended discussion of dietary fiber and its relation to health and disease. Historically, avoidance of nuts, seeds, and hulls has been recommended, but current literature indicates this is not required.[26-29]

Constipation

A common disorder, usually of short duration, constipation is characterized by retention of feces in the colon beyond normal emptying time. It is a problem for which Americans spend a quarter of a billion dollars each year on laxatives. However, "regularity" of elimination is highly individual, and it is not necessary to have a bowel movement every day to be healthy. Usually this common, short-term problem results from various sources of nervous tension, worry, and changes in social setting. Such situations include vacations and travel with alterations in usual routines. In addition, it may be caused by prolonged use of laxatives or cathartics, low-fiber diets, inadequate fluid intake, or lack of exercise, all of which can contribute to a decreased intestinal muscle tone. Increasing activity and improving dietary intake to include adequate fiber (goal of 25 to 35 g/day) and fluid are usually sufficient strategies to remedy the situation. If chronic constipation persists, however, then agents that increase stool bulk may be necessary. These bulking agents include bran or more soluble forms of fiber. Taking laxatives or enemas on a regular basis should be avoided. The problem of constipation occurs in all age-groups but is almost epidemic in older adults. In all cases, a personalized approach to management of constipation is fundamental.

DISEASES OF THE GASTROINTESTINAL ACCESSORY ORGANS

Three major accessory organs—(1) the liver, (2) the gallbladder, and (3) the pancreas (Figure 20-12)—lie adjacent to the GI tract and produce important digestive agents that enter the intestine and aid in processing of food substances. Specific enzymes are produced for each of the major nutrients, and bile is added to assist in enzymatic digestion of fats. Diseases of these organs can easily affect GI function and cause problems in the normal handling of specific types of food.

Viral Hepatitis

Cause

Viral hepatitis (inflammation of the liver) is a major public health problem throughout the world, affecting hundreds of millions of people. It causes considerable illness and death

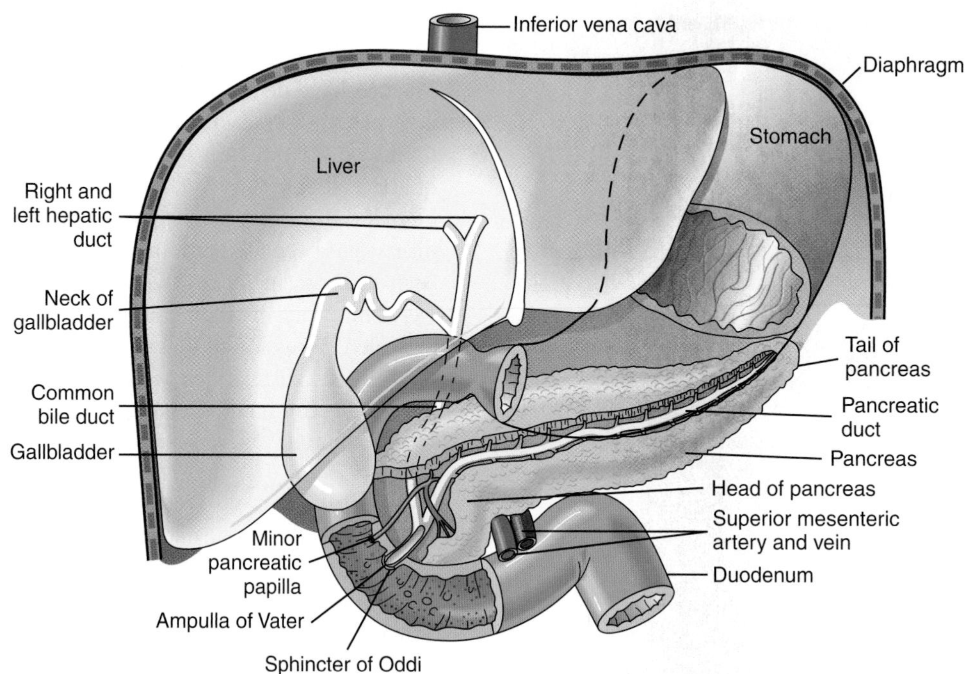

FIGURE 20-12 Liver, pancreas, and gallbladder. (From Copstead LE, Banasik JL: *Pathophysiology,* ed 4, Philadelphia, 2009, Saunders.)

in human populations from acute infection or its effects, which may include chronic active hepatitis, cirrhosis, and primary liver cancer. During the past few years, knowledge of viruses causing different types of hepatitis has grown rapidly. Currently, six unrelated human hepatitis viruses, A, B, C, D, and E, have been isolated and described. The two most common and well known are A and B, which serve as examples, as follows:

1. *Hepatitis A virus (HAV):* HAV is transmitted via the classic oral-fecal route through contaminated food and water. It is a prevalent infection worldwide, especially where overcrowding and poor hygiene or sanitation exists. An HAV vaccine has been developed that is far more effective than the former large and painful injection of gamma globulins, antibodies isolated from the blood. This vaccine protects travelers to developing countries, where the virus is endemic and may easily contaminate water and food.[30]
2. *Hepatitis B virus (HBV):* HBV is mainly spread via parenteral contact with infected blood or blood products, including contaminated needles, and sexual contact.[26] It has now been implicated worldwide as the major cause of chronic liver disease and associated liver cancer. HBV infection is closely related to the body's immune system. Approximately 10% to 20% of those who become infected with HBV become chronic carriers. Of this number, approximately 20% acquire chronic hepatitis eventually progressing to cirrhosis and, later in some, liver cancer.[30] Universal immunization is recommended for persons of any age, but particularly for the following high-risk groups: male homosexuals, Alaska Natives, immigrants from highly endemic areas, illicit drugs users, domestic associates of HBV carriers, hemodialysis patients, residents of institutions, medical and dental personnel, patients needing frequent transfusions, and those planning to reside in high-risk areas (e.g., Far East and sub-Saharan Africa).[30]

Clinical Symptoms

Viral agents of hepatitis produce diffuse injury to liver cells, especially parenchymal cells. In milder cases, liver injury is largely reversible, but with increasing severity, more extensive necrosis occurs. In some cases, massive necrosis may lead to liver failure and death. A cardinal symptom of hepatitis is anorexia, contributing to risk of malnutrition. Varying clinical symptoms appear depending on the degree of liver injury. Jaundice, a major symptom, may or may not be obvious, depending on severity of the disease, and it can have nutritional and psychologic effects. In an outbreak of hepatitis, many infected persons may be nonicteric and thus go undiagnosed and untreated because jaundice has not developed sufficiently to be seen. Malnutrition and impaired immunocompetence contribute to spontaneous infections and continuing liver disease. General symptoms, in addition to anorexia, include malaise, weakness, nausea and vomiting, diarrhea, headache, fever, enlarged and tender liver, and enlarged spleen. When jaundice develops, it usually occurs for a preicteric period of 5 to 10 days, deepens for 1 to 2 weeks, then levels off and decreases. After this crisis point, a sufficient recovery of injured cells occurs, and a convalescence of 3 weeks to 3 months follows. Optimal care during this time is essential to avoid relapse.

General Treatment

Bed rest is essential. Physical activity and exercise increases severity and duration of the disease. A daily intake of 3000 to 3500 mL of fluid guards against dehydration and gives a general sense of well-being and improved appetite. However, optimal nutrition is the major therapy. It provides the essential foundation for recovery of the injured liver cells and overall return of strength.

Nutrition Therapy

A complete nutrition assessment and initial personal history provide the basis for planning care. Nutrition therapy principles relate to the liver's function in metabolizing each of the nutrients, as follows[31]:

- *Adequate protein:* Protein is essential for liver cell regeneration, as well as for maintaining all essential bodily functions. It also provides lipotropic agents such as methionine and choline for conversion of fats to lipoproteins and removal from the liver, thus preventing fatty infiltration. The daily diet should supply 1.0 to 1.2 g/kg of actual body weight (ABW) of high-quality protein. This amount is usually enough to achieve a positive nitrogen balance.
- *Low fat:* Less than 30% of calories should come from fat in case of steatorrhea.
- *Four to six small feedings:* To promote adequate intake and minimize loss of muscle, at least three meals and a bedtime snack are recommended.
- *Sodium:* If fluid retention is present, then limit sodium to 90 mEq/day (approximately 2000 mg).

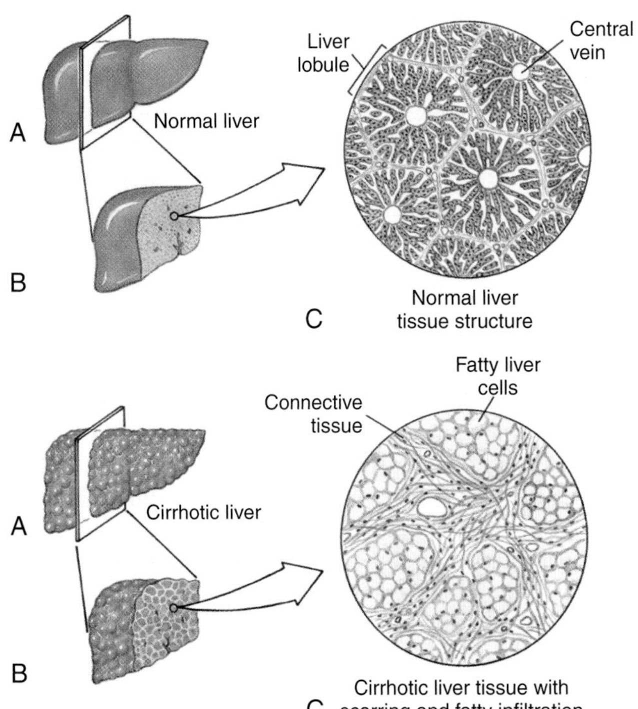

FIGURE 20-13 Comparison of normal liver and liver with cirrhotic changes. **A,** Anterior view of organ. **B,** Cross-section. **C,** Tissue structure. (Medical and Scientific Illustration.)

Meals and Feedings

The problem of supplying a diet adequate to meet increased nutritional demands of a patient with an illness that makes food almost repellent calls for creativity and supportive encouragement. As the patient improves, appetizing and attractive food is needed. Because nutrition therapy is key to recovery, a major nutrition and nursing responsibility requires devising ways to encourage the increased amounts of food intake needed. The clinical dietitian and nursing staff should work together to achieve mutual goals planned for the patient. All staff attendants must observe appropriate precautions in handling patient trays to prevent spread of the infection.

Cirrhosis

Cirrhosis is the general term used for advanced stages of liver disease, regardless of the initial cause of the disease. Among all digestive diseases, cirrhosis of the liver, caused by chronic alcohol abuse, is the leading nonmalignant cause of death in the United States and most of the developed world. The majority of deaths occur among young and middle-aged adults. The French physician René Laënnec (1781-1826) first used the term *cirrhosis* (from the Greek work *kirrhos,* meaning orange-yellow) to describe the abnormal color and rough surface of the diseased liver. The cirrhotic liver is a firm, fibrous, dull-yellowish mass with orange nodules projecting from its surface (Figure 20-13).

Cause

Some forms of cirrhosis result from biliary obstruction, with blockage of the biliary ducts and accumulation of bile in the liver.[32] Other cases may result from liver necrosis from undetermined causes or, in some cases, from previous viral hepatitis. A common problem is fatty cirrhosis, associated with the complicating factor of malnutrition. Continuing fatty infiltration causes cellular destruction and fibrotic tissue changes.

Clinical Symptoms

Early signs of cirrhosis include GI disturbances such as nausea, vomiting, loss of appetite, distention, and epigastric pain. In time, jaundice may appear, with increasing weakness, edema, ascites, and anemia from GI bleeding, iron deficiency, or hemorrhage. A specific macrocytic anemia from folic acid deficiency is also frequently observed. Steatorrhea is a common symptom. Major symptoms are caused by a basic protein deficiency and its multiple metabolic

KEY TERMS

endemic Characterizing a disease of low morbidity that remains constantly in a human community but is clinically recognizable in only a few.

parenchymal cells Functional cells of an organ, as distinguished from the cells constituting its structure or framework.

necrosis Cell death caused by progressive enzyme breakdown.

icteric Alternative term for jaundice (*nonicteric* indicates absence of jaundice and *preicteric* indicates a state before development of icterus, or jaundice).

immunocompetence The ability or capacity to develop an immune response, that is, antibody production or cell-mediated immunity (or both), after exposure to antigen.

problems: (1) plasma protein levels fall, leading to failure of the capillary fluid shift mechanism (see Chapter 2), causing ascites; (2) lipotropic agents are not supplied for fat conversion to lipoproteins, and damaging fat accumulates in the liver tissue; (3) blood-clotting mechanisms are impaired because factors such as prothrombin and fibrinogen are not adequately produced; and (4) general tissue catabolism and negative nitrogen balance continue the overall degenerative process.

As the disease progresses, increasing fibrotic scar tissue impairs blood circulation through the liver, resulting in portal hypertension.[32] Contributing further to the problem is continuing ascites. Impaired portal circulation with increasing venous pressure may lead to esophageal varices, with danger of rupture and fatal massive hemorrhage.

Drug therapy includes use of broad-spectrum antibiotics to limit growth of intestinal bacteria and laxatives to speed intestinal transit time, limiting the amount of time available for bacteria to produce ammonia in the GI tract. Lactulose, a synthetic derivative of lactose consisting of one molecule of galactose and one molecule of fructose, is a laxative that is used in the treatment of hepatic encephalopathy. Lactulose is ionized, cannot diffuse across the colon membrane, and is excreted in the stool. Lactulose can reduce blood ammonia levels by 25% to 50%. Diuretics may be given to reduce fluid retention and prevent ascites.

Nutrition Therapy

When alcoholism is an added underlying problem, treatment is difficult. Each patient requires supportive care. Therapy is usually aimed at correcting fluid and electrolyte problems and providing as much nutrition support as possible for hepatic repair. In any case, guidelines for nutrition therapy for cirrhosis of the liver should include the following principles[2,33]:

- *Energy:* 40 to 50 kcal/kg body weight. Fluid retention, if present, will affect the accuracy of estimating kcalorie needs. As muscle tissue is wasted, it is often replaced by fluid weight. An estimated dry weight (postparacentesis of ascites or well diuresed) should be used when feasible to estimate kcalorie needs.
- *Protein intake:* 1 to 1.5 g/kg body weight. Intake should be adequate to regenerate liver cells and prevent infections but not excessive to the point of aggravating ammonia buildup and inducing hepatic coma. Protein estimations should be based on dry weight whenever possible.
- *Sodium:* Intake is usually restricted to less than 2000 mg/day to help reduce fluid retention. A sodium intake level of less than 2000 mg/day is considered quite restrictive, and palatability of food is usually a problem. It may be necessary to liberalize the sodium restriction to improve intake.
- *Texture:* If esophageal varices develop, then it may be necessary to give soft foods that are smooth in texture to prevent the danger of rupture and hemorrhage.
- *Carbohydrate:* Adequate intake is needed to prevent catabolism of body protein for energy, which would further increase blood ammonia. Intestinal bacteria make ammonia from undigested proteins (proteins from shed mucosal cells, protein from GI tract bleed, and dietary proteins).
- *Fat:* Fat restriction should be less than 30% of calories (with or without MCT supplements) in patients with steatorrhea.
- *Vitamins and minerals:* The central role of the liver is to metabolize and store vitamins and minerals. Usually all people with advanced liver disease require supplementation of some vitamins, minerals, and trace elements. Nutrient supplementation is determined by monitoring serum levels and checking for clinical signs of deficiencies.
- *Alcohol:* To protect the liver from further injury, abstinence from alcohol is mandatory.
- *Personalized food plan:* Adequate intake is more likely, thus hastening recovery, if the food plan is developed based on the likes and dislikes and real-life schedule of the patient. If appetite is a problem, then several small meals per day instead of full meals may be required.
- *Fluids:* Fluids should be encouraged unless ascites or edema is present. Water is the fluid of choice. Calorie-dense beverages such as juicelike drinks and soft drinks provide excess calories with little nutrient, often taking the place of nutrient-dense foods.

Hepatic Encephalopathy

The term *encephalopathy* refers to any disease or disorder that affects the brain, especially chronic degenerative conditions. Effect on the brain in hepatic encephalopathy is a major serious complication of end-stage liver disease. Accumulation of toxic substances in the blood as a result of liver failure impairs consciousness and contributes to memory loss, personality change, tremors, seizures, stupor, and coma.

Cause

As cirrhotic changes continue in the liver, portal blood circulation diminishes and liver functions begin to fail. The normal liver has a major function of removing ammonia from blood by converting it to urea for excretion. The failing liver can no longer inactivate or detoxify substances or metabolize others. A key factor involved in the progressive disease process is an elevated blood level of ammonia, although it is by no means the sole agent. Resulting hepatic encephalopathy brings changes in consciousness, behavior, and neurologic status.

Clinical Symptoms

Typical response involves disorders of consciousness and alterations in motor function. Apathy, confusion, inappropriate behavior, and drowsiness is seen, progressing to coma. Speech may be slurred or monotonous. A coarse, flapping tremor known as *asterixis* is observed in the outstretched hands, caused by a sustained contraction of a group of muscles. Breath may have a fecal odor, *fetor hepaticus.*

Basic Treatment Objectives

Fundamental objectives of treatment are twofold: (1) removal of sources of excess ammonia and (2) provision of nutrition support. Parenteral fluid and electrolytes are used to restore normal balances. Lactulose and neomycin may be used to control ammonia levels. Neomycin is an antibiotic that reduces the population of urea-splitting organisms within the bowel that produce ammonia.

Nutrition Therapy

General nutrition support for hepatic encephalopathy is based on the following three principles of dietary management[34]:

1. *Alcohol:* Abstinence is necessary.
2. *Energy:* Moderately high energy intake (25 to 40 kcal/kg) is needed to prevent breakdown of body tissue. Moderate fat intake of 30% of total kcal or less is encouraged unless steatorrhea is present. In the case of steatorrhea, fat intake can be reduced. Carbohydrates provide the majority of energy intake.
3. *Protein:* Generally protein intake is limited to 1.0 to 1.5 g/kg unless encephalopathy is seen. If encephalopathy is present, then protein should be limited to 60 g/day. Protein intake can be increased gradually as patient improves. Plant protein seems to be better tolerated than animal protein by some patients.
4. *Meals:* Small frequent meals are better tolerated than large, less frequent meals. Soft foods that are low in fiber help prevent bleeding from esophageal varices.
5. *Supplements:* Water-soluble and fat-soluble vitamin supplements are often necessary.

Liver Transplantation

Liver transplantation is the treatment of choice for patients with end-stage liver disease who have not responded to conventional treatment. Patients being considered for liver transplantation undergo extensive physiologic and psychologic evaluations to detect possible contraindications to the procedure.[2]

As with all major surgery, aggressive nutrition support reduces risks. Careful pretransplantation nutrition assessment and support helps prepare the patient for the surgery. The general goal of posttransplant nutrition therapy is as follows[2]:

- *Energy:* 35-45 kcal/kg
- *Protein:* 1.0-1.2 g/kg
- *Other nutrients:* individualized based on immunosuppressant drug regimen (Complex carbohydrate should provide 50% to 60% of total kcalories. Use of corticosteroids results in the need for sodium to be restricted to 2 to 4 g/day. Cyclosporin and tacrolimus may require potassium restriction. Other minerals and electrolytes should be monitored.)
- *Vitamins:* Dietary Reference Intake (DRI) provided to encourage proper wound healing

Gallbladder Disease

Metabolic Function

Basic function of the gallbladder is to concentrate and store the bile produced in its initial watery solution by the liver. The liver secretes about 600 to 800 mL of bile per day, which the gallbladder normally concentrates fivefold to tenfold to accommodate this daily bile production in its small capacity of 40 to 70 mL. Through the cholecystokinin (CCK) mechanism, presence of fat in the duodenum stimulates contraction of the gallbladder with release of concentrated bile into the common duct and then into the small intestine.

Cholecystitis and Cholelithiasis

The prefix *chole* of the two terms *cholecystitis* and *cholelithiasis* comes from the Greek word *chole*, which means bile. Thus cholecystitis is an inflammation of the gallbladder, and cholelithiasis is the formation of gallstones. Incidence of gallstones is associated with age, gender, and an assortment of medical factors (Box 20-4).

Inflammation of the gallbladder usually results from a low-grade chronic infection and may occur with or without gallstones. However, in 90% to 95% of patients, acute cholecystitis is associated with gallstones and is caused by the obstruction of the cystic duct by stones, resulting in acute inflammation of the organ. Gallstones can be classified into the following two main groups: (1) *cholesterol stones* and (2) *pigment stones*[35]:

1. *Cholesterol stones:* In the United States and most Western countries, more than 75% of gallstones are cholesterol stones. The infectious process produces changes in gallbladder mucosa, which affects its absorptive powers. The main ingredient of bile is cholesterol, which is insoluble in water. Normally, cholesterol is kept in solution by other ingredients in bile. However, when the absorbing mucosal tissue of the gallbladder is inflamed or infected, changes occur in the tissue. Absorptive powers of the gallbladder may be altered, affecting solubility of the bile ingredients. Excess water or excess bile acid may be absorbed. Under these abnormal absorptive conditions, cholesterol may precipitate, forming gallstones of almost pure cholesterol.
2. *Pigment stones:* Black and brown pigment gallstones, although they differ in chemical composition and clinical features, are colored by the presence of *bilirubin*, the pigment in red blood cells. They are associated with chronic

BOX 20-4 RISK FACTORS FOR GALLBLADDER DISEASE

- Female gender
- Ethnicity: Native American, particularly Pima Indians of North America
- High-cholesterol diet
- Use of oral contraceptives
- Obesity (body mass index [BMI] >30)
- Ileal resection or disease
- Diabetes mellitus
- Rapid weight loss (in obese persons)
- Positive family history
- Some medications (e.g., lipid-lowering agents)
- Gallbladder hypomobility

Data from Sartin JS: Alterations in function of the gallbladder and exocrine pancreas. In Copstead LC, Banasik JL: *Pathophysiology,* ed 4, St Louis, 2009, Saunders.

hemolysis in conditions such as sickle cell disease, thalassemia, cirrhosis, long-term TPN, and advancing age. Pigment stones are often found in bile ducts and may be related to a bacterial infection with *Escherichia coli.*

Clinical Symptoms

When inflammation, stones, or both are present in the gallbladder, contraction from the cholecystokinin-pancreozymin (CCK-PZ) mechanism causes pain. Sometimes the pain is severe. Fullness, distention after eating, and particular difficulty with fatty foods are noted.

General Treatment

Surgical removal of the gallbladder, a cholecystectomy (Figure 20-14), is usually indicated. If the patient is obese, then some weight loss before surgery is advisable if surgery can be delayed. Supportive therapy is largely nutritional. Several nonsurgical treatments for removing the stones, using chemical dissolution or mechanical stone fragmentation, have been developed. These methods provide effective alternatives to surgery in some cases.[35]

Nutrition Therapy

Basic principles of nutrition therapy for gallbladder disease include the following:

- *Fat:* Because dietary fat is the principal cause of contraction of the diseased organ and subsequent pain, it is poorly tolerated. Energy should come primarily from carbohydrates, especially during acute phases. Control of fat will also contribute to weight control, a primary goal because obesity and excess food intake have been repeatedly associated with the development of gallstones.
- *Kcalories:* If weight loss is indicated, then kcalories will be reduced according to need. Principles of weight management are discussed in Chapter 6. Usually such a diet will have a relatively low percentage of calories from fat, meeting the needs of the patient for fat moderation.
- *Cholesterol and "gas formers":* Two additional modifications usually found in traditional diets for gallbladder disease concern restriction of foods containing cholesterol and foods labeled *gas formers.* Neither modification has a valid rationale. The body synthesizes more cholesterol per day than is present in an average diet. Thus restriction of dietary cholesterol has little effect in reducing gallstone formation. Total dietary fat reduction is more important. As for the use of gas formers, such as legumes, cabbage, or fiber, blanket restriction seems unwarranted because food tolerances in any circumstances are highly individual.

Diseases of the Pancreas

Pancreatitis

Acute inflammation of the pancreas (pancreatitis) is caused by digestion of the organ tissues by enzymes it produces, principally *trypsin.* Normally, enzymes remain in inactive form until pancreatic secretions reach the duodenum through the common duct. However, gallbladder disease may cause a gallstone to enter the common bile duct and obstruct flow from the pancreas or cause a reflux of these secretions and bile from the common duct back into the pancreatic duct. This mixing of digestive materials activates powerful pancreatic enzymes within the gland. In such activated form, they begin their damaging effects on pancreatic tissue itself, causing acute pain. Sometimes infectious

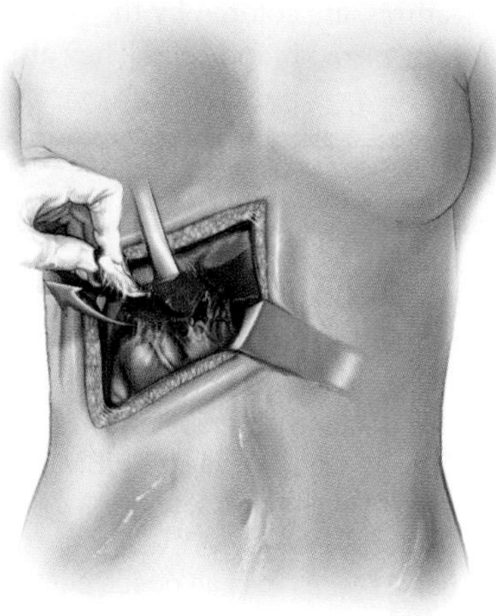

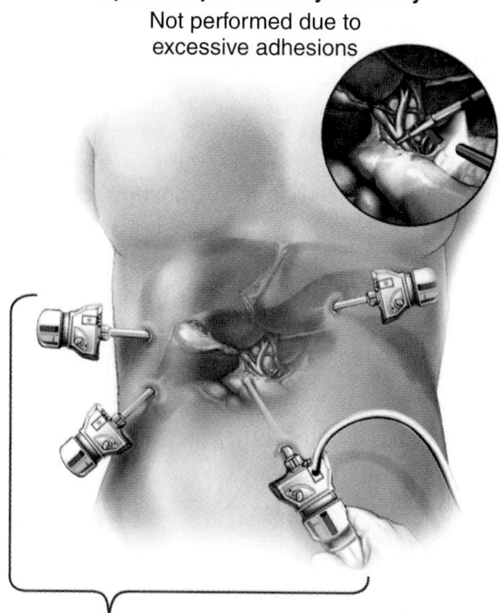

FIGURE 20-14 Open and laparoscopic cholecystectomy. (Medical Illustration Copyright © 2006 Nucleus Medical Art, All rights reserved. www.nucleusinc.com.)

pancreatitis may occur as a complication of mumps or a bacterial disease. Mild or moderate pancreatitis may subside completely, but it has a tendency to recur. Alcohol in Western societies and malnutrition worldwide are the major causes of chronic pancreatitis.

General Treatment

Initial care consists of measures recommended for acute disease involving shock. These measures include intravenous feeding at first, replacement therapy of fluid and electrolytes, blood transfusions, antibiotics and pain medications, and gastric suction.

Nutrition Therapy

In early stages (i.e., acute pancreatitis), oral feedings are withheld because entry of food into the intestines stimulates pancreatic secretions and usually causes pain. Nutritional status is maintained by intravenous fluids or jejunal enteral feeding with peptide-based or elemental EN formulas. Most patients with pancreatitis are able to resume oral feeding in 2 to 5 days.[34]

PN is generally not recommended in pancreatitis unless a patient fails an enteral feeding trial. Pseudocysts, intestinal and pancreatic fistulas, pancreatic abscesses, and pancreatic ascites may make enteral feeding impossible.

HEALTH PROMOTION

A single layer of cells maintains a barrier between toxins and infections in the GI tract. At the same time, this same layer of cells absorbs macronutrients, micronutrients, and water and puts them into circulation. If that is not enough, then these cells also regulate bodily functions via hormonal and immunologic mechanisms. It is plain to see why we would want to keep this remarkable organ healthy!

In 1998, Hasler[36] summarized research that identified foods that provide several physiologic benefits. Among the findings are the following:

- People consuming diets high in fruits and vegetables have only one half the cancer risk of those who consume very little of these foods.
- Intake of lycopene, the primary carotenoid found in tomatoes, is inversely associated with reduced risk of digestive tract cancer, among other cancers.
- Garlic and onions *might* offer a protective effect on cancers of the GI tract.
- Probiotics (fermented dairy products, such as yogurt) reduce risk of various cancers, particularly colon cancer.
- Prebiotics (fermentable carbohydrates, such as starches, dietary fibers, other nonabsorbable sugars, sugar alcohols, and oligosaccharides) stimulate growth and activity of one or more of the "friendly" bacteria that live in the gut.

In addition to how we eat, how we live plays an important role in GI health. Strong evidence indicates that physical activity reduces risk of colon cancer by half. Physical activity might also reduce risk of cholelithiasis, constipation, diverticulosis, GI hemorrhage, and IBD.[37] Washing the hands for a minimum of 20 seconds (the amount of time it takes to sing "Happy Birthday") with hot, soapy water will reduce risk of oral-fecal contamination that could cause foodborne illnesses and certain types of hepatitis.

This information can be summed up very simply: Mom was right when she asked you to do the following:

- Eat your fruits and vegetables.
- Go out and play (get plenty of physical activity).
- Wash your hands before eating.

TO SUM UP

Nutrition therapy for GI disease is based on careful consideration of the following four major factors:

1. Secretory functions, providing chemical agents and environment necessary for digestion to occur
2. Neuromuscular functions required for motility and mechanical digestion
3. Absorptive functions, enhancing entry of nutrients into the circulatory system
4. Psychologic factors reflected by changes in GI function

Esophageal problems vary widely from simple dysphagia to serious diseases or obstruction. Nutrition therapy and mode of intake vary according to degree of dysfunction.

PUD is a common GI problem affecting millions of Americans. It is an erosion of the mucosal lining, mainly in the duodenal bulb and less commonly in the lower antrum portion of the stomach. PUD results in increased gastric tone and painful hunger contractions on an empty stomach, as well as nutrition problems such as low plasma protein levels, anemia, and weight loss. Current medical management consists of acid and infection control with a coordinated system of drugs, rest, and a regular diet (with few food and drink considerations) to supply essential nutrition support for tissue healing.

Intestinal diseases are classified as (1) *anatomic changes,* such as development of small tubular sacs branching off the main alimentary canal in diverticular disease; (2) *malabsorption,* from multiple maldigestive and malabsorptive conditions; (3) *IBD,* resulting from mucosal changes and infectious processes, as seen in UC and Crohn's disease; or (4) *SBS,* resulting from surgical resection of parts of the intestine. Nutrition therapy involves fluid and electrolyte replacement, modifications in the diet's protein and energy content and food texture, and increased vitamins and minerals, with continuous adjustment of the diet according to changes in toleration for specific foods. Allergic responses to common food allergens, as well as missing cell enzymes in genetic disease, may also contribute to GI and metabolic problems from related food intolerances.

Accessory organs to the GI tract—liver, gallbladder, and pancreas—have important functions related to nutrient digestion, absorption, and metabolism, and their diseases interfere with these normal functions. Common liver disorders include hepatitis, usually caused by viral infection, and cirrhosis, an advanced liver disease leading to hepatic encephalopathy and progressive liver failure. The nutrient and energy levels required vary with each condition.

Diseases of the gallbladder include cholecystitis, inflammation that interferes with the absorption of water and bile acids, and cholelithiasis, or gallstone formation. Treatment involves a generally reduced-fat diet and surgical removal of the gallbladder. Diseases of the pancreas include acute and chronic forms of pancreatitis, in which alcohol abuse can be a primary cause. Other causes include biliary disease, malnutrition, drug reactions, abdominal injury, and genetic predisposition. In acute pancreatitis, pain is severe because of pancreatic enzyme reflux with self-digestion of pancreatic tissue by its own enzymes. PN support is used to avoid enzyme stimulus, with gradual return to small, frequent meals as the attack subsides. In chronic pancreatitis, which is caused by alcoholism in Western societies and malnutrition worldwide, maldigestion from lack of enzymes because of pancreatic insufficiency creates nutrition problems. Nutrition care focuses on a nourishing diet with enzyme replacement and vitamin-mineral supplementation.

QUESTIONS FOR REVIEW

1. What is the basic principle of diet planning for patients with esophageal problems? Outline a general nutrition care plan for a patient with GERD complicated by a hiatal hernia.
2. In current practice, what are the basic principles of diet planning for patients with PUD? How do these principles differ from former traditional therapy?
3. Outline a course of nutritional management for a person with PUD, based on the current approaches to medical management. How would you plan nutrition education for continuing self-care and avoidance of recurrence?
4. Describe the cause, clinical signs, and treatment of each of the following intestinal diseases: malabsorption and diarrhea, IBD, diverticular disease, IBS, and constipation.
5. Compare the basics of food intolerances resulting from food allergy with those resulting from a specific genetic disease such as CF.
6. How are the major metabolic functions of the liver affected in liver disease? Give some examples.
7. What is the rationale for treatment in the spectrum of liver disease—hepatitis, cirrhosis, and hepatic encephalopathy?
8. Develop a 1-day food plan for a 45-year-old man, 183 cm (6 feet, 1 inch) tall, weighing 90 kg (200 lb), with infectious hepatitis. Develop another plan for a similar patient with cirrhosis of the liver. What principles of diet therapy apply for each?
9. What are the principles of nutrition therapy for gallbladder disease? Write a 1-day meal plan for a 30-year-old woman, 165 cm (5 feet, 6 inches) tall, weighing 81 kg (180 lb), who has an inflamed gallbladder with stones and is scheduled for a cholecystectomy.
10. Compare acute and chronic forms of pancreatitis in terms of cause, symptoms, and nutrition therapy. What role does special EN and PN support play in this therapy?

REFERENCES

1. Fisichella PM, Patti MG: *Achalasia*, Omaha, Neb, 2008, eMedicine.com, Inc. Retrieved April 24, 2009, from www.emedecine.com.
2. Nelms MN, Sucher K, Long S: *Understanding nutrition therapy and pathophysiology*, Belmont, Calif, 2007, Wadsworth/Thomson Learning.
3. Blaser MJ: The bacteria behind ulcers, *Sci Am* 274(2):104, 1996.
4. Marchetti M, Arico B, Burroni D, et al: Development of a mouse model of *Helicobacter pylori* infection that mimics human disease, *Science* 267(5204):1655, 1995.
5. Division of Bacterial and Mycotic Disease, Centers for Disease Control and Prevention: *Helicobacter pylori and peptic ulcer disease*, Atlanta, 2005, Centers for Disease Control and Prevention. Retrieved December 15, 2005, from www.cdc.gov/ulcer/.
6. Merck & Co, Inc: *The Merck manual of diagnosis and therapy: Helicobacter pylori infection*, Whitehouse Station, NJ, 2007, Merck & Co, Inc. Retrieved April 24, 2009, from www.merck.com.
7. American Dietetic Association: *Nutrition care manual: peptic ulcers: nutrition prescription*, Chicago, Author. Retrieved April 24, 2009, from www.nutritioncaremanual.org.
8. Sartin JS: Gastrointestinal disorders. In Copstead LC, Banasik JL, editors: *Pathophysiology*, ed 4, Philadelphia, 2009, Saunders.
9. Trier JS: Celiac sprue, *N Engl J Med* 325(24):1709, 1991.
10. Beyer P: Medical nutrition therapy for lower gastrointestinal tract disorders. In Mahan LK, Escott-Stump S, editors: *Krause's food, nutrition, and diet therapy*, ed 12, Philadelphia, 2007, Saunders.
11. Mariné M, Fernández-Bañares F, Alsina M, et al: Impact of mass screening for gluten-sensitive enteropathy in working population, *World J Gastroenterol* 15(11):1331, 2009.
12. U.S. National Library of Medicine, National Institutes of Health: *Medline Plus medical encyclopedia: celiac disease—sprue*, Bethesda, Md, 2005, National Institutes of Health. Retrieved April 24, 2009, from www.nlm.nih.gov/medlineplus/ency/article/000233.htm.
13. American Dietetic Association: Nutrition care manual: celiac disease: nutrition care FAQs, Chicago, Author. Retrieved April 24, 2009, from www.nutritioncaremanual.org.
14. Merck & Co, Inc: *The Merck manual of diagnosis and therapy: cystic fibrosis*, Whitehouse Station, NJ, 2008, Merck & Co, Inc. Retrieved April 24, 2009, from www.merck.com.

15. American Dietetic Association: *Nutrition care manual: cystic fibrosis: nutrition intervention*, Chicago, Author. Retrieved April 24, 2009, from ww.nutritioncaremanual.org.
16. Merck & Co, Inc: *The Merck manual of diagnosis and therapy: inflammatory bowel disease*, Whitehouse Station, NJ, 2007, Merck & Co, Inc. Retrieved April 24, 2009, from www.merck.com.
17. Merck & Co, Inc: *The Merck manual of diagnosis and therapy: Crohn's disease (regional enteritis; granulomatous ileitis or ileocolitis)*, Whitehouse Station, NJ, 2008, Merck & Co, Inc. Retrieved April 24, 2009, from www.merck.com.
18. Merck & Co, Inc: *The Merck manual of diagnosis and therapy: ulcerative colitis*, Whitehouse Station, NJ, 2008, Merck & Co, Inc. Retrieved April 24, 2009, from www.merck.com.
19. American Dietetic Association: *Nutrition care manual: Crohn's and ulcerative colitis: nutrition intervention*, Chicago, Author. Retrieved April 24, 2009, from www.nutritioncaremanual.org.
20. Merck & Co, Inc: *The Merck manual of diagnosis and therapy: short bowel syndrome*, Whitehouse Station, NJ, 2008, Merck & Co, Inc. Retrieved April 24, 2009, from www.merck.com.
21. Weseman RA: Adult small bowel transplantation. In Hasse JM, Blue LS, editors: *Comprehensive guide to transplant nutrition*, Chicago, 2002, American Dietetic Association.
22. Merck & Co, Inc: *The Merck manual of diagnosis and therapy: gas-related complaints*, Whitehouse Station, NJ, 2007, Merck & Co, Inc. Retrieved April 24, 2009, from www.merck.com.
23. Drossman DA: The functional gastrointestinal disorders and the Rome II process, *Gut* 45:1, 1999.
24. International Foundation for Functional Gastrointestinal Disorders: *About irritable bowel syndrome (IBS)*, Milwaukee, 1999–2010, International Foundation for Functional Gastrointestinal Disorders. Retrieved April 24, 2009, from www.aboutibs.org.
25. Merck & Co, Inc: *The Merck manual of diagnosis and therapy: irritable bowel syndrome*, Whitehouse Station, NJ, 2007, Merck & Co, Inc. Retrieved April 24, 2009, from www.merck.com.
26. Sheth AA, Longo W, Floch MH: Diverticular disease and diverticulitis, *Am J Gastroenterol* 103(6):1550, 2008.
27. Strate LL, Liu YL, Syngal S, et al: Nut, corn, and popcorn consumption and the incidence of diverticular disease, *JAMA* 300(8):907, 2008.
28. Eglash A, Lane CH: What is the most beneficial diet for patients with diverticulosis? *J Fam Pract* 55(9):813, 2006.
29. Jacobs DO: Diverticulitis, *N Engl J Med* 357(20):2057, 2007.
30. Merck & Co, Inc: *The Merck manual of diagnosis and therapy: irritable bowel syndrome*, Whitehouse Station, NJ, 2007, Merck & Co, Inc. Retrieved April 24, 2009, from www.merck.com.
31. American Dietetic Association: *Nutrition care manual: hepatitis: nutrition prescription*, Chicago, Author. Retrieved April 24, 2009, from www.nutritioncaremanual.org.
32. Merck & Co, Inc: *The Merck manual of diagnosis and therapy: cirrhosis*, Whitehouse Station, NJ, 2007, Merck & Co, Inc. Retrieved April 24, 2009, from www.merck.com.
33. American Dietetic Association: *Nutrition care manual: cirrhosis: nutrition prescription*, Chicago, Author. Retrieved April 24, 2009, from www.nutritioncaremanual.org.
34. Moore MC: *Pocket guide to nutrition assessment and care*, ed 6, St Louis, 2009, Mosby.
35. Sartin JS: Alterations in function of the gallbladder and exocrine pancreas. In Copstead LC, Banasik JL, editors: *Pathophysiology*, ed 4, Philadelphia, 2009, Saunders.
36. Hasler CM: Scientific status summary: functional foods—their role in disease prevention and health promotion, *Food Technol* 52(11):63, 1998.
37. Peters HPF, De Vries WR, Vanberge-Henegouw G, et al: Potential benefits and hazards of physical activity and exercise on the gastrointestinal tract, *Gut* 48:435, 2001.

FURTHER RESOURCES

Websites of Interest

Celiac Sprue

Ask the Dietitian: *Gluten and celiac sprue*. www.dietitian.com/gluten.html.
Celiac Disease Foundation: www.celiac.org.
Celiac Sprue Association: www.csaceliacs.org.

Cirrhosis

American Gastroenterological Association: *Cirrhosis of the liver*, www.gastro.org.
American Liver Foundation: www.liverfoundation.org.
National Institute of Diabetes and Digestive and Kidney Diseases: www.niddk.nih.gov.

Dysphagia

Dysphagia Resource Center: www.dysphagia.com.
Dysphagia-Diet.com: www.dysphagia-diet.com.
Dysphagiaonline.com: www.dysphagiaonline.com.

Gastroesophageal Reflux Disease (GERD)

About GERD: www.aboutgerd.org.
American Gastroenterological Association: www.gastro.org.
GERD Information Resource Center: www.gerd.com.

Celiac Disease (CD)

Celiac Disease Foundation: www.celiac.org.
Medline Plus: *Celiac disease*. www.nlm.nih.gov/medlineplus/celiacdisease.html.
National Digestive Diseases Information Clearinghouse: *Celiac disease*. www.digestive.niddk.nih.gov/ddiseases/pubs/celiac/.

Cystic Fibrosis (CF)

Canadian Cystic Fibrosis Foundation: www.ccff.ca.
Cystic Fibrosis Foundation: www.cff.org/home/.
CysticFibrosis.com: www.cysticfibrosis.com.

Irritable Bowel Syndrome (IBS)

About IBS: www.aboutibs.org.
Irritable Bowel Syndrome Self Help and Support Group: www.ibsgroup.org.

Pancreatitis

eMedicine (search for *pancreatitis* for a number of resources): www.emedicine.com.
National Institute of Diabetes and Digestive and Kidney Diseases: www.niddk.nih.gov.
Tummyhealth.com: www.tummyhealth.com.

Peptic Ulcer Disease

National Institute of Diabetes and Digestive and Kidney Diseases: www.niddk.nih.gov.
National Library of Medicine: *Helicobacter pylori in Peptic Ulcer Disease*. www.nlm.nih.gov/archive/20040830/pubs/cbm/pepulcer.html.

21

Diseases of the Heart, Blood Vessels, and Lungs

Sara Long Roth

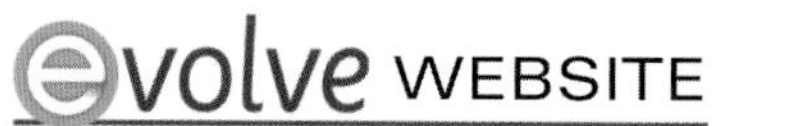

http://evolve.elsevier.com/Williams/essentials/

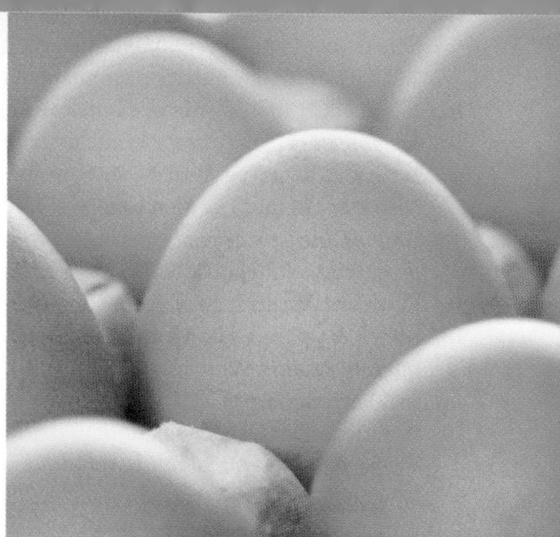

OUTLINE

In this chapter, we consider interrelated diseases of the circulatory system—heart, blood vessels, and lungs. In recent decades, these diseases of modern civilization have become the major causes of death of men and women in the United States and most other Western societies. One out of every three deaths is caused by heart disease; more than cancer, accidents, and acquired immunodeficiency syndrome (AIDS) combined. The magnitude of this overall health care problem is enormous.

CORONARY HEART DISEASE

Atherosclerosis

Underlying Disease Process

Atherosclerosis, the major arteriosclerosis disease and underlying pathologic process in coronary heart disease (CHD), is paramount in ongoing study in modern medicine. It is not a solitary disease entity but somewhat a pathologic progression that can involve vascular systems throughout the body, resulting in an extensive variety of clinical manifestations.[1]

An inflammatory process, the characteristic lesions involved are raised fibrous plaques (Figure 21-1) resulting from injury on the interior surface (intima) of blood vessels.[1] Once injury has occurred, plaques first appear as discrete lumps elevated above unaffected surrounding tissue and ranging in color from pearly gray to yellowish gray. Possible causes of injury are as follows[1]:

- Smoking
- Hypertension
- Diabetes
- Increased serum levels of low-density lipoprotein (LDL) cholesterol
- Decreases serum levels of high-density lipoprotein (HDL) cholesterol
- High levels of homocystine
- Elevated C-reactive protein
- Increased serum fibrinogen
- Insulin resistance
- Oxidative stress
- Infection
- Periodontal disease

Additional risk factors are shown in Box 21-1 (see also the *Focus on Culture* box, “Is Cardiovascular Disease an Equal Opportunity Disease?”).

About 90% of CHD patients have elevated levels of serum cholesterol, hypertension, smoke, or have diabetes.[2] The major risk factor for plaque development is a lipoprotein, LDL cholesterol, that carries cholesterol in the blood.[3] Oxidation of LDL cholesterol is the principal step in this process of atherogenesis. Inflammation with oxidative stress and activation of macrophages is the principal method of this step. The oxidized LDL cholesterol is toxic to the intima, initiates smooth muscle propagation, and triggers further immune and inflammatory responses causing formation of lesions called *fatty streaks.*[1]

This fatty degeneration and thickening narrow the vessel lumen and may allow a blood clot, an embolus, to develop from its irritating presence. Eventually the clot may cut off blood flow in the involved artery. If the artery is a critical one, such as a major coronary vessel, then a heart attack occurs. Tissue area serviced by the involved

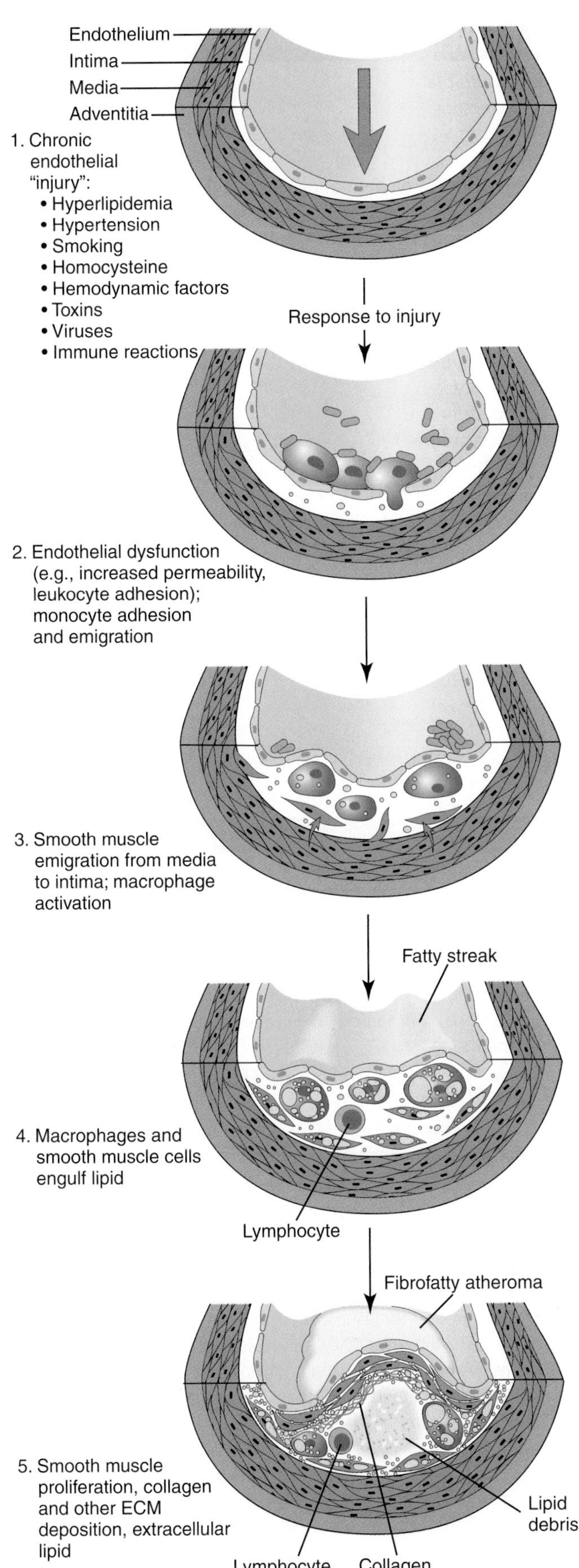

FIGURE 21-1 Raised fibrous plaques. (From Kumar V, Cotran R, Robbins S: *Robbins basic pathology*, ed 7, Philadelphia, 2003, Saunders.)

artery is deprived of its vital oxygen and nutrient supply, a condition called **ischemia**, and the cells die. The localized area of dying or dead tissue is called an **infarct**. Because the artery involved supplies cardiac muscle, the *myocardium*, the result is called an *acute myocardial infarction (AMI)*. The two major coronary arteries, with their many branches, are so named because they lie across the brow of the heart muscle and resemble a crown (Figure 21-2). Figure 21-3 shows the anterior internal view of the normal human heart.

Cholesterol, Lipoproteins, and Lipids

Cholesterol is a soft, fatlike substance found in all cell membranes and blood and is a precursor of bile acids and steroid hormones. Cholesterol and triglycerides cannot dissolve in blood and must be transported to and from cells by individual components containing lipid and proteins (lipoproteins). The following five types of lipoproteins (Figure 21-4) are classified according to fat content and thus their density, with those having the highest fat content possessing the lowest density[5]:

1. Chylomicrons have the highest lipid content and lowest density and are composed mostly of dietary triglycerides, with a small amount of carrier protein. They accumulate in portal blood after a meal and are efficiently cleared from the blood by the specific enzyme lipoprotein lipase.
2. Very low-density lipoproteins (VLDLs) still carry a large lipid (triglyceride) content but include about 20% cholesterol. These lipoproteins are formed in the liver from endogenous fat sources.

KEY TERMS

atherosclerosis Common form of arteriosclerosis, characterized by the gradual formation—beginning in childhood in genetically predisposed individuals—of yellow cheese-like streaks of cholesterol and fatty material that develop into hardened plaques in the intima or inner lining of major blood vessels, such as coronary arteries, eventually in adulthood cutting off blood supply to the tissue served by the vessels; the underlying pathologic process of coronary heart disease (CHD).

arteriosclerosis Blood vessel disease characterized by thickening and hardening of artery walls, with loss of functional elasticity, mainly affecting the intima (inner lining) of the arteries.

intima General term indicating an innermost part of a structure or vessel; inner layer of the blood vessel wall.

plaque Thickened deposits of fatty material, largely cholesterol, within the arterial wall that eventually may fill the lumen and cut off blood supply to the tissue served by the damaged vessel.

ischemia Deficiency of blood to a particular tissue, resulting from functional blood vessel constriction or actual obstruction of walls in atherosclerosis.

infarct An area of tissue necrosis caused by local ischemia, resulting from obstruction of blood circulation to that area.

BOX 21-1 MAJOR RISK FACTORS IN CARDIOVASCULAR DISEASE

Lipid Risk Factors
- Low-density lipoprotein (LDL) cholesterol >130 mg/dL
- High-density lipoprotein (HDL) cholesterol <40 mg/dL
- Total cholesterol >200 mg/dL
- Triglycerides >150 mg/dL

Nonlipid Risk Factors
Modifiable
- Tobacco smoke and exposure to tobacco smoke
- Hypertension (>140/90 mm Hg)
- Physical inactivity
- Obesity (body mass index [BMI] >30 kg/m^2) and overweight (BMI 25.0 to 29.9 kg/m^2)
- Diabetes mellitus
- Atherogenic diet (high intakes of saturated fats and cholesterol)
- Thrombogenic state
- Excessive alcohol consumption (>1 drink per day for women and >2 drinks per day for men)
- Individual response to stress and coping
- Some illegal drugs (cocaine and intravenous drug abuse)

Nonmodifiable
- Male gender
- Age (men >45 years, women >55 years)
- Heredity (including race)
- Family history of premature coronary heart disease (CHD) (myocardial infarction [MI] or sudden death <55 years of age in father or other male first-degree relative, or <65 years of age in mother or other female first-degree relative)

Probable Risk Factors (Emerging)
- Lipoprotein (a)
- Small LDL particles (pattern B)
- HDL subtypes
- Apolipoprotein B
- **Homocysteine**
- Fibrinogen
- High-sensitivity **C-reactive protein**
- Impaired fasting glucose (100 to 125 mg/dL)

Data from *National Cholesterol Education Program (NCEP): Third report of the NCEP Expert Panel on Detection, Evaluation, and Treatment of High Blood Cholesterol in Adults (Adult Treatment Panel III), full report,* Washington, DC, 2002, National Institutes of Health, National Heart, Lung, and Blood Institute. Retrieved December 20, 2005, from www.nhlbi.nih.gov/guidelines/cholesterol/atp3_rpt.htm; Banasik JL: Alterations in cardiac function. In Copstead LC, Banasik JL, editors: *Pathophysiology,* ed 3, St Louis, 2005, Saunders.

FOCUS ON CULTURE

Is Cardiovascular Disease an Equal Opportunity Disease?

"Race and ethnicity in the United States are associated with health status."

Marian E. Gornick: Disparities in Medicare services: Potential causes, plausible explanations, and recommendations. *Health Care Financing Reviews,* 21(4), 2000.

The Pfizer Journal Panel[1] states the following:

> The system of health care that exists in this country was developed at a time when life expectancy was short, diseases generally came on quickly and were all too frequently fatal, and patients needed lifesaving interventions at a relatively young age. The system has not changed, yet individuals who need health care now live a very long life, develop diseases that are chronic and disabling, and need prevention during a longer lifespan. One hundred million Americans have at least one chronic condition, and half of them have more. Among Americans older than age 65, 88% have one or more chronic illnesses, and one quarter of them have at least four conditions that should be treated.

After controlling for differences in age, health insurance status, disease severity, and other health problems, the following research findings might not be surprising but nonetheless are disheartening:

- African Americans, Hispanics, and other minorities on average have more underlying risk factors for cardiovascular disease (CVD), including hypertension, obesity, smoking, physical inactivity, higher level of body mass index (BMI), and non–high-density lipoprotein (HDL) cholesterol.
- After minority patients develop CVD, they are less likely to receive higher-quality care and as a result are more likely to die.
- African Americans receive clot-reducing drugs after a heart attack less than Caucasians.
- Approximately 18% of African-American patients have angioplasty surgery within 48 hours of a heart attack or stroke, compared with almost 30% of Caucasian patients.
- African-American women are "less familiar" with early warning signs of CVD.
- CVD deaths are highest among African Americans at all ages.
- All low-income and less-educated U.S. residents have higher mortality rates for heart disease and stroke than other residents.

During the past 30 years, CVD mortality rates have been decreasing across all racial and ethnic groups, but decline has been much greater for Caucasian Americans. African Americans have mortality rates for CVD about 50% higher than those of Caucasian Americans. Hispanic Americans are substantially more likely to be uninsured than Caucasian Americans, and Hispanic Americans are far more likely to lack a usual source of health care than any other group. Research has also found some immigrant families who assimilate into the United States, many of whom are Hispanic, experience deteriorating health status in subsequent generations.

So there is more to CVD than just risk factors. It may not be enough to teach prevention to the masses. Different life experiences attributed to different ethnic groups, as well as economic, time, and residential constraints, may compete with

FOCUS ON CULTURE

Is Cardiovascular Disease an Equal Opportunity Disease?—cont'd

heart-healthy behaviors to increase risk of CVD. So if you are a college student reading this information, then be thankful. You have just decreased your risk of CVD simply by being educated.

REFERENCES

1. Pfizer Journal Panel: The quality of health care in the United States: building quality into the health care system, *Pfizer Journal* 9(9):1, 2005. Retrieved December 20, 2005, from www.thepfizerjournal.com/default.asp?a=journal&n=tpj41.

BIBLIOGRAPHY

Cook NL, Ayanian JZ, Orav EJ, et al: Differences in specialist consultations for cardiovascular disease by race, ethnicity, gender, insurance status, and site of primary care, *Circulation* 119:1–8, 2009. Retrieved May 20, 2009, from circ.ahajournals.org.

De Lew N, Weinick RM: An overview: eliminating racial, ethnic, and SES disparities in health care, *Health Care Financ Rev* 21(4):1, 2000.

Gornick ME: Disparities in Medicare services: potential causes, plausible explanations, and recommendations, *Health Care Financ Rev* 21(4):23, 2000.

The Henry J. Kaiser Family Foundation: Racial/ethnic differences in cardiac care: the weight of the evidence, *USAID Highlights* October 2002. Retrieved July 1, 2010 from http://www.kff.org/uninsured/20021009c-index.cfm.

McWilliams JM, Meara E, Zaslavsky AM, et al: Differences in control of cardiovascular disease and diabetes by race, ethnicity, and education: U.S. trends from 1999 to 2006 and effects of Medicare coverage, *Ann Intern Med* 150:505, 2009.

Thomas AJ, Eberly LE, Smith GD, et al: Race/ethnicity, income, major risk factors, and cardiovascular disease mortality, *Am J Public Health* 95(8):1417, 2005.

Winkleby MA, Kraemer HC, Ahn DK, et al: Ethnic and socioeconomic differences in cardiovascular disease risk factors: findings for women from the Third National Health and Nutrition Examination Survey, 1988–1994, *JAMA* 280(23):1989, 1998.

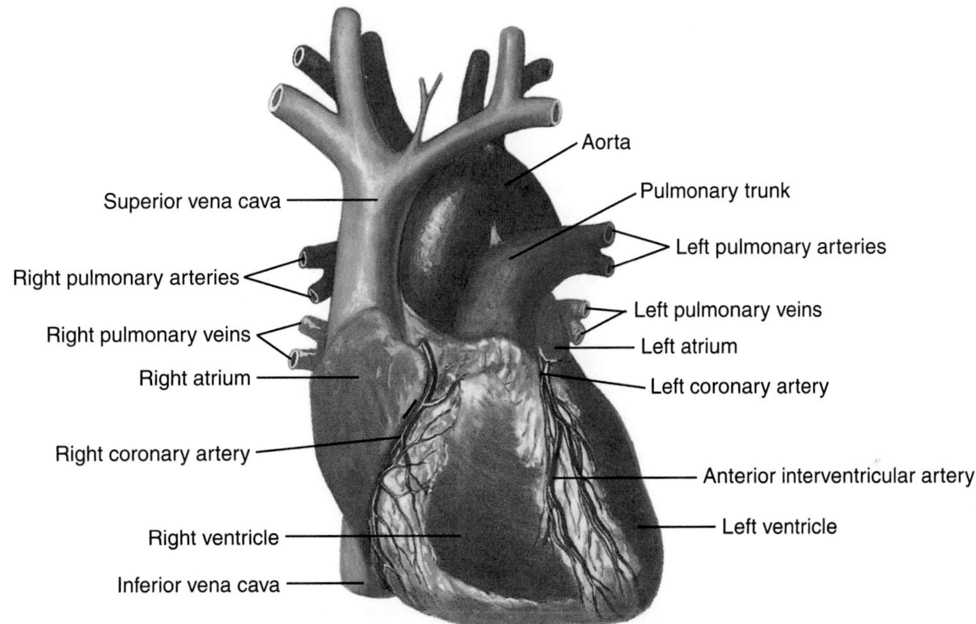

FIGURE 21-2 Coronary blood circulation. (From Seely RR, Stephens TD, Tate P: *Anatomy and physiology,* ed 3, St Louis, 1995, McGraw Hill.)

3. Intermediate-density lipoproteins (IDLs) continue the delivery of endogenous triglycerides to cells and carry about 40% cholesterol.
4. LDLs carry, in addition to other lipids, about two thirds or more of total plasma cholesterol formed in blood serum from catabolism of VLDL. Because LDL carries cholesterol to cells for deposit in tissues, it is considered the main agent in elevated serum cholesterol levels, or the "bad" cholesterol.
5. HDLs carry less total lipid and more carrier protein. They are formed in the liver from endogenous fat sources. Because HDL carries cholesterol from tissues to the liver for catabolism and excretion, higher serum levels of this "good" cholesterol form are considered protective against cardiovascular disease (CVD). A value of 60 mg/dL or more contributes definite protection and decreased risk.

Characteristics of these classes of lipoproteins are summarized in Table 21-1.

KEY TERMS

homocysteine An amino acid produced in the human body; high serum homocysteine levels can damage the linings of the arteries and possibly make it easier for blood to clot. Most individuals with high homocysteine levels have low dietary intakes of folic acid, vitamin B_6, or vitamin B_{12}.

C-reactive protein A protein found in the blood; levels rise in response to inflammation.

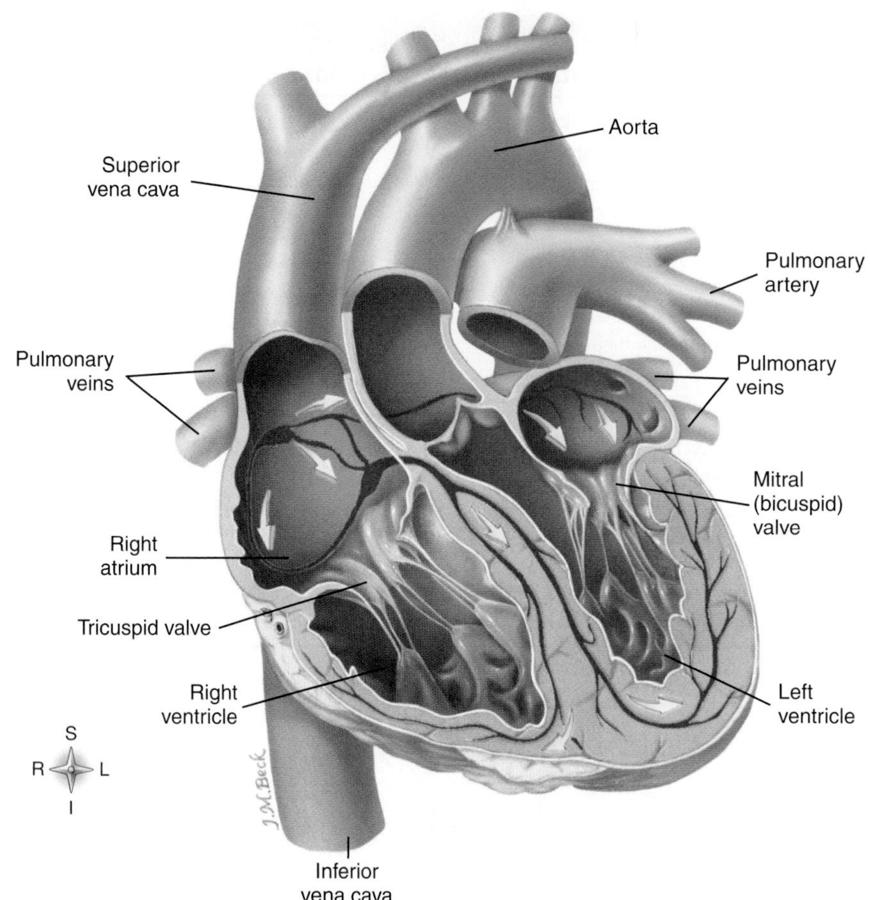

FIGURE 21-3 The normal human heart. Anterior internal view showing cardiac circulation. (From Thibodeau GA, Patton KT: *Anatomy and physiology,* ed 6, St Louis, 2007, Mosby.)

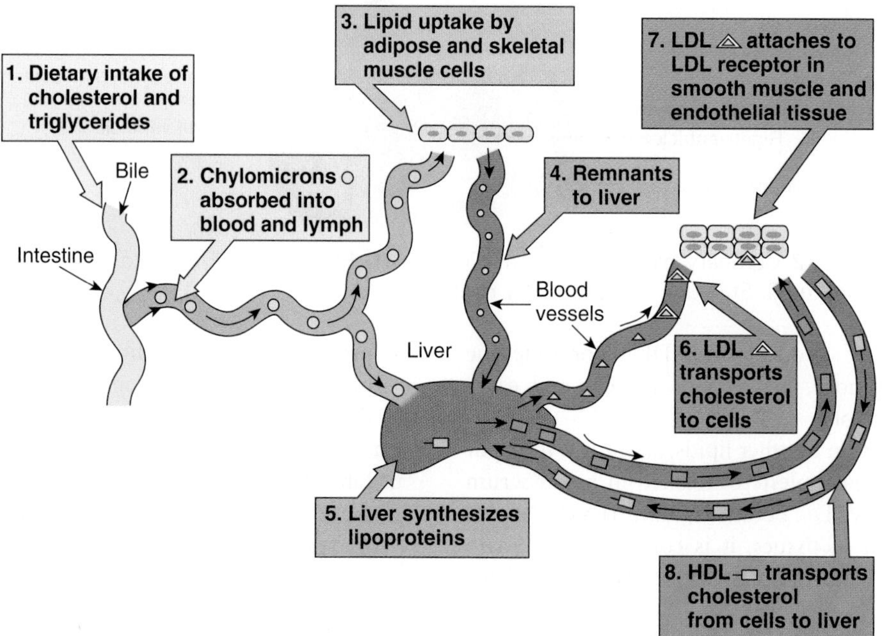

FIGURE 21-4 Composition of lipoproteins and transport of lipoproteins in blood. (From Gould BE: *Pathophysiology for the health professionals,* ed 3, Philadelphia, 2006, Saunders.)

TABLE 21-1 CHARACTERISTICS OF THE CLASSES OF LIPOPROTEINS

CHARACTERISTIC	CHYLOMICRONS	VERY LOW-DENSITY LIPOPROTEINS (VLDL)	INTERMEDIATE-DENSITY LIPOPROTEINS (IDL)	LOW-DENSITY LIPOPROTEINS (LDL)	HIGH-DENSITY LIPOPROTEINS (HDL)
Composition					
Triglycerides	85%, diet, exogenous	55%, endogenous	30%, endogenous	5%, endogenous	5%, endogenous
Cholesterol	5%	20%	40%	55%	20%
Phospholipid	3%-6%	15%-20%	20%	15%-22%	25%-30%
Protein	1%-2%	5%-10%	10%	20%	50%
Function	Transport dietary triglycerides to plasma and tissues, cells	Transport endogenous triglycerides to cells	Continue transport of endogenous triglycerides to cells	Transport cholesterol to peripheral cells	Transport free cholesterol from membranes to liver for catabolism
Place of synthesis	Intestinal wall	Liver	Liver	Liver	Liver
Size and Density					
Description	Largest, lightest	Next largest, next lightest	Intermediate size, lighter	Smaller, heavier	Smaller, densest, heaviest
Density	0.095	0.095-1.006	1.00-1.03	1.019-1.063	1.063-1.210
Size in nanometers (nm)	80-1000	30-80	25-40	15-20	5-10

Functional Classification of Lipid Disorders

Current clinical practice is based on a useful functional classification that reveals two important factors: (1) recognition of genetic factors involved and (2) focus on the role of **apolipoproteins** in the course of lipoprotein formation, transport, or destruction. Both factors will be encountered in readings and in clinical work with patients. Thus the outline provided in this discussion is useful in understanding clinical problems involved and in counseling patients.

Apolipoproteins. The term *apolipoprotein* refers to a major protein part of a combined metabolic product, in this case a specific protein part of a combined lipid-protein molecule. For example, apolipoprotein B is a common attachment to LDL and serves two basic functions: (1) it aids transport of lipids in a water medium (i.e., blood), and (2) it transports lipids into cells for metabolic purposes. When apolipoprotein B-100, a single large protein molecule, attaches to one pole of the LDL, it provides a recognition site for LDL receptors on the cell, causing the entire LDL to be transported by pinocytosis into the cell for use in cell metabolism.[5] Various types of LDL have specific receptor sites for particular apolipoproteins to which the apolipoprotein is attracted and that in large measure determine function.

Function. When lipoproteins are synthesized in the intestinal wall, liver, and blood serum, the protein component is made up of varying kinds of apolipoprotein parts. These genetically determined components influence the structure, receptor binding, and metabolism of lipoproteins. It is an apolipoprotein component that helps form special spherical droplets of lipid material for transport in the bloodstream (see Chapter 4). Apolipoprotein determination is currently a useful laboratory tool for identifying persons at high risk for CHD.[3]

Defects in Synthesis of Apolipoproteins. Current functional approach classifies lipid disorders into four major groups based on the underlying functional problem: (1) defects in apolipoprotein synthesis, (2) enzyme deficiencies, (3) LDL-receptor deficiency, and (4) other inherited hyperlipidemias.[3]

General Principles of Nutrition Therapy

Basic Guidelines. The National Cholesterol Education Program (NCEP) periodically publishes revised guidelines for clinical management of high serum cholesterol. The Adult Treatment Panel I (ATP I) delineated strategy for primary prevention of CHD in persons with high levels of LDL cholesterol (160 mg/dL) or those with borderline-high LDL cholesterol (130 to 159 mg/dL) and two or more risk factors. The Adult Treatment Panel II (ATP II) substantiated these strategies and made further recommendations for intensive management of LDL cholesterol in persons with established CHD. A new lower LDL cholesterol of 100 mg/dL was established. The Adult Treatment Panel III (ATP III) report identified more intensive LDL-lowering therapy. The ATP III[3] suggests a comprehensive lifestyle approach to reducing risk

KEY TERMS

apolipoproteins Separate protein compounds that attach to specific receptor sites on particular lipoproteins and activate certain functions, such as protein synthesis of a related enzyme. For example, apolipoprotein C-II is an apolipoprotein of high-density lipoprotein (HDL) and very low-density lipoprotein (VLDL) that functions to activate the enzyme lipoprotein lipase.

TABLE 21-2 ESSENTIAL COMPONENTS OF THERAPEUTIC LIFESTYLE CHANGES

COMPONENT	RECOMMENDATION
LDL-raising nutrients	
Saturated fats	<7% of total energy intake
Dietary cholesterol	<200 mg/day
Therapeutic options for LDL lowering	
Plant stanols/sterols	2 g/day
Soluble fiber	10-25 g/day
Total energy (kilocalories)	Adjust total energy intake to maintain desirable body weight/prevent weight gain
Physical activity	Include enough moderate exercise to expend at least 200 kcal/day
Trans fats	Avoid
Limit sodium to 2400 mg per day	When indicated

Data from National Cholesterol Education Program (NCEP): *Third report of the NCEP Expert Panel on Detection, Evaluation, and Treatment of High Blood Cholesterol in Adults (Adult Treatment Panel III), full report,* Washington, DC, 2002, National Institutes of Health, National Heart, Lung, and Blood Institute. Retrieved May 19, 2009 from www.nhlbi.nih.gov/guidelines/cholesterol/atp3_rpt.htm; American Dietetic Association: *Nutrition care manual,* Chicago, 2005, American Dietetic Association. Retrieved May 19, 2009, from www.nutritioncaremanual.org.
LDL, Low-density lipoprotein.

TABLE 21-3 NUTRIENT COMPOSITION OF THE THERAPEUTIC LIFESTYLE CHANGES DIET

COMPONENT	RECOMMENDATION
Polyunsaturated fat, including omega-3 fatty acids	Up to 10% total energy intake
Monounsaturated fat	Up to 20% total energy intake
Total fat	25%-35% total energy intake*
Carbohydrate†	50%-60% total energy intake
Dietary fiber	20-30 g/day
Protein	Approximately 15% total energy intake

Data from National Cholesterol Education Program (NCEP): *Third report of the NCEP Expert Panel on Detection, Evaluation, and Treatment of High Blood Cholesterol in Adults (Adult Treatment Panel III), full report,* Washington, DC, 2002, National Institutes of Health, National Heart, Lung, and Blood Institute. Retrieved May 19, 2009 from www.nhlbi.nih.gov/guidelines/cholesterol/atp3_rpt.htm; American Dietetic Association: *Nutrition care manual,* Chicago, 2005, American Dietetic Association. Retrieved May 19, 2009, from www.nutritioncaremanual.org.
*Adult Treatment Panel III (ATP III) allows for increase of total fat to 35% total energy intake and reduction in carbohydrate to 50% for persons with the metabolic syndrome. Any increase in fat intake should be in the form of either polyunsaturated or monounsaturated fat.
†Carbohydrates should come primarily from foods rich in complex carbohydrates, including grains—especially whole grains—fruits, and vegetables.

for CHD called *therapeutic lifestyle changes (TLC)* and incorporates the following components[2,3]:

- Reduced intake of saturated fats and cholesterol
- Therapeutic dietary options for enhancing LDL lowering (plant stanols and sterols and increased soluble fiber)
- Weight reduction
- Increased regular physical activity

Components of TLC are outlined in Table 21-2. The ATP III also suggests ranges for other macronutrients in the TLC Diet (Table 21-3).

Components of the Therapeutic Lifestyle Changes Diet.

Saturated fat and cholesterol. In view of the fact that the major LDL-raising nutrient components are saturated fat and cholesterol, reducing saturated fat (<7% of total energy intake) and cholesterol (<200 mg/day) in the diet is the foundation of the TLC Diet. The strongest nutritional influence on serum LDL cholesterol levels is saturated fats.[3] In fact, a "dose-response relationship" exists between saturated fats and LDL cholesterol levels. For every 1% increase in kilocalories (kcalories or kcal) from saturated fats as a percentage of total energy, serum LDL cholesterol increases approximately 2%. On the other hand, a 1% decrease in saturated fats will lower serum cholesterol by approximately 2%.[3] Although weight reduction by itself, even of a few pounds, will reduce LDL cholesterol levels, weight reduction attained using a kcalorie-controlled diet low in saturated fats and cholesterol will improve and maintain LDL cholesterol lowering. Although dietary cholesterol does not have the same influence as saturated fat on serum LDL cholesterol levels, high cholesterol intakes raise LDL cholesterol levels. Therefore reducing dietary cholesterol to less than 200 mg/day decreases serum LDL cholesterol in most persons.[3]

Monounsaturated fat. The TLC Diet recommends substitution of monounsaturated fat for saturated fats at an intake level of up to 20% of total energy intake because monounsaturated fats lower LDL cholesterol levels relative to saturated fats without decreasing HDL cholesterol or triglyceride levels. It is recommended that plant oils and nuts be used because they are the best sources of monounsaturated fats.[3]

Polyunsaturated fats. Polyunsaturated fats, in particular linoleic acid, reduce LDL cholesterol levels when used instead of saturated fats. However, they can also bring about small reductions in HDL cholesterol when compared side by side with monounsaturated fats. The TLC Diet recommends liquid vegetables oils, semiliquid margarines (soft, tub margarines), and other margarines low in trans fatty acids be used because they are the best sources of polyunsaturated fats; intakes can range up to 10% of total energy intake.[3]

Trans fatty acids. Two types of trans fatty acids exist: (1) those appearing naturally in foods (mostly meat products) and (2) those produced by the process of hydrogenation of unsaturated fats. Trans fats from partially hydrogenated fats are more harmful than naturally occurring trans fats[4] raising serum LDL cholesterol and lowering serum HDL cholesterol.

Total fat. In view of the fact that only saturated fats and trans fatty acids increase LDL cholesterol levels,[4] serum levels of LDL cholesterol are unrelated to total fat intake per se. For that reason, the ATP III suggests it is not crucial to limit total fat intake for the specific goal of reducing LDL cholesterol levels, provided saturated fats are decreased to goal levels.[2]

Carbohydrates. When saturated fats are replaced with carbohydrates, LDL cholesterol levels are reduced. On the other hand, very high intakes of carbohydrates (>60% of total energy intake) are associated with a reduction in HDL cholesterol and an increase in serum triglyceride. Increasing soluble fiber intake can sometimes reduce these responses. On average, increasing soluble fiber to 10 to 25 g/day is accompanied by an approximately 5% reduction in LDL cholesterol.[2]

Protein. Despite the fact that dietary protein as a rule has an insignificant effect on serum LDL cholesterol level, replacing animal protein with plant-based protein has been reported to decrease LDL cholesterol.[2] This may be the result of plant-based foods providing good sources of proteins (legumes, dry beans, nuts, whole grains, and vegetables) containing less saturated fat than many animal proteins and no cholesterol. This is not to say animal proteins cannot be low in saturated fat and cholesterol. Fat-free and low-fat dairy products, egg whites, fish, skinless poultry, and lean cuts of beef and pork are also low in saturated fat and cholesterol. All foods of animal origin will contain cholesterol.

Further dietary options for reducing LDL cholesterol. Adding 5 to 10 g of soluble fiber (oats, barley, psyllium, pectin-rich fruit, and beans) per day is associated with approximately a 5% reduction in LDL cholesterol and is regarded as a therapeutic option to enhance reduction of LDL cholesterol. Plant sterols present an additional therapeutic option.[2] Daily intakes of 2 to 3 g plant stanol and sterol esters (isolated from soybean and tall pine tree oils) have been shown to lower LDL cholesterol by 6% to 15%.[2]

General Approach to Therapeutic Lifestyle Changes

The ATP III[2] suggests patients at risk for CHD or with CHD be referred to registered dietitians (RDs) or other qualified nutritionists for the duration of all stages of nutrition therapy (NT). After 6 weeks of TLC, LDL cholesterol should be measured to evaluate response to TLC. If the LDL cholesterol target has been realized or an improvement in LDL lowering has occurred, then NT should be uninterrupted. If the goal has not been attained, then the physician can select from a number of alternatives. First, NT can be reexplained and reinforced. Next, therapeutic dietary options can be integrated into TLC. Response to NT should be assessed in an additional 6 weeks. If the LDL cholesterol target is achieved, then the current intensity of NT should be continued indefinitely. If downward movement is seen in LDL cholesterol measures, then thought should be given to continuing NT before adding LDL-lowering medications. If it looks unlikely the LDL target will be realized with NT, then medications should be considered.[2] The "Guide to Therapeutic Lifestyle Changes: Healthy Lifestyle Recommendations for a Healthy Heart" is shown in Box 21-2.

Metabolic syndrome is the name for a group of metabolic risk factors that increase risk for heart disease, type 2 diabetes, peripheral vascular disease (PVD), and stroke. Any one of these risk factors may develop, but they tend to occur together. Although no well-accepted criteria exist for diagnosis of metabolic syndrome, it is identified by the presence of at least three of the following:

- Abdominal obesity
  - Men: ≥40 inches (102 cm)
  - Women: ≥35 inches (88 cm)
- Elevated triglycerides (≥150 mg/dL)
- Reduced HDL cholesterol
  - Men: <40 mg/dL
  - Women: <50 mg/dL
- Elevated blood pressure (≥130/85 mm Hg)
- Elevated fasting blood glucose (≥100 mg/dL)

Data from American Heart Association: *Metabolic syndrome: information for professionals,* Dallas, Tex, 2009, American Heart Association. Retrieved July 8, 2009, from www.americanheart.org/presenter.jhtml?identifier=534; National Institutes of Health, National Heart, Lung, and Blood Institute: *Diseases and conditions index: metabolic syndrome,* Washington, DC, 2010. National Institutes of Health, National Heart, Lung, and Blood Institute. Retrieved July 8, 2009, from www.nhlbi.nih.gov/health/dci/Diseases/ms/ms_whatis.html.

Drug Therapy

Although use of TLC will attain LDL cholesterol target goal for many, a segment of the population will need LDL-lowering medications to achieve the prescribed goal for LDL cholesterol. If treatment with TLC alone is unsuccessful after 3 months, then the ATP III recommends initiation of drug treatment. When drugs are used, however, TLC also should continue to be used concomitantly. NT affords further CHD risk reduction beyond drug efficacy.[2] Actions of combined use of TLC and LDL cholesterol–lowering medications may include the following[4]:

- Intensive LDL lowering with TLC, including therapeutic dietary options
  - May prevent need for drugs
  - Can augment LDL-lowering medications
  - May allow for lower doses of medications
- Weight control plus increased physical activity
  - Reduces risk beyond LDL cholesterol lowering
  - Constitutes principal management of metabolic syndrome (see margin box above)
  - Raises HDL cholesterol
- Initiating TLC before medication consideration
  - For most people a trial of NT of about 3 months is advised before initiating drug therapy

KEY TERMS

trans fatty acids Fatty acids that have been hydrogenated to be used in margarine and in the food industry; have been shown to increase low-density lipoprotein (LDL) cholesterol and lower high-density lipoprotein (HDL) cholesterol.

BOX 21-2 GUIDE TO THERAPEUTIC LIFESTYLE CHANGES: HEALTHY LIFESTYLE RECOMMENDATIONS FOR A HEALTHY HEART

Food Items to Choose More Often

Breads and Cereals

- Six servings per day, adjusted to caloric needs
- Breads, cereals, especially whole grains; pasta; rice; potatoes; dry beans and peas; low-fat crackers and cookies

Vegetables

Three to five servings per day fresh, frozen, or canned, without added fat, sauce, or salt

Fruits

Two to four servings per day fresh, frozen, canned, dried

Dairy Products

Two to three servings per day fat-free, ½%, 1% milk, buttermilk, yogurt, cottage cheese, fat-free and low-fat cheese

Eggs

Less than two egg yolks per week; egg whites or egg substitute

Meat, Poultry, Fish

Five ounces per day

Lean-cut beef tenderloin, ground round, extra-lean hamburger; cold cuts made with lean meat or soy protein; skinless poultry; fish

Fats and Oils

Amount adjusted to caloric level: unsaturated oils; soft or liquid margarines and vegetable oil spreads; salad dressings, seeds, and nuts

Therapeutic Lifestyle Changes (TLC) Diet Options

Stanol/sterol-containing margarines; soluble-fiber food sources: barley, oats, psyllium, apples, bananas, berries, citrus fruits, nectarines, peaches, pears, plums, prunes, broccoli, brussels sprouts, carrots, dry beans, soy products (tofu, miso)

Food Items to Choose Less Often

Breads and Cereals

- Many baked products, including doughnuts, biscuits, butter rolls, muffins, croissants, sweet rolls, Danish, cakes, pies, coffee cakes, cookies
- Many grain-based snacks, including chips, cheese puffs, snack mix, regular crackers, buttered popcorn

Vegetables

Vegetables fried or prepared with butter, cheese, or cream sauce

Fruits

Fruits fried or served with butter or cream

Dairy Products

Whole milk, 2% milk, whole-milk yogurt, ice cream, cream, cheese

Eggs

Egg yolk, whole eggs

Meat, Poultry, Fish

Higher-fat meat cuts: ribs, T-bone steak, regular hamburger, bacon, sausage; cold cuts: salami, bologna, hot dogs; organ meats: liver, brains, sweetbreads; poultry with skin; fried meat; fried poultry; fried fish

Fats and Oils

Butter, shortening, stick margarine, chocolate, coconut

Recommendations for Weight Reduction

Weigh Regularly

Record weight, body mass index (BMI), and waist circumferences

Lose Weight Gradually

Goal: lose 10% of body weight in 6 months; lose ½-1 lb per week

Develop Healthy Eating Patterns

- Choose healthy foods (see "Food Items to Choose More Often").
- Reduce your intake of foods in "Food Items to Choose Less Often."
- Limit the number of eating occasions.
- Avoid second helpings.
- Identify and reduce hidden fat by reading food labels to choose products lower in saturated fat and calories, and ask about ingredients in ready-to-eat foods prepared away from home.
- Identify and reduce sources of excess carbohydrates such as fat-free and regular crackers, cookies and other desserts, snacks, and sugar-containing beverages.

Recommendations for Increased Physical Activity

Make Physical Activity Part of Daily Routines

- Reduce sedentary time.
- Walk or bike ride more and drive less.
- Take the stairs instead of an elevator.
- Get off the bus a few stops early and walk the remaining distance.
- Mow the lawn with a push mower, rake leaves, and work in a garden.
- Push a stroller.
- Clean your house.
- Do exercises or pedal a stationary bike while watching television.
- Play actively with children.
- Take a brisk 10-minute walk or bike ride before work, during your work break, and after dinner.

Make Physical Activity Part of Exercise or Recreational Activities

- Walk or jog.
- Ride a bicycle or use an arm pedal bicycle.
- Swim or do water aerobics.
- Play basketball.
- Join a sports team.
- Play wheelchair sports.
- Play golf, pulling or carrying clubs.
- Go canoeing, cross-country skiing, or dancing.
- Take part in an exercise program at work, at home, at school, or at the gym.

Data from U.S. Department of Health and Human Services, Public Health Service, National Institutes of Health, National Heart, Lung, and Blood Institute: *Your guide to lowering your blood pressure with DASH,* NIH Pub No 06-4082, Bethesda, Md, 2006, U.S. Government Printing Office. Retrieved May 19, 2009, from www.nhlbi.nih.gov.

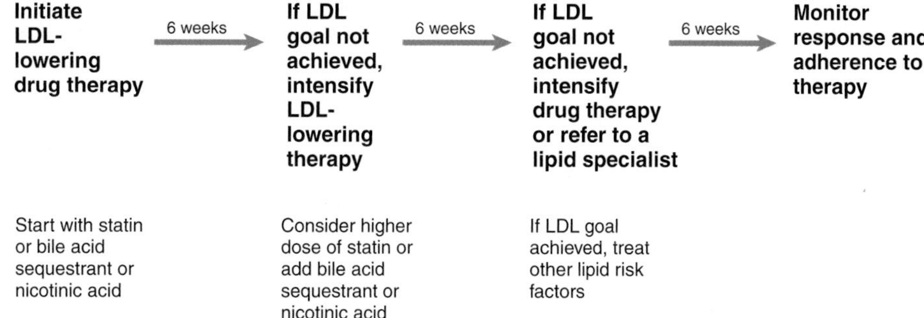

FIGURE 21-5 Progression of drug therapy. (From the National Cholesterol Education Program [NCEP]: *Third report of the NCEP Expert Panel on Detection, Evaluation, and Treatment of High Blood Cholesterol in Adults [Adult Treatment Panel III], full report,* Washington, DC, 2001, National Institutes of Health, National Heart, Lung, and Blood Institute.)

- Ineffective trials of NT exclusive of medications should not be protracted for indefinite period if goals of therapy are not approached in reasonable time (Medication should not be withheld if it is needed to reach targets in persons with high short-term or long-term CHD risk.)
- Initiating drug therapy simultaneously with TLC
  - For severe hypercholesterolemia in which NT alone cannot attain LDL cholesterol targets
  - For those with CHD or CHD risk equivalents in whom NT alone will not attain LDL cholesterol targets

The general strategy for initiation and progression of drug therapy is outlined in Figure 21-5. (For information about particular herbs and supplements that affect the cardiovascular system, see the *Complementary and Alternative Medicine [CAM]* box, "It Does a Heart Good... or Does It?" and the *Diet-Medications Interactions* box, "Possible Interactions Between Cardiovascular Diseases and Natural Therapies.")

Acute Cardiovascular Disease: Myocardial Infarction

Medical Management

Initial medical treatment of myocardial infarction (MI), or heart attack, usually includes strong analgesics (usually morphine sulfate) for severe unremitting pain, oxygen therapy, intravenous nitroglycerine for ischemic discomfort, control of hypertension or management of pulmonary congestion, and aspirin to produce a rapid antithrombotic effect.[5] This protocol is sometimes referred to as *MONA* (morphine, oxygen, nitroglycerine, and aspirin).

Nutritional Management

In the initial acute phase of CVD, an MI requires close attention to dietary modifications. The basic clinical objective is cardiac rest to allow the healing process to begin. All care is directed toward this basic need for cardiac rest so that the damaged heart can be restored to normal functioning. In addition to TLC (see Table 21-3), sodium may be restricted to 2 to 4 g for hypertension or to control edema[2] (see the *Case Study* box, "The Patient with Myocardial Infarction").

Metabolic Syndrome

If the patient has metabolic syndrome, further attention must be given to the following[5]:

- Weight management
- Gradual increase in physical activity under physician's supervision
- Limiting alcohol intake

Chronic Coronary Heart Disease: Congestive Heart Failure

In chronic CHD a condition of congestive heart failure (CHF) may develop over time. Each year more than 550,000 new cases are diagnosed.[1] The progressively weakened heart muscle, the *myocardium,* is unable to maintain an adequate cardiac output to sustain normal blood circulation. Resulting fluid imbalances cause edema, especially **pulmonary edema,** to develop. This condition brings added problems in breathing called *respiratory distress* or *dyspnea,* which places added stress on the laboring heart. The most common cause of CHF is myocardial ischemia from coronary artery disease, hypertension, and cardiomyopathy. About half of CHF patients suffer diastolic dysfunction, whereas systolic function is preserved. This is more likely to develop in older adults, women, and those without history of MI.[1]

Etiology: Relationship to Sodium and Water

Fluid congestion of chronic heart disease relates to imbalances in the body's capillary fluid shift mechanism and its resulting hormonal effects, as follows:

- *Imbalance in capillary fluid shift mechanism:* As the heart fails to pump out returning blood fast enough, venous return is delayed. This causes a disproportionate amount of blood to accumulate in the vascular system working with the right side of the heart. Venous pressure rises, a sort of "backup" pressure effect, and overcomes the balance of filtration pressures necessary to maintain

KEY TERMS

pulmonary edema Accumulation of fluid in tissues of the lung.

COMPLEMENTARY AND ALTERNATIVE MEDICINE (CAM)

It Does a Heart Good… or Does It?

Herbs are used by many to treat "what ails them." Although research is constantly being undertaken to test the efficacy of herbs, available information remains limited. The following table reviews the efficacy of herbal medicines that affect the cardiovascular system. In an effort to simplify the information, herbs are classified under the primary diseases they treat. However, please keep in mind most herbal medicines have multiple, overlapping cardiovascular effects. It is also important to remember that herbs sold in the United States are not standardized doses or preparations; therefore no regulation exists regarding the safety of herbal products.

CARDIOVASCULAR DISORDER	COMMONLY USED HERB/ SUPPLEMENT	EFFICACY OF HERB/SUPPLEMENT
Congestive heart failure (CHF)	Coenzyme Q_{10} (CoQ_{10}) (mitoquinone, ubidecarenone, ubiquinone)	Reasonably good evidence supports use of CoQ_{10} as adjunct therapy; thought to work by improving efficiency of cardiac muscle
	Hawthorn (*Crataegus laevigata, C. monogyna, C. oxyacantha, C. pentagyna*)	No evidence hawthorn reduces CHF morbidity or mortality
	Carnitine	Improves myocardial contractility and relaxation and cardiac pump function in patients with ventricular dysfunction
	Taurine	Might be useful in adjuvant therapy in class II, III, and IV CHF
	Arginine	Might improve some CHF symptoms
	Creatine	Might improve skeletal muscle exercise tolerance in patients with CHF
	Vitamin B_1 (thiamin)	Slight evidence that intravenous thiamin followed by oral supplementation could improve heart function in patients with CHF
	Vitamin E (α-tocopherol)	Ineffective for treatment of CHF
	Garlic (*Allium* spp, including *Allium sativum*)	Might mildly reduce blood pressure (approximately 10 mm Hg systolic and 5 mm Hg diastolic)
High blood pressure	CoQ_{10}	Adjunctive treatment with 120 mg CoQ_{10} daily has been shown to reduce average blood pressure by about 9%; might prolong hypotensive effects of enalapril and nitrendipine without changing their maximal effect
	Fish oils (alternative names/supplement forms: docosahexaenoic acid [DHA], eicosapentaenoic acid [EPA], omega-3 fatty acids, omega-3 oils)	Might have slight antihypertensive effect
	Hawthorn	Might increase exercise tolerance
	Carnitine	Might increase exercise tolerance; decrease number of premature ventricular contractions (PVCs); might decrease need for some medications such as nitroglycerides, β-blockers, antihypertensives, diuretics, anticoagulants, antiarrhythmics, and hypolipidemics
	Inositol hexaniacinate (a form of niacin)	Might improve walking distance
	L-carnitine	Improves muscle energy use
	Mesoglycans	Might improve walking distance
	Policosanol	Improves walking distance
	Oxerutins	In combination with compression stockings, effective in reducing leg edema
	Diosmin/hesperidin (citrus bioflavonoids)	Significantly improves symptoms
	Butcher's broom *(Ruscus aculeatus)*	Improves symptoms of venous insufficiency
	Grape leaf	Dose-dependent improvements in symptoms
	Oligomeric proanthocyanidin complexes (OPCs)	Provide significant benefit in chronic venous insufficiency
	Gotu kola *(Centella asiatica)*	Dose-dependent improvements in symptoms
Angina pectoris	*N*-acetylcysteine (NAC) (modified form of the dietary amino acid cysteine)	Given in combination with nitroglycerine is more effective than either drug alone in preventing death, myocardial infarction (MI), or need for revascularization; unfortunately, combined treatment also associated with high rate of severe headache
Hypertension	Stevia	Might posses antihypertensive effects; considered safe when used at recommended doses
Peripheral vascular disease (PVD) (intermittent claudication)	Ginkgo *(Ginkgo biloba)*	Modest improvement in pain-free walking
Venous insufficiency	Horse chestnut *(Aesculus hippocastanum)*	Used in combination with compression stockings, useful treatment for pain, itching, leg fatigue, and feelings of tension in the legs

BIBLIOGRAPHY

Bratman S, Girman AM: *Mosby's handbook of herbs and supplements and their therapeutic uses,* St Louis, 2003, Mosby.

Kuhn MA, Winston D: *Herbal therapy and supplements: a scientific and traditional approach,* Philadelphia, 2001, Lippincott Williams & Wilkins.

Springhouse Corporation: *Professional guide to complementary and alternative therapies,* Baltimore, 2001, Springhouse.

DIET-MEDICATIONS INTERACTIONS

Possible Interactions Between Cardiovascular Diseases and Natural Therapies

PHARMACEUTICAL CLASS	NATURAL THERAPY	INTERACTION
Warfarin	Coenzyme Q_{10} (CoQ_{10})	Concurrent use could reduce effectiveness of drug; might increase excretion or metabolism of warfarin
Angiotensin-converting enzyme (ACE) inhibitors	Arginine, potassium	Possible hyperkalemia
	Dong quai *(Angelica polymorpha sinensis),* St. John's wort *(Hypericum perforatum)*	Possible increased risk of photosensitivity
	Iron	Mutual absorption interference; possible reduction of ACE inhibitor–induced cough
	Licorice (natural)	Antagonism of drug action
	Zinc	Correction of possible drug-induced depletion
Digitoxin, digoxin	*Eleutherococcus* (Siberian ginseng)	Interference with laboratory measurement of digoxin levels
	Hawthorn *(Crataegus laevigata, C. monogyna, C. oxyacantha, C. pentagyna)*	Might interfere with effects of digoxin or serum monitoring
	Horsetail, licorice (natural)	Possible hypokalemia leading to increased drug toxicity
	Magnesium	Absorption interference
	St. John's wort	Decreased serum levels of drug with possible rebound toxicity if herb is stopped
Loop diuretics	Dong quai, St. John's wort	Possible increased risk of photosensitivity
	Licorice (natural)	Potentiation of hypokalemic action of drug
Potassium-sparing diuretics	Arginine	Possible increased risk of hyperkalemia
	Licorice (natural)	Antagonism of drug action
	Magnesium	Risk of hypermagnesemia
	White willow *(Salix alba)*	Possible interference of salicylate content with spironolactone action
	Zinc	Excessive zinc levels with spironolactone
Thiazide diuretics	Calcium	Potential risk of hypercalcemia
	Dong quai, St. John's wort	Possible increased risk of photosensitivity
	Licorice (natural)	Potentiation of hypokalemic action of drug
Fluoroquinolones, tetracyclines	Calcium	Mutual absorption interference
Levothyroxine	Calcium	Possible absorption interference
Calcium channel blockers (CCBs)	Combined high-dose calcium and vitamin D, grapefruit juice	Possible antagonism of drug action
Anticoagulant and antiplatelet agents	Fish oil	Possible increased risk of bleeding complications
	Vitamin C	Possible antagonism of drug action
	Garlic, ginkgo, high-dose vitamin E, policosanol	Possible increased risk of bleeding complications
	Horse chestnut, oligomeric proanthocyanidin complexes (OPCs)	Possible increased risk of bleeding complications

Continued

DIET-MEDICATIONS INTERACTIONS

Possible Interactions Between Cardiovascular Diseases and Natural Therapies—cont'd

PHARMACEUTICAL CLASS	NATURAL THERAPY	INTERACTION
Amiloride	Magnesium	Possible hypermagnesemia
β-blockers	Calcium	Absorption interference
	Chromium	Increased high-density lipoprotein (HDL) levels
Nitrates	*N*-acetylcysteine (NAC)	Increase of headache side effects

BIBLIOGRAPHY

Bratman S, Girman AM: *Mosby's handbook of herbs and supplements and their therapeutic uses*, St Louis, 2003, Mosby.

Kuhn MA, Winston D: *Herbal therapy and supplements: a scientific and traditional approach*, Philadelphia, 2001, Lippincott Williams & Wilkins.

Springhouse Corporation: *Professional guide to complementary and alternative therapies*, Baltimore, 2001, Springhouse.

CASE STUDY

The Patient with Myocardial Infarction

Edward is a 37-year-old sedentary executive who was seen for an annual physical examination 6 months ago. He had no complaints other than feeling the "everyday pressures" of his job as a corporate attorney and head of the legal division. He admitted smoking two packs of cigarettes a day as a means of relieving stress.

Edward is 175 cm (5 feet, 9 inches). At the time of his examination, he weighed 83 kg (185 lb). His blood pressure was 148/90 mm Hg, and his serum cholesterol level was 285 mg/dL. He was advised to quit smoking, exercise daily at a moderate pace, and lose 9 kg (20 lb).

Edward arrived in the hospital emergency department 3 months later complaining of severe chest pains and difficulty breathing. His wife reported that he had appeared pale that evening, had broken out into a cold sweat, and had vomited shortly after arriving home from work. Once regular breathing was restored by the emergency medical team and his pain subsided, a number of laboratory tests were ordered. These tests included serum glutamic-oxaloacetic transaminase (SGOT), lactate dehydrogenase (LDH), prothrombin time (PT), lipid panel plus high-density lipoprotein (HDL) cholesterol, sedimentation rate, coagulation times, fasting plasma glucose (FPG), blood urea nitrogen (BUN), and complete blood count (CBC). An electrocardiogram (ECG) was also ordered. The patient was then transferred to the coronary care unit for closer monitoring.

The following tests results were elevated: SGOT, LDH, LDL, as well as total cholesterol, triglycerides, glucose, PT, white blood cell count, and sedimentation rate. HDL level was low. The ECG revealed an infarction of the posterior wall of the myocardium. The diagnosis was myocardial infarction (MI), with underlying familial hypercholesterolemia.

In consultation with the hospital's registered dietitian (RD), the cardiologist ordered a liquid diet, increasing it to a soft diet with low saturated fats 2 days later. The RD noted continued improvement in the patient's appetite accompanying recovery and recommended changing the diet order to the therapeutic lifestyle changes (TLC) diet.

One week later, Edward was discharged. During his convalescence, the RD and nurse met with him and his wife several times to discuss his continuing care at home. At each follow-up clinic visit with the physician and nutritionist, Edward showed good general recovery and enjoyment of his new modified fat and cholesterol food habits.

Questions for Analysis

1. What predisposing factors in Edward's lifestyle place him in the high-risk category for coronary heart disease (CHD)?
2. Why was moderate, consistent exercise originally recommended?
3. Explain the causes for Edward's initial symptoms.
4. How does each laboratory test ordered in the emergency department relate to cell metabolism? Why were the results elevated?
5. Explain the association between the final diet order and his lipid disorder.
6. What nondietary needs might Edward have while convalescing at home? What community agencies might be of assistance?

the normal capillary fluid shift mechanism (see Chapter 7). Fluid that would normally flow between interstitial spaces and blood vessels is held in the tissue spaces rather than recirculated.

- *Hormonal mechanisms:* Two hormonal mechanisms are involved in fluid balance in normal circulation. In this instance, both of the following contribute to cardiac edema:

1. *Aldosterone mechanism:* This mechanism, described more completely by its full name, *the renin-angiotensin-aldosterone mechanism,* is normally a lifesaving sodium- and water-conserving mechanism that ensures essential fluid balances. In this case, however, it only compounds the edema problem. As the heart fails to propel blood circulation forward, deficient cardiac output effectively

reduces blood flow through kidney nephrons. Decreased renal blood pressure triggers the renin-angiotensin system. Renin is an enzyme from the renal cortex that combines in blood with its substrate, angiotensinogen, which is produced in the liver, to produce in turn angiotensin I and II. Angiotensin II acts as a stimulant to the adrenal glands to produce aldosterone. This hormone in turn effects a reabsorption of sodium in an ion exchange with potassium in the distal tubules of the nephrons, and water reabsorption follows. Ordinarily this is a lifesaving mechanism to protect the body's vital water supply. In CHF, however, it only adds to the edema problem. The mechanism reacts as if the body's total fluid volume is reduced, when in truth the fluid is excessive; it is just that it is not in normal circulation but is being retained in the body's tissues.

2. *Antidiuretic hormone (ADH) mechanism:* This water-conserving hormonal mechanism also adds to edema. Cardiac stress and reduced renal flow cause the release of ADH, also known as vasopressin, from the pituitary gland. ADH then stimulates still more water reabsorption in nephrons of the kidney, further increasing the problem of edema.

Increased Cellular Free Potassium

As reduced blood circulation depresses cell metabolism, cell protein is broken down and releases its bound potassium in the cell. As a result, the amount of free potassium inside the cell is increased, which increases intracellular osmotic pressure. Sodium ions in fluid surrounding the cell then also increase in number to balance increased osmotic pressure within the cell and to prevent cell dehydration. In time, the increased sodium outside the cell causes still more water retention.[6]

Nutritional Management

Basis for all care of the person with CHF is improving cardiac output while reducing workload of the heart and minimizing congestive symptoms. Medical treatment involves oxygen therapy, decreased physical activity, and drug therapy with (1) diuretic and vasodilator agents to control fluid congestion in the lungs; (2) digitalis drugs to strengthen contractions of the heart muscle; and (3) sympathetic antagonists, angiotensin-converting enzyme (ACE) inhibitors, nitrate, and vasodilators to decrease workload of the heart.[8] Nutrition support involves the following[7]:

- *Sodium* is usually restricted to 2 g/day and may be adjusted upwards to 3 g/day if necessary to promote food and nutrient intake.
- *Fluids* may be restricted to 1500 mL/day, if necessary.
- *Texture* may be modified to soft foods so that little physical effort is needed.
- *Meals* may be divided into smaller feedings to also decrease effort necessary for eating.
- *Alcohol* is generally limited to one drink per day. If alcohol is thought to be a causative factor in the heart disease, then abstinence is mandatory.

Cardiac Cachexia

Etiology

Sometimes with prolonged myocardial insufficiency and heart failure an extreme clinical condition of cardiac cachexia develops. Progressive, profound malnutrition results from an insufficient oxygen supply that cannot meet demands of red blood cell formation by bone marrow or energy needs for basic breathing. The enlarged, laboring heart is unable to maintain a sufficient blood supply to the body tissues, and nutrient delivery to cells is impaired. Edema, unpalatable sodium-restricted diets, drug reactions, and postoperative complications of cardiac surgery all worsen the anorexia and reduce food intake. In addition, the individual has probably become hypermetabolic and hypercatabolic. It should be no surprise that the incidence of nosocomial (hospital induced) cardiac cachexia is a common occurrence.

Nutrition Therapy

The goal is to help restore heart-lung function as much as possible and to rebuild body tissue. Team care involving the physician, clinical dietitian, nurse, patient, and family is essential. Nutrition support focuses on energy, nutrients, supplements, and feeding plan, as follows[5]:

- *Energy:* Sufficient kcalories are needed to cover basal energy needs, as well as energy for minimal activity and the hypermetabolism of severe CHF; more kcalories may be needed if major surgery is planned. Depending on the extent of malnutrition indicated by nutrition assessment, an increase of 30% to 50% of basal needs may be indicated.
- *Fluids:* Sufficient but not excessive fluid intake is needed, at a rate of about 0.5 mL/kcal/day or 1000 to 1500 mL/day.
- *Protein:* Approximately 1.0 to 1.5 g/kg body weight is needed to replace tissue losses and cover malabsorption.
- *Sodium:* Sodium restriction varies with individual status, usually in a range of 1 to 2 g/day, with attention to multiple alternate seasonings to enhance palatability of food.
- *Mineral-vitamin supplementation:* May need to supplement intake with folate, magnesium, thiamin, zinc, and iron depending on serum levels. Increasing vitamins E, B_6, B_{12}, and thiamin may be beneficial.
- *Feeding plan:* Small, frequent feedings are better tolerated. Large meals add to the risk of carbon dioxide (CO_2) accumulation and respiratory failure.
- *Enteral nutrition (EN) and parenteral nutrition (PN) support:* Tube feedings or PN may be appropriate. Several EN feeding formulas are available that have a low volume with a high density of kcalories. These are suitable for patients requiring fluid restriction.

KEY TERMS

antidiuretic hormone (ADH) Water-conserving hormone from posterior lobe of pituitary gland; causes resorption of water by kidney nephrons according to body need.

vasopressin Alternative name of antidiuretic hormone (ADH).

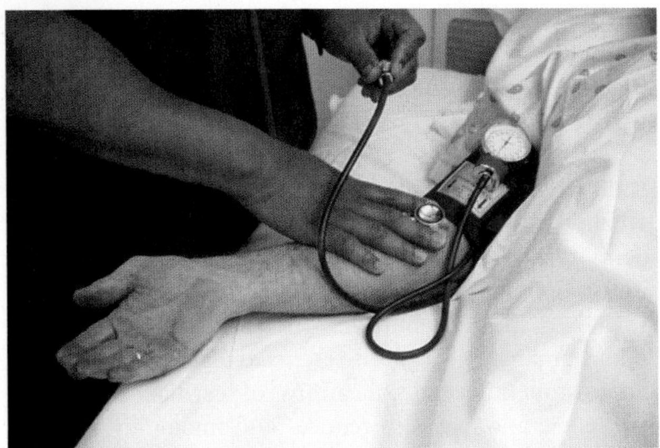

FIGURE 21-6 Monitoring blood pressure. (From Potter PA, Perry AG: *Basic nursing: essentials for practice,* ed 5, St Louis, 2003, Mosby.)

ESSENTIAL HYPERTENSION AND VASCULAR DISEASE

Hypertension

High blood pressure is one of the most prevalent vascular diseases worldwide. As the population ages, prevalence of hypertension will increase. It is a major factor in the development of stroke, heart attack, heart failure, and kidney disease.[7] At least 95% of these persons have essential hypertension, meaning its cause is unknown, although a strong familial predisposition exists, with its onset in young teenage years. It has often been called the *silent disease* because it carries no overt signs, but it can have serious implications if not treated and controlled.[9] The large United States study—Dietary Approaches to Stop Hypertension (DASH)—has clearly indicated that a diet rich in fruits, vegetables, and low-fat dairy foods and with reduced saturated and total fat can substantially lower blood pressure.[10] Individual treatment uses current antihypertensive drugs as needed.

Blood Pressure Controls

Arterial Pressure. As commonly measured, blood pressure is an indication of arterial pressure in vessels of the upper arm. This measure is obtained by an instrument for determining force of the pulse (Figure 21-6). This instrument is called a *sphygmomanometer,* from the Greek words *sphygmos* (meaning pulse), *manos* (meaning thin), and *metron* (meaning measure). Pulse pressure is measured in millimeters of mercury (mm Hg) rise or in equivalent values read on gauges or digital indicators. The higher, or upper, value recorded is systolic pressure from contraction of the heart muscle. The lower value recorded is diastolic pressure, produced during the relaxation phase of the cardiac cycle.

Several factors contribute to maintaining fluid dynamics of normal blood pressure: (1) increased pressure on forward blood flow; (2) increased resistance from containing blood vessels; and (3) increased viscosity of blood itself, making movement through vessels more difficult. Of these factors, increased viscosity is a rare event. Thus in discussing high blood pressure in general terms, we are dealing with the first two factors: (1) pumping pressure of the heart muscle propelling blood forward and (2) resistance to this forward flow presented by blood vessel walls normally or by any abnormal added constriction or thickening.

Muscle Tone of Blood Vessel Walls. In hypertension the body's finely tuned mechanisms designed to maintain fluid dynamics are not operating effectively. Normally these systems include several agents that act to variously dilate and constrict blood vessels to meet whatever need is present at a given time. In a person with hypertension, however, dilation or constriction of blood vessels does not occur in the normal manner. If not effectively treated, then uncontrolled elevated blood pressure results. Body systems that operate to help maintain normal blood pressure include (1) neuroendocrine functions of the sympathetic nervous system, mainly mediated by chemical neurotransmitters, such as norepinephrine; (2) hormonal systems such as the renin-angiotensin-aldosterone mechanism and its vasopressor effect; and (3) enzyme systems such as the kallikrein-kinin mechanism (sometimes operating with prostaglandins), which controls substances that act to dilate or constrict smooth muscle as needed.

Classifications of Blood Pressure

Hypertension is defined as systolic blood pressure of 140 mm Hg or higher, diastolic blood pressure of 90 mm Hg or higher or taking antihypertensive medication. The objective of identifying and treating hypertension is to reduce morbidity and mortality. For that reason, classification of adult (>18 years of age) blood pressure (Table 21-4) provides a mechanism for identifying high-risk individuals and provides guidelines for follow-up and treatment.[8]

Prevention and Treatment

The goal of prevention and management of hypertension is to reduce morbidity and mortality by the least intrusive means possible.[8] Lifestyle modifications (Table 21-5) offer potential for preventing hypertension, have been shown capable of lowering blood pressure, and can reduce cardiovascular risk factors at minimal cost and risk.[8]

Nutritional Management of Hypertension

Taste for a given amount of salt with food is an acquired one, not a physiologic necessity. Sufficient sodium for the body's need is provided as a natural mineral in foods consumed. Some persons salt their foods heavily and thus form high salt taste levels. Others form lighter tastes by using smaller amounts. Common daily adult intakes of sodium range widely from about 2 to 4 g, with lighter tastes to as high as 10 to 12 g with heavier use. Salt (sodium chloride [NaCl]) intakes are about twice these amounts because sodium makes up about 40% of the NaCl molecule. The large amount of salt in the American diet, estimated to be about 6 to 15 g of sodium per day (260 to 656 mEq), is largely a result of the

TABLE 21-4 CLASSIFICATION OF BLOOD PRESSURE FOR ADULTS

BLOOD PRESSURE (BP) CLASSIFICATION	SYSTOLIC (in mm Hg)*	DIASTOLIC (in mm Hg)	LIFESTYLE MODIFICATION	INITIAL DRUG THERAPY: WITHOUT COMPELLING INDICATION	INITIAL DRUG THERAPY: WITH COMPELLING INDICATION†
Normal‡	<120	And <80	Encourage	No antihypertensive drug indicated	None
Prehypertension	120-139	Or 80-89	Yes	No antihypertensive drug indicated	Drug(s) for compelling indications§
Stage 1 hypertension¶	140-159	Or 90-99	Yes	Thiazide-type diuretics for most; consider ACEI, ARB, BB, CCB, or combinations	Drug(s) for the compelling indications§ Other antihypertensive drugs (diuretics, ACEI, ARB, BB, CCB) as needed
Stage 2 hypertension¶	>160	Or >100	Yes	Two-drug combination for most§	

Data from National High Blood Pressure Program: *The seventh report of the Joint National Committee on Prevention, Detection, Evaluation, and Treatment of High Blood Pressure (JNC 7), National Institutes of Health, National Heart, Lung, and Blood Institutes,* NIH Pub No 04-5230, Washington, DC, 2004, U.S. Government Printing Office. Available from http://www.nhlbi.nih.gov/guidelines/hypertension/jnc7full.htm.
ACEI, Angiotensin-converting enzyme inhibitor; *ARB,* aldosterone receptor blocker; *BB,* β-blocker; *CCB,* calcium channel blocker.
*Treatment determined by highest blood pressure category.
†Heart failure, post-MI, high coronary disease risk, chronic kidney disease, recurrent stroke prevention.
‡Optimal blood pressure with respect to cardiovascular risk is less than 120/80 mm Hg. However, unusually low readings should be evaluated for clinical significance.
§Initial combined therapy should be used cautiously in those at risk for orthostatic hypotension.
¶Based on the average of two or more readings taken at each of two or more visits after initial screening.

TABLE 21-5 LIFESTYLE MODIFICATIONS TO MANAGE HYPERTENSION*†

SBP MODIFICATION (RANGE)	RECOMMENDATIONS	APPROXIMATE SBP REDUCTION (RANGE)
Weight reduction	Maintain normal body weight (BMI 18.5-24.9 kg/m^2).	5-20 mm Hg per 10 kg weight loss
Adapt DASH eating plan	Consume a diet rich in fruits and vegetables and low in fat.	8-14 mm Hg
Dietary sodium reduction	Reduce dietary sodium intake to no more than 2.4 g sodium or 6 g sodium chloride (NaCl).	2-8 mm Hg
Physical activity	Engage in regular aerobic physical activity such as brisk walking (at least 30 minutes per day, most days of the week).	4-9 mm Hg
Moderation of alcohol consumption	Limit consumption to no more than two drinks (1 oz or 30 mL ethanol [e.g., 24 oz beer, 10 oz wine, or 3 oz 80-proof whiskey]) per day in most men and to no more than one drink per day in women and lighter-weight persons.	2-4 mm Hg

Data from National High Blood Pressure Program: *The seventh report of the Joint National Committee on Prevention, Detection, Evaluation, and Treatment of High Blood Pressure, National Institutes of Health, National Heart, Lung, and Blood Institutes,* NIH Pub No 04-5230, Washington, DC, 2004, U.S. Government Printing Office.
SBP, Systolic blood pressure; *BMI,* body mass index; *DASH,* Dietary Approaches to Stop Hypertension.
*For overall cardiovascular risk reduction, stop smoking.
†The effects of implementing these modifications are dose and time dependent and could be increased for some individuals.

increased use of many processed food products. The main source of dietary sodium is food processing (about 75%). Approximately 10% to 11% occurs naturally in foods, about 15% is discretionary (half of which is contributed by table salt and half by cooking), and less than 1% comes from water.

KEY TERMS

essential hypertension An inherent form of hypertension with no specific discoverable cause and considered to be familial; also called *primary hypertension.*

Other nutrients that affect blood pressure are potassium and calcium. High potassium intake from food sources (see the *Perspectives in Practice* box, "Dietary Approaches to Stop Hypertension [DASH] Diet Pattern") such as fresh fruits and vegetables may protect against developing hypertension and improve blood pressure control in those who do have hypertension.[8] Calcium in the form of low-fat dairy products (which are also low in saturated and total fat) is also recommended to reduce blood pressure. Moderate consumption of alcohol (equivalent to two drinks per day for men and one drink per day for women) is also known to reduce blood pressure.[8]

PERSPECTIVES IN PRACTICE

Dietary Approaches to Stop Hypertension (DASH) Diet Pattern

The following list indicates the number of recommended daily servings from each food group, with examples of food choices (based on the 2000-kcal reference diet). The number of servings may increase or decrease, depending on individual calorie needs, and can be found on the DASH website: *www.nhlbi.nih.gov/health/public/heart/hbp/dash/*.

FOOD GROUP	DAILY SERVING (EXCEPT WHERE NOTED)	SERVING SIZES	EXAMPLES AND NOTES	SIGNIFICANCE TO THE DASH DIET PATTERN
Grains and grain products	7-8	1 slice of bread 1 oz of dry cereal* ½ cup of cooked rice, pasta, or cereal	Whole wheat bread, English muffin, pita bread, bagel; cereals; grits; oatmeal	Major source of energy and fiber
Vegetables	4-5	1 cup of raw, leafy vegetables ½ cup of cooked vegetables 6 oz of vegetable juice	Tomatoes, potatoes, carrots, peas, squash, broccoli, turnip greens, collard greens, kale, spinach, artichokes, beans, sweet potatoes	Rich sources of potassium, magnesium, and fiber
Fruits	4-5	6 oz of fruit juice 1 medium fruit ¼ cup of dried fruit ½ cup of fresh, frozen, or canned fruit	Apricots, bananas, dates, grapes, oranges, orange juice, tangerines, strawberries, mangoes, melons, peaches, pineapple, prunes, raisins	Important sources of potassium, magnesium, and fiber
Low-fat or nonfat dairy foods	2-3	8 oz of milk 1 cup of yogurt 1½ oz of cheese	Fat-free or 1% milk, fat-free or low-fat buttermilk; nonfat or low-fat yogurt; part-nonfat mozzarella cheese, nonfat cheese	Major sources of calcium and protein
Meat, poultry, and fish	<2	3 oz of cooked meats, poultry, or fish	Select only lean meats; trim away visible fats; broil, roast, or boil, instead of frying; remove skin from chicken	Rich sources of protein and magnesium
Nuts, seeds, and legumes	4-5/wk	1½ oz or ½ cup of nuts ½ oz or 2 tbsp of seeds ½ cup of cooked legumes	Almonds, filberts, mixed nuts, peanuts, walnuts, sunflower seeds, kidney beans, lentils	Rich sources of energy, magnesium, potassium, protein, and fiber
Fats and oils†	2-3	1 tsp of soft margarine 1 tbsp of low-fat mayonnaise or salad dressing 2 tbsp of light salad dressing 1 tsp of vegetable oil	Soft margarine, low-fat mayonnaise, light salad dressing, vegetable oil (e.g., olive, corn, canola, safflower)	DASH has 27% of calories as fat, including that in or added to foods
Sweets	5/wk	1 tbsp of sugar 1 tbsp of jelly or jam ½ oz of jelly beans 8 oz of lemonade	Maple syrup, sugar, jelly, jam; fruit-flavored gelatin, jelly beans, fruit punch, sorbet, ices, hard candy	Sweets should be low in fat

PERSPECTIVES IN PRACTICE

Dietary Approaches to Stop Hypertension (DASH) Diet Pattern—cont'd

Strategies for Adopting DASH

Dietary changes are best achieved through small changes in food selections. Use this list of tips as a way to initiate discussion and dietary compliance to reduce hypertension among your clients.

Tips on Eating the DASH Way

- Change gradually.
- If you now eat one or two vegetables a day, then add a serving at lunch and another at dinner.
- If you do not eat fruit now or have only juice at breakfast, then add a serving to your meals or have it as a snack.
- Gradually increase your use of fat-free and low-fat dairy products to three servings a day. For example, drink milk with lunch or dinner instead of soda, sugar-sweetened tea, or alcohol. Choose low-fat (1%) or fat-free (skim) dairy products to reduce your intake of saturated fat, total fat, cholesterol, and kcalories.
- Read food labels on margarines and salad dressings, and choose those lowest in unsaturated fat. Some margarines are now trans fat free.
- Treat meat as one part of the whole meal instead of the focus.
- Limit meat to 6 oz a day (two servings)—all that is needed (3 to 4 oz is about the size of a deck of cards).
- If you now eat large portions of meat, cut them back gradually—by one half or one third at each meal.
- Include two or more vegetarian-style (meatless) meals each week.
- Increase servings of vegetables, rice, pasta, and dry beans at meals. Try casseroles, pasta, and stir-fry dishes that have less meat and more vegetables, grains, and dry beans.
- Use fruit or other foods low in saturated fat, cholesterol, and kcalories as desserts and snacks.
- Fruits and other low-fat foods offer great taste and variety. Use fruits canned in their own juices. Fresh fruits require little or no preparation. Dried fruits are a good choice to carry with you or to have ready in the car.
- Try these snacks ideas: unsalted pretzels or nuts mixed with raisins, graham crackers, low-fat and fat-free yogurt and frozen yogurt, popcorn with no salt or butter added, and raw vegetables.

Try these additional tips:

- Choose whole grain foods to get added nutrients such as minerals and fiber. For example, choose whole wheat bread and whole grain cereals.
- If you have trouble digesting dairy products, then try taking lactase enzyme pills or drops (available at drugs and grocery stores) with the dairy foods or buy lactose-free milk or milk with lactase enzyme added to it.
- Use fresh, frozen, or no-salt-added canned vegetables.

BIBLIOGRAPHY

U.S. Department of Health and Human Services, Public Health Service, National Institutes of Health, National Heart, Lung, and Blood Institute: *Your guide to lowering your blood pressure with DASH,* NIH Pub No 06-4082, Bethesda, Md, 2006, U.S. Government Printing Office. Retrieved May 19, 2009, from www.nhlbi.nih.gov.

*Equals ½ to ¼ cup, depending on cereal type. Check the product's nutrition label.

†Fat content changes serving counts for fats and oils. For example, 1 tbsp of regular salad dressing equals 1 serving; 1 tbsp of low-fat dressing equals ½ serving; 1 tbsp of fat-free dressing equals 0 servings.

Cerebrovascular Accident

Arteriosclerotic vascular injury and hypertension may also affect blood vessels in the brain. A cerebrovascular accident (CVA), or stroke, occurs when a blood vessel carrying oxygen and nutrients to the brain ruptures (hemorrhagic stroke) or is clogged by a blood clot (ischemic stroke), interrupting blood flow to an area of the brain. When any part of the brain does not receive blood and oxygen, nerve cells in the affected area die, resulting in loss of control of abilities that area of the brain once controlled. During the past 20 years, with the declining U.S. early death rate from heart disease, stroke stands in third place as a leading cause of death of adults ages 25 to 65 years.[11] Nearly 170,000 Americans die annually of stroke, meaning someone in the United States experiences a stroke every 45 seconds.[2] Among all U.S. population groups, the incident rate for first stroke among African Americans is almost double that of European Americans.[12]

Four main types of stroke exist; two are caused by blood clots, and two are caused by ruptured blood vessels. Cerebral thrombosis and cerebral embolism account for approximately 70% to 80% of all strokes. Cerebral thrombosis, the most common stroke, occurs when a thrombus forms and blocks blood flow in an artery bringing blood to part of the brain. They usually occur at night or first thing in the morning when blood pressure is low. They are often preceded by a transient ischemic attack (TIA), or "ministroke." Cerebral embolism occurs when an embolus forms away from the brain, usually in the heart. The clot is carried in the bloodstream until it lodges in an artery leading to or in the brain and blocks the flow of blood.[2] A subarachnoid hemorrhage occurs when a blood vessel on the brain's surface ruptures and bleeds into the space between the brain and skull. A cerebral hemorrhage occurs when a defective artery in the brain bursts, flooding the surrounding tissue with blood.[2]

Nutrition Therapy

Paralysis and other problems may occur, depending on the site and extent of brain damage resulting from a stroke. Patients who experience left-sided CVA most commonly experience sight and hearing losses, including ability to see where food is on plates or trays. Right-hemisphere, bilateral, or brainstem CVA causes significant problems with feeding and swallowing, in addition to speech problems.[8]

Dysphagia often occurs, and foods that cause choking or that are hard to manage should be avoided (dry or crisp foods, peanut butter, thinly pureed foods, raw vegetables, to mention a few). If the patient has problems with saliva production, then foods can be moistened with small amounts of liquid (au jus or gravy). Because thin liquids are often difficult to swallow, thickeners are used to make semisolid foods from soups, beverages, and juices.[8]

Peripheral Vascular Disease

Peripheral vascular disease (PVD) is characterized by narrowing of blood vessels in the legs and sometimes the arms. Blood flow is restricted and causes pain in affected area. Contributory risk factors include hypertension and diabetes mellitus. However, the greatest risk factor is cigarette smoking, which constricts blood vessels. More than 90% of patients with PVD are or were moderate to heavy smokers.

Symptoms and Complications

As arteries gradually narrow because of atherosclerosis (the most common cause), an aching, tired feeling occurs in leg muscles when walking. Resting the leg for a few minutes relieves pain, but it recurs shortly when walking is resumed. For this reason the symptom is called intermittent claudication. Sometimes a sudden arterial blockage occurs when a blood clot develops on the top of a plaque or a clot formed in the heart is carried to a peripheral artery and blocks it. The blockage causes sudden severe pain in the affected area, which becomes cold and either pale or blue and has no pulse. Movement and sensation are lost.

Treatment

By far the most important treatment for the patient is to stop smoking. As with coronary vessels, surgery on diseased vessels is sometimes required: (1) arterial reconstructive surgery to bypass them, (2) endarterectomy to remove obstructing fatty deposits on inner linings, or (3) balloon angioplasty to widen vessels. Drug therapy may include antiplatelet or anticoagulant agents to prevent blood clotting. NT consists of regular fat and cholesterol modifications described for CHD. Exercise is also important. The person should walk every day with medical clearance, gradually increasing to about 1 hour—stopping whenever intermittent pain occurs and resuming when it stops. Regular inspection of feet, daily washing and stocking change, good-fitting shoes to avoid pressure, and scrupulous foot care (ideally by a podiatrist) are essential to prevent infection.

PULMONARY DISEASES

Chronic Obstructive Pulmonary Disease

Clinical Characteristics

Progressive CHF contributes to lung disease and risk of respiratory failure. Malnutrition is common with the debilitating condition of chronic obstructive pulmonary disease (COPD). This term describes a group of disorders in which airflow in the lungs is limited and respiratory failure develops. Two main interrelated COPD conditions are (1) chronic bronchitis and (2) emphysema. Malnutrition usually accompanies COPD, and its presence increases illness and death rates associated with the disease process. Anorexia and significant weight loss reflect a growing inability to maintain adequate nutritional status, which in turn severely compromises pulmonary function. Progression of the disease process, with its increasing shortness of breath, prevents the person from living a normal life, and prognosis is poor. Eventually, in progressive respiratory failure, the patient becomes dependent on a mechanical respirator and controlled oxygen supply. A poor prognosis is associated with a compromised nutritional status in these patients.

Nutritional Management

Respiratory failure is actually a failure of pulmonary exchange of oxygen and CO_2. Thus its common manifestations are hypoxemia, deficient oxygenation of blood, and hypercapnia, excess CO_2 in the blood. Patients with COPD have increased energy requirements, which will vary for each individual. Requirements for carbohydrate, protein, and fat will be determined by the underlying lung disease, oxygen therapy, medications, weight status, and any acute fluid fluctuations.[5] A balanced proportion of protein (15% to 20% total kcalories) with fat (30% to 45% total kcalories) and carbohydrate (40% to 55% total kcalories) is necessary to maintain appropriate respiratory quotient (RQ) from substrate use.[5] Although it is important not to overfeed patients with COPD (especially too much carbohydrate), these patients often have difficulty taking in sufficient amounts of food because of fatigue (food preparation, shortness of breath, the act of eating) and lose weight. Commonly, other coexisting diseases (CVD, diabetes mellitus, renal disease, or cancer) may be present, thereby influencing total amount and kind of carbohydrate, protein, and fat prescribed.[5]

Pneumonia

The term *pneumonia* comes from the Greek word *pneuma,* meaning breath. It is an acute inflammation of the lung caused by an infectious agent and can stem from three sources: (1) aspiration of normal bacterial flora, gastric contents, or both in oropharyngeal secretions; (2) inhalation of contaminants (e.g., virus); or (3) contamination from systemic circulation. A common disorder, community-acquired pneumonia is the most lethal infectious disease in the United States and the sixth leading cause of death.[13]

Symptoms

Generally the immune response, cough with or without sputum production, sneezing, and mucociliary clearance (pulmonary defense mechanisms) guard against pneumonia.[13] Community-acquired pneumonia is usually bacterial in origin and produces exudate that is hard to expectorate. Viral pneumonia does not produce exudate.[13] Hospital-acquired, or nosocomial, pneumonia develops in up to

5% of hospitalized patients.[13] Nosocomial pneumonia and community-based pneumonia are caused by different pathogens. Aspiration of infected pharyngeal or gastric secretions delivers bacteria straight to the lungs. This is promoted by exogenous factors such as contamination by dirty hands and equipment, treatment with broad-spectrum antibiotics that promote emergence of drug-resistant organisms, and patient factors such as malnutrition, smoking, preexisting lung disease, advanced age, swallowing disorders, and chest or upper abdominal surgery. Signs and symptoms are nonspecific; however, fever, purulent sputum, and leukocytosis are present in most patients.[13]

Treatment

Sputum and blood specimens are cultured before antibiotic treatment. Usual treatment is with a broad-spectrum penicillin antibiotic. Erythromycin may be added if the presence of an atypical organism is suspected. Oxygen therapy is often used, and in severe cases the patient may be ventilated. Nosocomial pneumonia is treated more aggressively with broad-spectrum antibiotics and tailored to specific clinical setting because of the high mortality rate.[13]

Nutritional Management

Sufficient fluids (3 to 3.5 L) should be given daily if not contraindicated. Frequent small meals may be better tolerated. A multivitamin and mineral supplement may be beneficial, and fiber should be encouraged to avoid constipation. Adequate fruit and fruit juice intake will supply necessary potassium.[8]

Tuberculosis

Tuberculosis (TB), caused by *Mycobacterium tuberculosis*, is one of the world's more widespread and deadly diseases. It occurs disproportionately among disadvantaged populations such as the malnourished, the homeless, and those living in overcrowded and substandard housing. *M. tuberculosis* is an airborne disease, and strains resistant to one or more first-line antituberculosis drugs are increasing.[13]

Symptoms

Typical symptoms of TB are malaise, anorexia, weight loss, fever, and night sweats. Chronic cough is the most universal pulmonary symptom. It may be dry at first but becomes productive of purulent sputum as the disease progresses. More often than not, the sputum is blood streaked. Patients appear chronically ill and malnourished.[3,11]

Treatment

The basic goals of TB treatment are as follows[13]:

- Administer multiple drugs to which organisms are susceptible.
- Add at least two new antitubercular agents to a regimen when treatment failure is suspected.
- Provide the safest, most effective therapy in the shortest period of time.
- Ensure adherence to therapy.

Nonadherence (because of adverse drug reaction) to treatment is a major cause of treatment failure, continued transmission of TB, and development of drug resistance. Hospitalization for initial therapy of TB is not necessary for most patients,[13] but hospitalization has increased because of increasing resistance of the organism to treatment and an increasing number of cases.[5]

Nutritional Management

The objective of nutritional management is to maintain weight or prevent weight loss. If febrile, then patients will be hypermetabolic. A well-balanced diet with liberal amounts of protein and adequate kcalories is usually necessary. Ensure the patient is consuming adequate amounts of calcium, iron, vitamin C, and B-complex vitamins.[5]

HEALTH PROMOTION

ADDED FOOD FACTORS IN CORONARY HEART DISEASE THERAPY

The primary focus of NT for CHD is on control of lipid factors, including cholesterol and saturated fats. Two other food factors, however, play a different role. In varying ways they help to protect us from the development of CHD.[3]

Dietary Fiber

Studies indicate water-soluble types of dietary fiber have significant cholesterol-lowering effect. Soluble fiber includes gums, pectin, certain hemicelluloses, and the body's storage polysaccharide, glycogen. Foods rich in soluble fiber include oat bran and dried beans, with additional amounts in barley and fruits. Oat bran, for example, contains a primary water-soluble gum, β-glucan, which is a lipid-lowering agent. Soluble dietary fiber has the following properties:

- Delays gastric emptying
- Slows intestinal transit time
- Slows glucose absorption
- Is fermented in colon into short-chain fatty acids that may inhibit liver cholesterol synthesis and help clear LDL cholesterol

On the other hand, insoluble dietary fiber—cellulose, lignin, and many hemicelluloses—found in vegetables, wheat, and most other grains does not have these lipid-lowering effects. Thus an increased use of soluble fiber food sources, especially oat bran and legumes, would have beneficial effects.

KEY TERMS

dysphagia Difficulty in swallowing, commonly associated with obstructive or motor disorders of the esophagus.

intermittent claudication A symptomatic pattern of peripheral vascular disease (PVD), characterized by the absence of pain or discomfort in a limb, usually the legs, when at rest, which is followed by pain and weakness when walking, intensifying until walking becomes impossible, and then disappearing again after a rest period; seen in occlusive arterial disease.

hypoxemia Deficient oxygenation of the blood, resulting in hypoxia, reduced oxygen supply to tissue.

hypercapnia Excess carbon dioxide (CO_2) in the blood.

Omega-3 Fatty Acids

Studies indicate omega-3 fatty acids, eicosapentaenoic acid (EPA) and docosahexaenoic acid (DHA) (see Chapter 4), found mostly in seafood and marine oils, also have protective functions. They can do the following:

- Change pattern of plasma fatty acids to alter platelet activity and reduce platelet aggregation that causes blood clotting, thus lowering the risk of coronary thrombosis
- Decrease the synthesis of VLDL
- Increase antiinflammatory effects

It would seem, then, factors in foods such as oats, dried beans, and fatty fish would provide valuable lipid-lowering additions to our diets.

KEY TERMS

hyperlipoproteinemia Elevated level of lipoproteins in the blood.

TO SUM UP

CHD remains the leading cause of death in the United States. Atherosclerosis, its underlying pathologic process, involves the formation of plaque, a fatty substance that builds up along the interior surfaces of blood vessels, interfering with blood flow and damaging blood vessels. If this buildup becomes severe, then it cuts off blood supplies of oxygen and nutrients to tissue cells, which in turn begin to die. When this occurs in a coronary artery, the result is an MI, or heart attack. When it occurs in a brain vessel, the result is a CVA, or stroke.

Risk for atherosclerosis increases with amount and type of blood lipids (lipoproteins) available. The apolipoprotein portion of lipoproteins is an important genetically determined part of the disease process. Elevated serum LDL cholesterol level is a primary factor in atherosclerosis development.

Initial dietary recommendations for acute CVD (heart attack) include caloric restriction, soft-textured foods, and small, frequent meals to reduce the metabolic demands of digestion, absorption, and metabolism of foods and their nutrients. Maintenance of a lean body weight is important. Persons with chronic CHD (i.e., CHF) and those with essential hypertension benefit from weight management, exercise, and sodium restriction to overcome cardiac edema and to help control elevated blood pressure.

Current dietary recommendations to help prevent CHD involve maintaining a healthy weight; limiting fats to 25% to 30% of all kcalories, with the majority being unsaturated food forms; limiting sodium intake to 2 to 3 g/day; and increasing exercise.

Concerted efforts are needed to combat development of cardiac cachexia in progressive heart failure. In addition, atherosclerotic plaques may occur in the extremities, usually the legs, causing PVD and the pain of intermittent claudication when walking. Progressive respiratory failure interferes with normal exchange of blood gases, oxygen and CO_2, and results in COPD, for which changed ratios of the fuel macronutrients are sometimes indicated.

QUESTIONS FOR REVIEW

1. Which types of hyperlipoproteinemia occur most often? Identify lipids that are elevated in each case, as well as predisposing factors. Describe the types of diet recommended for each.
2. Identify four dietary recommendations that should be made for the person with a heart attack. Describe how each recommendation helps recovery.
3. What dietary changes can the average American make to reduce saturated fats and to substitute polyunsaturated fats?
4. What does the term *essential hypertension* mean? Why would weight management and sodium restriction contribute to its control?
5. Outline NT for cardiac cachexia, and discuss the rationale for each aspect of the feeding plan.
6. Discuss cause and treatment of PVD.
7. Outline NT for COPD, and discuss the rationale for the fuel macronutrient adjustments.

REFERENCES

1. Brashers VL: Alterations of cardiovascular function. In McCance KL, Huether SE, editors: *Pathophysiology: the biologic basis for disease in adults and children*, ed 3, St Louis, 2006, Mosby.
2. American Heart Association: *Heart disease and stroke statistics*, Dallas, Tex, 2009, American Heart Association. Retrieved May 16, 2009, from www.americanheart.org.
3. National Cholesterol Education Program (NCEP): *Third report of the NCEP Expert Panel on Detection, Evaluation, and Treatment of High Blood Cholesterol in Adults (Adult Treatment Panel III), full report*, Washington, DC, 2002, National Institutes of Health, National Heart, Lung, and Blood Institute. Retrieved May 14, 2009 from www.nhlbi.nih.gov/guidelines/cholesterol/atp3_rpt.htm.
4. Mozaffarian D, Katan MB, Ascherio A, et al: Trans fatty acids and cardiovascular disease, *N Engl J Med* 354(15):1601, 2006.
5. Mahan LK, Escott-Stump S, editors: *Krause's food & nutrition therapy*, ed 12, St Louis, 2008, Saunders.
6. Banasik JL: Alterations in cardiac function. In Copstead LC, Banasik JL, editors: *Pathophysiology*, ed 3, St Louis, 2005, Saunders.

7. Antman EM, Anbe DT, Armstrong PW, et al: ACC/AHA guidelines for the management of patients with ST-elevation myocardial infarction—executive summary: a report of the ACC/AHA Task Force on Practice Guidelines (Committee to Revise the 1999 Guidelines on the Management of Patients With Acute Myocardial Infarction), *Circulation* 110:588, 2004.
8. Banasik JL: Heart failure and dysrhythmias: common sequelae of cardiac diseases. In Copstead LC, Banasik JL, editors: *Pathophysiology*, ed 3, St Louis, 2005, Saunders.
9. National High Blood Pressure Program: *The seventh report of the Joint National Committee on Prevention, Detection, Evaluation, and Treatment of High Blood Pressure, National Institutes of Health, National Heart, Lung, and Blood Institutes*, NIH Pub No 04-5230, Washington, DC, 2004, U.S. Government Printing Office.
10. Sachs FN, Svetkey LP, Vollmer WM, et al: Effects on blood pressure of reduced dietary sodium and the Dietary Approaches to Stop Hypertension (DASH), *N Engl J Med* 344:3, 2001.
11. National Center for Health Statistics, Centers for Disease Control and Prevention: *Stroke/cerebrovascular disease*, Hyattsville, Md, 2009, Centers for Disease Control and Prevention. Retrieved May 18, 2009, from www.cdc.gov/nchs/fastats/stroke.htm.
12. American Heart Association: *Stroke statistics*, Dallas, Tex, 2005, American Heart Association. Retrieved August 8, 2009, from www.americanheart.org.
13. Schumann L: Restrictive pulmonary disorders. In Copstead LC, Banasik JL, editors: *Pathophysiology*, ed 3, St Louis, 2005, Saunders.

FURTHER RESOURCES

Websites of Interest

American Heart Association: www.americanheart.org. *[Information for health professionals and consumers regarding cardiovascular diseases and stroke.]*

Centers for Disease Control and Prevention: *Health Topic: Heart Disease.* http://www.cdc.gov/heartdisease/index.htm. *[This website provides credible and reliable health information for consumers, health professionals, policy makers, and the media.]*

MedlinePlus: *Heart Diseases.* www.nlm.nih.gov/medlineplus/heartdiseases.html. *[This is the National Institutes of Health web site for consumers. It is produced by the National Library of Medicine to provide reliable, up-to-date health information about diseases, conditions, and wellness issues.]*

Womenshealth.gov: *Heart Health and Stroke.* http://www.womenshealth.gov/heart-stroke/heart-disease-stroke-prevention/index.cfm. *[The Office of Women's Health is housed in the U.S. Department of Health and Human Services to promote health equity for women and girls through sex/gender-specific approaches.]*

World Health Organization (WHO): *Cardiovascular Diseases.* www.who.int/cardiovascular_diseases/en/. *[Part of the United Nations, WHO is responsible for providing leadership on global health matters.]*

22

Diabetes Mellitus

Sara Long Roth

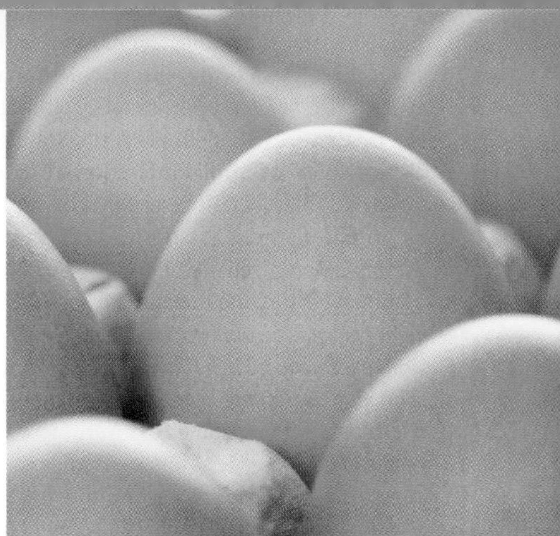

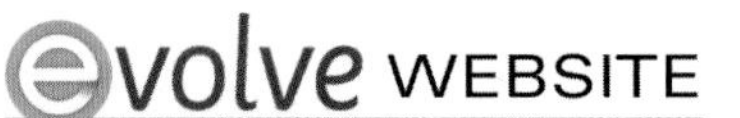

http://evolve.elsevier.com/Williams/essentials/

OUTLINE

In this chapter of our continuing clinical nutrition series, we look at the problem of diabetes. We seek to understand its nature and how it can be managed to maintain good health and avoid complications.

Diabetes is a serious, costly, and increasingly common chronic disease. In the United States, 23.6 million (7.8%) of the population have diabetes. An estimated 18 million Americans have diagnosed diabetes, and an additional 5.7 million have undiagnosed diabetes. Approximately 1.6 million new cases of diabetes are diagnosed each year.[1] Diabetes can be diagnosed on the basis of two fasting glucose readings of 126 mg/dL or higher or a random glucose level of 200 mg/dL or higher and symptoms such as polyuria, polydipsia, and unexplained weight loss.[2]

Although elevation of blood glucose level is the hallmark characteristic of diabetes, it is a group of metabolic disorders resulting from a defect in insulin secretion, insulin action, or both. These defects interfere with normal cellular uptake of glucose and use of glucose within cells. Restoring normal metabolic function is the goal in the early diagnosis and treatment of diabetes. Restoration of normal metabolism can prevent many of the short-term complications such as hyperglycemia and hypoglycemia and the longer-term microvascular, macrovascular, and neurologic complications that affect multiple body systems.

Direct and indirect health costs of diabetes are estimated to exceed $174 billion a year in the United States (or one out of every five health care dollars).[3] The death rate among middle-aged people with diabetes is double the death rate of those who do not have diabetes. Diabetes causes preventable complications that can be life threatening, including heart disease. Lifestyle changes can delay the progression of diabetes, as can controlling blood glucose, lipids, and blood pressure.

NATURE OF DIABETES

History

The metabolic disease we know today as diabetes mellitus has been with us for a long time. Ancient records describe its devastating effects as observed by early healers. In the first century ad, the Greek physician Aretaeus wrote of a malady in which the body "ate its own flesh" and gave off large quantities of urine. He gave it the name *diabetes,* from the Greek word meaning siphon or to pass through. Much later, in the seventeenth century, the word *mellitus,* from the Latin word for honey, was added because of the sweet nature of the urine. This addition also distinguished it from diabetes insipidus (*insipid,* meaning tasteless, or not sweet), another disorder, although uncommon, in which the passage of copious amounts of urine had been observed. Today, use of the single name diabetes always means diabetes mellitus.

As medical knowledge began to grow, early clinicians—such as Rollo in England and Bouchardat in France—observed that diabetes became less severe in overweight patients who lost weight. Later another French physician, Lancereaux, and his students described two kinds of diabetes: (1) diabète gras ("fat diabetes") and (2) diabète maigre ("thin diabetes").[4] All of these observations preceded any knowledge about insulin or any relation to the pancreas. During these times, which have aptly been called the *diabetic dark ages,* individuals with diabetes had short lives and were maintained on a variety of semistarvation diets.[5]

Later, evidence began to point to the pancreas as a primary organ involved in the disease process. Paul Langerhans (1847-1888), a young German medical student, found special clusters—or islets—of cells scattered throughout the human pancreas that were different from the rest of the tissue. Although their function was still unknown, these special islet cells were named for their young discoverer: the *islets of Langerhans.* Research at that time focused on the pancreas. Finally, in 1921 and 1922 a University of Toronto team discovered and successfully used the controlling agent from the "island cells," naming it *insulin* for its source.[6]

Classification

The American Diabetes Association classifies diabetes into the four categories[2]:

1. Type 1 diabetes (T1DM), formerly called insulin-dependent diabetes mellitus
2. Type 2 diabetes (T2DM), formerly called noninsulin-dependent diabetes mellitus
3. Gestational diabetes mellitus (GDM)
4. Impaired glucose tolerance (IGT) and impaired fasting glucose (IFG) (sometimes called prediabetes)

The terms *insulin-dependent diabetes mellitus* (IDDM) and *noninsulin-dependent diabetes mellitus* (NIDDM), should no longer be used because they are confusing and have often resulted in classifying patients based on treatment rather than cause of their diabetes.[2]

T1DM is characterized by sudden, severe insulin deficiency requiring insulin therapy to prevent ketoacidosis, coma, and death. T1DM generally appears during childhood or adolescence and accounts for 5% to 10% of the cases of diabetes. However, T1DM can occur at any age, and almost half of new cases are diagnosed after 20 years of age. Two forms of T1DM exist: (1) immune-mediated diabetes and (2) idiopathic diabetes. Immune-mediated diabetes results from a cellular-mediated autoimmune destruction of the beta cells of the pancreas.[7] Idiopathic diabetes has no known cause.

Onset of T1DM is often rapid, accompanied by classic symptoms of weight loss and increased urination and thirst, especially if a viral infection or other stress increases the need for insulin. Onset may be less acute, or a "honeymoon period" of 6 to 12 months may occur in which the diabetes may appear to be "cured" after an initial acute onset and initiation of insulin therapy. Destruction of the beta cells in the pancreas and loss of insulin production are usually gradual, accounting for the honeymoon period after insulin therapy restores normal glucose and metabolic stress is resolved.

T2DM is associated with insulin resistance and obesity combined with inadequate insulin produced in the pancreatic beta cells to compensate for the insulin resistance or an insulin secretory defect with insulin resistance.[2] T2DM accounts for 90% to 95% of all cases of diabetes, and symptoms may include poor wound healing, blurred vision, or recurrent gum or bladder infections. Many individuals are not symptomatic, and the diabetes may be detected as the result of a routine blood test. Obesity and physical inactivity are strong risk factors for T2DM.[8-10] A large waist circumference is considered to be a biomarker for insulin resistance and the metabolic syndrome associated with diabetes, hypertension, and dyslipidemia (typically low high-density cholesterol and elevated triglyceride levels).[11] Although T2DM is associated with insulin resistance and is typically diagnosed after 40 years of age, it is occurring in epidemic proportions in younger populations, including children and adolescents. Most children diagnosed with T2DM have a family history of T2DM, are overweight or obese, are insulin resistant, or have physical signs of insulin resistance such as acanthosis nigricans.[10] Undiagnosed, these young people may be at early risk for cardiovascular disease (CVD).[10] Current testing criteria and diabetes risk factors to help identify T2DM before the onset of complications has been developed by the American Academy of Pediatrics and the American Dietetic Association (ADA).[11]

GDM is defined as carbohydrate intolerance of variable severity with onset or first recognition during pregnancy. GDM develops in 2% to 5% of all pregnancies, and 30% to 40% of women with GDM are likely to develop T2DM.[12] In T2DM and GDM, a relative insulin deficiency exists because the pancreas fails to produce the level of insulin needed to compensate for insulin resistance.

If cross-sectional data were applied to the 2007 U.S. population, about 57 million adults (20 years or older) would have IFG, suggesting at least 57 million adults in the United States had prediabetes in 2007.[1] *Prediabetes* is a term used to distinguish people at increased risk of developing diabetes. People are considered to have prediabetes if they have IFG

KEY TERMS

diabetes insipidus A condition of the pituitary gland and insufficiency of one of its hormones, vasopressin (antidiuretic hormone); characterized by a copious output of a nonsweet urine, great thirst, and sometimes a large appetite. However, in diabetes insipidus these symptoms result from a specific injury to the pituitary gland, not a collection of metabolic disorders as in diabetes mellitus. The injured pituitary gland produces less vasopressin, a hormone that normally helps the kidneys reabsorb adequate water.

insulin Hormone formed in the beta cells of the islets of Langerhans in the pancreas. It is secreted when blood glucose and amino acid levels rise and assists their entry into body cells. It also promotes glycogenesis and conversion of glucose into fat and inhibits lipolysis and gluconeogenesis (protein breakdown). Commercial insulin is manufactured from pigs and cows; new "artificial" human insulin products have recently been made available.

or IGT; some people have both conditions.[1] IFG is identified through fasting blood glucose, and IGT is identified by an oral glucose tolerance test (OGTT).[11] Formerly called *borderline diabetes,* IFG, IGT, and prediabetes are associated with metabolic syndrome that includes abdominal obesity, dyslipidemia (high triglycerides, low high-density lipoprotein (HDL) cholesterol, or both), and hypertension.[1] Research has shown lifestyle interventions can reduce the rate of progression to T2DM.[13,14] Table 22-1 outlines criteria used to diagnose diabetes.

TABLE 22-1 CRITERIA FOR DIAGNOSING DIABETES

DIABETES TYPE	FORMER TERMS	ETIOLOGY	CRITERIA
Type 1 diabetes (T1DM)*: immune-mediated or idiopathic	Insulin-dependent diabetes mellitus (IDDM), type I diabetes, juvenile-onset diabetes, ketosis-prone diabetes, brittle diabetes	Beta cell destruction, usually leading to absolute insulin deficiency	Symptoms† of diabetes mellitus and casual plasma glucose ≤200 mg/dL (*Casual* is defined as any time of day without regard to last meal.)
			or
Type 2 diabetes (T2DM) (adults)	Noninsulin-dependent diabetes mellitus (NIDDM), type II diabetes, adult-onset diabetes, maturity-onset diabetes, ketosis-resistant diabetes, stable diabetes	Insulin resistance with insulin secretory defect	Fasting plasma glucose (FPG) ≤126 mg/dL (*Fasting* is defined as no kcalorie intake for at least 8 hr.)
			or
			2-hr postprandial plasma glucose (PPG) ≤200 mg/dL during oral glucose tolerance test (OGTT) (performed as described by the World Health Organization [WHO] using glucose load containing the equivalent of 75 g anhydrous glucose dissolved in water)
T2DM (children)			Overweight (body mass index [BMI] >85th percentile for age and gender, weight for height >85th percentile, or weight >120% of ideal for height)
			plus
			Any two of the following: • Family history of T2DM in first- or second-degree relative • Native American, African American, Latino, Asian American, Pacific Islander • Signs of insulin resistance or conditions associated with insulin resistance (acanthosis nigricans, hypertension, dyslipidemia, or polycystic ovary syndrome [PCOS])
Gestational diabetes (GDM)			*One-step approach:* diagnostic OGTT *Two-step approach:* initial screening to measure plasma or serum glucose concentration 1 hr after 50 g oral glucose load (glucose challenge test [GCT]) and perform diagnostic OGTT on those women exceeding glucose threshold value on GCT (glucose threshold >140 mg/dL identifies >80% of women with GDM)
Impaired glucose tolerance (IGT)	Borderline diabetes, chemical diabetes		2-hr PPG >140 mg/dL and <200 mg/dL

Modified from American Diabetes Association: Standards of medical care in diabetes—2008. *Diabetes Care* 31(suppl 1):S12, 2008, with permission from The American Diabetes Association.

*Patients with any form of diabetes may require insulin treatment at some stage of their disease. Such use of insulin does not classify the patient as having T1DM.

†Symptoms include polyuria, polydipsia, and unexplained weight loss.

Contributing Causes

Genetics

For some time, early insulin assay tests developed to measure level of insulin activity in blood found insulin-like activity in diabetes to be two or three times normal insulin levels. It is now evident that diabetes is a syndrome with multiple forms, resulting from (1) lack of insulin or (2) insulin resistance (or from both).[2]

Diabetes has long been associated with body weight, since the early observations of differences in "fat diabetes" and "thin diabetes."[4] Current research has reinforced the relation of overweight state to development of T2DM. Obesity can increase circulating insulin levels, which will ultimately lead to increased insulin resistance. In addition, individuals with a family history may have mutations on genes that control insulin production or may inherit insulin resistance not directly related to obesity. Thus multiple genetic mutations may interact to increase the risk of T2DM.

Environmental Role: "Thrifty Gene"

Environmental factors apparently play a role in unmasking the underlying genetic susceptibility—a "thrifty" diabetic genotype that probably developed during primitive times. This theory indicates diabetes may be associated with past genetic modifications for survival during varying periods of food availability. Gene mutations and the thrifty trait associated with T2DM facilitated more efficient use of limited food during times of difficult survival conditions. As food supplies became more plentiful, negative aspects of the thrifty trait began to appear. Such is indeed the case, for example, with the experience of Pima Indians in Arizona, as earlier studies and recent archaeological excavations have indicated.[15] In earlier times this group ate a limited diet mainly of carbohydrate foods harvested through heavy physical labor in a primitive agricultural climate. Now, however, with the "progress" of civilization, Pimas have become obese, and half of the adults have T2DM (the highest reported rate of this type of diabetes in the world). Native Americans develop diabetes at almost three times the rate of Caucasians. This same pattern is seen among populations of now-urbanized Pacific Islanders, South Asians, Asian Indians, and Creoles, although less is known about the exact numbers.[8,9] Other at-risk populations include Hispanic and Latino Americans, who are 1.5 times as likely to develop diabetes as Caucasians, and African Americans, who develop diabetes at 1.6 times the rate of Caucasians.[1] Thus evidence suggests that these groups have a genetic susceptibility to T2DM (diabetic genotype) and that the disease is triggered by environmental factors, including obesity (see the *Focus on Culture* box, "Type 2 Diabetes: An Equal Opportunity Disease?"). Several specific genes involved in energy metabolism are thought to increase the risk for developing obesity, T2DM, or both. As we commonly observe, lifestyle (dietary and physical activity habits) can interact with genetics in the development of T2DM.

Symptoms

Symptoms of T1DM in its uncontrolled state include the following:

- Increased thirst (polydipsia)
- Increased urination (polyuria)
- Increased hunger (polyphagia)
- Weight loss (more common with T1DM)
- Fruity smell to breath (symptom of ketoacidosis)
- Fatigue or weakness

These symptoms occur because in an insulin-deficient state, blood glucose levels and renal filtration of glucose are increased beyond the kidney's threshold for reabsorption; as the level of glucose excreted increases, urine volume increases. Without adequate glucose use, fat mobilization increases, and an increased breakdown of fat leads to excess ketone formation.

T2DM may be asymptomatic, or symptoms may be more subtle and may include the following:

- Poor wound healing or recurrent infections
- Blurred vision (result of effects of hyperglycemia on shape of the cornea, which is returned to normal after glucose levels are stabilized)
- Skin irritation or infection
- Recurrent gum or bladder infections

Classic symptoms of diabetes are the result of short-term effects of hyperglycemia. These symptoms are reversible if blood glucose levels are returned to a normal or near-normal level.

Metabolic Pattern of Diabetes

Overall Energy Balance and Energy Nutrients

Because initial symptoms of glycosuria and hyperglycemia are related to excess glucose, historically diabetes was called a *disease of carbohydrate metabolism.* However, as more becomes known about the intimate interrelationships of carbohydrate, fat, and protein metabolism, we view it in more general terms. It is a metabolic disorder resulting from lack of insulin (absolute, partial, or unavailable) affecting more or less each basic energy nutrient. It is especially related to metabolism of the two fuels—(1) carbohydrate and (2) fat—in the body's overall energy system.

Normal Blood Glucose Control

Control of blood glucose level within its normal range of 70 to 120 mg/dL (3.9 to 6.7 mmol/L) is vital to normal overall fuel metabolism and other metabolic functions. A knowledge of factors involved in maintaining a normal blood glucose level is essential to understanding the impairment of these factors (see Chapters 3 and 4). An overview of these normal balancing controls is illustrated in Figure 22-1.

Sources of Blood Glucose

Two sources of blood glucose ensure a constant supply of this primary body fuel: (1) diet, energy nutrients in our food

FOCUS ON CULTURE

Type 2 Diabetes: An Equal Opportunity Disease?

Type 2 diabetes (T2DM) occurs disproportionately in people of color throughout the United States. Rates of T2DM are two to six times higher in Native Americans, Alaska Natives, African Americans, and Hispanic Americans than in the non-Hispanic Caucasian population. In addition, people of color experience onset at an earlier age, and their complications are more harsh. Although the cause for these ethnic disparities has not been identified, it is hypothesized that the differences may lie in the interaction of inherent susceptibility and modifiable risk factors such as physical inactivity and poor diet.

ETHNIC GROUP	PREVALENCE (AGES 20+)	ADDITIONAL INFORMATION
Non-Hispanic Caucasians	6.6%	
Native Americans	16.5% of the population: 6.0% among Alaska Natives, 29.3% among Native Americans	Diagnosis 2.2 times more likely than Caucasians Pima tribe has highest rate of diabetes in the world: 50% Complications of diabetes are major causes of death and health problems in most Native American populations
African Americans	11.8%	Diagnosis 1.6 times more likely; 25% between ages 65 and 74 have diabetes, 1 in 4 women older than age 55 has diabetes
Latinos/Hispanics	10.4%	Diagnosis 1.5 times more likely Approximately 11.9% of Mexican Americans have diabetes Approximately 12.6% of Puerto Rican Americans have diabetes Approximately 8.2% of Cuban Americans have diabetes

BIBLIOGRAPHY

Brown TL: Ethnic populations. In Ross TA, Boucher JL, O'Connell BS, editors: *American Dietetic Association guide to diabetes medical nutrition therapy and education*, Chicago, 2005, American Dietetic Association.

Centers for Disease Control and Prevention: *National diabetes fact sheet: general information and national estimates on diabetes in the United States, 2007*, Atlanta, 2008, U.S. Department of Health and Human Services, Centers for Disease Control and Prevention. Retrieved July 13, 2010, from www.cdc.gov/diabetes/pubs/pdf/ndfs_2007.pdf.

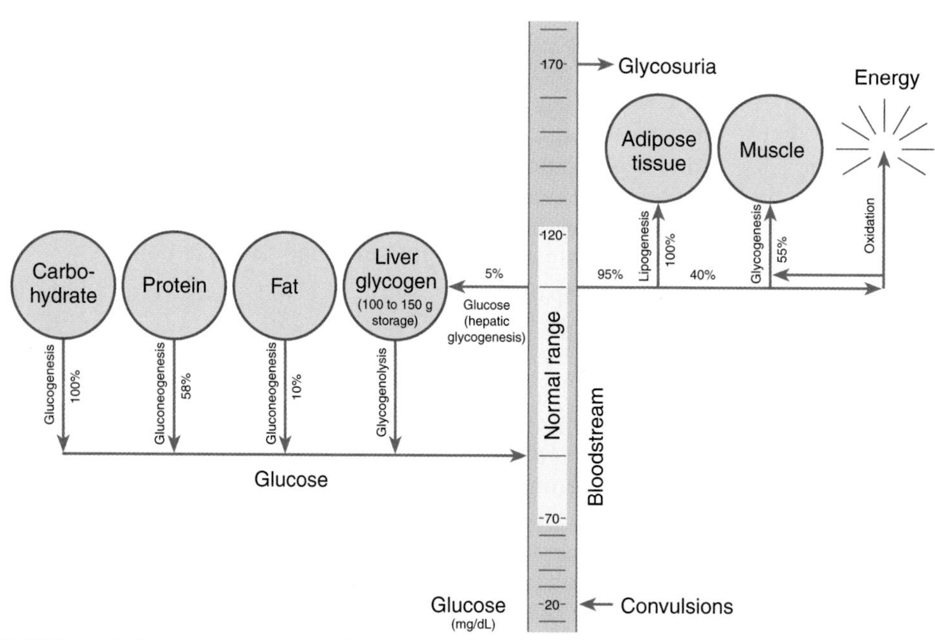

FIGURE 22-1 Sources of blood glucose (food and stored glycogen) and normal routes of control.

(i.e., dietary carbohydrate, protein, fat), and (2) glycogen, the backup source from constant turnover of "stored" liver glycogen by a process called glycogenolysis.

Uses of Blood Glucose

To prevent continued rise of blood glucose beyond normal limits, several basic uses for blood glucose are constantly available according to need. These include the following: (1) glycogenesis, conversion of glucose to glycogen for storage in liver and muscle; (2) lipogenesis, conversion of glucose to fat and storage in adipose tissue; and (3) glycolysis, cell oxidation of glucose for energy.

Pancreatic Hormonal Controls

The following three types of islet cells scattered in clusters throughout the pancreas (islets of Langerhans) provide hormones closely interbalanced in the regulation of blood glucose levels.

1. *Alpha cells:* Arranged around the outer rim of the islets are alpha cells, one to two cells thick, making up about 30% of the total cells. These cells synthesize glucagon.
2. *Beta cells:* The largest portion of islets is occupied by beta cells filling the central zone or about 60% of the gland. These primary cells synthesize insulin.
3. *Delta cells:* Interspersed between alpha and beta cells—or occasionally between alpha cells alone—are delta cells, the remaining 10% of total cells. These cells synthesize somatostatin.

This specific arrangement of human islet cells is illustrated in Figure 22-2.

Interrelated Hormone Functions

Juncture points of the three types of islet cells act as sensors of blood glucose concentration and its rate of change. They constantly adjust and balance the rate of secretion of insulin, glucagon, and somatostatin to match whatever conditions prevail at any time. Each of the following three hormones has specific interbalanced functions:

1. *Insulin:* Although precise mechanisms are not entirely clear in every case, insulin has a profound effect on glucose control. It functions extensively in the metabolism of all three energy nutrients, as follows:
   - Insulin facilitates transport of glucose through cell membranes by way of special insulin receptors. These receptors are located on the membrane of insulin-sensitive cells, including those in adipose tissue, muscle tissue, and monocytes. These insulin receptors mediate all metabolic effects of insulin. Research has shown that cells of obese persons with diabetes have fewer than the normal number of insulin receptors. Weight loss in obese individuals and physical exercise increase the number of these receptors. The insulin receptor also appears to control several metabolic steps within the cell.
   - Insulin enhances conversion of glucose to glycogen and its consequent storage in the liver (glycogenesis). Insulin also, then, inhibits the breakdown of glycogen to glucose and its release into the body.
   - Insulin stimulates conversion of glucose to fat (lipogenesis) for storage as adipose tissue.
   - Insulin inhibits fat breakdown (lipolysis) and the breakdown of protein.
   - Insulin promotes uptake of amino acids by skeletal muscles, thus increasing protein synthesis.
   - Insulin influences glucose oxidation through the main glycolytic pathway.
2. *Glucagon:* The hormone glucagon functions as a balancing antagonist to insulin. It rapidly causes breakdown of liver glycogen, and—to a lesser extent—fatty acids from adipose tissue to serve as body fuel. This action raises blood glucose levels to protect the brain and other body tissues. It helps maintain normal blood glucose levels during fasting hours of sleep. A lowering of the blood glucose concentration, increased amino acid concentrations, or sympathetic nervous system stimulation triggers glucagon secretion.
3. *Somatostatin:* Although pancreatic islet delta cells are the major source off somatostatin, this hormone is also

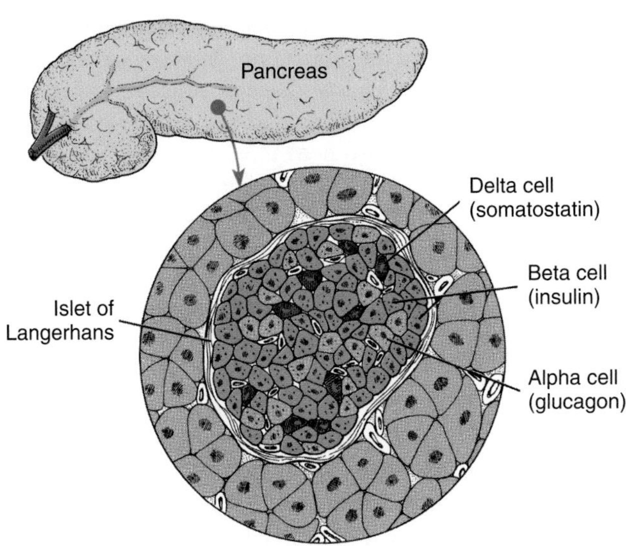

FIGURE 22-2 Islets of Langerhans, located in the pancreas.

KEY TERMS

glycogenolysis Production of blood glucose from liver glycogen.

glycogenesis Synthesis of glycogen from blood glucose.

lipogenesis Synthesis of fat from blood glucose.

glycolysis Cell oxidation of glucose for energy.

glucagon A polypeptide hormone secreted by the alpha cells of the pancreatic islets of Langerhans in response to hypoglycemia; has an opposite balancing effect to that of insulin, raising the blood sugar, and thus is used as a quick-acting antidote for the hypoglycemic reaction of insulin. It stimulates the breakdown of glycogen (glycogenolysis) in the liver by activating the liver enzyme phosphorylase and thus raises blood sugar levels during fasting states to ensure adequate levels for normal nerve and brain function.

somatostatin A hormone formed in the delta cells of the pancreatic islets of Langerhans and the hypothalamus. It is a balancing factor in maintaining normal blood glucose levels by inhibiting insulin and glucagon production in the pancreas as needed.

synthesized and secreted in different regions of the body, including the hypothalamus. It acts in balance with insulin and glucose to inhibit their interactions as needed to maintain normal blood glucose levels. It also helps regulate blood glucose levels by inhibiting the release of a number of other hormones as needed.

Metabolic Changes in Diabetes

In uncontrolled diabetes, insulin is lacking to facilitate operation of normal blood glucose controls; abnormal metabolic changes occur, as follows, that affect glucose, fat, and protein and account for symptoms of diabetes:

- *Glucose:* Blood glucose cannot be oxidized properly through the main glycolytic pathway in the cell to furnish energy (see Chapter 8), and a lack of insulin allows the breakdown of hepatic glycogen and the release of glucose; therefore glucose builds up in the blood (hyperglycemia).
- *Fat:* Formation of fat (lipogenesis) is curtailed, and fat breakdown (lipolysis) increases. This leads to excess formation and accumulation of ketones (ketoacidosis). Appearance of the major ketone, acetone, in urine indicates development of ketoacidosis.
- *Protein:* Tissue protein is also broken down in an effort to secure energy. This causes weight loss and nitrogen excretion in the urine.

GENERAL MANAGEMENT OF DIABETES

Treatment Goals: Basic Objectives

The diabetes care team—the physician, dietitian, nurse, and person with diabetes—are guided by the following three basic objectives:

1. *Maintain optimal nutrition:* The first objective is to fulfill the basic nutritional requirement for health, growth and development, and a desirable body weight.
2. *Prevent hypoglycemia or hyperglycemia:* This second objective is designed to keep the person relatively free of hypoglycemia or insulin reaction, which requires immediate countermeasures, and hyperglycemia, which, if untreated, contributes to more serious ketoacidosis or diabetic coma.
3. *Prevent complications:* The third objective recognizes the increased risk a person with diabetes faces for developing complicating problems that reflect the damaging effects of chronic diabetes on tissues of small and large blood vessels and peripheral nerves. These damages may occur in tissues such as eyes (retinopathy), nerves (neuropathy), and kidneys (nephropathy). In addition, coronary artery disease occurs in persons with diabetes about four times as often as in the general population. Peripheral vascular disease (PVD) occurs about 40 times as often.

In all of these areas, evidence indicates that consistent, well-planned food habits and exercise, balanced as needed with early aggressive insulin therapy, can significantly help normalize metabolism and thereby reduce risks of these potentially serious complications.[16]

This aggressive insulin therapy consists of multiple daily injections or continuous subcutaneous infusion by an insulin pump (Figure 22-3). Self-monitoring of blood glucose (SMBG) levels is used to guide decisions to improve glycemic control. The added cardiovascular risk associated with diabetes is reflected in having blood pressure and lipid goals for diabetes management that are similar to those used in treating individuals who have diagnosed CVD (Table 22-2).

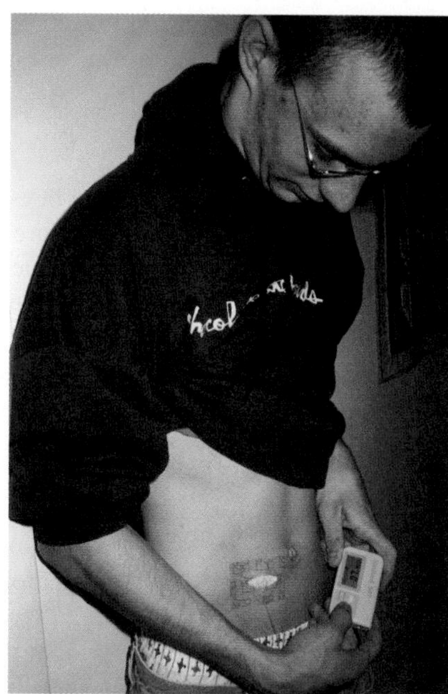

FIGURE 22-3 Insulin injecting using an insulin pump. (From Peckenpaugh NJ: *Nutrition essentials and diet therapy,* ed 11, St Louis, 2010, Saunders.)

Self-Care Role of the Person with Diabetes

To effectively control diabetes, the person with diabetes must play a central role. Daily self-discipline and informed self-care, supported by a skilled and sensitive health care team, are required for sound diabetes management. Ultimately, all persons with diabetes must treat themselves. This is especially true with the stricter normal blood glucose control currently being used, with frequent SMBG and multiple insulin injections or an insulin infusion pump. Thus even greater need now exists for comprehensive diabetes education programs that encourage self-monitoring and self-care responsibility. Diabetes-related issues also need to be addressed as an integral component of primary care. Weight, activity, variety, and excess are themes that are relevant for assessing basic needs and providing basic recommendations.

RATIONALE FOR DIABETES NUTRITION THERAPY

Nutrition therapy (NT) for diabetes is multifaceted. Physicians and nurses can no longer rely on preprinted diet sheets to assume they are providing nutrition care for patients.[17] No standard American Diabetes Association or diabetic diet exists. The American Diabetes Association does not sanction any single meal plan or specific percentages

TABLE 22-2 METABOLIC GOALS IN DIABETES MANAGEMENT

INDICATOR	NORMAL VALUE	GOAL	ADDITIONAL ACTION SUGGESTED*
Plasma values (mg/dL)			
Average preprandial glucose	<110	90-130	>90/<150
Average bedtime glucose	<120	110-150	>110/<180
Whole blood values† (mg/dL)			
Average preprandial glucose	<100	80-120	>80/<140
Average bedtime glucose	<110	100-140	>100/<160
Hemoglobin A_{1c} (HbA_{1c}) (%)	<6	<7	<8
Low-density lipoprotein (LDL) cholesterol		<100 mg/dL	
High-density lipoprotein (HDL) cholesterol		*Men:* >55 mg/dL	
		Women: >55 mg/dL	
Triglycerides		<150 mg/dL	
Blood pressure		<130/80 mm Hg	

Modified from American Diabetes Association: Standards of medical care in diabetes—2008, *Diabetes Care* 31(suppl 1):S12, 2008, with permission from The American Diabetes Association.
*Depends on individual patient circumstances.
†Measurement of capillary blood glucose.

of nutrients.[18] It is essential that persons with diabetes are assessed by a registered dietitian (RD) to determine an appropriate nutrition prescription and plan for self-management education.[11] In addition, diet orders such as *no sugar added, no concentrated sweets, low sugar, and liberal diabetic* are not considered suitable because they do not reflect diabetes nutritional recommendations and pointlessly restrict sucrose. Such meal plans support the erroneous concept that simply limiting sucrose-sweetened foods will enhance blood glucose control.[18]

NT should be individualized, taking usual eating habits and other lifestyle factors into consideration.[19] Consistency within an eating pattern will result in better glycemic control than abiding by an arbitrary eating style. Nutrition recommendations are the same for individuals with diabetes as for the general population in regard to total fat, saturated fat, cholesterol, fiber, vitamins, and minerals. Recommendations for protein, carbohydrates, sucrose, and alcohol are modified, depending on the nature of diabetes in relation to carbohydrate metabolism or effects of complications.[17]

Type 1 Diabetes Mellitus

Recognizing the need for a more comprehensive program of care of diabetes, based on the individual metabolic balance concept and designed to help delay or avoid life-threatening complications of this chronic disease, a national U.S. clinical research study supported by the National Institutes of Health was organized. The Diabetes Control and Complications Trial (DCCT)[16] involved 1441 subjects in 29 clinical centers across the country for approximately 10 years. The study was designed to compare the effects of intensive insulin therapy aimed at achieving blood glucose levels as close as possible to the normal nondiabetic range with effects of conventional therapy on early microvascular complications of T1DM. The DCCT demonstrated that lowering hemoglobin A_{1c} (HbA_{1c}) from 9% to 7% in the intensively treated group reduced the risk of the development or progression of eye, kidney, and neurologic complications by 50% to 75%.[11,20] Dietary strategies played an important role in achieving control in the intensively treated group.[21] Reduction in complications was linearly related to improvement in glycemic control, indicating risk reduction can be achieved even if intensification of treatment fails to achieve a near-normal HbA_{1c}.[17,22] Adverse effects of intensive therapy included a twofold to threefold increase in severe hypoglycemia and a weight gain of 10 lb (4.5 kg).[16] Initial weight was considerably higher, but providing consultation about overeating to prevent or treat hypoglycemia appears to attenuate the weight gain.

KEY TERMS

retinopathy Noninflammatory disease of the retina—the visual tissue of the eye—characterized by microaneurysms, intraretinal hemorrhages, waxy yellow exudates, "cotton wool" patches, and macular edema; a complication of diabetes that may lead to proliferation of fibrous tissue, retinal detachment, and blindness.

neuropathy General term for functional and pathologic changes in the peripheral nervous system; in diabetes, a chronic sensory condition affecting mainly the nerves of the legs, marked by numbness from sensory impairment, loss of tendon reflexes, severe pain, weakness, and wasting of muscles involved.

nephropathy Disease of the kidneys; in diabetes, renal damage associated with functional and pathologic changes in the nephrons, which can lead to glomerulosclerosis and chronic renal failure.

Type 2 Diabetes Mellitus

The United Kingdom Prospective Diabetes Study (UKPDS) evaluated effects of treatments to improve glycemic control and cardiovascular risk factors in individuals with newly diagnosed diabetes. Glycemic control and cardiovascular risk reduction therapies reduced rates of macrovascular and microvascular complications. The UKPDS confirmed DCCT findings with respect to preventing microvascular complications of diabetes and provided evidence that a comprehensive risk reduction approach could also reduce macrovascular complications.[23–26] The major cause of morbidity and mortality in persons with diabetes is CVD. T2DM and its common coexisting conditions (e.g., hypertension, dyslipidemia) are considered to be independent risk factors for macrovascular disease.[11]

Gestational Diabetes Mellitus

For women with preexisting diabetes or GDM, risks of fetal abnormalities and mortality are increased in the presence of hyperglycemia. Maternal insulin does not cross the placenta, but glucose does, causing the fetus's pancreas to increase insulin production if the mother becomes hyperglycemic. This increased production of insulin causes macrosomia—the most typical characteristic of babies born to women with diabetes. Other problems such as hyperinsulinemia and hyperglycemia may occur.[27] Therefore every effort should be made to control blood glucose levels.[11] All women with GDM should receive counseling by a RD when possible.[28] Individualized MNT, contingent on maternal weight and height, should include provision of adequate kilocalories (kcalories or kcal) and nutrients to meet the needs of the pregnancy and be consistent with established maternal blood glucose goals.[28] At the start, SMBG should be planned four times a day (fasting and 1 or 2 hours postprandial). Frequency can be decreased once glycemic control is established. Blood glucose goals during pregnancy are as follows[28]:

- *Fasting:* ≤105 mg/dL
- *1 Hour postprandial:* ≤155 mg/dL
- *2 Hours postprandial:* ≤130 mg/dL

IMPLEMENTING NUTRITION THERAPY

Nutrition intervention is governed by consideration of treatment goals and lifestyle changes the person with diabetes is ready to make, preferably to predetermined energy levels and percentages of carbohydrates, protein, and fat. The objective of NT is to support and facilitate individual lifestyle and behavior changes that will lead to improved glycemic control. Cultural and ethnic preferences should be taken into consideration, and persons with diabetes should be included in the decision-making process.[17]

Current nutrition principles and recommendations focus on lifestyle goals and strategies for treatment of diabetes. For the first time, the 2002 evidence-based nutrition recommendations purposely address lifestyle approaches to diabetes prevention, because MNT for treating and managing diabetes may not necessarily be the same for preventing or delaying onset of diabetes.[17] Goals of NT that apply to all persons with diabetes are as follows[17]:

- Attain and maintain optimal metabolic outcomes, including the following:
  - Blood glucose levels in the normal (or near-normal) range
  - Lipid and lipoprotein profiles that reduce risk for macrovascular diseases
  - Blood pressure levels that reduce risk for vascular disease
- Prevent and treat chronic complications.
- Improve health through healthy food choices and physical activity.
- Address individual nutritional needs, taking into consideration personal and cultural preferences and lifestyle while respecting individuals' wishes and willingness to change.

Additional, more specific medical nutrition goals include the following[17]:

- *Youth with T1DM:* NT goals for children and adolescents with T1DM should ensure provision of sufficient energy for normal growth and development. Insulin regimens should be integrated into usual eating and physical activity habits.
- *T2DM in children and adolescents:* Goals for NT for children and adolescents with T2DM should facilitate changes in eating and physical activity habits to decrease insulin resistance and enhance metabolic status.
- *Pregnant and lactating women:* NT goals for pregnant and lactating women should provide adequate energy and nutrients necessary for optimal pregnancy outcomes.
- *Older adults:* Nutritional and psychosocial needs of an aging individual should be provided in NT goals.
- *Individuals treated with insulin or insulin secretagogues:* Self-management education for treatment and prevention of hypoglycemia, acute illness, and exercise-related blood glucose problems should be included in MNT goals for individuals treated with insulin or insulin secretagogues.
- *Individuals at risk for diabetes:* For those at risk for developing diabetes, physical activity should be encouraged and food choices that facilitate moderate weight loss (or at least prevent weight gain) should be promoted.

In addition, any medications a person has been prescribed should be considered as well; certain foods and drinks may interfere with them (see the *Diet-Medications Interactions* box, "Interactions with Diabetes Drugs").

ISSUES RELATED TO MEDICAL THERAPY

Blood Glucose Control

Insulin Therapy

The management goal for persons with T1DM is to maintain a normal blood glucose level as closely as possible. Strong evidence from the DCCT, as well as accumulating practice experience, indicates that maintaining such

KEY TERMS
macrosomia Unusually large size.

DIET-MEDICATIONS INTERACTIONS

Interactions with Diabetes Drugs

DRUG CLASS	DRUG NAMES	INTERACTIONS/INSTRUCTIONS
α-Glucosidase inhibitor agents	Acarbose: Precose Miglitol: Glyset	Take with first bite of main meal Limit alcohol
Biguanide agents	Metformin: Glucophage Metformin and glibenclamide: Glucovance, Glucophage, Glyburide	Take with meals to decrease GI distress May cause anorexia Avoid alcohol
DPP-4 inhibitors	Sitagliptin: Januvia Saxagliptin: Onglyza	Does not cause hypoglycemia when used as a single agent Increases insulin release after meals; lowers glucagon release
Insulin and related agents	Insulin mixtures, intermediate acting, long acting, rapid acting, short acting	May increase weight Should use alcohol with caution and under advice from physician (alcohol increases hypoglycemic effect of insulin) Large weight gain increases insulin needs
Meglitinide agents (nonsulfonylurea insulin releasers)	Nateglinide: Starlix Repaglinide: Prandin	Take 15-30 minutes before meals May increase weight Tooth disorders Nausea/vomiting Diarrhea/constipation Limit alcohol May increase risk of hypoglycemia in malnutrition
Sulfonylurea agents	Acetohexamide: Dymelor Tolazamide: Tolinase Tolbutamide: Orinase Chlorpropamide: Diabinese	Take with first meal of the day Nausea Avoid alcohol Increased risk of hypoglycemia in geriatric or malnourished patients
Sulfonylurea agents—second generation	Glimepiride: Amaryl Glyburide: DiaBeta, Micronase, Glynase PresTabs	Take 30 minutes before first meal of the day Hyperglycemia with high doses of nicotinic acid May increase or decrease appetite Increased weight Dyspepsia, nausea Constipation/diarrhea Avoid alcohol Possible hypoglycemia in geriatric or malnourished patients
Thiazolidinedione agents	Pioglitazone: Actos Rosiglitazone: Avandia	Take once a day without regard to food Increased weight
Pramlintide agent	Symlin	Used with insulin, an increased risk of insulin-induced severe hypoglycemia, particularly in patients with T1DM; seen usually within 3 hours of injection
Exenatide	Byetta	Hypoglycemia can occur when combined with sulfonylureas, or Byetta combined with metformin and a sulfonylurea

BIBLIOGRAPHY

American Diabetes Association: Living with Diabetes: What are my options? Alexandria, Va, American Diabetes Association. Retrieved July 13, 2010, from http://www.diabetes.org/living-with-diabetes/treatment-and-care/medication/oral-medications/what-are-my-options.html.

Pronsky ZM: *Food medication interactions*, ed 16, Birchrunville, Penn, 2010, Food-Medication Interactions.

Drugs A-Z: *Rancho*, Santa Fe, Calif, 2005, RxList. Retrieved May 24, 2009, from www.rxlist.com.

GI, Gastrointestinal; *T1DM*, type 1 diabetes.

a "normoglycemic" state helps prevent the chronic complications of long-term uncontrolled hyperglycemia.[29] To achieve this goal, more intensive insulin therapy with the different types of insulin now available is being used. Insulin is increasingly being used as adjunctive therapy in T2DM.

Types of Insulin. A number of insulin preparations are available for therapeutic use, and new ones are constantly being developed to meet medical care needs for individual patients and market changes. Individual responses to these insulins are highly variable. According to time of action, they are as follows:

1. *Rapid-acting insulins:* These insulins have various names, depending on the manufacturer (e.g., Humulin R, Semilente, Velosulin R). Rapid-acting insulins have their onset of action within approximately ½ hour after injection and stay in the body for less than 5 hours. This type of insulin peaks about 2 hours after injection. Human insulin analogue, Humalog (generic name, insulin lispro), has the shortest time-action curve of any insulin currently available. Short-acting insulins have their onset of action in ½ to 1 hour and have a 6- to 8-hour duration. Short-acting insulins peak around 3 hours. A number of variables influence absorption rate, such as site of injection, physical activity, skin temperature, and any circulating antiinsulin antibodies. Effect on blood glucose can be detected in about 1 hour, peaks at 4 to 6 hours, and lasts about 12 to 16 hours.
2. *Intermediate-acting insulins:* These insulins include Humulin L, Lente, NPH, Insulatard N, and Insulatard. Effect is detected in about 2 hours, peaks at about 11 hours, and lasts about 20 to 29 hours.
3. *Long-acting insulins:* These insulins include Humulin U. Its duration is somewhat longer than that of intermediate-acting insulins. It can be difficult to use because basal insulin is difficult to predict or control when the insulin peaks. Insulin glargine rDNA, which was first released in 2001, is a recombinant deoxyribonucleic acid (rDNA) insulin analogue specifically formulated to provide a long, flat response. However, insulin glargine rDNA (trade name, Lantus) cannot be mixed with other insulins, and two injections are needed to combine the action with a short-acting insulin. It is a long-acting insulin that works slowly during 24 hours and may not be used in combination with another type of insulin or an oral hypoglycemic medication to keep blood glucose regulated. Treatment algorithms are developed to adjust insulin on the basis of lifestyle and SMBG.

The process of intensifying T1DM management occurs in several stages. The initial dose of insulin is usually calculated based on current body weight with 0.5 to 0.6 unit of insulin/kg/day, with approximately half being for basal needs and half being as boluses for meals. During this initial phase a consistent carbohydrate intake is needed to identify a blood glucose pattern. Next, the client can move on to more complex planning using monitoring results to achieve better glycemic control and a more flexible lifestyle. Bolus requirement varies widely, but the initial dose is often estimated to provide 1 unit of short-acting insulin per 15 g of carbohydrate. Gradually the client learns to adjust insulin for changes in food or activity using a ratio of carbohydrate intake to insulin dose. A similar approach is used for insulin therapy in other forms of diabetes. In the treatment of T2DM, insulin may be used alone or in conjunction with an oral agent.

Insulin and Exercise Balance. Exercise benefits all persons with diabetes through its action in increasing the number of insulin receptors on muscle cells, thus increasing insulin efficiency. However, physical activity must be regular to be effective. A detailed history of personal activity and exercise habits provides information that is needed to help a client plan a wise program of regular moderate exercise. Guidelines for extra food to cover periods of heavier exercise, athletic practice, or competition can be included (Table 22-3).

Insulin Delivery Systems. Intensive insulin therapy for maintaining more normal blood glucose control requires multiple injections of rapid-acting insulin, alone or in combination with basal intermediate-acting insulin. This is accomplished either by regular injection with disposal syringes or with an insulin pump. The pump is not for everyone, but for many it has made life easier to use an insulin pump to achieve a basal insulin infusion and bolus insulin for meals. It is a small device that is easily worn on the belt with a subcutaneous needle in the abdomen and buttons the wearer pushes to obtain a fixed programmed flow of insulin

TABLE 22-3 MEAL-PLANNING GUIDE FOR ACTIVE PEOPLE WITH TYPE 1 DIABETES MELLITUS

EXCHANGE NEEDS	SAMPLE MENUS
Moderate Activity	
30 Minutes	
1 bread *or*	1 bran muffin *or*
1 fruit	1 small orange
1 Hour	
2 bread + 1 meat *or*	Tuna sandwich *or*
2 fruit + 1 milk	½ cup fruit salad + 1 cup milk
Strenuous Activity	
30 Minutes	
2 fruit *or*	1 small banana *or*
1 bread + 1 fat	½ bagel + 1 tsp cream cheese
1 Hour	
2 bread + 1 meat + 1 milk *or*	Meat and cheese sandwich + 1 cup milk *or*
2 bread + 2 meat + 2 fruit	Hamburger + 1 cup orange juice

in balance with food intake. Frequent monitoring is needed to adjust insulin dose with either multiple injections or the insulin pump.

Oral Antidiabetic Drugs

Five classes of oral antidiabetic drugs are used to treat hyperglycemia in T2DM: (1) sulfonylurea, (2) biguanide, (3) thiazolidinedione, (4) meglitinide, and (5) α-glucosidase inhibitor. When lifestyle changes alone cannot normalize metabolism, MNT should help optimize metabolic control and reduce potential medication side effects. Table 22-4 provides a brief review of insulin and oral antidiabetic drugs (see the *Complementary and Alternative Medicine [CAM]* box, "Herbs and Supplements Commonly Used in Diabetes Mellitus").

TABLE 22-4 MEDICATIONS USED TO TREAT DIABETES

DRUG CLASS	DRUG NAMES	ACTION	TARGET ORGANS	SIDE EFFECTS	HOW TAKEN
α-Glucosidase inhibitor agents	Acarbose: Precose Miglitol: Glyset	Delays absorption of glucose from GI tract	Small intestine	Excess flatulence, diarrhea (particularly after high-carbohydrate meal), abdominal pain; may interfere with iron absorption	Must be taken with meals three times/day
Biguanide agents	Metformin: Glucophage	Decreases hepatic glucose production and intestinal glucose absorption; improves insulin sensitivity	Liver, small intestine, and peripheral tissues	Less likely to gain weight; may lose weight; anorexia, nausea, diarrhea, metallic taste; may reduce absorption of vitamin B_{12} and folic acid; rarely suitable for adults <80 yr	Take with first main meal
Insulin and related agents	Insulin mixtures: Humulin 50/50, Humulin 70/30, Novolin 70/30	Exogenous insulin preparations	Cells	Hypoglycemia, fatigue, hunger, nausea, muscular weakness or trembling, headache, sweating, blurred vision, fainting, weight gain, skin irritation	Subcutaneous injection
	Intermediate acting: Humulin L, Humulin N, Iletin II Lente, Iletin II NPH, Novolin L, Novolin N	Exogenous insulin preparations		Hypoglycemia, fatigue, hunger, nausea, muscular weakness or trembling, headache, sweating, blurred vision, fainting, weight gain, skin irritation	Subcutaneous injection
	Long acting: Humulin U, Lantus (insulin glargine)	Exogenous insulin preparations		Hypoglycemia, fatigue, hunger, nausea, muscular weakness or trembling, headache, sweating, blurred vision, fainting, weight gain, skin irritation	Subcutaneous injection
	Rapid acting: Humalog, insulin lispro, insulin aspart	Exogenous insulin preparations		Hypoglycemia, fatigue, hunger, nausea, muscular weakness or trembling, headache, sweating, blurred vision, fainting, weight gain, skin irritation	Subcutaneous injection, intramuscular or intravenous in special situations

Continued

TABLE 22-4 MEDICATIONS USED TO TREAT DIABETES—cont'd

DRUG CLASS	DRUG NAMES	ACTION	TARGET ORGANS	SIDE EFFECTS	HOW TAKEN
	Short acting: Humulin R, Iletin II Regular, Novolin R, Novolin BR	Exogenous insulin preparations		Hypoglycemia, fatigue, hunger, nausea, muscular weakness or trembling, headache, sweating, blurred vision, fainting, weight gain, skin irritation	Subcutaneous injection, intramuscular or intravenous in special situations
Meglitinide agents (nonsulfonylurea insulin releasers)	Nateglinide: Starlix Repaglinide: Prandin	Stimulates secretion of insulin	Pancreatic beta cells	Hypoglycemia and weight gain; repaglinide (Prandin) has a slightly increased risk for cardiac events	Take with meals
Sulfonylurea agents—first generation	Acetohexamide: Dymelor Tolazamide: Tolinase Tolbutamide: Orinase Chlorpropamide: Diabinese	Stimulates secretion of insulin	Pancreatic beta cells	Hypoglycemia and weight gain; tolbutamide may be associated with cardiovascular complications; chlorpropamide (Diabinese) can cause hyponatremia; should not be used by women who are pregnant, who are nursing, or those individuals allergic to sulfa drugs; sulfonylurea interacts with many other drugs (prescription, OTC, and alternative); *Diabinese:* avoid alcohol	Take before or with meals
Sulfonylurea agents—second generation	Glimepiride: Amaryl Glyburide: DiaBeta, Micronase, Glynase PresTabs				
Thiazolidinedione agents	Pioglitazone: Actos Rosiglitazone: Avandia	Improves insulin sensitivity	Activates genes involved with fat synthesis and carbohydrate metabolism	Possible liver damage, weight gain, mild anemia	Once or twice daily

Data from Nelms MN, Sucher K, Lacey L, Long S: *Nutrition therapy and pathophysiology,* ed 2, Belmont, Calif, 2010, Thomson Cengage; Mahan LK, Escott-Stump S, editors: *Krause's food & nutrition therapy,* ed 12, St Louis, 2008, Saunders.
GI, Gastrointestinal; *OTC,* over the counter.

Insulin is often used in T2DM as adjunctive therapy when oral agents are not achieving glycemic control. A nighttime dose of insulin is commonly used to help reduce fasting glucose levels, especially if fasting levels are 13.9 mmol/L (250 mg/dL) or higher. Insulin therapy is also commonly used as adjunctive therapy when glycemic control is not achieved with oral agent monotherapy or combination therapy.

Adjunctive Therapies

Two new injectable drugs have been approved by the U.S. Food and Drug Administration (FDA). Exenatide (Byetta) is first in its class of drugs for treatment of T2DM for patients taking metformin, a sulfonylurea, or a combination of metformin and a sulfonylurea. This class of drugs is referred to as *incretin mimetics.* Isolated from the saliva of Gila monsters, exenatide works to lower blood glucose levels by increasing insulin

COMPLEMENTARY AND ALTERNATIVE MEDICINE (CAM)

Herbs and Supplements Commonly Used in Diabetes Mellitus

HERB/ SUPPLEMENT	COMMON USES	EFFICACY	SAFETY	DRUG/HERB INTERACTIONS	INTERACTION
Chromium	Glycemic control	Improved glycemic control	No adverse effects reported	Hyperglycemic agents and any other agent used for glycemic control	Possible risk of hypoglycemia
Cinnamon (*Cinnamomum verum*)	Glycemic control	Increases use of endogenous insulin	Large amounts increase heart rate and intestinal motility, followed by sleepiness and depression As a spice, long-term use safe	None known	
Ginseng (*Panax ginseng*)	Glycemic control	Improved glycemic control	Possible overstimulation and insomnia	Hyperglycemic agents and any other agent used for glycemic control May enhance effect of stimulants, antibiotics, MAOIs Antagonism of warfarin; might falsely elevate digoxin levels Increases alcohol clearance; might decrease diuretic effect of furosemide Might potentiate effects of hormones and anabolic steroid therapies	Possible risk of hypoglycemia Estrogenic effects of ginseng may cause vaginal bleeding and breast nodules
Evening primrose oil (*Oenothera biennis*)	Peripheral neuropathy	May be helpful	No adverse effects reported	Phenothiazines	Might increase risk of seizures
Lipoic acid	Neuropathy	Slight evidence intravenous lipoic acid can reduce symptoms of peripheral neuropathy in the short term Evidence for oral lipoic acid inadequate	No adverse reactions documented	Some concern that lipoic acid potentiates effects of insulin, but has not been documented in formal studies	None noted
Vanadium	Glycemic control	May improve glycemic control	Usually well tolerated, but GI disturbances can occur Studies suggest excess is toxic (hepatotoxicity, nephrotoxicity, teratogenicity, and developmental/ reproductive toxicity)	Might cause hypoglycemia if used in conjunction with effective antidiabetic regimen	None noted

BIBLIOGRAPHY

Bratman S, Girman AM: *Mosby's handbook of herbs and supplements and their therapeutic uses,* St Louis, 2003, Mosby.

Contributors and Consultants: *Professional guide to complementary and alternative therapies,* Springhouse, Penn, 2001, Springhouse.

Kuhn MA, Winston D: *Herbal therapy and supplements: a scientific and traditional approach,* Philadelphia, 2001, Lippincott Williams & Wilkins.

MAOIs, Monoamine oxidase inhibitors; *GI,* gastrointestinal.

secretion. It only has this effect in the presence of elevated blood glucose levels; therefore it does not tend to increase risk of hypoglycemia on its own.

Pramlintide (Symlin) is a synthetic form of the hormone amylin. Amylin and insulin are produced by the beta cells in the pancreas. Amylin, insulin, and glucagon work together to maintain normal blood glucose levels. Pramlintide injections taken with meals modestly improve HbA_{1c} levels by slowing gastric emptying rate without altering overall absorption of nutrients. In addition, pramlintide suppresses glucagon secretion from the liver and regulates food intake because of centrally mediated modulation of appetite.

Testing Methods for Monitoring Results

Frequent testing of blood glucose levels is necessary for successful tight control of T1DM and to reduce risk of complications.

Self-Monitoring of Blood Glucose. For insulin doses to be administered in sufficient time intervals and amounts to maintain normal blood glucose, close monitoring of immediate blood glucose levels is mandatory. Small, lightweight, easy-to-use, hand-sized meters, easily carried in pockets and handbags, are available for convenient use. A reagent test strip is inserted into the blood glucose meter, a drop of capillary blood from the finger obtained with an automatic lancer is placed on the reagent test strip, and a digital reading of the blood glucose level appears on the meter. Frequency of monitoring varies according to need for control and goal of care. More frequent self-monitoring is indicated for unstable forms of diabetes, persons using insulin pumps, and those who want close control and freedom of movement. Usually two to eight before- and after-meal tests are performed daily. During pregnancy, postprandial monitoring is performed at 1 hour after meals. Glucose goals are lower during pregnancy because of the dilution effect of having increased blood volume.

Glycated Hemoglobin. The most common glycated hemoglobin (Hb) test is the HbA_{1c}. Glycated Hb molecules are relatively stable within the red blood cell. During the 120-day life of the red blood cell, glucose molecules attach themselves to Hb. This irreversible glycosylation of Hb depends on the concentration of blood glucose. Glycosylation of proteins in various body systems appears to play a role in the development of diabetic complications. The greater the level of circulating glucose is during the life of the red blood cells, the greater is the concentration of glycohemoglobin. Thus measurement of HbA_{1c} relates to the level of blood glucose during a longer period. It provides an effective tool for evaluating the long-term management of diabetes and degree of control.[11] Because glucose attaches to Hb during the life of the red blood cell, the test gives an accumulated history of glucose levels across time, providing an effective management tool for evaluating progress and making decisions about treatment changes. Obtaining a HbA_{1c} level every 6 to 8 weeks can be used to monitor the overall glucose control.

Physical Activity Habits

In counseling clients with diabetes, a detailed history of personal activity and physical exercise habits should be discussed. This information is then used as a basis for planning a wise program of regular moderate exercise. Guidelines for extra food to cover periods of heavier exercise or athletic practice and competition are included (see Table 22-3). Self-monitoring is a regular procedure now used by most persons with T1DM and T2DM. It is a helpful means of determining the balance needed at any point in time between exercise, insulin, and food.

Gestational Diabetes

Occasionally the stress of pregnancy may bring about GDM, which is a form of glucose intolerance that has onset during pregnancy and is resolved on parturition.[30] Risk of fetal abnormalities and mortality are increased in the presence of hyperglycemia; therefore every effort should be made to control blood glucose levels. All women with GDM should receive nutrition counseling by a RD when possible.[28]

Changes that take place during pregnancy greatly affect insulin use. Some hormones and enzymes produced by the placenta are antagonistic to insulin, thus reducing its effectiveness. Maternal insulin does not cross the placenta, but glucose does, causing the fetal pancreas to increase insulin production if maternal blood glucose levels get too high. Increased production of insulin causes the most predictable characteristic of infants born to women with diabetes, macrosomia, in addition to other problems such as respiratory difficulties, hypocalcemia, hypoglycemia, hypokalemia, and jaundice.[27]

Individualization of NT based on maternal weight and height is recommended.[28] MNT should include the provision of adequate kcalories and nutrients to meet pregnancy needs and should be consistent with accepted maternal blood glucose goals.[28] SMBG provides important information about the effect of food on blood glucose levels. At the beginning of the pregnancy, minimal daily SMBG should be planned four times a day (fasting and 1 or 2 hours after each meal). Blood glucose goals during pregnancy are fasting, less than 105 mg/dL; 1 hour postprandial, 155 mg/dL; and 2 hours postprandial, less than 130 mg/dL.[28] Frequency of SMBG may be decreased once blood glucose control is established. However, some monitoring should continue throughout pregnancy.

Recommended weight gains and nutrient requirements are the same as for established pregnancy guidelines, as follows[27]:

- Underweight (body mass index [BMI] <18.5): 28 to 40 lb
- Normal/healthy weight (BMI 18.5 to 24.9): 25 to 35 lb
- Overweight (BMI 25 to 29.9): 15 to 25 lb
- Obesity (class 1) (BMI 30 to 34.9): greater than 15 lb
- Obesity (class 2) (BMI 35 to 39.9): not available
- Obesity (class 3) (BMI >40): not available

No kcalorie modifications are needed for the first trimester.[17] During the second and third trimesters, increased energy intake of approximately 180 kcal/day is suggested.[27]

High-quality protein should be increased by 25 g/day. As with any pregnancy, 600 mcg/day of folic acid is recommended for prevention of neural tube defects (NTDs) and other congenital abnormalities.[27] Alcohol consumption is not recommended in any amount.

Kcaloric restriction must be considered with care. A minimum of 1700 to 1800 kcal/day of carefully selected foods has been shown to prevent ketosis. Intakes less than this level are not advised.[28] Weight gain goals are established using prepregnancy BMI. Weight gain should still occur even if patients have gained substantial weight before the onset of GDM. Each patient with GDM should be evaluated individually by a RD, should have care plans fine-tuned, and should have patient education provided as required to realize weight goals.

Impaired Fasting Glucose and Impaired Glucose Tolerance

The terms *IFG* and *IGT* refer to a metabolic stage somewhere between normal glucose homeostasis and overt diabetes. Although not clinical entities in their own right, these conditions are risk factors for future diabetes and CVD.[2,11] Lifestyle interventions should be consistent with current guidelines for overweight and obesity and address cardiovascular risk factors and common concomitant conditions. The Da Qing IGT and Diabetes Study provided preliminary evidence that diet and exercise intervention can lower the conversion to overt diabetes during the 6-year period.[14] The Finnish Diabetes Prevention Study demonstrated that a lifestyle change program could reduce the risk for developing T2DM by 58% during a 3-year period.[13] In the United States, the Diabetes Prevention Program (DPP) has confirmed the findings of the Finnish trial in a highly diverse American population with IGT. The DPP addressed how an intensive diet and exercise intervention compares with metformin in a three-arm randomized clinical trial that uses placebo as the third arm.

MANAGEMENT OF DIABETES NUTRITION THERAPY

Counseling Process in Nutrition Therapy for Diabetes

NT for diabetes is highly individualized. The American Diabetes Association recommendations clearly state that no one diabetic or American Diabetes Association diet exists. Today the recommended diet is a dietary prescription based on individual nutrition assessment and treatment goals.[19] This model emphasizes actions of the diabetes team clinical dietitian in an individualized, integrated four-point approach: (1) assessment, (2) goal setting, (3) nutrition intervention, and (4) evaluation, as follows[31]:

1. *Assessment:* The first step involves a comprehensive assessment of the client's background. It includes clinical information, medical and lifestyle data such as personal SMBG, and dietary history. Interview follow-up tools such as questionnaires and food records assess general food patterns and nutrient intake.
2. *Nutrition diagnosis:* The second step identifies and labels problems the client may have.
3. *Nutrition intervention:* The third step guides the client in selecting and using the most appropriate meal-planning guide from the number that are now available, based on individual needs for knowledge and skills to change or maintain eating habits and daily living practices.
4. *Monitoring and evaluation:* Together the client and dietitian evaluate goals and nutrition intervention, as well as ongoing clinical data, to help the client succeed at the established individual program. They then make any desired adjustments, and the dietitian provides continuing counseling and education as needed.

Diabetes Meal-Planning Tools

Since the DCCT, growing emphasis has been placed on selecting a planning approach that meets the needs of each client from a wide array of meal-planning guides. Regardless of the diabetes NT management tool, the first vital principle in working with persons who have diabetes is to begin where they are physically, mentally, and emotionally. Any food-planning process must focus first on the unique individual rather than on the case or disease. Numerous planning approaches are used by skilled and sensitive clinical dietitians who tailor their actions to the person's learning needs and abilities, as well as his or her nutritional needs, personal needs, and lifestyle issues. Because of the widespread use of the exchange lists as a dietary management tool, they are outlined in Appendix B.

Carbohydrate Counting

Carbohydrate counting is one of the most commonly used methods of meal planning. Research shows carbohydrate is the primary nutrient affecting postprandial blood glucose level and consequently insulin requirements.[21,22] Carbohydrate quantity and distribution can affect metabolic control.[22] Carbohydrate counting can help people with diabetes become more aware of carbohydrate content of the foods they eat and consistency of food consumption at meals and when snacking.[19]

At an advanced level, carbohydrate counting is a tool that allows the person with diabetes to focus on adjustment of foods, medication, and activity based on patterns from daily food intake records and blood glucose records.[19] To use carbohydrate counting effectively, the dietetic professional and person with diabetes must have a good understanding of intensive insulin therapy.[22]

Carbohydrate content can be measured in grams of carbohydrate or servings: one carbohydrate serving equals 15 g

KEY TERMS

tight control Keeping blood glucose levels as close to normal as possible.

BOX 22-1 EQUIVALENTS TO ONE 15-g CARBOHYDRATE SERVING*

Grains, Breads, Cereals, Starches
- 1 slice bread
- ¾ cup dry cereal
- ½ cup cooked cereal
- ⅓ cup cooked rice or pasta

Milk and Yogurt
- 1 cup milk
- ⅓ cup (6 oz) unsweetened or sugar-free yogurt

Fruits
- 1 small fresh fruit
- ½ cup canned fruit (caned in juice)
- 1 cup melon or berries
- ¼ cup dried fruit
- ½ cup unsweetened fruit juice

Vegetables
- ½ cup cooked potatoes, peas, or corn
- 3 cups raw vegetables
- 1½ cups cooked vegetables
- (Small portions [½ cup] of nonstarchy vegetables are free.)

Sweets and Snack Foods
- ½ cup or ¾ oz snack food (pretzels, chips)
- 4 to 6 snack crackers
- 1 oz sweet snack (2 small cookies)
- ½ cup regular ice cream
- 1 tbsp sugar

From American Diabetes Association, American Dietetic Association: *Choose your foods: exchange lists for diabetes,* ed 6, Alexandra, Va/Chicago, 2008, American Diabetes Association, American Dietetic Association.

*Reproduction of the Exchange Lists in whole or part without permission of The American Dietetic Association or the American Diabetes Association, Inc. is a violation of federal law. This material has been modified from *Choose Your Foods: Exchange Lists for Diabetes,* which is the basis of a meal planning system designed by a committee of the American Diabetes Association and The American Diabetic Association. While designed primarily for people with diabetes and others who must follow special diets, the Exchange Lists are based on principles of good nutrition that apply to everyone.

carbohydrate. Most people find it easier to count the number of carbohydrate servings consumed rather than keeping track of grams of carbohydrate consumed.[22] Box 22-1 provides a brief outline of carbohydrate content of foods to equal one serving of carbohydrate.

Planning for Special Needs

Sick Days. When general illness occurs, food and insulin amounts must be adjusted accordingly. Texture may be modified as needed to use easily digested and absorbed liquid foods while still maintaining as many as possible glucose equivalents of the usual food plan.

Physical Activity. For any strenuous physical activity, the client with T1DM must make special advanced plans. This is particularly true of a young person with diabetes who is engaging in athletic practice or competition. Energy demands of exercise are discussed in Chapter 14.

Travel. When a trip is planned, the clinical dietitian must confer with the client to guide food choices according to what will be available. SMBG levels, insulin therapy equipment, and making food plans are just as important on a trip as they are at home. The traveler always needs to plan ahead with the health care team (see the *Perspectives in Practice* box, "Travel and Illness: 'Real-Life' Situations").

Dining Out. Provide similar guidelines and suggestions for various situations when the client eats meals away from home. As a general rule, the plan must be made ahead of time; therefore accommodations for what is eaten at home before and after the restaurant meal reflect the continuing balance needs of the day. Have the client get the menu ahead of time. Many restaurants are willing to fax their menus, or they may be available on websites.

Stress. Any form of emotional stress is reflected in variations of diabetes control.[22] These variations are caused by hormonal responses that act as antagonists to insulin. The clinical dietitian must help the client learn and practice a variety of useful stress reduction activities.

DIABETES EDUCATION PROGRAM

Goal: Person-Centered Self-Care

In past years the traditional medical model has guided diabetes education in its methods, language, and respective roles assumed. Professionals have viewed themselves as having major authoritative roles and have assigned to the person with diabetes the more passive role of patient. With notable exceptions in certain places, this model has been followed in most cases. However, with the increasing movement toward changing roles of practitioners and consumers in the health care system, persons with diabetes are assuming a more active voice in planning and conducting their own care. Several barriers in our traditional system stem from three sources: (1) our culture, (2) our health care delivery system, and (3) our professional training habits. Essentially, much of the core problem focuses on communication. For example, a list of words we use too commonly that may be objectionable to persons with diabetes, along with the preferred language, include the following:

- Diabetic used as a noun: The word diabetic is an adjective and should not be used alone as a noun. Instead, use the phrase person with diabetes.
- Compliance: The word compliance raises red flags in minds of persons with diabetes. It is a purely medical term and connotes an authoritative physician position. Instead, the word adherence should be used, which has been adopted by national committees and associations working in the field of diabetes. The word adherence indicates placement of more decision-making responsibility on the person with diabetes to determine courses of action in varying situations, which is, of course, the necessity.

PERSPECTIVES IN PRACTICE

Travel and Illness: "Real-Life" Situations

People do not stop living their lives just because they have diabetes. They still travel, and they still catch colds, influenza, and other common illnesses. Special considerations to all areas of diabetes management will enhance safe traveling, as well as the traveler's health. What kind of information does the person with diabetes need to know when traveling or if he or she becomes too ill to eat? The following are a few helpful hints you may want to offer clients for these situations.

Traveling Safely with Diabetes

General Tips

1. Ensure that you have sufficient medication (insulin or oral glucose-lowering medication) for the entire trip.
2. Carry some form of medical identification that includes type of diabetes, name, address, telephone number, emergency contact information, medications taken, physician's name and phone number, and additional relevant medical conditions. Preferably, this information should be worn on a necklace or bracelet (rather than carrying it in a wallet or purse).
3. Take extra snacks such as cereal bars, vanilla wafers, peanut butter crackers, or glucose tablets or gel.
4. Always keep insulin cool, especially when vacationing in warm climates.
5. Keep some money available for food purchases if necessary. Change for vending machines may not always be available.
6. Always carry blood glucose monitoring equipment. Blood glucose levels should be checked before beginning a trip, as well as every 2 hours. An extra check should be done whenever symptoms of hypoglycemia occur, even if recent blood glucose checks were acceptable.
7. Walking around and stretching every 2 to 4 hours helps stimulate circulation.
8. Whenever possible, travel with a companion.
9. Wear comfortable shoes.
10. Plan for time zone changes. Meal schedules may need to be revised to balance with insulin activity pattern.
11. If traveling abroad, learn to say the following in the local language: "I have diabetes. Please give me something sweet to drink."
12. If travel is frequent, contact a registered dietitian (RD) or diabetes educator for ideas for healthful, portable meals and snacks.

Driving Tips

1. If diabetes medication has potential to cause hypoglycemia, medications and meals will need to be scheduled during a long trip.
2. If diabetes medications have potential to cause hypoglycemia, food should be eaten before leaving home or snacks should be taken in the automobile. Traffic may not be conducive to stopping at a favorite store or restaurant for a quick meal or snack.
3. Keep nonperishable, carbohydrate-containing foods in the automobile in case flat tires, traffic jams, or breakdowns occur. Handy, premeasured carbohydrate amounts may be beneficial to avoid overeating or undereating. Replenish the food supply as needed to avoid running out at inopportune times.
4. Always carry blood glucose monitoring equipment when driving. Blood glucose levels should be checked before the trip begins, as well as every 2 hours while driving. An extra check should be done if symptoms of hypoglycemia occur (even if recent blood glucose checks have been acceptable).
5. An extra glucose meter should not be kept in an automobile. Internal automobile temperatures can get very hot and very cold. Strips and meters exposed to extreme temperatures may not be accurate or function properly.
6. High blood glucose levels may cause the following symptoms that can affect driving:
   - Fatigue related to the body's inability to use glucose for energy
   - Increased urination, causing preoccupation, repeated stops, and a delay in arriving at destination
   - Blurry vision, which may impair ability to see road signs clearly; blurry vision may be especially problematic at night or while driving in rain or snow
   - Numbness or tingling in hands or feet, which may impair ability to steer, accelerate, and stop the vehicle
7. Prompt attention to hypoglycemia and treatment is necessary to prevent mental confusion and even losing consciousness. When blood glucose is low, the first organ affected is the brain! Keep appropriate sources of carbohydrates available in the automobile.
8. If driving hours at a time, it is important to stop the automobile, get out and stretch, and walk around every 2 to 4 hours.
9. Wear medical identification. Law enforcement officers may not be familiar with diabetes or symptoms of hypoglycemia or hyperglycemia. They can mistake impaired awareness and judgment for drunkenness.
10. Whenever possible, drive with a friend.
11. If driving for several hours, set an alarm as a reminder for blood glucose checks, meals, and even times to stretch and walk.
12. Visual disturbances can occur with either hyperglycemia or hypoglycemia.
13. If driving long distances, take twice as many diabetes supplies as thought to be needed. Be aware of all medicines taken (prescription and over-the-counter [OTC] medications).
14. Always carry money for toll booths, parking fees, and telephone calls. Consider keeping a cell phone to call for assistance.

Flying Tips

1. Call ahead to airlines to advise them of the diabetes and supplies needed.
2. Carry a copy of physician's prescription for insulin and other medications.
3. Carry a letter from the physician explaining the need to carry syringes/injection devices and insulin.
4. If problems are encountered, request to speak to a manager or supervisor.
5. Carry insulin onto the aircraft. Insulin should not be packed in luggage that will be stored in the hold of an airplane. Low temperatures can damage the insulin.

Continued

PERSPECTIVES IN PRACTICE

Travel and Illness: "Real-Life" Situations—cont'd

6. Notify the Transportation Security Administration (TSA) representative that you have diabetes and are carrying your supplies with you. The following are allowed through the checkpoint once screened:
   - Insulin and insulin-loaded dispensing products clearly marked and labeled
   - Unlimited number of unused syringes when accompanied by insulin or other injectable medication
   - Lancets, blood glucose meters, blood glucose meter test strips, alcohol swabs, meter-testing solutions
   - Insulin pump and supplies
   - Glucagon emergency kit clearly identified and labeled
   - Urine ketone test strips
   - Unlimited number of used syringes when transported in sharps disposal container or other similar hard-surfaced container

Sick Day Survival

1. Keep taking diabetes medications even if solid foods cannot be eaten.
2. For insulin users the physician may prescribe extra doses or increased amounts of insulin during an illness.
3. Blood glucose should be tested and recorded every 4 hours.
4. Test for ketones in urine if blood glucose level stays at or greater than 240 mg/dL for at least 4 hours.
5. Try to use regular meal plan and diet, but if that is not possible, soft foods or liquids can be consumed to take the place of carbohydrates usually eaten. Some easily digested foods to replace one serving (15 g) of carbohydrate include the following:
   - ⅓ to ½ cup fruit juice
   - ½ cup regular soft drink
   - ½ cup regular gelatin
   - ½ cup hot cereal
   - ½ cup vanilla ice cream
   - 1 cup broth-based soup
6. To prevent dehydration, sip 3 to 6 oz of noncaffeinated, sugar-free beverages or water every hour. Sugar-free fluids may be alternated with liquids containing sugar to help control blood glucose levels.
7. Keep a thermometer on hand to determine body temperature.
8. When buying OTC medicines, choose one that is sugar free. In addition to the word *sugar* on labels, *dextrose, fructose, lactose, sorbitol, mannitol, xylitol,* and *honey* indicate that a product contains sugar.
9. OTC cold medications containing epinephrine-like compounds (including ephedrine, pseudoephedrine, phenylpropanolamine, phenylephrine, and epinephrine) can raise blood glucose levels and should only be used with a physician's approval.
10. *Planning ahead:* Keep the following items on hand in case of colds, influenza, or other kinds of illnesses:
    - Thermometer
    - Urine test strips for ketones (check expiration date periodically)
    - Approved OTC cold and influenza medicines
    - Syringes or prescription for them (if insulin is not usually taken but is part of a sick day plan)
    - Short-acting insulin (keep refrigerated)
    - Extra prescriptions for all medications usually taken (or have on file at pharmacy)
    - Nonperishable foods such as noncaffeinated soft drinks (regular and diet), regular gelatin, Popsicles, sport drinks, saltines, and canned fruit juices
11. Call the physician if any of the following occurs:
    - Vomiting for several hours
    - Diarrhea recurring within 6 hours
    - Difficulty breathing
    - Blood glucose levels greater than 240 mg/dL for 24 hours if using oral medications; blood glucose levels greater than 240 mg/dL for two consecutive tests (4 hours apart) after taking supplemental insulin
    - Blood glucose levels less than 60 mg/dL
    - Moderate to large amounts of ketones in urine and no improvement after at least 12 hours
    - Signs of dehydration such as dry skin or mouth, sunken eyes, or weight loss
    - Sickness that continues from 12 to 48 hours without improvement
    - Increased fatigue
    - Stomach or chest pain
    - Temperature that stays at higher than 101° F
    - Acute loss of vision
12. When calling the physician, he or she will want to know blood glucose levels and urine ketone levels, how long the illness has lasted, what medicines have been taken, temperature, how much has been eaten or drunk, and other symptoms that have been experienced.
13. If necessary to go to the emergency department, then staff should be informed of the diabetes.

In summary, in all cases the client must be advised to (1) maintain a steady intake of food every day, (2) replace the carbohydrate value of solid foods with that of liquid or soft foods as needed, (3) monitor blood and urine frequently for sugar and ketone levels, and (4) contact the physician if the illness lasts more than a day or so.

BIBLIOGRAPHY

American Diabetes Association: *Traveling with diabetes supplies,* Alexandria, Va, 2006, American Diabetes Association. Retrieved May 23, 2009, from www.diabetes.org/advocacy-and-legalresources/discrimination/public_accommodation/travel.jsp.

Diabetes Mall: FAA regulations for diabetes supplies, *Diabetes News* Oct 7, 2001. Retrieved May 23, 2009, from www.diabetesnet.com/news/news100701.php.

National Diabetes Information Clearinghouse: *What I need to know about eating and diabetes,* NIH Pub No 03-5043, Bethesda, Md, 2003, National Institute of Diabetes and Digestive and Kidney Diseases, National Institutes of Health.

- Patient: Instead of patient, the phrase person with diabetes should be used. Persons with diabetes are patients only when they are in the hospital or seeing a physician for an illness.
- Cheating: A particularly abusive word in the minds of many persons with diabetes, especially parents of children and young people with diabetes, is the word cheating, because it suggests dishonesty or failure to live up to an external code. By and large, persons with diabetes do not cheat. They may kid themselves, or they may be inaccurate in their reporting, but they do not cheat. Instead phrases such as having difficulty or having a problem with should be used.

Contents: Tools for Self-Care

A plan for diabetes education must recognize the need for building self-sufficiency and responsibility within persons with diabetes and their families. It should provide practical guidelines that build on necessary skills that a person with diabetes must have for the best possible control, as well as additional surrounding factors related to life situations and psychosocial needs. Content areas include needs in relation to the nature of diabetes, nutrition and basic meal planning, insulin (or oral medication) effects and how to regulate them, monitoring of blood glucose, how to deal with illness, and, if relevant, urine ketones (see the *Case Study* box, "The Woman with Type 2 Diabetes Mellitus").

Educational Materials: Person-Centered Standards

A broad, confusing array of diabetes education materials are available. Some are excellent, and some should be discarded. Whatever is used should measure up to several basic person-centered requirements by doing the following:

- Give the intended receiver credit for having some intelligence and wanting new information
- Inform persons fully and completely, giving both sides when experts disagree (as they surely do on occasion)
- Appeal to various levels of audience, ranging from basic to sophisticated
- Never be patronizing, dehumanizing, or childish

HEALTH PROMOTION

Nutrition Questions from Persons with Diabetes

Persons with diabetes have many questions about their diets, especially when they are newly diagnosed and anxieties are high. They do not want just a yes-or-no answer. For any diet item of concern, they want to know if it can be used. If use of the diet item should be limited, then they want to know why this is so and exactly how often they can use it.

Alcohol and Diabetes: Do They Mix?

Questions about alcohol and various sweeteners are common. People with diabetes should follow the same sensible drinking guidelines as people without diabetes, as follows[17,32,33]:

- Use alcohol only in moderation (one drink/day for women, two drinks/day for men).
  - One drink = 12 oz regular beer, 5 oz wine, or 1.5 oz of 80-proof distilled spirits (whiskey, scotch, rye, vodka, brandy, cognac, rum).
- Never drink alcohol on an empty stomach.
- Some medications may not mix with alcohol; check with physician or pharmacist.

CASE STUDY

The Woman with Type 2 Diabetes Mellitus

Angela is a 35-year-old woman diagnosed 2 years ago with type 2 diabetes mellitus (T2DM). She has three children whose birth weights were in the range of 4.5 to 5 kg (10 to 11 lb). The children, now teenagers, show no signs of diabetes, and their weights are reported to be within normal limits despite their mother's fondness for cooking. Her husband, an underpaid construction worker, is slightly overweight.

Approximately 6 months ago, Angela was seen with a complaint of a series of infections that lasted longer than usual during the past 2 months. At that time she was measured as 165 cm (5 feet, 5 inches) and 71 kg (156 lb). Her glucose tolerance test was positive. She was seen for follow-up twice during the next month, each time showing hyperglycemia and glycosuria. At the second follow-up, an oral antidiabetic medication was prescribed, and she was referred for medical nutrition therapy (MNT).

Angela did not keep this appointment or her subsequent medical appointment. She was not seen again until 1 month ago, when she arrived at the emergency department with ketoacidosis. She responded well to treatment and was placed on a 1200-kcal diet and a mixture of intermediate- and rapid-acting insulin given in two injections a day. Her discharge plan included a referral for a MNT consultation session and diabetes education classes.

Questions for Analysis

1. What factors do you think contributed to the ketoacidosis?
2. What relation do these factors have to diabetes control?
3. Why did Angela first appear to have T2DM?
4. Assume that Angela administers insulin before breakfast and before the evening meal. What additional information is necessary to develop an individualized meal plan?
5. Identify any personal factors that may affect Angela's adherence to her treatment plan. Do you anticipate any problems?
6. If so, then how would you attempt to help her solve them?
7. Outline a diabetes education plan for Angela.

- Never drink and drive.
- Never drink if pregnant or trying to become pregnant.
- Above all, use common sense.

Having diabetes should not prevent consumption of alcohol; however, some considerations must be made. Alcoholic beverages, depending on amount and type, can cause hyperglycemia and hypoglycemia. Alcohol moves very quickly from the stomach into the bloodstream; it does not require digestion or metabolism. Approximately 30 to 90 minutes after an alcoholic drink is consumed, alcohol in the bloodstream is at its highest concentration. Because the liver plays the biggest role in removing alcohol from the blood, it stops making glucose while cleansing alcohol from the body. If blood glucose levels are falling during the same time, then hypoglycemia can occur very quickly. For those taking insulin or oral hypoglycemic agents, they too are lowering blood glucose levels. This is why two shots of whiskey on an empty stomach lowers blood sugar dramatically.

Alcoholic beverages can be high in kcalories (and low in food value) and can raise blood glucose, especially if mixed with sweet mixers, fruit juices, or ice cream. Two ounces of 90-proof alcohol contain almost 200 kcal. Wine coolers, liqueurs, and port wines are also high in sugar and kcalories. This can interfere with weight loss goals and practicing tight control. Alcohol also increases serum cholesterol levels, although this effect is transient. In addition, it can lead to hyperlipoproteinemia, with high triglyceride levels in susceptible persons, including persons with diabetes, when it is excessive. Alcohol can also make neuropathy and retinopathy worse.

For clients who choose to use alcohol, they should ask themselves the following three basic questions:

1. Is my diabetes under control?
2. Does my health care provider agree that I am free from any health problems that alcohol can make worse (e.g., high blood pressure, neuropathy)?
3. Do I know how alcohol can affect me and my diabetes?

If the answer to all three questions is *yes*, then the client can have an occasional drink. In addition to the sensible drinking guidelines listed earlier, the following recommendations should also be considered:

- Discuss the use of alcohol with your physician or dietitian.
- Drink with caution, and carry identification.
- Choose drinking buddies wisely. (Make sure at least one friend or trusted companion knows that you have diabetes and is aware of what should be done in case of hypoglycemia.)
- Have a snack before going to bed to prevent hypoglycemia during sleep.
- Do not drink if you are practicing tight control (because alcohol impairs judgment); have neuropathy, hypertriglyceridemia, or hypertension; or are taking Diabinese (which causes nausea, flushing, headache, or dizziness when mixed with alcohol); or Glucophage (which can cause lactic acidosis).
- Always sip alcoholic drinks slowly.
- If you are a man and taking insulin, you can include two alcoholic beverages in addition to your regular meal plan. If you are a woman taking insulin, then you can include one alcoholic beverage. Do not omit food in exchange for an alcoholic drink.
- If you are not taking insulin (and watching your weight), you can substitute alcohol for fat choices and in some cases extra starch choices (sweet wines, sweet vermouth, and wine coolers).

Can I Use Fructose in My Diabetic Diet?

How would you answer this question from your diabetic client? Fructose has been touted as a sweetener for persons with diabetes because it is a naturally occurring sugar that is as much as 1.0 to 1.5 times as sweet as sucrose. However, can the person with diabetes use it safely?

Although fructose as a sweetener is not for all persons with diabetes, generally you can reply, "Yes, but with qualifications." The following should be considered:

- Advertising claims promoting fructose are sometimes so misleading that many consumers mistakenly believe that it can be used as a "free" food. However, fructose has the same nutritive value as other sugars—4 kcal/g. Persons with T1DM should especially be instructed to use fructose as carefully as they use any other food with a caloric and carbohydrate value.
- The quantity must be limited. If used, then the maximum amount is 75 g/day.
- Consumption of fructose in large amounts may have adverse effects on plasma lipids. It may also cause loose stools and gas when consuming amounts greater than approximately 25 g/serving.
- The sweetness of fructose varies with temperature, acidity, and dilution. It has been used satisfactorily in some cooked desserts. However, with high temperatures, a rise in pH, and increased concentration of solution, its sweetness is reduced.

TO SUM UP

Whatever methods or materials we use, one central fact remains: The person who has diabetes is the most important and a fully equal member of the diabetes care team. Interdisciplinary approaches and strategies that involve this recognition can be developed.

Diabetes mellitus is a syndrome composed of many metabolic disorders collectively characterized by hyperglycemia and other symptoms. Treatment relies heavily on a basic type of therapy—a carefully controlled diet. Diabetes is classified in four categories: (1) *T1DM,* (2) *T2DM,* (3) *GDM,* and (4) *prediabetes.*

Blood glucose levels are controlled primarily by hormones of pancreatic islet cells: insulin, which facilitates passage of glucose through cell membranes via special membrane receptors; glucagon, which ensures adequate levels of glucose to prevent hypoglycemia; and somatostatin, which controls the actions of insulin and glucagon to maintain normal blood glucose levels. Diabetes results from inadequate insulin secretion or insulin resistance from too few receptor sites. Symptoms range from polydipsia, polyuria, polyphagia, and signs of abnormal energy metabolism to fluid and electrolyte imbalances, acidosis, and coma in seriously uncontrolled conditions.

T1DM affects about 5% to 10% of all persons with diabetes. It often develops during childhood or adolescence. Treatment involves blood glucose self-monitoring, insulin administration, and regular meals and exercise to balance insulin activity. T2DM occurs mostly in adults, particularly those who are overweight. Acidosis is rare. Treatment consists of weight management and exercise. The food plan for both types of diabetes should be low in saturated fats and cholesterol to reduce cardiovascular risk. Moderate regular exercise increases efficiency of insulin and aids in weight management. GDM occurs in 2% to 5% of all pregnancies.

QUESTIONS FOR REVIEW

1. Describe the major characteristics of T1DM and T2DM. Explain how these characteristics influence differences in NT. List and describe medications used to control these conditions.
2. Identify and explain symptoms of uncontrolled diabetes mellitus.
3. Describe three major complications of uncontrolled diabetes and therapy used in the DCCT designed to achieve and maintain normal blood glucose levels and help avoid these complications.
4. Glenn just found out that he has diabetes mellitus. He is a sedentary, 45-year-old man who is 170 cm (5 feet, 8 inches) tall and weighs 94 kg (210 lb). No medications were prescribed for him. What is his BMI? If he decides to drink, then how much alcohol could be allowed and how should he fit it into his diet? Defend your answer. Glenn wants to help his children reduce their chances of developing diabetes. What advice would you offer?

REFERENCES

1. Centers for Disease Control and Prevention: *National diabetes fact sheet: general information and national estimates on diabetes in the United States, 2007*, Atlanta, 2008, U.S. Department of Health and Human Services, Centers for Disease Control and Prevention. Retrieved May 23, 2009, from www.cdc.gov/diabetes/pubs/pdf/ndfs_2007.pdf.
2. American Diabetes Association: Diagnosis and classification of diabetes mellitus, *Diabetes Care* 32(Suppl 1):S62, 2009.
3. American Diabetes Association: *The cost of diabetes*, Alexandria, Va, 2007, American Diabetes Association. Retrieved July 13, 2010, from http://www.diabetes.org/advocate/resources/cost-of-diabetes.html.
4. Whitehouse FW: Classification and pathogenesis of the diabetes syndrome: a historical perspective, *J Am Diet Assoc* 81(3):243, 1982.
5. Nestle M: A case of diabetes mellitus, *N Engl J Med* 81:127, 1982.
6. Bliss M: *The discovery of insulin*, Chicago, 1982, University of Chicago Press.
7. Atkinson MA, Maclaren NK: The pathogenesis of insulin dependent diabetes, *N Engl J Med* 331:1428, 1994.
8. McKeigue PM, Shah B, Marmot MG: Relation of central obesity and insulin resistance with high diabetes prevalence and cardiovascular risk in South Asians, *Lancet* 337:382, 1991.
9. Dowse GK, Zimmet PZ, Gareeboo H, et al: Abdominal obesity and physical inactivity as risk factors for NIDDM and impaired glucose tolerance in Indian, Creole, and Chinese Mauritians, *Diabetes Care* 14(4):271, 1991.
10. National Diabetes Education Program: *Overview of diabetes in children and adolescents*, Washington, DC, May 2008, U.S. Department of Health and Human Services. Retrieved May 23, 2009 from www.ndep.nih.gov/diabetes/youth/youth_FS.htm#IdentifyingType2.
11. American Diabetes Association: Standards of medical care in diabetes—2008, *Diabetes Care* 31(Suppl 1):S12, 2008.
12. Dabelea D, Snell-Bergeon JK, Heartsfield CL, et al: Increasing prevalence of gestational diabetes mellitus (GDM) over time and by birth cohort, *Diabetes Care* 28:579, 2005.
13. Tuomilehto J, Lindstrom J, Eriksson JG, et al: Prevention of type 2 diabetes mellitus by changes in lifestyle among subjects with impaired glucose tolerance, *N Engl J Med* 344:1343-1350, 2001.
14. Pan XR, Li GW, Hu YH, et al: Effects of diet and exercise in preventing NIDDM in people with impaired glucose tolerance: the Da Qing IGT and Diabetes Study, *Diabetes Care* 20:537, 1997.
15. Wendorf M, Goldfine ID: Archeology of NIDDM—excavation of the thrifty genotype, *Diabetes* 40:161, 1991.
16. Diabetes Control and Complications Trial Research Group: The effect of intensive treatment of diabetes on the development and progression of long-term complications in insulin-dependent diabetes mellitus, *N Engl J Med* 329:977, 1993.
17. Franz MJ, Bantle JP, Beebe CA, et al: Evidence-based nutrition principles and recommendations for the treatment and prevention of diabetes and related complications, *Diabetes Care* 25:148, 2002.
18. American Diabetes Association: Translation of the diabetes nutrition recommendations for health care institutions, *Diabetes Care* 25(Suppl):S61, 2002.
19. American Diabetes Association: Nutrition recommendations and interventions for diabetes, *Diabetes Care* 31(Suppl):S61, 2008.
20. American Diabetes Association: Implications of the Diabetes Control and Complications Trial (position statement), *Diabetes Care* 25:S25, 2002.
21. Delahanty LM, Halford BN: The role of diet behaviors in achieving improved glycemic control in intensively treated patients in the Diabetes Control and Complications Trial, *Diabetes Care* 16:1453, 1993.

22. Harris MI, Eastman RC: Is there a glycemic threshold for mortality risk? *Diabetes Care* 21:331, 1998.
23. The Oxford Center for Diabetes, Endocrinology and Metabolism Diabetes Trials Unit: *UK prospective diabetes study*, Oxford, England, 1998, Oxford Center for Diabetes, Endocrinology and Metabolism. Retrieved January 17, 2006, from http://www.dtu.ox.ac.uk/ukpds_trial/index.php.
24. Robertson KE: What the UKPDS really says about cardiovascular disease and glycemic control, *Clin Diabetes* 17:109, 1999.
25. Ousman Y, Sharma M: The irrefutable importance of glycemic control, *Clin Diabetes* 19:71, 2001.
26. American Diabetes Association: Implications of the United Kingdom Prospective Diabetes Study (position statement), *Diabetes Care* 25:S28, 2002.
27. Thomas AM, Gutierrez YM: *American Dietetic Association guide to gestational diabetes mellitus*, Chicago, 2005, American Dietetic Association.
28. American Diabetes Association: Gestational diabetes mellitus (position statement), *Diabetes Care* 27(Suppl):88S, 2004.
29. Anderson EJ, Richardson M, Castle G, et al: The DCCT Research Group: nutrition interventions for the intensive therapy in the Diabetes Control and Complications Trial, *J Am Diet Assoc* 93(7):768, 1993.
30. Metzger BE, Coustan DR, editors: *Proceedings of the Fourth International Workshop Conference on Gestational Diabetes Mellitus, Diabetes Care*, vol 21 (Suppl), 1998, p 1B.
31. Ross TA, Boucher JL, O'Connell BS: *American Dietetic Association guide to diabetes medical nutrition therapy and education*, Chicago, 2005, American Dietetic Association.
32. American Diabetes Association: *Alcohol*, Alexandria, Va, American Diabetes Association. Retrieved July 13, 2010, from http://www.diabetes.org/food-and-fitness/food/what-can-i-eat/alcohol.html.
33. Joslin Diabetes Center: *Managing diabetes: fitting alcohol into your meal plan*, Boston, 2006, Joslin Diabetes Center. Retrieved May 29, 2009, from http://www.joslin.org/info/Fitting_Alcohol_Into_Your_Meal_Plan.html.

FURTHER READINGS AND RESOURCES

Websites of Interest

American Association of Diabetes Educators (AADE). As a multidisciplinary organization of health professionals who teach about diabetes, the AADE and its website provide information about the scope of practice and standards related to diabetes education; the website also has information and AADE publications: www.aadenet.org.

American Diabetes Association. The American Diabetes Association publishes many health professional and client materials in addition to its scientific journals; in an annual supplement to *Diabetes Care,* the American Diabetes Association reissues its practice guidelines that address a wide array of clinical issues, including nutrition; these guidelines can be downloaded from the American Diabetes Association website free of charge; local information about American Diabetes Association activities can be obtained from either the website or the 800 number; diabetes self-management educational programs that are reviewed and receive American Diabetes Association "recognition" are covered by Medicare and other third-party payers: www.diabetes.org (1-800-DIABETES).

Centers for Disease Control and Prevention, National Center for Chronic Disease Prevention and Health Promotion, Diabetes Public Health Resource. This site has information about the Diabetes Control Program in each state and diabetes-related statistics such as the rise in the prevalence and incidence of diabetes; the National Diabetes Fact Sheet *CDC Information* is available as a downloadable file: www.cdc.gov/diabetes (1-877-CDC-DIAB).

Diabetes Care and Education (DCE) Practice Group of the American Dietetic Association (ADA). The DCE publishes *On the Cutting Edge*, a theme-centered newsletter on timely topics related to nutrition and diabetes; educational materials developed by the DCE are available for purchase from the American Diabetes Association; the DCE website provides information about the Medicare MNT benefits for persons with diabetes, Health Care Financing Administration (HFCA) rules for American Diabetes Association Education Recognition Programs reimbursement, and Current Procedural Terminology (CPT) codes for MNT; the website also provides information about the DCE publications and e-mail listserv: www.dce.org. www.eatright.org.

National Diabetes Education Program (NDEP). The NDEP is a federally sponsored initiative that involves public and private partnerships to improve the treatment and outcomes for people with diabetes through a variety of activities; the NDEP publications include a newsletter, materials for people with diabetes (in several languages), materials for health care providers, materials for organizations, and media kits; single copies of most materials are available free of charge or can be downloaded from the NDEP website: www.ndep.nih.gov (1-800-860-8747).

National Institutes of Diabetes and Digestive and Kidney Diseases (NIDDK), National Diabetes Information Clearinghouse (NDIC). The NIDDK website provides information about its diabetes-related clinical trials and other research programs, a directory of diabetes organizations, health education programs, and diabetes-related topics; downloadable files include *Diabetes Dateline,* a NIDDK newsletter; client education materials; and information for health professionals; the NIDDK website also includes the National Diabetes Information Clearinghouse, which disseminates information about online and print materials and provides access to database searches for diabetes-related references: www.niddk.nih.gov.

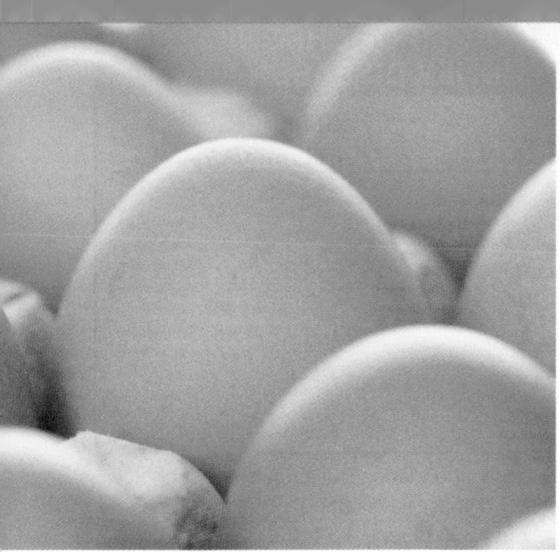

23

Renal Disease

Sara Long Roth

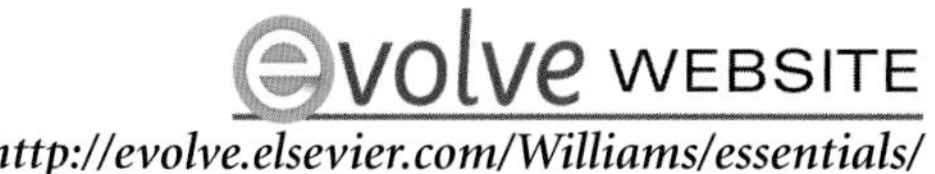

http://evolve.elsevier.com/Williams/essentials/

OUTLINE

This chapter reviews basic kidney function and pathophysiology of kidney diseases. Nutrition assessment methodology and nutritional recommendations for chronic kidney disease (CKD), maintenance dialysis therapy, postrenal transplantation, acute renal failure (ARF), renal stones, and urinary tract infection (UTI) are discussed.

BASIC KIDNEY FUNCTION

Main functions of the kidney are excretory, regulatory, and endocrine. The excretory function serves to remove potentially toxic metabolic waste products such as urea, major end product of protein metabolism, from the blood. The regulatory function controls electrolyte, acid-base, and fluid balance. The result is maintenance of proper serum concentrations of sodium, potassium, calcium, phosphorus, chloride, bicarbonate, and hydrogen ions. The endocrine functions include conversion of the biologically inactive form of vitamin D (25-hydroxycholecaliciferol) to the biologically active vitamin D (1,25-dihydroxycholecalciferol), synthesis of erythropoietin (needed for red blood cell production in the bone marrow), and synthesis and release of renin, which regulates systemic blood pressure.[1]

These functions are accomplished by the unique architecture of the **nephron**, the basic functioning unit of the kidney. Each human adult kidney consists of approximately 1 million nephrons (Figure 23-1). The key structures of the nephron are the glomerulus and the tubules.

Glomerulus

At the head of each nephron, blood enters in a single capillary and then branches into a group of collateral capillaries. This tuft of collateral capillaries is held closely together in a cup-shaped membrane. This cup-shaped capsule is named *Bowman's capsule* for the young English physician Sir William Bowman. In 1843 Bowman established the basis of plasma filtration and consequent urine secretion from the interrelationship of blood-filled glomeruli and enveloping membrane. The filtrate formed here is cell free and virtually protein free.

> **KEY TERMS**
>
> **nephron** Microscopic anatomic and functional unit of the kidney that selectively filters and resorbs essential blood factors, secretes hydrogen ions as needed for maintaining acid-base balance, and then resorbs water to protect body fluids and forms and excretes a concentrated urine for elimination of wastes. The nephron includes the renal corpuscle (glomerulus), the proximal convoluted tubule, the loop of Henle, the distal convoluted tubule, and the collecting tubule, which empties the urine into the renal medulla. The urine passes into the papilla and then to the pelvis of the kidney. Urine is formed by filtration of blood in the glomerulus and by the selective reabsorption and secretion of solutes by cells that constitute the walls of the renal tubes. Approximately 1 million nephrons exist in each kidney.

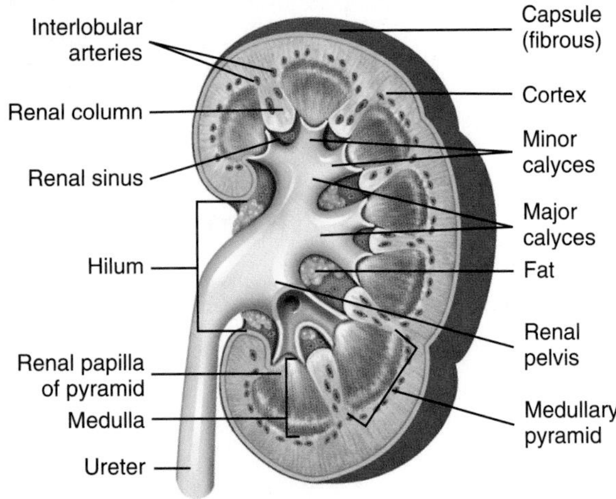

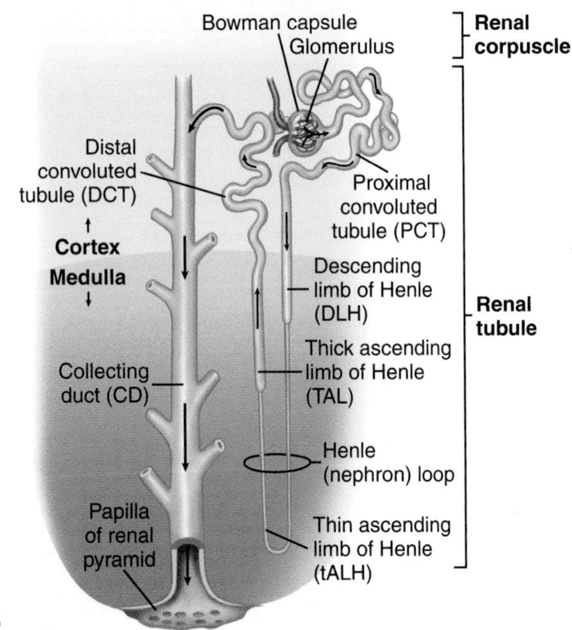

FIGURE 23-1 A, Kidney structure. **B,** Components of nephron. (From Thibodeau GA, Patton KT: *Anatomy & physiology,* ed 7, St Louis, 2010, Mosby.)

Tubules

Continuous with the base of Bowman's capsule, nephron tubules wind in a series of convolutions toward their terminal in the renal pelvis. The following list details specific reabsorption functions performed by the four sections of the tubule:

1. *Proximal tubule:* In the first section nearest the glomerulus, major nutrient reabsorption occurs. Essentially, 100% of the glucose and amino acids and 80% to 85% of the water, sodium, potassium, chloride, and most other substances are reabsorbed. Only 15% to 30% of the filtrate remains to enter the next section.
2. *Loop of Henle:* This narrowed midsection of the renal tubule is named for the German anatomist Friedrich Henle, who in 1845 first demonstrated its unique structure and function in creating the necessary fluid pressures for ultimately forming concentrated urine. At this narrowed midsection, the thin loop of the tubule dips into the central renal **medulla.** Here, through a balanced system of water and sodium exchange through sodium pumps in the limbs of the loop (the countercurrent system), important fluid density is created surrounding the loop. This area of increased density in the central part of the kidney is important to concentrate urine through osmotic pressure because the lower collecting tubule later passes through this same area of the kidney.
3. *Distal tubule:* This latter portion of tubule functions primarily in providing acid-base balance through secretion of ionized hydrogen. It also conserves sodium by reabsorbing it under the influence of the hormones aldosterone and vasopressin (also called *antidiuretic hormone* [ADH]).
4. *Collecting tubule:* In this final widened section of the tubule, filtrate is concentrated to save water and form urine for excretion. Water is absorbed under the influence of pituitary hormone vasopressin (ADH) and osmotic pressure of the denser surrounding fluid in this central part of the kidney. Resulting volume of urine, now concentrated and excreted, is only 0.5% to 1% of the original water and solutes filtered at the beginning in Bowman's capsule.

It is through these specialized anatomic components that the kidney serves to maintain homeostasis of the body's internal environment.[1]

TABLE 23-1 STAGES OF CHRONIC KIDNEY DISEASE*

STAGE	DESCRIPTION	GFR RANGE (mL/min/1.73 m²)
1	Kidney damage with normal or ↑ GFR	≥90
2	Kidney damage with mild ↓ GRF	60-89
3	Moderate ↓ GFR	30-59
4	Severe ↓ GFR	15-29
5	Kidney failure	<15 (or dialysis)

Modified from National Kidney Foundation: K/DOQI clinical practice guidelines for chronic kidney disease: evaluation, classification and stratification, *Am J Kidney Dis* 399 (suppl 1):S1, 2002.
GFR, Glomerular filtration rate; *CKD,* chronic kidney disease.
*CKD is defined as either kidney damage or GFR <60 mL/min/1.73 m² for ≥3 months. Kidney damage is defined as pathologic abnormalities or markers of damage, including abnormalities in blood or urine tests or imaging studies.

CHRONIC KIDNEY DISEASE

CKD is a syndrome in which progressive, irreversible losses of excretory, endocrine, and metabolic capacities of the kidney occur as a result of kidney damage (Table 23-1). Determination of renal function requires evaluation of glomerular filtration rate (GFR), which is accomplished through clearance tests. Clearance tests measure the rate at which substances are cleared from the plasma by the glomerulus.

CASE STUDY

The Patient with Chronic Renal Failure

Mr. Steinberg is 45 years old, married, and works as a city planner for a large municipal government. He cited a recent history of nausea, anorexia, **hematuria,** and swollen ankles during a physical examination. His wife reported that he had been tiring more easily than usual during the past year. A history of prior illnesses proved negative, except for a severe case of influenza with sore throat 10 years before during an epidemic when he was stationed with the Army overseas. Tests were ordered, and the patient was advised to return in 1 week for review of the test results (and sooner if any changes in his symptoms were noted).

Mr. Steinberg did return, with additional symptoms of headaches and occasionally blurred vision. At that time his blood pressure was 160/98 mm Hg, his temperature was 37.5° C (99.6° F), and he had lost 4 kg (8¾ lb). Laboratory tests showed albumin and red and white blood cells in the urine, with an elevated **blood urea nitrogen (BUN);** a phenolsulfonphthalein (PSP) test indicated a reduced filtration rate. The diagnosis was chronic renal failure.

The physician discussed the diagnosis and its serious prognosis with Mr. and Mrs. Steinberg, giving them benefits and disadvantages of **hemodialysis** and kidney transplantation. Antihypertensive medication was prescribed along with other drugs to minimize discomfort.

During the following weeks Mr. Steinberg continued to lose weight, had increasing joint pain, and became anemic. He found it increasingly difficult to maintain his hectic schedule of frequent meetings, conferences, and public speeches because of gastrointestinal (GI) bleeding, increasing nausea, and occasional muscle spasms. Small mouth sores made eating very difficult.

Finally the Steinbergs informed the physician of their decision to accept the kidney transplant as a means of controlling the disease process. They were referred to the registered dietitian (RD) for renal diet counseling to control protein, sodium, potassium, phosphate, and fluids, as well as to ensure adequate kilocalorie (kcalories or kcal) intake. After discussing these needs for nutritional maintenance before surgery, the RD helped them develop a meal plan based on Mr. Steinberg's food preferences. Food selection and preparation were discussed in detail, with many ideas for building in as much variety and taste appeal as possible.

The Steinbergs follow-up with the food plan was excellent. One month later the laboratory values were almost normal, blood pressures averaged 140/88 mm Hg, the headaches and blurred vision had virtually disappeared, and Mr. Steinberg had gained 3.2 kg (7 lb) of his lost weight. The nutrient supplements, including the amino acid analogues, were taken each day as instructed.

Fortunately a kidney donor was soon found, and with the aid of drug control of immune responses the transplant surgery was apparently a success. Mr. Steinberg convalesced well at home, kept all follow-up visits with the health care team, and has continued to be asymptomatic 1 year after surgery.

Questions for Analysis

1. Identify a metabolic imbalance caused by chronic renal failure that may account for each symptom presented by Mr. Steinberg.
2. What factors affect the amount of protein needed by persons with chronic renal failure? What amounts are usually used? Why? What are the amino acid analogues used with the low-protein diet, and why are they used?
3. What factors affect the amount of sodium needed by persons with chronic renal failure? How much is usually recommended?
4. Why is it important to control potassium levels? How much is recommended? What clinical signs presented by Mr. Steinberg may indicate that he had not been getting enough potassium?
5. Why is control of phosphate important in the diet for chronic renal failure? What additional means may be used to control it?
6. What factors affect fluid balance in chronic renal failure? How much is usually allowed?
7. Outline a general teaching plan you would use to instruct the Steinbergs about the presurgical and postsurgical dietary needs.

In clinical practice, GFR is best approximated by using prediction equations and factoring in serum creatinine concentration, age, gender, race, and body size. Recommended prediction equations for adults are the Modification of Diet in Renal Disease (MDRD) study and Cockcroft-Gault equations.[2] A normal GFR is 125 mL/min/1.73 m^2. As kidney disease progresses, GFR falls. Chronic renal failure progresses slowly over time and may include periods during which kidney function remains stable. However, once the disease progresses to stage 5 kidney failure, continuance of life requires initiation of maintenance **dialysis** therapy or subsequent kidney transplantation[3] (see the *Case Study* box, "The Patient with Chronic Renal Failure").

CKD is a public health problem. Incidence and prevalence of end-stage renal disease (ESRD) have increased 20% to 25% in the United States during the past decade.[4] Of the group being treated by dialysis, 97 per million were older than age 70, compared with 2.1 per million who were children[5] (see the *Focus on Culture* box, "Kidney Failure: Another Equal

KEY TERMS

medulla Inner tissue substance of the kidney.

hematuria The abnormal presence of blood in the urine.

blood urea nitrogen (BUN) The nitrogen component of urea in the blood; a measure of kidney function; elevated levels of BUN indicate a disorder of kidney function.

hemodialysis Removal of certain elements from the blood according to their rates of diffusion through a semipermeable membrane (e.g., by a hemodialysis machine).

dialysis Process of separating crystalloids and colloids in solution by the difference in their rates of diffusion through a semipermeable membrane; crystalloids pass through readily, and colloids pass through only very slowly or not at all.

FOCUS ON CULTURE

Kidney Failure: Another Equal Opportunity Disease?

Of the millions of Americans currently living with kidney disease, a disproportionate number are African American. This reflects an incidence rate fourfold greater than that of their European-American counterparts and is most commonly attributed to increased prevalence of high blood pressure, diabetes, and a familial history of the disease. However, not only are African Americans at an increased risk for developing kidney disease but also they seem to acquire it earlier in life, with almost half not knowing they have the condition until dialysis is required.

This is a startling realization, considering early interventions can limit damage done to the kidneys. Later diagnosis of kidney disease can result in increased rates of chronic problems, dialysis dependency, and need for transplantation. The difficulty is that relatively few African Americans receive screening or intervention. Adding to the problem, with diabetes being the primary risk factor for kidney disease, one third of the cases of diabetes among African Americans go undiagnosed, demonstrating the need for further screening.

According to the National Kidney Foundation, African Americans represent 13% of the American population but make up 35% of those on kidney transplant waiting lists. Consequently, although an increased kidney transplant demand exists for African Americans, a moderately low donorship rate is seen from this group, compounding the problem.

The following five primary reasons influence low African-American kidney donorship:

1. Lack of transplant awareness
2. Religious myths and misconceptions
3. Distrust of the medical community
4. Fear of premature declaration of death after signing a donor card
5. Fear of potential preference for races other than African Americans

Whether the increased rate of kidney disease in African Americans stems from lack of awareness, lack of health care, or genetic factors, the fact remains that African Americans possess many risk factors affecting renal health. Screenings and education about blood glucose and blood pressure control at a younger age, along with lifestyle and medication interventions, have been shown to have dramatic results in kidney health. Unfortunately, only a small percentage actually receives these screenings or treatment. This problem is a major one that is made all the more disheartening by the unnecessary suffering involved. It is hoped that with increased attention brought to kidney disease, the incidence rate in the African-American population will decline.

BIBLIOGRAPHY

Freedman B, Spray BJ, Tuttle AB, et al: The familial risk of end-stage renal disease in African Americans, *Am J Kidney Dis* 21(4):387, 1993.

National Kidney Foundation: *Diabetes, chronic kidney disease and special populations*, New York. Available at http://www.kidney.org/professionals/tools/diabetesandckd.cfm.

National Kidney and Urologic Diseases Information Clearinghouse, National Institute of Diabetes and Digestive and Kidney Diseases, National Institutes of Health: *Strategic plan on minority health disparities*, Bethesda, Md. Available at http://www2.niddk.nih.gov/AboutNIDDK/ReportsAndStrategicPlanning/Strategic_Plan_Minority_Health_Disparities.htm.

Reif M, Hall P: *Kidney failure among African Americans*, Cincinnati, Ohio, 2001, Net Wellness. Retrieved June 19, 2009, from www.netwellness.org/healthtopics/kidney/faq2.cfm.

Tarver-Carr M, Powe NR, Eberhardt MS, et al: Excess risk of chronic kidney disease among African-American versus white subjects in the United States: a population-based study of potential explanatory factors, *J Am Soc Nephrol* 13:2363, 2002.

Opportunity Disease?"). The total cost for the CKD program continues to increase.

The most common causes of CKD are diabetic nephropathy and hypertension. Other common causes of kidney failure include glomerulonephritis, cystic kidney disease, and urologic disease.[4] Table 23-1 outlines the stages of chronic kidney disease.

PATHOPHYSIOLOGY OF GLOMERULAR DISEASE

The majority of nondiabetic glomerular diseases are the result of immune-mediated mechanisms. Although renal injury induced by antibody alone is known to occur, mechanisms involved in renal injury resulting from antigen-antibody complex formation are better understood. Antigen-antibody complex formation occurs as a result of antibody reacting either to circulating antigens or to native kidney antigens expressed on renal cell membranes. Immune complex deposition may occur within the glomerular basement membrane (GBM), between the GBM and epithelial cell (subepithelial), between the GBM and endothelial cell (subendothelial), or within the mesangial matrix. The pattern of immune complex deposition within the glomerulus is helpful diagnostically because different diseases have characteristic patterns.[4,8] For example, membranous nephropathy is characterized in part by subepithelial immune complex deposition (Figures 23-2 and 23-3).

Deposition of immune complexes leads to activation of the complement system, which mediates injury

KEY TERMS

glomerulonephritis A form of nephritis affecting the capillary loops in an acute short-term infection. It may progress to a more serious chronic condition leading to irreversible renal failure.

complement A complex series of enzymatic proteins occurring in normal serum that interact to combine with and augment (fill out, complete) the antigen-antibody complex of the body's immune system, producing lysis when the antigen is an intact cell; composed of 11 discrete proteins or functioning components, activated by the immunoglobulin factors IgG and IgM.

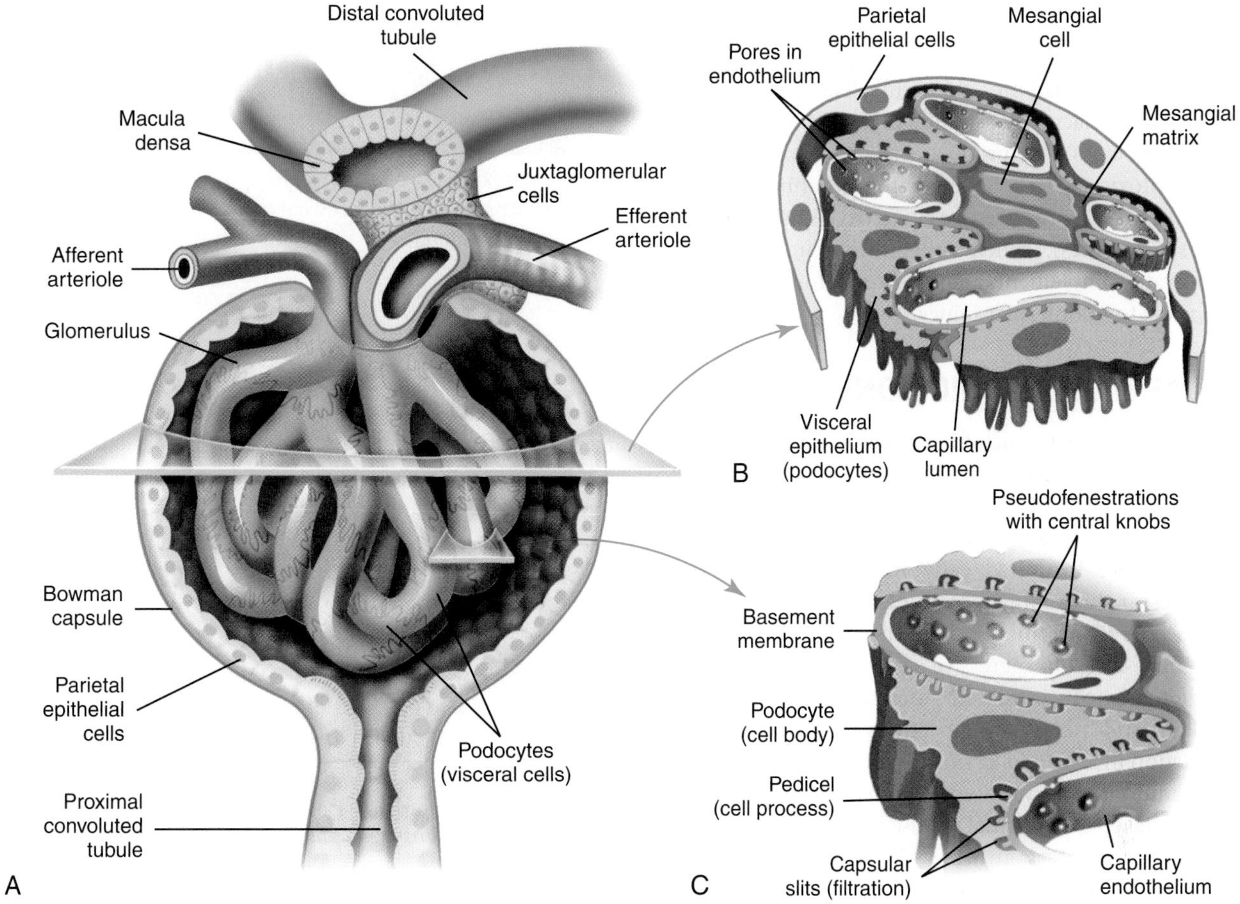

FIGURE 23-2 Anatomy of the glomerulus and juxtaglomerular apparatus. **A,** Longitudinal cross-section of glomerulus and juxtaglomerular apparatus. **B,** Horizontal cross-section of glomerulus. **C,** Enlargement of glomerular capillary filtration membrane. (From McCance K, Huether S: *Pathophysiology: the biologic basis for disease in adults and children,* ed 5, St Louis, 2006, Mosby.)

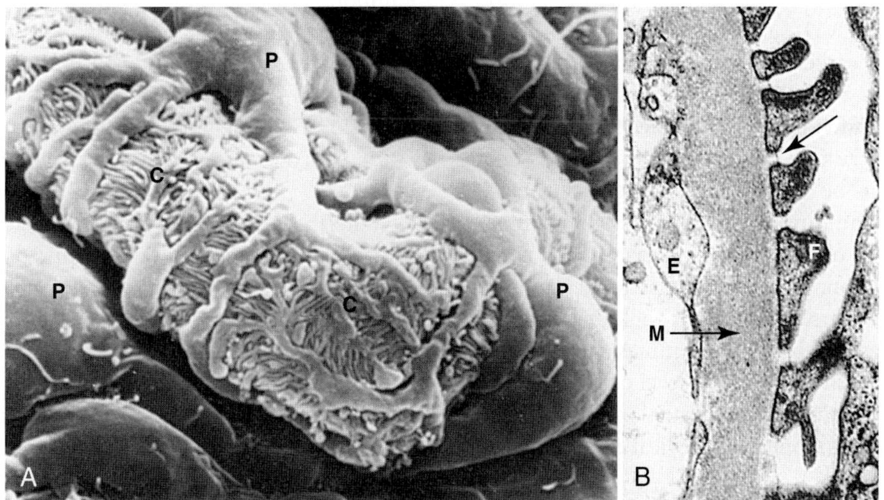

FIGURE 23-3 Glomerular capillary. **A,** Scanning electron micrograph of normal glomerular capillary *(C)* enclosed by podocytes *(P)* with primary processes and interdigitating foot processes. **B,** Glomerular capillary wall showing foot processes of endothelial podocytes *(F)*, filtration slit membrane (*arrow*), basement membrane *(M)*, and fenestrated endothelium *(E)* (magnification, ×40,000). (From Kissane JM, editor: *Anderson's pathology,* ed 9, St Louis, 1990, Mosby.)

through inflammatory or noninflammatory mechanisms. Chemotactic complement components formed as products of the activated complement cascade result in the migration of inflammatory cells into glomeruli. These cells, which include platelets, macrophages, and polymorphonuclear neutrophils (leukocytes), all produce products that are either directly cytotoxic or serve as mediators for further cell or matrix injury (e.g., proteases, reactive oxygen species, lipid mediators, cytokines). When subepithelial immune complexes activate complement, a noninflammatory mechanism is responsible for glomerular injury.[7]

TREATMENT OF CHRONIC KIDNEY DISEASE

The approach to treatment of CKD has shifted focus from diagnosis and treatment of established kidney diseases to detection and treatment at much earlier stages.[5] The clinical course of this disease can be significantly improved if specific interventions are instituted early in development of the disease. These include annual screening for microalbuminuria (>30 mg/day or 20 mcg/min of albumin in the urine); improving glycemic control; aggressive antihypertensive therapy with angiotensin-converting enzymes or angiotensin receptor blockers; and lifestyle modifications that include weight loss, reduction in salt and alcohol intake, and exercise.[6]

Less traditional interventions that have been explored for their beneficial effects on renal disease include nutrients such as amino acids and carbohydrates. A class of nutrients that continues to be investigated for potential benefits on progression of renal disease is omega-3 fatty acids (see Health Promotion later in this chapter).

Through their initiative, titled *K/DOQI: Kidney Disease Outcomes Quality Initiative,* the National Kidney Foundation recently published clinical practice guidelines for evaluation, classification, and stratification of CKD.[5] A main rationale for development of these clinical guidelines was accumulation of evidence that adverse effects of CKD including kidney failure, cardiovascular disease (CVD), and premature death can be prevented or delayed by earlier testing and treatment of CKD.[5]

K/DOQI guidelines for CKD recommend that during health evaluations all individuals be evaluated as to whether they are at increased risk of having or developing renal disease. Patients are to be considered at risk if they have diabetes, hypertension, autoimmune diseases, systemic infections, exposure to drugs or procedures associated with acute decline in kidney function, recovery from acute kidney failure, age greater than 60 years, family history of kidney disease, or reduced kidney mass.[5] Table 23-1 identifies the stages of disease and associates each stage with a level of GFR. As the GFR falls below 60 mL/min/1.73 m^2, nutrition intervention becomes an important component of medical care.

NUTRITION ASSESSMENT OF PATIENTS WITH CHRONIC KIDNEY DISEASE

Malnutrition is a significant comorbidity of CKD, including patients on hemodialysis or peritoneal dialysis therapy.[8] Life-threatening malnutrition is present in 5% to 10% of patients, and moderate malnutrition is present in an additional 20% to 40%.[9] Factors contributing to malnutrition in patients with renal failure are listed in Box 23-1.

BOX 23-1 FACTORS CONTRIBUTING TO THE PRESENCE OF MALNUTRITION IN PATIENTS WITH CHRONIC RENAL FAILURE

1. Anorexia as a result of the following:
   - Nausea, emesis, medications
   - Uremia/uremic state of metabolism
   - Underdialysis
   - Accumulation of uremic toxins not completely removed by dialysis
2. Metabolic acidosis
3. Endocrine disorders (insulin resistance, hyperparathyroidism, impaired response to insulin-like growth factor I)
4. Comorbidity (infections, intercurrent illnesses)
5. Reduced nutrient intake
6. Dialysis related to the following:
   - Inadequate dose of dialysate
   - Catabolism (bioincompatible membrane)
   - Loss of amino acids and protein to the dialysate
   - Dialysate reused with bleach
7. Psychosocial
   - Depression
   - Inability to purchase or prepare food adequately
   - Loss of or poorly fitting dentures

From Wolfson M: Causes, manifestations, and assessment of malnutrition in chronic renal failure. In Kopple JD, Massry SG, editors: *Nutrition management of renal disease,* ed 2, Philadelphia, 2004, Lippincott Williams & Wilkins.

Evaluating and monitoring nutritional status are vital components of nutrition care of patients with kidney disease. High prevalence of malnutrition, large number of aberrations in normal metabolism, and complications including anorexia and catabolism all indicate need for consistent monitoring. Nutrition assessment is best completed by a registered dietitian (RD) who has received special training in renal nutrition care.

When completing a nutrition assessment, an array of indexes, each representing a specific data category, are mea-

KEY TERMS

peritoneal dialysis Dialysis through the peritoneum into and out of the peritoneal cavity.

hyperparathyroidism Abnormally increased activity of the parathyroid gland, resulting in excessive secretion of parathyroid hormone (PTH), which usually helps regulate serum calcium levels in balance with vitamin D hormone; excess secretion occurs when the serum calcium level falls below normal, as in chronic renal disease or in vitamin D deficiency.

TABLE 23-2 **NUTRITION ASSESSMENT PARAMETERS IN CHRONIC KIDNEY DISEASE**

PARAMETER	WHAT IT MEASURES	COMPONENTS
History and physical examination	Past and present nutritional status; areas that should be addressed when developing a plan of care	Review of medical record Patient, family, and/or caregiver interview Psychosocial history Ability to obtain, prepare, ingest, and enjoy food Mental status Educational level Functional status Person responsible for shopping/preparing food Patient's functional status (activities of daily living) Diet histories: usual food intake, food intake patterns, and factors affecting intake Religious/cultural beliefs Use of supplements and alternative or complementary therapies Past diet restrictions (and education) Patient's ability to chew, swallow, taste, and smell foods Changes in appetite and eating pattern Food preferences, allergies, and intolerances Use of alcohol Practice of pica
Anthropometric assessment	Weight status; nutritional status; distribution of body fat, lean muscle mass, and bone	Body weight (can be difficult to determine because of fluid retention) Estimated dry weight or edema-free body weight Hemodialysis: weight postdialysis Peritoneal dialysis: weight after drainage of dialysate with peritoneum empty Interdialytic weight gains Fluid gains between hemodialysis treatments Height Initial measurement essential Recumbent bed height, arm span, or knee height may be used if patient cannot stand Estimation of frame size Body mass index Estimate of body composition Skinfold thicknesses
Energy and nutrient requirements	Must be individually assessed based on type of dialysis, cause of kidney disease, and other comorbidities	Kcalories per kg formulas
Subjective global assessment	Useful measure of protein-energy nutritional status in maintenance dialysis patients	4-item, 7-point scale Medical history Weight change during previous 6 months Dietary intake Gastrointestinal symptoms Physical examination Visual assessment of subcutaneous tissue and muscle mass
Biochemical parameters	Monitored on ongoing basis to assess nutritional status	See Table 23-3

Data from Barbá PD, Goode JL: Nutrition assessment in chronic kidney disease. In Byham-Gray L, Wiesen K, editors: *A clinical guide to nutrition care in kidney disease,* Chicago, 2004, American Dietetic Association.

sured independently and then evaluated collectively to ascertain nutritional status of the renal patient. Table 23-2 lists the data categories that encompass the nutrition assessment of the renal patient. Specific indexes used to evaluate biochemical values are listed in Table 23-3. Following is a review of indexes most commonly measured from each data category.[10]

TABLE 23-3 BIOCHEMICAL PARAMETERS FOR ASSESSING NUTRITIONAL STATUS

PARAMETER	SUBSTANCE	NORMAL RANGE	CKD RANGE
Visceral protein stores	Albumin	3.5-5.0 g/dL	WNL for laboratory or >4.0 g/dL
	Prealbumin (transthyretin)	15-36 mg/dL	>30 mg/dL
	Transferrin	Female subjects: 15%-50% Male subjects: 20%-50%	WNL
	C-reactive protein (CRP)	0.8 mg/dL	2-15 mg/dL
Static (somatic) protein reserves	Serum creatinine	Female subjects: 0.5-1.1 mg/dL Male subjects: 0.6-1.2 mg/dL	2-15 mg/dL
Other estimates of protein reserves	Nitrogen balance		
Fluid, electrolyte, and acid-base status	Sodium	135-145 mEq/L	WNL
	Potassium	3.5-5.0 mEq/L	3.5-6.0 mEq/L
	Calcium	WNL for laboratory	Normal: 8.4-10.2 mg/dL; preferably at low end of normal (8.4-9.5 mg/dL)
	Phosphorus	3.0-4.5 mg/dL	3.5-5.5 mg/dL
	CO_2		22-25 mEq/L
	Glucose	70-105 mg/dL	WNL <200 nonfasting before dialysis; intake has influence
Indirect indices of renal function and dialysis adequacy	Serum creatinine	Female subjects: 0.5-1.1 mg/dL Male subjects: 0.6-1.2 mg/dL	2-15 mg/dL
	Blood urea nitrogen (BUN)	10-20 mg/dL	60-80 mg/dL in anuric; well dialyzed and eating adequate protein
	Kt/V (hemodialysis)	N/A	1.2
	Kt/V (peritoneal dialysis)	N/A	2.0-2.2
Anemia	Hemoglobin (Hb)	Female subjects: 12-16 g/dL Male subjects: 14-18 g/dL	Variable: 11-12 g/dL
	Ferritin	Female subjects: 10-150 mg/mL Male subjects: 12-300 mg/mL	≥100 ng/mL, but no know benefit >800
	Serum iron	Female subjects: 50-170 mcg/dL Male subjects: 60-175 mcg/dL	WNL
Hyperlipidemia	Serum cholesterol	<200 mg	WNL <150 mg, evaluate for nutrient deficit
	Triglycerides	Female subjects: 35-135 mg/dL Male subjects: 40-160 mg/dL	WNL <200 mg/dL
Renal osteodystrophy	Calcium	WNL for laboratory	Normal: 8.4-10.2 mg/dL; preferably at low end of normal (8.4-9.5 mg/dL)
	Alkaline phosphatase	30-85 U/mL	WNL for laboratory
	Parathyroid hormone (PHT) (i) intact	10-65 pg/mL	150-300 pg/mL
	Biointact (third generation)	60-140 pg/mL	80-160 pg/mL

Data from Barbá PD, Goode JL: Nutrition assessment in chronic kidney disease. In Byham-Gray L, Wiesen K, editors: *A clinical guide to nutrition care in kidney disease,* Chicago, 2004, American Dietetic Association; Wilkens KG: Medical nutrition therapy for renal disorders. In Mahan LK, Escott-Stump S, editors: *Krause's food & nutrition therapy,* ed 12, St Louis, 2008, Saunders.
CKD, Chronic kidney disease; *WNL,* within normal limits.

History and Physical Examination

Medical History

The medical record should include information concerning comorbid conditions, medications, past hospitalizations, weight history, socioeconomic status, and functional status, as well as information from the physical examination. Record of any major organ or GI diseases, surgeries, or previous symptoms of malabsorption or other digestive problems, including nausea, vomiting, and diarrhea, should be noted. Impairment in fluid and electrolyte balance, hypertension and hypotension, proteinuria, and any previous symptoms of uremia that affect appetite, food intake, digestion, or nutritional status should also be noted.

Psychosocial History

This evaluates patients' mental status, as well as factors regarding economics, education level, physical home environment, food shopping and preparation capabilities, and available support systems. The goal is to create an individualized intervention the patient or patient's support system can understand and apply. Factors that might compromise nutritional status include depression or improper food preparation and storage equipment. This component of the assessment process helps identify patients requiring social services to assist with economic needs or special services to provide regular access to food and medications.

Demographics

Information on age, marital status, gender, and ethnicity is needed to assess nutritional status. Many reference standards used to classify clinical indexes adjust for gender and age. Knowledge of ethnicity affects ability to individualize nutrition therapy; marital status helps identify support systems.

Physical Activity

Assessment of the patient's physical capabilities is needed to maintain activities of daily living (ADLs) and proper level of physical exercise for psychologic and physical therapeutics. The following questionnaires have been validated for the purpose of measuring physical activity and physical functioning in the ESRD patient population: the Stanford 7-Day Physical Activity Recall, Physical Activity Scale for the Elderly, Human Activity Profile, and Medical Outcomes Study Short-Form 36-Item Questionnaire.

Current Medical and Surgical Issues

Identification of nutritional implications of medical and surgical problems is imperative for the nutrition assessment procedure. For the patient with chronic, progressive disease, this requires acknowledgment of any newly diagnosed medical and surgical illnesses.

Diet and Food Intake

This category relies on subjective patient reporting to evaluate qualitative and quantitative aspects of food intake. One of the most useful outputs from this category is calculation of nutrient intake. Other outputs include information related to past and current food intake (qualitative and quantitative), eating patterns, and specific food preferences. This information allows an approximation of the diet's adequacy. It also helps to identify nutrient factors that may be contributing to medical problems. Qualitative data are essential for formulation of individual diet therapy, including meal plans and menus.

Diet History

Nutrition history is usually obtained at the initial meeting. It is an all-inclusive collection of some objective, but primarily subjective, information concerning the patient's food consumption, such as aversions, allergies, preferences, and intake. Information on previous and current diet intake assists in devising interventions to improve diet or devising an acceptable therapeutic meal plan. The most commonly used tools to obtain food intake information differ in approach to data collection, retrospective versus prospective, and whether the information is a qualitative description of intake versus a quantitative one.

Food Record. A food record provides qualitative and approximate quantitative food intake information that is best collected prospectively. The minimal time recommended for data collection is 3 days; a reasonable maximum is 5 days. The patient should provide intake information for weekends and weekdays so that variability can be determined. For the dialysis patient, it is strongly recommended the food record include intake for dialysis, as well as nondialysis days, in addition to weekend versus weekday pattern. A difference in food intake between dialysis and nondialysis days has been noted in type and amount of food selected.

The patient should be provided with instructions on how to approximate food portion sizes and servings of fluid to ensure accurate reporting. Use of food models is very helpful. The food record should include time of day of any intake (meals and snacks), names of foods eaten, approximate amount of food ingested, method of preparation, and special recipes or steps taken in the food preparation. The same instructions apply to fluid intake. Brand names are requested when available.

Some patients find it is more convenient to record food intake at the end of the day. This is an inferior method because the data collection becomes retrospective and more subject to error. Calculation of intake of total protein, protein quality, carbohydrate, fat, fatty acid classes, and other selected nutrients is best completed by a computerized nutrient analysis program.

24-Hour Food Recall. The 24-hour food recall is an interactive tool in which the clinician assists the patient in remembering qualitative and quantitative food intake via prompting. The clinician can sit with a patient during dialysis and slowly help the patient recall the previous day's intake of food and fluid. Food models or drawings can be used to help the patient identify portion size. One 24-hour recall, however, does not provide sufficient information to ascertain total food intake.

A variation of the 24-hour recall for a dialysis patient is to meet with the patient during three consecutive treatments, or at least four sessions within a 2-week period, and obtain one 24-hour recall at each visit. Effort should be made to obtain a recall for a weekend day, a dialysis day, and a nondialysis day. To obtain a total food intake on a dialysis day, the practitioner can ask the patient what he or she had to eat so far that day and record it. The patient or family member can finish recording for the rest of the day, or the clinician can meet with the patient at the next session to help him or her recall what

KEY TERMS

proteinuria The presence of an excess of serum proteins, such as albumin, in the urine.

was eaten for the rest of that day. Calling the patient's home on a daily basis to obtain the needed information is an option but is not practical.

Food Frequency Questionnaires. Food frequency questionnaires (FFQs) approximate nutrient intake by identifying periodicity of intake of specific foods within food groups that are significant sources of a particular nutrient or nutrients (e.g., dairy products are a good source of calcium, vitamin D, and protein). A food frequency consists of listing foods according to group, such as vegetables, fruits, dairy, protein, and so forth. The patient is questioned as to how often he or she eats this food per day, per week, and per month. An approximation of adequacy of intake of specific nutrients can be calculated from the results.

Biochemical Values

Serum biochemical values are used to assess and monitor nutritional status over time. Selected serum values pertain to visceral protein stores, static protein reserves, overall protein nutriture, immune competence, iron stores, as well as vitamin, mineral, and trace element status. In addition to these components, nutrition assessment involves evaluating fluid, electrolyte, and acid-base status; renal function; dialysis adequacy for the patient receiving replacement therapy; serum lipid levels; and bone health.

Visceral Protein Stores

Serum Albumin. Albumin, the most abundant plasma protein, functions to maintain plasma oncotic pressure and serves as a major carrier protein for drugs, hormones, enzymes, and trace elements. Clinically significant hypoalbuminemia occurs with different types of malnutrition besides kidney disease (e.g., protein-energy kwashiorkor, uncomplicated) in children and adults. In these conditions, hypoalbuminemia usually indicates other metabolic derangements, as well as a poor prognosis. From these observations, serum albumin became a part of routine nutrition assessment of the hospitalized patient and subsequently the renal patient.

Although serum albumin levels have been used extensively in clinical practice, research studies, and nutritional surveys to assess nutritional status of the CKD population, reliability and sensitivity of this parameter have been questioned. Concerns are independent of conditions that change serum albumin as a marker of visceral protein stores. Use of albumin for assessment purposes has been criticized because of its long half-life, averaging 14 to 20 days, and large body pool, 4 to 5 mg/kg, making albumin slow to respond to changes in visceral protein stores. It is therefore a late marker of malnutrition.

Prealbumin (Thyroxine-Binding Prealbumin, Transthyretin). Prealbumin is a carrier protein for retinol-binding protein (RBP) and thus has a major role in transport of thyroxine. Its short half-life of 2 to 3 days and its small body pool make it more sensitive than albumin to changes in protein status. This was the first visceral protein found to be low in healthy children who were eating marginal amounts of protein. In primates, prealbumin reflects overall nitrogen balance during starvation and refeeding. Decreases in serum levels occur independently of nutritional status when acute metabolic stress is seen, including trauma, minor stress, and inflammation. Serum concentration has also been observed to decrease in liver disease and with iron supplementation. Prealbumin can be useful as a nutritional marker after acute metabolic stress.

The low molecular weight of prealbumin (approximately 54,980 daltons) precludes its use as a marker of nutritional status in patients with CKD who have a decreased GFR. Prealbumin levels have been reported to be elevated in the euvolemic patient with chronic renal failure. In hemodialysis patients, high levels have been observed and are attributed to decreased renal catabolism. A decline in the proportion of circulating free prealbumin versus that complexed with RBP may explain the diminished catabolism and therefore elevated levels. A concentration of less than 30 mg/dL (normal range, 10 to 40 mg/dL) may indicate malnutrition in the hemodialysis patient and has recently been associated with an increased risk of death. These studies indicate prealbumin level may serve as a better nutrition assessment tool and predictor of patient outcome than the traditionally used serum albumin in the dialysis population.

Transferrin (Siderophilin). The main function of transferrin is to bind ferrous iron and to transport iron to the bone marrow. Its half-life of 8 to 10 days and small body pool enable it to respond more rapidly to short-term changes in protein status, compared with albumin. Its value is influenced by iron pool status and needs to be assessed in conjunction with this value.

C-Reactive Protein. CRP mirrors the acute-phase response to inflammation. Increases are regulated by the rise in circulating cytokines and tumor necrosis factor-α (TNF-α), very powerful determinants of albumin levels in CKD patients.

Body Weight

Initial assessment of body weight and monitoring of weight change over time represent critical components of the nutrition assessment process. Weight loss in excess of 5% to 10%, depending on the patient's overall nutritional status, or substandard weight for height should be considered a risk factor for malnutrition. Interrelationships between weight loss over time and outcome in the renal patient population have not yet been reported.

Body mass index (BMI), current weight, usual weight, ideal body weight (IBW), percent usual weight, percent IBW, and particularly percent weight change over a defined time period are important parameters of body weight. A database or sheet in the patient's chart committed to record body weight is recommended for every patient.

ALTERED NUTRIENT REQUIREMENTS WITH CHRONIC KIDNEY DISEASE

Nutrition intervention for patients with CKD includes modifications for sodium, fluid, potassium, phosphorus, calcium, vitamin D, iron, calories, and protein. Although global recommendations are available, nutrition care must be individualized based on serum chemistry levels, fluid balance, and nutritional status. These concerns are addressed in the following discussion (see the *Diet-Medications Interactions* box, "Common Drugs Used for Renal Disorders and Potential Food-Drug Interactions").

Sodium and Potassium

As kidney function declines, ability of the nephrons to maintain sodium balance through sodium excretion diminishes. However, an adaptive mechanism results in undamaged nephrons being able to excrete an increased percentage of filtered sodium, with the effect being a decrease in the fractional reabsorption and an increase in fractional excretion of sodium by renal tubules. As GFR falls to 10 mL/min, a 2.0- to 3.0-g sodium restriction may be required to maintain sodium and fluid balance. Clinical symptoms of excessive sodium intake include shortness of breath, hypertension, congestive heart failure (CHF), and edema.

Kidney regulation of potassium balance is obtained by renal excretion of potassium in an amount equal to that absorbed by the gastrointestinal (GI) tract. Potassium

DIET-MEDICATIONS INTERACTIONS

Common Drugs Used for Renal Disorders and Potential Food-Drug Interactions

DRUGS	POTENTIAL FOOD DRUG INTERACTIONS, SIDE EFFECTS, AND RECOMMENDATIONS
Pyelonephritis and Urinary Tract Infections	
Ceftriaxone and gentamicin	Sufficient water and fluids should be consumed Monitor glucose changes in persons with diabetes mellitus Avoid use with alcohol
Sulfisoxazole (Gantrisin)	Can deplete folacin and vitamin K
Trimethoprim (Trimpex), trimethoprim/sulfamethoxazole (Bactrim, Septra, Cotrim)	May cause diarrhea, gastrointestinal (GI) distress, stomatitis
Nitrofurantoin (Furadantin, Macrodantin)	Sufficient fluid intake necessary
Quinolones: ofloxacin (Floxin), norfloxacin (Noroxin), ciprofloxacin (Cipro), trovafloxacin (Trovan)	Should be taken with food or milk Adequate dietary protein necessary Nausea, vomiting, anorexia common Milk, yogurt, and calcium supplements should be avoided when taking Cipro; caffeine intake should be limited Floxin should be taken separately from vitamin supplements; nausea one side effect
Urolithiasis/Nephrolithiasis (Kidney Stones)	
Allopurinol (Zyloprim) and probenecid (usually used instead of or in conjunction with purine-restricted diet)	Drink 10-12 glasses of fluid daily Avoid concomitant intake of vitamin C supplements Should maintain alkaline urine Side effects include nausea, vomiting, diarrhea, abdominal pain
Thiazide diuretics	Increase intake of high-potassium foods Control sodium intake Increase magnesium intake Dry mouth or GI distress may occur
D-Penicillamine	Requires vitamin B_6 and zinc supplementation Increase fluid intake with cystinuria Take 1 to 2 hours before/after meals Stomatitis, diarrhea, nausea, vomiting, abdominal pain may occur
Demerol and similar medications	Dry mouth, constipation, nausea, vomiting can occur
Acute Renal Failure	
Exchange resins (Kayexalate)	Take separately from calcium and antacids by several hours
Sorbitol	Bloating, flatulence, diarrhea may occur

Continued

DIET-MEDICATIONS INTERACTIONS

Common Drugs Used for Renal Disorders and Potential Food-Drug Interactions—cont'd

DRUGS	POTENTIAL FOOD DRUG INTERACTIONS, SIDE EFFECTS, AND RECOMMENDATIONS
Chronic Kidney Disease	
Phosphate binders: calcium acetate or calcium carbonate	Nausea/vomiting may occur
Ergocalciferol (vitamin D analogue)	Additional water necessary to prevent constipation Monitor fluids carefully if urine output decreased Avoid long-term use
Recombinant human erythropoietin (r-HuEPO)	Iron supplements necessary Do not take iron supplement at same time as calcium
Hemodialysis	
Kayexalate	Take separately from calcium supplements or antacids
Transplantation (patients are usually on three to four of the five drugs listed following)	
Corticosteroids (Prednisone, Solu-Cortef)	Increased catabolism or proteins Negative nitrogen balance Hyperphagia Ulcers Decreased glucose tolerance Sodium and fluid retention Impaired calcium absorption and osteoporosis Cushing's syndrome Obesity Muscle wasting Increased gastric secretion
Cyclosporine	Nausea, vomiting, diarrhea Hyperlipidemia and hyperkalemia may occur Elevated glucose and lipids
Immunosuppressants (Muromonab, Orthoclone [OKT3], antithymocyte globulin [ATG])	Nausea, anorexia, diarrhea, vomiting
Azathioprine (Imuran)	Fever Stomatitis Leucopenia, thrombocytopenia Oral and esophageal sores Macrocytic anemia Pancreatitis Vomiting, diarrhea Folate supplementation may be needed Dietary modifications (liquid or soft diet, use of oral supplements) may be needed
Tacrolimus (Prograf, FK506)	GI distress, nausea, vomiting, diarrhea Hyperglycemia

Data from Escott-Stump S: *Nutrition and diagnosis-related care,* ed 6, Philadelphia, 2007, Lippincott Williams & Wilkins.

balance is dependent on the ability of the tubules to continue to secrete potassium into the ultrafiltrate. This ability will decrease as kidney failure progresses. As serum potassium levels increase to more than 5.0 mg/dL, dietary potassium restriction to approximately 3 to 4 g/day may be needed.[11]

Phosphorus, Calcium, and Vitamin D

The consequence of abnormalities of calcium, phosphorus, and vitamin D metabolism seen in CKD is development of bone diseases, which are referred to as *renal osteodystrophy*. Diagnoses include osteoporosis, osteosclerosis, osteomalacia, and osteitis fibrosa. The healthy kidney filters about 7 g of

TABLE 23-4 RECOMMENDED DIETARY NUTRIENT INTAKE FOR PATIENTS WITH CHRONIC KIDNEY DISEASE

NUTRIENT	STAGES 1 AND 2	STAGE 3	STAGE 4	STAGE 5
Protein (g/kg/day)	0.75	0.75	0.6	0.6-0.75
Energy (kcal/kg/day)	Based on energy expenditure	Based on energy expenditure	30-35 kcal/kg/day	30-35 kcal/kg/day
Sodium (mg/day)	1-4 g/day, depending on comorbidities	1-4 g/day, depending on comorbidities	1-4 g/day, depending on comorbidities	1-4 g/day, depending on comorbidities
Potassium (mEq/day)	Usually no restriction unless serum level high	Usually no restriction unless serum level high	Usually no restriction unless serum level high	Usually no restriction unless serum level high
Phosphorus (mg/kg/day)	Monitor and restrict if serum levels >4.6	8-12 mg/g protein or 800-1000 mg/day	8-12 mg/g protein or 800-1000 mg/day	8-12 mg/g protein or 800-1000 mg/day
Calcium (mg/day)	1.2-1.5 mg/day; serum calcium should be maintained on lower end	1.2-1.5 mg/day; serum calcium should be maintained on lower end	Same as stages 1-3, but not to exceed 2000 mg/day	Same as stages 1-3, but not to exceed 2000 mg/day
Vitamins and minerals	Dietary Reference Intakes (DRIs) for all	DRIs for B complex and C; individualize D, zinc, and iron	DRIs for B complex and C; individualize D, zinc, and iron	DRIs for B complex and C; individualize D, zinc, and iron

Modified from Fedje L, Karalis M: Nutrition management in early stages of chronic kidney failure. In Byham-Gray L, Wiesen K, editors: *A clinical guide to nutrition care in kidney disease*, Chicago, 2004, American Dietetic Association.

phosphorus per day, of which 80% to 90% is reabsorbed by the renal tubules and the remaining 10% is excreted into urine. Phosphorus balance can be maintained until the GFR falls below 20 mL/min. At that point, phosphorus accumulation occurs in the serum. In addition, conversion of vitamin D to the active form 1,25-dihydrocholecalciferol is diminished, resulting in low serum calcium levels and elevated parathyroid hormone (PTH) levels. Dietary intervention for bone disease management is dietary phosphorus restriction to 8 to 12 mg of phosphorus per kilogram of body weight per day. In addition to dietary phosphate restriction, most patients require oral calcium, oral or intravenous vitamin D, or vitamin D analogues (or a combination of these therapies). Serum PTH, calcium, and phosphorus levels must be monitored closely to avoid excesses and deficiencies that can exacerbate the bone disease.[11]

Iron

Because of the diminished ability of the failing kidney to synthesize adequate amounts of erythropoietin, most patients with chronic renal failure develop anemia if left untreated. Recommended levels for hematocrit are 33% to 36%; for hemoglobin (Hb), 11 to 12 g/dL. These target levels are accomplished through administration of recombinant human erythropoietin (r-HuEPO) and 10 to 18 mg oral iron. Doses are individualized. If left untreated, then adverse clinical events can occur, including increased mortality rates, malnutrition, angina, cardiac enlargement, and impaired immunologic response.

Calories and Protein

K/DOQI guidelines for CKD recommend 0.6 g protein per kilogram of body weight per day when GFR is less than 25 mL/min and the patient is not on dialysis. For individuals who do not want to observe this diet or are unable to maintain adequate caloric intake, a diet providing protein in the amount of 0.75 g/kg/day should be considered. At this same level of GFR, caloric intake for patients younger than 60 years is recommended to be 35 kcal/kg/day; for those 60 years or older, 30 to 35 kcal/kg/day.[12] Other diet recommendations that integrate current data concerning protein, calories, fatty acids, vitamins, and minerals until additional data are available are listed in Table 23-4.

MEDICAL NUTRITION THERAPY

Chronic Kidney Disease Stages 1 to 4

Nutrition goals for CKD stages 1 to 4 should center on comorbid states (diabetes, hypertension, and hyperlipidemia) and slowing development of potential CVD[5,12]:

- Protein 0.60 g/kg to 0.75 g/kg of body weight, ≥50% high biologic value (HBV) protein
- Energy 35 kcal/kg of body weight for <60 years; 30 kcal/kg to 35 kcal/kg of body weight for >60 years
- Sodium 1 g/day to 3 g/day
- Potassium usually unrestricted unless serum level is high
- Phosphorus 800 mg/day to 1000 mg/day when serum phosphorus >4.6 mg/dL or parathyroid hormone (PTH) is elevated
- Calcium 1.0 g/day to 1.5 g/day, not to exceed 2 g/day with binder load
- Fluid: no restriction

KEY TERMS

osteodystrophy Defective bone formation.

- Vitamins/minerals: Daily Reference Intakes (DRIs) for B complex and vitamin C; individualize vitamin D, iron, and zinc

Chronic Kidney Disease Stage 5

A patient requiring maintenance hemodialysis usually requires two or three treatments per week, with each treatment lasting 2½ to 5 hours. During treatment the patient's blood circulates through the dialysis solution in an artificial kidney (the dialyzer), maintaining normal blood levels of life-sustaining substances the patient's own kidneys can no longer accomplish. An alternative form of peritoneal dialysis is practical for long-term ambulatory therapy at home.

Diet of a patient on kidney dialysis is a vital aspect of maintaining biochemical control. Several basic objectives govern each individually tailored diet, designed to (1) maintain adequate protein and calorie intake, (2) prevent dehydration or fluid overload, (3) maintain normal serum potassium and sodium blood levels, and (4) maintain acceptable phosphate and calcium levels[5,12]:

- Protein ≥1.2 g/kg of body weight, ≥50% HBV protein (At least 50% of dietary protein should come from HBV protein [meats, poultry, game, fish, eggs, soy and dairy].)
- Energy 35 kcal/kg of body weight for patients <60 years old; 30 kcal/kg to 35 kcal/kg of body weight for patients >60 years old
- Sodium 1 g/day to 3 g/day
- Potassium 2 g/day to 3 g/day; adjust based on serum levels
- Phosphorus 800 mg/day to 1000 mg/day when serum phosphorus >5.5 mg/dL or PTH is elevated
- Calcium ≤2 g/day; include binder load
- Fluid: urine output +1000 cc
- Vitamins/minerals:
  - Vitamin C: 60 mg/day to 100 mg/day
  - Vitamin B_6: 2 mg/day
  - Folate: 1 mg/day
  - Vitamin B_{12}: 3 mcg/day
  - DRIs for all other water-soluble vitamins
  - Vitamin E: 15 IU/day
  - Zinc: 15 mg/day
  - Iron and vitamin D: individualize

Stage 5: Peritoneal Dialysis

An alternative form of dialysis, peritoneal dialysis, allows dialysate solutions to flow directly through a catheter port established through the abdominal wall into the abdominal cavity. The solution is typically a dextrose-salt solution. High osmolality of the solution causes waste materials to diffuse across the saclike peritoneum lining the abdominal cavity (see the *Perspectives in Practice* box, "Peritoneal Dialysis"). Then this dialysate collection of waste materials flows back into the dialysate bag for disposal. The peritoneal membrane serves as the filtering mechanism.[13]

Two main types of peritoneal dialysis exist:

1. Continuous ambulatory peritoneal dialysis (CAPD), in which a dialysis solution in a plastic pouch is infused and drained via gravity each day (24 hours), five times at 4-hour intervals
2. Continuous cyclic peritoneal dialysis (CCPD), in which three or four machine-delivered exchanges are given at night, about 3 hours each, leaving about 2 L of dialysate solution in the peritoneal cavity for 12 to 15 hours during the day

Nutritional concerns specific to peritoneal dialysis involve calories contributed by the dialysate, which are usually 1.5%, 2.5%, or 4.25% dextrose in 1.5 to 2 L of solution, and the concern that fluid and potassium intake can be liberalized compared with hemodialysis because of the enhanced clearance of potassium.

- Protein ≥1.2 g/kg to 1.3 g/kg of body weight, ≥50% HBV
- Energy 35 kcal/kg of body weight for patients <60 years old; 30 kcal/kg to 35 kcal/kg of body weight for patients >60 years old, including dialysate calories
- Sodium 2 g/day to 4 g/day; monitor fluid balance
- Potassium 3 g/day to 4 g/day; adjust to serum levels
- Phosphorus 800 mg/day to 1000 mg/day when serum phosphorus >5.5 mg/dL or PTH elevated
- Calcium ≤2 g/day; include binder load
- Fluid: maintain balance
- Vitamins/minerals:
  - Vitamin C: 60 mg/day to 100 mg/day
  - Vitamin B_6: 2 mg/day
  - Folate: 1 mg/day
  - Vitamin B_{12}: 3 mcg/day
  - Vitamin B_{12}: may need 1.5 mg/day to 2 mg/day because of dialysis losses
  - DRIs for all other B vitamins
  - Vitamin E: 15 IU/day
  - Zinc: 15 mg/day
  - Iron and vitamin D: individualize

Table 23-5 summarizes dietary recommendations for patients receiving hemodialysis and peritoneal dialysis.

Kidney Transplantation

Nutritional care of kidney transplant recipients is divided into three phases: (1) pretransplantation, (2) acute posttransplantation, and (3) chronic posttransplantation. Pretransplant nutrition concerns are based on current renal replacement therapy, if any, along with assessment of nutritional status.[14]

The nutritional challenges of the acute posttransplant period are most often related to posttransplantation medications (see

KEY TERMS

peritoneum A strong smooth surface—a serous membrane—lining the abdominal and pelvic walls and the undersurface of the diaphragm, forming a sac enclosing the body's vital visceral organs within the peritoneal cavity.

PERSPECTIVES IN PRACTICE

Peritoneal Dialysis

A variety of types of peritoneal dialysis exist, with the two main types being continuous ambulatory peritoneal dialysis (CAPD) and continuous cyclic peritoneal dialysis (CCPD). Similar to the decision to choose hemodialysis or peritoneal dialysis, the choice of which type of peritoneal dialysis to perform depends on lifestyle and clinical considerations. CAPD is an ambulatory dialysis procedure that introduces dialysate directly into the peritoneal cavity. Solutes and water flow across the peritoneal membrane into dialysate fluid. This is accomplished by attaching a disposable bag containing dialysate to a catheter permanently inserted into the peritoneal cavity, waiting an individually prescribed amount of time (i.e., "dwell time") for solution exchange, and then lowering the bag to allow the force of gravity to cause the waste-containing fluid to drain into it. When the bag is empty, it can be folded around the waist or tucked into a pocket, allowing the user mobility.

The exchange takes place via osmosis and diffusion, with the rate being determined in part by the amount of dextrose in the solution. The most common dialysate solutions are 1.5%, 2.5%, or 4.25% dextrose in 1.5 to 2 L of solution. Actual rate of solute transport, type and number of peritoneal dialysis exchanges, and solution dwell times vary among patients. Each patient is prescribed an individualized dialysis prescription that includes the number and type of dialysate solutions to use each day and the length of dwell times. A method to determine membrane function and the optimal peritoneal dialysis method for each patient is the peritoneal equilibration test. Peritoneal solute and solvent movement rates vary among patients and over time can vary even within the same patient. Therefore clinical monitoring of dialysis adequacy is important. Patients using CAPD as a renal replacement therapy have better mobility than those on hemodialysis. In addition, they typically have a more liberal diet in regard to dietary potassium, phosphorus, and total fluid intake due in large part to the more continuous nature of the therapy. Protein requirement is increased and can be a challenge for some patients. Table 23-5 lists the nutritional recommendations for patients on peritoneal dialysis. Special nutrient considerations are as follows:

- *Protein and amino acid* losses average 5 to 15 g/24 hours; amino acid losses average 3 g/day (see Table 23-5 for protein requirements).
- *Potassium* requirements depend on the number of solution exchanges, whether the patient has any residual renal function, and the individual clearance characteristics of the patient's peritoneal membrane. On average, potassium recommendation is 3 to 4 g/day. Some patients will require potassium supplementation.
- *Phosphorus-binding antacids* are not as needed because of improved control of phosphorus blood levels with CAPD use.
- *Dietary sodium* is usually restricted to 2 to 4 g/day. The recommendation must be individualized in accordance to the patient's fluid status, blood pressure, and thirst.
- *Fluid* requirements depend on weight, blood pressure, and residual renal function.

CAPD poses nutrition-related problems related to weight gain from the dialysate and, on the other end of the spectrum, anorexia because of glucose absorption from the dialysate.

One method available to calculate glucose absorption in an individualized manner is the D/D_0 formula: grams of glucose absorbed.

$$\text{Glucose (g)} = (1 - D/D_0)x_i$$

where D_0 is initial dextrose in the dialysate at zero hours (g); D is remaining dextrose in the dialysate after an appropriate dwell time (g); D/D_0 is the fraction of glucose remaining in the dialysate; and x_i is initial glucose instilled:

13 g/L for 1.5% dextrose
22 g/L for 2.5% dextrose
38 g/L for 4.25% dextrose

In addition to posing possible weight management problems, extra dextrose can lead to elevated triglycerides and low-density lipoprotein (LDL) levels and depressed levels of protective high-density lipoproteins (HDLs), thus increasing risk of coronary heart disease in long-term users.

Nutritionists and nurses who counsel patients being transferred from hemodialysis to CAPD regimen may find that patients need guidance in adjusting to their new diet. The following guidelines may be helpful:

- Increase potassium intake by eating a wide variety of fruits and vegetables each day.
- Encourage liberal fluid intake to prevent dehydration.
- Encourage complex carbohydrates while avoiding overindulging in concentrated sweets to help control triglyceride and HDL levels.
- Maintain lean body weight by incorporating the kcalories provided by the dialysate into the total meal plan (to be calculated and explained to the patient by the renal dietitian).

BIBLIOGRAPHY

National Kidney Foundation: K/DOQI clinical practice guidelines for nutrition in chronic renal failure, *Am J Kidney Dis* 35(Suppl 2):S9, 2000.

National Kidney Foundation: Kidney disease outcomes quality initiative (K/DOQI): practice guidelines for peritoneal dialysis adequacy, *Am J Kidney Dis* 37(Suppl 1):S55, 2001.

Passadakis T, Vagemezis V, Oreopoulos D: Peritoneal dialysis: better than, equal to, or worse than hemodialysis? Data worth knowing before choosing a dialysis modality, *Perit Dial Int* 21:25, 2001.

Valderrabano F, Lopez-Gomez J: Quality of life in end-stage renal disease patients, *Am J Kidney Dis* 38(3):443, 2001.

Wiggins K: *Guidelines for nutrition care of renal patients,* ed 3, Chicago, 2002, American Dietetic Association.

TABLE 23-5 NUTRITIONAL RECOMMENDATIONS FOR PATIENTS ON HEMODIALYSIS AND PERITONEAL DIALYSIS THERAPY

NUTRIENT	HEMODIALYSIS	PERITONEAL DIALYSIS
Protein (g/kg)*	1.2 average weight (50% HBV)	1.2-1.3 SBW or adjusted BW (>50% HBV)
Energy (kcal/kg)*	30 kcal/kg if <60 years of age and 30-35 kcal/kg if >60 years of age or obese	30-35 if >60 years of age and 35 if <60 years of age
If patient <90% or >115% of median standard weight, use aBW_{ef}		
Phosphorus	800-1000 mg/day or <17 mg/kg IBW or SBW	800-1000 mg or 10-15 mg phosphorus/g protein
Sodium	2-4 g if fluid output ≥1 L 2 g if fluid output ≤1 L 2 g if anuria	2-4 g
Potassium	40 mg/kg IBW or SBW	2-4 g (considered consistent with unrestricted diet)
Fluid	2 L if fluid output ≥1 L 1-1.5 L if fluid output ≤1 L 1 L if anuria	1-3 L/day
Calcium	Individualized	< 2000 mg including diet and binders

From Biesecker R, Stuart N: Nutrition management of the adult hemodialysis patient. In Byham-Gray L, Wiesen K, editors: *A clinical guide to nutrition care in kidney disease*, Chicago, 2004, American Dietetic Association; McCann L: Nutrition management of the adult peritoneal dialysis patient. In Byham-Gray L, Wiesen K, editors: *A clinical guide to nutrition care in kidney disease*, Chicago, 2004, American Dietetic Association.
*For continuous ambulatory peritoneal dialysis (CAPD) and automated peritoneal dialysis (APD) include dialysate calories.
HBV, High biologic value; *SBW*, standard body weight; *BW*, body weight; BW_{ef}, edema-free body weight; *IBW*, ideal body weight.

TABLE 23-6 NUTRITIONAL GUIDELINES FOR ADULT KIDNEY TRANSPLANT RECIPIENTS

NUTRIENT	ACUTE PERIOD	CHRONIC PERIOD
Protein	1.3-2.0 g/kg	0.8-1.0 g/kg; limit with chronic graft dysfunction
Calories	30-35 kcal/kg or BEE × 1.3 (may need to be increased with postoperative complications)	Maintain desirable body weight
Carbohydrates	Limit simple carbohydrate intake if intolerance evident	Emphasize complex carbohydrate and distribution
Fats	Remainder of kcal; emphasize PUFA and MUFA	Emphasize PUFA and MUFA
Potassium	2-4 g if hyperkalemic	Unrestricted unless hyperkalemic
Sodium	2-4 g	2-4 g with hypertension
Calcium	1200-1500 mg	1200-1500 mg
Phosphorus	DRIs; may need supplementation to normalize serum levels	DRIs
Fluids	Limited only by graft function	Limited only by graft function (generally unrestricted)

Modified from Cochran CC, Kent PS: Nutrition management of the renal transplant patient. In Byham-Gray L, Wiesen K, editors: *A clinical guide to nutrition care in kidney disease*, Chicago, 2004, American Dietetic Association.
BEE, Basal energy expenditure; *PUFA*, polyunsaturated fatty acids; *MUFA*, monounsaturated fatty acids; *DRIs*, Dietary Reference Intakes.

the *Evidence-Based Practice* box, "Kidney Transplantation"). Hyperlipidemia, weight gain, and abnormal blood glucose levels can result, often because of side effects of the antirejection medications such as corticosteroids and cyclosporin A.[15] Foodborne infections can be life-threatening for transplant patients receiving immunosuppressive medications; therefore food safety education should be routinely included.

During the chronic posttransplant period, overnutrition may lead to complications such as obesity, dyslipidemias, diabetes mellitus, and hypertension. Nutritional goals are to provide adequate nutrition, prevent infection, and manage long-term nutritional complications.[14] A summation of nutritional guidelines for this patient group is provided in Table 23-6.

ACUTE RENAL FAILURE

The catabolic ARF patient, most frequently encountered in the intensive care setting, presents a management challenge to the entire team of physicians, nurses, dietitians, respiratory therapists, dialysis staff, pharmacists, and other technicians. These patients are in negative nitrogen balance and generate much urea resulting from the catabolic process. Infection is a major threat, and it aggravates the existing malnutrition.

EVIDENCE-BASED PRACTICE

Kidney Transplantation

Thousands await transplantation every year. Others cannot consider a transplant because of medical or psychosocial issues (or because of both). Overall, kidney transplantation remains the treatment of choice for the majority of patients with CKD. Advances in solid organ transplantation and immunosuppressive therapy have resulted in improved patient survival and improved viability of transplanted kidneys.

Nearly 50% of all kidney transplant recipients will be alive with a successful functioning transplant 10 years after transplantation. One-year cadaver kidney success rates are 89%, and 5-year success rates are 65%. In comparison, success rates for recipients of living donor kidneys are 97% at 1 year and 78% at 5 years. A patient who is trouble free for the first 3 months after the transplantation has an excellent prognosis. Most common causes of death after the first year are cardiovascular disease (CVD), infection, and cancer.

The patient who receives a kidney transplant has a challenging first year. Visits to the transplant team occur an average of two or three times per week during the first month and once per week for up to 3 months after the surgery. Visits then drop to once monthly during the first year if no problems occur. After the first year it is recommended that patients have their laboratory parameters monitored every 1 to 2 months.

Medication regimens are challenging for the transplant recipient. Immunosuppressive agents, lipid-lowering drugs, antihypertensives, and hypoglycemic agents are needed for quite some time. Significant side effects can occur from these medicines, and adherence to the rigid medication schedule is critical for successful allograft survival. Medical problems that can develop during the first year include infections such as cytomegalovirus, hyperlipidemia, bone disease, diabetes, CVD, hypertension, and dental problems. Weight gain as a side effect of medications can also become a problem (see Table 23-6 for nutritional recommendations for the kidney transplant recipient).

Morbidity and mortality rates for kidney transplantation are clinically significant. These statistics should improve as advances in the technology of the surgery and pharmacologic management occur over time. Not every patient will medically qualify for transplantation, and every candidate must be assessed for his or her ability to meet the demands of the posttransplantation period. In addition, evidence suggests that living kidney donors have survival similar to nondonors, and their risk of CKD is not increased.

In the future, perhaps availability of organs for transplantation will be increased by improvements in living-related surgeries, development of artificial organs, and most optimistically, finding a cure for progressive kidney disease.

BIBLIOGRAPHY

Baiardi F, Degli Esposti E, Cocchi R, et al: Effects of clinical and individual variables on quality of life in chronic renal failure patients, *J Nephrol* 15(1):61, 2002.

Braun WE: Update on kidney transplantation: increasing clinical success, expanding waiting lists, *Cleve Clin J Med* 69(6):501, 2002.

Centers for Medicare and Medicaid Services: 2001 Annual report: End Stage Renal Disease Clinical Performance Measures Project, *Am J Kidney Dis* 39(Suppl 2):S1, 2002.

Ibrahim HN, Foley R, Tan L, et al: Long-term consequences of kidney donation, *N Engl J Med* 360(5):459, 2009.

Matas AJ, Halbert RJ, Barr ML, et al: Life satisfaction and adverse effects in renal transplant recipients: a longitudinal analysis, *Clin Transplant* 16(2):113, 2002.

Disease Process

Renal failure may occur acutely with sudden shutdown of renal function after some metabolic insult or traumatic injury to normal kidneys. It is typically characterized by retention of nitrogenous waste products, fluid overload, acid-base disturbances, electrolyte imbalance, and hemodynamic instability. ARF is linked with major in-hospital morbidity and mortality.[16] Immediate and continuing nutrition support is essential.

ARF may have various causes: (1) severe injury such as extensive burns or crushing injuries that cause widespread tissue destruction; (2) infectious diseases such as peritonitis; (3) traumatic shock after surgery on the abdominal aorta; (4) toxic agents in the environment such as carbon tetrachloride or poisonous mushrooms; or (5) immunologic drug reactions in allergic or sensitive persons, such as penicillin reaction.[16]

Clinical Symptoms

The major sign of ARF is **oliguria**, *diminished* urine output, often accompanied by proteinuria or hematuria. This diminished urine output is brought on by underlying tissue problems that characterize ARF. Usually blockage of tubules is seen, caused by cellular debris from tissue trauma or urinary failure with backup retention of filtrate materials.[16]

Oliguria

Diminished urinary output is a cardinal symptom, often with proteinuria or hematuria accompanying the small output. Water balance becomes a crucial factor. The course of the disease is usually divided into an oliguric phase followed by a diuretic phase. The urinary output during the oliguric phase varies from as little as 20 mL/day to 200 mL/day.

Anorexia, Nausea, and Lethargy

During this initial phase of ARF, the patient may be lethargic and anorectic and experience nausea and vomiting. Blood pressure elevation and signs of uremia may be present. Oral intake is usually difficult in this catabolic period.[16]

Increasing Serum Urea Nitrogen and Creatinine Levels

During the initial catabolic period after injury, surgery, or some other metabolic dysfunction, the serum urea nitrogen level increases along with the creatinine level. These increases

KEY TERMS

oliguria Secretion of a very small amount of urine in relation to fluid intake.

result from tissue breakdown of muscle mass. Blood potassium, phosphate, and sulfate levels also increase, and sodium, calcium, and bicarbonate levels decrease.[16]

Basic Treatment Goals

Treatment must be individualized, adjusted according to the progression of the illness, the type of treatment being used, and the patient's response. In general, however, basic therapy objectives are as follows[16]:

- Reduce and minimize protein breakdown.
- Prevent protein catabolism, and minimize uremic toxicity.
- Prevent dehydration or overhydration.
- Correct acidosis carefully.
- Correct electrolyte depletions, and avoid excesses.
- Control fluid and electrolyte losses from vomiting and diarrhea.
- Maintain optimal nutritional status.
- Maintain appetite, general morale, and sense of well-being.
- Control complications—hypertension, bone pain, nervous system problems.

Nutritional Requirements for Patients with Acute Renal Failure

The ARF patient nutrition requirements are directly influenced by type of renal replacement therapy (if any), nutritional and metabolic status, and degree of hypercatabolism. Current recommendations for protein and calories for this patient population are defined in the following discussion.

When energy requirements cannot be measured directly, calorie requirements can usually be met by providing 25 to 35 kcal/kg IBW, reserving the upper limit of the range for patients who are severely catabolic and whose nitrogen balance does not improve at lower intakes.[16] Protein sources containing essential and nonessential amino acids should be provided. For patients whose ARF is expected to resolve in a few days and who are not catabolic and will not need dialysis, 0.8 to 1.2 g of protein is recommended. The patient's nutritional and metabolic status and renal diagnosis determine exact dose. For patients who are catabolic, receiving acute hemodialysis, or both, the recommendation is 1.2 to 1.5 g of protein.[16]

Total fluid intake for any patient depends on the amount of residual renal function (i.e., if the patient is oliguric or anuric) and fluid and sodium status. In general, fluid intake can be calculated by adding 500 mL (for insensible losses) to the 24-hour urine output. During dieresis, fluids should be increased to prevent dehydration.[16]

Although the diet should be as liberal as possible to support sufficient intake, nutrient needs should be frequently reevaluated because requirements may change as a consequence of resumption of kidney function, use of dialysis, and anabolism. Sodium needs may increase to restore losses from diuresis, but the general recommendation is 2 to 3 g per day. Potassium requirements depend on lab valued and degree of hyperkalemia. In general, 2 to 3 g/day is suggested, but requirements may possibly increase with dialysis, restoration of kidney function, and anabolism. Phosphate binders may be necessary, along with a restriction of 8 to 15 mg/kg body weight per day. Requirements may increase with daily dialysis, return of kidney function, and anabolism.[16]

UROLITHIASIS (CALCULI OR KIDNEY STONES)

Disease Process

Kidney stone disease is an ancient medical problem. Since the days of Hippocrates, records of its incidence have appeared in medical documents. It continues to be a prevalent health problem. Multiple stone attacks affect 12% of American men and 5% of women during their lifetimes.[17]

Kidney stone disease appears to be chronic and recurrent. Calculi form when excessive amounts of reasonably insoluable salts are found in the urine or when inadequate fluid intake creates highly concentrated urine. When any solid substance forms, sediment continues to build up. The salts that form crystals can grow to form stones.[17] Immobility can also cause calculi because of stasis of urine and ensuing chemical alterations.[17,18] Existence of stones typically becomes evident only when they obstruct the flow of urine.[18]

Although the basic cause of kidney stones remains unknown, many factors contribute directly or indirectly to their formation. These factors relate to the nature of the urine itself or to conditions of the urinary tract environment. Risk for urinary calculi development is affected by a number of factors, including age, gender, race, geographic location, seasonal factors, fluid intake, diet, and occupation. Geographic locations effect stone formation as the result of indirect factors such as average temperature, humidity, and rainfall, and their influence on fluid and dietary patterns.[17] According to the concentration of urinary constituents, roughly 75% of major stones formed are calcium stones. The rest consist chiefly of uric acid, struvite, or cystine (Figure 23-4).[18]

Major Types of Stones

Calcium Stones

Calcium stones are composed of calcium compounds, usually calcium oxalate, calcium carbonate, or calcium phosphate. Calcium stones form as a result of hypercalciuria that can result from alkaline urine, inadequate fluid intake, high levels of dietary oxalate (see Appendix C), prolonged immobilization, or parathyroid tumor.[17,18] Oxalates occur naturally only in a few food sources and individual absorption and excretion rates influence availability. Only eight foods cause a significant increase in urinary oxalate excretion: (1) spinach, (2) rhubarb, (3) beets, (4) nuts, (5) chocolate, (6) tea, (7) wheat bran, and (8) strawberries. Nutrition therapy for stone-forming individuals may be limited to restriction of these eight foods, with results monitored by laboratory analysis of urine composition.

- *Animal protein:* A diet high in animal protein, such as the typical American diet, has been linked to increased excretions of calcium, oxalate, and urate. A vegetarian type of diet has been recommended by some investigators as a wise choice for stone-forming persons.
- *Dietary fiber:* Added dietary fiber has been found to reduce risk factors for stone formation, especially calcium stones.

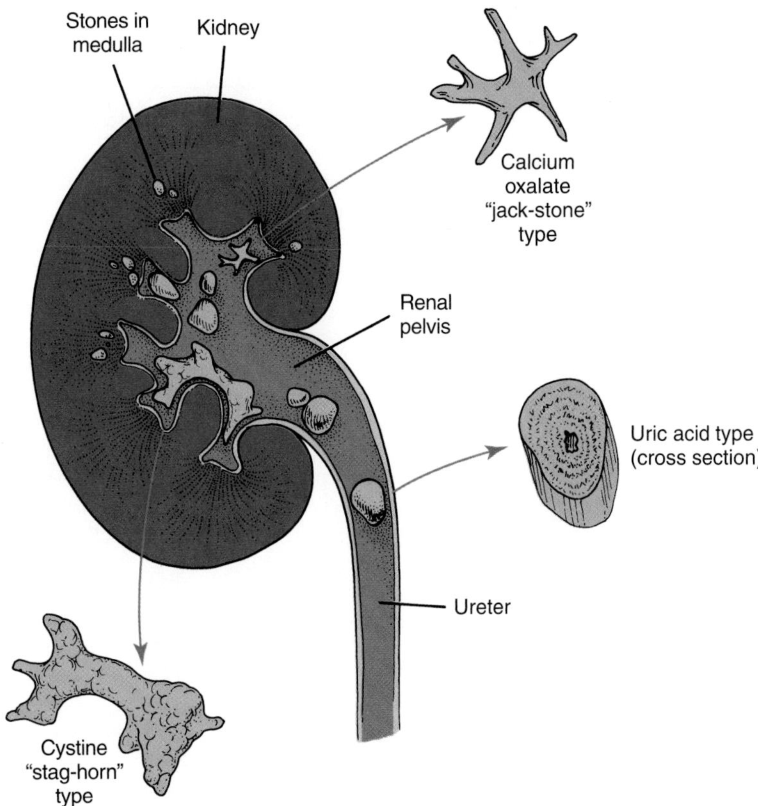

FIGURE 23-4 Renal stones in kidney, pelvis, and ureter.

Struvite Stones

Next to calcium stones in frequency are struvite stones, composed of a single compound—magnesium ammonium phosphate ($MgNH_4PO_4$). These are often called *infection stones* because they are associated with UTIs. The offending organism in the infection is *Proteus mirabilis.* This is a urea-splitting bacterium that contains urease, an enzyme that hydrolyzes urea to ammonia. Thus urinary pH becomes alkaline. In the ammonia-rich environment, struvite precipitates and forms large, "staghorn" stones.[17] Surgical removal is usually indicated.

Uric Acid Stones

Excess uric acid excretion may be caused by an impairment in intermediary metabolism of purine, as occurs in gout. Cancer chemotherapy may also cause urine to be acidic, which aids in hyperuricemia.

Cystine Stones

A heredity metabolic defect in renal tubular reabsorption of the amino acid cystine causes this substance to accumulate in urine. This condition is called *cystinuria.* Because this is a genetic disorder, it is characterized by early onset and a positive family history. This is one of the most common metabolic disorders associated with kidney stones in children before puberty.

Clinical Symptoms

Severe pain and numerous urinary symptoms may result, with general weakness and sometimes fever. Laboratory examination of urine and chemical analysis of any stone passed help determine treatment.

General Treatment

Fluid Intake

Large fluid intake produces a more dilute urine and is a foundation of therapy. Dilute urine helps to prevent concentration of stone constituents.

Urinary pH

An attempt to control solubility factor is made by changing urinary pH to an increased acidity or alkalinity, depending on the chemical composition of the stone formed. An exception is calcium oxalate stones because solubility of calcium oxalate in urine is not pH dependent. Conversely, however, calcium phosphate is soluble in an acid urine.

Stone Composition

When possible, dietary constituents of the stone are controlled to reduce the amount of the substance available for precipitation.

Binding Agents

Materials that bind stone elements and prevent their absorption in the intestine cause fecal excretion. For example, sodium phytate is used to bind calcium, and aluminum gels are used to bind phosphate. Glycine and calcium have a similar effect on oxalates.

Alternative Remedies

A number of herbs are also used to help prevent the development of kidney stones (see the *Complementary and Alternative Medicine [CAM]* box, "Common Herbal Treatments for Kidney Stones").

COMPLEMENTARY AND ALTERNATIVE MEDICINE (CAM)

Common Herbal Treatments for Kidney Stones

Patients interested in complementary and alternative medicine may also be interested in knowing low fluid intake greatly increases risk of developing all types of kidney stones.

HERB	EFFICACY	SIDE EFFECTS AND/OR RISKS	DRUG INTERACTION
Citrate	Might help prevent oxalate and acid stones by binding with calcium in urine, reducing the amount of calcium available to form calcium oxalate stones. It also alkalizes urine, inhibiting development of calcium oxalate and uric acid stones.		Increases serum levels of ephedra, flecainide, mecamylamine, and methamphetamine. Decreases serum levels of lithium, methotrexate, salicylates, sulfonylureas, and tetracyclines. Hyperkalemia can occur when taking ACE inhibitors and potassium-sparing diuretics.
Calcium	Calcium supplements might slightly increase kidney stone risk, whereas dietary calcium reduces risk of kidney stones.	Increased intakes are associated with increased risk of prostate cancer.	Concurrent use of calcium with pheasant's eye *(Adonis vernalis)* increases risk of cardiac toxicity. CCBs can be affected by combinations of calcium supplements and high doses of vitamin D. Might decrease blood level of atenolol (β-blocker) and possibly other β-blockers. Interferes with absorption of tetracyclines and levothyroxine. Excess intake can interfere with absorption of iron, zinc, magnesium, iodine, manganese, and copper.
Magnesium (magnesium oxide or magnesium hydroxide)	No strong evidence that magnesium prevents calcium oxalate stones.	Should not be taken by those with severe heart or kidney disease without consultation with a health care provider.	Might decrease absorption of psyllium.
Vitamin B_6 (pyridoxamine)	Weak evidence indicates that vitamin B_6 might help prevent calcium oxalate stones.	Vitamin B_6 deficiency increases the amount of oxalate in urine. Large doses may cause nausea, vomiting, and potential risk of neurotoxicity.	None were found.
GLA (omega-6 oils, omega-6 fatty acids, evening primrose oil, black currant oil, borage oil)	No evidence is available.	No adverse effects have been noted.	Increases bleeding time when used with anticoagulant therapy. GLA is synergistic with paclitaxel.

BIBLIOGRAPHY

Bratman S, Girman AM: *Mosby's handbook of herbs and supplements and their therapeutic uses*, St Louis, 2003, Mosby.

Herr SM: *Herb-drug interaction handbook*, ed 2, Nassau, NY, 2002, Church Street Books.

ACE, Angiotensin-converting enzyme; *CCBs*, calcium channel blockers; *GLA*, γ-linolenic acid.

Nutrition Therapy

Manipulation of single nutritional components is usually not effective. General nutrition recommendations for kidney stones entails the following[19]:

- Protein: not to exceed the DRI of 0.8-1.0 g/kg body weight/day
- Calcium: should not restrict; balance intake throughout the day
- Fluids: 12-16 cups to produce urine volume >2.5 L/day
- Oxalate: <40-50 mg/day
- Sodium: decrease intake to 2300 (100 mEq) to 3450 (250 mEq) mg/day
- Energy: level to maintain healthy weight
- Vitamin and mineral supplement: vitamin C should be restricted to DRI; B vitamins have not been shown to be harmful

URINARY TRACT INFECTION

Disease Process

The term *UTI* refers to a wide variety of clinical infections in which a significant number of microorganisms are present in any portion of the urinary tract. A common form is cystitis, an inflammation of the bladder that is very prevalent in young women. At least 20% of women experience a UTI during their lifetime, of which the vast majority are cases of uncomplicated cystitis.[17,18] The condition is called *recurrent UTI* if three or more bouts are experienced in 1 year.

The majority of cases are caused by aerobic members of the fecal flora, especially *Escherichia coli.* Presence of these organisms in urine is termed *bacteriuria.* Urine produced by the normal kidney is sterile and remains so as it travels to the bladder. In UTI, however, the normal urethra has microbial flora; therefore any voided urine generally contains many bacteria. Bacteriuria is present when the quantity of organisms is more than 100,000/mL of urine. The female anatomy is more conducive to entry of these bacteria into the urinary tract. Recurrent cystitis occurs mostly in young and otherwise healthy women who have infections that usually correspond with sexual activity and continued diaphragm use. In most cases, simply changing to another birth control method will solve the problem. Cystitis is characterized by frequent voiding and burning on urination.

Treatment

Although regular consumption of cranberry juice can help prevent UTIs, it is not effective for treatment. Intake of adequate fluids helps to produce a dilute urine. Control of UTI is an important measure because it is a risk factor in stone formation.

RESOURCES

The renal diet is complex and presents a challenge to practitioners and even more so to patients. A basic resource, the *National Renal Diet* educational series, provides valuable guides. These standardized guidelines for nutrition intervention and patient education in renal disease have been developed by the collaborative work of renal dietitians from the American Dietetic Association Renal Dietitians Dietetic Practice Group and the National Kidney Foundation Council on Renal Nutrition. The *Professional Guide* can be used in conjunction with other guides from the American Dietetic Association (ADA) for the care of renal disease patients. Because dietary management must be tailored to the stage of the disease and method of treatment, the series of materials contains a professional guide and six client booklets, each designed with special food lists to meet specific needs of the various renal disease requirements. These ADA resources give the practitioner a comprehensive basis for individualizing dietary instructions and provide the patient and family with a practical guide for everyday decisions and plans for food choices.

The Council on Renal Nutrition of the National Kidney Foundation is an expert resource for information. Membership includes a subscription to the *Journal of Renal Nutrition,* a quarterly publication geared toward nutritionists, scientists, and physicians interested and working in the fields of nephrology and renal nutrition. (For contact information, see the Websites of Interest section at the end of this chapter.)

Importance of nutritional status and care has been documented to have a role in patient outcomes; therefore interest in renal nutrition and the number of online resources have substantially increased. (See the Websites of Interest section for a listing of websites that provide excellent information and links to other sites pertaining to renal nutrition and nephrology.)

HEALTH PROMOTION

OMEGA-3 FATTY ACIDS AND RENAL DISEASE

Despite countless research efforts, mechanisms responsible for the progressive nature of renal disease remain elusive. Historically, nutrition science has been an inherent component of research directed toward identifying nutrient manipulations that ameliorate kidney disease, metabolic abnormalities associated with chronic renal insufficiency, and mechanisms by which nutrients modulate factors involved in promoting exacerbation of existing disease. In all of these research areas, dietary protein, phosphorus, and caloric deprivation have been more widely studied than other nutrients. However, more recently, research interest has become directed toward dietary essential fatty acids (EFAs). This shift is in response to a growing body of evidence indicating that fatty acid substitution of cell membrane phospholipids modulates biochemical pathways implicated in the pathophysiology of progressive kidney disease and CVD, so prominent in the renal patient population.

It has been demonstrated that altering availability of EFAs can influence the natural course of several important diseases in the mammalian organism. For example, epidemiologic studies of the Dutch, Japanese, and native Greenland Eskimo populations attribute their low incidence of heart disease to a fish diet high in omega-3 fatty acids. Beneficial observations have included an improved lipid profile, prolonged survival, and improved renal function.

Dietary EFAs are direct precursors to the biologically diverse and potent class of compounds called *eicosanoids.* EFAs can also modulate cellular production of interleukins (ILs). Several chronic inflammatory and renal diseases are characterized in part by an overproduction of eicosanoids and ILs. These facts suggest manipulation of dietary fatty acids might contribute a therapeutic influence by altering proinflammatory and other activated pathways in disease processes.

TO SUM UP

Through its unique functional units, the nephrons, the kidneys act as a filtration system, reabsorbing substances the body needs, secreting additional hydrogen ions to maintain a proper pH balance in the blood, and excreting unnecessary materials in a concentrated urine.

Renal function may be impaired by a variety of conditions. These include inflammatory and degenerative diseases, infection and obstruction, chronic diseases such as hypertension and diabetes, environmental agents such as insecticides and solvents and other toxic substances, and some medications and trauma. Some clinical conditions affecting structure and function include glomerulonephritis, ARF and chronic renal failure, renal calculi, and UTI.

Stage 5 of CKD is treated by dialysis—hemodialysis or peritoneal dialysis—and kidney transplantation. The diet for CKD needs to include ample calories and protein with restrictions for GFR of less than 25 mL/min/1.73 m^2 only if the patient is able to maintain adequate caloric intake. Dialysis patients must be monitored closely for calories, protein, fluid, and electrolyte balance. All of the diets need to be individualized to ensure overall nutritional adequacy and adherence. Monitoring of nutritional status is important for all patients.

QUESTIONS FOR REVIEW

1. For each of the following conditions, outline nutritional components of therapy, explaining effect of each on kidney function: glomerulonephritis, ARF (renal insufficiency), and chronic renal failure.
2. Identify four clinical conditions that impair renal function. Give an example of each, describing its effect on various structures in the kidney.
3. List nutritional factors that must be monitored in individuals undergoing renal dialysis.
4. Summarize the rationale and nutrient recommendations for patients who have received a renal transplant.
5. Outline nutrition therapy used for patients with various types of kidney stones. Describe each type of stone and explain the rationale for each aspect of therapy.
6. For what condition is a UTI a predisposing factor? What general nutrition principles are recommended in the treatment of such infections?

REFERENCES

1. Huether SE: Structure and function of the renal and urologic systems. In Huether SE, McCance KL, editors: *Understanding pathophysiology*, ed 4, St Louis, 2008, Mosby.
2. National Kidney Foundation: K/DOQI clinical practice guidelines and clinical practice recommendations for diabetes and chronic kidney disease, *Am J Kidney Dis* 49(Suppl 2):S12, 2007.
3. National Kidney Foundation: K/DOQI clinical practice guidelines for chronic kidney disease: evaluation, classification and stratification, *Am J Kidney Dis* 39(Suppl 1): S1, 2002.
4. U.S. Renal Data System, USRDS 2008 Annual Report: *Atlas of chronic kidney disease and end-stage renal disease in the United States*, Bethesda, Md, 2008, National Institutes of Health, National Institute of Diabetes and Digestive and Kidney Diseases.
5. National Kidney Foundation: K/DOQI clinical practice guidelines for chronic kidney disease: evaluation, classification and stratification, *Am J Kidney Dis* 39(Suppl 1): S1, 2002.
6. American Diabetes Association: Diabetic nephropathy, *Diabetes Care* 25(Suppl 1):S85, 2002.
7. Gray M, Huether SE, Forshee BA: Alterations of renal and urinary tract function. In McCance KL, Huether SE, editors: *Pathophysiology. The biologic basis for disease in adults and children*, ed 5, St Louis, 2006, Saunders.
8. Beekley MD: Update on nutrition and chronic kidney disease. In *Medscape Nephrology, Chronic Kidney Disease Expert Column*, July 2007. Retrieved June 2, 2009, from www.medscape.com.
9. Chertow G, Lazarus M: Malnutrition as a risk factor for morbidity and mortality in maintenance patients. In Kopple J, Massry S, editors: *Nutritional management of renal disease*, Philadelphia, 1997, Williams & Wilkins.
10. Barbá PD, Goode JL: Nutrition assessment in chronic kidney disease. In Byham-Gray L, Wiesen K, editors: *A clinical guide to nutrition care in kidney disease*, Chicago, 2004, American Dietetic Association.
11. Fedje L, Karalis M: Nutrition management in early stages of chronic kidney failure. In Byham-Gray L, Wiesen K, editors: *A clinical guide to nutrition care in kidney disease*, Chicago, 2004, American Dietetic Association.
12. National Kidney Foundation: K/DOQI clinical practice guidelines for nutrition in chronic renal failure, *Am J Kidney Dis* 35(Suppl 2):S9, 2000.
13. Biesecker R, Stuart N: Nutrition management of the adult hemodialysis patient. In Byham-Gray L, Wiesen K, editors: *A clinical guide to nutrition care in kidney disease*, Chicago, 2004, American Dietetic Association.
14. Cochran CC, Kent PS: Nutrition management of the renal transplant patient. In Byham-Gray L, Wiesen K, editors: *A clinical guide to nutrition care in kidney disease*, Chicago, 2004, American Dietetic Association.
15. Weil SE: Nutrition in the kidney transplant recipient. In Danovitch GM, editor: *Handbook of kidney transplantation*, ed 2, Boston, 1996, Little, Brown.
16. Bickford A, Schatz SR: Nutrition management in acute renal failure. In Byham-Gray L, Wiesen K, editors: *A clinical guide to nutrition care in kidney disease*, Chicago, 2004, American Dietetic Association.
17. Huether SE, Gray M: Alterations of renal and urinary tract functions. In Huether SE, McCance KL, editors: *Understanding pathophysiology*, ed 4, St Louis, 2008, Mosby.
18. Gould BE: *Pathophysiology for the health professions*, ed 3, St Louis, 2006, Mosby.
19. American Dietetic Association: *Nutrition care manual. Celiac disease: nutrition care FAQs*, Chicago, 2009, Author. Retrieved June 11, from www.nutritioncaremanual.org.

FURTHER RESOURCES

Websites of Interest

American Dietetic Association. Website of the world's largest food and nutrition professionals organization providing information regarding nutrition and health through research, education, and advocacy: www.eatright.org.

American Journal of Kidney Diseases. Website of the official journal of the National Kidney Foundation: www.ajkd.org.

Da Vita. Provider of dialysis services and education for patients with CKD: www.davita.com.

Hypertension, Dialysis and Clinical Nephrology (HDCN). Provides up-to-date, selected information on renal disorders and their treatment: www.hdcn.com.

Journal of the American Society of Nephrology: www.jasn.org.

Journal of Renal Nutrition. This site also provides links to the homepage of the National Kidney Foundation and the Council on Renal Nutrition: www.jrnjournal.org.

National Kidney Foundation: www.kidney.org.

Nephrology News and Issues Online (NephrOnline): www.nephronline.com.

24

Acquired Immunodeficiency Syndrome (AIDS)

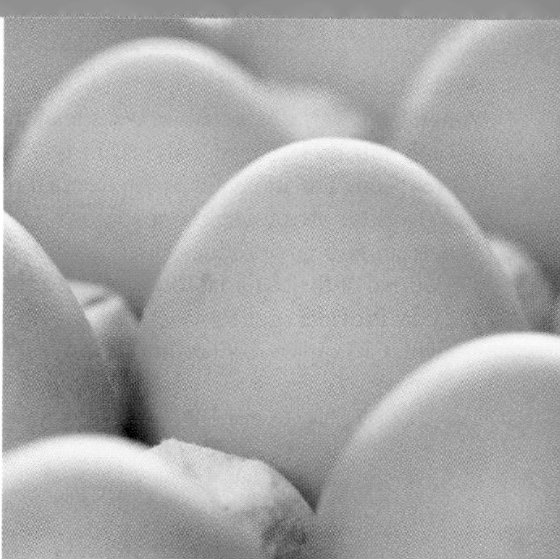

Sara Long Roth

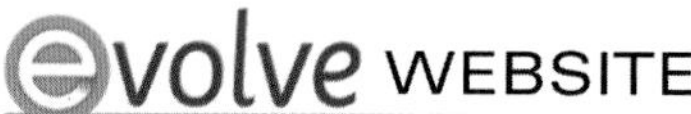

http://evolve.elsevier.com/Williams/essentials/

OUTLINE

The human immunodeficiency virus (HIV), the virus that causes acquired immunodeficiency syndrome (AIDS), is found in all regions of the world, making it one of the greatest public health challenges of the past 30 years. Countless numbers of infected adults and children have died in its wake.

Here we examine the background of the AIDS epidemic and nature of the human immunodeficiency virus-1 (HIV-1). We review the current state of medical management and its relation to nutritional status in the course of the disease. As knowledge of the disease process has grown, it has become increasingly evident that nutrition support plays a vital role in the care of HIV-infected and AIDS patients.

EVOLUTION OF HIV AND THE AIDS EPIDEMIC

The first cases of AIDS in the United States were reported in June of 1981.[1] Since then, AIDS has become one of the greatest epidemics in history,[2] claiming the lives of more than 22 million people worldwide, including more than 500,000 in the United States.[1] The majority of cases of AIDS are found in sub-Saharan Africa, the Caribbean, and Latin America, with the number of new cases increasing in Asia.[2,3]

Although awareness of AIDS came to attention in the United States as being related to homosexual activity, the most common method of transmission in the rest of the world is by heterosexual contact. Worldwide, more than half of all persons living with HIV/AIDS are women. In the United States, like the rest of the world, the principal mode of transmission to women is via heterosexual contact, making the numbers of those infected with HIV/AIDS escalate faster in female subjects than in male subjects, particularly in teenagers. Children also develop the disease, generally from their mothers across the placenta, through contact with infected blood during delivery, or through breast milk.[3]

HIV attacks the central processes involved in development of the immune response. It infects and destroys helper T cells essential for the maturation of plasma cells and cytotoxic T cells. By doing so, HIV suppresses the immune response against itself and creates a generalized immune deficiency, making the body unable to immunologically respond against other pathogens and opportunistic infections.[4]

Transmission

HIV is a bloodborne pathogen and is transmitted through direct contact with infected body fluids via unprotected heterosexual and homosexual intercourse; intravenous drug abuse (needle sharing); and mother-to-child transmission before (pregnancy), during (delivery), or after birth (breastfeeding)[2,4] (see the *Focus on Culture* box, "Special Considerations for Children with AIDS"). Risk of transmission is comparative to the viral load in the fluid, which reflects the amount of virus in the body. The virus is prone to be transmitted in the course of acute HIV infection, when high viral replication occurs.[2] The predominant means of transmission worldwide is through sexual contact.[4]

Disease Progression

Primary HIV Infection

HIV is classified as a retrovirus. Retroviruses carry genetic information in the form of ribonucleic acid (RNA) instead of deoxyribonucleic acid (DNA) (Figure 24-1) using a viral enzyme (reverse transcriptase) to change RNA into

FOCUS ON CULTURE

Special Considerations for Children with AIDS

Malnutrition, particularly inadequate calories and protein, and dehydration are serious issues in children with AIDS. In adults, the disease affects nutritional status. In children, not only is nutritional status affected but also growth and development can be significantly impaired, resulting in growth failure. A strong relationship exists between early nutritional status—poor growth, cachexia, poor oral intake, decreased absorption of nutrients, and increased energy expenditure—and mortality risk.

Nutrition assessments should be performed routinely in all children with AIDS so that any problems can be identified and treated as they occur and nutritional deficits can be minimized. Assessments should include evaluation of anthropometrics, visceral protein stores, red blood cell indexes, and electrolytes. Appetite, intake, and feeding ability should also be assessed. Developmental delays can also increase the risk for developing failure to thrive.

Providing adequate calories to maintain linear growth and support weight gain can be difficult as a result of chronic infections, fever, and medications. In 1994 the Centers for Disease Control and Prevention (CDC) revised the criteria for wasting in HIV-infected children younger than age 13 to the following:

- Persistent weight loss of more than 10% of baseline
- Decrease of at least two percentiles on the weight-for-age chart in children younger than 1 year of age *or*
- Two consecutive measurements more than 30 days apart of less than the fifth percentile on the weight-for-height chart and chronic diarrhea (more than two loose stools daily for >30 days) or documented or constant fever for more than 30 days

Diarrhea and malabsorption can result in dehydration, which can be very serious in infants and young children, and the onset may occur suddenly. To prevent dehydration, offer Popsicles, Jell-O, juices, and other beverages frequently. Oral rehydration fluids, such as Pedialyte, will also help to replace electrolytes lost with acute or chronic diarrhea.

The following list contains suggestions to provide supplemental calories and nutrient intake:

- Use a calorie-dense formula (24 to 27 kcal/oz) for infants. Add glucose polymers or medium-chain triglycerides (MCTs) to formulas, or reduce the amount of water added to powdered formulas to boost calories.
- Try liquid medical nutritional supplements, such as PediaSure, to provide supplemental calories.
- Add fats such as butter, margarine, or mayonnaise to foods to boost calories.
- Encourage nutrient-dense snacks such as raisins and peanuts or peanut butter.
- For the older, lactose-tolerant child, add skim milk powder to whole milk to boost calories and proteins.
- Make adjustments in diet consistency and temperatures to overcome eating difficulties associated with disease complications and any other eating problems.
- For lactose-intolerant children with AIDS, use soy-based infant formulas instead of milk.
- Add Lactaid (the enzyme lactase) to milk for better tolerance and digestion.
- Use low-lactose dairy foods such as yogurt and mild cheddar cheese, if tolerated.

Vitamin and mineral supplements in amounts one or two times the Recommended Dietary Allowance (RDA) may ensure adequate intake of these nutrients and contribute to meeting increased requirements that occur during hypermetabolic states. Attention should also be given to drug-nutrient interactions and other effects of these drugs on nutritional status.

Caregivers need to be particularly careful about food safety and sanitation. Safe food preparation is as important for children as it is for adults with HIV/AIDS, and the same food safety guidelines also apply.

Proper procedures and sanitary formula preparation must be followed for infants being bottle-fed. Infants should not be put to bed with a bottle of milk or juice, because they are easily contaminated. Unpasteurized milk and milk products should never be given, because they may be a source of *Salmonella* and other microorganisms that can cause intestinal infections.

Children should never be fed any food directly from a jar to avoid possible bacterial contamination of the remaining food from the child's mouth. Fruits and vegetables should be peeled or cooked, and meat, chicken, and fish should be well cooked. All utensils and dishes should be washed in a dishwasher or in hot, soapy water.

BIBLIOGRAPHY

American Dietetic Association: Position of the American Dietetic Association and Dietitians of Canada: nutrition intervention in the care of persons with human immunodeficiency virus infection, *J Am Diet Assoc* 104:1425, 2004.

Ball CS: Global issues in pediatric nutrition: AIDS, *Nutrition* 14(10):767, 1998.

Beisel WR: Nutrition in pediatric HIV infection, *J Nutr* 126(Suppl 10): 2611S, 1996.

Fields-Gardner C: HIV and children: the nutrition story. II. Nutrition in pediatric HIV disease, *BETA* July: 37, 1998. Retrieved June 29, 2009, from www.sfaf.org/treatment/beta/b37/b37kids2.html.

Grossman M: Special problems in the child with AIDS. In Sande MA, Volberding PA, editors: *The medical management of AIDS*, ed 2, Philadelphia, 1990, Saunders.

Raiten DJ: Nutrition and HIV infection: a review and evaluation of the extant knowledge of the relationship between nutrition and HIV infection, *Nutr Clin Pract* 6(3):S1, 1991.

KEY TERMS

virus Minute infectious agent, characterized by lack of independent metabolism and by the ability to reproduce with genetic continuity only with living host cells. They range in decreasing size from about 200 nm to 15 nm. (A nanometer [nm] is a linear measure equal to one billionth of a meter; it is also called a *millimicron*.) Each particle (virion) basically consists of nucleic acids (genetic material) and a protein shell, which protects and contains the genetic material and any enzymes present.

retrovirus Any of a family of single-strand ribonucleic acid (RNA) viruses having an envelope and containing a reverse coding enzyme that allows for a reversal of genetic transcription from RNA to deoxyribonucleic acid (DNA), rather than the usual DNA to RNA, the newly transcribed viral DNA then being incorporated into the host cell's DNA strand for the production of new RNA retroviruses.

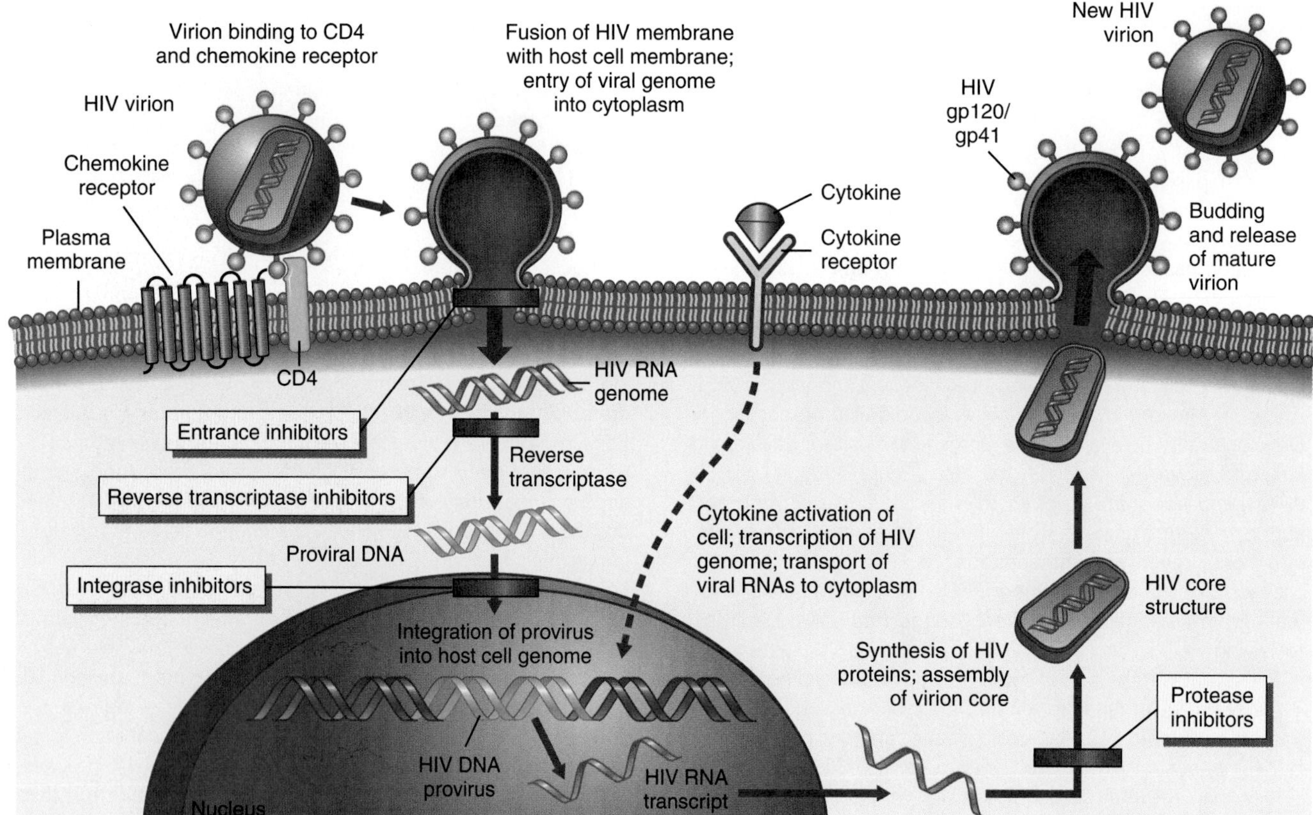

FIGURE 24-1 Life cycle and possible sites of therapeutic interventions of human immunodeficiency virus (HIV). (From Huether SE, McCance KL, editors: *Understanding pathophysiology,* ed 4, St Louis, 2008, Mosby.)

double-stranded DNA. The new DNA is inserted into the infected cell's genetic material by means of a second viral enzyme (integrase). Contained inside the cell, the new DNA may continue to be dormant, or it may be activated. If activated, then the viral information may be translated, causing the cell to break open and die, shedding infectious HIV particles. If the cell remains dormant, then the viral genetic material may remain dormant for years and is probably present for the life of the individual.[3]

Asymptomatic Phase

The individual clinical course of HIV infection varies substantially, but typically 3 to 6 weeks after the primary infection, most individuals experience varying degrees of nonspecific symptoms of fatigue, sore throat, muscle pain, fever, night sweats, and enlarged lymph nodes.[2,3] This stage of AIDS is self-limiting and is known as *acute HIV infection*. It may last days or weeks.[2] Antibody tests for HIV do not usually test positive at this time. This brief response corresponds to the process of *seroconversion,* the development of antibodies to the viral infection. Subsequent HIV testing will be positive. An extended asymptomatic period usually continues for the next 10 to 12 years.[2] However, this seemingly inactive period of relative wellness can be deceiving.

Antibodies typically appear within 4 to 7 weeks after infection through blood products but may remain seronegative for 6 to 14 months after sexual transmission. This phase between infection and manifestation of antibody is referred to as the *window period.*[3] During the asymptomatic stage of infection, viral replication continues and cellular destruction takes place in many tissues and organs of the body.[4] The virus continues to proliferate during this phase.[3]

Latent Phase

During this protracted phase, many individuals will still not exhibit clinical signs of the infection, whereas others have generalized enlarged lymph nodes. Viral replication appears to be reduced during this time. Helper-CD4+ T-cell count decreases, resulting in a weaker immune response.[5]

Final Acute Phase

Immune deficiency becomes evident in this phase, manifested by numerous serious complications such as gastrointestinal (GI) effects, neurologic effects, secondary infections, and manifestations (AIDS-related complex [ARC]) (see the *Case Study* box, "AIDS in a Young Man"). Individuals with HIV may demonstrate more effects in one or two categories, as well as minor changes in other body symptoms. CD4+ T-cell count is very low.[5]

CASE STUDY

AIDS in a Young Man

David is a 32-year-old man who was recently admitted to the hospital with a history of weight loss, painful difficulty swallowing, and watery diarrhea. He has been in a long-term, monogamous relationship with his partner for 6 years. David works as an accountant at a large firm. Six months ago, David started to notice he was losing weight involuntarily and he began having large-volume, loose stools. He developed thrush in his mouth about 3 months before admission, which caused the odynophagia. About 1 week before admission, a high temperature developed in David that did not respond to analgesics. He also complained of shortness of breath, chest tightness, and a dry cough. Physical examination revealed a weight loss of 11.3 kg (25 lb) and oral candidiasis; the chest radiographic examination was positive for *Pneumocystis carinii* pneumonia (PCP). David was admitted to receive intravenous antibiotics (trimethoprim-sulfamethoxazole [TMP-SMX]) and intravenous fluconazole, an antifungal. A stool culture revealed cytomegalovirus (CMV), and therefore intravenous ganciclovir, an antiviral agent, was initiated. David's oral intake was noted to be extremely poor; he also developed severe nausea and vomiting as a result of the medications and the infectious processes. His average daily volume of diarrhea also increased to 1800 mL/day. Results of the nutrition assessment were as follows:

Height	177.8 cm
Weight	61.4 kg
Usual weight	72.7 kg
Percentage weight loss	15.5%
Body weight (percentage of usual)	84%
Triceps skinfold	25th percentile
Midarm muscle circumference	25th percentile
$CD4^+$ cell count	118
Serum potassium	3.1 mEq/dL
Blood glucose	70 mg/dL
Blood urea nitrogen (BUN)	32 mg/dL
Creatinine	0.4 mg/dL
Serum albumin	2.8 mg/dL
Serum osmolality	325 mOsm/kg
Calculated basal energy expenditure (BEE)	2450 kcal/day

Questions for Analysis

1. Name and describe nutritional complications of oral candidiasis, gastrointestinal (GI) CMV infection, and PCP. How does treatment affect nutritional status?
2. Based on laboratory and anthropometric data, does David appear to be malnourished? What is your specific, objective evidence? What type of malnutrition does he exhibit?
3. Assess David's hydration status. What data could help you determine this?
4. What are the acute or immediate nutrition goals? What about long-term goals?
5. What type of nutrition support (enteral nutrition [EN] or parenteral nutrition [PN]) would you administer to David to prevent further nutritional depletion?

Diagnosis of HIV Infection

Testing Procedures

HIV infection is diagnosed by detection of the virus or serologic response to the virus. HIV infection can be identified by the detection of specific antibodies, as is done in the routine screening of blood and blood products for transfusion and in most epidemiologic studies. The recommended procedure for virus detection is a two-step process. The first step is enzyme-linked immunosorbent assay (ELISA) screening. Second, suspected positive samples from the ELISA screening are followed with Western blot testing for confirmation. Both tests are highly sensitive and specific, and both are used to confirm the results before informing the individual. Because a positive test is such a personal and life-changing event, most experienced physicians caring for HIV-infected patients repeat all positive tests again, even when they have been confirmed by Western blotting, before informing the individual.

Viral load assays are used to assess prognosis, determine the need for antiretroviral therapy and type of antiretroviral therapy to use, and monitor the progression of the disease. Viral load is inversely correlated with the $CD4^+$ cell count.

Clinical Symptoms and Illnesses

Early clinical symptoms that may follow initial exposure to the virus add further confirmation to the HIV-seropositive testing procedures. These initial symptoms, as well as possible associated illnesses and diseases that characterize later HIV stages, have been generally described earlier in discussion of basic disease progression. Some examples of these common opportunistic infections that manifest depending on $CD4^+$ cell count range are listed in Table 24-1.

MEDICAL MANAGEMENT

Elimination of HIV is not possible at this time.[6] The treatment regimen for HIV is a combination of drugs called *highly active antiretroviral therapy (HAART)*. HAART is a three-drug combination antiretroviral therapy. The combination includes reverse transcriptase inhibitors and protease inhibitors (PIs). Although resistant variants to these medications have been recognized, the death rate from AIDS-related diseases has been significantly decreased from the time of its introduction.[5]

HAART is used to achieve long-term viral suppression (measured by HIV viral load) and immunologic restoration (measured by CD4+ T-cell count) as a means to decrease HIV-related morbidity and mortality and improve quality of life.[6] This is frequently complicated because retroviruses incorporate into the genetic material of the host and may never be removed by antimicrobial therapy. Therefore medications to manage HIV are typically prescribed for the lifetime of the infected individual. Furthermore, HIV can survive in regions of the body where the antiviral drugs are not as effective, for instance the central nervous system (CNS).[5]

TABLE 24-1 COMMON INFECTIOUS COMPLICATIONS OF AIDS

MICROORGANISM	NUTRITIONAL IMPLICATIONS
Parasites	
Pneumocystis carinii	Dyspnea, fever, weight loss
Toxoplasma gondii	Fever
Cryptosporidium	Malabsorption, diarrhea
Isospora belli	Diarrhea
Microspora	Malabsorption, diarrhea
Entamoeba histolytica	Diarrhea
Giardia lamblia	Diarrhea
Acanthamoeba	Meningoencephalitis
Bacteria	
Campylobacter	Abdominal pain, cramping, bloody diarrhea, fever
Legionella	Fever
Listeria monocytogenes	Fever
Mycobacterium-avium-intracellulare	Fever, weight loss, diarrhea, malabsorption
Salmonella	Diarrhea, bacteremia
Shigella	Abdominal pain, bloody diarrhea, fever
Fungi	
Aspergillus	Fungemia, fevers, weight loss
Candida albicans	Thrush, stomatitis, esophagitis, nausea
Cryptococcus neoformans	Fever, nausea, vomiting
Histoplasma capsulatum	Fever, weight loss, dysphagia
Viruses	
Cytomegalovirus	Esophagitis, colitis, diarrhea
Herpes simplex virus	Ulcerative mucocutaneous lesions, stomatitis, esophagitis, pneumonia
Epstein-Barr virus	Oral hairy leukoplakia
Hepatitis B	Nausea, vomiting, fever
Herpes zoster	Mucocutaneous lesions

Data from American Dietetic Association: *Manual of clinical dietetics*, ed 6, Chicago, 2000, Author; Gold JWM: HIV-1 infection: diagnosis and management, *Med Clin North Am* 76(1):1, 1992; Bernard EM, Sepkowitz KA, Telzak EE, et al: Pneumocystosis, *Med Clin North Am* 76(1):107, 1992; and Ralten DJ: Nutrition and HIV infection: a review and evaluation of the extent of knowledge of the relationship between nutrition and HIV infection, *Nutr Clin Pract* 6(3):1S, 1991.

Indications for starting HAART predominantly centers around the CD4+ T-cell count (<350 cells/mm^3) and viral load (>100,000 copies/mL). Antiretroviral therapy is recommended for pregnant women, those with HIV-associated nephropathy, and individuals coinfected with hepatitis B virus (HBV) regardless of CD4+ T-cell count.[6,7] Adherence to this drug regime can be demanding for the HIV-infected individual and health care providers. Motivation to begin lifelong medication therapy should be considered in advance of initiating HAART. Furthermore, dosing convenience, drug safety profiles, and drug-drug interactions ought to be contemplated for each individual.[6]

Once-daily regimens and fixed-dose combinations of antiretroviral medications have radically reduced the number of pills taken daily from as many as 10 to 20 pills to as few as one or two tablets per day. On the whole, individuals tolerate HAART; however, drug toxicities can be common and should be evaluated in contrast to benefits of favorable virologic and immunologic responses.[6]

Classes of Drugs

More than 20 antiretroviral agents, from five classes of drugs, exist[6,7]:

- Nucleoside/nucleotide reverse transcriptase inhibitors (NRTIs)
- Nonnucleoside reverse transcriptase inhibitors (NNRTIs)
- PIs
- Entry inhibitors (fusion and CCR5 entry inhibitors)
- Integrase inhibitors

Although many of these drugs are available as fixed-dose combinations, the majority are formulated as individual medications. This makes treatment regimens easier, lessens pill burden, and optimistically increases patient medication compliance (Table 24-2).[6] Many side effects occur from these drugs, which may contribute to noncompliance with drug regimens as listed in the *Diet-Medications Interactions* box, "Protease Inhibitor Drug-Nutrient Side Effects and Interactions." Side effects such as nausea and diarrhea may require diet modifications (see Chapter 19).

NUTRITION THERAPY

Basic Role of Nutrition in HIV Disease Process

Nutrition support plays a vital role in three basic areas throughout the HIV disease process. First, it is a vital component of care for the involuntary weight loss and body tissue wasting caused by disease effects on metabolism, reflected in the severe state of protein-energy malnutrition (PEM). Second, and fundamental in all conditions associated with the body's basic immune system, nutrition is an intimate and integral component of care through specific roles of key nutrients in maintaining the body's immunocompetence. Furthermore, for many associated diseases, individual nutritional status influences the effect of morbidity and mortality regardless of disease process. Third, many drug therapies, especially PIs, cause lipodystrophy, reduced levels of high-density lipoprotein (HDL) cholesterol, hypertriglyceridemia, hyperglycemia, and insulin resistance. Long-term consequences include an elevated risk of cardiovascular disease (CVD) in this population.

Nutrition Assessment

The initial nutrition assessment for an HIV-infected patient is an important beginning point for continuing nutrition care that is to follow. A registered dietitian (RD) should conduct

TABLE 24-2 ANTIRETROVIRAL DRUGS USED TO TREAT HIV/AIDS

GENERIC (ABBREVIATION)	TRADE NAME	FREQUENCY OF DOSING	TIMING CONSIDERATIONS AND COMMON ADVERSE NUTRITION CONSEQUENCES
Nucleoside Reverse Transcriptase Inhibitors*			
(As a general rule, these agents may lead to anemia, loss of appetite, low vitamin B_{12}, low copper, low zinc, and low carnitine)			
Abacavir (ABC)	Ziagen	Once daily	Take without regard to meals; snacks may reduce gastrointestinal (GI) upset; alcohol can increase drug levels; nausea, vomiting, diarrhea, and loss of appetite possible
Didanosine (ddl)	Videx/Videx EC	Once daily	Take 30 min before or 2 hr after meal; do not mix with acidic liquid (e.g., grapefruit juice, oranges, other citrus; tomatoes or tomato juice); do not take antacids with magnesium or aluminum within 2 hr; nausea possible
Emtricitabine (FTC)	Emtriva	Once daily	Take without regard to meals; snacks may reduce GI upset
Lamivudine (3TC)	Epivir	Once daily	Take without regard to meals; snacks may reduce GI upset
Stavudine (d4T)	Zerit	Twice daily	Take without regard to meals; snacks may limit GI upset; mouth/esophageal ulcers possible
Tenofovir disoproxil fumarate (TDF)	Viread	Once daily	Take without regard to meals; diarrhea, nausea, vomiting, and flatulence possible
Zidovudine (AZT, ZDV)	Retrovir	Twice daily	Take without regard to meals; constipation, taste alterations possible; macrocytic anemia or neutropenia possible
Nonnucleoside Reverse Transcriptase Inhibitors*			
Delavirdine (DLV)	Rescriptor	Three times daily	Take without regard to meals; avoid St. John's wort; constipation, diarrhea, dry mouth, and flatulence possible; decreased appetite possible
Efavirenz (EFV)	Sustiva	Once daily	High-fat/high-calorie meals increase peak plasma concentrations; take on empty stomach; take at bedtime to decrease adverse effects; taste alterations, potential loss of appetite, and flatulence possible
Etravirine (ETR)	Intelence	Twice daily	Take after a meal; nausea possible
Nevirapine (NVP)	Viramune	Twice daily	Take without regard to meals; snacks may limit GI upset; nausea and loss of appetite possible
Protease Inhibitors†			
Amprenavir (APV)	Agenerase	Twice daily	Take on empty stomach; low fat limits GI upset (avoid high fat meals); avoid grapefruit juice; increase fluid intake; avoid taking antacids within 2 hr; nausea, vomiting, gas, and diarrhea possible
Atazanavir (ATV)	Reyataz	Once daily	Take with food; avoid taking simultaneously with antacids or H_2 blockers
Darunavir (DRV)	Prezista	Twice daily	Take with food; diarrhea and nausea possible
Fosamprenavir (FPV)	Lexiva	Twice daily	Take without regard to meals; diarrhea, nausea, and vomiting possible
Indinavir (IDV)	Crixivan	Three times daily	Avoid grapefruit juice; avoid St. John's wort; *(unboosted)* take 2 hr before or 2 hr after meals; take on empty stomach, but if not tolerated may take with nonfat milk; eat low-fat meals and light snacks; *(ritonavir [RTV] boosted)* timing of food intake not a consideration; loss of appetite, nausea, and metallic taste possible
Lopinavir + ritonavir (LPV/r)	Kaletra	Twice daily	Time of food not a consideration; nausea, vomiting, and diarrhea possible
Nelfinavir (NFV)	Viracept	Twice daily	Diarrhea possible
Ritonavir (RTV)	Norvir	Twice daily	Take with food if possible (may improve tolerability); nausea, vomiting, diarrhea, and taste changes possible
Saquinavir (SQV) (hard gel) Fortovase (FTV) (soft gel)	Invirase	Twice daily	Take within 2 hr of a meal; GI intolerance, nausea, and diarrhea possible
Tipranavir (TPV)	Aptivus	Twice daily	Take with fatty meal

Continued

TABLE 24-2 **ANTIRETROVIRAL DRUGS USED TO TREAT HIV/AIDS—cont'd**

GENERIC (ABBREVIATION)	TRADE NAME	FREQUENCY OF DOSING	TIMING CONSIDERATIONS AND COMMON ADVERSE NUTRITION CONSEQUENCES
Entry and Fusion Inhibitors‡			
Enfuvirtide (T-20)	Fuzeon	Twice daily (subcutaneously)	Not applicable
CCR5 Antagonists			
Maraviroc (MVC)	Selzentry	Twice daily	No food effect; take with or without food; abdominal pain possible
Integrase Inhibitors§			
Raltegravir (RAL)	Isentress	Twice daily	Take with or without food; nausea and diarrhea possible

Data from Dong KR, Mangili A: Highly active antiretroviral therapy (HAART). In Hendricks KM, Dong KR, Gerrior JL, editors: *Nutrition management of HIV and AIDS*, Chicago, 2009, American Dietetic Association; Panel on Antiretroviral Guidelines for the use of antiretroviral agents in HIV-1-infected adults and adolescents, Washington, DC, 2008, Department of Health and Human Services. Retrieved July 14, 2010, from http://www.aidsinfo.nih.gov/contentfiles/adultandadolescentgl.pdf.
*Nucleoside/nucleotide reverse transcriptase inhibitors (NRTIs) and nonnucleoside reverse transcriptase inhibitors (NNRTIs) prevent reverse transcriptase from making more copies of the human immunodeficiency virus (HIV) genome.
†Protease inhibitors (PIs) prevent protease from breaking apart long strands of viral proteins to make the smaller, active proteins HIV needs to reproduce.
‡Fusion inhibitors are specific types of entry inhibitors that prevent fusion between HIV's outer envelope and the cell's outer membrane.
§Integrase inhibitors prevent integrase from inserting HIV's genetic material into an infected cell's genetic material.

DIET-MEDICATIONS INTERACTIONS

Protease Inhibitor Drug-Nutrient Side Effects and Interactions

PROTEASE INHIBITOR DRUGS	DRUG SIDE EFFECTS	COMMENTS
Saquinavir (Invirase)	Diarrhea, nausea, abdominal cramps	Take after high-kcalorie, high-fat meal for best absorption; grapefruit juice decreases absorption
Indinavir (Crixivan)	Taste changes, nausea, vomiting, diarrhea, elevated blood cholesterol, hypertriglyceridemia, and hyperglycemia	Best absorbed on empty stomach or nonfat light snack Increase fluids to about 24 oz/day (consider weight and age) High-kcalorie diet
Ritonavir (Norvir)	Diarrhea, nausea, vomiting; elevated liver function tests, anorexia, abnormal feelings in mouth (burning, prickling); hypercholesterolemia, hypertriglyceridemia	Take with high-kcalorie, high-fat foods
Nelfinavir (Viracept)	Nausea, diarrhea, loose stools	Take with food
Amprenavir (Agenerase)	Nausea, vomiting, diarrhea, flatulence	Do not take with a high-fat meal
Nevirapine* (Viramune)	Skin rash, mouth sores, general fatigue; elevated liver function tests	May take with food or on empty stomach

Data from Heller LS, Shattuck L: Nutrition support with children with HIV/AIDS, *J Am Diet Assoc 97*(5):473, 1997; AIDS Project Los Angeles: *Nutritional considerations for protease inhibitors*, Los Angeles, 2009, AIDS Project Los Angeles. Retrieved June 30, 2009, from www.apla.org.
*Nevirapine is in the drug category of nonnucleoside reverse transcriptase inhibitors (NNRTIs).
Note: All protease inhibitors (PIs) have the potential for causing hypercholesterolemia, hypertriglyceridemia, and hyperglycemia, along with body composition changes (lipodystrophy).
Note: A high-fat/high-calorie meal is defined as 1006 kcal, 48 g protein, 57 g fat, 60 g carbohydrate (the nutritional breakdown for this meal for the best absorption rates).

this work, which provides necessary baseline information for planning practical individual nutrition support. More importantly, it establishes the essential provider-patient relationship, the human context within which this continuing nutrition care and support will be provided as needed. The basic nutrition assessment will provide a practical guide for HIV-infected patients, as outlined in the following sections.[8]

Clinical Assessment

- Medical history
- Physical parameters related to nutrition care
- Existing nutrition-related issues:
  - Hepatitis
  - Diabetes
  - Oral health issues
  - Bone disorders

COMPLEMENTARY AND ALTERNATIVE MEDICINE (CAM)

Are Persons with HIV and AIDS Vulnerable to Nutritional Quackery?

People with chronic diseases, such as acquired immunodeficiency syndrome (AIDS), who lack curative therapy and have poor prognoses are susceptible to claims of unproved therapies and nutrition quackery. The following questionable practices are some of the nutritional quackery being touted as treatments for human immunodeficiency virus (HIV) infection.

Megadoses of Nutrients

Large doses of vitamins A and C, selenium, and zinc have been recommended to restore cell-mediated immunity by increasing T-cell number and activity. The value of such large doses has not been established in controlled clinical studies. In fact, the opposite is true; megadoses of these nutrients can be dangerous. Chronic intakes of vitamin A in excess of 25,000 IU/day can be toxic, especially to the liver. Doses of vitamin C greater than 2000 mg can cause diarrhea, nausea, and gastrointestinal (GI) upset; increase the risk of kidney stones; and cause a urine test to test falsely positive for diabetes. Chronic intakes of excess zinc, as little as 25 mg/day, can cause GI distress, nausea, and impaired immune function. Selenium is also toxic in high chronic doses. It is recommended that persons with HIV/AIDS take two multivitamin-mineral supplements per day to ensure intake of 200% of the Recommended Dietary Allowance (RDA) for vitamins and minerals.

Dr. Berger's Immune Power Diet

In his 1985 book, Stuart M. Berger[1] states that poor health is caused by "immune hypersensitivity" to many foods such as milk, wheat, corn, yeast, soy, sugar, and eggs. He suggests a 21-day elimination diet for foods believed to cause allergies, followed by a reintroduction phase and then a maintenance diet, to prevent food sensitivities and "revitalize" the immune system. The usefulness of this diet has not been tested or proved by scientific studies. The diet promoted in Berger's book (high in fruits and vegetables and low in fat and calcium) may cause malnutrition, and the suggestion that moldy food be consumed to test for allergy to molds is dangerous to persons who are immunocompromised. His claims are unsubstantiated.

Antiviral AL 721

This compound, developed in Israel and approved by the U.S. Food and Drug Administration (FDA) for clinical trials, is composed of "active lipids" (ALs) mixed in a ratio of 70% neutral lipid, 20% lecithin, and 10% phosphatidylethanolamine—hence the 721 designation. It has been hypothesized that AL 721 can reduce or inhibit HIV infection. Clinical trials found little toxicity but no consistent trends in T-cell quantification or HIV cultures. AL 721 made at home from soy or egg yolk lecithin or obtained already mixed may be impure and can spoil easily if stored improperly.

Yeast-Free Diet (Anticandidiasis Diet)

Candida infection, which causes oral and esophageal thrush, is common in individuals who are immunocompromised. Authors of this diet suggest that certain persons have "candidiasis hypersensitivity" and that by observing the diet (restricted in carbohydrates, yeast, sugar, processed foods, fruits [initially], and milk), this disorder can be successfully treated. The American Academy of Allergy, Asthma, and Immunology has been strongly critical of these concepts. Because the diet is limited in carbohydrates, an individual may develop ketosis, which can cause nausea and headache. This diet may also be too low in calories for individuals with HIV/AIDS.

Colonic Therapy

Colonic irrigation is touted to detoxify the large intestine to reduce poisons and wastes in the body. This procedure is expensive and the FDA has not approved it for "cleansing" the body of wastes. Colon cleansing is only approved and medically indicated before a colonoscopy or sigmoidoscopy. Great potential exists for harm because colonic irrigation can cause severe cramps, pain, perforation of the large intestine resulting in serious infection, and electrolyte losses, especially potassium. No medically substantiated reason exists for a person with HIV/AIDS (or anyone, for that matter) to have a colonic irrigation.

Macrobiotic Diet

A macrobiotic diet is based on an Eastern philosophy that it will restore balance and harmony between yin and yang forces and thereby improve health. However, it is very low in fat and high in fiber: 50% (by volume) whole grain cereals, 20% to 30% vegetables, 10% to 15% cooked beans or seaweed, and 5% miso (fermented soy paste) or tamari broth soup. This regimen can produce protein-calorie malnutrition and provides inadequate intake of riboflavin, niacin, and calcium in adults, as well as pyridoxine and vitamins B_{12} and D in children (in addition to those nutrients mentioned for adults).

These diets and other alternative therapies require further study in controlled clinical trials.

REFERENCES

1. Berger SM: *Dr. Berger's immune power diet*, New York, 1985, New American Library Trade.

BIBLIOGRAPHY

Jarvis WT: *Colonic irrigation, Peabody*, Mass, 1995, National Council Against Health Fraud.

Raiten DJ: Nutrition and HIV infection: a review and evaluation of the extant knowledge of the relationship between nutrition and HIV infection, *Nutr Clin Pract* 6(3):S1, 1991.

- Family history of nutrition-related issues
- Weight history
- Usual level of physical activity
- GI complications
- Medications:
  - Potential food and drug interactions
  - Nutrition-related adverse effects
- Use of any complimentary therapies (see the *Complementary and Alternative Medicine [CAM]* box, "Are Persons With HIV and AIDS Vulnerable to Nutritional Quackery?")
- Presence of opportunistic infections that may affect intake or metabolism
- Anthropometric measurements:
  - Weight
  - Body mass index (BMI)
  - Subcutaneous fat stores

Biochemical Assessment

- Albumin
- Hemoglobin (Hb)
- Serum iron
- Magnesium
- Vitamin levels
- Blood lipids
- Renal function
- Liver enzyme levels

Diet Intake Assessment

- Usual intake, current intake, restrictions, modifications (use 24-hour recall and food diaries)
- Ethnic and cultural food practices
- Limitations in food access, food preparation, or both
- Food intolerances, allergies, or both
- Use of macronutrient or micronutrient supplements (or use of both)
- Patient's goals for improving his or her intake
- Use of fraudulent nutrition products or fads

Psychosocial Issues Related to Nutrition

- Living situation, personal support
- Food environment, types of meals, eating assistance needed
- History of eating disorders or body image concerns
- Housing status
- Access to safe food and water

Goals of Nutrition Therapy

Quality and length of life can be enhanced by nutrition intervention. Nutritional status is directly linked to survival rate of individuals with HIV. Furthermore, nutrition therapy (NT) has been shown to reduce morbidity, improve health outcomes, reduce cost, and shorten hospital stays. Goals of nutrition intervention include the following[8]:

- Early assessment and treatment of conditions leading to malnutrition
- Maintenance of nutrition status:
  - Weight
  - Protein stores
- Management of comorbid conditions:
  - Obesity
  - Diabetes
  - Hyperlipidemia
- Management of nutrition-related side-effects from HIV or disease treatment

Nutrient Requirements

As in any disease process, sufficient intake of nutrients is vital to restoration and preservation of health. In addition, although the benefits of providing adequate amounts of energy, protein, and micronutrients for individuals living with HIV are clear,[8,9] the exact amount of each nutrient needed is less clear.[8]

Energy

Individuals' energy needs will vary depending on numerous factors, including nutrient malabsorption, altered metabolism, nutrient depletion, severity of disease, and opportunistic infections. Adequate energy intake is important to prevent weight loss and loss of lean body mass. Care should be taken to estimate recommendations for daily energy intake, although no standard level of energy intake has been established.[8]

Protein

For asymptomatic HIV-positive individuals, the Dietary Reference Intakes (DRIs) or 0.8 g protein/kg body weight will most likely be sufficient. For those who have suffered wasted lean body mass, increased protein intake up to 1.2 to 2.0 g protein/kg body weight may be beneficial. Animal and plant sources of protein may be used. Strict vegetarians should consume an extensive variety of foods to make certain sufficient intake of essential amino acids is achieved, and they may benefit from additional protein, calorie, iron, and vitamin B_{12} supplementation.[8]

Fat

Fat requirements of individuals with HIV do not seem to be different from the general population. Some medications, therapies for HIV, symptoms of infections (i.e., diarrhea), and malabsorption syndromes possibly will necessitate modification in timing, quality, and type of fat intake for some. It is crucial to work with each individual closely to determine his or her needs.[8]

Micronutrients

Currently, the complete function of micronutrients in treatment of HIV is not completely known. However, individuals are sure to benefit from a varied diet rich in micronutrients.[8]

Food and Water Safety

The compromised immune system of individuals with AIDS puts them at great risk for foodborne or waterborne illnesses. Fortunately, nearly all cases of foodborne and waterborne illnesses can be reduced or prevented with appropriate safety measures including safe food handling and use of safe water sources (Box 24-1). It is essential for the RD to stress food and water safety in nutrition counseling for individuals living with HIV, their significant others, and their caretakers.[8]

According to the Centers for Disease Control and Prevention (CDC), boiling municipal tap water and use of bottled water are not essential unless a local public health department has issued notice that public drinking water is not safe for individuals living with HIV.[10] Box 24-2 outlines precautions of particular importance for individuals living in areas without a municipal water source. Ice and fountain drinks in restaurants are often made from municipal water and should be avoided if safety of the water is unknown.[8] Food and water sanitation may not be adequate when traveling abroad. Guidelines for choosing safer beverages are outlined in Box 24-3.

HAART-Associated Metabolic and Body Composition Changes

Although HAART has revolutionized medical treatment of HIV and AIDS and reduced incidence of malnutrition and infections, adverse effects of HAART continue to be a major obstacle to patient compliance and a limiting factor that drives the cost-benefit ratio for pharmacologic therapy. Lipodystrophy and its related fat distribution complications have become the major nutrition issues in patients being treated with PIs. Lipodystrophy syndrome consists of changes in body shape that are caused by abnormal redistribution of fat. Fat accumulates in the abdominal area (truncal and visceral obesity), in the axillary pads, and in the dorsocervical pads ("buffalo hump") but decreases in the legs, arms, and nasolabial and cheek pads.[11] Lipodystrophy,

BOX 24-1 FOOD SAFETY PRECAUTIONS FOR INDIVIDUALS LIVING WITH HIV

Purchasing Food
- Do not eat food that has passed the expiration date or purchase past the "sell by" date.
- Make sure all dairy products (including cheeses) and juices have been pasteurized or made with pasteurized ingredients.
- When shopping, put packaged meat, poultry, and fish in separate plastic bags to ensure juices do not drip on other foods.
- Do not purchase food that has been displayed in unsafe or unclean conditions (e.g., meat that has been unrefrigerated or cooked shrimp that is displayed with raw shrimp).
- Do not purchase cans that are dented, leaking, or bulging.

Preparing and Serving Food
- Wash hands with warm soapy water before and after preparing and eating foods. Also wash hands before and after using the bathroom, handling pets, or changing diapers.
- Wash counter surfaces, cutting boards, can openers, and utensils with hot soapy water before and after use. Sanitize kitchen surfaces, using a commercial sanitizing product or a mixture of 1 teaspoon of chlorine bleach per 1 quart of water.
- Avoid cross-contamination of foods.
- Do not eat raw or undercooked meat, eggs, poultry, fish, or shellfish. (This includes hotdogs, types of sushi and sashimi that contain raw fish, and foods that contain raw eggs.)
- Use an appropriate food thermometer to ensure that all foods reach the proper internal temperature before serving.

Storing Foods
- Store raw meat, poultry, and seafood in separate containers on the bottom shelf of the refrigerator
- Freeze fresh meat, poultry, and seafood that you do not plan to use within a few days. Do not refreeze previously frozen foods and thawed foods, especially meat, poultry, and seafood.
- Use refrigerator and freezer thermometers to ensure foods are stored at appropriate temperatures (freezer at 0° F and refrigerator at 40° F).

Eating Out
- Choose "well done" meats, fish, and poultry. Make sure they are served hot.
- Avoid raw or undercooked eggs. Order fried eggs cooked "hard" and avoid eggs that are "sunny-side-up." Scrambled eggs should not be runny.
- If you aren't sure about the ingredients in a dish or how it is cooked, ask your wait staff before you order.
- Avoid open salad bars in public places.

Reprinted with permission from Vining L: General nutrition issues for healthy living with HIV infection. In Hendricks KM, Dong KR, Gerrior JL, editors: *Nutrition management of HIV and AIDS*, Chicago, 2009, American Dietetic Association.

BOX 24-2 EXTRA PRECAUTIONS TO ENSURE SAFE WATER

- Do not drink water straight from lakes, rivers, streams, springs, or the ocean.
- Boil tap water (bring to rolling boil for 1 minutes, then store in a clean container) or distill or filter using a filter that is effective down to 1 micron.*
- Choose bottled water (ensure water has been filtered using a filter that is effective down to 1 micron).
- Use boiled, distilled, or filtered tap water for home use (including making ice, brushing teeth, etc.).

*Current recommendations from the Centers for Disease Control and Prevention (CDC) state that use of bottled water and/or boiling of municipal tap water are not necessary unless the local public health department has issued warnings that public drinking water is not safe for persons living with HIV.

Reprinted with permission from Vining L: General nutrition issues for healthy living with HIV infection. In Hendricks KM, Dong KR, Gerrior JL, editors: *Nutrition management of HIV and AIDS*, Chicago, 2009, American Dietetic Association.

BOX 24-3 CHOOSING SAFER BEVERAGES

Beverages That Are Safer	Beverages That May Not Be Safe
• Carbonated beverages ("sodas") that come in cans or bottles (check seal to ensure safety)	• Fountain drinks or drinks served over ice
• Fruit drinks that come in cans or bottles (check seal to ensure safety)	• Drinks made by mixing frozen concentrate with water
• Steaming hot tea or coffee	• Iced tea or coffee
• Pasteurized milk and other dairy products	• Unpasteurized milk and other dairy products
• Pasteurized juices	• Fresh fruit juices (e.g., unpasteurized cider, fresh-squeezed orange juice)

Reprinted with permission from Vining L: General nutrition issues for healthy living with HIV infection. In Hendricks KM, Dong KR, Gerrior JL, editors: *Nutrition management of HIV and AIDS*, Chicago, 2009, American Dietetic Association.

although not life threatening, can cause varying degrees of depression, anxiety, social withdrawal, and low self-esteem, which can ultimately lead to poor medication compliance. Many patients discontinue therapy, risking progression of HIV infection. HAART can also cause hyperlipidemia (especially hypertriglyceridemia and hypercholesterolemia) and insulin resistance, which can significantly increase the risk of developing CVD. This is a major concern and potentially a major deterrent to early or continuous therapy. Overall, the risk of myocardial infarction (MI) in HIV-infected patients taking PIs appears to be twofold to threefold greater than in the general population.[12] Persons on HAART are also at increased risk of developing diabetes, hypertension, and osteoporosis.

Obtaining baseline anthropometrics (waist-hip ratio, bioelectric impedance analysis, skinfold measurements) and serial measurements (i.e., at each clinic visit) is important for monitoring changes in body composition. In addition, baseline measurements of triglycerides, total cholesterol and lipoproteins (HDL, low-density lipoprotein [LDL], very low-density lipoprotein [VLDL]), blood glucose, and blood pressure should be obtained (also at each clinic visit to monitor for changes). Diet, exercise, and pharmacologic agents are useful in the treatment of lipodystrophy syndrome. Patients with abnormal LDL, HDL, and total cholesterol levels may benefit from observing the therapeutic lifestyle changes (TLC) diet (see Chapter 21 for details), which emphasizes grains, cereals, legumes, fruits, vegetables, lean meats, poultry, fish, and low-fat dairy products. Diet-resistant hyperlipidemia may need to be controlled with lipid-lowering agents. Currently researchers are trying to determine which drugs can be used safely and effectively in persons on anti-HIV drugs. Individuals with insulin resistance and hyperglycemia will need counseling for carbohydrate counting (see Chapter 22). An individual with hypertriglyceridemia will need to limit intake of simple carbohydrates and alcohol. Exercise, especially weight training, may help prevent muscle wasting in the arms, legs, and buttocks, whereas aerobic exercise may help control abdominal visceral fat accumulation. Clinical trials are ongoing to determine actual benefits.

Use of Anabolic Agents in HIV and AIDS

Use of anabolic agents has been recommended as an effective way of improving gains in lean body mass. Anabolic agents such as oxandrolone and nandrolone decanoate are known to promote protein anabolism and are generally safe when taken as prescribed.[13] Recombinant human growth hormone (rhGH) (trade name, Serostim) is the most extensively studied anabolic agent; it has also been shown to significantly improve lean body mass and nitrogen balance in treatment of HIV/AIDS wasting.[14] Human growth hormone therapy may help control some of the body composition changes seen in some individuals with lipodystrophy. However, many potential side effects exist for anabolic agents, including gynecomastia, testicular atrophy and decreased fertility, salt retention, lipid and carbohydrate abnormalities, and acne. In addition, anabolic agents are frequently very expensive (approximately $18,000 per year); however, Medicaid has approved reimbursement for this treatment.[15] Resistance or weight training is strongly recommended as a safe and effective method for maintaining and improving lean body mass in all individuals who are physically able to exercise.

Nutrition Counseling, Education, and Supportive Strategies

An adolescent client once aptly defined a counselor as "someone to talk to while I make up my mind." Client-centered counseling in the care of persons with HIV infection and AIDS must be just that. Professionals and patients must remain involved throughout the progressive course of the disease, because the patient's wishes and needs are ultimately paramount in various treatments and decisions about care. The basic goal of nutrition counseling is to make the fewest possible changes in the person's lifestyle and food patterns necessary to promote optimal nutritional status while providing maximal comfort and quality of life. In this person-centered care process, several counseling principles are particularly pertinent, as follows:

- *Motivation:* Changed behavior in any area requires motivation, desire, and ability to achieve one's goals. Until the patient perceives food patterns and behaviors as appropriate goals, it is best to wait for a better time and begin with establishing a general supportive climate in which to continue working together. Any specific obstacle raised by the patient, such as time, physical limitations, money, or increased anxiety, can be met with related suggestions for the patient to consider. Priorities among needs should be recognized in the care plan, and items should be introduced according to order of importance and immediacy of the patient's nutrition problems.
- *Rationale:* Any diet or food behavior change, with possible benefits and risks, must be clearly explained to the patient. The reason *why* something is being done is important to everyone.
- *Provider-patient agreement:* In the best interests of all concerned, the patient and health care provider must agree to the change. Any change should be structured around daily routines and include any caregivers as needed. The nutrition counselor should provide any needed information and encouragement throughout the process.
- *Manageable steps:* All information given and actions agreed on should proceed in manageable steps, as small as necessary, in order of complexity and difficulty. Information overload can discourage anyone, and the particular stress load at any point can be intolerable for the patient. At such points of stress, patients are more vulnerable to the lure of unproved HIV/AIDS therapies.

TO SUM UP

The viral evolution and current worldwide spread of HIV infection have reached epidemic proportions and are still growing. Disease progression follows three distinct stages: (1) HIV infection; (2) AIDS-related complex (ARC), with associated opportunistic illnesses; and (2) full-blown AIDS, with complicating diseases leading to death. This overall disease progression from initial infection to death lasts about 10 to 12 years. The Public Health Service and the CDC are responsible for monitoring the disease and providing leadership in research and treatment development, based on collaborative information exchange with scientists worldwide.

During the initial decade of the epidemic in the 1980s, scientists learned the nature and life cycle of the new mutation of HIV, as well as its transmission modes and population groups at risk. Development of diagnostic-testing procedures has enabled population surveillance, individual detection of disease, and personal care to proceed. The important role of nutrition support in the personal care of HIV-infected individuals has become evident.

Medical management of HIV infection, which is without a vaccine or cure, involves supportive treatment of associated illnesses and complicating diseases. In the terminal HIV stage, the virus eventually gains sufficient strength to destroy white blood cells of the host's immune system and death follows.

Current ongoing research involves study of the role of micronutrients in oxidation processes in the cell. Nutritional management focuses on providing personal individual nutrition support to counteract the severe body wasting and malnutrition characteristic of the disease. The process of nutrition care involves comprehensive nutrition assessment and evaluation of personal needs, planning care with each patient and his or her caregivers, and meeting practical food needs. Throughout the care process, nutrition counseling, education, and strategic services also help provide psychosocial support to each patient.

QUESTIONS FOR REVIEW

1. Describe the evolutionary history of HIV-1 and its current worldwide epidemic spread. How is it transmitted, and why do you think it has spread so rapidly? Identify major population groups at risk.
2. Describe the nature of the AIDS virus and its action in the human body. What is a retrovirus?
3. Describe the progression of HIV infection in terms of its stages of development from initial infection to death.
4. Identify the drugs currently used in the medical management of HIV/AIDS, and describe any associated actions, side effects, or toxicities that may relate to dietary management.
5. Discuss the causes of HIV wasting and its medical and nutrition therapies.
6. Outline the basic parts of a comprehensive initial nutrition assessment of a patient with HIV/AIDS.
7. Describe the general process of planning nutrition care based on patient assessment information and the main types of nutrition problems in patients with HIV/AIDS. Devise a related plan of action for each type of problem. Can you give an example of how you might follow up to determine what parts of your plan worked and what parts did not work? List any adjustments that should be made to your original nutrition care plan based on that follow-up.

REFERENCES

1. Centers for Disease Control and Prevention: Twenty-five years of HIV/AIDS—United States, 1981-2006, *MMWR Morb Mortal Wkly Rep* 55(21):585, 2008.
2. Wanke C, Khalil S, Gerrior JL: Overview of HIV/AIDS today. In Hendricks KM, Dong KR, Gerrior JL, editors: *Nutrition management of HIV and AIDS*, Chicago, 2009, American Dietetic Association.
3. Rote NS: Hypersensitivities, infection, and immune efficiencies. In Huether SE, McCance KL, editors: *Understanding pathophysiology*, ed 4, St Louis, 2008, Mosby.
4. Rote NS: Alterations in immunity and inflammation. In McCance KL, Huether SE, editors: *Pathophysiology: the biologic basis for disease in adults and children*, ed 5, St Louis, 2006, Mosby.
5. Gould BE: *Pathophysiology for the health professions*, ed 3, St Louis, 2006, Mosby.
6. Dong KR, Mangili A: Highly active antiretroviral therapy (HAART). In Hendricks KM, Dong KR, Gerrior JL, editors: *Nutrition management of HIV and AIDS*, Chicago, 2009, American Dietetic Association.
7. Panel on Antiretroviral Guidelines for Adults and Adolescents: *Guidelines for the use of antiretroviral agents in HIV-1-infected adults and adolescents*, Washington, DC, 2008, Department of Health and Human Services. Retrieved July 14, 2010, from http://www.aidsinfo.nih.gov/contentfiles/adultandadolescentgl.pdf.
8. Vining L: General nutrition issues for healthy living with HIV infection. In Hendricks KM, Dong KR, Gerrior JL, editors: *Nutrition management of HIV and AIDS*, Chicago, 2009, American Dietetic Association.
9. American Dietetic Association: Position of the American Dietetic Association and Dietitians of Canada: nutrition intervention in the care of persons with human immunodeficiency virus infection, *J Am Diet Assoc* 104:1425, 2004.
10. Centers for Disease Control and Prevention: *You can prevent cryptosporidiosis*, Atlanta, 2007, Centers for Disease Control and Prevention. Retrieved June 30, 2009, from http://www.cdc.gov/hiv/resources/brochures/crypto.htm.
11. Kotler DP: In *Lipodystrophy—it just gets more complicated*, Paper presented at the Eighth Annual Conference on Retroviruses and Opportunistic Infections, Chicago, Feb 6, 2001.
12. Scerola D, Di Matteo A, Uberti F, et al: Reversal of cachexia in patient treated with potent antiviral therapy, *AIDS Read* 10(6):365, 2000.
13. Loss JC: The use of anabolic agents in HIV disease, *Support Line* 21(3):23, 1999.
14. Schambelan M, Mulligan K, Grunfeld C: Recombinant growth hormone in patients with HIV-associated wasting: a randomized, placebo-controlled trial, *Ann Intern Med* 125:873, 1996.
15. FDC Reports: *Serono Serostim required on state Medicaid formularies, HCFA says*, vol 66, Chevy Chase, Md, 1999, FDC Reports.

FURTHER RESOURCES

Websites of Interest

AIDS.org News: www.aids.org/news.html. *[This organization provides education to help prevent HIV infections and improve the lives of those affected by HIV and AIDS.]*

American Dietetic Association: www.eatright.org. *[Website of the world's largest food and nutrition professionals organization providing information regarding nutrition and health through research, education, and advocacy.]*

Centers for Disease Control and Prevention, Division of HIV/AIDS Prevention (DHAP): www.cdc.gov/hiv/dhap.htm. *[This website provides information regarding treatment, care, and support for persons living with HIV/AIDS.]*

Medscape: www.hiv.medscape.com. *[Provides news and research regarding the fight against HIV/AIDS.]*

National AIDS Treatment Advocacy Project: www.natap.org. *[This non-profit corporation educates individuals about HIV and hepatitis treatments.]*

National Association of People With AIDS: www.napwa.org.

National Institute of Allergy and Infectious Diseases (NIAID), Division of Acquired Immunodeficiency Syndrome: www.niaid.nih.gov/daids/default.htm. *[Develops and implements the national research agenda to address the HIV/AIDS epidemic.]*

National Institutes of Health Office of AIDS Research: www.oar.nih.gov/. *[Coordinates scientific, budgetary, legislative, and policy components of NIH AIDS research.]*

The Foundation for AIDS Research (amFAR): www.amfar.org. *[Leading non-profit foundation for AIDS-related research, HIV prevention, treatment, and education.]*

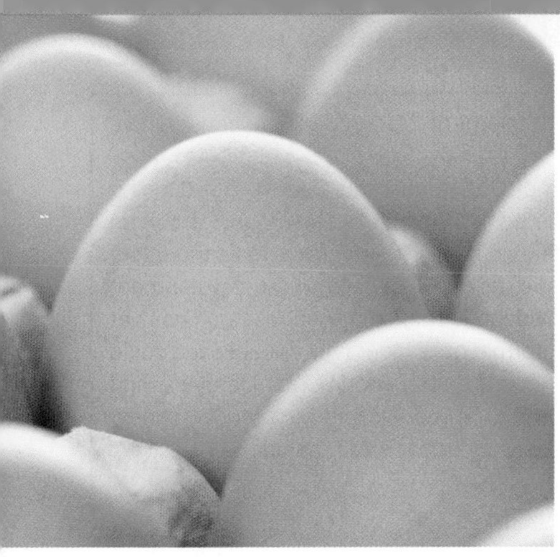

25

Cancer

Kenneth Byrne

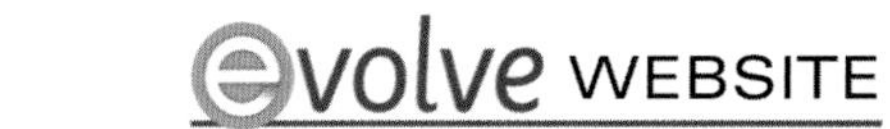

http://evolve.elsevier.com/Williams/essentials/

OUTLINE

This chapter focuses on cancer, one of the major diseases in the Western world. We examine the nature of the cancer process and its treatments and seek to relate these processes to nutritional factors involved.

Here we look at nutrition and cancer in two basic areas: (1) the role of nutrition in cancer development and prevention and (2) its role in cancer therapy and rehabilitation. Cancer development and its prevention are discussed in relation to the interplay of environment, the body's defense system, and nutritional factors that govern each. During medical therapy for the disease process, nutrition support plays a large role in the effectiveness of therapy and quality of life. To understand these nutritional relationships, we must understand the nature of cancer as a growth process, the physiologic basis of cancer and structure and function of cells, and the body's defense systems in immunity and in the healing process.

PROCESS OF CANCER DEVELOPMENT

Multiple Forms of Cancer

The health toll of cancer continues to extract its price in human disease and death, despite ongoing efforts by the scientific and health care communities. In 1971 the United States first initiated a nationwide moratorium to fight the disease with the National Cancer Act. In 1995 the Assistant Secretary for Health and the Surgeon General chaired an initiative called *Healthy People 2000*. This program, co-coordinated by the U.S. Department of Health and Human Services (USDHHS) and the National Cancer Institute of the National Institutes of Health (NIH), began a national initiative on health goals and objectives. It sought to focus the attacks on cancer into several priority areas. Building on these initiatives, *Healthy People 2010* was launched in 1999. It is a set of health objectives for the nation to achieve during the first decade of the new century.[1]

In its latest report the NIH statistical cancer review program Surveillance, Epidemiology, and End Results (SEER) has indicated an overall decline in the incidence of cancer by 0.8% per year between 1990 and 1997.[2] However, when reported in aggregate, due in large part to an older and expanding population, the incidence expressed in numbers of cases of overall cancer deaths continues to increase.[3]

The American Cancer Society estimated that in the year 2008 approximately 565,560 Americans died from cancer. In its multiple forms, cancer has become one of our major health problems, second only to heart disease, and accounts for approximately 23% of the total deaths in the United States each year (see the *Focus on Culture* box, "Americancer?").[3]

Breast cancer is the most common form of cancer among women in the United States. The incidence of breast cancer has continued to rise for the past 2 decades.[5] Prostate cancer

> **KEY TERMS**
> **cancer** A malignant cellular tumor with properties of tissue invasion and spreading to other parts of the body.

FOCUS ON CULTURE

Americancer?

America has long been seen as a destination for those hoping to start a new life. Since the days when immigrants poured through Ellis Island, the dream of becoming an American citizen has been idealized as a way of life that provides immense opportunities and personal freedom. However, could immigrants to the United States be putting themselves and their children at risk for developing cancer?

Over the last couple of decades, several researchers have investigated the increased cancer risk facing immigrants who assimilate to the American way of life. First-generation immigrants gave researchers a unique view on the effects that American customs, dietary patterns, and environments have on the development of various forms of cancer. Unpredictably, these immigrants showed little discrepancy from their native counterparts in cancer rates; it was only in subsequent generations that variances were of consequence. It seemed first-generation immigrants were more likely to adhere to traditions from their homeland and accordingly remained in sync with their native health history.

This phenomenon is important because it shows that external factors play a considerable role in increasing cancer risk. Although genetic predisposition to cancer is also a factor, diet and other lifestyle choices made by Americans can be examined for shortcomings through these migrant studies. Moreover, preventative characteristics of immigrants' culture can be examined and implemented for a possible constructive effect on cancer risk.

Because assimilation of U.S. immigrants into the surrounding culture encourages the corresponding development of certain "negative" diet and lifestyle habits, this trend reveals the effect that domestic habits, such as diet, can have on the development of cancer in these individuals. Although much research has yet to be concluded, this information is incredibly valuable and could potentially help identify particular environments, lifestyles, and dietary practices that could be modified to help reduce cancer risk and fight the national cancer crisis in America.

BIBLIOGRAPHY

Herrington J, Stanford JL, Schwartz SM, et al: Ovarian cancer: incidence among Asian migrants to the United States and their descendants, *J Natl Cancer Inst* 86:1336, 1994.

Karagas TM: *Migrant studies: cancer epidemiology and prevention*, New York, 1996, Oxford University Press.

King S, Schottenfeld D: The "epidemic" of breast cancer in the U.S.—determining the factors, *Oncology* 10:4, 1996.

Li F, Pawlish K: Cancers in Asian-Americans and Pacific Islanders: migrant studies, *Asian Am Pac Isl J Health* 8(2):123, 1998.

McCredie M: What have we learned from studies of migrants? *Cancer Causes Control* 9:1, 1998.

is the leading cancer diagnosed among men in the United States.[5] Cancer of the lung is the second most common cancer and leading cause of cancer death among men and women.[5]

Difficulties in the study of cancer have arisen from its varying nature and multiple forms. The word *cancer* is a general term used to designate any one of many malignant tumors, or **neoplasms** (new growths), forming in various body tissue sites. Many different forms of cancer exist, varying worldwide and changing with population migrations. Multiple causes exist, and often conflicting research results because of the large number of variables involved. We would be more correct, then, to use the plural term *cancers* in discussing this great variety of neoplasms.

To better understand cancer development we should view it as a growth process that has its physiologic basis in the structure and function of cells. Because nutrition is fundamental to all tissue growth, we need to look briefly at the cancer cell to understand the relationship of nutritional factors to cancer. This "misguided cell" and its tumor tissue represent normal cell growth that has gone wild.

Cancer Cell

Molecular mechanisms that influence conversion of a normal cell into a cancerous cell have been extensively studied and continually evolve on the basis of new scientific theories. It was originally thought that the scientific basis of all cancers was a single metabolic disturbance in cell replication caused by some sort of mutation. However, in the latter half of the twentieth century it was determined that because the normal cell cycle of division and replication is governed by multiple signals, loss of the controlled state as it occurs during neoplastic development must proceed through multiple steps.[6] In fact, it is now generally understood that cancer develops through a series of four distinct steps: (1) initiation, (2) promotion, (3) development, and (4) progression.[7]

In adult humans about 3 to 4 million cells complete the normal life-sustaining process of cell division every second, in large part without mistake, guided by a genetic code unique to each living being. How are the process and rate of cell reproduction maintained so precisely in normal cells? More important, why is this normal, precise regulation of cell reproduction and function lost in cancer cells, and why do cancer cells then remain mutant and malformed, functionally imperfect, and incapable of normal cell life?

The first part of the answer lies in the nature of the cell's genetic material and its regulating components. Specific genetic material in the cell's nucleus is arranged as chromosomes, containing deoxyribonucleic acid (DNA). Specific sites along chromosome threads are called *genes.* Each gene carries specific information that controls synthesis of specific proteins and transmits genetic heritage. A single chromosome thread is made up of hundreds of genes arranged end to end, and each gene of DNA is made up of about 600 to several thousand smaller subunits called *nucleotides.* The nucleic acids, DNA and its companion ribonucleic acid (RNA), compose the controlling system by which the cell and thus the organism sustain life. The structure of DNA is that of a very large polynucleotide made up of many individual mononucleotides, each one of which has three parts: (1) a sugar (deoxyribose), (2) a phosphate, and (3) a

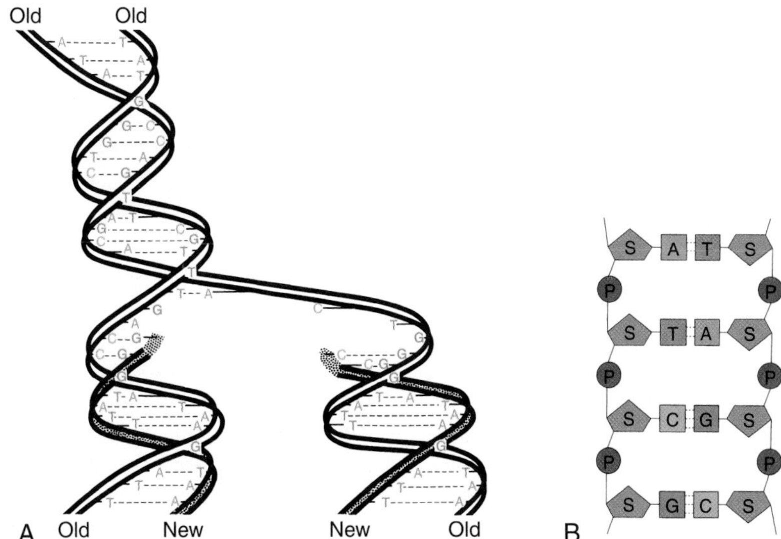

FIGURE 25-1 DNA structure. **A,** The "unzipping" of deoxyribonucleic acid (DNA) to form new ribonucleic acid (RNA) strands. Note the cross-links connecting the strands: *A,* adenine; *T,* thymine; *C,* cytosine; *G,* guanine. **B,** Diagram of a portion of DNA structure. An enlargement of a four-bar twist of the DNA molecule.

specific nitrogenous base—adenine, cytosine, guanine, or thymine. It is the ladderlike pairing of these nitrogenous bases (as shown in Figure 25-1) that incorporates the "genetic code" and enables the DNA to transmit messages to guide protein structure. DNA appears as a twisted ladder or spiral staircase in structure and thus is called a *helix,* the Greek word that means *coil.*

Gene Control of Cell Reproduction and Function

Normal Cell

New cells are created by division of preexisting cells, a process in which the preexisting cell's genetic pattern is exactly replicated in the new cell. Normally each particular cell's structure and function operate in an orderly manner under gene control, directing the cell's specific processes of protein synthesis. Gene action, however, may be switched on and off, depending on the position of a cell in the body, the stage of body development, and the external environment. Specific regulator genes control such function by producing a repressor substance as needed to regulate operator genes and structural genes. This orderly regulation of induction and repression in cell activity, however, may be lost with mutation of these regulatory genes. Control is also lost when a specific gene for some reason moves from its position to another location on the chromosome. Four types of such mutated genes are presently thought to contribute to tumor development: (1) oncogenes, (2) tumor suppressor genes, (3) DNA repair genes, and (4) genes that influence programmed cell death.[6]

Cancer Cell

A cell may become malignant when one of these potentially cancer-causing genes is translocated and reinserted into a highly active part of the DNA. This has been shown to occur, for example, in patients with Burkitt's lymphoma and the blood cancer acute nonlymphocytic leukemia (i.e., the cancer cell appears to be derived from a normal cell that has mutated and lost control over cell reproduction).

Cancer Tumor Types

On this basis of cell nature and differentiation, it is possible to classify cancer tumor types according to the type of originating tissue; for example, those arising from connective tissues are called sarcomas, and those arising from epithelial tissues are called carcinomas. We can also classify tumor types by extent or degree of cell tissue change. Tumor stages are defined in relation to rate of growth, degree of autonomy, and invasiveness.

Relation to the Aging Process

Because the incidence of cancer increases with age, a relationship exists between cancer development and the aging process in cells, tissues, and organ systems.

Causes of Cancer Cell Development

It is thus evident the basic cause of cancers is a mutation of genes that govern normal cell reproduction.

KEY TERMS

neoplasms Any new tissue growth that is abnormal, uncontrolled, and progressive.

oncogenes Any of various genes that, when activated as by radiation or a virus, may cause a normal cell to become cancerous; viral genetic material carrying the potential of cancer and passed from parent to offspring.

sarcomas A tumor, usually malignant, arising from connective tissue.

carcinomas Malignant new growths made up of epithelial cells, infiltrating the surrounding tissue and spreading to other parts of the body.

Chemical and Environmental Carcinogens

One of the first indications that chemical carcinogens exist in the environment came from a British investigator, Percival Pott, when he discovered chimney sweeps had an increased incidence of scrotal cancer; it was determined the common denominator among cancer victims was exposure to soot.[8] Chemical carcinogens interfere with structure or function of regulatory genes by binding to DNA bases in such a way that the likelihood it will undergo a mutation during DNA repair or replication is increased. This mutation can thus lead to neoplastic transformation.[8] Exposure to such agents may be by individual choice, as in cigarette smoking. Smoking causes cancer in primary sites such as the larynx, oral cavity, and oropharynx. Smoking contributes to cancer of the upper respiratory tract, esophagus, bladder, and pancreas, with the degree of malignancy depending on the frequency of smoking and duration of the habit, especially when started at a young age.

Other exposure comes via general environmental substances, such as pesticide residues, water and air pollutants, food additives and contaminants, and occupational hazards. However, many of our natural environmental agents can carry more hazard potential, depending on the dose. The principle that "the dose makes the poison" applies to all substances, including carcinogens, natural or synthetic. These potentially carcinogenic substances may cause cancer either by mutation, altering the regulation of gene function, or by activating a dormant virus.

Radiation

Radiation sufficient to damage DNA causes breakage and incorrect rejoining of chromosomes. Such radiation damage may be ionizing, such as from x-rays, radioactive materials, and atomic exhausts or wastes, or it may be nonionizing, such as from sunlight. Ultraviolet radiation in sunlight is one of the most prominent sources of environmental carcinogens. It is highly genotoxic but does not penetrate the skin. Our longtime pursuit of the bronzed-god look has taken a large toll: sun-related skin cancer rates have risen rapidly in the United States and Europe, afflicting younger and younger persons. The common forms on the head and neck—basal cell carcinoma and squamous cell carcinoma—are easily cured by surgical removal. However, a far more lethal form, malignant melanoma, occurs in skin cells that produce the pigment melanin and accounted for approximately 7800 deaths in 2001 alone.[3] In the United States the incidence varies with latitude, with an increased number occurring in the southern states. It is thought exposure to high levels of sunlight in childhood is a strong determinant of risk for development of melanoma; however, sun exposure in adulthood also plays a role.[9] The rising incidence probably results from increased recreational exposure to sunlight and tanning beds, as well as the potential "greenhouse effect" of decreased protective ozone layers.[10]

Oncogenic Viruses

Although oncogenes were first found in viruses, their evolutionary history indicates they are also present and functioning in normal vertebrate cells in the form of proto-oncogenes. It is their abnormal expression, or activation by mutation, that can lead to cancerous growth. Viruses may be thought of as a major risk factor for cancer development, exceeded only by tobacco use.

A virus is little more than a packet of genetic information encased in a protein coat (see Chapter 24). It contains a small chromosome, DNA or RNA, with a relatively small number of genes, usually fewer than five and never more than several hundred. In contrast, cells of complex organisms have tens of thousands of genes. Generally, when viruses produce disease, they act as parasites, taking over the cell machinery to replicate themselves. Numerous oncogenic, or tumor-producing, viruses have been identified. A tumor virus is a type of transforming virus capable of producing tumors only in hosts in which the virus can replicate. They transform cells by integrating a DNA copy of the virus (termed a *provirus*) into the host cell genome. If a proto-oncogene is contained in the region, then the provirus integration alters the structure or function of the proto-oncogene and thereby promotes tumor development.[8] Human papillomavirus (HPV) is now recognized as the main cause of cervical cancer.[11] Retroviruses are implicated in a number of mammary tumors and skin cancer.[12] Other viruses implicated in the causes of cancer include the Epstein-Barr virus (lymphomas), hepatitis B and C (hepatocellular carcinoma), and human immunodeficiency virus (HIV) (Kaposi's sarcoma).

Epidemiologic Factors

Studies of cancer distribution and occurrence in relation to such factors as race, diet, region, sex, age, heredity, and occupation show variable and conflicting results. It is becoming increasingly clear, for example, that racial differences in cancer incidence between African Americans and Caucasians in the United States are great, with more cancer cases occurring among African Americans than among Caucasians. However, it is also clear that these differences have nothing to do with race but have much to do with poverty, which has implications for nutritional status, health care, education, and resources. World incidence of cancer greatly varies from country to country, and the rate of specific cancer types varies from six- to 300-fold, with incidence rates in the United States being appreciably greater than those in many other countries.

In addition, racial incidence of cancer seems to change as population groups migrate and acquire the different cancer characteristics of the new population. Although specific dietary factors have been hard to pinpoint in the cause of cancer, worldwide epidemiologic studies show significant correlation of death from breast cancer, for example, with the consumption of fat in the diet and of liver cancer with the consumption of alcohol.

Stress Factors

The idea that emotions may play a part in malignancy is not new. Galen, a second-century Greek physician, wrote of such relationships, as have many different kinds of "healers" since that time. However, these relationships are difficult to measure. Even with great technologic and scientific advances, Western medicine holds fast to its basic tenet that a thing must be measurable under controlled conditions to be said to exist.

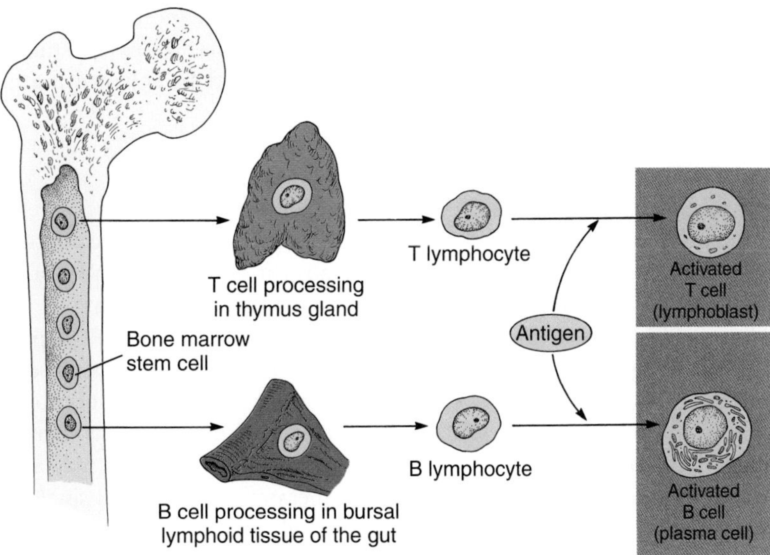

FIGURE 25-2 Development of the T and B cells, lymphocyte components of the body's immune system.

Nonetheless, increasing observations are being made of relationships between cancer and less measurable factors of stress. Clinicians and researchers have reported psychic trauma, especially the loss of a central relationship, seems to carry with it a strong cancer correlation. Cause of a possible relationship between such trauma and cancer may lie in two physiologic areas: (1) damage to the thymus gland and immune system and (2) neuroendocrine effects mediated through the hypothalamus, pituitary, and adrenal cortex. This automatic "cascade of physiologic events" triggered by stress may well provide the neurologic currency that converts anxiety to malignancy. Such a stressful state may also make a person more vulnerable to other factors that are present, influencing integrity of the immune system, food behaviors, and nutritional status. Once cancer occurs, however, patients with cancer have many options for easing their distress and improving the quality of their lives through supportive relations and current positive medical approaches to pain management.[13,14]

BODY'S DEFENSE SYSTEM

Components of the Immune System

The human body's defense system is remarkably efficient and complex. Several components of special type cells protect not only against external invaders such as bacteria and viruses but also against internal "aliens" such as malignant tumor cells. These malignant cells from developing tumors in the body can spread invading cells into other body tissues and form secondary tumors, or metastases, that become life threatening.

Two major populations of cells provide the immune system's primary line of defense for detecting and destroying malignant cells that arise daily in the body. These cells mediate specific cellular immunity and humoral immunity, as well as providing supportive backup biologic systems. These two populations of lymphoid cells, or lymphocytes, a type of white blood cell, develop early in life from a common stem cell in fetal liver and bone marrow (Figure 25-2). They then differentiate and populate peripheral lymphoid organs during latter stages of gestation. One type, T cells, is traced from thymus-derived cells. The other type, B cells, is preprocessed by the liver and bone marrow.

T Cells

After precursor cells migrate to the thymus, the T-cell population is differentiated in this small gland, which lies posterior to the sternum and anterior to the great vessels partially covering the trachea. The majority of the circulating small lymphocytes in blood, lymph, and certain areas of the lymph nodes and spleen are T cells. These cells recognize invading antigens by means of specific specialized receptors on their surfaces. When T cells meet an antigen—a foreign intruder, a "nonself," or an alien substance such as abnormal cancer cells—they proliferate and initiate specific cellular immune responses, as follows:

- They activate phagocytes, special cells that have intracellular killing and degrading mechanisms for destroying invaders.
- They cause an inflammatory response through chemical mediators released by the antigen-stimulated T cells.

In the early 1970s, Burnet[15] proposed the theory of immune surveillance of cancer wherein most cancer tumors are rejected by the immune system and occasional failure to do so leads

KEY TERMS

radiation A highly controlled treatment for cancer, using radioactive substances in limited, controlled exposure to kill cancerous cells.

malignant melanoma A tumor tending to become progressively worse, composed of melanin (the dark pigment of the skin and other body tissues), usually arising from the skin and aggravated by excessive sun exposure.

to cancer development. It was subsequently discovered that most tumors express tumor antigens that can then be targets for rejection responses. Furthermore, T cells recognize these antigens in a different way than antibodies recognize them.[16] Harnessing this ability in the patient with cancer, scientists developed gene therapy, which has been used to create these cytotoxic T lymphocytes specific for specific tumor types. Many strategies are being developed to deploy this immune-mediated destruction of tumors. For example, bone marrow transplantation has developed to infuse T cells from healthy donors against well-defined tumor antigens into the blood of patients with cancer with that specific tumor type.

B Cells

The B-cell population matures first in bone marrow and then, after migration, in the solid peripheral lymphoid tissues of the body—lymph nodes, spleen, and gut. These cells are responsible for synthesis and secretion of specialized protein known as *antibodies*. When the B cells contact an antigen, they increase and initiate specific humoral immune responses, as follows:

- They produce specific antibodies or immunoglobulins in the blood.
- They produce a particular antibody secretion, immunoglobulin A, in the bowel and upper respiratory mucosa.

This combination of antigen and antibody then activates the complement system, which attracts phagocytes and initiates the inflammatory response for healing.

Relation to Nutrition

Immune System

Integrity of the body's immune system components requires nutrition support. Acute starvation causes thymic atrophy and has immunosuppressive effects.[17,18] Severely malnourished persons show changes in structure and function of the immune system with atrophy of the liver, bowel wall, bone marrow, spleen, lymphoid tissue, and diaphragm muscles.[19] Sound nutrition can help to maintain normal immunity and combat sustained attacks in malignancy. Early use of vigorous nutrition support for patients with cancer may help to provide recovery of normal nutritional status, including immunocompetence, thereby improving their response to therapy and prognosis.[20]

Healing Process

Tissue integrity, essential for the healing process, is maintained through protein synthesis. Such strength of tissue is a front line of the body's defense system. This process of healing requires optimal nutritional intake to support (1) cell function and structure of all its parts involving DNA, RNA, amino acids, and proteins and (2) integrity of all of the immune system components.

EFFECT OF CANCER THERAPY ON NUTRITION

Current cancer therapy takes four major forms: (1) surgery, (2) radiation, (3) chemotherapy, and (4) bone marrow transplantation. Medical treatments for cancer entail physiologic stress. These results include toxic tissue effects, often with damage to cell DNA structure and changes in normal body function. Thus the benefit achieved is not without attendant problems. Nutrition support seeks to alleviate these problems and to enhance the potential success of cancer therapy.

Surgery

Operable Tumors

Early diagnosis of operable tumors has led to successful surgical treatment of a large number of patients with cancer. Success of any surgery depends in large measure on sound nutritional status of the patient (see Chapter 17); this is especially true of patients with cancer because their general condition may be weakened. Prevention of problems through early detection and surgical treatment has significantly increased cancer cure rates. Surgical treatment may also be used with other forms of therapy for removal of single metastases or for prevention and alleviation of symptoms. Optimal nutritional status preoperatively and maximal nutrition support postoperatively are fundamental to the healing process.

Medical Nutrition Therapy of the Oncology Surgery Patient

Two goals exist for nutrition therapy for patients with cancer who are undergoing surgery:

1. To support the general healing process and overall body metabolism
2. To modify the diet or feeding regimen in appropriate ways to compensate for the surgical site involved

Beyond regular nutritional needs surrounding any surgical procedure and its healing process, gastrointestinal (GI) surgery poses special problems for normal eating and digesting and absorbing of food nutrients (Table 25-1). Clinical examples include esophageal and stomach resections, as follows:

- *Head and neck surgery*, or resections in the oropharyngeal area, is sometimes necessitated by presence of cancer. In such cases, food intake is greatly affected. A creative variety of food forms and semiliquid textures, as well as modes of feeding, must be devised. Often mechanical problems of food ingestion make long-term tube feeding necessary (see Chapter 18).
- *Gastrectomy* may cause numerous postgastrectomy "dumping" problems requiring frequent, small, low-carbohydrate feedings (see Chapter 20). Vagotomy contributes to gastric stasis. Various intestinal resections or tumor excisions may cause steatorrhea because of general malabsorption, fistulas, or stenosis.
- *Pancreatectomy* causes loss of digestive enzymes with ensuing malabsorption and weight loss; it also induces insulin-dependent diabetes mellitus.

Radiation

After discovery of radiation in the nineteenth century, scientists soon found it could damage body tissue. Continued study of its use and control revealed normal tissue could largely withstand an amount of radiation that would damage and destroy cancer tissue. The subsequent role of radiation in cancer treatment has developed around controlled use with two types of tumors: (1) those responsive to radiation

TABLE 25-1 NUTRITION-RELATED SIDE EFFECTS OF CANCER TREATMENT

TREATMENT MODALITY	NUTRITION-RELATED SIDE EFFECTS
Upper Gastrointestinal (GI) Surgery	
Radical resection of oropharyngeal area	Chewing and swallowing difficulties
Esophagectomy	Gastric stasis, hypochlorhydria, steatorrhea, and diarrhea secondary to vagotomy, early satiety, regurgitation
Gastrectomy	Dumping syndrome, malabsorption, achlorhydria, lack of intrinsic factor and R protein, hypoglycemia, and early satiety
Intestinal Resection	
Jejunum	Decreased efficiency of absorption and many nutrients
Ileum	Vitamin B_{12} deficiency, bile salt losses with diarrhea or steatorrhea, hyperoxaluria and renal stones, calcium and magnesium depletion, and fat-soluble vitamin deficiencies
Massive bowel resection	Life-threatening malabsorption, malnutrition, metabolic acidosis, and dehydration
Ileostomy and colostomy	Complication of salt and water balance
Blind loop syndrome	Vitamin B_{12} malabsorption
Pancreatectomy	Malabsorption and diabetes mellitus
Radiation Therapy	
Oropharyngeal area	Destruction of sense of taste and smell, xerostomia and odynophagia, oral mucositis and ulceration, loss of teeth, and osteonecrosis
Thorax and mediastinum	Esophagitis with dysphagia; fibrosis with esophageal stricture
Abdomen and pelvis	Bowel damage, acute and chronic, with diarrhea, malabsorption, stenosis and obstruction, ulceration, and fistula formation

Modified from Shils ME, editor: *Modern nutrition in health and disease,* ed 10, Philadelphia, 2006, Lippincott Williams & Wilkins.

therapy, or radiotherapy, within a dose level tolerable to health of normal tissue and (2) those that can be targeted without damage to overlying vital organ tissue.

Forms of Radiation Therapy

Radiation therapy damages the DNA of cells; therefore cells cannot continue to divide and grow. Radiation used in cancer therapy is produced from three main sources:

1. In external beam irradiation (or x-ray), radiation is directed at the patient externally from a linear accelerator. This type of radiation frequently causes nutrition-related side effects.
2. In brachytherapy, highly radioactive isotopes, such as cobalt 60, are placed directly into or next to the tumor to deliver a highly localized dose. Nutritional side effects do not generally occur from this type of radiotherapy.
3. In stereotaxis, radiation is delivered in a narrow beam to difficult-to-reach places such as brain tumors.

Medical Nutrition Therapy of the Radiation Oncology Patient

Radiotherapy may be used alone or in conjunction with other therapies for curative and palliative care for approximately 50% of all patients with cancer at some time during the course of the disease. Radiation enteritis will influence nutritional status and therapy a great deal, depending on the site and intensity of treatment. Clinical examples include irradiation to head, neck, and abdominal cavity, as follows:

- *Head and neck* irradiation will affect oral mucosa and salivary secretions, as well as the esophagus, influencing taste sensations and sensitivity to food temperature and texture. Common side effects include mucositis, xerostomia, loss of taste, and alteration in or loss of smell. Other means of tempting appetite through food appearance and aroma, as well as texture, must be developed. Nutritional management may be further compounded by the curtailment of food intake caused by anorexia and nausea. Esophagitis from head and neck radiation may be so severe as to cause esophageal fibrosis or stricture. In this scenario, dilation of the esophagus is sometimes attempted to create a passageway large enough to swallow a bolus of food; if unsuccessful, then a feeding tube often becomes necessary for nutrition support.
- *Abdomen* irradiation may produce denuded bowel mucosa, loss of villi, and absorbing surface area with tissue edema and congestion; vascular changes occur as a result of intimal thickening, thrombosis, ulcer formation, or inflammation. In the intestinal wall, fibrosis, stenosis, necrosis, or ulceration may occur. General malabsorption or fistulas may develop, as well as hemorrhage, obstruction, and diarrhea, all contributing to nutrition problems.

Chemotherapy

Drug Development

Chemotherapy refers to use of chemical agents to treat cancer in a systemic manner; these agents are delivered intravenously and therefore elicit their effects throughout

KEY TERMS

palliative Care affording relief but not cure; useful for comfort when cure is still unknown or obscure.

the body. Many of the most effective chemotherapy agents currently in use have been developed only within the past few years. Therapeutic use of a chemotherapy agent is based on two general principles related to rate and mode of action.

Rate of Action

The so-called cell or log (logarithm)-kill hypothesis of the action of chemotherapeutic agents on tumors indicates a single dose can be only as much as 99.9% effective in killing the tumor cells. Thus if as large a tumor as is compatible with life can be treated with a drug tolerable at a toxicity level that is 99.9% effective, then the tumor is gradually reduced with successive doses that cause "fractional killing" with each dose. This process finally brings the tumor within the capability of the body's own immune system to take over and make the final kill and cure. The smaller the tumor is, either because of early detection or initial treatment by surgery or radiation, the greater is the possible effectiveness of the chemotherapeutic agents. In addition, the following two other principles of dosage rate for increased effectiveness are important:

- Aggressive use of maximal tolerable doses in repeated series
- Use of several drugs combined for a synergistic effect

Many malignancies such as leukemias, lymphomas, and testicular cancer are now successfully treated by such combination therapy.[21] However, most common cancers, such as breast, lung, colorectal, and prostate, require an overall program that involves surgery and radiation for a maximal cure rate.

Mode of Action

Chemotherapeutic agents are effective because they disrupt normal processes in the cell responsible for cell growth and reproduction. Some agents interfere with DNA synthesis. Others disrupt DNA structure and RNA replication. Others prevent cell division through mitosis, cause hormonal imbalances, or make unavailable specific amino acids necessary for protein synthesis. It is this diversity in mode of action that provides a basis for grouping drugs into certain classes of chemotherapeutic agents, as follows:

- Alkaloid agents
- Alkylating agents
- Antibiotic agents
- Antimetabolite agents
- Enzymal agents
- Hormonal agents

They are usually used in combined therapy or as adjuvant therapy in conjunction with surgery or radiation.

Toxic Effects

Chemotherapeutic agents have the same effects on rapidly reproducing normal cells as they do on the rapidly reproducing cancer cells. Interference with normal function is most apparent in normal cells of the bone marrow, GI tract, and hair follicles, accounting for a number of the toxic side effects and problems in nutritional management, as follows:

- *Bone marrow effects* include interference with production of red blood cells (anemia), white blood cells (infections), and platelets (bleeding). Many health care practitioners subscribe to the use of a neutropenic diet during these instances, in which potentially microbially contaminated food ingredients, such as raw, unwashed vegetables and other foods, are eliminated.
- *GI effects* include nausea and vomiting, stomatitis, anorexia, ulcers, and diarrhea.
- *Hair follicle effects* include alopecia (baldness) and general hair loss.

Modes of Drug Use

Chemotherapy may be used alone or in conjunction with other treatments such as surgery or radiotherapy to increase the cure rate.

Chemotherapy Research

Researchers are working to find substances, in either food or drugs that can prevent or halt cancer development. Their goal is to develop drugs or modify foods as a preventive strategy for people at high risk for cancer.[22] Considerable evidence suggests that many plant-derived extracts contain compounds that can inhibit the process of carcinogenesis effectively.[23] These chemical compounds produced by plants or in persons eating the plants are now termed *phytochemicals* (see discussion in Chapter 6). For example, members of this group of compounds include α- and β-carotene found in carrots; β-cryptoxanthin found in oranges, peaches, and tangerines; and lutein found in vegetables such as tomatoes, green beans, spinach, and other green vegetables. The many phytochemicals found in a wide variety of vegetables and fruits provide specific health benefits. Another group, called *disease-preventive agents,* is being studied. This group—the dithiolethiones found in cruciferous vegetables such as broccoli, cauliflower, and cabbage—are potential preventive agents.[23] Phytochemicals can inhibit carcinogenesis by inhibiting phase I and II enzymes, scavenging DNA reactive agents, suppressing the abnormal proliferation of preneoplastic lesions, and inhibiting certain properties of the cancer cell.[24,25] Moreover, ingestion of specific beneficial bacteria, known as *probiotics,* may have anticarcinogenic effects in colon cancer.[26]

Major nutritional concerns during chemotherapy relate to (1) GI symptoms caused by the effect of toxic drugs on rapidly developing mucosal cells, (2) anemia associated with bone marrow effects, and (3) general systemic toxicity effect on appetite (see the *Diet-Medications Interactions* box, "Nutritional Side Effects of Chemotherapeutic Agents"). Stomatitis, nausea, diarrhea, and malabsorption contribute to many food intolerances. Antiemetic drugs such as prochlorperazine (Compazine) may be used (Table 25-2); such drugs act on the vomiting center in the brain to prevent the nausea response. Prolonged vomiting seriously affects fluid and electrolyte balance, especially in older adult patients, and needs to be controlled. In patients with breast cancer, relief from nausea has been achieved with use of the antiemetic drug megestrol acetate (Megace), a synthetic

DIET-MEDICATIONS INTERACTIONS

Nutritional Side Effects of Chemotherapeutic Agents

SIDE EFFECTS	CHEMOTHERAPY AGENTS
Nausea and vomiting	Bleomycin Busulfan Cisplatin Cyclophosphamide Doxorubicin Ifosfamide Interferon-α Interleukin Fludarabine Flutamide Leuprolide Methotrexate Mitomycin 5-Fluorouracil Vincristine Vinorelbine Paclitaxel Rituximab Tamoxifen citrate Trastuzumab Docetaxel
Anorexia	Bleomycin Busulfan Cisplatin Cyclophosphamide Doxorubicin Ifosfamide Interferon-α Interleukin Fludarabine Mitomycin Methotrexate 5-Fluorouracil Vincristine Vinorelbine Paclitaxel Docetaxel
Diarrhea	Fludarabine Methotrexate 5-Fluorouracil Flutamide Vincristine Vinorelbine Paclitaxel Docetaxel Doxorubicin
Oral ulceration	Fludarabine Methotrexate Mitomycin Bleomycin Doxorubicin Dactinomycin 5-Fluorouracil Vincristine Vinorelbine Paclitaxel Docetaxel
Gastrointestinal (GI) ulceration	Methotrexate Ara-C Procarbazine hydrochloride
Abdominal or epigastric pain	Methotrexate Cyclophosphamide Dactinomycin Prednisone Dexamethasone
Constipation	Vincristine

Data from Coulston AM, Rock CL, Monsen ER, editors: *Nutrition in the prevention and treatment of disease,* San Diego, 2001, Academic Press; McCallum PD, Polisena CG, editors: *The clinical guide to oncology nutrition,* Chicago, 2000, American Dietetic Association; Shils ME: Nutrition and diet in cancer. In Shils ME, Young VR, editors: *Modern nutrition in health and disease,* Philadelphia, 1988, Lea & Febiger.

female sex hormone similar to the natural hormone progesterone. However, results have shown that although megestrol acetate can increase appetite and weight gain in patients with cancer, it has no effect on lean body mass; rather weight gain appears to be related solely to increases in fat mass.[27,28] Two drugs that act as serotonin blockers, granisetron hydrochloride (Kytril) and ondansetron hydrochloride (Zofran), administered in combination therapy with dexamethasone, an adrenal cortical steroid, have been shown to control episodic nausea and vomiting.[29]

In some cases of chronic long-term drug therapy, special nutritional management restricting conditioned, or learned, food aversions to odors and colors has been effective. For example, patients receiving periodic treatments of the drug cisplatin (Platinol), who had a special diet of three meals a day of plain colorless, odorless foods, including items such as cottage cheese, applesauce, vanilla ice cream, and other predetermined foods, experienced little nausea and increased

KEY TERMS

stomatitis Inflammation of the oral mucosa, especially the buccal tissue lining the inside of the cheeks, but it also may involve the tongue, palate, floor of mouth, and the gums.

TABLE 25-2 MEDICATIONS USED TO CONTROL NAUSEA AND VOMITING IN PATIENTS RECEIVING CHEMOTHERAPY

ANTIEMETICS

		ROUTE						
CLASS	**DRUG**	**ORAL**	**RECTAL**	**INJECTABLE**	**MECHANISM OF ACTION**	**SITE OF ACTION**	**SIDE EFFECTS**	**COMMENTS**
Phenothiazine agents	Perphenazine (Trilafon)	X		X	DA	CTZ	EPS, sedation, hypotension	Prochlorperazine is most effective agent in this class; perphenazine may be effective with high IV doses; prochlorperazine is available in sustained released capsule that should not be crushed
	Prochlorperazine (Compazine)	X	X	X				
	Promethazine (Phenergan)	X	X	X				
	Thiethylperazine (Torecan)	X	X	X				
Butyrophenone agents	Droperidol (Inapsine)	X		X	DA	CTZ	EPS, sedation	
	Haloperidol (Haldol)	X	X	X				
Substituted benzamide	Metoclopramide (Reglan)	X	X	X	DA or 5-HT3 in high doses	CTZ	EPS, sedation, fatigue, diarrhea, nausea	Also used in early satiety and anorexia
Serotonin antagonist agents	Dolasetron (Anzemet)	X		X	5-HT3	CTZ, PGSEC	Headache, diarrhea, constipation, ECG changes, somnolence	Increased effect with corticosteroid agents
	Granisetron (Kytril)	X		X			Headache, diarrhea, constipation, somnolence	
	Ondansetron (Zofran)	X		X				
Benzodiazepine agents	Lorazepam (Ativan)	X		X	BDZ	Unknown	Sedation, confusion, amnesia, slurred speech	Effective for anticipatory nausea/anxiety; lorazepam may be placed under tongue
	Diazepam (Valium)	X		X				
Corticosteroid agents	Dexamethasone (Decadron)	X		X	Unknown	Unknown	Increased appetite, mood change, anxiety, euphoria, headache, metallic taste, hyperglycemia	Most effective when used with 5-HT3
Anticholinergic agents	Scopolamine (Transderm Scop)		Patch		ACH	Emetic center	Urinary retention, dry eyes, constipation	Effective for nausea related to motion
Cannabinoid agent	Dronabinol (Marinol)	X			Unknown	CNS	Mood changes, increased appetite, hypotension, tachycardia	Well tolerated in younger patients; may crush

From Kennedy LD: Common supportive drug therapies used with oncology patients. In MacCallum PD, Polisena CG, editors: *The clinical guide to oncology nutrition,* Chicago, 2000, American Dietetic Association.

DA, Dopamine antagonist; *CTZ,* chemoreceptor trigger zone; *EPS,* extrapyramidal side effects; *IV,* intravenous; *5-HT3*, serotonin (5-hydroxytryptamine) antagonist; *PGSEC,* peripheral gastrointestinal stimulation to emetic center; *ECG,* electrocardiographic; *BDZ,* benzodiazepine; *ACH,* anticholinergic; *CNS,* central nervous system.

food intake.[30] The potential for development of conditioned food aversions while on long-term chemotherapy is diminished by the use of food with little or no odor or color; drug-related dysgeusia (i.e., perverted sense of taste) and dysosmia (i.e., impaired sense of smell) are correlated with visual olfactory stimulation factors.[30,31]

Certain chemotherapeutic drugs also have special effects. For example, monoamine oxidase inhibitors (MAOIs) may be used for pretreatment relief of mental and emotional depression or for palliative therapy. These antidepressant drugs cause well-known pressor effects when used with tyramine-rich foods (see Appendix M on the Evolve website). Thus these foods should be avoided when using such drugs.

NUTRITION THERAPY

Therapeutic Goals

In general, nutrition therapy deals with two types of cancer-related issues:

1. Those alterations in nutritional status related to the disease process itself
2. Those related to medical treatment of the disease

Basic objectives of nutrition therapy in cancer are (1) to meet increased metabolic demands of the disease and prevent catabolism as much as possible and (2) to alleviate symptoms resulting from the disease and its treatment through adaptations of food and the feeding process.

Alterations in Nutritional Status Related to the Disease Process

In patients with cancer, the basic feeding challenges of nutrition therapy are the result of (1) general systemic effects of the neoplastic disease process and (2) specific responses related to the type of cancer.

General Systemic Effects of the Neoplastic Disease Process Affecting Nutrition Therapy

Malnutrition is the most common secondary diagnosis in patients with cancer and is a prognostic indicator for poor response to cancer therapy and shortened survival time.[32] The disease process causes three basic systemic effects—(1) anorexia, (2) altered metabolic state, and (3) negative nitrogen balance—which are often accompanied by a continuing weight loss. These effects may vary widely with individual patients, according to type and stage of the disease, from mild, scarcely discernible responses to the extreme forms of debilitating cachexia seen in advanced disease, and they are estimated to cause more than 50% of the cancer deaths.[33,34]

Cachexia is not a local effect but rather arises from distant metabolic effects (i.e., it is a type of paraneoplastic syndrome). Although some have suggested tumor and host compete for nutrients, this is unlikely, given that some patients with cancer with very large tumors show no signs of cachexia.[34] This extreme weight loss and weakness are caused by abnormalities in fat, muscle, and glucose metabolism, mediated in part by natural body defense substances such as tumor necrosis factor and cytokines. First, evidence indicates that the cancer's catabolic effects may result in an increase in fat breakdown, brought about by tumor necrosis factor.[34] Second, a reduced rate of somatic protein synthesis and an increased rate of protein degradation have been noted, also brought about by tumor necrosis factor. Third, evidence indicates that the wasting in patients with cancer is caused in part by abnormalities in metabolism of glucose.[34] The drug hydrazine sulfate seems to correct this metabolic error, allowing patients to conserve more energy and show modest improvements in survival, but no remissions have been documented.[35]

Anorexia is frequently accompanied by depression or discomfort during normal eating. This contributes further to a limited nutrient intake at the very time the disease process causes an increased metabolic rate and nutrient demand. Often this imbalance of decreased intake and increased demand creates a negative nitrogen balance, an indication of body tissue wasting. Sometimes a true tissue loss of protein is masked by outward nitrogen equilibrium as the growing tumor retains nitrogen at the expense of the host, further compounding the problem.

Nutritional Effects Related to the Type of Cancer

In addition to the generalized wasting syndrome known as *cachexia* discussed here, specific nutrition problems individually present themselves depending on the site or organ involved. Of foremost significance are tumors that cause obstruction or lesions in the GI tract or adjacent tissue. In fact, the cancer may reduce intake or absorption of nutrients via (1) altered oral intake, (2) malabsorption of nutrients and subsequent diarrhea, (3) functional and motility problems arising from surgical procedures or tumor growth, (4) fluid and electrolyte imbalances, (5) hormonal imbalances (e.g., pancreatectomy for pancreatic cancer has caused diabetes), and (6) anemia.

Abdominal radiation may cause intestinal damage, with tissue edema and congestion, decreased peristalsis, or endarteritis in small blood vessels.[36] The liver is somewhat more resistant to damage from radiation in adults, but children are more vulnerable than adults.

Individualizing Nutrition Therapy for Cancer

Two important principles of nutrition therapy, vital in any sound nutrition practice but especially essential in care of patients with cancer, provide the basis for planning the nutrition care of each patient, as follows (see also the *Case Study* box, "Patient with Cancer"):

1. Personal nutrition assessment
2. Vigorous nutrition therapy to maintain good nutritional status and support medical treatment

Nutrition Screening and Assessment

It is far more difficult to replenish a nutritionally depleted patient than to maintain a good nutritional status from the outset of the disease process. Therefore a primary goal in nutrition therapy is to prevent a depleted state. Initial assessment for baseline data and regular monitoring thereafter during treatment are necessary. A detailed personal history is essential to determine individual needs, desires, and tolerances. To be valid the interview should be conducted as a conversation, using verbal and nonverbal probes and pauses rather than a barrage of separate questions and answers (see Chapter 16).

Nutrition Therapy and Plan of Care

Based on careful individual nutrition diagnosis, the registered dietitian (RD) conducts a thorough nutrition assessment and prepares a nutrition diagnosis for optimal nutrition therapy to meet needs. This nutrition therapy outline is then incorporated into the nutrition care plan as the RD works with other members of the health care staff to accomplish their mutual goals. Primary care provided by a dietitian and nurse on a regular basis is a necessary part of oncology team practice. This early, vigorous care often makes the difference in the success rate of medical therapy. Thus working closely with the oncology nurse and physician, the RD assesses personal needs, determines nutritional requirements, plans and manages nutrition care, monitors progress and responses to therapy, and makes adjustments in care according to status and tolerances.

CASE STUDY

Patient with Cancer

Catherine is a 35-year-old mother of three young children. She was admitted to the hospital with multiple enterocutaneous fistulas 3 weeks ago at which time she weighed 52 kg (116 lb). She is 165 cm (5 feet, 5 inches) tall. Catherine has a history of recurrent cervical cancer for which she had a hysterectomy 4 months before admission. During chemotherapy that followed, she had regular bouts of nausea and anorexia. Surgery was performed again. Her fistulas continued to drain for 2 weeks postoperatively, during which time she tolerated clear liquids only. An intravenous drip of 10% glucose and 45% normal saline was ordered to supplement fluids and kilocalories (kcalories or kcal). This week she developed peritonitis and has had a fever with a maximum temperature of 39° C (102° F) during the past 24 hours. Her weight has dropped to 41 kg (90 lb); drainage from the fistulas has become odorous. The patient was placed in isolation today and was advised by her physician that he intended to start her on total parenteral nutrition (TPN) and conduct more tests to determine her progress.

Questions for Analysis

1. What types of nutrition assessment procedures would be used by the TPN team for planning Catherine's nutrition therapy? Explain the purpose of each.
2. Calculate Catherine's energy and protein needs, and account for increased needs.
3. Why did Catherine develop nausea and anorexia during chemotherapy? What are the implications of this for recovery? Outline a plan for evaluating and controlling nausea and vomiting in patients undergoing chemotherapy.
4. What personal concerns would you expect Catherine to have? What resources would you use to help her obtain the personal and physical support she probably needs?

Determining Nutritional Needs

Each nutrient factor related to tissue protein synthesis and energy metabolism requires careful attention. Increased needs for energy, protein, vitamins and minerals, and fluid are based on demands made by the disease and its treatment. Individual needs and food tolerances vary, but general guidelines are the same.

Energy. Great energy demands may be placed on the patient with cancer. These demands result from a hypermetabolic state that exists in some patients with cancer and from tissue-healing requirements. Of this total dietary kcalories value, sufficient carbohydrate (at least 45% to 50% of total calories) to spare protein for vital tissue synthesis is essential. For the adult patient with good nutritional status, approximately 25 to 30 kilocalories (kcalories or kcal)/kg body weight/day will provide for maintenance needs. A more malnourished patient may require more calories, depending on the degree of malnutrition and body trauma. Carbohydrate should supply the majority of energy intake, with fat making up about 30% of total calories.

Providing a malnourished patient with cancer with nutrition support must be done with caution. Overfeeding must be avoided to minimize the risk of "refeeding syndrome," in which severe intracellular electrolyte and fluid shifts may occur.

Dietary Fat. In deciding whether to alter components of the diet of the patient with cancer, it is important to note the patient's usual intake and recent intake and relative efficacy of this diet change at the particular stage of disease of the patient. Certainly in early stages of cancer a reduction in fat may be beneficial; however, in later states of disease, a primary goal of therapy is to increase the caloric density of the diet, and limiting fat will be counterproductive to that end.

Protein. Tissue protein synthesis, a necessary component of healing and rehabilitation, requires essential amino acids and nitrogen. Efficient protein use, which depends on an optimum protein-to-calorie ratio, promotes tissue building, prevents tissue wastage (catabolism), and helps make up tissue deficits. An adult patient with good nutritional status will need about 0.8 to 1.2 g/kg/day of protein to meet maintenance needs and ensure anabolism. A malnourished patient may need up to two times more protein to replenish tissue and restore positive nitrogen balance.

Vitamins and Minerals. Adequate intakes of vitamins and trace elements are important for normal tissue function and healing and for maintenance of immune function. However, care must be given to avoiding megavitamin and trace mineral alternative therapy in cancer treatment. Excessive doses of vitamins can have deleterious health effects, may interfere with immune function, and may accelerate rate of growth of some cancers.[39] Key vitamins and minerals control protein and energy metabolism through their roles in cell enzyme systems. They also play a necessary part in structural development and tissue integrity. B-complex vitamins in general serve as necessary coenzyme agents in energy and protein metabolism. Vitamins A and C are necessary for development and integrity of body tissues. Vitamin A also has a significant role in protective immunity and cell differentiation; vitamin C has significant antioxidant, enzymatic, and immune biologic functions related to cancer.[40,41] Increased dietary consumption of vegetables and fruits is the best way to obtain these vitamins. Vitamins A, E, and D may alter expression of certain oncogenes.[42] Vitamin D hormone ensures proper calcium and phosphorus metabolism in bone and blood serum. Vitamin E protects the integrity of cell wall materials and hence tissue integrity. Many minerals function in structural and enzymatic roles in vital metabolic and tissue-building processes. Thus an optimal intake of vitamins and minerals, at least to the Recommended Dietary Allowance (RDA) levels but frequently augmented with supplements according to individual patient nutritional status, is indicated.

Fluids. Most adults require water in the amount of approximately 35 mL/kg/day, or between 1500 and 2000 mL/day. Adequate fluid intake is important for two reasons:

1. To replace GI losses or losses caused by infection and fever
2. To help the kidneys dispose of metabolic breakdown products from destroyed cancer cells, as well as from toxic drugs used in treatment

For example, some toxic drugs such as cyclophosphamide (Cytoxan) require as much as 2 to 3 L of forced fluids daily to prevent hemorrhagic cystitis.

Alternative Therapy with Herbal Products. In recent years many patients with cancer have turned toward herbal therapy as an alternative to chemotherapy, radiation, or surgery. Many herbal therapies have not been adequately tested and have been found to have toxic effects (see the *Complementary and Alternative Medicine [CAM]* box, "Alternative Therapy: Commonly Recommended Herbal Products").

The health care practitioner must have some basic understanding of therapeutic claims and dangers of some of these herbal products. Although many patients with cancer should not have all hopes for a cure dashed, it behooves the health care team to caution patients about the use of these products and to point out those products that are unproven and could be unsafe.

COMPLEMENTARY AND ALTERNATIVE MEDICINE (CAM)

Alternative Therapy: Commonly Recommended Herbal Products

Patients diagnosed with cancer often develop a sense of desperation resulting from feelings of helplessness. Lack of knowledge regarding what is happening in their bodies can lead them to seek out alternative methods to combat their cancer. When patients take an active role in their treatment, it has been shown to have a positive therapeutic effect. However, results are less than encouraging for certain complementary and alternative medicine (CAM) treatments. In fact, for the most part, alternative cancer treatments are unproven, unscientific, and ineffective methods that in some cases interfere with lifesaving proven treatments.

It is easy to see why CAM would be an attractive substitute for traditional chemotherapy or radiation treatments, because those traditional methods are taxing on the body and are not 100% effective. However, it is important for patients to understand the severity and results of the alternative therapies they use. Although some treatments are as harmless (and possibly helpful) as prayer and touch therapy, others involve invasive risky procedures. Each therapy should be judged on a case-by-case basis as it relates to the condition of the patient. The following list contains a few examples and information about some more well-known CAM treatments.

HERB	CLAIM	EFFICACY	SAFETY	CURRENT RECOMMENDATIONS
Chaparral	Analgesic agent Expectorant agent Diuretic agent Emetic agent Antiinflammatory agent	Studies have shown no anticancer effect.	Long-term use in rats led to lesions in mesentery, lymph nodes, and kidneys. One documented case of liver disease in humans exists. Removed from the generally recognized as safe (GRAS) list.	Not recommended for use.
Echinacea	Immune stimulant, wound healer	Widely used in Germany to treat the common cold and respiratory and urinary tract infections (UTIs). More research is needed.	Significant side effects have not been observed. Allergies are always possible.	May be used with caution. Not recommended to be used for longer than 8 consecutive weeks. Not recommended for use during pregnancy or lactation.
Essiac	Anticancer agent (Developed by Canadian nurse Rene Cassie.)	No anticancer effects have been reported.	Not safe for consumption, and is illegal to distribute in the United States.	Not recommended for use.
Ginger	Digestive aid Stimulant agent Diuretic agent Antiemetic agent	Found to be useful in treating motion sickness. Antiemetic properties are the result of the local action on the stomach, not on the central nervous system (CNS).	No toxicities have been reported. Very large overdoses may cause CNS depression and cardiac arrhythmias. Thrombocytopenia has been reported in people taking large doses.	May be used for temporary relief of nausea.

Continued

COMPLEMENTARY AND ALTERNATIVE MEDICINE (CAM)

Alternative Therapy: Commonly Recommended Herbal Products—cont'd

HERB	CLAIM	EFFICACY	SAFETY	CURRENT RECOMMENDATIONS
Hoxey herbs	Anticancer agent	No benefit has ever been documented. Note that the originator Harry Hoxey died of prostate cancer while treating himself with his formula.	Not recommended for use.	Not recommended for use.
Kombucha tea (Manchurian tea or Kargasok tea)	Immune system stimulator agent	Claims of antitumor activity are unsubstantiated.	Home-brewed "mushroom" usually passed to friends and family members. Susceptible to microbial contamination. Acidosis, aspergillosis, nausea, vomiting, and jaundice have been reported.	Not recommended for use.
Milk thistle	Liver protector agent (Active ingredient is silymarin.)	Appears to protect undamaged liver cells from toxins. Might be helpful in cirrhosis and hepatitis.	No adverse effects have been noted.	Safe for use. May have beneficial effects.
Mistletoe (American and European)	American—stimulates smooth muscle, increases blood pressure, increases uterine and intestinal contractions. European—decreases blood pressure and acts as antispasmodic and calmative agent.	Extracts of the European form have been used as a palliative cancer treatment. Little evidence supports its effectiveness.	Berries are poisonous, and some evidence suggests that the leaves may also be poisonous.	Not recommended for use.
Pau d'arco	Powerful tonic Blood builder Anticancer agent Also used to treat diabetes, rheumatism, and ulcers.	Has been shown to have activity against cancer in animals but causes severe side effects in humans.	Toxic—induces nausea, vomiting, anemia, and bleeding in humans.	Not recommended for use.
Peppermint	Digestive aid Antispasmodic agent	Stimulates bile flow. Stimulates tonus of the lower esophageal sphincter (LES). Appetite stimulant effects have been reported.	Safe for adults. Not recommended for children because of increased choking reflex with menthol.	Safe for adults. Not recommended for children.
Pokeroot	Cathartic agent Emetic agent Narcotic agent Anticancer agent Dyspepsia treatment Glandular swelling treatment	No efficacy has been demonstrated for any claim except that it is a strong emetic and cathartic agent.	Extremely toxic. Causes gastroenteritis, hypotension, and hyporespiration. Fatal in children.	Not recommended for use.

The despair that cancer triggers can lead many to look for additional treatment regimens, some safe and some potentially dangerous. The act of finding and using these alternative or complementary treatments has been proven a therapeutic practice and can give the patient a sense of control in an otherwise chaotic process. Even so, the bottom line remains that patients should be urged to provide total disclosure of all alternative treatments so that any adverse side effects can be discussed and prevented.

NAME	WHAT IT IS	CLAIMS AND RISKS
CanCell (Protocel, crocinic acid, Cantron)	This treatment (a dark liquid initially produced by a chemist who received its formulation in a dream) is sometimes used in place of traditional cancer medications.	Although promoted as a cure to all cancers and even AIDS, no studies support this claim. Formulation of CanCell is not totally known, partially because of the fact different manufacturers use different names and ingredients. Although banned, this therapy is still sold and used as a dietary supplement under various names. Possible interactions, flulike symptoms, fatigue, and lack of other treatments could pose considerable risks to the patient using this method.

COMPLEMENTARY AND ALTERNATIVE MEDICINE (CAM)

Alternative Therapy: Commonly Recommended Herbal Products—cont'd

NAME	WHAT IT IS	CLAIMS AND RISKS
Colon therapy (colonic, enema irrigation)	This treatment involves cleansing the large intestine through water or some other liquid formulation.	Touted as a prevention method, colon therapy is literally the removal of waste and "toxins" from the large intestine. No scientific evidence supports any claims of colon therapy or even that toxins accumulate in the large intestine. Procedures are rather invasive and can result in electrolyte imbalance, fluid overload, allergic reactions, intestinal tears, and even death.
Spirituality, religion, and prayer	This is generally a belief in something greater than oneself that exhibits control over lives and events.	Although prayer and other religious methods are therapeutic to many, clinical trials of effectiveness are sketchy at best. However, virtually no risk of side effects exists unless the patient refuses traditional treatments in lieu of religious practices.
Heat therapy	This treatment involves exposing parts or all of the body to high temperatures to increase effectiveness of other treatments.	Some evidence supports the claims of this therapy; however, more research is needed. The high death rate relating to whole-body heat therapy has been cause for some concern, as well as burns and blisters stemming from the localized heat treatments.

Data from American Cancer Society: *Complementary and alternative therapies,* Atlanta, 2006, American Cancer Society. Retrieved February 23, 2006, from www.cancer.org/docroot/ETO/ETO_5.asp; Molseed L: Alternative therapies in oncology. In MacCallum PD, Polisena CG, editors: *The clinical guide to oncology nutrition,* Chicago, 2000, American Dietetic Association; Edzard E, Casselith B: The prevalence of complementary/alternative medicine in cancer, *Cancer* 83(4):777, 1998.
AIDS, Acquired immunodeficiency syndrome.

NUTRITIONAL MANAGEMENT OF SELECTED CANCER-RELATED SYMPTOMS

The specific feeding method used depends on the individual patient's condition. However, the classic dictum of nutritional management should prevail: "If the gut works, use it." Details of available enteral and parenteral modes of nutrition support are provided in Chapter 19. If at all possible, then an oral diet with supplementation is the most desired form of feeding. A carefully designed personal plan of care based on nutrition assessment data and including adjustments in texture, temperature, food choices, and tolerances, as well as family food patterns, can often meet needs (see the *Perspectives in Practice* box, "Promoting Oral Intake in Patients with Cancer"). Often the hospitalized patient's diet can be supplemented with familiar foods from home as the clinical nutritionist plans with the family. Personal food tolerances will vary according to the current treatment and nature of the disease. A number of adjustments in food texture, temperature, amount, timing, taste, appearance, and form can be made to help alleviate symptoms stemming from common problems in successive parts of the GI tract.

Difficulties in eating may be caused by loss of appetite, problems in the mouth, or swallowing problems.

PERSPECTIVES IN PRACTICE

Promoting Oral Intake in Patients with Cancer

Encouraging and maintaining adequate oral intake for patients with cancer represents one of the most difficult aspects of cancer treatment. It is time consuming and often frustrating but may be one of the most rewarding experiences in patient care. By identifying feeding problems, initiating appropriate interventions, and providing individual education, adequate oral nutrition is promoted. The registered dietitian (RD) is the key figure for coordinating the nutrition program, but its success requires the full support and cooperation of the entire health care team, especially the nurse.

The patient interview is one of the most important parts of nutrition assessment. Information that helps identify adequacy of current nutritional intake and potential nutrition problems is obtained during the interview. The following list of questions may assist in gathering accurate information about the patient's ability to obtain oral nutrition:

- How would you describe your appetite?
- Has it changed recently?
- Are you eating differently than you have most of your life?
- Do you usually eat three meals each day? Has this changed recently?
- Are you nauseated or experiencing vomiting? Is this food or medication related? How long have you been experiencing this? How often do you vomit or feel nauseated?
- Do you have a bowel movement every day? Has this changed?
- Do you have diarrhea? If so, then do you think this may be food related?
- Do food smells or cooking odors bother you?
- Do you have difficulty chewing?
- Do your dentures (if any) fit? Do you wear them?
- Do you have difficulty swallowing?
- Is your mouth dry? Does your saliva seem to be different? Is it thicker or decreased in amounts?
- Do you find it easier to drink liquids than to eat solid foods?
- What were you able to eat yesterday? (Obtain a brief 24-hour dietary recall.)
- Are you unable to eat certain foods right now?

Continued

PERSPECTIVES IN PRACTICE

Promoting Oral Intake in Patients with Cancer—cont'd

- Do some foods taste different to you? Can you give an example?
- Have you ever taken any high-kcalorie, high-protein supplements? When? What kind? How often? Were you able to tolerate them?
- Do you take a multivitamin supplement?
- Do you have any food allergies or intolerances? Are these new, or have you always experienced these intolerances?
- Do you prepare your own meals? If so, then do you ever feel too tired to prepare something to eat?

The success of the interview depends on the RD's professional competence, interviewing skills, and bedside manner. If the RD establishes a feeling of comfort and trust with the patient, then the opportunity to accomplish successful dietary interventions is greatly increased.

BIBLIOGRAPHY

Bloch AS: Nutrition and cancer: the paradox, *Diet Curr* 23(2):1, 1996.

Marian M: Cancer cachexia: prevalence, mechanisms, and interventions, *Support Line* 20(2):3, 1998.

Nahikian-Nelms ML: Encouraging oral intake. In Bloch AS, editor: *Nutrition management of the cancer patient*, Rockville, Md, 1990, Aspen.

Loss of Appetite

Anorexia is a major problem and curtails food intake when it is needed most. It is a general systemic effect of the cancer disease process itself, often further induced by cancer treatment and progressively enhanced by personal anxiety, depression, and stress of the illness. Such a vicious cycle, if not countered by much effort, can lead to more malnutrition and the well-recognized starvation "cancer cachexia," a syndrome of emaciation, debilitation, and malnutrition (Table 25-3).[34]

A vigorous program of eating, not dependent on appetite for stimulus, must be planned and maintained with patient and family. It is helpful sometimes to develop protein and caloric goals, discussing the role of nutrients and key foods in combating the disease and providing support for therapy. With such support, the patient and his or her family are better able to build a positive mental attitude toward the diet as an integral part of treatment; thus they are more inclined to accept responsibility for this aspect of therapy. Often this positive attitude of the vital role patients play in their own treatment is a means of gaining some sense of control of their own lives, a sense frequently lost in the bewildering world of cancer and its therapy.

The overall goal is to provide food with as much nutrient density as possible so that every bite will count. If appetite is better in the morning, then a good breakfast should be emphasized. Food texture may be varied as tolerated, with appeal to sensory perceptions of color, aroma, and taste. A series of small meals with a wide variety of foods is better tolerated than regular larger meals. Getting some exercise before meals and maintaining surroundings that reduce stress may also help in the eating process.

Mouth Problems

Eating difficulties may stem from sore mouth, stomatitis, or taste changes. Sore mouth often results from chemotherapy or from radiation to the head and neck area. It is increased by any state of malnutrition or from infections such as candidiasis (thrush), with numerous ulcerations of the oral and throat mucosa. Frequent small meals and snacks—soft in texture, bland in nature, and cool or cold in temperature—are often better tolerated. Alterations may also be seen in the tongue's taste buds, causing taste distortion ("taste blindness") and inability to distinguish the basic tastes of salt, sweet, sour, or bitter, with consequent food aversions. Because the aversion is often toward basic protein foods, a high-protein, high-energy liquid drink supplement may be needed. Dental problems may also contribute to mouth difficulties and should be corrected. Salivary secretions are also affected by cancer treatment; therefore foods with a high liquid content should be used. Solid foods may be swallowed more easily with the use of sauces, gravies, broth, yogurt, or salad dressings. A food processor or blender can render foods in semisolid or liquid forms and make them easier to swallow. If the swallowing problem is especially severe because of tumor growth or therapy, then guides for a special swallowing training program, including progressive food textures, exercises, and positions, can be followed.

Gastrointestinal Problems

Eating difficulties may include nausea and vomiting, general indigestion, bloating, or specific surgery responses such as the postgastrectomy "dumping" syndrome (see Chapter 17). Nausea is often enhanced by foods that are hot, sweet, fatty, or spicy; these can be avoided according to individual tolerance. Other lower GI problems may include general diarrhea, constipation, flatulence, or specific lactose intolerance or surgery responses, such as occur with intestinal resections and various ostomies. Helpful guidance for patients with colostomies, ileostomies, or ileoanal reservoirs is necessary (see Chapter 17). The effect of chemotherapy or radiation treatment on mucosal cells secreting lactase contributes to lactose intolerance. In such cases a nutrient supplement formula that is lactose free or a soy milk formula should be used.

A number of commercial nutrient supplement products are available. A comparative review of these products will provide the basis for developing a formulary in the hospital setting for a limited number of such products (see Chapter 19). A food processor or blender can be used at home to produce creative solid and liquid food combinations from regular foods for interval liquid supplementation.

TABLE 25-3 DIETARY MODIFICATIONS FOR NUTRITION-RELATED SIDE EFFECTS OF CANCER

SIDE EFFECT	SUGGESTED DIETARY MODIFICATIONS
Anorexia	Provide small, frequent meals. Offer high-calorie, high-protein, nutrient-dense foods. Encourage consumption of the highest-calorie, highest-protein foods first. Suggest commercially available nutritional supplements, as tolerated. Avoid foods with offensive odors. Encourage favorite foods.
Altered perception of taste and odor	Maximize use of herbs and seasonings to enhance flavor of foods. If the flavor and aroma of red meats are offensive, avoid these foods and use alternative protein-rich foods such as chicken, fish, cheese, eggs, and milk. Serve cold foods and beverages more often than hot foods and beverages. Vary appearance (i.e., color, texture) of foods. Prepare and serve food in glass or porcelain rather than metal pans or dishes.
Stomatitis and mucositis	Provide foods in liquid, semisolid, or pureed form. Avoid tart, citric, or acidic foods and beverages. Avoid extremes in temperature. Avoid excessively seasoned and spicy foods. Avoid dry, coarse foods; serve foods with sauces or gravies. Encourage foods that melt or are liquid or soft textured at room temperature. Avoid carbonated beverages.
Xerostomia	Moisten foods with sauces, gravies, liquid, melted butter, mayonnaise, or yogurt. Encourage naturally soft, moist foods. Encourage sipping of liquids throughout the day. Avoid alcohol.
Dysphagia	Provide foods in liquid, semisolid, or pureed form. Maximize calorie and protein density of food as much as possible. Use commercially available liquid nutritional supplements.
Nausea and vomiting	Give small, frequent meals. Give dry foods without added fats or sauces, such as dry toast. Give liquids only between meals. Avoid greasy, fried, high-fat foods. Avoid foods with strong odors.
Diarrhea	Provide small, frequent meals. Encourage plenty of liquids to prevent dehydration. Avoid greasy, fried, high-fat foods. Consider limiting dietary lactose if these foods exacerbate symptoms. Avoid high-fiber foods. Avoid gassy, cruciferous vegetables, such as broccoli and cauliflower. Avoid caffeine.

Modified from Dobbin M, Harmuller VW: Suggested management of nutrition-related symptoms. In MacCallum PD, Polisena CG, editors: *The clinical guide to oncology nutrition,* Chicago, 2000, American Dietetic Association.

Patients with cancer need plenty of encouragement and a feeling of autonomy or personal control for the optimal success of a dietary plan. Sometimes it becomes necessary to make small attainable goals of specific foods and amounts to be consumed. If the patient can be made to view food as important as medication in the daily routine, then better success is likely.

Feeding in Terminal Illness

Although many advances have been made in detection and treatment of cancer, mortality rates for some cancers have not declined and have actually increased for some cancers.[3] In working with patients with cancer, one can automatically see that the progressive weight loss and malnutrition that occur—caused by the primary tumor and its spread—lead to profound nutritional depletion and cause a great deal of personal turmoil, increased morbidity, and overall reduced quality of life. For some patients a time comes when spread of the disease overcomes the body's capacity to combat it.

KEY TERMS

candidiasis Infection with the fungus of the genus *Candida,* generally caused by *C. albicans,* so named for the whitish appearance of its small lesions; usually a superficial infection in moist areas of the skin or inner mucous membranes.

When the patient is no longer able to eat, enteral tube feeding or parenteral feeding may be considered. Ultimately, however, ethical questions about continued feeding efforts are faced in many cases (see the *Evidence-Based Practice* box, "Examination of Lessons Learned, Ethics, and End-of-Life Nutrition"). Answers lie with the patient, as long as possible, and with the family. However, sensitive and supportive counseling is needed from the cancer team members, especially the RD and nurse responsible for administering the continued feeding and for personal care.

NUTRITION AND CANCER: THE FINAL ANALYSIS

What, then, are our overall final conclusions? As Bloch, an experienced oncology nutrition specialist, has well reminded us, nutrition has a dual role in relation to cancer—both as prevention and as therapy.[29]

Preventive Role

Nutrition and health professionals have a major role in maintaining health and preventing illness, especially in relation to cancer. This role is embodied in the American Cancer Society's dietary guidelines, as follows[43]:

1. Choose most of the foods you eat from plant sources.
   - Eat five or more servings of fruits and vegetables each day.
   - Eat other foods from plant sources, such as breads, cereals, grain products, rice, pasta, or beans, several times each day.
2. Limit your intake of high-fat foods, particularly from animal sources. Choose foods low in fat. Limit consumption of meats, especially high-fat meats.
3. Be physically active; achieve and maintain a healthy weight. Be at least moderately active for 30 minutes or more on most days of the week. Stay within your healthy weight range.
4. Limit consumption of alcoholic beverages, if you drink at all.

EVIDENCE-BASED PRACTICE

Examination of Lessons Learned, Ethics, and End-of-Life Nutrition

Topic

The decision to reject nutrition support creates many ethical and legal questions for the patient and the registered dietitian (RD), as well as for others interested in the patient's welfare. Understanding the complex nature of such decisions (both morally and legally) requires knowledge of past experiences involving these decisions, rules and guidelines set forth by the local institution, as well as requirements set forth by law.

Findings

The American Dietetic Association (ADA) recently released a position paper on ethical and legal issues in nutrition, hydration, and feeding. This paper provides recommendations on ethical deliberation including a suggested deliberative process that highlights the importance of critical thinking, furthering information, determining options, and above all, respecting the wishes and best interests of the patient. The position paper examines ethical decision-making processes in a variety of instances including dementia, terminal illness, terminally ill children, and persistent vegetative state (PVS). They found that medical decisions involving children are the responsibility of parents or guardians. For adults, the decision should follow the wishes set forth by the patient. They also reported that it is widely accepted that a difference exists between withdrawing medically inappropriate treatment and physician-assisted suicide. The official position of the ADA is to make treatment patient centered within the limits of the law.

In 2005 the *Annals of Internal Medicine* published findings from a multisociety task force set out to determine criteria for diagnosing PVS in the Terri Shiavo case. Terri Shiavo experienced severe hypoxia for several minutes in early 1990 and never recovered. The task force examined case series totaling 603 adults and 151 children with and without traumatic brain injury who were diagnosed with PVS. They found that the probability of good recovery or recovery with moderate disability was 1% after 3 months and 0% after 6 months of diagnosis. No reports exist of anyone recovering from PVS. The task force also determined criteria for artificial nutrition and hydration, stating that (1) these procedures are the same as other medical procedures; (2) these procedures, when not providing any benefit to a patient or his or her family, may be discontinued; and (3) patients diagnosed with PVS receive no benefit from these procedures. Terri Shiavo had been diagnosed with PVS 15 years before the final decision to remove feeding. After her death an autopsy revealed that she suffered from irreversible PVS. After examination of the proceedings and diagnosis of Terri Shiavo, the article concludes that due process was upheld and the order to cease nutrition support was moral and in accordance with what Terri Shiavo would have wanted had she been able to decide.

Conclusion

The wishes and rights of the patient should be upheld primarily, but laws governing the extent of rights vary from state to state. It is the RD's responsibility to work with patients to determine what course of action is most beneficial to the patient while still upholding the patient's rights and local legislation. Artificial nutrition and hydration are like any other medical procedure; when neither medically beneficial nor in accordance with the desires of the patient, they may be withheld. However, moral and ethical controversy still exists with regard to this topic and ultimately the care provider will be responsible for his or her actions. For this reason it is difficult to make an evidence-based decision on an ethical topic.

BIBLIOGRAPHY

Maillet JO: Position of the American Dietetic Association: ethical and legal issues in nutrition, hydration, and feeding, *J Am Diet Assoc* 108:874–882, 2008.

Perry JE, Churchill LR, Kirsher HS: The Terri Shiavo case: legal, ethical, and medical perspectives, *Ann Intern Med* 143:744–748, 2005.

These guidelines are similar to the overall *Dietary Guidelines for Americans 2005* (see Chapter 1). They are displayed in the 2005 *MyPyramid Food Guidance System* and emphasized in national and state health initiatives, including encouraging Americans to eat more servings of fruits and vegetables every day.[44] This emphasis stems from certain compounds found in plants, called *phytochemicals* (i.e., plant chemicals), which ongoing research indicates have promising effects in chemoprevention of cancer.[23] As indicated, these compounds include food nutrients—vitamins A (and its analogues), C, and E—as well as nonnutritive substances such as indoles, isothiocyanates, dithiolthiones, and organosulfur.[24,25]

Therapeutic Role

For the patient with cancer, the RD must shift into a therapeutic role, in which the patient is central in diet planning during disease stages and therapy effects. Nutrition therapy must now focus constantly on proactive assessment, with early and continuing preventive measures to intervene wisely before malnutrition occurs. For example, the RD should anticipate possible GI needs or psychosocial situations that relate to appetite, eating various foods, or drug effects. In addition, he or she should provide information concerning mouth care, symptoms experienced, or drug actions and effects. The cancer diagnosis need not be a ticket to starvation. With appropriate pain control and treatment for chemotherapy- and radiation-induced side effects, patients with cancer can continue to eat well through the latter stages of their disease. The RD and health care team should work closely with the patient to plan meals and snacks based on food preferences and dislikes, subjective intolerance of certain foods, and difficulties in chewing and swallowing.

HEALTH PROMOTION

Toward the Prevention of Cancer

Studies of geographic, socioeconomic, chronologic, and immigration patterns of cancer distribution indicate the vast majority of cancer cases are primarily caused by environmental factors. The logical conclusion is that reduction of these causative factors[23] may reduce or eliminate most forms of cancer.[45–51]

The American Cancer Society suggests that two thirds of all cases of cancer in the United States are caused by only two factors: (1) inhaled smoke and (2) ingested food. Tobacco, alone or in combination with alcohol, remains the most important cause of cancer, accounting for about one of every three cancer deaths in the United States. Cigarettes are the most important cause of tobacco-related cancer, but other forms of tobacco (chewing tobacco and snuff) are also established carcinogens. Cancer risk of ex-smokers remains elevated compared with lifetime nonsmokers. However, quitting smoking, even late in life after heavy long-term abuse, greatly reduces cancer risk when compared with the risk of continued smoking. Despite the rhetoric of tobacco companies, even regular smokers of low-tar cigarettes have a much increased cancer risk than nonsmokers.[45–51]

Alcohol, in addition to its synergistic effects with tobacco, increases risk of cancers of the oral cavity, pharynx, liver, and esophagus. Alcohol use has also been consistently linked to colorectal cancer and female breast cancer. Liquor, wine, and beer seem to be equal in effect on cancer risk.

Major incriminating dietary factors that appear now to be carcinogenic are the food changes that contrast current Western diets with those of our Paleolithic hunter-gatherer ancestors. We have reduced the amount of energy we obtain from starchy foods by one half to two thirds. We have decreased our intake of dietary fiber by 75%. We have more than doubled the proportion of energy we derive from fat and changed from mostly unsaturated fats to saturated fats. We have increased our salt intake fivefold, and sugar now accounts for one fifth of our total energy intake. The diet of our ancestors was energy dilute, whereas our modern diet is energy dense.[45–51]

Many studies link what we eat and do not eat to development of cancer. Direct relationships between preserved or salty foods and nasopharynx and stomach cancer have been consistently observed in case-control and correlational studies. Generous ingestion of fresh fruits and vegetables has consistently been found to decrease the risk of stomach cancer. Epidemiologic studies suggest a relation between high–animal fat, low-fiber intakes and colorectal cancer. The basis for this relationship lies in decreased transit time through the colon associated with high-fiber diets and increased water content in the intestinal lumen that dilutes other nutrients such as animal fat.

Considerable, although not yet conclusive, evidence exists that ascorbic acid has a protective effect against cancer of the esophagus, larynx, and oral cavity. Nutrients such as vitamin A, β-carotene, vitamin E, and ascorbic acid are thought to lower cancer risk in patients with elevated risk for cancers of the lung, esophagus, colon, and skin. Clinical and laboratory studies support findings that adequate intakes of vitamin D and calcium are associated with reduced incidence of colorectal cancer. These studies did not necessarily use supplemental amounts of these nutrients in addition to the RDAs but were based more on low levels of intake of these nutrients, which would parallel the low levels of fresh fruit and vegetable intakes that are prevalent in our society.

The majority of the causes of cancer—such as tobacco, alcohol, animal fat, obesity, and ultraviolet light—are associated with lifestyle (i.e., personal choices and not environmental causes). This fact reinforces the basic truth that the best cure is prevention. Lifestyle changes, including regular exercise, are the best prevention.[45–51]

TO SUM UP

Cancer is a term applied to abnormal, malignant growths in various body tissue sites. The cancerous cell is derived from a normal cell that loses control over cell reproduction. Cancer cell development occurs via mutation, carcinogens, radiation, and oncogenic viruses. It is also influenced by many epidemiologic factors such as diet, alcohol use, and smoking, as well as physical and psychologic stress factors. Cell development is mediated by the body's immune system, primarily its T cells, a type of white blood cell found in blood, lymph, and certain parts of the lymph nodes and spleen, and B cells, which manufacture and secrete antibodies.

Cancer therapy consists primarily of surgery, radiation, and chemotherapy. Supportive nutrition therapy for the patient with cancer should be highly individualized and depends on the response of each body system to the disease and to the treatment itself. It is based on a thorough nutrition assessment and provided by a number of routes—oral, tube feeding, peripheral vein, and total parenteral nutrition (TPN). If at all possible, then the oral route is preferred. Nutrient requirements and feeding mode must be designed for the specific physical and psychologic needs of individual patients.

QUESTIONS FOR REVIEW

1. What is cancer? Identify and describe several major causes of cancer cell formation.
2. How does your body attempt to defend itself against cancer? What nutritional factors may diminish this ability?
3. List and describe the rationale and mode of action of the types of therapies used to treat cancer.
4. Differentiate those factors challenging cancer recovery that are associated with the disease versus the type of therapy used.
5. Outline the general procedure for the nutritional management of a patient with cancer.

REFERENCES

1. U.S. Department of Health and Human Services: *Healthy people 2010: with understanding and improving health and objectives for improving health*, ed 2, Washington, DC, 2000, U.S. Government Printing Office.
2. Ries LAG, Wingo PA, Miller DS, et al: The annual report to the nation on the status of cancer, with a special section on colorectal cancer, 1973-1997, *Cancer* 88:2398, 2000.
3. Greenlee RT, Hill-Harmon MB, Murray T, et al: Cancer statistics 2001, *CA Cancer J Clin* 51:15, 2001.
4. Reference deleted in proofs.
5. Centers for Disease Control and Prevention: *United States cancer statistics: 2004 incidence and mortality*, 2007. Accessed July 27, 2010, from http://wonder.cdc.gov/wonder/help/cancer/USCS_2004.pdf.
6. Klein G: Fould's dangerous ideas revisited: the multistep development of tumors 40 years later, *Adv Cancer Res* 72:1, 1998.
7. Reif AE, Hearen T: Consensus on synergism between cigarette smoke and other environmental carcinogens in the causation of lung cancer, *Adv Cancer Res* 76:161, 1999.
8. Ross J: Structure and function of the gene. In Abeloff MD, Armitage JO, Niederhuber JE, et al, editiors: *Clinical oncology*, ed 2, New York, 2000, Churchill Livingstone.
9. Whiteman DC, Whiteman CA, Green AC: Childhood sun exposure as a risk factor for melanoma: a systematic review of epidemiologic studies, *Cancer Causes Control* 12:69, 2001.
10. deGruijl FR: Skin cancer and solar UV radiation, *Eur J Cancer* 35:1999, 2003.
11. Franco EL, Duarte-Franco E, Ferenczy A: Cervical cancer: epidemiology, prevention and the role of human papillomavirus infection, *CMAJ* 164:1017, 2001.
12. Sourvinos G, Tsatsanis C, Spandidos DA: Mechanisms of retrovirus-induced oncogenesis, *Folia Biol (Praha)* 46:226, 2000.
13. Holland JC: Cancer's psychological challenges, *Sci Am* 275(3):158, 1996.
14. Foley KM: Controlling the pain of cancer, *Sci Am* 275(3):164, 1996.
15. Burnet FM: Immunologic surveillance in neoplasia, *Transplant Rev* 7:3, 1971.
16. Boon T, et al: T-lymphocyte response. In Abeloff MD, Armitage JO, Niederhuber JE, et al, editiors: *Clinical oncology*, ed 2, New York, 2000, Churchill Livingstone.
17. Matarese G: Leptin and the immune system: how nutritional status influences immune response, *Eur Cytokine Netw* 11:7, 2000.
18. Carlson GL: The influence of nutrition and sepsis upon wound healing, *J Wound Care* 8(9):471, 1999.
19. Dureil B, Matuszczak Y: Alteration in nutritional status and diaphragm muscle function, *Reprod Nutr Dev* 38:175, 1998.
20. Bozzetti F, Gavazzi C, Miceli R, et al: Perioperative total parenteral nutrition in malnourished gastrointestinal cancer patients: a randomized clinical trial, *JPEN J Parenter Enteral Nutr* 24:7, 2000.
21. Hellman S, Vokes EE: Advancing current treatments for cancer, *Sci Am* 275(3):118, 1996.
22. Watzl B, Watson RR: Role of alcohol abuse in nutrition immunosuppression, *J Nutr* 122:733, 1992.
23. Greenwald P: Chemoprevention of cancer, *Sci Am* 275(3):96, 1996.
24. Kelloff GJ, Crowell JA, Steele VE, et al: Progress in cancer chemoprevention: development of diet-derived chemopreventive agents, *J Nutr* 467S:130, 2000.
25. Walaadkhan AR, Clemens MR: Effect of dietary phytochemicals on cancer development, *Int J Mol Med* 1(4):742, 1998.
26. Vanderhoof JA: Probiotics: future directions, *Am J Clin Nutr* 73(Suppl):1152S, 2001.
27. Aulas JJ: Alternative cancer treatments, *Sci Am* 275(3):162, 1996.
28. Loprinzi CL, Schaid DJ, Dose AM, et al: Body composition changes in patients who gain weight while receiving megestrol acetate, *J Clin Oncol* 11:152, 1993.
29. Bloch AS: Nutrition and cancer: the paradox, *Diet Curr* 23(2):1, 1996.

30. Menashiam L, Flam M, Douglas-Paxton D, et al: Improved food intake and reduced nausea and vomiting in patients given a restricted diet while receiving cisplatin chemotherapy, *J Am Diet Assoc* 92(2):58, 1992.
31. Darbinian J, Coulston A: Impact of chemotherapy on the nutritional status of the cancer patient. In Bloch AS, editor: *Nutrition management of the cancer patient*, Rockville, Md, 1990, Aspen.
32. Wilson RL: Optimizing nutrition for patients with cancer, *Clin J Oncol Nurs* 4(1):23, 2000.
33. Tayek JA, Chlebowski RT: Metabolic response to chemotherapy in colon cancer patients, *JPEN J Parenter Enter Nutr* 16(Suppl 6): 65, 1992.
34. Shaw JHF, Humberstone DA, Douglas RG, et al: Leukine kinetics in patients with benign disease, non-weight losing cancer and cancer cachexia: studies at the whole body level and the response to nutritional support, *Surgery* 109:37, 1991.
35. Tisdale MJ: Wasting in cancer, *J Nutr* 129(1):243S, 1999.
36. Polisena GG: Nutrition concerns in the radiation therapy patient. In McCallum PD, Polisena CG, editors: *The clinical guide to oncology nutrition*, Chicago, 2000, American Dietetic Association.
37. Reference deleted in proofs.
38. Reference deleted in proofs.
39. Molseed L: Alternative therapies in oncology. In McCallum PD, Polisena CG, editors: *The clinical guide to oncology nutrition*, Chicago, 2000, American Dietetic Association.
40. Ross C: Vitamin A and protective immunity, *Nutr Today* 27(4):18, 1992.
41. Henson DE, Block G, Levine M, et al: Ascorbic acid: biologic functions and relation to cancer, *J Natl Cancer Inst* 83(8):547, 1991.
42. Prasad KN, Edwards-Prasad J: Expressions of some molecular cancer risk factors and their modification by vitamins, *J Am Coll Nutr* 9(1):28, 1990.
43. American Cancer Society: *Guidelines for nutrition in cancer prevention*, Atlanta, 1999, American Cancer Society.
44. Foerster SB, Kizer KW, Disogra LK, et al: California's "5-a-Day-For Better Health" campaign: an innovative population-based effort to effect large-scale dietary change, *Am J Prev Med* 11:124, 1995.
45. Garland CF, Garland FC, Gorham ED: Can colon cancer incidence and death rates be reduced with calcium and vitamin D? *Am J Clin Nutr* 54:193S, 1991.
46. Henderson BE, Ross RK, Pike MC: Toward the primary prevention of cancer, *Science* 254:1131, 1991.
47. Kalman DS, Villani LJ: Exercise and the cancer patient, *On-Line* 6(1):1 American Dietetic Association.
48. Leffell DJ, Brash DE: Sunlight and skin cancer, *Sci Am* 275(1):52, 1996.
49. Trichopoulos D, Li FP, Hunter DJ: What causes cancer? *Sci Am* 275(3):80, 1996.
50. Willett WC, Colditz GA, Mueller NE: Strategies for minimizing cancer risk, *Sci Am* 275(3):88, 1996.
51. Wynder EL: Primary prevention of cancer: planning and policy considerations, *J Natl Cancer Inst* 83(7):475, 1991.
52. Reference deleted in proofs.
53. Reference deleted in proofs.

FURTHER READINGS AND RESOURCES

Readings

Bloch AS, editor: *Nutrition management of the cancer patient*, Rockville, Md, 1990, Aspen. *[This helpful reference by an experienced oncology dietitian and her contributors provides a comprehensive background for a better understanding of the complexities of caring for patients with cancer.]*

Bloch AS, Thomson CA: Position of the American Dietetic Association: phytochemicals and functional foods, *J Am Diet Assoc* 95(4):493, 1995. *[This statement provides important information for nutrition counseling.]*

Kalman D, Villani LJ: Nutritional aspects of cancer-related fatigue, *J Am Diet Assoc* 97(6):650, 1997. *[This article describes the fatigue associated with cancer and its treatment and ways in which all cancer team members may contribute to using nutritional management to minimize these side effects and broaden the patient's nutritional limits and food choices.]*

Steinmetz KA, Potter JD: Vegetables, fruit, and cancer prevention: a review, *J Am Diet Assoc* 96(10):1027, 1996. *[This statement provides important information regarding the role of certain foods in cancer prevention.]*

Websites of Interest

American Association for Cancer Research: www.aacr.org/. *[Resources for scientists, survivors, and the public.]*

American Cancer Society: www.cancer.org/docroot/home/index.asp. *[Excellent resource for the public and medical personnel.]*

Breastcancer.org: www.breastcancer.org/. *[This non-profit organization's website provides reliable, complete, and up-to-date information about breast cancer.]*

M.D. Anderson Cancer Center (University of Texas): www.mdanderson.org/. *[One of the world's most-respected medical centers devoted entirely to care of cancer patients, research, and cancer prevention.]*

National Cancer Institute: www.cancer.gov/. *[Part of the National Institutes of Health (NIH), this is the principle government agency for cancer research and training.]*

OncoLink (University of Pennsylvania): www.oncolink.com/. *[Founded by Penn cancer specialists to help cancer patients, families, health care professionals, and the general public.]*

WebMD: www.webmd.com/diseases_and_conditions/cancer.htm. *[Part of the WebMD medical information network, Cancer Health Center provided information regarding cancer.]*

APPENDIXES

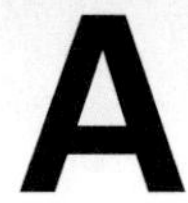

Body Mass Index: Obesity Values (Second of Two BMI Tables)*

HEIGHT (INCHES)	BODY WEIGHT (POUNDS)																		
BMI	**36**	**37**	**38**	**39**	**40**	**41**	**42**	**43**	**44**	**45**	**46**	**47**	**48**	**49**	**50**	**51**	**52**	**53**	**54**
58	172	177	181	186	191	196	201	205	210	215	220	224	229	234	239	244	248	253	258
59	178	183	188	193	198	203	208	212	217	222	227	232	237	242	247	252	257	262	267
60	184	189	194	199	204	209	215	220	225	230	235	240	245	250	255	261	266	271	276
61	190	195	201	206	211	217	222	227	232	238	243	248	254	259	264	269	275	280	285
62	196	202	207	213	218	224	229	235	240	246	251	256	262	267	273	278	284	289	295
63	203	208	214	220	225	231	237	242	248	254	259	265	270	278	282	287	293	299	304
64	209	215	221	227	232	238	244	250	256	262	267	273	279	285	291	296	302	308	314
65	216	222	228	234	240	246	252	258	264	270	276	282	288	294	300	306	312	318	324
66	223	229	235	241	247	253	260	266	272	278	284	291	297	303	309	315	322	328	334
67	230	236	242	249	255	261	268	274	280	287	293	299	306	312	319	325	331	338	344
68	236	243	249	256	262	269	276	282	289	295	302	308	315	322	328	335	341	348	354
69	243	250	257	263	270	277	284	291	297	304	311	318	324	331	338	345	351	358	365
70	250	257	264	271	278	285	292	299	306	313	320	327	334	341	348	355	362	369	376
71	257	265	272	279	286	293	301	308	315	322	329	338	343	351	358	365	372	379	386
72	265	272	279	287	294	302	309	316	324	331	338	346	353	361	368	375	383	390	397
73	272	280	288	295	302	310	318	325	333	340	348	355	363	371	378	386	393	401	408
74	280	287	295	303	311	319	326	334	342	350	358	365	373	381	389	396	404	412	420
75	287	295	303	311	319	327	335	343	351	359	367	375	383	391	399	407	415	423	431
76	295	304	312	320	328	336	344	353	361	369	377	385	394	402	410	418	426	435	443

From NIH/National Heart, Lung, and Blood Institute: Appendix V: Body mass index chart (chart 2), Clinical guidelines on the identification, evaluation, and treatment of overweight and obesity in adults, NIH Publication No. 98-4083, Bethesda, Md, September 1998, National Institutes of Health.

To use the table, find the appropriate height in the left-hand column. Move across to a given weight. The number at the top of the column is the BMI of that height and weight. Pounds have been rounded off.

*__Note:__ For lower body mass index values, see Table 8-4 on p. 177.

Choose Your Foods: Exchange Lists for Diabetes*

HOW THIS EXCHANGE LIST WORKS WITH MEAL PLANNING

There are three main groups of foods in this exchange list. They are based on the three major nutrients: carbohydrates, protein (meat and meat substitutes), and fat. Each food list contains foods grouped together because they have similar nutrient content and serving sizes. Each serving of a food has about the same amount of carbohydrate, protein, fat, and calories as the other foods on the same list.

- Foods on the **Starch** list, **Fruits** list, **Milk** list, and **Sweets, Desserts, and Other Carbohydrates** list are similar because they contain 12 to 15 grams of carbohydrate per serving.
- Foods on the **Fat** list and **Meat and Meat Substitutes** list usually do not have carbohydrate (except for the plant-based meat substitutes such as beans and lentils).
- Foods on the Starchy Vegetables list (part of the **Starch** list and including foods (such as potatoes, corn, and peas) contain 15 grams of carbohydrate per serving.
- Foods on the **Nonstarchy Vegetables** list (such as green beans, tomatoes, and carrots) contain 5 grams of carbohydrate per serving.
- Some foods have so little carbohydrate and calories that they are considered "free," if eaten in small amounts. You can find these foods on the **Free Foods** list.
- Foods that have different amounts of carbohydrates and calories are listed as **Combination Foods** (such as lasagna) or **Fast Foods.**

Foods are listed with their serving sizes, which are usually measured after cooking. When you begin, measuring the size of each serving will help you learn to "eyeball" correct serving sizes. The following chart shows the amount of nutrients in one serving from each list:

FOOD LIST	CARBOHYDRATE (grams)	PROTEIN (grams)	FAT (grams)	CALORIES
Carbohydrates				
Starch: breads, cereals and grains, starchy vegetables, crackers and snacks, and beans, peas, and lentils	15	0-3	0-1	80
Fruits	15	—	—	60
Milk				
Fat-free, low-fat, 1%	12	8	0-3	100
Reduced fat, 2%	12	8	5	130
Whole	12	8	8	150
Sweets, desserts, and other carbohydrates	15	Varies	Varies	Varies
Nonstarchy Vegetables	5	2	—	25
Meat and Meat Substitutes				
Lean	—	7	0-3	45
Medium-fat	—	7	4-7	75
High-fat	—	7	8+	100
Plant-based proteins	Varies	7	Varies	Varies
Fats	—	—	5	45
Alcohol	Varies	—	—	100

*The Exchange Lists are the basis of a meal-planning system designed by a committee of the American Diabetes Association and The American Dietetic Association. While designed primarily for people with diabetes and others who must follow special diets, the Exchange Lists are based on principles of good nutrition that apply to everyone.

STARCH

Cereals, grains, pasta, breads, crackers, snacks, starchy vegetables, and cooked beans, peas, and lentils are starches. In general, 1 starch is:

- ½ cup of cooked cereal, grain, or starchy vegetable
- ½ cup of cooked rice or pasta
- 1 oz of a bread product, such as 1 slice of bread
- ¾ oz to 1 oz of most snack foods (some snack foods may also have extra fat)

Nutrition Tips

1. A choice on the **Starch** list has 15 grams of carbohydrate, 0-3 grams of protein, 0-1 grams of fat, and 80 calories.
2. For maximum health benefits, eat three or more servings of whole grains each day. A serving of whole grain is about ½ cup of cooked cereal or grain, 1 slice of whole-grain bread, or 1 cup of whole-grain cold breakfast cereal.

Selection Tips

1. Choose low-fat starches as often as you can.
2. Starchy vegetables, baked goods, and grains prepared with fat count as 1 starch and 1fat.
3. For many starchy foods (bagels, muffins, dinner rolls, buns), a general rule of thumb is 1 oz equals 1 serving. Always check the size you eat. Because of their large size, some foods have a lot more carbohydrate (and calories) than you might think. For example, a large bagel may weigh 4 oz and equal 4 carbohydrate servings.
4. For specific information, read the Nutrition Facts panel on the food label.

FOOD	SERVING SIZE
Bread	
Bagel, large (about 4 oz)	¼ (1 oz)
Biscuit, 2½ inches across†	1
Bread	
Reduced-calorie*	2 slices (1½ oz)
White, whole-grain, pumpernickel, rye, unfrosted raisin	1 slice (1 oz)
Chapatti, small, 6 inches across	1
Cornbread, 1¾ inch cube†	1 (1½ oz)
English muffin	½
Hot dog bun or hamburger bun	½ (1 oz)
Naan, 8 inches by 2 inches	¼
Pancake, 4 inches across, ¼ inch thick	1
Pita, 6 inches across	½
Roll, plain, small	1 (1 oz)
Stuffing, bread†	⅓ cup
Taco shell, 5 inches across†	2
Tortilla, corn, 6 inches across	1
Tortilla, flour, 6 inches across	1
Tortilla, flour, 10 inches across	⅓ tortilla
Waffle, 4-inch square or 4 inches across†	1
Cereals and Grains	
Barley, cooked	⅓ cup
Bran, dry	
Oat*	¼ cup
Wheat*	½ cup
Bulgar (cooked)*	½ cup
Cereals	
Bran*	½ cup
Cooked (oats, oatmeal)	½ cup
Puffed	1½ cup
Shredded wheat, plain	½ cup
Sugar-coated	½ cup
Unsweetened, ready-to-eat	¾ cup
Couscous	⅓ cup
Granola	
Low-fat	¼ cup
Regular†	¼ cup
Grits, cooked	½ cup
Kasha	½ cup
Millet, cooked	⅓ cup
Muesli	¼ cup
Pasta, cooked	⅓ cup
Polenta, cooked	⅓ cup
Quinoa, cooked	⅓ cup
Rice, white or brown, cooked	⅓ cup
Tabbouleh (tabouli), prepared	½ cup
Wheat germ, dry	3 Tbsp
Wild rice, cooked	½ cup
Starchy Vegetables	
Cassava	⅓ cup
Corn	½ cup
On cob, large	½ cob (5 oz)
Hominy, canned*	¾ cup
Mixed vegetables with corn, peas, or pasta*	1 cup
Parsnips*	½ cup
Peas, green*	½ cup
Plantain, ripe	⅓ cup
Potato	
Baked with skin	¼ large (3 oz)
Boiled, all kinds	½ cup or ½ medium (3 oz)
Mashed, with milk and fat†	½ cup
French fried (oven-baked)	1 cup (2 oz)
Pumpkin, canned, no sugar added*	1 cup
Spaghetti/pasta sauce	½ cup
Squash, winter (acorn, butternut)*	1 cup
Succotash*	½ cup
Yam, sweet potato, plain	½ cup

*The Exchange Lists are the basis of a meal-planning system designed by a committee of the American Diabetes Association and The American Dietetic Association. While designed primarily for people with diabetes and others who must follow special diets, the Exchange Lists are based on principles of good nutrition that apply to everyone.

FOOD	SERVING SIZE
Crackers and Snacks	
Animal crackers	8
Crackers	
Round-butter type†	6
Saltine-type	6
Sandwich-style, cheese or peanut butter filling†	3
Whole-wheat regular†	2-5 (¾ oz)
Whole-wheat lower fat or crispbreads*	2-5 (¾ oz)
Graham cracker, 2½-inch square	3
Matzoh	¾ oz
Melba toast, about 2-inch by 4-inch piece	4 pieces
Oyster crackers	20
Popcorn (microwave popped)	3 cups
With butter†*	3 cups
No fat added*	3 cups
Lower fat*	3 cups
Pretzels	¾ oz
Rice cakes, 4 inches across	2
Snack chips	
Fat-free or baked (tortilla, potato), baked pita chips	15-20 (¾ oz)
Regular (tortilla, potato)†	9-13 (¾ oz)
Beans, Peas, and Lentils	
The choices on this list count as 1 starch + 1 lean meat.	
Baked beans*	⅓ cup
Beans, cooked (black, garbanzo, kidney, lima, navy, pinto, white)*	½ cup
Lentils, cooked (brown, green, yellow)*	½ cup
Peas, cooked (black-eyed, split)*	½ cup
Refried beans, canned‡*	½ cup

*More than 3 grams of dietary fiber per serving.
†Extra fat, or prepared with added fat. (Count as 1 starch + 1 fat.)
‡480 milligrams or more of sodium per serving.

FRUITS

Fresh, frozen, canned, and dried fruits and fruit juices are on this list. In general, 1 fruit choice is:

- ½ cup of canned or fresh fruit or unsweetened fruit juice
- 1 small fresh fruit (4 oz)
- 2 tablespoons of dried fruit

Nutrition Tips

1. A choice on the **Fruits** list has 15 grams of carbohydrate, 0 grams of protein, 0 grams of fat, and 60 calories.
2. Fresh, frozen, and dried fruits are good sources of fiber. Fruit juices contain very little fiber. Choose fruits instead of juices whenever possible.
3. Citrus fruits, berries, and melons are good sources of vitamin C.

Selection Tips

1. Use a food scale to weigh fresh fruits. Practice builds portion skills.
2. The weight listed includes skin, core, seeds, and rind.
3. Read the Nutrition Facts on the food label. If 1 serving has more than 15 g of carbohydrate, you may need to adjust the size of the serving.
4. Portion sizes for canned fruits are for the fruit and a small amount of juice (1 to 2 tablespoons).
5. Food labels for fruits may contain the words *no sugar added* or *unsweetened*. This means that no sucrose (table sugar) has been added; it *does not* mean the food contains no sugar.
6. Fruit canned in *extra light syrup* has the same amount of carbohydrate per serving as the *no sugar added* or the *juice pack*. All canned fruits on the **Fruits** list are based on one of these three types of pack. Avoid fruit canned in heavy syrup.

The weight listed includes skin, core, seeds, and rind.

FOOD	SERVING SIZE
Fruit	
Apple, unpeeled, small	1 (4 oz)
Apples, dried	4 rings
Applesauce, unsweetened	½ cup
Apricots	
Canned	½ cup
Dried	8 halves
Fresh*	4 whole (5½ oz)
Banana, extra small	1 (4 oz)
Blackberries*	¾ cup
Blueberries	¾ cup
Cantaloupe, small	⅓ melon or 1 cup cubed (11 oz)
Cherries	
Sweet, canned	½ cup
Sweet fresh	12 (3 oz)
Dates	3
Dried fruits (blueberries, cherries, cranberries, mixed fruit, raisins)	2 Tbsp
Figs	
Dried	1½
Fresh*	1½ large or 2 medium (3½ oz)
Fruit cocktail	½ cup

Continued

*The Exchange Lists are the basis of a meal-planning system designed by a committee of the American Diabetes Association and The American Dietetic Association. While designed primarily for people with diabetes and others who must follow special diets, the Exchange Lists are based on principles of good nutrition that apply to everyone.

FOOD	SERVING SIZE
Fruit—cont'd	
Grapefruit	
Large	½ (11 oz)
Sections, canned	¾ cup
Grapes, small	17 (3 oz)
Honeydew melon	1 slice or 1 cup cubed (10 oz)
Kiwi*	1 (3½ oz)
Mandarin oranges, canned	¾ cup
Mango, small	½ fruit (5½ oz) or ½ cup
Nectarine, small	1 (5 oz)
Orange, small*	1 (6½ oz)
Papaya	½ fruit or 1 cup cubed (8 oz)
Peaches	
Canned	½ cup
Fresh, medium	1 (6 oz)
Pears	
Canned	½ cup
Fresh, large	½ (4 oz)
Pineapple	
Canned	½ cup
Fresh	¾ cup
Plums	
Canned	½ cup
Dried (prunes)	3
Small	2 (5 oz)
Raspberries*	1 cup
Strawberries*	1¼ cup whole berries
Tangerines, small*	2 (8 oz)
Watermelon	1 slice or 1¼ cups cubes (13½ oz)
Fruit Juice	
Apple juice/cider	½ cup
Fruit juice blends, 100% juice	⅓ cup
Grape juice	⅓ cup
Grapefruit juice	½ cup
Orange juice	½ cup
Pineapple juice	½ cup
Prune juice	⅓ cup

*More than 3 grams of dietary fiber per serving.

MILK

Different types of milk and milk products are on this list. However, 2 types of milk products are found in other lists:

- Cheeses are on the **Meat and Meat Substitutes** list (because they are rich in protein).
- Cream and other dairy fats are on the **Fats** list.

Milks and yogurts are grouped in 3 categories (fat-free/low-fat, reduced-fat, or whole) based on the amount of fat they have. The following chart shows you what 1 milk choice contains:

	CARBOHYDRATE (grams)	PROTEIN (grams)	FAT (grams)	CALORIES
Fat-free (skim), low-fat (1%)	12	8	0-3	100
Reduced-fat (2%)	12	8	5	130
Whole	12	8	8	150

Nutrition Tips

1. Milk and yogurt are good sources of calcium and protein.
2. The higher the fat content of milk and yogurt, the more saturated fat and cholesterol it has.
3. Children over the age of 2 and adults should choose lower-fat varieties such as skim, 1%, or 2% milks or yogurts.

Selection Tips

1. 1 cup equals 8 fluid oz or ½ pint.
2. If you choose 2%, or whole-milk foods, be aware of the extra fat.

*The Exchange Lists are the basis of a meal-planning system designed by a committee of the American Diabetes Association and The American Dietetic Association. While designed primarily for people with diabetes and others who must follow special diets, the Exchange Lists are based on principles of good nutrition that apply to everyone.

FOOD	SERVING SIZE	COUNT AS
Milk and Yogurts		
Fat-free or low-fat (1%)		
Milk, buttermilk, acidophilus milk, Lactaid	1 cup	1 fat-free milk
Evaporated milk	½ cup	1 fat-free milk
Yogurt, plain or flavored with an artificial sweetener	⅔ cup (6 oz)	1 fat-free milk
Reduced-fat (2%)		
Milk, acidophilus milk, kefir, Lactaid	1 cup	1 reduced-fat milk
Yogurt, plain	⅔ cup (6 oz)	1 reduced-fat milk
Whole		
Milk, buttermilk, goat's milk	1 cup	1 whole milk
Evaporated milk	½ cup	1 whole milk
Yogurt, plain	8 oz	1 whole milk
Dairy-Like Foods		
Chocolate milk		
Fat-free	1 cup	1 fat-free milk + 1 carbohydrate
Whole	1 cup	1 whole milk + 1 carbohydrate
Eggnog, whole milk	½ cup	1 carbohydrate + 2 fats
Rice drink		
Flavored, low-fat	1 cup	2 carbohydrates
Plain, fat-free	1 cup	1 carbohydrate
Smoothies, flavored, regular	10 oz	1 fat-free milk + 2½ carbohydrates
Soy milk		
Light	1 cup	1 carbohydrate + ½ fat
Regular, plain	1 cup	1 carbohydrate + 1 fat
Yogurt		
And juice blends	1 cup	1 fat-free milk + 1 carbohydrate
Low carbohydrate (less than 6 grams carbohydrate per choice)	⅔ cup (6 oz)	½ fat-free milk
With fruit, low-fat	⅔ cup (6 oz)	1 fat-free milk + 1 carbohydrate

SWEETS, DESSERTS, AND OTHER CARBOHYDRATES

You can substitute food choices from this list for other carbohydrate-containing foods (such as those found on the **Starch, Fruit,** or **Milk** lists) in your meal plan, even though these foods have added sugars or fat.

Common Measurements

Dry:
3 tsp = 1 Tbsp
4 oz = ½ cup
8 oz = 1 cup
Liquid:
4 Tbsp = ¼ cup
8 oz = ½ pint

Nutrition Tips

1. A carbohydrate choice has 15 grams of carbohydrate, variable grams of protein, variable grams of fat, and variable calories.
2. The foods on this list do not have as many vitamins, minerals, and fiber as the choices on the **Starch, Fruits,** or **Milk** lists. When choosing sweets, desserts, and other carbohydrate foods, you should also eat foods from other food lists to balance out your meals.
3. Many of these foods don't equal a single choice. Some will also count as one or more fat choices.
4. If you are trying to lose weight, choose foods from this list less often.
5. The serving sizes for these foods are small because of their fat content.

Selection Tips

1. Read the Nutrition facts on the food label to find the serving size and nutrient information.
2. Many sugar-free, fat-free, or reduced-fat products are made with ingredients that contain carbohydrate. These types of food usually have the same amount of carbohydrate as the regular foods they are replacing. Talk with your RD and find out how to fit these foods into your meal plan.

*The Exchange Lists are the basis of a meal-planning system designed by a committee of the American Diabetes Association and The American Dietetic Association. While designed primarily for people with diabetes and others who must follow special diets, the Exchange Lists are based on principles of good nutrition that apply to everyone.

FOOD	SERVING SIZE	COUNT AS
Beverages, Soda, and Energy/Sports Drinks		
Cranberry juice cocktail	½ cup	1 carbohydrate
Energy drink	1 can (8.3 oz)	2 carbohydrates
Fruit drink or lemonade	1 cup (8 oz)	2 carbohydrates
Hot chocolate		
Regular	1 envelope added to 8 oz water	1 carbohydrate + 1 fat
Sugar-free or light	1 envelope added to 8 oz water	1 carbohydrate
Soft drink (soda), regular	1 can (12 oz)	2½ carbohydrates
Sports drink	1 cup (8 oz)	1 carbohydrate
Brownies, Cake, Cookies, Gelatin, Pie, and Pudding		
Brownie, small, unfrosted	1¼-inch square, ⅞ inch high (about 1 oz)	1 carbohydrate + 1 fat
Cake		
Angel food, unfrosted	1/12 of cake (about 2 oz)	2 carbohydrates
Frosted	2-inch square (about 2 oz)	2 carbohydrates + 1 fat
Unfrosted	2-inch square (about 2 oz)	1 carbohydrate + 1 fat
Cookies		
Chocolate chip	2 cookies (2¼ inches across)	1 carbohydrate + 2 fats
Gingersnap	3 cookies	1 carbohydrate
Sandwich, with crème filling	2 small (about ⅔ oz)	1 carbohydrate + 1 fat
Sugar-free	3 small or 1 large (¾ -1 oz)	1 carbohydrate + 1-2 fats
Vanilla wafer	5 cookies	1 carbohydrate + 1 fat
Cupcake, frosted	1 small (about 1¾ oz)	2 carbohydrates + 1-1½ fats
Fruit cobbler	½ cup (3½ oz)	3 carbohydrates + 1 fat
Gelatin, regular	½ cup	1 carbohydrate
Pie		
Commercially prepared fruit, 2 crusts	⅙ of 8-inch pie	3 carbohydrates + 2 fats
Pumpkin or custard	⅛ of 8-inch pie	1½ carbohydrates + 1½ fats
Pudding		
Regular (made with reduced-fat milk)	½ cup	2 carbohydrates
Sugar-free or sugar- and fat-free (made with fat-free milk)	½ cup	1 carbohydrate
Candy, Spreads, Sweets, Sweeteners, Syrups, and Toppings		
Candy bar, chocolate/peanut	2 "fun size" bars (1 oz)	1½ carbohydrates + 1½ fats
Candy, hard	3 pieces	1 carbohydrate
Chocolate "kisses"	5 pieces	1 carbohydrate + 1 fat
Coffee creamer		
Dry, flavored	4 tsp	½ carbohydrate + ½ fat
Liquid, flavored	2 Tbsp	1 carbohydrate
Fruit snacks, chewy (pureed fruit concentrate)	1 roll (¾ oz)	1 carbohydrate
Fruit spreads, 100% fruit	1½ Tbsp	1 carbohydrate
Honey	1 Tbsp	1 carbohydrate
Jam or jelly, regular	1 Tbsp	1 carbohydrate
Sugar	1 Tbsp	1 carbohydrate
Syrup		
Chocolate	2 Tbsp	2 carbohydrates
Light (pancake type)	2 Tbsp	1 carbohydrate
Regular (pancake type)	1 Tbsp	1 carbohydrate
Condiments and Sauces		
Barbeque sauce	3 Tbsp	1 carbohydrate
Cranberry sauce, jellied	¼ cup	1½ carbohydrates
Gravy, mushroom, canned‡	½ cup	½ carbohydrate + ½ fat
Salad dressing, fat-free, low fat, cream-based	3 Tbsp	1 carbohydrate
Sweet and sour sauce	3 Tbsp	1 carbohydrate

*The Exchange Lists are the basis of a meal-planning system designed by a committee of the American Diabetes Association and The American Dietetic Association. While designed primarily for people with diabetes and others who must follow special diets, the Exchange Lists are based on principles of good nutrition that apply to everyone.

FOOD	SERVING SIZE	COUNT AS
Doughnuts, Muffins, Pastries, and Sweet Breads		
Banana nut bread	1-inch slice (1 oz)	2 carbohydrates + 1 fat
Doughnut		
Cake, plain	1 medium (1½ oz)	1½ carbohydrates + 2 fats
Glazed	3¾ inches across (2 oz)	2 carbohydrates + 2 fats
Muffin (4 oz)	¼ muffin (1 oz)	1 carbohydrate + ½ fat
Sweet roll or Danish	1 (2½ oz)	2½ carbohydrates + 2 fats
Frozen Bars, Frozen Desserts, Frozen Yogurt, and Ice Cream		
Frozen pops	1	½ carbohydrate
Fruit juice bars, frozen, 100% juice	1 bar (3 oz)	1 carbohydrate
Ice cream		
Fat-free	½ cup	1½ carbohydrates
Light	½ cup	1 carbohydrate + 1 fat
No sugar added	½ cup	1 carbohydrate + 1 fat
Regular	½ cup	1 carbohydrate + 2 fats
Sherbet, sorbet	½ cup	2 carbohydrates
Yogurt, frozen		
Fat-free	⅓ cup	1 carbohydrate
Regular	½ cup	1 carbohydrate + 0-1 fat
Granola Bars, Meal Replacement Bars/Shakes, and Trail Mix		
Granola or snack bar, regular or low-fat	1 bar (1 oz)	1½ carbohydrates
Meal replacement bar	1 bar (1⅓ oz)	1½ carbohydrates + 0-1 fat
Meal replacement bar	1 bar (2 oz)	2 carbohydrates + 1 fat
Meal replacement shake, reduced calorie	1 can (10-11 oz)	1½ carbohydrates + 0-1 fat
Trail mix		
Candy/nut-based	1 oz	1 carbohydrate + 2 fats
Dried fruit-based	1 oz	1 carbohydrate + 1 fat

‡480 mg or more of sodium per serving.

NONSTARCHY VEGETABLES

Vegetable choices include vegetables in this **Nonstarchy Vegetables** list and the Starchy Vegetables list found within the **Starch** list. Vegetables with small amounts of carbohydrate and calories are on the **Nonstarchy Vegetables** list. Vegetables contain important nutrients. Try to eat at least 2 to 3 nonstarchy vegetable choices each day (as well as choices from the Starchy Vegetables list). In general, 1 nonstarchy vegetable choice is:

- ½ cup of cooked vegetables or vegetable juice
- 1 cup of raw vegetables

If you eat 3 cups or more of raw vegetables or 1½ cups of cooked vegetables in a meal, count them as 1 carbohydrate choice.

Nutrition Tips

1. A choice on this list (½ cup cooked or 1 cup raw) equals 5 grams of carbohydrate, 2 grams of protein, 0 grams of fat, and 25 calories.
2. Fresh and frozen vegetables have less added salt than canned vegetables. Drain and rinse canned vegetables to remove some salt.
3. Choose dark green and dark yellow vegetables each day. Spinach, broccoli, romaine, carrots, chilies, squash, and peppers are great choices.
4. Brussels sprouts, broccoli, cauliflower, greens, peppers, spinach, and tomatoes are good sources of vitamin C.
5. Eat vegetables from the cruciferous family several times each week. Cruciferous vegetables include bok choy, broccoli, brussels sprouts, cabbage, cauliflower, collards, kale, kohlrabi, radishes, rutabaga, turnip, and watercress.

Selection Tips

1. Canned vegetables and juices are also available without added salt.
2. A 1-cup portion of broccoli is a portion about the size of a regular light bulb.
3. Starchy vegetables such as corn, peas, winter squash, and potatoes that have more calories and carbohydrates are on the Starchy Vegetables section in the **Starch** list.
4. The tomato sauce referred to in this list is different from spaghetti/pasta sauce, which is on the Starchy Vegetables list.

*The Exchange Lists are the basis of a meal-planning system designed by a committee of the American Diabetes Association and The American Dietetic Association. While designed primarily for people with diabetes and others who must follow special diets, the Exchange Lists are based on principles of good nutrition that apply to everyone.

Nonstarchy Vegetables

Amaranth or Chinese spinach
Artichoke
Artichoke hearts
Asparagus
Baby corn
Bamboo shoots
Beans (green, wax, Italian)
Bean sprouts
Beets
Borscht‡
Broccoli
Brussels sprouts*
Cabbage (green, bok choy, Chinese)
Carrots*
Cauliflower
Celery
Chayote*
Coleslaw, packaged, no dressing
Cucumber
Eggplant
Gourds (bitter, bottle, luffa, bitter melon)
Green onions or scallions
Greens (collard, kale, mustard, turnip)
Hearts of palm
Jicama
Kohlrabi
Leeks
Mixed vegetables (without corn, peas, or pasta)
Mung bean sprouts
Mushrooms, all kinds, fresh
Okra
Onions
Oriental radish or daikon
Pea pods
Peppers (all varieties)*
Radishes
Rutabaga
Sauerkraut‡
Soybean sprouts
Spinach
Squash (summer, crookneck, zucchini)
Sugar pea snaps
Swiss chard*
Tomato
Tomatoes, canned
Tomato sauce‡
Tomato/vegetable juice‡
Turnips
Water chestnuts
Yard-long beans

*More than 3 grams of dietary fiber per serving.
‡480 milligrams or more of sodium per serving.

MEAT AND MEAT SUBSTITUTES

Meat and meat substitutes are rich in protein. Foods from this list are divided into 4 groups based on the amount of fat they contain. These groups are lean meat, medium-fat meat, high-fat meat, and plant-based proteins. The following chart shows you what one choice includes:

	CARBOHYDRATE (grams)	PROTEIN (grams)	FAT (grams)	CALORIES
Lean meat	—	7	0-3	45
Medium-fat meat	—	7	4-7	75
High-fat meat	—	7	8+	100
Plant-based protein	Varies	7	Varies	Varies

Nutrition Tips

1. Read labels to find foods low in fat and cholesterol. Try for 5 grams of fat or less per serving.
2. Read labels to find "hidden" carbohydrate. For example, hot dogs actually contain a lot of carbohydrate. Most hot dogs are also high in fat, but are often sold in lower-fat versions.
3. Whenever possible, choose lean meats.
   a. Select grades of meat that are the leanest.
   b. Choice grades have a moderate amount of fat.
   c. Prime cuts of meat have the highest amount of fat.
4. Fish such as herring, mackerel, salmon, sardines, halibut, trout, and tuna are rich in omega-3 fats, which may help reduce risk for heart disease. Choose fish (not commercially fried fish fillets) two or more times each week.
5. Bake, roast, broil, grill, poach, steam, or boil instead of frying.

Selection Tips

1. Trim off visible fat or skin.
2. Roast, broil, or grill meat on a rack so that the fat will drain off during cooking.
3. Use a nonstick spray and a nonstick pan to brown or fry foods.
4. Some processed meats, seafood, and soy products contain carbohydrate. Read the food label to see if the amount of carbohydrate in the serving size you plan to eat is close to 15 grams. If so, count it as 1 carbohydrate choice and 1 or more meat choice.
5. Meat or fish that is breaded with cornmeal, flour, or dried bread crumbs contain carbohydrate. Count 3 Tbsp of one of these dry grains as 15 grams of carbohydrate.

*The Exchange Lists are the basis of a meal-planning system designed by a committee of the American Diabetes Association and The American Dietetic Association. While designed primarily for people with diabetes and others who must follow special diets, the Exchange Lists are based on principles of good nutrition that apply to everyone.

FOOD	AMOUNT
Lean Meats and Meat Substitutes	
Beef: Select or Choice grades trimmed of fat: ground round, roast (chuck, rib, rump), round, sirloin, steak (cubed, flank, porterhouse, T-bone), tenderloin	1 oz
Beef jerky‡	1 oz
Cheeses with 3 grams of fat or less per oz	1 oz
Cottage cheese	¼ cup
Egg substitutes, plain	¼ cup
Egg whites	2
Fish, fresh or frozen, plain: catfish, cod, flounder, haddock, halibut, orange roughy, salmon, tilapia, trout, tuna	1 oz
Fish, smoked: herring or salmon (lox)‡	1 oz
Game: buffalo, ostrich, rabbit, venison	1 oz
Hot dog with 3 grams of fat or less per oz‡ (8 dogs per 14 oz package) *(Note: May be high in carbohydrate)*	1
Lamb: chop, leg, or roast	1 oz
Organ meats: heart, kidney, liver *(Note: May be high in cholesterol)*	1 oz
Oysters, fresh or frozen	6 medium
Pork, lean	
Canadian bacon‡	1 oz
Rib or loin chop/roast, ham, tenderloin	1 oz
Poultry, without skin: Cornish hen, chicken, domestic duck or goose (well-drained of fat), turkey	1 oz
Processed sandwich meats with 3 grams of fat or less per oz: chipped beef, deli thin-sliced meats, turkey ham, turkey kielbasa, turkey pastrami	1 oz
Salmon, canned	1 oz
Sardines, canned	2 small
Sausage with 3 grams of fat or less per oz‡	1 oz
Shellfish: clams, crab, imitation shellfish, lobster, scallops, shrimp	1 oz
Tuna, canned in water or oil, drained	1 oz
Veal, loin chop, roast	1 oz

‡480 milligrams or more of sodium per serving

FOOD	AMOUNT
Medium-Fat Meat and Meat Substitutes	
Beef: corned beef, ground beef, meatloaf, Prime grades trimmed of fat (prime rib), short ribs, tongue	1 oz
Cheeses with 4-7 grams of fat per oz: feta, mozzarella, pasteurized processed cheese spread, reduced-fat cheeses, string	1 oz
Egg *(Note: High in cholesterol, so limit to 3 per week)*	1
Fish, any fried product	1 oz
Lamb: ground, rib roast	1 oz
Pork: cutlet, shoulder roast	1 oz
Poultry: chicken with skin; dove, pheasant, wild duck, or goose; fried chicken; ground turkey	1 oz
Ricotta cheese	2 oz or ¼ cup
Sausage with 4-7 grams of fat per oz‡	1 oz
Veal, cutlet (no breading)	1 oz

‡480 milligrams or more of sodium per serving.

The following foods are high in saturated fat, cholesterol, and calories and may raise blood cholesterol levels if eaten on a regular basis. Try to eat 3 or fewer servings from this group per week.

High-Fat Meat and Meat Substitutes

FOOD	AMOUNT
Bacon	
Pork‡	2 slices (16 slices per lb or 1 oz each, before cooking)
Turkey‡	3 slices (½ oz each before cooking)
Cheese, regular: American, bleu, brie, cheddar, hard goat, Monterey jack, queso, and Swiss	1 oz
Hot dog: beef, pork, or combination (10 per lb-sized package)‡†	1
Hot dog: turkey or chicken (10 per lb-sized package)‡	1
Pork: ground, sausage, spareribs	1 oz
Processed sandwich meats with 8 grams of fat or more per oz: bologna, pastrami, hard salami	1 oz
Sausage with 8 grams fat or more per oz: bratwurst, chorizo, Italian, knockwurst, Polish, smoked, summer‡	1 oz

†Extra fat, or prepared with added fat. (Add an additional fat choice to this food.)
‡480 milligrams or more of sodium per serving.

*The Exchange Lists are the basis of a meal-planning system designed by a committee of the American Diabetes Association and The American Dietetic Association. While designed primarily for people with diabetes and others who must follow special diets, the Exchange Lists are based on principles of good nutrition that apply to everyone.

Because carbohydrate content varies among plant-based proteins, you should read the food label.

FOOD	AMOUNT	COUNT AS
Plant-Based Proteins		
"Bacon" strips, soy-based	3 strips	1 medium-fat meat
Baked beans*	⅓ cup	1 starch + 1 lean meat
Beans, cooked: black, garbanzo, kidney, lima, navy, pinto, white*	½ cup	1 starch + 1 lean meat
"Beef" or "sausage" crumbles, soy-based*	2 oz	½ carbohydrate + 1 lean meat
"Chicken" nuggets, soy-based	2 nuggets (1½ oz)	½ carbohydrate + 1 medium-fat meat
Edamame*	½ cup	½ carbohydrate + 1 lean meat
Falafel (spiced chickpea and wheat patties)	3 patties (about 2 inches across)	1 carbohydrate + 1 high-fat meat
Hot dog, soy-based	1 (1½ oz)	½ carbohydrate + 1 lean meat
Hummus*	⅓ cup	1 carbohydrate + 1 high-fat meat
Lentils, brown, green, or yellow*	½ cup	1 carbohydrate + 1 lean meat
Meatless burger, soy-based*	3 oz	½ carbohydrate + 2 lean meats
Meatless burger, vegetable- and starch-based*	1 patty (about 2½ oz)	1 carbohydrate + 2 lean meats
Nut spreads: almond butter, cashew butter, peanut butter, soy nut butter	1 Tbsp	1 high-fat meat
Peas, cooked: black-eyed and split peas*	½ cup	1 starch + 1 lean meat
Refried beans, canned‡*	½ cup	1 starch + 1 lean meat
"Sausage" patties, soy-based	1 (1½ oz)	1 medium-fat meat
Soy nuts, unsalted	¾ oz	½ carbohydrate + 1 medium-fat meat
Tempeh	¼ cup	1 medium-fat meat
Tofu	4 oz (½ oz)	1 medium-fat meat
Tofu, light	4 oz (½ oz)	1 lean meat

*More than 3 grams of dietary fiber per serving.
‡480 milligrams or more of sodium per serving.

FATS

Fats are divided into 3 groups, based on the main type of fat they contain:

- **Unsaturated fats** (omega-3, monounsaturated, and polyunsaturated) are primarily vegetable and are liquid at room temperature. These fats have good health benefits.
  - **Omega-3 fats** are a type of polyunsaturated fat and can help lower triglyceride levels and the risk of heart disease.
  - **Monounsaturated fats** also help lower cholesterol levels and may help raise HDL (good) cholesterol levels.
  - **Polyunsaturated fats** can help lower cholesterol levels.
- **Saturated fats** have been linked with heart disease. They can raise LDL (bad) cholesterol levels and should be eaten in small amounts. Saturated fats are solid at room temperature.
- ***Trans* fats** are made in a process that changes vegetable oils into semi-solid fats. These fats can raise blood cholesterol levels and should be eaten in small amounts. Partially hydrogenated and hydrogenated fats are types of man-made *trans* fats and should be avoided. *Trans* fats are also found naturally occurring in some animal products such as meat, cheese, butter, and dairy products.

Nutrition Tips

1. A choice on the **Fats** list contains 5 grams of fat and 45 calories.
2. All fats are high in calories. Limit serving sizes for good nutrition and health.
3. Limit the amount of fried foods you eat.
4. Nuts and seeds are good sources of unsaturated fats if eaten in moderation. They have small amounts of fiber, protein, and magnesium.
5. Good sources of omega-3 fatty acids include:
   a. Fish such as albacore tuna, halibut, herring, mackerel, salmon, sardines, and trout
   b. Flaxseeds and English walnuts
   c. Oils such as canola, soybean, flaxseed, and walnut.

Selection Tips

1. Read the Nutrition Facts on food labels for serving sizes. One fat choice is based on a serving size that has 5 grams of fat.
2. The food label also lists total fat grams, saturated fat, and *trans* fat grams per serving. When most of the calories come from saturated fat, the food is part of the Saturated Fats list.

*The Exchange Lists are the basis of a meal-planning system designed by a committee of the American Diabetes Association and The American Dietetic Association. While designed primarily for people with diabetes and others who must follow special diets, the Exchange Lists are based on principles of good nutrition that apply to everyone.

3. When selecting fats, consider replacing saturated fats with monounsaturated fats and omega-3 fats. Talk with your RD about the best choices for you.
4. When selecting regular margarine, choose those that list liquid vegetable oil as the first ingredient. Soft or tub margarines have less saturated fat than stick margarines and are a healthier choice. Look for *trans* fat-free soft margarines.
5. When selecting reduced-fat or lower-fat margarines, look for liquid vegetable oil (*trans* fat-free). Water is usually the first ingredient.

Fats and oils have mixtures of unsaturated (polyunsaturated and monounsaturated) and saturated fats. Foods on the Fats list are grouped together based on the major type of fat they contain. In general, 1 fat choice equals:

- 1 teaspoon of regular margarine, vegetable oil, or butter
- 1 tablespoon of regular salad dressing

FOOD	SERVING SIZE
Unsaturated Fats—Monounsaturated Fats	
Avocado, medium	2 Tbsp (1 oz)
Nut butters (*trans* fat-free): almond butter, cashew butter, peanut butter (smooth or crunchy)	1½ tsp
Nuts	
Almonds	6 nuts
Brazil	2 nuts
Cashews	6 nuts
Filberts (hazelnuts)	5 nuts
Macadamia	3 nuts
Mixed (50% peanuts)	6 nuts
Peanuts	10 nuts
Pecans	4 halves
Pistachios	16 nuts
Oil: canola, olive, peanut	1 tsp
Olives	
Black (ripe)	8 large
Green, stuffed	10 large
Polyunsaturated Fats	
Margarine: lower-fat spread (30%-50% vegetable oil, *trans* fat-free)	1 Tbsp
Margarine: stick, tub (*trans* fat-free), or squeeze (*trans* fat-free)	1 tsp
Mayonnaise	
Reduced-fat	1 Tbsp
Regular	1 tsp
Mayonnaise-style salad dressing	
Reduced-fat	1 Tbsp
Regular	2 tsp
Nuts	
Walnuts, English	4 halves
Pignolia (pine nuts)	1 Tbsp
Oil: corn, cottonseed, flaxseed. grape seed, safflower, soybean, sunflower	1 tsp
Oil: made from soybean and canola oil—Enova	1 tsp
Plant stanol esters	
Light	1 Tbsp
Regular	2 tsp

FOOD	SERVING SIZE
Salad dressing	
Reduced-fat (Note: May be high in carbohydrate)‡	2 Tbsp
Regular‡	1 Tbsp
Seeds	
Flaxseed, whole	1 Tbsp
Pumpkin, sunflower	1 Tbsp
Sesame seeds	1 Tbsp
Tahini or sesame paste	2 tsp
Saturated Fats	
Bacon, cooked, regular or turkey	1 slice
Butter	
Reduced-fat	1 Tbsp
Stick	1 tsp
Whipped	2 tsp
Butter blends made with oil	
Reduced-fat or light	1 Tbsp
Regular	1½ tsp
Chitterlings, boiled	2 Tbsp (½ oz)
Coconut, sweetened, shredded	2 Tbsp
Coconut milk	
Light	⅓ cup
Regular	1½ Tbsp
Cream	
Half and half	2 Tbsp
Heavy	1 Tbsp
Light	1½ Tbsp
Whipped	2 Tbsp
Whipped, pressurized	¼ cup
Cream cheese	
Reduced-fat	1½ Tbsp (¾ oz)
Regular	1 Tbsp (½ oz)
Lard	1 tsp
Oil: coconut, palm, palm kernel	1 tsp
Salt pork	¼ oz
Shortening, solid	1 tsp
Sour cream	
Reduced-fat or light	3 Tbsp
Regular	2 Tbsp

‡480 milligrams or more of sodium per serving.

*The Exchange Lists are the basis of a meal-planning system designed by a committee of the American Diabetes Association and The American Dietetic Association. While designed primarily for people with diabetes and others who must follow special diets, the Exchange Lists are based on principles of good nutrition that apply to everyone.

FREE FOODS

A "free" food is any food or drink choice that has less than 20 calories and 5 grams or less of carbohydrate per serving.

Selection Tips

1. Most foods on this list should be limited to 3 servings (as listed here) per day. Spread out the servings throughout the day. If you eat all 3 servings at once, it could raise your blood glucose level.
2. Food and drink choices listed here without a serving size can be eaten whenever you like.

FOOD	SERVING SIZE
Low Carbohydrate Foods	
Cabbage, raw	½ cup
Candy, hard (regular or sugar-free)	1 piece
Carrots, cauliflower, or green beans, cooked	¼ cup
Cranberries, sweetened with sugar substitute	½ cup
Cucumber, sliced	½ cup
Gelatin	
Dessert, sugar-free	
Unflavored	
Gum	
Jam or jelly, light or no sugar added	2 tsp
Rhubarb, sweetened with sugar substitute	½ cup
Salad greens	
Sugar substitutes (artificial sweeteners)	
Syrup, sugar-free	2 Tbsp
Modified Fat Foods with Carbohydrate	
Cream cheese, fat-free	1 Tbsp (½ oz)
Creamers	
Nondairy, liquid	1 Tbsp
Nondairy, powdered	2 tsp
Margarine spread	
Fat-free	1 Tbsp
Reduced-fat	1 tsp
Mayonnaise	
Fat-free	1 Tbsp
Reduced-fat	1tsp
Mayonnaise-style salad dressing	
Fat-free	1 Tbsp
Reduced-fat	1 tsp
Salad dressing	
Fat-free or low-fat	1 Tbsp
Fat-free, Italian	2 Tbsp
Sour cream, fat-free or reduced-fat	1 Tbsp
Whipped topping	
Light or fat-free	2 Tbsp
Regular	1 Tbsp
Condiments	
Barbecue sauce	2 tsp
Catsup (ketchup)	1 Tbsp
Honey mustard	1 Tbsp
Horseradish	
Lemon juice	
Miso	1½ tsp
Mustard	
Parmesan cheese, freshly grated	1 Tbsp
Pickle relish	1 Tbsp
Pickles	
Dill‡	1½ medium
Sweet, bread and butter	2 slices
Sweet, gherkin	¾ oz
Salsa	¼ cup
Soy sauce, light or regular‡	1 Tbsp
Sweet and sour sauce	2 tsp
Sweet chili sauce	2 tsp
Taco sauce	1 Tbsp
Vinegar	
Yogurt, any type	2 Tbsp

‡480 milligrams or more of sodium per serving.

Free Snacks

These foods in these serving sizes are perfect free-food snacks:

- 5 baby carrots and celery sticks
- ¼ cup blueberries
- ½ oz sliced cheese, fat-free
- 10 goldfish-style crackers
- 2 saltine-type crackers
- 1 frozen cream pop, sugar-free
- ½ oz lean meat
- 1 cup light popcorn
- 1 vanilla wafer

Drinks/Mixes

Any food on this list—without a serving size listed—can be consumed in any moderate amount:

- Bouillon, broth, consommé‡
- Bouillon or broth, low-sodium
- Carbonated or mineral water
- Club soda
- Cocoa powder, unsweetened (1 Tbsp)
- Coffee, unsweetened or with sugar substitute
- Diet soft drinks, sugar-free
- Drink mixes, sugar-free

*The Exchange Lists are the basis of a meal-planning system designed by a committee of the American Diabetes Association and The American Dietetic Association. While designed primarily for people with diabetes and others who must follow special diets, the Exchange Lists are based on principles of good nutrition that apply to everyone.

- Tea, unsweetened or with sugar substitute
- Tonic water, diet
- Water
- Water, flavored, carbohydrate free

Seasonings

Any food on this list can be consumed in any moderate amount:

- Flavoring extracts (for example, vanilla, almond, peppermint)
- Garlic
- Herbs, fresh or dried
- Nonstick cooking spray
- Pimento
- Spices
- Hot pepper sauce
- Wine, used in cooking
- Worcestershire sauce

COMBINATION FOODS

Many of the foods you eat are mixed together in various combinations, such as casseroles. These "combination" foods do not fit into any one choice list. This is a list of choices for some typical combination foods. This list will help you fit these foods into your meal plan. Ask your RD for nutrient information about other combination foods you would like to eat, including your own recipes.

FOOD	SERVING SIZE	COUNT AS
Entrees		
Casserole type (tuna noodle, lasagna, spaghetti with meatballs, chili with beans, macaroni and cheese)‡	1 cup (8 oz)	2 carbohydrates + 2 medium-fat meats
Stews (beef/other meats and vegetables)‡	1 cup (8 oz)	1 carbohydrate + 1 medium-fat meat + 0-3 fats
Tuna salad or chicken salad	½ cup (3½ oz)	½ carbohydrate + 2 lean meats + 1 fat
Frozen Meals/Entrees		
Burrito (beef and bean)‡*	1 (5 oz)	3 carbohydrates + 1 lean meat + 2 fats
Dinner-type meal‡	Generally 14-17 oz	3 carbohydrates + 3 medium-fat meats + 3 fats
Entree or meal with less than 340 calories‡	About 8-11 oz	2-3 carbohydrates + 1-2 lean meats
Pizza		
Cheese/vegetarian, thin crust‡	¼ of a 12 inch (4½ -5 oz)	2 carbohydrates + 2 medium-fat meats
Meat topping, thin crust‡	¼ of a 12 inch (5 oz)	2 carbohydrates + 2 medium-fat meats + 1½ fats
Pocket sandwich‡	1 (4½ oz)	3 carbohydrates + 1 lean meat + 1-2 fats
Pot pie‡	1 (7 oz)	2½ carbohydrates + 1 medium-fat meat + 3 fats
Salads (Deli-Style)		
Coleslaw	½ cup	1 carbohydrate + 1½ fats
Macaroni/pasta salad	½ cup	2 carbohydrates + 3 fats
Potato salad‡	½ cup	1½ -2 carbohydrates + 1-2 fats
Soups		
Bean, lentil. or split pea‡	1cup	1carbohydrate + 1 lean meat
Chowder (made with milk)‡	1 cup (8 oz)	1 carbohydrate + 1 lean meat + 1½ fats
Cream (made with water)‡	1 cup (8 oz)	1 carbohydrate + 1 fat
Instant‡	6 oz prepared	1 carbohydrate
With beans or lentils‡	8 oz prepared	2½ carbohydrates + 1 lean meat
Miso soup‡	1 cup	½ carbohydrate + 1 fat
Oriental noodle‡	1 cup	2 carbohydrates + 2 fats
Rice (congee)	1 cup	1 carbohydrate
Tomato (made with water)‡	1 cup (8 oz)	1 carbohydrate
Vegetable beef, chicken noodle, or other broth-type‡	1 cup (8 oz)	1 carbohydrate

*More than 3 grams of dietary fiber per serving.
‡600 milligrams or more of sodium per serving (for combination food main dishes/meals).

* The Exchange Lists are the basis of a meal-planning system designed by a committee of the American Diabetes Association and The American Dietetic Association. While designed primarily for people with diabetes and others who must follow special diets, the Exchange Lists are based on principles of good nutrition that apply to everyone.

FAST FOODS

The choices in the **Fast Foods** list are not specific fast food meals or items, but are estimates based on popular foods.

You can get specific nutrition information for almost every fast food or restaurant chain. Ask the restaurant or check its website for nutrition information about your favorite fast foods.

FOOD	SERVING SIZE	COUNT AS
Breakfast Sandwiches		
Egg, cheese, meat, English muffin‡	1 sandwich	2 carbohydrates + 2 medium-fat meats
Sausage biscuit sandwich‡	1 sandwich	2 carbohydrates + 2 high-fat meats + 3½ fats
Main Dishes/Entrees		
Burrito (beef and beans)‡*	1 (about 8 oz)	3 carbohydrates + 3 medium-fat meats + 3 fats
Chicken breast, breaded and fried‡	1 (about 5 oz)	1 carbohydrate + 4 medium-fat meats
Chicken drumstick, breaded and fried	1 (about 2 oz)	2 medium-fat meats
Chicken nuggets‡	6 (about 3½ oz)	1 carbohydrate + 2 medium-fat meats + 1 fat
Chicken thigh, breaded and fried‡	1 (about 4 oz)	½ carbohydrate + 3 medium-fat meats + 1½ fats
Chicken wings, hot‡	6 (5 oz)	5 medium-fat meats + 1½ fats
Oriental		
Beef/chicken/shrimp with vegetables in sauce‡	1 cup (about 5 oz)	1 carbohydrate + 1 lean meat + 1 fat
Egg roll, meat‡	1 (about 3 oz)	1 carbohydrate + 1 lean meat + 1 fat
Fried rice, meatless	½ cup	1½ carbohydrates + 1½ fats
Meat and sweet sauce (orange chicken)‡	1 cup	3 carbohydrates + 3 medium-fat meats + 2 fats
Noodles and vegetables in sauce (chow mein, lo mein)‡*	1 cup	2 carbohydrates + 1 fat
Pizza		
Cheese, pepperoni, regular crust‡	⅛ of a 14 inch (about 4 oz)	2½ carbohydrates + 1 medium-fat meat + 1½ fats
Cheese/vegetarian, thin crust‡	¼ of a 12 inch (about 6 oz)	2½ carbohydrates + 2 medium-fat meats + 1½ fats
Sandwiches		
Chicken sandwich, grilled‡	1	3 carbohydrates + 4 lean meats
Chicken sandwich, crispy‡	1	3½ carbohydrates + 3 medium-fat meats + 1 fat
Fish sandwich with tartar sauce	1	2½ carbohydrates + 2 medium-fat meats + 2 fats
Hamburger		
Large with cheese‡	1	2½ carbohydrates + 4 medium-fat meats + 1 fat
Regular	1	2 carbohydrates + 1 medium-fat meat + 1 fat
Hot dog with bun‡	1	1 carbohydrate + 1 high-fat meat + 1 fat
Submarine sandwich		
Less than 6 grams fat‡	6-inch sub	3 carbohydrates + 2 lean meats
Regular‡	6-inch sub	3½ carbohydrates + 2 medium-fat meats + 1 fat
Taco, hard or soft shell (meat and cheese)	1 small	1 carbohydrate + 1 medium-fat meat + 1½ fats
Salads		
Salad, main dish (grilled chicken type, no dressing or croutons)‡*	Salad	1 carbohydrate + 4 lean meats
Salad, side, no dressing or cheese	Small (about 5 oz)	1 vegetable
Sides/Appetizers		
French fries, restaurant style†	Small	3 carbohydrates + 3 fats
	Medium	4 carbohydrates + 4 fats
	Large	5 carbohydrates + 6 fats
Nachos with cheese‡	Small (about 4½ oz)	2½ carbohydrates + 4 fats
Onion rings‡	1 serving (about 3 oz)	2½ carbohydrates + 3 fats
Desserts		
Milkshake, any flavor	12 oz	6 carbohydrates + 2 fats
Soft-serve ice cream cone	1 small	2½ carbohydrates + 1 fat

*More than 3 grams of dietary fiber per serving.
†Extra fat, or prepared with extra fat.
‡600 milligrams or more of sodium per serving (for fast food main dishes/meals).

* The Exchange Lists are the basis of a meal-planning system designed by a committee of the American Diabetes Association and The American Dietetic Association. While designed primarily for people with diabetes and others who must follow special diets, the Exchange Lists are based on principles of good nutrition that apply to everyone.

ALCOHOL

Nutrition Tips

1. In general, 1 alcohol choice (½ oz absolute alcohol) has about 100 calories.

Selection Tips

1. If you choose to drink alcohol, you should limit it to 1 drink or less per day for women, and 2 drinks or less per day for men.
2. To reduce your risk of low blood glucose (hypoglycemia), especially if you take insulin or a diabetes pill that increases insulin, always drink alcohol with food.
3. While alcohol, by itself, does not directly affect blood glucose, be aware of the carbohydrate (for example, in mixed drinks, beer, and wine) that may raise your blood glucose.
4. Check with your RD if you would like to fit alcohol into your meal plan.

ALCOHOLIC BEVERAGE	SERVING SIZE	COUNT AS
Beer		
Light (4.2%)	12 fl oz	1 alcohol equivalent + ½ carbohydrate
Regular (4.9%)	12 fl oz	1 alcohol equivalent + 1carbohydrate
Distilled spirits: vodka, rum, gin, whiskey 80 or 86 proof	1½ fl oz	1 alcohol equivalent
Liqueur, coffee (53 proof)	1 fl oz	1 alcohol equivalent + 1 carbohydrate
Sake	1 fl oz	½ alcohol equivalent
Wine		
Dessert (sherry)	3½ fl oz	1 alcohol equivalent + 1carbohydrate
Dry, red or white (10%)	5 fl oz	1 alcohol equivalent

*The Exchange Lists are the basis of a meal-planning system designed by a committee of the American Diabetes Association and The American Dietetic Association. While designed primarily for people with diabetes and others who must follow special diets, the Exchange Lists are based on principles of good nutrition that apply to everyone.

APPENDIX C

Food Sources of Oxalates

FRUITS

- Berries, all
- Concord grapes
- Currants
- Figs
- Fruit cocktail
- Plums
- Rhubarb
- Tangerines

NUTS

- Almonds
- Cashews
- Peanut butter
- Peanuts

BEVERAGES

- Chocolate
- Cocoa
- Draft beer
- Tea

VEGETABLES

- Baked beans
- Beans, green and wax
- Beet greens
- Beets
- Celery
- Chard, Swiss
- Chives
- Collards
- Eggplant
- Endive
- Kale
- Leeks
- Mustard greens
- Okra
- Peppers, green
- Rutabagas
- Spinach
- Squash, summer
- Sweet potatoes
- Tomatoes
- Tomato soup
- Vegetable soup

OTHER

- Grits
- Soy products
- Tofu
- Wheat germ

APPENDIX

D

Calculation Aids and Conversion Tables

In 1799 a group of French scientists set up the metric system of weights and measures. Today, with refinements over years of use, it is called the "Système International" (SI) and is used in most countries throughout the world. The United States continues to follow the British/American system of weights and measures. Given below are a few conversion factors to help you make these transitions in your necessary calculations.

METRIC SYSTEM OF MEASUREMENT

Like our money system, this is a simple decimal system based on units of 10. It is uniform and used internationally.

Weight Unit

1 kilogram (kg) = 1000 grams (gm or g)

1 g = 1000 milligrams (mg)

1 mg = 1000 micrograms (mcg or μg)

Length Units

1 meter (m) = 100 centimeters (cm)

1000 m = 1 kilometer (km)

Volume Units

1 liter (L) = 1000 milliliters (mL)

1 ml = 1 cubic centimeter (cc)

Temperature Units

The Celsius (C) scale is based on 100 equal units between 0° C (freezing point of water) and 100° C (boiling point of water). This scale is used entirely in all scientific work.

Energy Units

Kilocalorie (kcal) = Amount of energy required to raise 1 kg water 1° C

Kilojoule (kJ) = Amount of energy required to move 1 kg mass 1 m by a force of 1 newton

1 kcal = 4.184 kJ

BRITISH/AMERICAN SYSTEM OF MEASUREMENT

Our customary system is made up of units having no uniform relationships. It is not a decimal system but rather a collection of different units brought together in usage and language over time. It is predominately used in America.

Weight Units

1 pound (lb) = 16 ounces (oz)

Length Units

1 foot (ft) = 12 inches (in)

1 yard (yd) = 3 feet (ft)

Volume Units

3 teaspoons (tsp) = 1 tablespoon (tbsp)

16 tbsp = 1 cup

1 cup = 8 fluid ounces (fl oz)

4 cups = 1 quart (qt)

5 cups = 1 imperial quart (qt), Canada

Temperature Units

The Fahrenheit (F) scale is based on 180 equal units between 32° F (freezing point of water) and 212° F (boiling point of water) at standard atmospheric pressure.

CONVERSIONS BETWEEN MEASUREMENT SYSTEMS

Weight

1 oz = 28.35 g

2.2 lb = 1 kg

Length

1 in = 2.54 cm

1 ft = 30.48 cm

39.37 in = 1 m

Volume

1.06 qt = 1 L

0.85 imperial qt = 1 L (Canada)

Temperature

Boiling point of water: 100° C; 212° F

Body temperature: 37° C; 98.6° F

Freezing point of water: 0° C; 32° F

Interconversion Formulas

Fahrenheit temperature (°F) = $\frac{9}{5}$ (°C) + 32

Celsius temperature (°C) = $\frac{5}{9}$ (°F − 32)

Approximate Metric Conversions

WHEN YOU KNOW	MULTIPLY BY	TO FIND
Weight		
Ounces	28	Grams
Pounds	0.45	Kilograms
Length		
Inches	2.5	Centimeters
Feet	30	Centimeters
Volume		
Teaspoons	5	Milliliters
Tablespoons	15	Milliliters
Fluid ounces	30	Milliliters
Cups	0.24	Liters
Pints	0.47	Liters
Quarts	0.95	Liters

E

Cultural Dietary Patterns and Religious Dietary Practices

Only foods that are specifically associated with these cultural groups are noted. Individuals may also consume typical American foods, as dietary adaptations are common. Assumptions of dietary patterns cannot be made, but knowledge of these unique foods provides a common understanding of the range of possible food choices.

CULTURAL DIETARY PATTERNS

CULTURE	BREAD, CEREAL, RICE, AND PASTA GROUP	VEGETABLE GROUP	FRUIT GROUP	MILK, YOGURT, CHEESE GROUP	MEAT, POULTRY, FISH, DRY BEANS, EGGS, AND NUTS GROUPS	FATS, OILS, AND SWEETS GROUP
Native American	Blue corn flour (ground dried blue corn kernels) used to make corn bread, mush dumplings; fruit dumplings (walakshi); fry bread (biscuit dough deep fried); ground sweet acorn; hominy; tortillas; wheat and rye products; wild rice	Artichokes, cacti, chili, mushrooms, nettles, onions, potatoes, pumpkin, squash, sweet potatoes, tomatoes, wild greens, turnips, and yucca	Dried wild berries, cherries and grapes; berries, elderberries, persimmons, plums, and rhubarb	None in traditional diet	Bear, buffalo, deer, elk, moose, rabbit, and squirrel Duck, goose, quail, and wild turkey A variety of fish, legumes, nuts, and seeds	Tallow and lard Maple sugar and pine sugar
Northern European	Barley, hops, oat, rice, rye, and wheat products	Artichokes, asparagus, beets, brussels sprouts, cabbage, carrots, cauliflower, celery, cucumbers, eggplant, fennel, green peppers, kale, leeks, mushrooms, olives, onions, peas, potatoes, radishes, spinach, turnips, and watercress	Apples, apricots, cherries, currants, gooseberries, grapes, lemons, melons, oranges, peaches, pears, plums, prunes, raspberries, rhubarb, and strawberries	Cheese (made from cow, sheep, and goat milk), cream, milk, sour cream, and yogurt	Beef, lamb, oxtail, pork, rabbit, veal, and venison Chicken, duck, goose, pheasant, pigeon, quail, and turkey A wide variety of fish, legumes, and nuts	Butter, lard, margarine, olive oil, vegetable oil, and salt pork Honey and sugar
Southern European	Cornmeal, rice, and wheat products	Arugula, artichokes, asparagus, broccoli, cabbage, cardoon, cauliflower, celery, chicory, cucumber, eggplant, endive, escarole, fennel, kale, kohlrabi, mushrooms, mustard greens, olives, pimentos, potatoes, radicchio, Swiss chard, turnips, and zucchini	Apples, apricots, bananas, cherries, citron, dates, figs, grapefruit, grapes, lemons, medlars, oranges, peaches, pears, pineapples, prunes, pomegranates, quinces, raisins, and tangerines	Cheese (made from cow, sheep, buffalo, and goat milk), and milk	Beef, goat, lamb, pork, and veal Chicken, duck, goose, pigeon, turkey, and woodcock A variety of fish, shellfish, legumes, and nuts	Butter, lard, olive oil, and vegetable oil Honey and sugar
Central European and Russian	Barley, buckwheat, corn, millet, oats, potato starch, rice, rye, and wheat products	Asparagus, beets, brussels sprouts, cabbage, carrots, cauliflower, celery, chard, cucumbers, eggplant, endive, kohlrabi, leeks, mushrooms, olives, onions, parsnips, peppers, potatoes, radishes, sorrel, spinach, and turnips	Apples, apricots, a variety of berries, currants, dates, grapes, grapefruit, lemons, melons, oranges, peaches, pears, plums, prunes, quinces, raisins, rhubarb, and strawberries	Buttermilk, cheese, cream, milk, sour cream, and yogurt	Beef, boar, hare, lamb, pork, sausage, veal, and venison Chicken, Cornish hen, duck, goose, grouse, partridge, pheasant, quail, squab, and turkey A variety of fish, shellfish, legumes, and nuts	Butter, bacon, chicken fat, flaxseed oil, lard, olive oil, salt pork, and vegetable oil Honey, sugar, and molasses

African American (Southern United States)	Biscuits; corn bread as spoon bread, cornpone, hush puppies, or grits; and rice	Broccoli, cabbage, corn; leafy greens including dandelion greens, kale, mustard greens, collard greens, and turnips. Okra, pumpkin, potatoes, spinach, squash, sweet potatoes, tomatoes, and yams	Apple, banana, berries, fruit juices, peaches, and watermelon	Buttermilk and some cheese	Beef; pork and pork products including scrapple (cornmeal and pork), chitterlings (pork intestines), bacon, pig feet and ears Fried meats and poultry, organ meats (kidney, liver, tongue, and tripe) Fish (catfish, crawfish, salmon, shrimp, and tuna) Frogs, rabbit, squirrel A variety of legumes and nuts	Butter and lard Honey, molasses, and sugar
Mexican	Corn (tortillas, masa harina), wheat, and rice products; sweet bread	Cactus (nopales), calabaza criolla, chili peppers, corn, jicama, onions, peas, plantains, squashes (chayote, pumpkin, etc.), tomatillos, tomatoes, yams, and yucca root (cassava or manioc)	Avocadoes, bananas, cactus fruit, carambola, casimiroa, cherimoya, coconut, granadilla, guanabana, guava, lemons, limes, mamey, mangoes, melon, oranges, papaya, pineapple, strawberries, sugar cane, and zapote	Cheese, flan, sour cream, and milk	Beef, goat, and pork Chicken and turkey Firm-fleshed fish, shrimp, and a variety of legumes	Bacon fat, lard (manteca), salt pork, and dairy cream Sugar and panocha (raw brown cane sugar)
Central American	Corn (tamales, tortillas), rice, and wheat products	Asparagus, beets, cabbage, calabaza, chayote, chili peppers, corn, cucumbers, eggplant, hearts of palm, leeks, loroco flowers, onions, pacaya buds, plantains, pumpkin, spinach, sweet peppers, tomatillos, watercress, yams, yucca, and yucca flowers	Apples, avocadoes, bananas, breadfruit, cherimoya, coconut, grapes, guava, mameys, mangoes, nances, oranges, papaya, passion fruit, pejibaye, pineapples, prunes, raisins, tamarind, tangerines, and zapote	Cheese, cream, and milk	Beef, iguana, lizards, pork, and venison Chicken, duck, and turkey A variety of fish, shellfish, and legumes	Butter, lard, vegetable oils, and shortening Honey, sugar, and sugar syrup

Continued

CULTURAL DIETARY PATTERNS—cont'd

CULTURE	BREAD, CEREAL, RICE, AND PASTA GROUP	VEGETABLE GROUP	FRUIT GROUP	MILK, YOGURT, CHEESE GROUP	MEAT, POULTRY, FISH, DRY BEANS, EGGS, AND NUTS GROUPS	FATS, OILS, AND SWEETS GROUP
Caribbean Islands	Cassava bread; cornmeal (surrulitos); oatmeal; rice, and wheat products	Arracacha, arrowroot, black-eyed peas, cabbage, calabaza, callaloo, cassava, chilis, corn, cucumbers, eggplant, malangas, okra, onions, palm hearts, peppers, radishes, spinach, squashes, sweet potatoes, taro, and yams	Acerola cherries, akee, avocadoes, bananas, breadfruit, caimito, cherimoya, citron, coconuts, cocoplum, gooseberries, granadilla, grapefruit, guanabana, guava, jackfruit, kumquats, lemons, limes, mamey, mangoes, oranges, papayas, pineapples, plantains, pomegranates, raisins, sapodilla, sugar cane, and tamarind	Cheese and milk	Beef, goat, and pork Chicken, turkey, and a variety of fish, shellfish, and legumes	Butter, coconut oil, lard, and olive oil Sugar cane products
Cuban and Puerto Rican	Rice; starchy green bananas, usually fried (plantain)	Beets, breadfruit, chayote, chili peppers, eggplant, onion, tubers (yucca), white yams (boniato)	Coconuts, guava, mango, oranges (sweet and sour), prune and mango paste	Flan, hard cheese (queso de mano)	Chicken, fish, (all kinds and preparations including smoked, salted, canned, and fresh), shellfish, legumes (all kinds especially black beans), pork (fried), sausage (chorizo), calf brain, beef tongue	Olive and peanut oil, lard Coconut
South American	Amaranth (corn, rice, quinoa) and wheat products	Ahipa, arracacha, calabaza, cassava, green peppers, hearts of palm, kale, okra, oca, onions, rosella, squash, sweet potatoes, yacon, and yams	Avocado, abiu, acerola, apples, banana, caimito, casimiroa, cherimoya, feijoa, guava, grapes, jackfruit, jabitocaba, lemons, limes, lulo, mammea, mango, melon, olives, oranges, palm fruits, papaya, passion fruit, peaches, pineapple, pitanga, quince, sapote, and strawberries	Cheese and milk	Beef, frog, goat, guinea pig, llama, mutton, pork, and rabbit Chicken, duck, turkey, and a variety of fish, shellfish, and nuts	Palm oil, olive oil, and butter Sugar cane, brown sugar, and honey

Chinese	Rice and related products (flour, cakes, and noodles); noodles made from barley, corn, and millet; wheat and related products (breads, noodles, spaghetti, stuffed noodles [won ton] and filled buns [bow])	Bamboo shoots, cabbage (napa), celery, Chinese turnips (lo bok), dried day lilies, dry fungus (Black Juda's ear); leafy green vegetables including kale, cress, mustard greens (gai choy), chard (bok choy), amaranth greens (yin choy), wolfberry leaves (gou gay), and Chinese broccoli (gai lan); eggplant, lotus tubers, okra, snow peas, stir-fried vegetables (chow yuk), taro roots, white radish (daikon), yams, and yam beans	Apples, bananas, custard apples, coconuts, dates, longan, figs, grapes, kumquats, lime, litchi, mango, muskmelon, oranges, papaya, passion fruit, peaches, persimmons, pineapples, plums, pomegranates, pomelos, tangerines, and watermelon	Milk (cow's, buffalo, and soymilk)	Beef, lamb, and pork Chicken, duck, quail, squab, a large variety of fish and shellfish, in addition to legumes and nuts	Lard; peanut, soy, sesame, and rice oil Honey, rice or barley malt, palm sugar, sorghum sugar, and dehydrated cane juice
Japanese	Rice and rice products, rice flour (mochiko), noodles (comen/soba), buckwheat, and millet	Artichoke, asparagus, bamboo shoots (takenoko), burdock (gobo), cabbage (napa), eggplant, horseradish (wasabi), mizuna, mushrooms (shiitake, matsutake, nameko), Japanese parsley (seri), lotus root (renkon), pickled cabbage (kimchee), pickled vegetables, seaweed (laver, nori, wakame, kombu), snow peas, spinach, sweet potato, vegetable soup (mizutaki), watercress, white radish (daikon)	Pear-like apple (nasi), apricots, bananas, cherries, figs, grapefruit (yuzu), kumquats, lemons, limes, persimmons, pineapples, plums, strawberry, and tangerine (mikan)	Milk, butter, and ice cream	Beef, deer, lamb, pork, rabbit, and veal Fish and shellfish including dried fish with bones, raw fish (sashimi), and fish cake (kamaboko) A variety of poultry (chicken, duck, goose, turkey) and legumes (black beans, red beans, soybeans—as tofu, fermented soybean, and sprouts)	Lard; soy, sesame, rapeseed, and rice oil Honey and sugar
Korean	Barley, buckwheat, millet, rice, and wheat products	Bamboo shoots, bean sprouts, beets, cabbage, chives, chrysanthemum leaves, cucumber, eggplant, fern, green onion, green pepper, leeks, lotus root, mushrooms, onion, perilla, seaweed, spinach, sweet potato, turnips, water chestnut, watercress, and white radish	Apples, Asian pears, cherries, dates, grapes, melons, oranges, pears, persimmons, plums, and tangerines	Very little, if any, consumption	Beef, oxtail, pork, chicken, pheasant, and a variety of fish, shellfish, legumes, and nuts	Sesame oil and vegetable oil Honey and sugar

Continued

CULTURAL DIETARY PATTERNS—cont'd

CULTURE	BREAD, CEREAL, RICE, AND PASTA GROUP	VEGETABLE GROUP	FRUIT GROUP	MILK, YOGURT, CHEESE GROUP	MEAT, POULTRY, FISH, DRY BEANS, EGGS, AND NUTS GROUPS	FATS, OILS, AND SWEETS GROUP
Filipino	Noodles, rice, rice flour (mochiko), stuffed noodles (won ton), white bread (pan de sal)	Amaranth, bamboo shoots, beets, burdock root, cassava, Chinese celery, dark green leafy vegetables (malunggay and salvyot), eggplant, garlic, green peppers, hearts of palm, hyacinth bean, kamis, leek, mushrooms, okra, onion, sweet potatoes (camotes), turnips, and root crop (gabi)	Apples, avocado, banana, bitter melon (ampalaya), breadfruit, coconut, guavas, jackfruit, limes, mangoes, papaya, pod fruit (tamarind), pomelos, rambutan, rhubarb, star fruit, tangelo (naranghita), and watermelon	White cheese, evaporated cow or goat milk and soymilk	Beef, carabao, goat, pork, monkey, organ meats, and rabbit Fish, dried fish (dilis), egg roll (lumpia), fish sauce (alamang and bagoong) Legumes such as mung beans, bean sprouts, and chickpeas; soybean curd (tofu)	Coconut oil, lard, and vegetable oil Brown and white sugar, coconut, and honey
Pacific Islanders	Rice and wheat products	Arrowroot, bitter melon, burdock root, cabbage, carrot, cassava, daikon, eggplant, ferns, green pepper, horseradish, jute, kohlrabi, leeks, lotus root, mustard greens, green onions, seaweed, spinach, squashes, sweet potato, taro, water chestnuts, and yams	Acerola cherries, apples, apricot, avocado, banana, breadfruit, coconut, guava, jackfruit, kumquat, litchis, loquat, mango, melons, papaya, passion fruit, peach, pear, pineapple, plum, prune, strawberries, and tamarind	Very little, if any, consumption	Beef, pork, chicken, duck, squab, and turkey A variety of fish, shellfish, and legumes	Butter, coconut oil, lard, sesame oil, and vegetable oil Sugar
South Asian	Rice, wheat, buckwheat, corn, millet, and sorghum products	Agathi flowers, amaranth, artichokes, bamboo shoots, beets, bitter melon, brussels sprouts, cabbage, collard greens, cucumbers, drumstick plant, eggplant, lotus root, manioc, mushrooms, okra, pandanus, plantain flowers, sago palm, spinach, squash, turnips, water chestnuts, water convulus, water lilies, and yams	Apples, apricots, avocados, bananas, coconut, dates, figs, grapes, guava, jackfruit, limes, litchis, loquats, mangoes, melon, nongus, oranges, papaya, peaches, pears, persimmons, pineapple, plums, pomegranate, pomelos, star fruit, sugar cane, tangerines, and watermelon	Milk (evaporated and fermented products), cheese, and milk-based desserts	Beef, goat, mutton, pork, chicken, duck, and a variety of fish, seafood, legumes, and nuts	Coconut oil, ghee, mustard oil, peanut oil, sesame seed oil, and sunflower oil Sugar cane, jaggery, and molasses Chicken fat
Jewish (both cultural and religious customs)	Bagel, buckwheat groats (kasha), dumplings made with matzoh meal (matzoh balls or knaidelach), egg bread (challah), noodle or potato pudding (kugel), crepe filled with farmer cheese and/or fruit (blintz), unleavened bread or large cracker made with wheat flour and water (matzoh)	Potato pancakes (latkes); vegetable stew made with sweet potatoes, carrots, prunes, and sometimes brisket (tzimmes); beet soup (borscht)			A mixture of fish formed into balls and poached (gefilte fish); smoked salmon (lox)	

RELIGIOUS DIETARY PRACTICES

	SEVENTH-DAY ADVENTIST	BUDDHIST	EASTERN ORTHODOX	HINDU	JEWISH	MORMON	MUSLIM	ROMAN CATHOLIC
Beef		Avoided by most devout		Prohibited or strongly discouraged				
Pork	Prohibited or strongly discouraged	Avoided by most devout		Avoided by most devout	Prohibited or strongly discouraged		Prohibited or strongly discouraged	
All meat	Avoided by most devout	Avoided by most devout	Permitted but some restrictions apply	Avoided by most devout	Permitted but some restrictions apply		Permitted but some restrictions apply	Permitted but some restrictions apply
Eggs/dairy	Permitted but avoided at some observances	Permitted but avoided at some observances	Permitted but some restrictions apply	Permitted but avoided at some observances	Permitted but some restrictions apply			
Fish	Avoided by most devout	Avoided by most devout	Permitted but some restrictions apply	Permitted but some restrictions apply	Permitted but some restrictions apply			
Shellfish	Prohibited or strongly discouraged	Avoided by most devout	Permitted but avoided at some observances	Permitted but some restrictions apply	Prohibited or strongly discouraged			
Meat and dairy at same meal					Prohibited or strongly discouraged			
Leavened foods					Permitted but some restrictions apply			
Ritual slaughter of animals					Practiced		Practiced	
Alcohol	Prohibited or strongly discouraged			Avoided by most devout		Prohibited or strongly discouraged	Prohibited or strongly discouraged	
Caffeine	Prohibited or strongly discouraged						Prohibited or strongly discouraged	Avoided by most devout

Compiled by Staci Nix for *Williams' basic nutrition & diet therapy,* ed 12, St Louis, 2005, Mosby. Modified from Kittler PG, Sucher KP: *Food and culture,* ed 4, Belmont Calif, 2004, Brooks/Cole, a division of Thomson Learning (www.thomsonrights.com).

F

Federal Food Assistance Programs

Programs described below are funded by the U.S. government with state allocations based on population, numbers of eligible participants, or other factors. States may be required to provide some degree of match in support of the statewide program.

Special Nutrition Assistance Program (SNAP) (The Food Stamp Program)

Type of Program: Entitlement program

Supervising Agency: United States Department of Agriculture

Population Served: Individuals and families with incomes falling within 130% of the federal poverty line and assets within federal guidelines. SNAP eligibility and benefits take into consideration household income, household size, housing costs, total assets, and work registration requirements. Eligibility requirements and benefits are adjusted annually.

Benefits Provided/Nutrition Standards: Food stamps increase the amount of money participants have to spend for food. Recipients are given electronic benefit transfer cards (EBT) and at the time of purchase funds are transferred from the client's food stamp account to the retailer's account. Food stamps can be used to buy most foods as well as seeds and plants for raising food, although there are exceptions.

The following items cannot be purchased with food stamps:

- Hot, ready-to-eat foods
- Foods that will be eaten in the store
- Vitamin or mineral supplements
- Pet foods
- Cleaning supplies
- Tobacco items
- Alcoholic beverages

The average monthly SNAP benefit is about $101 per person and about $227 per household.

Number Served: About 31 million people benefit from food stamps (49% are children and 9% are older adults). More than one-third of the families with children are single-parent households.

Availability of Nutrition Education: Most states offer nutrition education in conjunction with their SNAP program, but not all families are reached and participation is voluntary. See the discussion of the Special Nutrition Assistance Education Program (SNAP-ED) on p. 605.

Commodity Foods Distribution Program/The Emergency Food Assistance Program (TEFAP)

Type of Program: Entitlement program

Supervising Agency: United States Department of Agriculture

Population Served: Individuals and families with incomes below the federal poverty guidelines or who qualify for food stamps. Commodity foods are also available to (1) schools for use in the National School Lunch and School Breakfast Programs, (2) congregate and home-delivered meals programs serving older adults, (3) Head Start and other child care programs, and (4) food pantries or soup kitchens serving the homeless and indigent populations.

Benefits Provided/Nutrition Standards: Market surpluses of perishable foods, including meat, poultry, fruits and vegetables, eggs, dried beans and peas, fats, and cheese.

Number Served: Unknown.

Availability of Nutrition Education: No formal mandate; may be provided at facilities or locations serving or distributing commodity foods (see below).

CHILD NUTRITION PROGRAMS

National School Lunch Program

Type of Program: Serves all children of school age who choose to participate. Free lunches are provided to children whose family income falls at or below 130% of the federal poverty level, and lunches are available at a reduced cost (students can be charged no more than 40 cents) to children whose family incomes fall between 130% and 185% of the federal poverty level.

Supervising Agency: United States Department of Agriculture

Population Served: Children in public schools, nonprofit private schools, and residential child care programs.

Benefits Provided/Nutrition Regulations: Nutritionally balanced lunches provide one third of the Dietary Reference Intakes (DRI) for protein, vitamin A, vitamin C, iron, calcium, and kcalories. No more than 30% of kcalories should be supplied by fat, and less than 10% should be supplied by saturated fat. Programs can chose to receive either commodity foods or cash reimbursement based on the number of students served.

Suggested School Lunch Pattern:

FOOD GROUP	SCHOOL LUNCH
Grains/Bread (includes whole grain or enriched bread, rolls, muffins, cereal, rice, macaroni, or noodles)	1 slice bread or 1 muffin or 1 roll and/or ½ cup rice, pasta, or macaroni for a total of 2 servings
Juice/Fruit/Vegetables (includes fruit, vegetables, fruit or vegetable juice)	½ cup fruit and ½ cup vegetable (minimum)
Milk (includes whole milk, low fat milk, nonfat milk, buttermilk)	1 cup
Meat or Meat Alternate (includes meat, poultry, fish, soy, cheese, egg, peanut butter, peas and beans, yogurt)	2 oz lean meat, poultry, fish, soy, or cheese or 1 egg or ½ cup peas or beans or 4 tbsp peanut butter or 1 cup yogurt

Number Served: More than 101,000 schools and child care institutions offer a school lunch program, and meals are served to 30.5 million children every school day. Since the program's inception in 1946, it has served over 219 billion meals.

Availability of Nutrition Education: A comprehensive nutrition education program called Team Nutrition contains educational materials and suggested activities for the school classroom, lunchroom, and after-school setting that encourage good food choices, portion control, and physical activity.

National School Breakfast Program

Type of Program: Serves all children of school age who choose to participate. Free breakfasts are provided to children whose family income falls at or below 130% of the poverty level, and breakfasts are available at a reduced cost to children whose family income falls between 130% and 185% of the poverty level.

Supervising Agency: United States Department of Agriculture

Population Served: Children in public schools, nonprofit private schools, and residential child care programs.

Benefits Provided/Nutrition Regulations: The school breakfast must provide one fourth of the DRI for protein, calcium, iron, vitamin A, vitamin C, and kcalories. As is recommended for the lunch meal, the breakfast meal should limit total fat to no more than 30% of total kcalories and saturated fat to less than 10% of total kcalories.

Suggested School Breakfast Pattern:

FOOD GROUP	SCHOOL BREAKFAST
Grains/Bread (includes whole grain or enriched bread, rolls, muffins, cereal, rice, macaroni, or noodles)	1 slice bread or 1 muffin or ¾ cup cereal
Juice/Fruit/Vegetables (includes fruit, vegetables, fruit or vegetable juice)	½ cup
Milk (includes whole milk, low fat milk, nonfat milk, buttermilk)	1 cup
Meat or Meat Alternate (includes meat, poultry, fish, soy, cheese, egg, peanut butter, peas and beans, yogurt)	1 oz meat, soy, or cheese or ½ egg or 2 tbsp peanut butter or ½ cup yogurt

Number Served: More than 87,000 schools offer a breakfast program, and about 10.5 million children receive a daily breakfast; 8.1 million children obtain their breakfast at a free or reduced price.

Availability of Nutrition Education: See National School Lunch Program above.

Summer Food Service Program

Type of Program: Entitlement where program is available.

Supervising Agency: United States Department of Agriculture

Population Served: Children meeting federal poverty guidelines.

Benefits Provided/Nutrition Regulations: Provides a noon meal during summer vacation periods for children who depend on the school breakfast and lunch programs for a significant portion of their nutrient intake. Nutritional guidelines are the same as for the school lunch program. These meals are usually offered as part of a summer school or camp experience sponsored by the local school district, recreation department, or other government or nonprofit community agency.

Number Served: Unknown.

Availability of Nutrition Education: May be offered as part of the educational program.

School Milk Program

Type of Program: Available to all children in participating schools or child care facilities.

Supervising Agency: United States Department of Agriculture

Population Served: Children in schools or child care facilities that do not offer a school breakfast or lunch program.

Benefits Provided/Nutrition Regulations: Cash reimbursement to school for milk provided free to children meeting income guidelines or sold at a nominal charge.

Number Served: Over 4600 schools participate in the special milk program; more than 85 million half-pints of milk are served each year.

Availability of Nutrition Education: Unknown.

Child and Adult Care Food Program

Type of Program: Available to all children and adults in participating programs and facilities.

Supervising Agency: United States Department of Agriculture

Population Served: Participants in child care programs serving children up to 12 years of age, adult day care programs serving persons age 60 and over, or programs caring for younger adults with disabilities. Such settings include child and adult day care centers, recreation centers, settlement houses, homeless shelters, and some Head Start programs.

Benefits Provided/Nutrition Regulations: Cash equivalents or commodity foods to the program or facility providing meals. Children and adults are eligible to receive two meals and one snack per day, with an additional meal or snack if care exceeds 8 hours.

Number Served: Unknown.

Availability of Nutrition Education: May be offered as part of the educational program.

Special Supplemental Nutrition Program for Women, Infants, and Children (WIC)

Type of Program: Not an entitlement program because income eligibility does not ensure benefits. Only those judged to be at the highest medical or nutritional risk can participate to the extent that resources are available.

Supervising Agency: United States Department of Agriculture; local programs are administered through State Health Departments

Population Served: Women falling within poverty guidelines who are pregnant, postpartum, or breastfeeding and infants and children up to 5 years of age who are found to be at nutritional risk. Postpartum mothers can receive supplementary food for 6 months, and breastfeeding mothers can receive supplementary food for 12 months.

Eligibility must be determined by a health professional based on the following criteria:

1. *Medically based risk:* anemia, underweight, overweight, poor prior pregnancy outcome, or history of pregnancy complications.
2. *Dietary risk:* mothers, infants, or children with nutrient deficiencies or nutrition-related medical conditions.

Benefits Provided/Nutrition Regulations: Participants receive vouchers to purchase designated foods that are rich sources of protein, calcium, iron, vitamin A, and vitamin C, or in some states receive food packages. Different types and amounts of food or vouchers are provided for different categories of participants. Vouchers may be used to purchase fresh fruits and vegetables at farmers' markets. Food packages were updated recently to comply more closely with the 2005 Dietary Guidelines for Americans.

Approved WIC Foods:

Infants

- Iron-fortified infant formula
- Iron-fortified infant cereal
- Baby food fruits and vegetables
- Baby food meat

Women and Children

- Vitamin C–rich fruit juice
- Vitamin C–rich vegetable juice
- Eggs
- Milk (soy beverage also available)
- Cheese
- Iron-fortified breakfast cereal
- Whole wheat bread (other grains such as brown rice, oatmeal, and whole wheat tortillas are also available)
- Peanut butter
- Dried or canned legumes
- Canned fish
- Fruits and vegetables

(The regulatory requirements for WIC food packages and the alternative choices available can be found at http://www.fns.usda.gov/wic/benefitsandservices/foodpkg.htm.)

Number Served: Of the 8.7 million individuals receiving monthly benefits, 4.3 million are children, 2.2 million are infants, and 2.2 million are women.

Availability of Nutrition Education: Public health nutritionists provide nutrition counseling at every WIC visit, and nutrition education is offered to individuals and groups. WIC also provides referrals to other needed medical or social services.

The WIC program has been shown to be cost effective in (1) reducing the number of premature and low-birth-weight infants, (2) producing savings of more than $3 in health care costs within the first 60 days after birth for every $1 paid out in benefits, and (3) lowering the number of children with anemia.

NUTRITION PROGRAM FOR THE ELDERLY

Type of Program: Available to all persons 60 years of age or over regardless of income, although the program targets those at risk based on income, frailty, and isolation (mandate of the Older Americans Act, As Amended). There is no set charge for the meal, but participants are encouraged to make a donation. Areas of high demand may have waiting lists for both congregate and home-delivered meals.

Supervising Agency: Administration on Aging, United States Department of Health and Human Services

Population Served: Congregate meals are offered at noon in community centers, churches, senior housing, or similar locations with familiarity and easy access to the aging population. Home-delivered meals are provided for those who cannot leave home as a result of illness, disability, or a dependent family member; certification for home-delivered meals must be renewed every 6 months by a health or social services professional.

Benefits Provided/Nutrition Regulations: A hot meal is provided on weekdays at noon at congregate meal sites; delivered noon meals may include a cold lunch for the evening meal or cold breakfast for the following day. As the costs of daily home delivery continue to rise, programs have experimented with weekly delivery of several frozen meals that can be defrosted and reheated as needed. Unfortunately, the occasional delivery of several frozen meals takes away the social aspect of a daily visitor, which can be important to a homebound and isolated senior. Each meal served or delivered should provide at least one third of the DRI for all nutrients as defined for persons above 50 years of age and should conform to the Dietary Guidelines for Americans in total fat, saturated fat, and sodium.

Number Served: More than 3 million older adults receive meals regularly.

Availability of Nutrition Education: May be offered as part of the educational program at congregate sites.

EXPANDED FOOD AND NUTRITION EDUCATION PROGRAM (EFNEP)/SPECIAL NUTRITION ASSISTANCE EDUCATION PROGRAM (SNAP-ED)

Type of Program: Services are directed toward individuals and families meeting the federal poverty guidelines and/or receiving food stamps, but participation is not mandatory.

Supervising Agency: United States Department of Agriculture

Population Served: Families with children, older adults, and youth. Individuals are recruited through neighborhood contacts, food stamp offices, and WIC.

Benefits Provided/Nutritional Regulations: EFNEP and SNAP-ED do not provide food but support limited-resource families through education, helping them obtain the knowledge and skills necessary for making healthy food choices. Youth and adult programs are delivered by Cooperative Extension agents, paraprofessionals, and volunteers. Paraprofessionals are indigenous to the communities and populations they serve.

Number Served: Over 380,000 youth and 158,000 adults are reached by EFNEP each year.

Availability of Nutrition Education: An experiential series of lessons offers hands-on opportunities to develop skills in food preparation, food safety, food budgeting, and wise shopping. Group classes, media methods, one-on-one instruction, and educational mailings are used to reach various audiences.

The EFNEP reporting system indicates that 84% of adults improve their food management practices (e.g., planning meals and shopping more wisely) and 74% of youth improve their food preparation and food safety skills.

Page numbers followed by *b* indicate boxes; *f*, figures; and *t*, tables.

C

E

F

G

H

O

P

Q

R

S